MW01040814

Developmental Juvenile Osteology

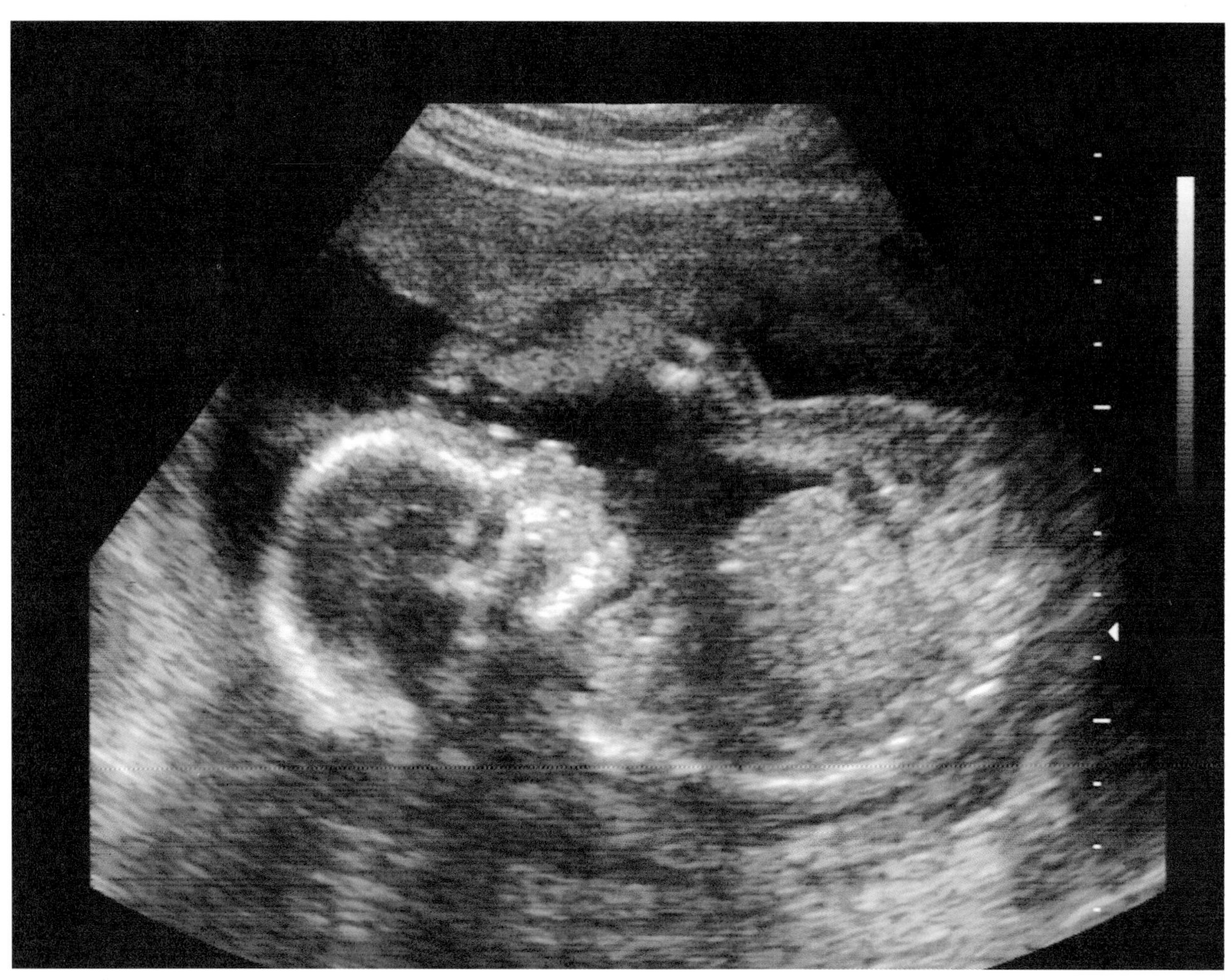

Ultrasound picture of a fetus *in utero* at 20 week's gestation.

Developmental Juvenile Osteology

Louise Scheuer
Department of Anatomy and Developmental Biology,
Royal Free and University College Medical School,
University College London, UK

Sue Black
Department of Forensic Medicine and Science,
University of Glasgow, UK

Illustrations by
Angela Christie

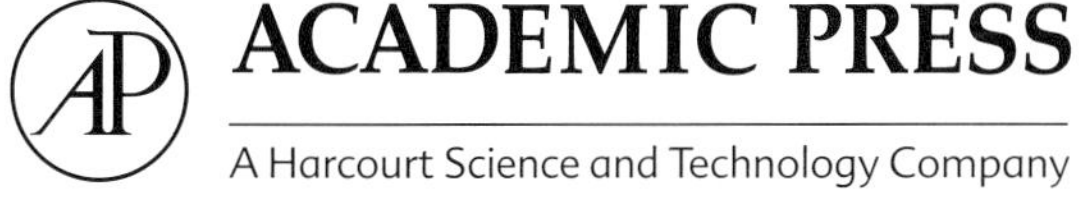

San Diego San Francisco New York Boston London Sydney Tokyo

Academic Press Limited
A Harcourt Science and Technology Company
Harcourt Place, 32 Jamestown Road
London NW1 7BY
http://www.academicpress.com

Academic Press
A Harcourt Science and Technology Company
525 B Street, Suite 1900, San Diego, California 92101-4495, USA
http://www.academicpress.com

Library of Congress Catalog Card Number: 99-67565

A catalogue record for the book is available from the British Library

ISBN 0-12-624000-0

Produced and typeset by Gray Publishing, Tunbridge Wells, Kent
Printed in Great Britain by Bath Press, Bath, Somerset
00 01 02 03 04 05 BP 9 8 7 6 5 4 3 2 1

Contents

Foreword: The Development of Juvenile Osteology

The importance of this volume will be immediately obvious to anyone who has been confronted with fetal or juvenile human osteological material in an archaeological, palaenotological, forensic or physical anthropological context. There is simply no currently available reference work that deals with the fetal and juvenile human skeleton in sufficient detail to be practically useful. Louise Scheuer and Sue Black have recognized a major gap in the field and have responded with a volume that is sure to become a classic wherever there is an interest in the identification and interpretation of the human fetal and juvenile skeleton.

It is perhaps easy, or relatively so, to recognize a need for a major reference work. It is much more difficult to fill that need. Both Scheuer and Black are highly experienced anatomists with many years of classroom and research experience. There is no doubt about their qualifications to carry out this task. But even so, I doubt if at the beginning they realized the enormity of the project they had set themselves or the length of time that would be needed to bring it to fruition. One major obstacle was their conviction that the book must be based on skeletal material of known age to avoid the circularity of discussing age-specific skeletal development on the basis of material that itself was aged using skeletal size or morphology. This proved to be difficult because such skeletal material is so rare and required considerable detective work to bring together. A second obstacle was the wealth of previously published material scattered in many disparate references relevant to many different disciplines and published in many different languages. The bibliography is large, spans 300 years and the information presented therein has been meticulously sorted and summarized. This in itself is a highly valuable contribution to the field. The absolute insistence on documentation and accuracy of both the skeletal and the contextual information in the book will ensure that it becomes a classic in the field.

In recent times, descriptive anatomy has taken a definite back seat to the various biochemical approaches to skeletal analysis. Among others, these new approaches include DNA analyses that have the potential to uncover the genetic basis of skeletal growth, the sex and possible familial and/or ethnic affiliation of skeletal material and the infectious diseases that the individual suffered in life. There is also the possibility, through stable isotope analysis, of determining the diet of the individual. In many academic departments, topographic anatomists live in the shadow of the perceived cutting-edge importance of these newer biochemical approaches to the understanding and interpretation of skeletal material. There is no doubt that these approaches are important, have enriched the disciplines that deal with the interpretation of skeletal material and have great potential to continue to do so. But there is still much to learn and understand through the study of whole organisms. Macro-anatomy gives much more than context and background for these newer biochemical techniques. It is here that this contribution will provide an invaluable and unparalleled resource.

Archaeologists, forensic pathologists and anthropologists will simply not be able to do without it in the context of recognizing and identifying fetal and juvenile material. It will also be invaluable to anyone interested in human growth and development. For example, in my own field of human palaeontology, there is a growing realization that there have been major changes in the tempo and mode of ontogeny in human evolution and that a good understanding of these ontogenetic patterns will provide significant insight into our own evolution. To date, this work has focused primarily on the dentition, but this volume will provide the necessary comparative context to facilitate the interpretation of skeletal growth and development in pre-human fetal and juvenile material.

Scheuer and Black have put considerable thought into the organization of this work, making it not only informative, but also accessible and practically useable. The meticulous descriptions of each individual bone are clearly written and logically presented. The 'practical notes' for identification of all bones are invaluable to the field worker, as are the clear and beautifully executed illustrations by Angela Christie. There is no doubt that this reference will outlive the current generation of researchers. The authors and artist should be congratulated on providing a resource that will facilitate the research of so many current and future scientists whose work touches on the analysis of human fetal and juvenile skeletal material. On behalf of all of us, I offer them a sincere and well-deserved thank you.

Professor Leslie C. Aiello
Head of Department of Anthropology
University College London

Preface

It has been our privilege for the past 20 years and more to be involved in both the undergraduate and postgraduate teaching of the anatomy of the developing juvenile skeleton. The motivation to write this book arose from our own personal awareness of the general inadequacy of textbook assistance and indeed the absence of a text that is dedicated solely to the subject. Although, like many of the basic aspects of biological studies, one is certain that the required information will be available somewhere, it is often extremely difficult, costly and time-consuming to track down these original details from individual papers. Many embryological, anatomical and osteological books do summarize some of the facts about the developing skeleton, but there is often a limited amount of additional information on other equally important aspects. Even after extensive literature searches, we are still unaware of a single text in the English language that amasses a reasonable volume of information on this subject.

Regrettably, fetal and juvenile osteology receives little attention in modern-day anatomical, medical, anthropological and forensic teaching. It has been suggested that this might have arisen partly through the profound paucity of suitable teaching specimens, compounded perhaps by a lack of experienced teachers. However, the lack of a dedicated text must be unquestionably one of the fundamental underlying reasons for this regrettable situation. As a result, the developing skeleton has been dubbed somewhat of a 'Cinderella' in the academic osteological world, although it is interesting and encouraging to note that in recent years there is some evidence of a resurgence of research in this area.

When we began to write this book we envisaged a slim field/laboratory manual with a limited amount of additional background information. However, as our literature searches progressed so the book has expanded beyond the boundaries of our initial intentions because we encountered so much information that was, in our opinion, either too important to be omitted or simply too interesting to be ignored.

Our primary aim was to bring together the vast literature on the topic of the developing skeleton and, along with illustrations from our own specimens, to chart the development of each bone from its embryological origin to its final adult form. It has always been our intention that the text will be primarily aimed at physical anthropologists, forensic pathologists, archaeologists and palaeontologists but we hope that it may perhaps prove both interesting and useful to a wider clinical and scientific audience.

While we have attempted to restrict our information to the field of anatomical and osteological details, information on the developing skeleton arises from many diverse literature sources including anatomy, embryology, physical anthropology, palaeontology, pathology, paediatrics, orthopaedics, radiology and orthodontics, to mention but a few. Where possible, we have attempted not to stray too far into the obviously related fields of auxology, biological anthropology or (palaeo) pathology but often this has proved somewhat difficult. During the searches of the literature, especially in the older texts, we have often come across 'little gems' that have fascinated or amused us and we have included these as footnotes throughout the book. In this way we hope that they will not interfere with the flow of the text but will add a little levity to what can often be a 'heavy' read.

We were acutely aware from the outset that the quality of the illustrations would be critical to the value of the text. We soon realized that they would in fact have to be hand-drawn, as photographs proved to be unacceptably inferior in quality due to the variability of the bone specimens in preservation, colour, etc. We were extremely fortunate to discover the exceptional talents of Angela Christie who painstakingly drew every halftone illustration in the text from actual bone specimens and subsequently made many adjustments at our exacting request. Uniquely, the majority of the material displayed in this text is of documented age at death and, where appropriate, such information is clearly stated in the legends. In some instances we have included photographs and radiographs, many of which arose from the research projects undertaken by our BSc students throughout the years. Credit is naturally given to their dissertations in the bibliography and although they may not be readily accessible for direct consultation, it is our hope that given time, the details of their work will find their way into the literature.

Apart from our students, there are many other people who have helped us throughout the production of this text. We are especially indebted to our friend and colleague, George Maat from Leiden University, who has read and commented upon the entire text. Leslie Aiello, Tim Cowan, Christopher Dean, Sheila Jones, Mike Moore, Robert Poelmann, Shelley Saunders, and Anthony Wright have also read and commented upon parts of the script and for this we express our most sincere thanks. Helen Liversidge generously gave permission for unpublished data to be quoted. We have also received help with information, specimens and photography from John Norton and Tjeu Gysbers at the Royal Free and University College School of Medicine, Martin Greig of Queen Mary and Westfield College, Sarah Smith of the United Medical and Dental Schools, Gus Alusi and João Campos of the Institute of Otology and Laryngology and Margaret Clegg at University College.

We are grateful to Jamanda Haddock of the Department of Radiology at the Royal Free Hospital for permission to use the ultrasound picture of the fetus *in utero* which was taken by Sally Blackmore.

We are particularly indebted to Detective Chief Superintendent John Bunn, Detective Superintendent Duncan Jarrett, forensic photographer Nick Marsh and Photographic Officers Matt Sprake and Neal Williams of New Scotland Yard for their permission to include some photographic specimens.

For their assistance and invaluable access to various skeletal collections we gratefully acknowledge Theya Molleson of the Natural History Museum, Canon John Oates of St Bride's Church, Professor Almaca and Luis Lopes of the Museu Bocage in Lisbon, Joanna Norris and particularly the St Barnabus excavation team – Joy Pollard, Sheila Gates, Jacqui Bowman, Gerry Doyle and Sarah Smith. Searching the literature has proved to be a monumental task in the production of this text and we wish to thank Professor Peter Vanezis and Maria Vanezis of the University of Glasgow, the librarians at the Royal Free Campus of the Royal Free and University College Medical School, Mark Wilmshurst at the Royal Society of Medicine library and Simon Barker at Aberdeen Royal Infirmary for their help and encouragement. Special thanks are issued to The Anderson Cars Group for invaluable assistance with many practical matters, including photocopying and printing.

We are indebted to Andrew Richford and Graham Allen of Academic Press and especially to Lesley Gray of Gray Publishing for their support and encouragement throughout the production of the text.

However, it is the constant support and encouragement of our husbands, Peter Scheuer and Tom Black, that deserve our most sincere gratitude.

Louise Scheuer
Sue Black

CHAPTER ONE

Introduction. A Guide to the Text

It must surely be clear that if we wish to safeguard the interests of our science (physical anthropology), and of those innocents who identify themselves with it, and who by so doing voluntarily condemn themselves to a precarious, albeit interesting life brachiating as it were from one lower income bracket to another, then it is our duty to see to it that they are properly equipped for the work which they wish to do and which so urgently requires to be done.

(Montagu, 1941)

The correct identification of the skeletal components of the juvenile skeleton is critical to the analysis of skeletal remains, regardless of whether they are of archaeological or forensic origin. Without such information it is virtually impossible to establish the number of individuals represented, let alone ascertain their identity. Indeed, a lack of familiarity with immature remains has led, on more than one occasion, to their identification as 'non-human'. Once the remains have been confirmed as human, the next step is usually an attempt to establish the four principal parameters of biological identity (sex, age at death, stature and ethnic affinity). However, with juvenile skeletal remains it is often only the determination of the age at death that can be established with any degree of reliability. Sex determination from juvenile remains is tentative at best and stature is so closely linked to the age of the individual that it is often used to predict it. Race is difficult to establish in the adult, so in the child it is virtually impossible, especially when only skeletal remains are presented.

The main purpose of this book is to describe each individual bone of the skeleton, or indeed different components of a bone, from its embryological origin to the final adult form. It is hoped that this systematic approach will assist the processes of both identification and age determination of the juvenile skeleton.

Chapters 2–4 form an introduction to the juvenile skeleton. **Chapter 2** deals with many of the fundamental issues concerning juvenile skeletal remains including the origin of such material, the various techniques by which it has been studied, the variability of child growth, the dilemma of biological versus chronological age and skeletal versus dental age. **Chapter 3** examines the more specific cellular and vascular nature of bone growth and development. It discusses the ontogenetic development of bone from its mesenchymal origins, through a cartilaginous or membranous template, to its eventual transformation into bone. Bone growth is considered, as is the influence of its vascularity. **Chapter 4** gives a very brief outline of the early embryological development of the human body as a whole, and sets the scene for the more specific developmental aspects of the skeleton that are discussed in subsequent chapters.

Chapters 5–11 form the core of the text and describe the morphological development of the immature skeleton in a way that permits the ready identification of each skeletal element and thus allows an evaluation of the age at death of the individual. The chapters are arranged in a topographical order, commencing with the axial skeleton and continuing with the upper and then the lower limb girdles and their associated appendages. Each section is essentially separated into four sections – the adult bone, early development, ossification and practical notes.

Each section begins with a description of the **adult bone(s)** but this is far from an exhaustive consideration of the subject as there are many excellent texts written specifically to fulfil this purpose. However, it was deemed necessary to include this section primarily to ensure consistency of terminology used in the subsequent sections on the development and ossification of the bone. Where possible, the accepted standard anatomical planes and terminology have been used throughout, although more commonly used names and others that reflect a historical origin have sometimes been included. Several anomalies of the adult skeleton have been included as this is an important concept that is diminishing as teaching moves away from more traditional methods towards computer models and plastic skeletal teaching aids (Willan and Humpherson, 1999). Whilst it is appreciated that these minor skeletal variants may be of limited clinical value, they can occasionally prove extremely important in the identification of the deceased. In anthropological terms of course, many of these anomalies are referred to as non-metric traits that may be considered indicative of potential genetic influences (Berry, 1975; Finnegan, 1978). A variety of relevant clinical conditions has also been introduced in this section where they have some bearing on the future development of the bone. Comment has often been made with regards to the value of that particular element in the determination of some parameters of biological identity (sex, race and stature). Whilst this is not the primary aim of this text, it serves only to direct the reader to other sources of reference.

The illustrations of the adult bones are represented by stippled line drawings with muscle attachments indicated. The illustrations throughout the book always depict the right-hand side of the body.

The **early development** of each bone is described directly after the discussion of the adult morphology. Each follows on from the stage previously outlined in Chapter 4 and deals with the specific embryological and early fetal development of that particular bone. This section charts its development from the blastemal condition up to the stage prior to the commencement of ossification. It also includes reference to various congenital conditions and anomalies that may arise during this period and which could subsequently alter the final adult morphology of the bone.

The section on **ossification** describes the development of the bone from the time of appearance of the first centre(s) of ossification up to the stage of final fusion of the epiphyses. In most chapters, this section is separated into three sections–primary centres, secondary centres and pattern of epiphyseal fusion. It is in this section of the book that the illustrations are most important as they not only highlight the earliest stage at which a particular element can be positively identified but also describe the morphological changes that occur in that bone throughout its development. However, it has not always been possible to illustrate a specific stage of development due to the limited availability of material. The illustrations in this section are half-tone drawings of actual bone specimens, many of which are of known age and sex and again only the right side of the body is depicted.

The final section within each chapter is headed '**Practical notes**'. It was thought that some readers may want to use this text as a field or laboratory manual and so a summary of a morphological timetable of events from the commencement of ossification to final epiphyseal fusion (or the attainment of final adult form) is presented. The practical notes include guidelines on the sideing of remains and how to orientate them to achieve correct identification of the skeletal element. In addition, there is a small section that offers suggestions on which other bones have a similar morphology that may cause some confusion and thus result in misidentification.

Finally, some tables of metric information are included that may prove useful in the determination of age at death. This includes only observations on individuals of *documented* age in order to remove the inherent errors of the circular argument that ensues when age is subsequently predicted on the basis of the accuracy of another method (see Chapter 2). Naturally, this dramatically reduces the number of studies that could be included but it may serve to highlight where further research could be pursued. Because so much information is available on the long bones from undocumented archaeological sources, a summary of these studies is included in Appendix 3.

By far the most comprehensive account of fetal bones is that published by Fazekas and Kósa (English translation of 1978) referring to a group of 136 fetuses ranging from 12–40 weeks gestation. However, the sample was essentially of undocumented age at death and age was assigned on the basis of its well-documented relationship with body length (Streeter, 1920; Scammon and Calkins, 1929; Schultz, 1929a). There is, however, no other detailed text on fetal osteology and given the fact that all fetal material must by necessity be of uncertain age (see Chapter 2) its inclusion was considered justified.

As each bone of the skeleton is considered from its earliest formation to its adult morphology, it is obvious that each would display its own idiosyncrasies and resist being forced into a standard chapter format. As a result, whilst an attempt has been made to adhere to an organized structure, each chapter is by necessity slightly different in terms of its layout. For example, in Chapter 5 (Head, Neck and Dentition) there is a general introduction to the early development of the skull as a whole to prevent needless repetition of material that is common to a structure composed of so many conjoined elements. Also, there is no section on secondary centres, as these do not occur in the skull. Similarly in Chapter 6, as the vertebral column is a midline structure, there is obviously no section on side identification and instead this is replaced by a section on identification of position within a series.

The main thrust of the book lies with the osseous development of the skeleton, but to leave out dental development in a book of this nature would be a serious omission. However, there are many excellent texts which discuss in detail the development and identification of the teeth and this section (in Chapter 5) has therefore been reduced to a general introduction and review of the subject, thereby directing readers to other reference sources.

In addition to the principal elements of the skeleton, other structures such as the larynx and costal cartilages have been included. Being composed of hyaline cartilage, these structures maintain the potential to ossify and may do so at an age when the remainder of the skeleton is still in its late developmental phase. For this reason it is important that the structures can be identified, as they may be encountered in the excavation or retrieval of immature remains. Whilst such ossifications have always tended to be considered entirely within the domain of the elderly, the inaccuracy of this assumption is highlighted. In fact, awareness of their existence can lead to an increase in successful retrieval rates.

No apology is made for the length of the **bibliography**; in fact, it is hoped that this may prove to be one of the values of this text. The quantity of literature differs for each bone and so by necessity some areas are more heavily referenced than others. Many of the most basic descriptions of bones were written many years ago and for this reason again no apology is made for the fact that the bibliography spans over 300 years. Wise (1995) accused many authors of ignoring the contributors of the past, stating that 'we may have stood on the shoulders of giants but we did not cite them'. He attributes this to authors becoming victims of technology, relying like a crutch on the use of information retrieval systems that tend not to extend to more than 10 years ago. Many of the older texts may also express views and descriptions that would not now be considered ethically acceptable. Titles of these papers have obviously been given as they stand and where appropriate the text has been quoted *verbatim* in the hope that accusations of political incorrectness may not be directed at this text. O'Rahilly (1996) raised the criticism that rather than seek out the original reference, many authors substitute reviews of the subject or even cite student textbooks where, in all fairness, original research is rarely published. In addition, he further accused authors of repeating information from one text to another without due recourse to the original work, which can of course lead to the perpetuation of errors. Where possible this text has attempted to avoid these pitfalls by extensive literature searches but it is inevitable that vital references, perhaps in another language, may have been omitted and errors may indeed have been unwittingly perpetuated. It is hoped that readers may identify these and make them known to the authors of this text so that due rectification can be made.

CHAPTER TWO

Skeletal Development and Ageing

The childhood shows the man
As morning shows the day

(John Milton, *Paradise Regained*)

This chapter outlines the basic principles on which the estimation of age from the juvenile skeleton is based. It also attempts to identify the major areas of study from which information on the development of the skeleton is drawn.

Growth

Growth is a general term applied to the progressive incremental changes in size and morphology that occur throughout the development of the individual. In general, overall growth is positively correlated with age, but the relationship is not a simple one. It consists of two components, increase in size and increase in maturity, and while these two elements are closely integrated, they do not necessarily advance in synchrony. As a result, individuals reach developmental milestones, or biological ages, along the maturity continuum at different chronological ages. For example, two boys, both aged 8 years, may differ considerably in height or similarly, two girls, aged 13, may both be at sexually and skeletally different stages of maturity. Generally speaking, growth in size is a regular process, although there are distinct increases in rate, possibly between 6 and 8 years in mid-childhood and at the adolescent growth spurt. However, the only consistent characteristic of growth is its variability.

There are variations in growth rate between different tissues and organs of the body in all individuals. The brain and head attain their adult size early in childhood, while the lymphoid system reaches its peak in late childhood. The reproductive system displays yet another rate and develops later in the adolescent period (Tanner, 1978). Growth also varies between the sexes, between individuals of the same population and between populations themselves. These differences are due to both genetic and environmental influences, the varying admixture of the two elements being the basis of the old 'nature versus nurture' argument. In spite of much research, the causal picture still remains unclear. On the one hand, it is almost impossible to study the effects of a single factor alone and on the other, the effects of a factor on an individual may vary, depending at which stage of development it acts. Thus the causes responsible for differences in any particular person are complex and difficult to isolate.

Rates of increase in size and increase in maturity differ between the sexes and this becomes evident before birth (Choi and Trotter, 1970; Pedersen, 1982). There are also differences in the timing of ossification of bones and mineralization of teeth (Garn *et al.*, 1966a; Mayhall, 1992). Postnatally, skeletal maturation is more advanced in girls than boys (Pyle and Hoerr, 1955; Brodeur *et al.*, 1981) but bone mineral density is significantly less in girls than boys, the latter having a higher mineral density and larger long bones (Maresh, 1970; Specker *et al.*, 1987; Miller *et al.*, 1991). At adolescence, differential hormone secretion increases sexual dimorphism. The growth spurt occurs later in boys than in girls and therefore has its greatest influence at a different critical phase of growth. It establishes more growth beforehand and results in a greater adult size, predominantly because muscle mass increases rapidly during this period, which affects overall skeletal robusticity (Tanner, 1978). As in childhood, bone mineral density and the rate of accumulation of peak bone mass varies between the sexes during puberty (Gordon *et al.*, 1991).

Genetic differences are the basis for differences between population groups and it is self-evident that the adults of different ethnic groups have overall size differences; witness a group of Japanese and a group of Dutch tourists. A comprehensive survey of variation in the growth of children world-wide can be found in Eveleth and Tanner (1990). The difference that the environment may make on this intrinsic genetic factor is complex and one interesting approach to its elucidation has been longitudinal growth studies on monozygotic and dizygotic twins and their siblings (Tanner, 1962). By far the most important environmental factors are those that can be grouped together under the umbrella of socio-economic influences and they may be subdivided into the effects of nutrition, disease and social status itself. Although all these factors dominate most strongly in infancy and childhood, their extremes can affect growth and development even before birth. The starvation conditions in both Russia and the Netherlands during World War II caused a significant decline in both birth weight and vitality of infants (Antonov, 1947; Smith, 1947). The effects on optimum size and weight at birth and poor growth in the early years have been shown to affect not only final adult size, but also susceptibility to disease (Frisancho *et al.*, 1970; Clark *et al.*, 1986; Barker *et al.*, 1993). Maternal undernutrition appears to be one of the links in the causal chain between socio-economic factors and fetal growth (Lechtig *et al.*, 1975). Nutrition and disease have long been accepted as factors in raised childhood morbidity and mortality rates in countries with low socio-economic levels. It has also been shown that in the USA, delayed postnatal ossification rates and tooth emergence times are related to low income levels (Garn *et al.*, 1973a, b).

Minor factors such as season and climate are also thought to affect rates of growth and maturity. It is known that growth in height and weight differs according to the time of year but it is debatable as to what extent climate affects these processes. Studies comparing ethnic minorities in their adopted countries to populations still living in their original homeland have often given contradictory results. Again, it is difficult to isolate climate from the many changes that have acted on the immigrant community.

Evidence has accumulated that over the past 150 years there has been an increase in height and weight of adults and a decrease in the age at which adult size is achieved in many west European and North American populations (Tanner, 1962; Floud *et al.*, 1990; Hoppa and Garlie, 1998). There has also been a marked tendency for menarche and the adolescent growth spurt to occur earlier (Tanner, 1978; Roede and Van Wieringen, 1985; Hoppa and Garlie, 1998). The reasons for this so-called 'secular trend' are difficult to disentangle from the overall one of improvement in socio-economic circumstances with its concomitant better nutrition and housing. In fact, Maresh (1972) failed to find such changes in a stable economic and educationally privileged group that was studied over a 45-year period in the USA.

The variability of growth and some of the factors responsible are discussed in detail in Tanner (1962, 1978), Sinclair (1978) and Eveleth and Tanner (1990). It is clear that the relationship between growth and age is far from simple and because of this variability, growth can never be considered a reliable indicator of the actual age of a child. However, growth is the marker by which society invariably measures development and maturity.

Age

There are many practical situations that require the establishment of the age of a child. For example, clinicians in specialties such as orthopaedic surgery, orthodontics or growth hormone treatment often need to establish the stage of skeletal or dental maturity of a child almost regardless of the actual chronological age. A critical window of time can then be identified for corrective treatment so that intervention does not impede future development and an optimum time may be left for catch-up growth. The judicial system demands that a child of unknown age be assigned an age to ensure that appropriate procedures are observed in the processing of a legal case. In some countries, permits for refugees lacking proper documents are dependent on the establishment of adult status. In some developing countries, the ages of children may not be accurately known or may, for personal reasons, be falsified. For example, parents are known to falsify the ages, particularly of their sons, to obtain preferential educational opportunities (Chagula, 1960; Eveleth and Tanner, 1990). Skeletal biologists use child death rates and life expectancies to construct a demographic profile of a population and need the estimated ages of juveniles in the sample. This is often used as a reflection of health in an attempt to reconstruct the lifestyle of past peoples, both in prehistoric and historic periods. Forensic scientists who are called to investigate immature skeletal remains may need to establish age at death as part of the procedure to discover the identity of a particular individual.

Many terms are used to designate different phases of the lifespan of an individual and while a few are established clinical definitions, others are not universally accepted and their usage varies in different contexts and in different countries. Some commonly used terms, including those adopted in the present text, can be found in Appendix 1.

Postnatally, chronological, or true calendar age is calculated from the day of birth. While this may appear to be rather obvious, as with all biological criteria it is not always accurate. Dates of birth are sometimes simply incorrectly recalled or may be falsified for personal reasons. Todd (1920) reported that, in the Terry Collection, the listed ages at death for adults displayed peaks around 5-year intervals, indicating that perhaps in later life people giving information tend to round to the nearest quinquennium. Lovejoy *et al.* (1985a), investigating the cadaver records for the Hamann–Todd collection (Cleveland, Ohio), discovered gross discrepancies between 'stated' and 'observed' ages at death.

In the prenatal period chronological age *per se* does not technically exist as it is not possible to establish a starting point (i.e. fertilization) with any certainty and in fact, obstetricians and embryologists record age slightly differently (O'Rahilly, 1997). In the clinical context, the only known date is usually that of the first day of the last menstrual period (LMP) of the mother but even the accuracy of this date may be affected by factors such as postfertilization bleeding, inconsistencies of maternal recollection or intentional falsification. The actual known date of insemination is rarely known and tends to be restricted to cases of rape or *in vitro* fertilization. In addition, the period between insemination and fertilization is itself slightly variable. Clinically, normal term is calculated as 280 days (40 weeks/10 lunar months). The ranges of weights and lengths of a baby at term are population-dependent but for forensic purposes in the UK are taken as 2550–3360 g, 28–32 cm crown–rump length (CRL) and 48–52 cm crown–heel length (CHL) (Knight, 1996). Gestational age is also frequently estimated in the live newborn infant by evaluation of its neurological maturity (Dubowitz *et al.*, 1970; Dubowitz and Dubowitz, 1977).

Developmental embryologists calculate age from the time of fertilization (postovulation) which takes place approximately two weeks after the first day of the last menstrual period and anatomical prenatal age averages 266 days (9.5 lunar months). This can vary with the interval between ovulation and fertilization and it is extremely rare to know the actual age of an embryo (Tucker and O'Rahilly, 1972). Studies of early human development were carried out on embryos obtained from spontaneous or elective abortions and while the latter may technically be considered to constitute a normal sample, the former may have exhibited abnormalities that would negate the usefulness of the data. Historically, age was expressed in terms of the crown–rump length, crown–heel length or foot length of the embryo (Streeter, 1920; Noback, 1922; Scammon and Calkins, 1923). Because of the variation that inevitably occurs when a single criterion such as age is used, it was difficult to make valid comparisons between embryos of the same size but of obviously different developmental stages. This problem was overcome in the human embryonic period and also in a number of commonly used laboratory animals, by a practice called staging. It entailed the division of the first 8 postovulatory weeks (the embryonic period proper) into 23 stages, originally called Streeter developmental horizons but now known as Carnegie stages. Each stage was characterized by a number of external and internal morphological criteria, which were independent of size but indicative of maturity. Staging was initiated by Streeter (1942, 1945, 1948, 1951) and continued by O'Rahilly and co-workers (O'Rahilly and Gardner, 1972, 1975; O'Rahilly and Müller, 1986; Müller and O'Rahilly, 1994, 1997). See also Appendix 2, Table 1.

In the fetal period (from 9 weeks to term), the stage of development is still usually expressed in terms of CRL or related data. CRL itself is a rather inexact measurement and actual sizes do vary considerably, although the morphological differences between fetuses become less obvious as term approaches. Therefore texts that provide equivalent ages also vary, but there is, nevertheless, an accepted correlation of ranges of CRL with age (Appendix 2, Table 2). The relationship between various measurements and gestational age were discussed by Birkbeck (1976). More recently, Croft *et al.* (1999) used obstetrical ultrasound to determine the most suitable parameters for ageing formalin-fixed human fetuses. They found that both foot length and head circumference were superior to CRL, which, after the first trimester, was inaccurate due to distortion of the spine caused by compression in storage. Source material representing the fetal stage includes both aborted fetuses and stillbirths.

The inherent levels of variability in growth and the uncertainty of establishing actual age in a number of situations means that the concept of biological age is used as an indicator of how far along the developmental continuum an individual has progressed. Biological age encompasses both skeletal and dental age. The estimation of skeletal age uses both the times of appearance and fusion of ossification centres and the size and morphology of bones. Dental age is expressed either as time of tooth emergence, or in terms of the state of maturation of the teeth assessed from various stages of mineralization.

Skeletal age

To establish the age of an individual from a bone, or bone element, it is necessary to identify it in one of its three phases of development. First, the time at which the ossification centre appears; second, the morphological appearance including the size of the centre and finally, where appropriate, the time of fusion of the centre with another separate centre of ossification. Because the various bones of the skeleton are very different in function, growth pattern and timescale of development, these three phases will not necessarily apply either to all bony elements, or to all situations that require estimation of age. The three phases will be considered in relation to the source material from which they are derived.

Appearance of ossification centres

Ossification centres form throughout the entire period of skeletal development. In their earliest stages, they are identified by their anatomical position rather than their distinctive morphology as they are mostly indistinguishable from each other. They require the presence of soft tissue to hold them in place and therefore establish their identity. In general, the majority of primary centres form in the embryonic and early fetal periods of life, whereas most of the secondary centres make their appearance after birth. However, research data recorded before birth are from an entirely different material source from those obtained postnatally. In addition, most observations on prenatal material use different techniques from those employed postnatally. Prenatal ossification studies were mainly based on embryos and fetuses obtained as a result of abortions or stillbirths. Age was therefore uncertain and estimated from size or morphological characteristics. In addition, embryos and fetuses may not have been normal (see above). A number of factors, including single or multiple fetal occupation of the uterus, nutrition of the mother, and the introduction of teratogenic components such as nicotine, alcohol, and other drugs can affect development and in most cases such information was unknown (Roberts, 1976). In contrast, the vast majority of postnatal observations were based on healthy living children by means of longitudinal or cross-sectional radiographic studies, although there are a few observations on amputated and postmortem limbs.

Prenatal ossification centres include those of the skull, the vertebral column, the ribs, sternum and the primary centres in the major long bones of the limbs, their girdles and the phalanges of the hands and feet. Some primary centres in the ankle and the secondary centres around the knee appear in the last few weeks before term. The times of appearance of primary centres of ossification as reported in the literature are quite variable on account of two main factors. First, as already discussed, age itself in the prenatal period is not easy to establish and second, the detection of ossification varies according to the technique of observation. Prior to 1895 observations on bone development in embryonic, fetal and perinatal infants were made from gross anatomical dissections. A review can be found in Noback (1943, 1944). Drawings of the fetal skeleton by Kerckring (1717), Albinus (1737) and Rambaud and Renault (1864) are still some of the best recordings taken from gross specimens and are a salutary lesson in detailed observation. Subsequently, three principal methods were used: histological examination of serial sections, clearing and staining with alizarin and radiological investigation, each of which had a different sensitivity for the detection of bone (Noback and Robertson, 1951; Meyer and O'Rahilly, 1958; O'Rahilly and Gardner, 1972).

Bone is a tissue that is defined in histological terms and therefore its critical detection must, by definition, be by histological techniques (O'Rahilly and Gardner, 1972). Although the examination of serial sections of embryos is a time-consuming and laborious technique, most of the classical papers describing the human embryonic skeleton, especially the skull, have been made by this method (Fawcett, 1910a; Macklin, 1914, 1921; Lewis, 1920; Grube and Reinbach, 1976; Müller and O'Rahilly, 1980, 1986, 1994; O'Rahilly and Müller, 1984a). It is the most sensitive way of detecting bone and observations using this method nearly always result in earlier reported times of appearance of an ossification centre.

The second method involved clearing of whole specimens by potassium hydroxide, usually followed by staining with alizarin red S. This method provided a good overall picture of ossification in whole embryos, especially the establishment of periosteal bone collars and mineralization in tooth germs (Zawisch, 1956; Meyer and O'Rahilly, 1958; Kraus and Jordan, 1965). Its disadvantages were that it destroyed the soft tissues and could only be employed in the early period, when the embryo or fetus was small enough to be transparent (O'Rahilly and Gardner, 1972). The method is not specific for bone, and because some accounts have used the first sign of osteoid to signify the beginning of ossification, this has increased the range of reported appearance times of centres. However, an early, detailed and useful account of the whole skeleton using this method on 136 embryos and fetuses was given by Noback and Robertson (1951).

Third, radiological examination of fetuses is simple and rapid and leaves the specimen intact for subsequent investigation by other methods. Even after enhancement by soaking in silver solutions, detection of calcification is delayed by comparison with the previous two methods until a sufficient quantity of material has accumulated to render the tissue radiopaque. Calcified cartilage and bone are both radiopaque and the only reliable evidence that bone is present radiographically is the presence of trabeculae (Roche, 1986). This is the least sensitive of the methods available and the time difference between the alizarin technique and radiological observation in indicating the appearance of bone is approximately 1 week (Noback, 1944). Meyer and O'Rahilly (1958) used all three methods in each of several specimens to examine the variation in reported timings. Some of the differences in the reported times of appearance of ossification centres are obviously due to the variety of observational techniques used and in consequence, this has led to confusion and controversies in the literature about the exact time of appearance of centres (Youssef, 1964; Wood *et al.*, 1969; O'Rahilly and Gardner, 1972).

The appearance of postnatal ossification centres occupies a wide timespan from immediately after birth through to early adult life. Centres may be divided into two main categories: primary centres of bones of the wrist and ankle and the secondary ossification centres of the epiphyses of the ribs, vertebral column, sternum, girdles and the long bones of the limbs. Nearly all the data on these two groups of bones have come from systematic, non-repeatable, longitudinal radiological growth studies of children. They were carried out between 1930 and 1960 before the full risk of repeated exposure to X-rays was appreciated. Large groups of children, mostly of white, middle-class origin, were radiographed, often three times during the first year of life and then at 6-monthly, and then yearly intervals until cessation of growth in height. These collections of normal growth data were originally compiled for clinical purposes. Screening programmes could then identify individuals at risk who might benefit from treatment and response could be evaluated by paediatricians. Larger groups of data were also used to reflect the general health of the population in particular communities or between social classes (Tanner, 1978).

Some of the published studies in the USA and UK include:

Institution	Main researchers*
The University of Colorado	Maresh, Hansman
The Brush Foundation, Case Western Reserve	Todd, Greulich, Hoerr, Pyle
The Fels Institute, Yellow Springs, Ohio	Garn and colleagues
The Harpenden Growth Study	Tanner and colleagues
The Oxford Child Health Survey	Hewitt, Acheson and colleagues

*See bibliography.

In addition to these large longitudinal surveys, there have been other studies either of a cross-sectional nature or, as often happens, a mixture of the two. Both offer a different type of information and have their merits and disadvantages (Tanner, 1962, 1978). The statistical methods and sampling problems encountered in large studies of this kind are discussed by Goldstein (1986), Healy (1986) and Marubini and Milani (1986). Briefly, a longitudinal study consists of following the same group of individuals over a period of time, whereas a cross-sectional study measures a number of people once only at a particular time in their development. Longitudinal studies, especially those that extend over a number of years, are expensive and time-consuming, and require great commitment on the part of both the investigators and subjects. They are the only way to reveal true individual differences in growth velocity such as those that occur in the adolescent growth spurt. As there is always a drop-out rate, longitudinal studies are rarely exclusively longitudinal, and therefore often include by necessity some cross-sectional data. Because cross-sectional data collection only requires a single measurement (or set of measurements) for each individual, it is potentially easier to include greater numbers. Essentially, it will give information about whether an individual has reached a certain stage of development compared with the mean for that age group.

Many of the large growth studies were used to compile reference atlases specific to a particular joint or topographical region. They consist of a series of standards, separate for males and females, usually at 6-monthly intervals, each of which was compiled from approximately 100 films judged to be the most representative of the anatomical mode. The atlas of the hand and wrist (Greulich and Pyle, 1959) illustrates development of the primary centres of the carpus, secondary centres for the metacarpals, phalanges and distal ends of the radius and ulna. The atlas of the foot and ankle (Hoerr *et al.*, 1962) shows development of the primary centres of the tarsus and secondary centres of the calcaneus, metatarsals, phalanges and distal ends of the tibia and fibula. Similarly the atlas of the elbow (Brodeur *et al.*, 1981) illustrates the development of the secondary centres in the distal humerus and proximal radius and ulna; and that of the knee (Pyle and Hoerr, 1955) shows the appearance of the patella and secondary centres of the distal femur and proximal tibia and fibula.

The skeletal age of an individual can be estimated by comparing the pattern of appearance of ossification centres on a radiograph of the relevant region with the maturity stages in the atlas. However, this inspectional technique suffers from a number of disadvantages. First, systematic and variable errors occur in evaluation (Mainland, 1953, 1954, 1957; Cockshott and Park, 1983; Cundy *et al.*, 1988). Second, there are methodological objections to this way of assessing maturation (Acheson, 1954, 1957). It presupposes a fixed pattern and order of development in the appearance of centres which is by no means the case in all individuals. There is also necessarily a certain time interval between standard films so that a distinction can be made between successive standards. However, this is often too long for good matching to take place. Finally, Garn and Rohmann (1963) and Garn *et al.* (1965a) warn that as a general rule, ossification centres appearing in early postnatal life tend not to be normally distributed but are particularly skewed. As the mean and median no longer coincide, data presented with percentiles are more accurate than those with means, and the atlas method cannot take this into account.

In summary, the formation times of ossification centres:

- are useful in a clinical context to rapidly establish the developmental status of an individual by reference to a standard maturity stage. Treatment of, for example, hormonal pathology may then be carried out at the optimum time
- may be employed to assign an estimated age to an individual of unknown age using maturity status as in the clinical context. A variety of circumstances could include a legal situation
- are of little use in the estimation of age at death of individuals forming part of a skeletal assemblage as the remains are usually disassociated. The only exception is perhaps the examination of mummified material by a variety of radiographic techniques
- may be of use in specific forensic situations. If the body is decomposed but intact, radiological and possibly histological techniques may be possible, although the latter could be of poor quality. The possible presence of ossification in the calcaneus, talus (and possibly the cuboid) and the appearance of secondary centres in the distal femur and proximal tibia usually signify a full-term fetus and are therefore of direct legal significance (Knight, 1996).

Morphology and size of ossification centres

During development, each ossification centre assumes its own unique morphology. This permits identification in isolation and does not therefore rely on the presence of soft tissue to maintain its anatomical position. The database for this stage of ossification includes information from disassociated skeletal remains and is therefore drawn from a much wider source of material than that for appearance of centres. Once a bone element is recognizable, age may then be assessed, either from its size or from the morphological stage of its development. This phase covers a wide age range, extending from midfetal life onwards to the adult stage.

The primary centres that appear in the early part of prenatal life are nearly all recognizable as specific bones, or bone elements, by midfetal life and certainly most are identifiable by the time of birth. They include the bones of the skull, vertebral column, sternum, ribs, pectoral and pelvic girdles and the major long bones of the limbs. Ribs and elements of the vertebral column cannot usually be assigned to their particular segment in the series until the perinatal period.

The study of fetal osteology by Fazekas and Kósa (1978) contains much valuable information, including measurements of most bones of the skeleton from three lunar months to term. However, the age/bone-size correlations involve an inherent circular argument as their material, being of forensic origin, was essentially of uncertain age. Fetuses were grouped according to crown–heel length, each group being assigned an age at half-lunar month intervals in accordance with the widely accepted correlation between body length and age (Scammon and Calkins, 1929) by using Haase's rule (Fazekas and Kósa, 1978). Their 'regression diagrams' (graphs) are of body length as the independent variable against bone length as the dependent variable. While there is undoubtedly a close correlation between fetal age and size, as grouping was based on crown–heel length, all the bones, especially those of the lower limb that actually contribute to body length, inevitably show a high correlation and lie very close to a straight line. 'Modified regression diagrams' show age in lunar months superimposed onto these graphs.

Most of the other available data from the prenatal period relate to lengths of the diaphyses of major long bones and there is a relatively large database for comparison of diaphyseal length with gestational age. Diaphyses have been measured directly on alizarin-stained fetuses, on dry bone, or by means of standard radiography and by ultrasound. Data from measurement of dry bones can be found in Balthazard and Dervieux (1921), Hesdorffer and Scammon (1928), Moss *et al.* (1955), Olivier and Pineau[1] (1960), Olivier (1974), Keleman *et al.* (1984) and Bareggi *et al.* (1994a, 1996). Data from radiographs can be found in Scheuer *et al.* (1980) and Bagnall *et al.* (1982). Any data obtained by measurement on aborted fetuses are, of necessity, cross-sectional and in addition may introduce some abnormal data. Starting from the early 1980s

[1] Huxley and Jimenez (1996) report an error in the regression formula for the radius.

there has been increasingly detailed data from ultrasound studies (Jeanty *et al.*, 1981; O'Brien *et al.*, 1981; Filly and Golbus, 1982; Jeanty *et al.*, 1982; Seeds and Cefalo, 1982; Bertino *et al.*, 1996). These 'ages' commence from conception and have to be adjusted if dates are established from LMP (McIntosh, 1998). Ultrasound norms are derived either from cross-sectional surveys or from longitudinal surveys that involve a limited number of observations per pregnancy (Bertino *et al.*, 1996).

In the postnatal period, data on lengths of diaphyses are drawn from the many cross-sectional and longitudinal surveys described above. The data most commonly used for comparison with archaeological collections are those from the University of Colorado reported by Maresh (1943, 1955, 1970), which extend from birth to the cessation of growth in length and cover all six major limb bones. Other studies, some limited to fewer bones and shorter time periods, are by Ghantus (1951), Anderson *et al.* (1964) and Gindhart (1973). Almost all the data are from white Europeans, or from individuals in the USA of European descent and there is a dearth of published data from other parts of the world. There are many studies from Africa, Europe and North America that have measured the long bones of undocumented archaeological populations where age has been estimated, usually from dental development. Some of these, together with the details of age ranges and bones studied can be found in Appendix 3.

Estimation of age is also possible from the morphological appearance of the ossification centre. However, apart from radiological appearances, which are usually limited to standard two-dimensional views of a limited number of bones, there is very little information concerning the morphological changes that occur during development. This is a neglected area of osteology and there appear to be few accounts of the changes that occur in the detailed bony anatomy of either primary or secondary centres of the juvenile skeleton, enabling identification at the different stages of their development.

In the clinical context, changes in the radiological appearance during development have been used to a limited extent as a method for the assessment of maturity. The bone age together with height of a child can then be used to predict adult height (Tanner, 1978). As the inspectional atlas technique was often considered unsatisfactory (see above), alternative methods using the wrist and knee were developed (Acheson, 1954, 1957; Tanner *et al.*, 1983). The metaphyseal ends of the long bones and the epiphyses of each region were awarded a score in units as each change in shape occurred during development. In this way, each individual bone element was allowed to make its own contribution to a total maturity score, regardless of the order of development of individual units. It thus avoided the assessor being compelled to match an individual's X-ray to a standard picture in an atlas and so circumvented the problem of a fixed order of development. As the ossification sequence is also sexually dimorphic (Garn *et al.*, 1966a), the 'score' method allowed direct comparison between the sexes because the units were those of maturity and not of time. It proved to be a more accurate, but obviously more time-consuming and laborious procedure than the direct inspectional method. The principle is similar to that used for assessing mineralization stages of tooth development in the estimation of dental age (see below and Chapter 5).

Apart from this clinical application, the changing morphological appearance of both primary centres and epiphyses has been used very little in attempts to estimate age. Fazekas and Kósa (1978) comment briefly on the union of major elements of the sphenoid, temporal and occipital bones and relate this to viability in the neonatal period and Redfield (1970) and Scheuer and MacLaughlin-Black (1994) have related the size and morphology of elements of the occipital bone to age. Otherwise, there appears to be no significant body of information except for isolated accounts in the clinical literature.

Most endochondral centres start ossification as spherical or ovoid nodules of bone near the centre of their cartilaginous template and then expand as ossification proceeds (Chapter 3). Therefore, each element must reach a critical morphological stage before it can be identified and so distinguished from other bones. This stage varies greatly, depending on the part of the skeleton under consideration. Most of the bones of the skull, vertebral centra and arches, ribs and the major long bones of the limbs are recognizable from midfetal life onwards. Some bones of the ankle and early developing long bone epiphyses may be identified in the first few years of life, whereas those of the carpus and later developing epiphyses do not reach a recognizable stage until well into the childhood years. There is yet another group of distinctive epiphyses belonging to the scapula and pelvis that develop in late adolescence.

Paucity of information on the anatomy of all these bony elements is undoubtedly due to the difficulty in obtaining juvenile skeletal material. Postmortem specimens are fortunately rare, and rightly difficult to obtain, because of the sensitivity and obvious emotional consequences of a child's death. In archaeological skeletal collections, epiphyses, especially those of the later developing group, are particularly rare. This is partly due to the age at death profile of most of these samples. Children succumb to adverse environmental circumstances in the early years of life but if they survive the first 5 years, few die in later childhood. Material from the ages of 6–12 years is particularly rare.

Those epiphyses that start development early and have a longer separate existence, principally those at the growing end of the long bones (Chapter 3), are more plentiful than the later appearing epiphyses, which have a shorter life. For example, it is fairly common to find epiphyses of the proximal humerus, distal radius, proximal and distal femur and tibia but elbow epiphyses are extremely rare. Improved knowledge of timing of skeletal development and the ability to recognize these small elements would undoubtedly result in a better retrieval rate during skeletal excavations. Even with adult material, Waldron (1987) commented that recovery of some parts of the skeleton was much lower than expected. It was suggested that one of the factors responsible was lack of awareness of the anatomy. It is hoped that the present text will add to the sparse accounts of the juvenile stage of development. Obviously, age estimation will be determined with greater accuracy using those bone elements that undergo distinct changes within a relatively short time range. Together with diaphyseal length, this aspect of evaluating maturity, could then improve accuracy of age estimation.

In summary, the size and morphology of ossification centres:

- are useful in a clinical context to assess maturity. This may be made directly from the lengths of long bone diaphyses or from morphological changes, which can be used to provide maturity scores. Evaluations of both lengths of bones and changes in shape are used to predict adult height. The most common application at the present time is the use of preterm ultrasound to monitor fetal development
- may be used in age estimation of juveniles in both archaeological and forensic assemblages.

Fusion of ossification centres

Timing of fusion varies greatly in different parts of the skeleton, partly in response to the function of the soft tissues with which that element is associated. For example, the parts of the skeleton that enclose the brain and spinal cord reach union either before birth or during early childhood, reflecting the precocious development of the central nervous system (Humphrey, 1998). Long bone diameters on the other hand, are among the last areas of the skeleton to reach maturity and this is in part due to the delayed spurt in muscle growth especially in the adolescent male.

Fusion in most postcranial bones takes place at a growth plate between a primary centre and a secondary centre, or epiphysis (Chapter 3). The definition of a secondary centre is one whose formation is separated in time from the much earlier primary centre, thus allowing a period for growth. The skull does not in general follow this type of pattern. Many of the bones develop from a single centre and later fuse at sutures, whereas other compound bones can be said to develop from several primary centres since they all appear within a relatively short time span. There are growth plates between individual bones such as the spheno-occipital synchondrosis and jugular growth plate, but there are no secondary centres in the same sense as in the postcranial skeleton. Most of the components of the sphenoid, temporal and squamous occipital bones join prenatally and the principal parts of the occipital bone and the vertebral centra and arches fuse during early childhood. They may be viewed radiologically or macroscopically on dry bone and provide convenient indicators of age during this early period of life (Chapters 5 and 6). Later in childhood and adolescence, major components of the sternum, scapula and pelvis unite (Chapters 7, 8 and 10). The epiphyses of the major long bones of the limbs, those of the hands and feet and the spheno-occipital synchondrosis of the skull are among the large number of centres that fuse during the adolescent period (Chapters 5, 9 and 11). Postadolescence, there is a further group of bones whose epiphyses fuse in the early adult age period. They include the jugular growth plate of the skull, the secondary centres of the vertebrae, scapula, clavicle, sacrum and pelvis (Chapters 5, 6, 8 and 10). Interestingly, the clavicle, which is regarded as the first long bone to show signs of ossification, has an epiphysis at its medial end that is probably the last of the secondary centres to fuse.

As with times of appearance of ossification centres, the reported times of fusion are very variable. This is partly due to the fact that variability increases with increasing age and in addition, as with the appearance of centres, different methods of observation affect the reported times. Fusion has been chiefly studied either radiographically or by observations on dry bone, although there are a few histological studies (see Chapters 3 and 5). Radiographic studies are either confined to atlases of regions as discussed above or appear as scattered reports in the clinical literature. As with appearance times, there is a similar problem of matching an individual to a particular atlas pattern.

Early studies of fusion in dry bone and on radiographs were carried out by Stevenson (1924), Todd (1930a) and Stewart (1934a). In their investigation of the Korean War dead, McKern and Stewart (1957) used Stevenson's (1924) categories of fusion and although their data were more extensive in number, their sample was necessarily restricted to males of active military age. As a result, their 'late union' group of epiphyses probably displayed the full range, although their 'early union' group was inevitably truncated at its lower end. Their conclusions pointed to a constant order irrespective of age and to the innominate bone as being the best indicator throughout the particular age range studied (17–23 years).

There are several methodological problems involved with reporting epiphyseal union. The distinction between different stages was difficult to identify and as expected, intra- and interobserver errors increase as the process of union is divided into an increasing number of stages. It is also difficult to associate observations from dry bone and from radiographs as the former is observed from bridges of bones seen at the periphery of the epiphyseal/metaphyseal junction, whereas the descriptions of the latter often describe fusion as beginning in the centre of the epiphyseal plate (see Chapter 3). Timing of fusion is much affected by variation in the onset of the adolescent growth spurt and not all accounts give total age ranges or gender differences. Because secondary sexual characters are not reflected in the skeleton until adolescent sexual dimorphism is well under way, the consequent inability to determine sex in juvenile skeletal remains complicates the use of fusion times to estimate age in this group. Webb and Suchey (1985) used large numbers of both sexes in a study of ageing from the anterior iliac crest and medial clavicle. The epiphyses of these bones are different from those of the long bones in that they fuse relatively soon after formation and so different staging categories were employed. Results showed that both these bones were useful, at least in the forensic situation, where a complete cadaver was present and therefore their first stage of 'no epiphysis present' was capable of confirmation. Again, the best indicators of age are those whose ranges of fusion are the most restricted in time.

In summary, timing of fusion of ossification centres:

- is useful in a clinical context to identify premature fusion as a sign of pathological growth disturbance, or the normal cessation of growth
- in age at death estimations from juvenile skeletal remains is complicated by the inability to assign sex. Age ranges are therefore wider than they need to be had sex been known
- may be used to estimate age of forensic remains if the sex is known from soft tissues or other factors. If skeletal remains only are present, then the same problems stated above are relevant.

Dental age

Dental age is the other major indicator of maturity in the juvenile and was used historically in the UK to estimate age in children before it became obligatory to register births (Saunders, 1837[2]) and it has several advantages over skeletal ageing. First, teeth survive inhumation well, which makes dental age especially relevant to palaeontologists and skeletal biologists. Teeth are often the only structures representing certain fossil species and in more recent skeletal assemblages they may be the least damaged. Second, the growth of the deciduous and permanent teeth takes place over the entire range of the juvenile life span, starting during the embryonic period and nearing completion during the late adolescent or early adult period. Finally, it is well recognized that in living populations, for a given chronological age, dental age exhibits less variability than does skeletal age (Lewis and Garn, 1960; Demirjian, 1986; Smith, 1991a). Dental development is less affected than bone formation by adverse environmental and physiological circumstances such as nutrition and disturbances in endocrine function and therefore approximates more closely to chronological age than does skeletal age (Garn *et al.*, 1959; Lewis and Garn, 1960; Garn *et al.*, 1965b, 1973a, b; Demirjian, 1986). In a population of known chronological age, the estimated dental age diverges less from actual age than does estimated skeletal age (Bowman *et al.*, 1992). The reasons for this are not entirely clear but one factor could be the protected prenatal milieu in which the development of nearly all the deciduous and some of the permanent teeth takes place.

Two aspects of dental development have been used in dental ageing: the eruption of the teeth and the stage of mineralization of the crowns and roots. Mineralization appears to be less affected than does eruption by both intrinsic and extrinsic conditions. Developmental processes are thought to be mainly genetically determined (Lewis and Garn, 1960; Tanner, 1962; Garn *et al.*, 1965c, 1973c), whereas eruption can be affected by systemic influences such as nutrition or local conditions for example, early loss of deciduous precursors or inadequate space in the jaws (Fanning, 1961; Haavikko, 1973; Brown, 1978).

[2]In the UK ageing from the teeth dates from early in the nineteenth century. For instance, Edwin Saunders, a dentist, was the author of a pamphlet 'The Teeth a Test of Age, considered with reference to the Factory Children' which was addressed to the members of both Houses of Parliament. Also Thomson (1836), a medicolegal expert, said 'if the third molar [first permanent molar] hath not protruded, you can have no hesitation in affirming that the culprit has not passed his seventh year'. This fortunately prevented children below the age of 7 from being subject to the severe penal code of the time.

Strictly speaking, eruption includes the whole process by which a tooth moves from the depths of the alveolar bone to the occlusal level but nearly all studies of eruption are actually confined to emergence of the teeth and are therefore wrongly referred to as eruption (Demirjian, 1986). Clinically, emergence is defined as the time at which any part of a tooth has pierced the gingiva or, in a radiographic image, alveolar emergence is said to occur when the supporting bone on the occlusal surface has resorbed. Obviously, in studies on dry bone, gingival emergence cannot be measured and tooth emergence is usually defined as the appearance of the tooth cusp at or above the level of the crestal alveolar bone.

The advantage of studying mineralization rather than emergence is that stages can be observed at any point during the lifespan of a tooth, whereas emergence is a single event whose exact time of occurrence is not usually accurately known. However, there is a large volume of literature on tooth emergence times and there are occasions, both in fieldwork and in a forensic situation, when tooth emergence may be the only practical means on which to base the age of an individual.

The development of much of the deciduous dentition takes place during the prenatal period and, as with the study of appearance of ossification centres of the bones, much of the detailed development has been studied by methods of gross dissection, alizarin staining and radiography using aborted fetuses. The development of the roots of the deciduous teeth and the early stages of crown formation of the permanent teeth take place postnatally. There are problems with studying the stages that occur during infancy and early childhood, mainly concerned with the difficulties of X-raying very young children. Studies of the developing permanent dentition have, for the most part, been by radiographic methods in living populations of children. Emergence of both deciduous and permanent teeth is of course observed directly on living children. In skeletal and fossil remains, both alveolar emergence and more detailed developmental stages have been studied radiographically. Discrepancies in results are often due to different statistical methods and sampling (Smith, 1991a). Both emergence and mineralization stages of teeth are considered in more detail in Chapter 5.

Skeletal remains

While it can be difficult to assign an age to a living child, the problem is greatly compounded when the child is dead and only bones or teeth remain. This can create special problems that are absent from the study of living populations.

One approach to the investigation into the lifestyle of a past population is to construct a demographic profile that will reveal death rates and life expectancies. The establishment of the ages at death and sex of the individuals that comprise the skeletal remains are normally one of the first tasks performed by the skeletal biologist. Another factor that has a bearing on building a realistic model is how far the remains that are available for analysis constitute a representative sample of the population of which they formed a part. Age and its relationship to growth has been discussed in some detail, but both documentation and representativeness, and the determination of sex of the immature component of the remains need to be considered briefly.

Documentation

The term 'documented' is usually applied to a skeletal collection that consists of the remains of individuals of known sex and age at death. In the majority of archaeological assemblages however, the biological identity of the individuals is unknown. Even the term documented is sometimes interpreted differently. For example, Ubelaker and Pap (1998) refer to a whole archaeological sample being documented in terms of knowing its overall historical dates and origins. Others refer to documentation as applied to a particular skeleton of known sex and age at death (Molleson and Cox, 1993; Cunha, 1995; Scheuer and Black, 1995) and there are a small number of these documented collections known to us in Europe, North America and South Africa. In the UK this material is restricted to the St Bride's and Spitalfields collections (Molleson and Cox, 1993; Scheuer and Black, 1995; Scheuer and Bowman, 1995; Scheuer, 1998). Documented material is available in the few UK Anatomy Departments that still dissect cadavers, but apart from some notable exceptions, it tends to be restricted to individuals of advanced years (MacLaughlin, 1987). In Canada, there is a subsample of the St Thomas's, Belleville cemetery (Saunders *et al.* 1993a). There are skeletal collections in Europe: Leiden, the Netherlands (MacLaughlin and Bruce, 1986) and Lisbon and Coimbra in Portugal (MacLaughlin, 1990b; Cunha, 1995); and South Africa: Witwatersrand University (Saunders and DeVito, 1991) and Cape Town University.

In the context of this book, documentation of an individual means that the remains of the deceased must be associated with some means of identification, such as a coffin plate that gives at least the name, and therefore sex, and also the age at death. Occasionally, there is additional information from birth and death certificates and from parish records of baptisms, marriages and burials. Often, in the case of infants and children, the date of birth is also on the coffin plate.

This emphasis on documented material does not imply that meaningful conclusions may not be drawn from undocumented archaeological samples, but there are many problems associated with this. The main difficulty lies in the choice of an appropriate sample with which to compare any markers that reflect defects of growth and development. Unless carefully chosen, there is a risk of squeezing the newly observed sample into a reflection of the comparison (Bocquet-Apel and Masset, 1982, 1985).

Sampling and representativeness

By its very nature, an archaeological skeletal sample is bound to be biased so that it does not fairly represent the population of which it once formed a part. It is necessarily cross-sectional in nature and therefore differs from a living sample, which is composed of selected individuals. In addition, burial in a particular place is affected by a variety of factors including social and economic conditions and religious beliefs. After burial, subsequent skeletonization and preservation of the bones are in turn affected by the physical conditions of the burial place and these may include temperature, type of soil, coffin design or disturbance by humans and predators. Even in a carefully planned excavation, it is not always possible to recover all the material from the ground in a good enough condition to contribute useful information towards sexing and ageing of individual skeletons. As a result, the true age profile of the original population will always remain uncertain. Some of the factors affecting sampling and their effects on recovery and reconstruction in general are discussed further by Boddington (1987), Henderson (1987) and Waldron (1994).

The juvenile component of the sample can be biased in particular ways that do not affect the adults. Johnston (1962) and Lampl and Johnston (1996) warned that skeletal samples usually contain some degree of inbuilt error as the juveniles in many populations of this type consist of individuals that were subject to illness, or deficiency of some sort and could not represent the normal healthy children that went on to constitute the adult population. However, this criticism may only apply if the individuals suffered from chronic disease or malnutrition, whereas many illnesses, for example plague and childhood infectious diseases, probably killed people before they had time to manifest effects on the skeleton. Saunders and Hoppa (1993) reviewed the literature for evidence of reduced or retarded growth in skeletal samples and the issue of biological mortality bias. They concluded that while the potential for bias exists, errors introduced by the larger methodological difficulties outweigh the small amount of error in interpretation of past population health.

Saunders and co-workers (1992, 1993a) also emphasized that some palaeoepidemiologists mistakenly refer to their long bone measurements as growth curves. They are not true growth curves, or measures of growth velocity as used by auxologists, because these can only be carried out on longitudinal follow-up studies. Saunders *et al.* (1993a) discussed methodology in relation to the production of so-called 'skeletal growth profiles' and have argued that confidence intervals rather than standard deviations should be used to report variation as they control sample size as well as variance.

Another factor which is often thought to bias the immature component of a skeletal sample is that the overall numbers of juveniles are lower than might be expected for the time and conditions of the period and this can seriously bias any conclusions drawn from death rates (Saunders and Melbye, 1990; Scheuer and Bowman, 1995; Cox, 1996). Occasionally, this supposition can be corroborated by documentary evidence. For example, it is clear from examination of burial registers that the proportion of adults to children interred in the crypt of St Bride's Church, Fleet Street and the cemetery of St Bride's are quite different. Therefore, any conclusions concerning the numbers of child deaths in the parish drawn from the age-at-death profile of the crypt collection alone would be invalid (Scheuer, 1998).

It has been argued that the low numbers, especially of infants, are due to the relative fragility and poor preservation of the remains (Kerley, 1976; Johnston and Zimmer, 1989; Goode *et al.*, 1993). Guy *et al.* (1997) suggested that the physicochemical properties of infant bones were responsible for the scarcity of very young remains in cemeteries. However, Sundick (1978) attributed the low retrieval rate of subadult material to bias at the time of excavation, rather than to the nature of the material. Deficiencies of skill and failure to recognize small unfused parts of the immature skeleton were thought to play a large part in the incompleteness of many juvenile remains. Although some of the bones, particularly those of the calvaria and face, often do not survive inhumation intact, many bones useful for estimating age such as the base of the skull, parts of the vertebrae and most long bones survive as well as those of the adult under similar conditions.

One known reason for the smaller than expected number of young juveniles in some assemblages was the widespread habit of excluding infants and young children from burial, so that they are under-represented in certain ossuaries. This selective process was sometimes dependent on a belief system of the community or due to economic circumstances. The prehistoric Iroquoians of southern Ontario often buried infants along pathways, believing that they could affect the fertility of passing women (Saunders, 1992). In St Albans, babies of the Romano–British period were found buried under the doorsteps of houses on the supposition that they could bring luck to the household (Molleson, pers. com.). Even in relatively recent historic time, it is clear that the numbers of infants and children found in crypt and cemetery samples are less than the documented records of their death (Cox, 1995; Scheuer and Bowman, 1995; Scheuer, 1998). Some of the reasons for these selective burial practices are unknown but undoubtedly economic factors must have played a part. In the eighteenth and nineteenth centuries, the cost of lead coffin burials, for example, was considerable, especially to families who may have lost many children in infancy.

Recently, various methods have been employed to make use of juvenile material previously thought to be too damaged to include in a skeletal analysis. Measurements of fragmentary long bones, other than total length, from Anglo-Saxon remains have been used successfully by Hoppa (1992) and the same method increased sample size by over 100% in an analysis of prehistoric Ontario remains (Hoppa and Gruspier, 1996). However, comparison between the two populations revealed significant differences and it was suggested that population-specific models would be necessary to make use of this method. Goode *et al.* (1993) have used a standardized method that would include any individual on a single plot, even if only represented by a single long bone.

Sex determination

Undoubtedly the largest single problem in the analysis of immature skeletal remains is the difficulty of sexing juveniles with any degree of reliability. Males and females mature at different times and different rates, especially in the adolescent period. The growth spurt occurs at different times, both in individuals of the same sex, (early and later maturers; Tanner, 1962) and also between girls and boys. As a result, any estimated age category is necessarily wider than it would be, had the sex been known. As quantitative differences of size and rate of growth between males and females are of little use in sexing skeletal remains, a large literature has accumulated on morphological differences, mostly centred on those regions that are most sexually dimorphic in adults, such as the pelvis and skull.

It is reported that the general shape of the pelvis, and particularly the greater sciatic notch and subpubic angle, shows that sexual dimorphism exists from an early age (for literature see Chapter 10). Fazekas and Kósa (1978) related the length of the greater sciatic notch to its depth and to the length of the ilium and femur and reported 70–80% success rates in sexing but Schutkowski (1987), using discriminant function analysis on the same data, achieved an accuracy of just 70%. More recently, Schutkowski (1993) has described differences in the greater sciatic notch and mandible in a documented collection but this has yet to be tested on a comparable series. Weaver (1980) proposed that the configuration of the auricular surface of the sacro-iliac joint might be useful in sex determination but tests of the method by Hunt (1990) and Mittler and Sheridan (1992) have shown that it may have a very limited use. Although there are undoubtedly skeletal morphological differences between the sexes from the intra-uterine stage onwards, it appears that they do not reach a sufficiently high level for reliable determination of sex until after the pubertal modifications take place. Some discrete traits of the orbit and mandible were scored to test determination of sex on a sample of adults and juveniles of known sex by Molleson *et al.* (1998). Sex was inferred correctly in almost 90% of adults and 78% of juveniles. When the same traits were scored in a large skeletal assemblage of unknown sex, there was a concordance between facial characters, pelvic sexing and size of the mandibular canines. This suggests that these traits could be useful in attempting to sex juveniles under carefully controlled conditions in a specific population, but more work is necessary should a larger assemblage of known sex become available.

An interesting approach to the problem of sexual dimorphism in archaeological populations has recently been developed and discussed by Humphrey (1998). Based on the concept that different parts of the skeleton vary in the proportion of adult size attained both at birth and postnatally, a method was introduced for analysing the sexual differences in the growth of the postcranial skeleton. It was demonstrated by analysis of separate male and female cross-sectional growth patterns that sexual dimorphism occurs in many parts of the skeleton that complete their growth prior to adolescence. This sort of approach may possibly provide an insight into a morphological method of distinguishing males and females during the childhood period.

As rates of dental development, particularly those of mineralization, show less sexual dimorphism than rates of skeletal maturation, dental and skeletal age estimates would be expected to show closer comparison in males than females (Lewis and Garn, 1960). Hunt and Gleiser (1955) estimated dental age from the mineralization of the first permanent molar and skeletal age from hand–wrist maturation standards and achieved between 73–81% correct diagnosis in living children. A modified method using mandibular teeth was tested by Bailit and Hunt (1964) and although 70% success rate was achieved if the chronological age of the child was known, only 58% of individuals were correctly sexed using developmental dental stages alone, which would not be acceptable in remains of unknown sex and age. This sort of approach might usefully be modified using a skeletal indicator such as the diaphyseal lengths of long bones, but the main obstacle to testing any of these methods is the lack of a sufficiently large sample of juvenile remains of documented age and sex.

Significant size dimorphism has been described in the permanent dentition of various populations, although the methodology of data collection may have influenced the reported levels (Mayhall, 1992). The canine shows the greatest amount of sexual dimorphism (Garn *et al.*, 1964, 1966b, 1967a; Moss and Moss-Salentijn, 1977) and in theory, this could be used from mid-childhood onwards. Garn *et al.* (1979) also reported that, using combinations of crown diameters and root lengths of the mandibular incisors, canine and second molar, successful sex discrimination reached 87%. However, this was at 16–17 years of age, when there are already skeletal morphological indicators. Owsley and Webb (1983) evaluated discriminant functions using verification procedures and have emphasized the advantages of using the permanent dentition when preservation of other parts is poor and osseous remains are damaged. The deciduous dentition has also been shown to be dimorphic but levels are even smaller than in the permanent dentition and intra- and interobserver error then becomes a significant methodological factor. Correct sexing can be as high as 85% in a holdout sample within a population (Black, 1978a; DeVito and Saunders, 1990) but this is of limited value as the degree and pattern of variation is population-dependent. Ditch and Rose (1972) and Rösing (1983) have reported successful discriminant function techniques for sexing from the dentition. These two studies were on archaeological populations of unknown sex, and are in fact concordances between dental and skeletal indicators and not tests of accuracy.

Further avenues that have been explored are methods for chemical and genetic identification. Saunders (1992) reported that, as chemical testing of citrate levels in bone relied on the differences that occur with the menstrual cycle, this is of use only during the adolescent period when, in any case, morphological features start to become useful. Since the isolation and amplification of DNA in archaeological bone (Hagelberg *et al.*, 1989; Hagelberg and Clegg, 1991), a more promising possibility is the sex-typing of genetic material (Naito *et al.*, 1994). Breakdown products of the amelogenins, the organic components of the enamel of teeth, are sometimes preserved in archaeological material. These proteins are produced by a gene with copies on the X and the Y chromosomes (Lau *et al.*, 1988; Slavkin, 1988), and have been used in sex determination (Stone *et al.*, 1996; Blondiaux *et al.*, 1998). Smith *et al.* (1993) have outlined guidelines based on histological and experimental evidence for the management and sampling of dental DNA. At the present time, genetic methods are limited by problems of contamination and degradation and are both time-consuming and expensive and are therefore unlikely to become available for routine archaeological use in the near future.

In conclusion, it would appear that better recognition of small, unfused parts of the immature skeleton would lead to the improved retrieval of the juvenile component of skeletal remains. Also, various methods that make use of previously discarded remains would enlarge the size of many subadult samples. The major problem in the skeletal analysis of juvenile remains still to be resolved is the ineffectiveness of most methods of sexing. New methods will undoubtedly be devised, but the material on which they are tested must be documented in nature. Any new method for sex determination and age estimation needs a rigorous standard against which to test its validity and reliability and this can only be achieved on a sample of known biological identity. While the majority of scholars do detail their sexing and ageing methods, there is a tendency to refer to confirmation of age and sex when both the original and the derived data were observed from anatomical parameters, thus resulting in a circular argument. The other main difficulty lies in the choice of an appropriate sample with which to compare any markers that might reflect defects of growth and development. For instance, caution must be used when applying standards derived from relatively recent material to ancient human remains because an archaeological sample may not show the same relationship between chronological and skeletal age as that displayed by the reference sample. Unless carefully chosen, there is also a risk of constraining the newly observed sample into a reflection of the comparison. In addition to these problems, there are many living populations on which there are no metric or morphological data, thus reducing the database for comparisons.

Truly documented samples are one of the most valuable resources to which a skeletal biologist has access. Such collections are obviously very limited and should be treasured and maintained in good order so that improved methods of establishing biological parameters of identity may be tested. Only then can relevant and reasonable conclusions be drawn from the skeletal remains of past peoples.

CHAPTER THREE

Bone Development

Bone is a tissue: Bones are organs.

(Weinmann and Sicher, 1947)

Mammalian bone arises from the differentiation of primitive mesenchymal tissue. At some sites this may involve the replacement of cartilage by bone and in others by the conversion of a more primitive membranous template. Perhaps with some justification, a great deal of weight has been placed on the distinction between a bone that is preformed in cartilage (**endochondral**) and one that arises from the transformation of a mesenchymal tissue (**intramembranous**). An interesting theory as to the origin of this dichotomy of formation has been voiced by both Holden (1882) and Last (1973). They suggested that intramembranous ossification results in more rapid bone formation in locations where it is urgently required in the embryo, perhaps for support and protection, e.g. the calvaria. Similarly, it was suggested that this compelling and almost impatient need for early bone formation is related to the importance of the future function of the bone. For example, it was reported that the mandible and ribs require to be fully formed from the moment of birth to facilitate the functions of both sucking and respiration, respectively (Holden, 1882). Bones that form via intramembranous ossification were also thought to be **dermal** in origin, being remnants of an evolutionary distant exoskeleton. In addition to this dichotomous pattern, the clavicle, mandible and sutural areas of the skull can display a third type of formation. Areas of these bones are reported to commence ossification in a membranous template which gradually acquires cartilaginous sites, thereby suggesting an intermediary form of bone formation. Certainly it is not clear why certain bones preform in cartilage and others in membrane, and some authors have claimed that it is almost irrelevant, as the final outcome is the same. However, recent research disputes such a statement as the cellular components of the two forms of bone appear to behave in distinctly different ways (Smith and Abramson, 1974; Zins and Whitaker, 1979, 1983; Kusiak *et al.*, 1985; Moskalewski *et al.*, 1988; Scott and Hightower, 1991; Sullivan and Szwajkun, 1991; Chole, 1993). An important clinical implication of such differences in cellular behaviour can be seen in the field of plastic and reconstructive facial surgery. In this situation, the successful grafting of bone to a new location relies heavily on the cells behaving and growing in a manner that is appropriate to their new development site, as unpredictable cellular behaviour could seriously compromise a successful surgical outcome.

The connective tissue precursor of the future bone generally commences osteogenesis at a constant locus which will subsequently expand in size until the precursor has been totally replaced by bone. The initial site of ossification is known as the **primary centre** and whilst the majority of these appear in the embryonic and fetal period, a few develop (e.g. the pisiform of the hand) in the pre-adolescent years of childhood. Despite the wide time span of appearance for these centres, the order and chronology of appearance is reasonably well documented for most (see Chapter 2). Although some bones commence ossification from a single centre, it is more common for several small areas to appear, which usually coalesce at an early stage to form a single centre. Most histology texts invariably describe the development of a long bone shaft (**diaphysis**) as the typical example of growth of a primary centre. Whilst this may adequately illustrate this type of formation, it does not demonstrate the pattern of growth and development in the majority of bones, which do not display a long bone morphology.

The primary centre of ossification does not always extend into the entire cartilaginous area of the precursor template and in some regions, separate **secondary centres** of ossification (epiphyses) will develop. In some instances these will develop into large areas of bone (distal femur) whilst in others they form simple flake-like slivers of bone (rib tubercles). Throughout the growth of the bone, the primary and secondary centres are separated by an organized region of rapid growth (**growth plate, epiphyseal plate, physis**). When the rate of cartilage proliferation is exceeded by the rate of osseous deposition, then the growth plate will start to narrow and eventually will be replaced by bone so that **epiphyseal fusion** will occur. This event marks the end of longitudinal bone growth and whilst the time of fusion is relatively well documented, it can show a considerable degree of variation. Last (1973) likened the times of appearance and fusion of centres of ossification to telephone numbers, being sufficiently haphazard that recourse to a book should always be recommended as it is impossible to keep them all in one's memory.

Epiphyses are not present in every developing bone and so in certain areas (skull, wrist, etc.) the primary centre will form the entire future adult bone. Secondary centres always appear later than their primary counterparts and, with some notable exceptions, they generally appear after birth. The distinction between what constitutes a primary or a secondary centre of ossification seems by definition to be little more than an arbitrary time lapse phenomenon.

Pressure epiphyses (e.g. head of femur) form at the articular ends of the bone and are involved in the cushioning of stresses across a joint, thereby permitting the continuation of longitudinal growth during weight bearing (Parsons, 1905; Smith, 1962a). They are found in some reptiles and birds as well as in mammals (Haines, 1938). **Traction** epiphyses occur only in mammals and are generally found at the site of muscle attachment, e.g. lesser trochanter of femur (Parsons, 1904, 1908; Barnett and Lewis, 1958). Consequently these often become the sites at which avulsion fractures occur in the developing skeleton. The third group of epiphyses seem to encompass all those that do not fall into the first two categories and they are termed **atavistic** epiphyses as they are thought to represent structures that might have been separate at earlier evolutionary stages, e.g. costal notch flakes (Haines, 1940).

Bone formation is closely linked with vascularity. Each bone has at least one nutrient artery that enters via a **nutrient foramen**. The number and direction of such foramina have excited a considerable amount of research, with the latter being considered an indicator of the **growing end** of the bone. This is obviously a misnomer as (in long bones in particular, where this description is generally levied) both ends of a bone grow, but one is generally dominant and therefore contributes to a greater percentage of the final adult length (Chapters 9 and 11). The nutrient foramen is directed away from the growing end of the bone so that, for example, in the long bones of the limbs the nutrient foramina are directed towards the elbow and away from the knee.[1] The faster-growing ends are therefore located at the shoulder and wrist in the upper limb and around the knee in the lower limb. It is generally true in all long bones of the limbs (with the exception of the fibula) that the epiphysis at the growing end is the first to form and generally the last to fuse. If only one extremity of a long bone bears an epiphysis (e.g. metacarpals), then the nutrient foramen is generally directed away from the epiphyseal end.

Pre-osseous development

Mesenchymal condensation

Mesenchyme is the meshwork of embryonic connective tissue from which all other connective tissues of the body are formed, including cartilage and ultimately bone (see Chapter 4). Mesenchymal cells migrate to sites of future osteogenesis and there differentiate into osteogenic cells as a result of cellular interactions and locally generated growth factors (Hall, 1988). This local instruction ensures that bone does not develop in inappropriate sites.

The first sign of future potential bone formation occurs in the early embryonic period as a localized condensation of the mesenchyme (skeletal blastema). Cellular condensations may arise as a result of either increased mitotic activity or an aggregation of cells drawn towards a specific site (Hall and Miyake, 1992). Signalling agents such as retinoids seem to be responsible for controlling *Hox* gene expression so that cells are given positional addresses (Tickle, 1994). For example, this results in a humerus developing in the arm and not in the foot.

As the mesenchyme begins to condense, the cells become more rounded, concomitant with a reduction in the amount of intercellular substance (Streeter, 1949). This stage is referred to as the precartilage blastema (Hamilton and Mossman, 1972; Glenister, 1976; Atchley and Hall, 1991). The formation of mesenchymal condensations has been associated with the formation of gap junctions that permit intercellular communication (Hall and Miyake, 1992). Each cell begins to secrete a basophilic matrix, rich in collagen filaments along with other substances including chondroitin sulphate, indicating a differentiation into chondroblasts. As development continues, the levels of hyaluron decrease following an increase in hyaluronidase. Hyaluron blocks chondrogenesis, so its

[1] Every old-fashioned teacher of anatomy is familiar with the rhyme 'to the elbow I go and from the knee I flee'. This memorable phrase was first coined by Bérard (1835) and so should technically read as 'Au coude je m'appuis, du genou je m'en fuis'.

removal permits cellular differentiation (Knudson and Toole, 1987). As the levels of hyaluron decrease, so the levels of chondroitin sulphate increase (Toole and Trelstad, 1971). It appears that hyaluron may be necessary for cellular aggregation and therefore essential for the accumulation of a sufficient number of precartilage cells to initiate the transition from mesenchyme to cartilage (Grüneberg, 1963; Ogden, 1979). A number of factors, such as a mutation or the introduction of a teratogen may be responsible for the reduction in size of a mesenchymal condensation. If this condensation does not reach a critical size/mass, then the onset of chondrification may be retarded or even aborted. There is a substantial volume of evidence from *in vitro* cultures to suggest the requirement of a minimum cell number before prechondrogenic cells can differentiate (Steinberg, 1963; Flickinger, 1974; Solursh, 1983). A similar requirement has also been documented for pre-osteogenic cells (Thompson *et al.*, 1989; Nakahara *et al.*, 1991). Interestingly, this may go some way towards an explanation for the phylogenetic loss of certain skeletal structures (Hall, 1984). The embryonic potential to produce certain skeletal structures that will ultimately be suppressed can be retained. For example, snakes retain the mesenchymal condensations that would indicate limb formation. However, they remain small and so may fail to meet the prerequisite cellular quantity threshold so that they ultimately regress. Occasionally some of these suppressed structures do develop beyond the condensation stage and are then classified as atavistic traits (Hall, 1984). Conversely, should a condensation become excessively large, it can subsequently lead to abnormally large skeletal elements (Hall and Miyake, 1992).

As the tissue continues to mature, there is a continued separation of the cells by matrix deposition and so the tissue soon takes on the appearance of early hyaline cartilage. Gardner (1963) reported that such cellular condensations, which will ultimately lead to cartilage formation, could be distinguished at a very early age from the predominantly fibrous condensations that lead to the formation of intramembranous bone. This ease of identification is partly due to the early presence of a well-defined perichondrium.

Chondrification

Chondrogenesis is initiated by a response to an extracellular matrix-mediated interaction either via a basal lamina or via an ectodermal–mesenchymal interaction (Syftestad and Caplan, 1984; Hall, 1988). For example, interaction with the basal lamina of the notochord and neural tube increases the rate of differentiation of the paraxial mesoderm. The production of type II collagen in mesenchymal cells is a clear indication of chondrogenic potential.

The cells at the periphery of the blastema condense to form a bilaminar perichondrium whose inner layer is host to chondroblasts that will be responsible for appositional growth of the developing cartilage anlage. Interstitial growth of the cartilage model continues via cellular division. Such growth can only be maintained whilst the matrix is sufficiently pliable to permit expansion (Serafini-Fracassini and Smith, 1974; Glenister, 1976).

The question of maintained nutrition to the deepest areas of a cartilage anlage is a well-documented scientific debate. Whilst many texts incorrectly state that cartilage is an avascular structure, it is equally well known that cartilages will maintain viability either by diffusion from a blood source (usually perichondral) or via vascular bundles travelling in cartilage canals (Fig. 3.1). The presence of vascular canals within a cartilaginous mass is not a new discovery, as Hunter first described them in 1743. Despite the production of an anti-angiogenic factor (Kuettner and Pauli, 1983) it is known that vascular canals are present from a very early age (Haines, 1933; Brookes, 1971; Moss-Salentijn, 1975). Interestingly, their presence is not restricted to large cartilage masses as one might expect if their function was simply to supplement nutrition, but they have also been found in, for example, the epiphyses of fetal phalanges (Gray *et al.*, 1957). The canal is formed by an inflection of the deep layer of the perichondrium and carries a small central artery or arteriole surrounded by numerous venules and perivascular capillaries (Hurrell, 1934; Wilsman and Van Sickle, 1972). The arteriole of a canal enters the cartilage matrix at a groove or sulcus and terminates by division into a capillary glomerulus. The capillaries are lined by fenestrated endothelium and the pericytes are thin, facilitating the transfer of nutrients and metabolites. The capillaries recombine to form a venule that rejoins the perichondral network via the same channel as the parent arteriole. The loose connective tissue that surrounds the blood vessels is continuous with the perichondrium and is rich in fibroblasts, connective tissue fibres, undifferentiated mesenchymal cells and macrophages. Also present are unmyelinated nerve fibres and lymphatic vessels and the entire cartilage canal is bathed in interstitial fluid, facilitating metabolic exchange throughout its entire length (Lufti, 1970; Wilsman and Van Sickle, 1972).

Given the production of anti-angiogenic factors, it is unlikely that embryonic chondrogenic condensations are in fact actively invaded by blood vessels, but

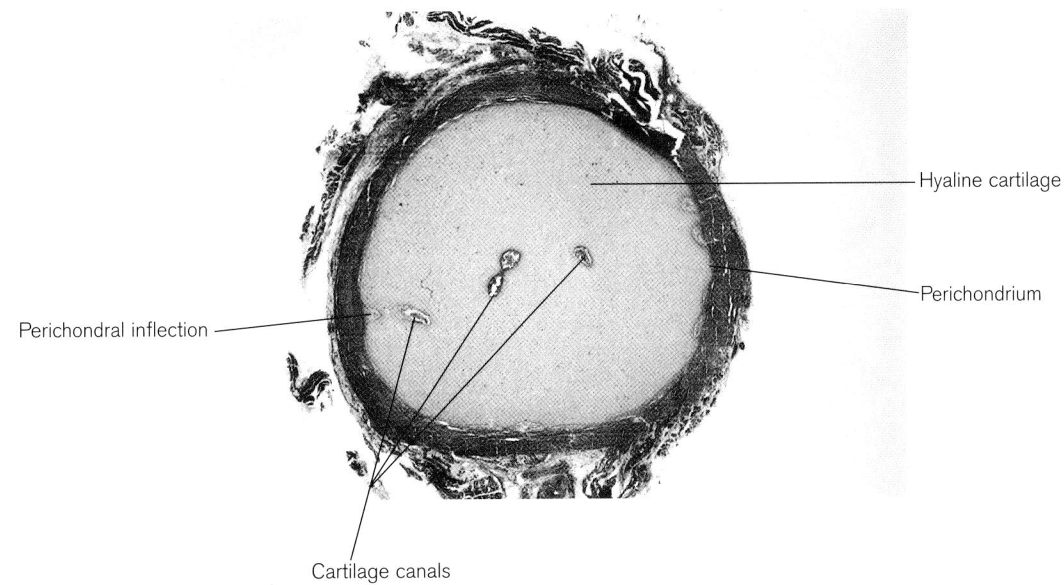

Figure 3.1 Transverse section of fetal costal cartilage canals (Masson's stain ×1 objective).

it is well established that osteogenic condensations are (Hall, 1983, 1988). Thompson *et al.* (1989) suggested that the pre-osteogenic condensation must release an angiogenic factor that encourages vascularization.

Engfeldt and Reinholt (1992) summarized the chondrification stage of development as beginning with a morphogenetic phase of development and ending with a cytodifferentiation phase. The former is characterized by migration of the mesenchymal cell populations, cellular division and proliferation and cellular interactions. The latter is characterized by synthesis and secretion of cartilaginous proteoglycans and type II collagen.

There is the additional matter of small regions of so-called 'secondary cartilage' to be considered. This seems to be temporary cartilage that is found in bones that will typically develop via intramembranous ossification, e.g. the mandible and the clavicle (de Beer, 1937; Koch, 1960; Andersen, 1963). The full significance of this cartilage is not clear but it does serve to emphasize the similarity of development between the mechanisms involved in intramembranous and endochondral ossification (Glenister, 1976). Small regions of cartilage also form in membranous bones wherever rapid development is taking place, e.g. cranial sutures and alveolar ridges, and they may arise in response to a requirement for a localized alteration in growth rate (Jones, personal communication).

Details of the histological structure and biochemical composition of hyaline cartilage can be found in many anatomical, orthopaedic, biochemical and physiological texts.

Ossification

De novo mineralization

The *de novo* mineralization of connective tissue is surrounded by a long tradition of controversial theories that have subsequently been upheld or refuted by the development of relatively new histo- and biochemical techniques. Two discoveries were of particular importance in this regard – the identification of matrix vesicles by Bonucci in 1967 (although not named as such until Anderson in 1969) and the process of epitactic nucleation that was first described by Neuman and Neuman (1953). Matrix vesicles are double-membrane bound, round or ovoid structures (0.1–0.2μm in diameter) that are often found between collagen fibrils in small clusters about halfway between adjacent chondrocytes (Bonucci, 1967, 1971; Boyan *et al.*, 1990). These small extracellular structures are the recognized induction sites of mineralization (Fig. 3.2). They develop as small buds from the plasma membrane of chondrocytes and are released following retraction of the supporting microfilament network (F-actin) of the cell surface microvilli (Hale and Wuthier, 1987; Wuthier, 1989; Sela *et al.*, 1992). Matrix vesicles are a universal phenomenon of mesenchymal tissues and this was implied, although not fully appreciated, as early as 1931 by Charles Huggins (cited in Anderson, 1990). Huggins found that if the transitional epithelium from a dog's bladder was transplanted into the rectus sheath of that same animal then bone would form wherever the mesenchymal cells of the sheath came into contact with the epithelium. It is thought that the matrix

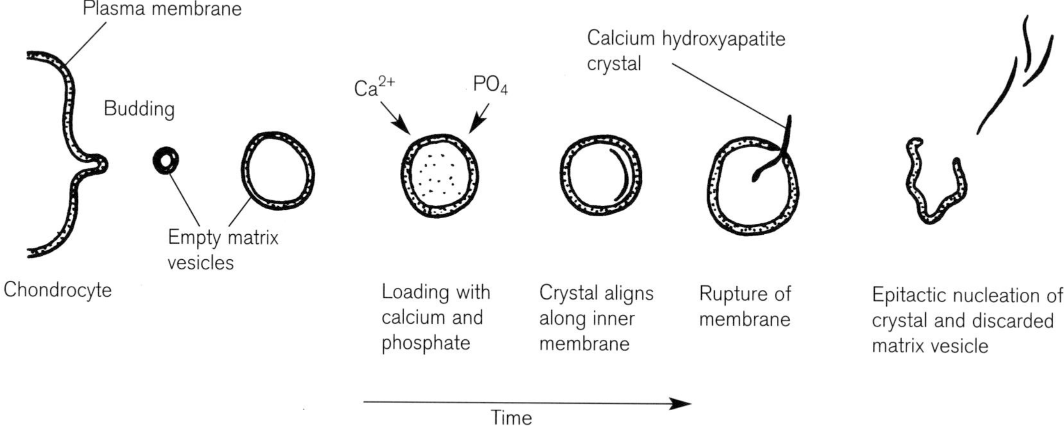

Figure 3.2 *De novo* mineralization via matrix vesicles (after Sela *et al.*, 1992).

vesicles may provide both the necessary enzymes and environment to concentrate both calcium and phosphates sufficiently to overcome the threshold for crystallization (Hunter, 1987). In cartilage, calcium is bound to anionic groups of proteoglycans and therefore not directly available for precipitation. A localized increase in phosphate levels serves to displace some of the calcium from the proteoglycans by ion-exchange mechanisms, thereby raising the calcium and phosphate product above the threshold for precipitation of calcium hydroxyapatite ($Ca_{10}[PO_4]_6[OH]_2$). It is known that the inner membrane of the matrix vesicle is rich in phosphatidylserine, a calcium-binding phospholipid (Wuthier, 1989). It has also been shown that to initiate the mineralization process *in vitro*, modest amounts of adenosine triphosphate (ATP) are required (Ali and Evans, 1973).

Initial mineralization occurs along the inner membrane of the matrix vesicle (Fig. 3.2). Calcium is attracted to this membrane by phosphatidylserine and various other calcium-binding proteins. A localized increase in phosphate levels occurs via the presence of phosphatases including alkaline phosphatase. Thus the initial phase of mineralization is brought about by a complex interaction between calcium-binding molecules and phosphate-metabolizing enzymes (Anderson and Morris, 1993). The initial nuclei of hydroxyapatite are thought to be somewhat unstable and so a protective micro-environment is required where the levels of calcium and phosphate can be both concentrated and controlled (Sauer and Wuthier, 1988). The crystallites of hydroxyapatite initially form as small needle or plate-like structures aligned along the inner membrane of the vesicle (Moradian-Oldak *et al.*, 1991; Akisaka *et al.*, 1998). As the crystals increase in size they rupture the membrane and so break free from the protective environment of the matrix vesicle (Eanes and Hailer, 1985). These 'seed' crystals are now exposed to the extracellular fluid and serve as templates for new crystal proliferation – epitactic nucleation (Neuman and Neuman, 1953). In this extravesicular phase, collagen provides a favourable environment for nucleation and propagation of the hydroxyapatite seeds (Arsenault, 1989). Although some authors believe that the crystallites are deposited at specific sites along the collagen fibrils, mainly in the spaces between the tropocollagen molecules, others consider that most lie outwith the confines of the fibrils in the extrafibrillar volume (Lees and Prostak, 1988; Weiner and Traub, 1989; Bonucci, 1992; Traub *et al.*, 1992; Mundy and Martin, 1993). As the matrix becomes heavily mineralized the matrix vesicles are fragmented and destroyed, as they serve no further purpose (Fig. 3.2). The histological appearance of *de novo* mineralization is illustrated in Fig. 3.3.

Intramembranous ossification

This is probably the more primitive of the two modes of ossification but it is certainly the first to commence formation and it continues throughout life. Indeed, this form of ossification is expressed in every bone in the human skeleton, although most texts tend to dwell only on the embryonic range of its spectrum. Its earliest stages of development are perhaps less complicated than its adult stages, which are represented by subperiosteal apposition and bone remodelling. Perhaps there is therefore some mileage in the suggestion that endochondral ossification is a more recent phylogenetic development that has been superimposed onto an existing intramembranous ossification framework (McLean and Urist, 1955). After all, many authors have referred to those bones that develop in this way as 'dermal' bones, in deference to their proposed phylogenetic origins as a protective exoskeleton.

Intramembranous ossification is defined as the direct mineralization of a highly vascular connective tissue membrane. It occurs in many of the plate-like bones of the vault of the skull, all of the facial bones, the mandible and the clavicle. The clavicle is probably the first bone in the human skeleton to show evidence of bone formation and osteoprogenitor cells can be detected in the differentiating mesenchyme from approximately day 39 in the sixth week of intra-uterine life. It is widely accepted that ossification commences via the process outlined above for *de novo* mineralization. The crystals expand spherically within the osteoid (the organic matrix of bone) thereby forming bone nodules which subsequently fuse to form seams of woven bone (Bernard and Pease, 1969; Marvaso and Bernard, 1977). Perhaps as a result of a breaching of a threshold potential, once a sufficient number of these nodules has been deposited in the mesenchymal matrix, there is evidence of vascular invasion. Proliferation of the centre of ossification does tend to be located around a capillary network (Hamilton and Mossman, 1972; Hansen, 1993) and it has been suggested by Thompson *et al.* (1989) that the osteogenic cells may in fact secrete an angiogenic factor that actively encourages vascular invasion. The intimate relationship between osteogenic cells and vascularity is further evidenced by the fact that the osteoblasts are always polarized so that they secrete with their 'backs' aligned next to a blood vessel.

Fine trabeculae of early bone can be detected between adjacent differentiating mesenchymal cells and these will extend and expand into a diffuse network of bony spicules. Intervascular sprouts of bone extend to enclose the blood vessels as more mesenchymal cells differentiate into osteoblasts. This primary spongiosa begins to thicken with the laying down of more osteoid on the surfaces of the trabeculae. The primary trabeculae radiate centrifugally from the centre of ossification and increase in length by accretion to their free ends (Weinmann and Sicher, 1947; Ogden, 1979). Small secondary trabeculae develop at right angles to the primary struts helping to enclose the vascular spaces, and as the rate of bone growth slows, primary osteonal systems form.

The mesenchyme on the surface of the developing bone begins to condense and form the fibrovascular periosteum that will remain actively osteogenic throughout life. As each successive layer of bone is laid down on the surface, osteoblasts become trapped in the matrix and are transformed into osteocytes occupying the lacunae in the interstitial bony substance. Some fetal and neonatal bones present with an incomplete cortex in which the underlying trabeculae are visible. This is not a pathological condition but is simply an intermittent stage, indicating as yet incomplete development of the periosteal layer of compact bone.

There is a delicate balance between bone formation and bone resorption during bone modelling and remodelling, with an abnormality in one or the other leading to extensive pathological change. Intramembranous subperiosteal apposition and resorption is a critical component of the ongoing remodelling of the skeleton throughout life (Enlow, 1963; Garn, 1970; Martin *et al.*, 1998). Not only is remodelling necessary to allow bone growth and development, but, of course, it is essential for repair following traumas, including fracture. It should therefore be born in mind

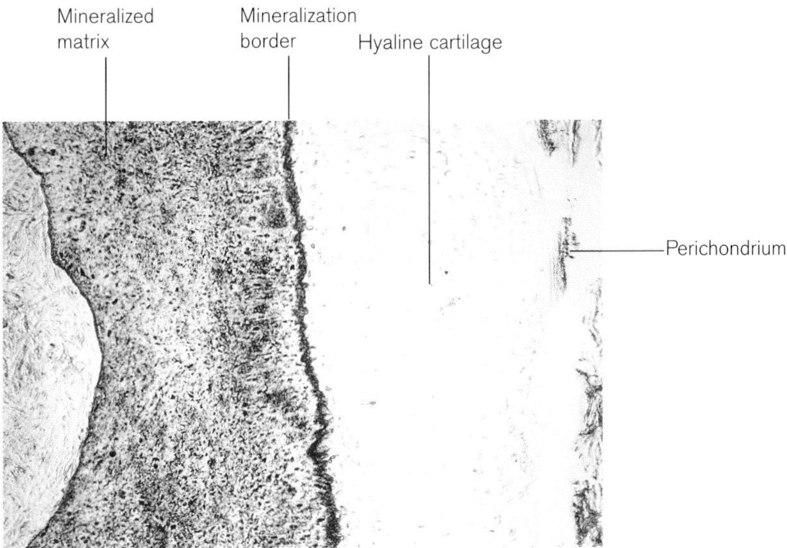

Figure 3.3 *De novo* mineralization of costal cartilage (ground section ×2.5 objective).

that continued subperiosteal apposition is a form of intramembranous ossification.

Endochondral ossification

The process of endochondral ossification is most frequently described in relation to the development of the long bones. However, the first step in this process is in fact intramembranous in nature, as there is no direct replacement of cartilage *per se*. The perichondrium in the region of the centre of the long bone diaphysis begins to thicken and the osteoprogenitor cells give rise to osteoblasts. Bruder and Caplan (1989) termed these 'stacked cells', and described them as a layer of 4–6 cells that completely surrounds the cartilage. Interestingly, they stated that the osteogenic differentiation in this region progressed independent of any chondrogenic activity in the cartilage anlage of developing bone. The osteoblasts surround capillaries from the perichondral arterial network and secrete osteoid, which is quickly mineralized (matrix vesicles have been identified in this location). In this way a discrete bone collar or constricting cuff forms around the midshaft region (Fig. 3.4). Above and below this region the perichondrium is continuous with the now appropriately named periosteum. Bruder and Caplan (1989) also suggested that such a restrictive bone collar would initiate a nutrient diffusion barrier that might be directly responsible for the hypertrophy of the chondrocytes in the centre of the cartilage model. The bone in this area will be remodelled as growth progresses, but in essence, it can be said that the compact bone of the mature diaphysis of each long bone is almost entirely periosteal and therefore intramembranous in origin. The periosteum retains its osteogenic potential throughout life but it has been noted that in the earlier years, bone formation can become somewhat exuberant such that excess new woven bone is formed at such a rate that its remodelling into more mature bone may be somewhat delayed (Shopfner, 1966). Such so-called 'periosteal reactions' are quite commonly found in immature bones (Malmberg, 1944; Caffey and Silverman, 1945; Tufts *et al.*, 1982; Aoki *et al.*, 1987; Anderson and Carter, 1994; Lewis and Roberts, 1997) and are not necessarily, as has been suggested, an indication of inflammatory reaction/infection, stress or even child abuse. They can be identified radiologically as a 'double contour' effect which is most commonly seen between 2–6 months of age in otherwise healthy children. These contours later disappear with no treatment or change in clinical management and are therefore probably normal (Glaser, 1949; Hancox *et al.*, 1951). Shopfner (1966) suggested that increased activity of the periosteum may arise when it is not tightly bound to the underlying cortex, perhaps as a result of sparse or shortened Sharpey's fibres. In 35% of his sample there was no evidence of any other clinical condition. It is also possible that this situation may arise following asynchrony in the rate of growth of the physis cartilage and the periosteum, resulting in periosteal tension and reactive apposition (Jones, personal communication).

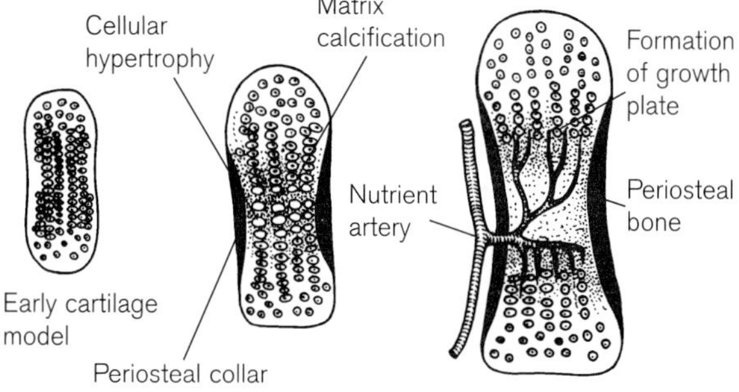

Figure 3.4 The early stages of long bone diaphyseal ossification.

True endochondral ossification occurs within the cartilage core of the anlage (template). The chondrocytes in the centre of the cartilage begin to enlarge and the cytoplasm becomes vacuolated (Fig. 3.4). The cells degenerate and the intercellular matrix becomes compressed into septae (primary areolae) that ultimately mineralize due to the presence and involvement of matrix vesicles. A vascular bud then penetrates the periosteal collar forming an **irruption canal**, thereby permitting osteogenic invasion of the cartilage core and the development of marrow spaces. Whilst several periosteal vessels may initially penetrate the bony ring, usually only one will become dominant and develop into the nutrient artery. The traditional view of subsequent events is that osteoid is laid down in the residual walls of the calcified cartilage and the newly introduced osteoprogenitor cells convert this into woven bone, thereby forming an internal trabecular network. It is not clear whether the function of such internal struts in the midshaft region is to provide support for the haemopoietic tissue of the developing marrow cavity or to provide an internal framework to underpin the developing cylindrical shaft. However, it is clear that following cortical drift in the midshaft region of the more mature thick compact bone of the diaphysis, short thick endosteal struts are all that are likely to remain of the endochondral element of diaphyseal ossification (Jones *et al.*, 1999). However, in the proximal and distal extremities of the more mature diaphysis, an abundance of cancellous struts are retained, presumably indicating that their presence is necessary/desirable for force dissipation. Bruder and Caplan (1989) forcefully stated that the embryonic cartilage model *does not* provide scaffolding for new bone formation but rather serves as a target for future bone marrow elements. It is at this stage, when a periosteal collar has been formed and endochondral ossification has commenced in the core, that the primary centre of ossification of a long bone is said to have developed.

Not only does endochondral ossification play a critical role with regards to the longitudinal growth of a long bone (growth plate – see below) but it is also the mode of ossification encountered in the epiphyses of the long bones, the centra of the vertebral column, sternebrae, carpals, tarsals and in fact almost any region of the skeleton that displays significant volumes of cancellous or trabecular bone. In these areas, the first sign of impending ossification occurs when isogenous cell groups in the centre of the cartilaginous mass begin to hypertrophy. Matrix vesicles have been identified in these locations and it is highly probably that they form the initial site of *de novo* crystallite formation. The region is subsequently invaded by osteogenic vascular mesenchyme, probably via the cartilage canals that have been identified even in the youngest human fetal epiphyses (Weinmann and Sicher, 1947; Brookes, 1958, 1971; Wilsman and Van Sickle, 1972). Arterial invasion normally occurs at a number of sites via a vascular arcade, which explains the multitude of nutrient foramina generally found in the non-articular regions of epiphyses (Brookes, 1971). Following the pattern of endochondral ossification seen in the long bone diaphyses, bone is laid down in these centres along the mineralized cartilage septae and subsequently remodelled into the characteristic thicker trabeculae of recognizable cancellous bone. Bone can only grow via accretion and so, as the ossification centre enlarges, its cartilaginous periphery becomes a proliferative zone permitting an increase in size in a radial direction. The cartilaginous cell columns are generally directed towards the growth plate.

Bone islands (enostoses) have been identified as benign lesions of mature compact bone that are probably congenital in origin and arise from a failure of resorption during the normal process of endochondral ossification (Greenspan, 1995; Forest, 1998). They are generally asymptomatic and usually found by accident. They can occur virtually anywhere in the skeleton but there is a higher prevalence in the pelvis, ribs and long bones.

The growth plate and bone growth

Due to the rigid nature of the matrix component of bone, osseous tissue cannot increase in size by interstitial development and so grows by a well-balanced process of apposition and resorption that constitute bone modelling. Shortly after formation of the primary centre of ossification, an organized region of rapid growth (growth plate) will develop between the epiphysis and the diaphysis, which is primarily responsible for the increase in length of the developing diaphysis (Rang, 1969). This region is often referred to as the epiphyseal plate or the physis and whilst the latter is appropriate as it is the Greek term for ‘growth’, the former is inappropriate as this plate does not play a part in the increase in size of the epiphysis (Siegling, 1941).

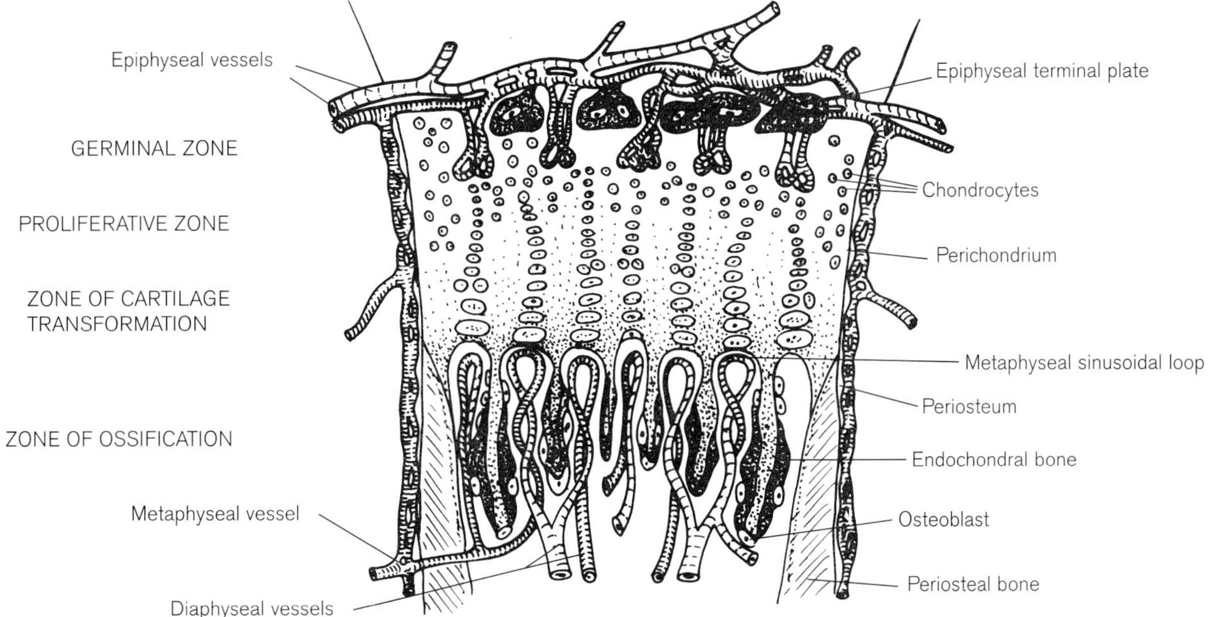

Figure 3.5 A summary of the major features of a diaphyseal growth plate.

The traditional description of a growth plate is that found at the extremities of a long bone diaphysis (Fig. 3.5). These are generally described as being discoid in shape and are responsible not only for the longitudinal growth of the shaft but also for its diametric expansion. The division of the growth plate into distinct zones is artificial but helpful for the appreciation of the histological appearance, although unfortunately the terminology used is not universal. However, it is the function of each zone that is important and not its name. The zone furthest away from the diaphysis and closest to the epiphysis is called the resting or **germinal zone**. In this area the chondrocytes are small, quiescent and randomly distributed. These cells receive a vascular supply from the epiphyseal vessels that penetrate the terminal plate (see below). In the adjacent **proliferative zone**, the chondrocytes increase in size as they accumulate glycogen. The cells exhibit mitotic division and become arranged in longitudinal pillars or palisades of initially wedge-shaped cells. These palisades make up almost half the height of a growth plate and are the sites of new cartilage formation that will ensure the continued longitudinal expansion of the diaphysis. Although the majority of mitotic divisions occur in a transverse plane, Lacroix (1951) and Serafini-Fracassini and Smith (1974) have explained the paradox of their contribution to the lengthening of the shaft. Following mitosis, the daughter cells do indeed lie side by side but the cells are wedge-shaped and orientated so that their narrow edges overlap considerably. As the cells migrate towards the metaphysis, the narrow edges expand so that the cell is ultimately rectangular and as a result the originally oblique intercellular septum becomes transverse and the cells align in a longitudinal direction.

The chondrocytes start to hypertrophy in the **zone of cartilage transformation**, in preparation for their replacement by bone. In this region there is a progressive degeneration of the cellular component, with an increase in hydroxyapatite deposition via matrix vesicles. Any intercellular connections are removed as the vascular invasion by metaphyseal sinusoidal loops advances. Rather than degenerating, some of the cells in this region may be released into the next zone where transformation into osteoblasts may occur. In the **zone of ossification**, osteoblasts form a layer of bone on the remnants of the mineralized cartilage of the preceding zone. This bone undergoes re-organization through osteoclastic activity and the subsequent addition of new bone.

As the primary ossification centre expands towards the epiphyses, the periosteal collar remains slightly in advance of the endochondral replacement, although it will eventually adopt a position level with the hypertrophic zone. This region, comprising the extremity of the periosteal collar, peripheral physis and fibrovascular tissue, is referred to as the zone of Ranvier and is important for diametric expansion (Ogden, 1979). Diametric or transverse expansion occurs by cell division and matrix expansion within the growth plate and by cellular addition from the periphery at the zone of Ranvier (Speer, 1982; Rodriguez *et al.*, 1992). This small, wedge-shaped zone of cells governs the control of relative diametric proportions between the expanding diaphysis and epiphysis. To maintain proportions within a bone, the diaphysis must remodel in the transverse plane as it expands longitudinally (see below). New layers of bone are laid down at the periosteal margin (apposition) whilst bone is removed from the endosteal surface (resorption). This complementary relationship ensures a relatively constant ratio between bone addition and bone loss. Obviously, when one or other of these processes no longer maintains that balance, then disorders of excess or insufficient cortical mass will ensue.

Appositional bone growth via the periosteum was discovered almost by accident around 1736 by Mr Belchier, a surgeon at Guy's Hospital (Holden, 1882). He was dining with a friend who happened to be a calico printer and they were eating a leg of pork when he noted that the bones were red and not white. On making further enquiries he found that the pig had been fed on the refuse from the dyeing vats, which contained a substantial quantity of madder (Eurasian vegetable dye from *Rubia tinctorum*). As a direct result of this fortuitous discovery, many of the earlier studies on bone growth and development were performed on animals that were fed on madder. More recently of course, this form of bone growth has been observed by tetracycline labelling and radioisotopes such as ^{85}Sr (Milch *et al.*, 1958; Shock *et al.*, 1972).

The typical physis described at the extremity of a long bone diaphysis is only one type of growth plate. The epiphysis (or indeed primary centre, e.g. in a carpal or tarsal bone) has its own growth plate, which is more appropriately described as a growth zone as it is approximately spherical in shape (Fig. 3.6). It is represented by a proliferative zone of cartilage cells that are modelled into cancellous bone by the progressive centrifugal expansion of endochondral ossification. In this situation the bony nucleus of the developing epiphysis is homologous with the metaphyseal region of a long bone and forms the initial osseous growth site. As the ossification centre expands in the epiphysis of a long bone, it is inevitable that it will eventually approximate to the growth plate of the diaphysis (Fig. 3.6). Juxtaposition of the epiphyseal spherical growth plate with the developing cartilaginous model of the diaphysis results in the

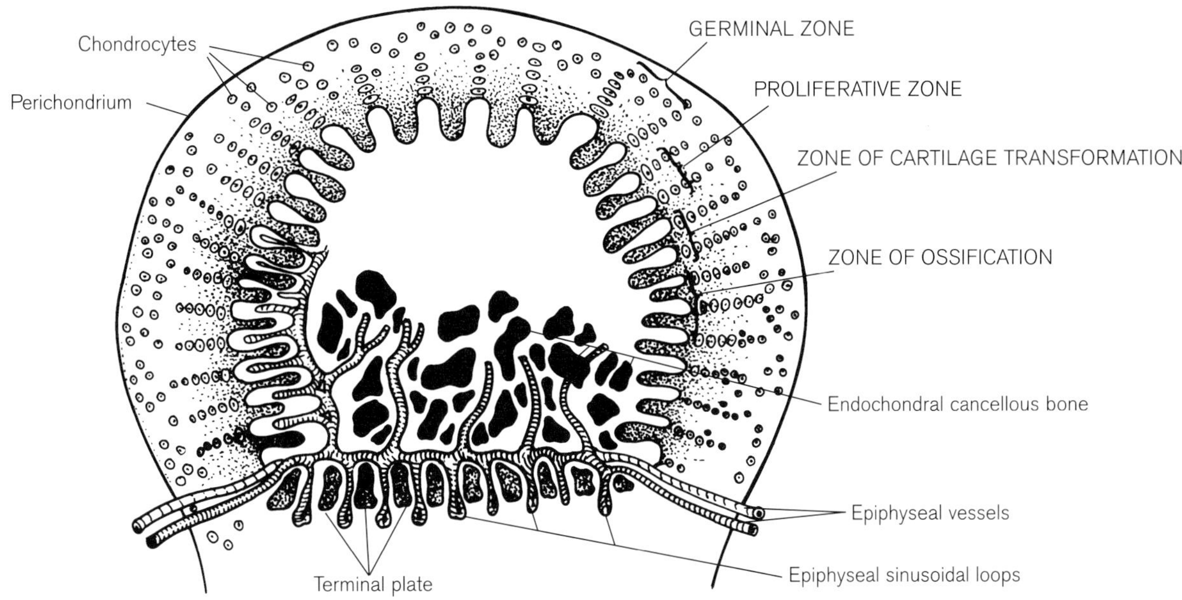

Figure 3.6 A summary of the major features of an epiphyseal (spherical) growth plate.

formation of a temporary bipolar physis (Ogden, 1979). The epiphyseal contribution is eventually replaced by a subchondral growth plate, which is also known as the **terminal plate**. This plate is formed when the trabeculae of the epiphysis unite to form a sealing plate that ensures the separate containment of the respective marrow spaces (Weinmann and Sicher, 1947).

Obviously, the spherical growth plate is also the means whereby small cancellous bones such as the carpals and tarsals increase in size. Expansional growth will cease when the interstitial expansion of the cartilage template no longer keeps pace with the advancing front of endochondral ossification and it comes into contact with the enveloping perichondrium. Via intramembranous ossification, the periosteum will then form a thin covering shell of compact bone. Further bone growth will, by necessity, involve the processes of apposition and resorption for continued remodelling (see below).

Much is made in the literature about the 'growing end' of a long bone. Obviously, this is an inappropriate description as both ends of a long bone exhibit growth. It actually refers to the fact that one extremity of the shaft may contribute to a larger proportion of the overall diaphyseal development than the other. It has been suggested that growth is equal at both ends until birth but that after that event one extremity becomes dominant (Brookes, 1963). In all long bones, except the fibula, the general rule is that the growing end is represented by the epiphysis that is the first to appear and the last to fuse. It is also recognized that the angles of obliquity of the nutrient foramina conform to this pattern so that in the upper limb they are directed towards the elbow and in the lower limb, away from the knee (Hughes, 1952; Mysorekar, 1967; Patake and Mysorekar, 1977). In this way, the nutrient foramen is said to be directed away from the growing end of the bone. Hales (1727) and later Hunter (1837) were probably the first to note and study the phenomenon of unequal growth in the extremities of long bones. Hales (1727) pierced two small holes in the tibia of a chick and sacrificed the animal 2 months later. He found that the distance between the marks had remained constant but that the shaft had grown in length and had increased more at one end than at the other. Many other researches have since repeated the experiment but probably the two most quoted are Bisgard and Bisgard (1935) on goats and the findings of Digby (1915) on human material.

An insult to the growth plate whether developmental, hereditary, disease- or trauma-related, may result in an abnormal growth rate which can either stimulate or inhibit growth at the plate. For this reason, precise surgical management of growth plate abnormalities are extremely important to ensure not only the continued bilateral symmetrical growth of the bones but also to safeguard against foreshortening of the limb (De Campo and Boldt, 1986; Young *et al.*, 1986; Nilsson *et al.*, 1987). There are many factors that can cause a disturbance of the normal functioning of the growth plate and the aetiology of such disorders is most conveniently considered under the somewhat traditional headings of congenital (genetically programmed disorders, chromosomal abnormalities and developmental disorders), infection, nutrition, trauma, physical injury, vascular factors, hormonal imbalance and neoplasm (Rang, 1969).

The growth plate represents a site of potential weakness in the bone, which subsequently decreases its resilience to withstand trauma. Approximately 15% of all fractures in children involve the growth plate (Salter and Harris, 1963; Ogden, 1981). Males tend to sustain physeal injuries more frequently than females and this may be due either to social factors (i.e. greater degree of physical activity) or to the extended duration of the physis in the male. Interestingly, distal growth plates tend to be affected more frequently than proximal ones in all long bones. The prognosis following physeal fracture is obviously highly dependent upon the nature and site of the fracture and the integrity of the blood supply (Adams and Hamblen, 1992).

Probably one of the best known indicators of growth arrest (delay) is the presence of radiodense lines or bands in the diaphyses of the growing long bones, although they are not solely restricted to this location (Sontag, 1938; Stammel, 1941). However, they are most frequently encountered in the proximal end of the tibia and the distal end of the femur (Kapadia, 1991; Kapadia *et al.*, 1992; Aufderheide and Rodriguez-Martin, 1998). First described by Wegner in 1874, they have been variously called Harris lines (Harris, 1926a, 1933), growth arrest lines (Ogden, 1984a) or even recovery lines (Park and Richter, 1953; Park, 1964) depending upon the considered mode of formation (Fig. 3.7). These radiopaque lines form as a result of stress, whether biological, mechanical or even psychological. The normal maladies of childhood such as measles, mumps and chickenpox can be sufficient to induce the formation of such a stress marker (Gindhart, 1969). As a result of the insult, it has been noted that the cartilaginous growth plate diminishes in size following decreased chondrogenesis, although the advancing front of mineralization continues (Eliot *et al.*, 1927). Whilst proliferation of the cartilage slows, the osteoblasts continue bone formation so that the undersurface of the cartilage plate becomes an almost impenetrable barrier. When normal growth is resumed or the restrictive factor is removed, the Harris line continues to thicken as there is a delay whilst osteoclastic activity penetrates the bony plate before a normal rate of activity can be resumed (Park and Richter, 1953). In cross-section, the radiopaque line appears as a latticework of trabeculae and is composed of discontinuous projections of compact bone that end in the marrow cavity (Garn *et al.*, 1968; McHenry, 1968).

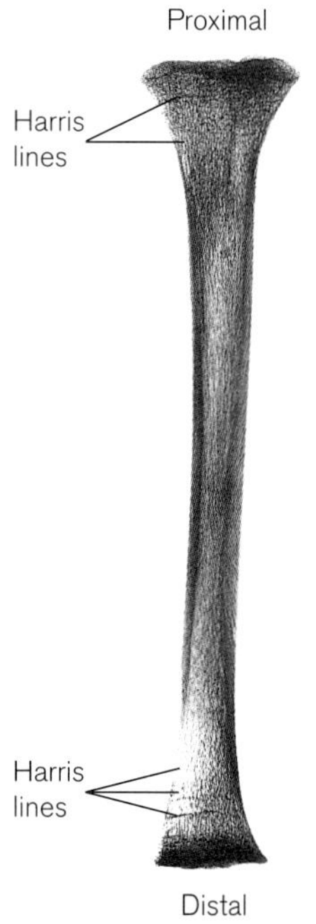

Figure 3.7 Harris lines at both the proximal and distal extremities of a juvenile tibial shaft.

Several studies have attempted to determine the age of formation of these lines using information on the percentage of growth that occurs at each end of the growing bone at a given age (Hunt and Hatch, 1981; Maat, 1984; Hummert and Van Gerven, 1985; Byers, 1991). It should be borne in mind of course that when the bone recommences its growth after cessation of the upset then such trabecular struts are susceptible to remodelling and therefore resorption (Kapadia, 1991; Kapadia *et al.*, 1992).

Epiphyseal union

When osteogenesis surpasses chondrogenesis so that the advancing ossification fronts of both the diaphysis and epiphysis become juxtaposed, then the process of epiphyseal union commences (Rang, 1969). The control and initiation of union is probably governed by hormonal influences, given the evidence that it occurs at a consistently earlier age in females than in males and it is known that oestrogen favours bone maturation whilst testosterone stimulates cartilaginous growth (Ogden, 1979). However, there must also be some additional local influence over growth plate closure, as if it were solely under systemic control, then every epiphysis would fuse at the same time within any one individual (Sidhom and Derry, 1931; Rang, 1969).

The degree of epiphyseal union is generally separated into at least four morphological phases – no fusion, commencement of fusion, advanced fusion and complete fusion (Stevenson, 1924; McKern and Stewart, 1957). However some authors have condensed this to only three stages (Hasselwander, 1910), whilst others have expanded it to five (MacLaughlin, 1990a) or even nine different stages (Todd, 1930a). From dry bone specimens it is obvious whether or not fusion has commenced and indeed whether or not external fusion is completed, but much of the research in this area has used radiographic images which have the distinct disadvantage of providing only two-dimensional information (Haines *et al.*, 1967). Epiphyseal union (epiphyseodesis) commences with the formation of a mineralized bridge and ends with the complete replacement of the cartilaginous growth plate (Haines, 1975). Although this entire process can extend over quite a considerable period of time, it can also occur quite rapidly within the space of a matter of months and so in this situation it is often quite difficult to capture a critical moment in dry bone specimens, let alone in radiographic images. Much of the detailed histological information is therefore extrapolated from animal models and so must be viewed with some caution when applying it to the human condition (Dawson, 1929; Smith and Allcock, 1960; Haines and Mohuiddin, 1962; Haines, 1975).

As bone maturity approaches, cartilage proliferation slows and the growth plate becomes quiescent and gradually thins. The juxtaposed subchondral bone of the epiphysis thickens, while a similar thickening occurs at the juxtaposed metaphyseal surface. In this way, dense parallel bone plates (sclerotic lines) begin to form on either side of the remaining physis (Ogden, 1979). This double layer of bone tends to persist throughout life (often beyond 70 years of age) in many of the long bones and can be detected radiographically, when it is known as the 'epiphyseal line, scar or ghost' (Cope, 1920; MacLaughlin, 1987; Martin *et al.*, 1998). There is rapid replacement of the cellular palisades by metaphyseal bone and vascular shoots will ultimately pierce the thin cartilaginous plate and unite with the epiphyseal vessels. Ossification occurs concomitant with this invasion, forming initial bony bridges that will ultimately lead to fusion of the diaphysis to the epiphysis. Depending upon the size of the bone, perforation may only occur at one site or in the cases of larger bones there may be many sites of vascular breakthrough. There seem to be few rules as to whether epiphyseal union commences peripherally or centrally and in fact it seems to be bone, and possibly even individual, dependent (Haines, 1975).

Vascularity

The normal growth and development of a bone is inextricably linked to its vascular, and in particular its arterial, supply. In fact, the onset and maintenance of ossification is dependent upon an uninterrupted nutritive flow. There are three principal arterial networks

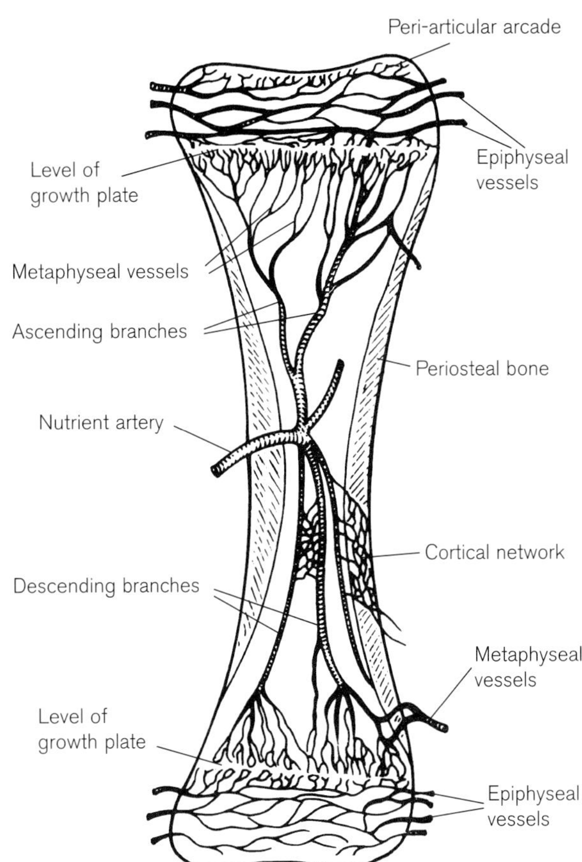

Figure 3.8 A summary of the main arterial supply to a developing long bone.

associated with the developing bone and each fulfils a different functional role (Fig. 3.8). The **diaphyseal** arteries are synonymous with nutrient arteries and are generally derived from an adjacent major systemic artery. They enter a bone via its nutrient foramen (Havers, 1691) which leads into a nutrient canal. There is no branching within the canal but once the vessel enters the medullary cavity it normally divides into ascending and descending medullary branches (Crock, 1996; Brookes and Revell, 1998). The direction and source of arterial blood flow in the cortex has been a long-standing topic of much debate. The historical views tended to support the theory that the cortex derives its superficial peripheral supply from periosteal vessels, while its deeper layers are supplied by medullary vessels (Lewis, 1956; Trueta and Morgan, 1960; Trueta and Cavadias, 1964; Skawina and Gorczyca, 1984). However, Brookes and Harrison (1957) suggested that in youth, the arterial input to the cortex is in fact predominantly medullary in origin. Modern research has confirmed that in the young (<35 years) there is no periosteal supply to the cortical bone, but it is entirely medullary in origin and therefore operates in a centrifugal manner (Dillaman, 1984; Skawina *et al.*, 1994; Bridgeman and Brookes, 1996; Brookes and Revell, 1998). However, it has been suggested that the cortical supply becomes increasingly periosteal in nature with advancing age due to medullary ischaemia brought on by atherosclerosis of the medullary vessels (Bridgeman and Brookes, 1996). In advancing years (70+) the cortical supply is reported to be almost entirely periosteal in nature.

The ascending and descending branches of the medullary vessel branch profusely throughout the cavity and terminate in helical loops in the vicinity of the metaphyseal zone. Here they anastomose with the **metaphyseal** vessels, which are also direct branches from adjacent systemic vessels. They are aligned vertical to the growth plate and are uniformly dispersed throughout the cancellous bone. The active metaphysis obtains its blood supply not only from the metaphyseal vessels but also from branches of the sinusoidal medullary loops in the zone of ossification. In fetal bone, the metaphyseal vessels support the entire width of the growth plate but in the postnatal years they tend to be responsible for maintenance of the cells in the zones of cartilage transformation and ossification (Brookes and Revell, 1998).

The **epiphyseal** arteries are derived from peri-articular vascular arcades that form on the non-articular bone surfaces. Branches of these vessels can be identified in the cartilage canals of the epiphyseal mass as early as the ninth fetal week (Haraldsson, 1962; Brookes and Revell, 1998). The epiphyseal mass is a discrete vascular zone with limited or no anastomoses occuring with the adjacent metaphyseal vessels. In postnatal long bones it has been shown that the epiphyseal vessels penetrate through the juxtaposed subchondral (terminal) plate to supply the germinal and proliferative zones of the growth plate (Brookes and Revell, 1998). Thus the overall viability of the growth plate to maintain normal bone growth and development is dependent upon the integrity of these vessels. Should damage occur to these arteries then growth arrest will occur. Whilst it has been shown that some degree of arterial anastomosis exists, it is generally insufficient to fully compensate when a major vessel is damaged (Brookes, 1957) and so an interruption to normal growth is unavoidable.

For more detailed information on the vascularity of bone, including its venous drainage, readers are directed to two particular texts (Crock, 1996; Brookes and Revell, 1998).

Bone modelling and remodelling

As a bone develops it must not only increase in length and width but also alter its shape and composition to accommodate the changing stresses and strains that are placed upon it in this dynamic stage. Bone **modelling** therefore involves the sculpting of a developing bone by the removal of bone is some locations with a concomitant addition in other places. Throughout bone development it is a continuous activity involving mutually dependent actions of bone-forming cells (osteoblasts) and bone removal cells (osteoclasts). Such geometric alterations are witnessed in almost all bones, irrespective of whether they form by intramembranous or endochondral ossification. Obviously, bone modelling is markedly reduced once the individual attains maturity.

Remodelling involves the removal of bone that was formed at an early time and its replacement with new bone. It has been estimated that approximately 5% of adult compact bone is renewed every year, and an astonishing 25% of cancellous bone (Martin *et al.*, 1998). Remodelling tends to occur more as a co-ordinated operation between bone formation and resorption, tends not to affect the overall size and shape of the bone, is episodic and continues throughout life (Enlow, 1963; Garn, 1970). The function of remodelling is thought to be essentially reparative in nature by the elimination of microscopic damage that could eventually lead to fatigue failure.

Haversian systems

Haversian systems (first identified by Clopton Havers in 1691) develop almost exclusively in compact bone (Cohen and Harris, 1958; Cooper *et al.*, 1966). Although they epitomize the microscopic appearance of adult bone they are also found in **woven bone**, which is the most immature type of developing bone and is typical of young fetal bones. Woven bone tends to be formed very quickly, is poorly organized and relatively weak. When viewed under polarized light it appears similar to the weave of fabric, hence its name. It is present in bones that are formed both by intramembranous and endochondral ossification and appears as a randomly interconnecting labyrinth that houses large vascular spaces. Osteoblast-mediated apposition of **concentric lamellae** on the walls of the vascular spaces reduces them to such an extent that eventually only a small canal persists around the central blood vessel. Thus a **primary osteon** (Haversian system) develops with its Haversian canal and associated neurovascular contents. At the periosteal surface, blood vessels become incorporated into the circumferential lamellar structure laid down by the periosteum and become surrounded by several layers of concentric lamellae, thereby forming a primary osteon in this location.

Lamellar bone is more mature, forms slowly, is well organized, consists of parallel layers and constitutes almost all of adult compact bone. It appears in two distinct patterns which have been likened to plywood architecture (Giraud-Guille, 1988). In the first of these, the collagen fibres are parallel in each lamella but change by 90° at the interface with the next lamella. In other regions, this can be replaced by a helicoidal arrangement where the collagen fibres constantly change their direction so that the individual identification of a lamella is almost impossible. Both of these patterns of collagen orientation lead to birefringence when a section is viewed under polarized light (Ascenzi and Bonucci, 1967). This alteration in fibre orientation imparts great resilience and strength to the tissue.

The **primary bone** that is formed by early primary Haversian systems is short-lived and is soon remodelled into a more complex tissue comprised of longitudinally orientated cylindrical secondary Haversian systems (secondary osteons). The existing primary bone is removed and replaced with new lamellar bone by osteoblasts and osteoclasts that operate together in a basic multicellular unit or BMU. This generally consists of approximately 9–10 osteoclasts and several hundred osteoblasts operating in unison (Jaworski *et al.*, 1981). A BMU operates in a predictable pattern – activation, resorption and formation (ARF – Jaworski *et al.*, 1983), although there are in fact six identifiable phases in the sequential development of a secondary osteon. These are as follows.

(1) Activation – this involves the recruitment of precursor cells to form the BMU. It has been reported that this phase can take up to 3 days to complete (Martin *et al.*, 1998).

(2) Resorption – in this stage the newly differentiated osteoclasts begin to resorb the primary bone at a rate of approximately 40–50 μm per day. This collection of 9–10 osteoclasts forms the so-called 'cutting cone'. The secretion of acids demineralizes adjacent bone and then enzymes dissolve the collagen. The tunnel that is cut by the osteoclasts is more or less longitudinal to the axis of the bone but there is some evidence to suggest that it spirals slightly at an angle of curvature of approximately 12° (Petrtyl *et al.*, 1996).

(3) Reversal – this marks the stage of transition between the leading osteoclastic cutting cone and the following osteoblastic region of bone formation.

(4) Formation – osteoblasts align along the periphery of the tunnel cut by the osteoclasts and begin to lay down concentric lamellae at a closing rate of approximately 1–2 μm per day and is commonly called the 'closing cone' (Polig and Jee, 1990). The tunnel is not completely infilled, as it is necessary to house a nutrient artery in the central Haversian canal. The average formation phase takes approximately 3 months to complete in the adult (Martin *et al.*, 1998).

(5) Mineralization – following deposition of the osteoid the process of mineralization commences by the growth of mineral crystals between the layers of collagen fibrils (Landis, 1995). Mineralization can continue for up to 6 months, so that newly formed osteons, can exhibit very different mechanical properties from more mature osteons, which will exhibit a greater proportion of mineralization.

(6) Quiescence – In this stage, the osteoclasts are no longer required and the remaining osteoblasts either convert into osteocytes or are removed. The secondary osteon is fully mature at this stage and able to fully participate in its primary roles of tissue metabolism and mechanics.

Remodelling of bone occurs throughout life and can be used as a means of determining the age of the bone. As the osteons are remodelled, so the proportion of bone 'debris' such as woven bone, primary osteons, osteon fragments, etc. to new osteons will alter. This has been utilized by anthropologists to establish an age at death using microscopic sections of compact bone. The usefulness of this technique lies in its ability to establish age in the adult when often there are few other methods available, although it cannot be undertaken by the amateur and does require a considerable laboratory facility. Whilst Amprino (1948) and Hattner and Frost (1963) recognized the relationship between bone turnover and age, Kerley (1965) is attributed with being the first to apply it to anthropological problems. Although revisions were made to his original technique (Kerley and Ubelaker, 1978), this work remains the ground-breaking research in the field and it has since been used by many investigators (Ahlqvist and Damsten, 1969; Singh and Gunberg, 1970; Bouvier and Ubelaker, 1977; Thompson, 1979; Ericksen, 1991; Stout *et al.*, 1994; Walker *et al.*, 1994; Cool *et al.*, 1995; Watanabe *et al.*, 1998).

Whilst most anthropologists recognize the value of this approach, there are certain limitations to be taken into consideration (Lazenby, 1984; Aiello and Molleson, 1993). For example, the accuracy of this approach will vary between different populations depending upon factors such as health, nutrition, etc. Factors such as the choice of bone, the sample site and the amount required must be carefully selected. However, these problems are not specific to this technique alone but apply to many methods of age determination. The true benefit of histological age determination probably lies in the ability to assign an age at death from relatively small fragments of bone, although the effect of diagenesis must be borne in mind (Bell, 1990; Bell *et al.*, 1996).

CHAPTER FOUR

Early Embryological Development

This chapter is a brief synopsis of very early embryogenesis, in order to prevent unnecessary repetition in the following chapters. For a fuller account the reader should refer to specific embryology texts (e.g. Larsen, 1993; Williams *et al.*, 1995). Details on early skeletal development of individual bones can be found in subsequent relevant chapters.

At the end of the second week following fertilization (stages 5 and 6), the cells that will form the embryo are arranged as a circular bilaminar embryonic disc of about 0.2 mm in diameter. The upper layer, or **epiblast**, consists of columnar cells that lie adjacent to the amniotic cavity. The lower layer of the disc, or **hypoblast**, is composed of cuboidal cells that form the roof of the secondary yolk sac. Both these layers are continuous peripherally outside the embryonic area with extra-embryonic tissues (Fig. 4.1).

Cells of the epiblast are involved in the process of gastrulation, which involves a complex re-arrangement of cell populations that begins with the formation of the **primitive streak**. By stage 6 (about day 15), a proliferative zone of cells called the **primitive groove** appears in the midline of the caudal part of the epiblast, which has become oval-shaped. At the presumptive cephalic end of the groove there is a raised area, the **primitive node** (Hensen's node), surrounding the **primitive pit** (Fig. 4.2). These three structures, which establish the bilateral symmetry of the embryo, constitute the primitive streak. Some cells of the epiblast become detached and ingress at the primitive streak into the space between the epiblast and the hypoblast. The first cells replace the hypoblast to form the definitive **endoderm** (Fig. 4.3). The remaining cells form intra-embryonic **mesoderm** between the other two layers and produce two midline structures between the epiblast and the endoderm, the **prechordal plate** and the **notochordal process**. The prechordal plate, anchored into the endoderm, is a localized, thickening cephalad to the notochordal process but its limits and fate remain uncertain (Williams *et al.*, 1995). The notochordal process is a rod-like bar of cells extending cranially from the primitive node to the prechordal plate. Its primary function is the induction of the neural plate and it goes through several changes before becoming the definitive notochord (stages 8–11). It takes part in the maintenance of the neural floor plate and is involved in signalling to the sclerotomal part of the paraxial mesoderm. Once the three germ layers are fully established, the remaining surface epiblast is known as the **ectoderm**. At the cranial and caudal ends of the embryo the ectoderm and endoderm fuse together to exclude the mesoderm and form the **buccopharyngeal** and **cloacal** membranes, respectively. These two membranes, which later break down, form the oral and cloacal ends of the gut tube (Fig. 4.2).

The establishment of the three germ layers of the embryo is fundamental to the subsequent development of the major systems of the body, although the notion of their separate development is an oversimplification. The study of morphogenetic mechanisms has revealed that there are complex interactions between cells from different layers and many structures have contributions from more than one layer.

By stage 9 (during the third week), the beginnings of the nervous system are seen as the thickened **neural plate**, which lies in the midline over the notochord from the primitive node to the prechordal plate, and laterally over the paraxial strip of mesoderm. The neural plate enlarges rapidly becoming pear-shaped in outline and develops a **neural groove** in the midline, while the margins become raised as **neural folds** (Fig. 4.4). The folds gradually meet over the top of the groove, beginning in the region of the future neck, and fusion proceeds both rostrally and caudally to form a hollow **neural tube**, which subsequently detaches itself from the surface ectoderm (Fig. 4.5a–c). This process is known as neurulation. Ante-

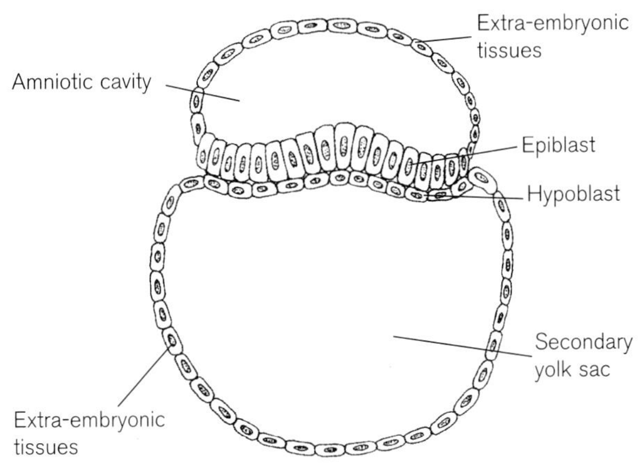

Figure 4.1 The bilaminar disc at the end of week 2.

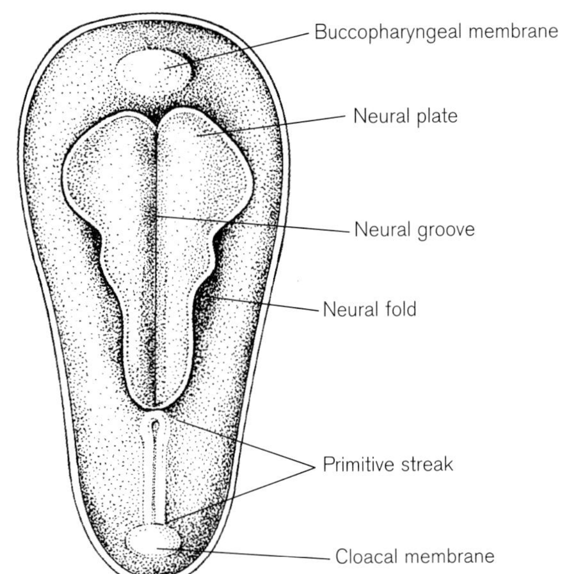

Figure 4.4 The position of the neural plate.

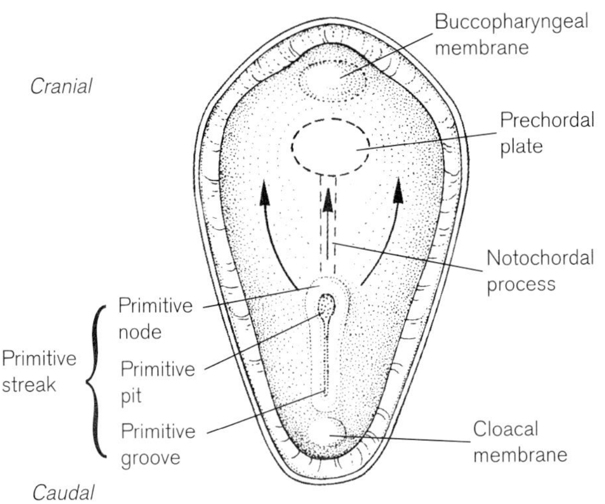

Figure 4.2 The primitive streak.

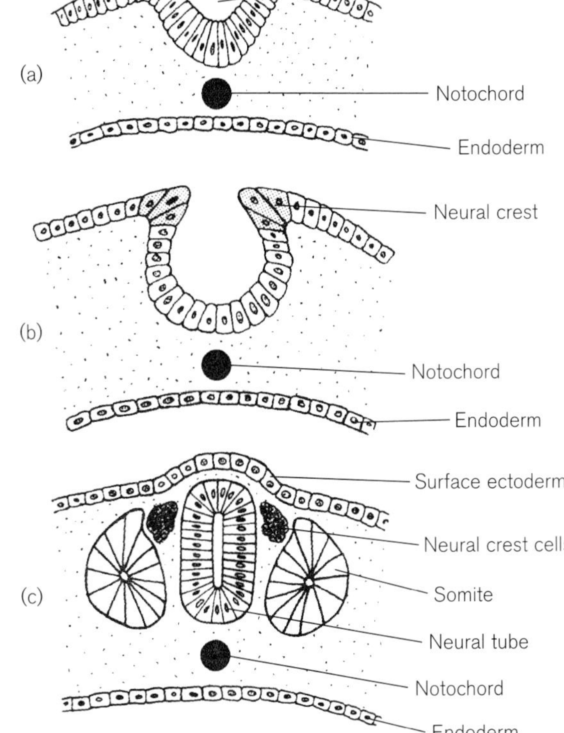

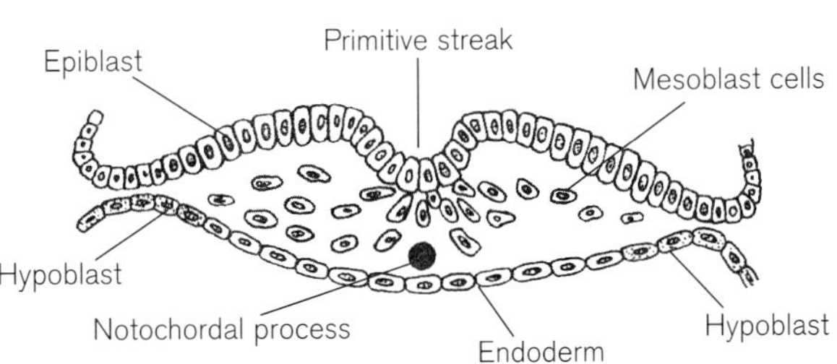

Figure 4.3 The trilaminar disc – stage 8 (3rd week).

Figure 4.5 Neurulation – stages 9–11 (4th week).

riorly, the tube enlarges to form three primary cerebral vesicles, which are the first indications of brain formation. The tube temporarily remains open at **anterior** and **posterior neuropores**, which eventually close by the middle and end of the fourth week, respectively (Fig. 4.6). The region at the lateral margins of the neural folds forms a special population called **neural crest** cells (ectomesenchyme), which differentiate first in the midbrain region and later more cranially and caudally. Neural crest cells detach from the epithelium and become mesenchymal and migratory in nature, invading the intra-embryonic mesoderm and contributing to a wide range of tissues, including those which form much of the skeleton of the head and neck.

As the neural folds are forming, the bilateral **paraxial mesoderm** alongside the notochord thickens, while laterally, it connects to a narrower band of **intermediate** mesoderm. This in turn is continuous with a flatter band called the **lateral plate** (Fig. 4.7). The paraxial mesoderm in the region of the hindbrain becomes subdivided lengthways into a series of rounded whorls of cells, which have been called **somitomeres** and this formation proceeds cephalocaudally as the embryo grows. The seven pairs rostral to the mid-myelencephalon are said to remain as somitomeres but caudal to this point, starting in the future occipital region at stage 9, they develop into discrete blocks or segments called **somites**, of which there are eventually 42–44 pairs, although several of the terminal pairs later regress. Each somite consists of three parts: a ventromedial **sclerotome**, which forms the basis of the future postcranial skeleton, a dorsolateral **dermatome** and a dorsomedial **myotome**, which will develop into the skin and muscles respectively of the body wall and limbs. The first four or five pairs of somites are incorporated into the occipital region, while the successive eight pairs form the cervical region with the most cranial of these also taking part in the formation of the occiput. The next 12 somite pairs form the thoracic vertebrae and the bones, striated muscles and dermis of the thorax. Some cells from the lower cervical and upper thoracic somites migrate laterally to form the structures of the upper limb buds. Of the next 10 somite pairs, the upper five form the lumbar column and the dermis and striated muscles of the abdominal wall, while the lower five form the sacrum and its associated structures. As with the upper limb, cells from the lumbar and upper sacral somites contribute to the development of the structures of the lower limb. The remainder of the somite pairs will form the region of the embryonic tail including the coccyx (for further details see Chapter 6).

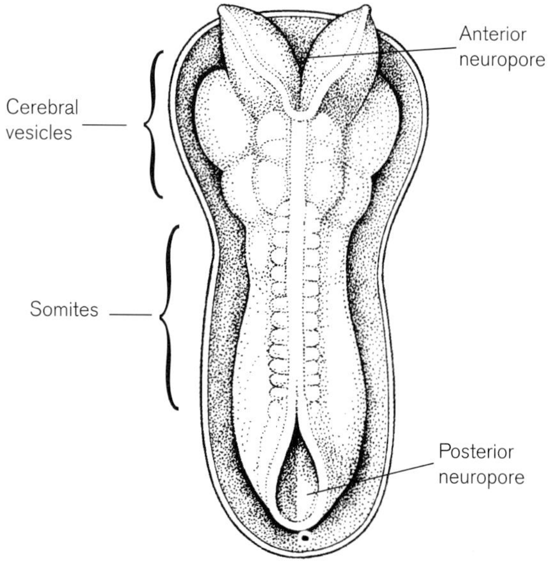

Figure 4.6 Embryo showing neuropores and somites – stage 10–11 (4th week).

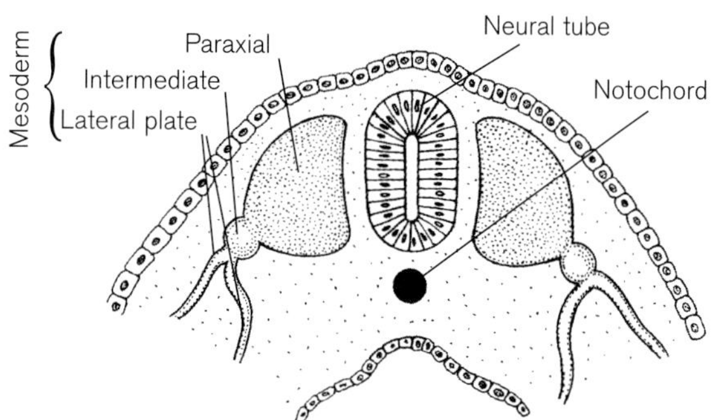

Figure 4.7 Divisions of the mesoderm.

During the third and fourth weeks, other fundamental changes are taking place in the embryo that are only outlined here. Differential growth causes a folding of the embryo both cephalocaudally and laterally to assume its definitive shape (Fig. 4.8). In the very early stages, the prechordal plate and cardiogenic area lie in front of the anterior tip of the notochord. The rapid overgrowth of the nervous system produces a head fold during which the buccopharyngeal membrane and pericardium tilt a full 180° ventrally in a process known as reversal. Thus, the future mouth (stomodeum) and pharyngeal region is bounded dorsally by the developing forebrain and notochord and below by the heart tube in its pericardial cavity. In a similar manner, during the formation of the tail fold, the cloacal membrane and connecting stalk, originally posterior, also come to lie ventrally (Fig. 4.8).

During the third, fourth and fifth weeks the first external signs of the formation of the ear, eye and nose

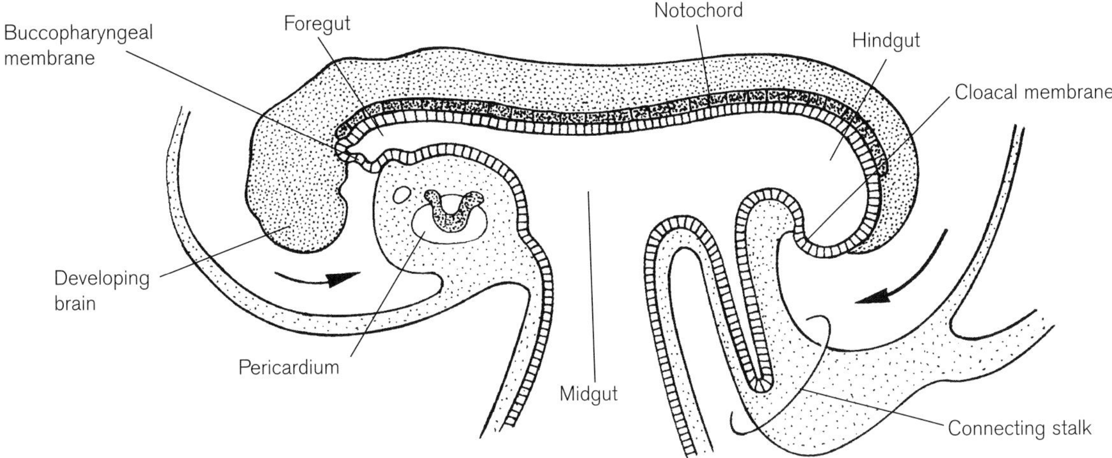

Figure 4.8 Folding of the embryo – stages 9–11 (4th week).

show as ectodermal thickenings. The **otic placodes**, which give rise to the inner ear, are situated lateral to the hindbrain region, the **lens placodes** are associated with the lateral aspects of the forebrain and the **nasal placodes** are found on the frontonasal process of the future face.

During the fourth and fifth weeks of development, a series of **pharyngeal** (branchial) **arches** are formed in the lateral walls of the pharyngeal region of the foregut. They develop in craniocaudal sequence during stages 10–13 (between the 22nd and 29th days) and form a series of bars, each with a mesodermal core covered by ectoderm and lined by endoderm. Between the bars lie the external **pharyngeal grooves** (clefts) and the internal **pharyngeal pouches**, where the ectoderm and endoderm are in contact. The arches are transient structures with the first four being fairly prominent and it appears from experimental evidence on animal models, that they contain contributions from the neural crest. The fifth arch is rudimentary and short-lived and this and the sixth arch cannot be recognized externally. Some of the skeletal structures derived from the arches develop in cartilage, which subsequently ossifies, while others develop directly from mesenchyme. Skeletal elements of the first (mandibular) arch form within the maxillary and mandibular processes and so contribute to the face, Meckel's cartilage in the mandible and the malleus and incus of the middle ear. The second (hyoid) arch gives rise to the styloid process of the temporal bone, part of the

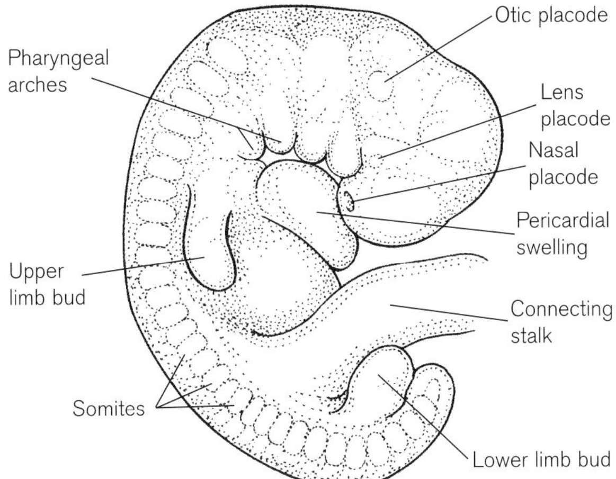

Figure 4.9 Embryo at stage 12–13 (about 5 weeks).

hyoid bone and the stapes of the middle ear. The rest of the hyoid bone forms from the third arch, while the fourth and sixth arches contribute to the cartilages of the larynx. The external auditory meatus, the tympanic cavity and the auditory (pharyngotympanic/Eustachian) tube are remnants of the first cleft and pouch (see Chapter 5).

At stages 12 and 13 (during the third and fourth weeks) the **limb buds** appear as small projections from a lateral ridge on the ventrolateral aspect of the trunk (Fig. 4.9). The early development of both limbs is similar, but the timing of the upper limb precedes that of the lower limb by 1 or 2 days (see Chapter 9).

CHAPTER FIVE

The Head, Neck and Dentition

In keeping with its traditional topographical title, this chapter includes not only the skull, mandible and dentition but also the hyoid and larynx. However, the cervical vertebrae are considered together with the rest of the column in Chapter 6.

The skull is the most complex region of the axial skeleton. It both supports and protects the brain and organs of special sense, as well as housing the first part of the respiratory and alimentary tracts. The **neurocranium** (braincase) consists of a base and a vault whose side walls and roof (calvaria) complete the bony protective covering. Attached anteriorly is the face, or **viscerocranium**, the upper part forming the skeleton of the orbits and nose, and the lower part, together with the mandible, constituting the jaws.

The terminology used in human cranial embryology is principally derived from the literature of comparative morphology, and a very brief synopsis of development of the vertebrate skull is introduced here so that the subsequent description of the early embryology of the human skull may be more easily appreciated. In the earliest forms of vertebrates there was both an inner (endo-) and an outer (exo-) skeleton. The **endoskeleton** consisted of a cartilaginous braincase, or **chondrocranium**, to which were attached capsules that surrounded organs of special sense, and a **jaw** skeleton composed of visceral (branchial/pharyngeal) arch cartilages which, in later forms, became secondarily attached to the skull. The **exoskeleton** developed in relation to the skin, hence the term dermal bone, and covered the anterior end of the body as a protective bony shield. During the course of vertebrate evolution, the basic pattern of the chondrocranium has been retained, albeit with additional new elements in higher vertebrates. On the other hand, the exoskeleton has been greatly reduced but some derivatives still exist in mammals.

The vertebrate chondrocranium consists of a basal plate of fused cartilages to which are attached three pairs of capsules that support and protect the organs of hearing, sight and smell. Posteriorly, the paired **parachordal cartilages** surround the anterior end of the notochord and have the **otic capsules** attached laterally. In front of the notochord, the plate is composed of paired **trabeculae cranii**, which, for descriptive purposes, can be divided into an **hypophyseal** area around the pituitary posteriorly and an **interobitonasal** element anteriorly, to which are attached the **nasal** and **optic** capsules. The side wall of the braincase was incomplete in early vertebrates, but, in subsequent mammalian evolution, which involved enlargement of the brain, a new element, the **ala temporalis** formed. The roof of the chondrocranium was also incomplete and consisted of three bands of cartilage called the synotic tecta connecting, from anterior to posterior, the orbital cartilages, the otic capsules and the posterior cartilages (Jarvik, 1980).

The second component of the endoskeleton is derived from a variable number of cartilaginous **pharyngeal** (visceral) **arches**, which develop in the floor and walls of the pharynx. In aquatic forms, they support the gills, but their function and subsequent development varies in different groups of land animals. In early jawed vertebrates, the first two arches were involved in the formation and support of the jaws, but in higher vertebrates they became incorporated into the skull, ear and skeleton of the neck. For instance, Meckel's cartilage is a prominent but transient structure from the lower element of the first (mandibular) arch seen in the embryos of all mammals. Reichert's cartilage, from the second (hyoid) arch, contributes to the temporal and hyoid bones, and parts of the posthyoid arches form the larynx.

Elements of the original dermal armour that comprised the exoskeleton have become highly modified and, in higher vertebrates, contribute to the cranial vault, the orbital and nasal cavities, the jaws and pectoral girdle. In higher vertebrates, most of these bones are not preformed in cartilage but develop directly in mesenchyme by intramembranous ossification.

Despite variations in different groups of vertebrates, the basic pattern of the chondrocranium has essentially been maintained throughout phylogeny and manifestations of this have fascinated biologists for several centuries. As early as 1820, Goethe proposed that the skull was composed of modified vertebrae (see Singh-Roy, 1967) and from this time to the present, the study of segmentation has continued (Goodrich, 1930; Gadow, 1933; de Beer, 1937; Romer, 1966, 1970; Jarvik, 1980). Metameric segmentation is clearly reflected in the trunk, where there is a common pattern in such tissues as the vertebral column, ribs, spinal cord and developing urogenital system. In the head and neck the situation is less clear, but there is evidence of segmentation in the cranial nerves, mesoderm of the caudal part of the skull and pharyngeal arches. Early studies resulted in elaborate theories of head segmentation, based on varying numbers of cranial and postcranial somites and this led to far-reaching assumptions about the homologies of head and trunk vertebrae in different groups of vertebrates. It proved impossible to envisage a single plan in which there were homologies for individual structures in different taxonomic groups (for example the alisphenoid, Presley and Steele, 1976, 1978). The idea of a unified plan for the head and trunk was never universally accepted and some authorities suggested that the embryology of the head was organized differently from that of the postcranial skeleton, although most agreed that, at least, the posterior part of the skull was segmented. The head segmentation theory is well reviewed by Moore (1981).

Resurgence of interest in head segmentation was stimulated by the work of Meier and colleagues (Meier, 1979, 1981; Meier and Tam, 1982; Jacobson and Meier, 1984). They described arrangements of cells prior to the formation of somites, which they called somitomeres. These are described as incompletely divided paraxial mesoderm, which condense to form properly segmented somites in the trunk but remain essentially unsegmented anterior to the mesencephalic region of the head. Although the actual physical existence of somitomeres has been disputed, there appears to be a consensus that they probably do exist (Alberch and Kollar, 1988). There is much debate about whether the neuronal, mesodermal and pharyngeal elements belong to a single series that is continuous with the segmentation seen in the trunk. This is partly because there is variability, both in branchial arch number in different species, and variation in time of development of various elements. The number of occipital somites contributing to the skull also varies between species, and the number of mesodermal segments anterior to the first somite is uncertain. However, some authorities believe that somites and somitomeres have the same range of developmental potential (Noden, 1988).

An alternative theory of head morphology (Gans and Northcutt, 1983; Northcutt and Gans, 1983), whilst accepting that the hind part of the skull is segmented, argues that the front part of the skull is an entirely new construction, not homologous with trunk structures. This 'new head' was envisaged as evolving in response to a shift from a passive mode of feeding found in the ancestral protochordates to an active role of predation in vertebrates. Recent experimental studies investigating possible mechanisms for chondrocranial patterning appear to support this theory. They have been carried out mainly on avian models and involve both following morphogenetic movements of cells and the study of tissue interactions, especially the role of the extracellular matrix. Fate mapping experiments in quail-chick chimeras indicate that, not only the anterior part of the skull and face, but most of the vault is derived from neural crest cells (Couly *et al.*, 1992, 1993). Crest cells (ectomesenchyme) migrate to large areas of the midfacial and visceral arch skeleton and their fate is thought to be determined very early in development, even before they leave the edges of the neural folds (Noden, 1983). Thus, they could act as important patterning agents for other skeletal forming tissues (Alberch and Kollar, 1988). A possible mechanism for how the chondrocranial pattern might be specified – the 'fly-paper' model – was proposed by Thorogood (1987, 1988). Much of the basic research on the genetic control of segmentation and regionalization has involved invertebrates, but recent research on homeobox-containing genes in mammals has opened up interesting possibilities of experimental investigation in vertebrate animal models (Holland, 1988; Holland and Hogan, 1988).

It is assumed that the avian and mammalian chondrocranium, vault and face are derived from homologous tissues and that therefore the human skull follows the general mammalian pattern. Some bones develop from a cartilaginous template (endochondral), others form directly in membrane (intramembranous), but there are several compound bones, principally the occipital, temporal and sphenoid, which contain portions with both intramembranous and endochondral origins (see Chapter 3). Much of the cranial base undergoes ossification during prenatal development, but cartilaginous synchondroses remain until early adult life, when growth ceases. Some cartilage is retained throughout life in the nasal alae, the external ear and part of the Eustachian tube. Fusion

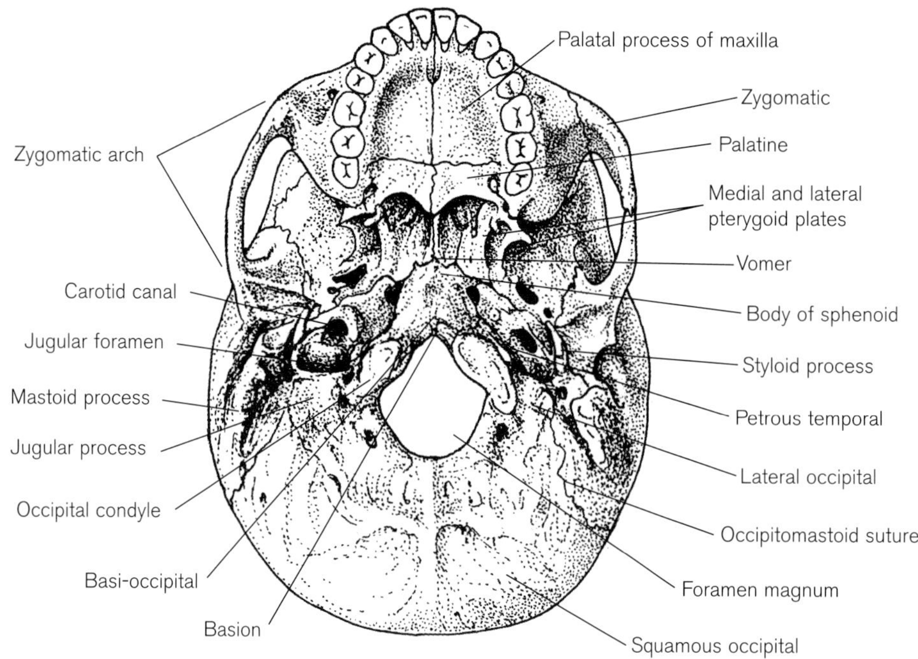

Figure 5.1 Basal view of the adult skull.

between parts of compound bones occurs over a wide time range extending from fetal life, through infancy to early childhood. Articulations between most of the bones of the vault and face are composed of fibrous sutures, most of which are well developed during infancy.

In summary, the **cranial base** and the major part of the **nose** are preformed in cartilage. This comprises the basal, lateral parts and lower squama of the occipital bone, the petromastoid parts of the temporals, the body, the lesser wings and medial parts of the greater wings of the sphenoid, and the ethmoid and inferior

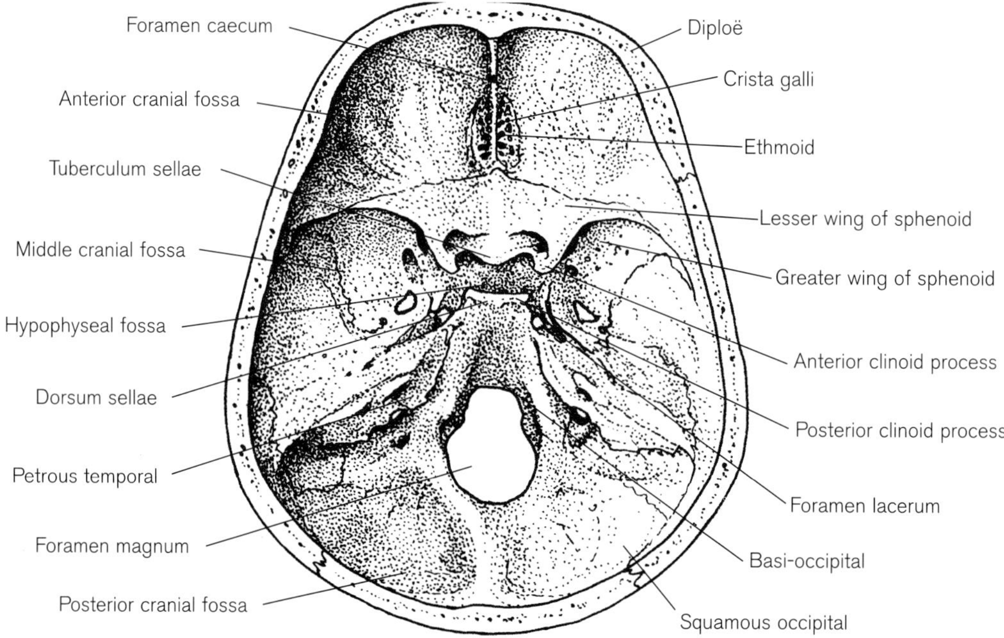

Figure 5.2 Intracranial view of base of adult skull.

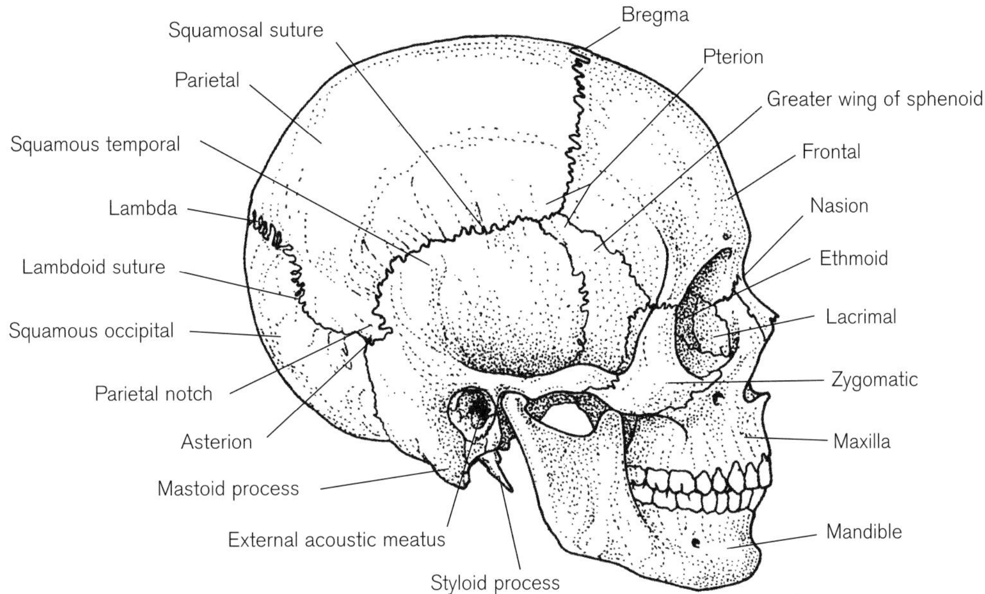

Figure 5.3 Lateral view of adult skull and mandible.

conchae (Figs. 5.1, 5.2 and 5.5). The bones of the **vault,** arise directly in membranous tissue to cover the rapidly expanding brain. They include the frontal, parietals, greater wings of the sphenoid, squamous parts of the temporals and the upper squama of the occipital bone (Figs. 5.3 and 5.4). Most of the remainder of the bones of the skull, which constitute the **face** and form around the nasal capsule, also develop directly in membrane. They are represented by the maxillae, palatines, nasals, lacrimals, zygomatics, and the vomer (Figs. 5.1, 5.3 and 5.5). Derivatives of the pharyngeal arches contribute to the maxilla, mandible, ear ossicles, styloid process of the temporal, hyoid bone and the skeleton of the larynx. Thus,

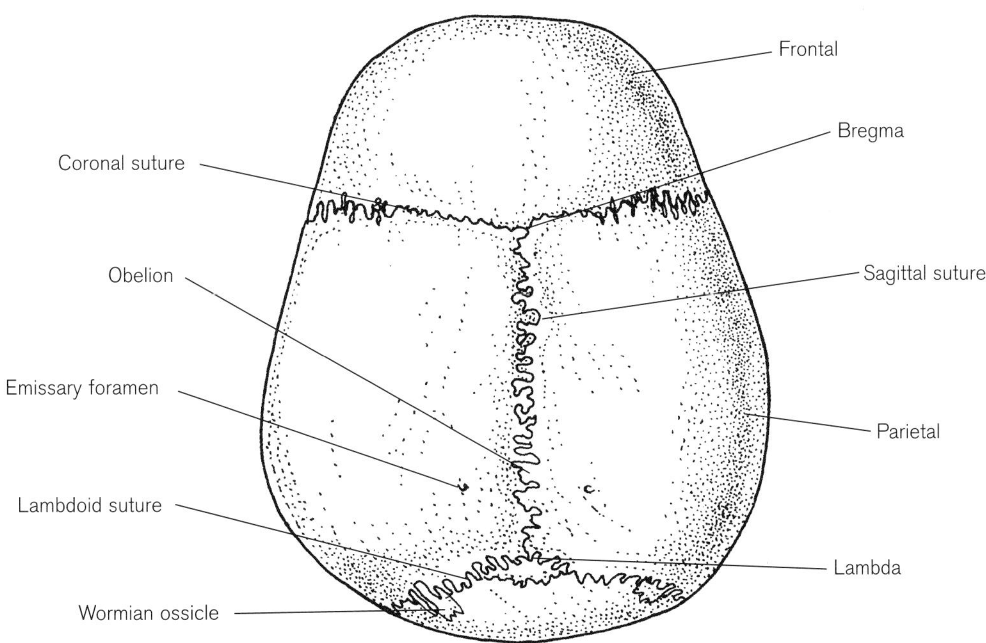

Figure 5.4 Superior view of adult skull.

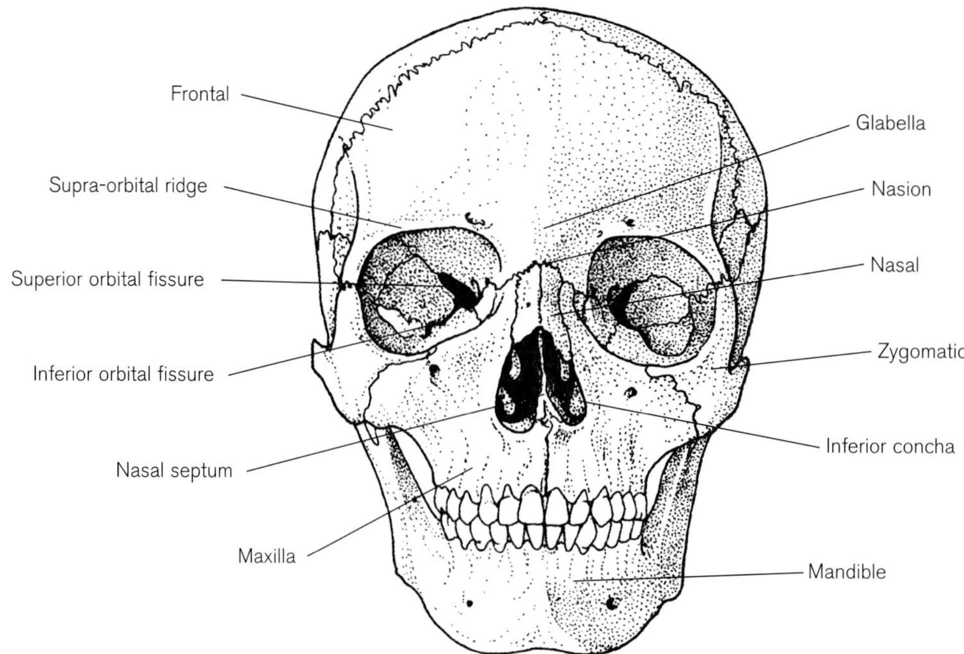

Figure 5.5 Anterior view of adult skull and mandible.

the neurocranium and viscerocranium have both cartilaginous and membranous components.

A full description of the adult skull is obviously outwith the context of this book and excellent descriptions may be found in other texts (Augier, 1931; Frazer, 1948; Williams *et al.*, 1995). Here, adult anatomy is limited to a description of the shape and articulations of each bone and details of anomalies are included where they have a bearing on development.

Early development of the human skull

Details of the early development of the human skull up to the end of the embryonic period may be found in Macklin (1914, 1921), Lewis (1920), Youssef (1964), Müller and O'Rahilly (1980, 1986, 1994) and O'Rahilly and Müller (1984a) and an outline is presented here. The **blastemal** skull develops in the embryonic mesenchyme, which surrounds the developing brain and primitive pharynx. The first signs of the **cranial base** are mesenchymal masses that appear in the occipital area during the fourth week of intrauterine life. These gradually spread anteriorly and by the beginning of the second month, encompass the pituitary region and then penetrate the territory of the nasal septum beneath the forebrain. The posterior part of the cranial base is penetrated obliquely by the notochord (Fig. 5.6), which leaves the dens of the axis and enters the basal plate where, at first, it lies dorsally between the hindbrain and the occipital mesenchyme. It then passes ventrally to lie in the dorsal wall of the pharynx and finally ends just in front of the region that is to become the dorsum sellae of the sphenoid (Müller and O'Rahilly, 1980; David *et al.*, 1998). At about the fifth week, the otic placodes, specialized neurepithelial cells, sink below the surface ectoderm and become encased in mesenchyme to form the **otic capsules**, which gain attachment to the occipital part of the basal plate. Meanwhile, the basic organization of the face is being laid down (see below).

At the beginning of the second month, transition to the **chondrocranium** begins as separate foci of cartilage gradually fuse and spread to form a continuous but incomplete cartilaginous mass, the basal plate (Fig. 5.7). Names given to the cartilages of the human cranial base vary, depending on the supposed derivation from the ancestral condition, but commonly accepted accounts may be found in Sullivan and Lumsden (1981) and Sperber (1989). The central stem (Fig. 5.6) is divided into chordal and prechordal parts that are angled in the region of the hypophyseal fossa. Although these terms have been applied to the human skull for some time (e.g. Müller and O'Rahilly, 1980), recent work on the development of the avian embryo using quail-chick chimeras has identified important differences of cellular derivation between the two parts and it is probable that this also applies to the

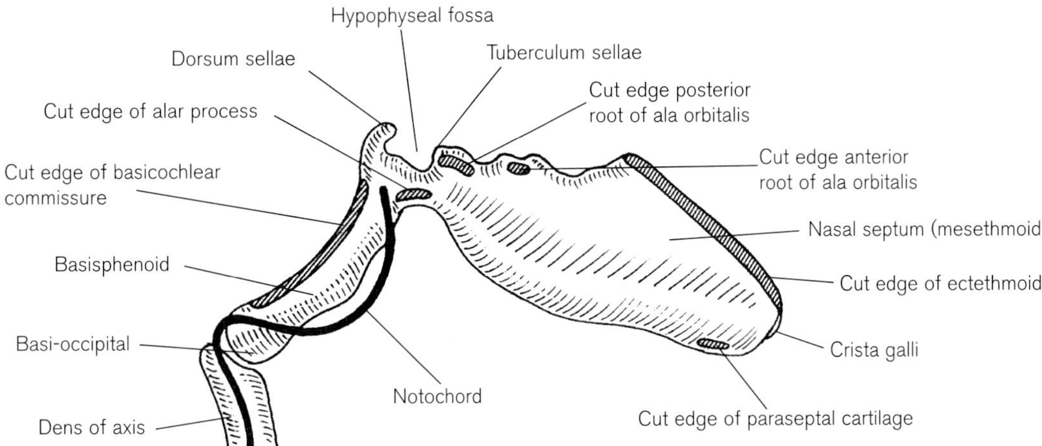

Figure 5.6 The central stem of the chondrocranium.

human skull. Couly *et al.* (1993) distinguish between the skull formed in front of the tip of the notochord, which incorporates most of the vault including the parietal and frontal bones and the region caudal to the notochord. The prechordal skull is derived entirely from the neural crest, while the chordal skull is formed from a complex mixture of crest and cephalic (somitic) mesoderm. Cranial base angulation, measured at the prechordal–chordal junction, by lines from nasion to sella (mid-hypophyseal fossa), and sella to basion (Figs. 5.2 and 5.5), changes rapidly during early fetal development, as reflected by the rapidly growing brain and the extension of the neck region. It flexes from about 130° in the 7 week embryo (cartilaginous stage) to 115°–120° at 10 weeks (pre-ossification stage) and then widens again to between 125° and 130° by 20 weeks as the cranial base ossifies. The prechordal cranial base increases in length and width sevenfold, while the posterior part grows only fivefold as these changes keep pace with the rate of develop-

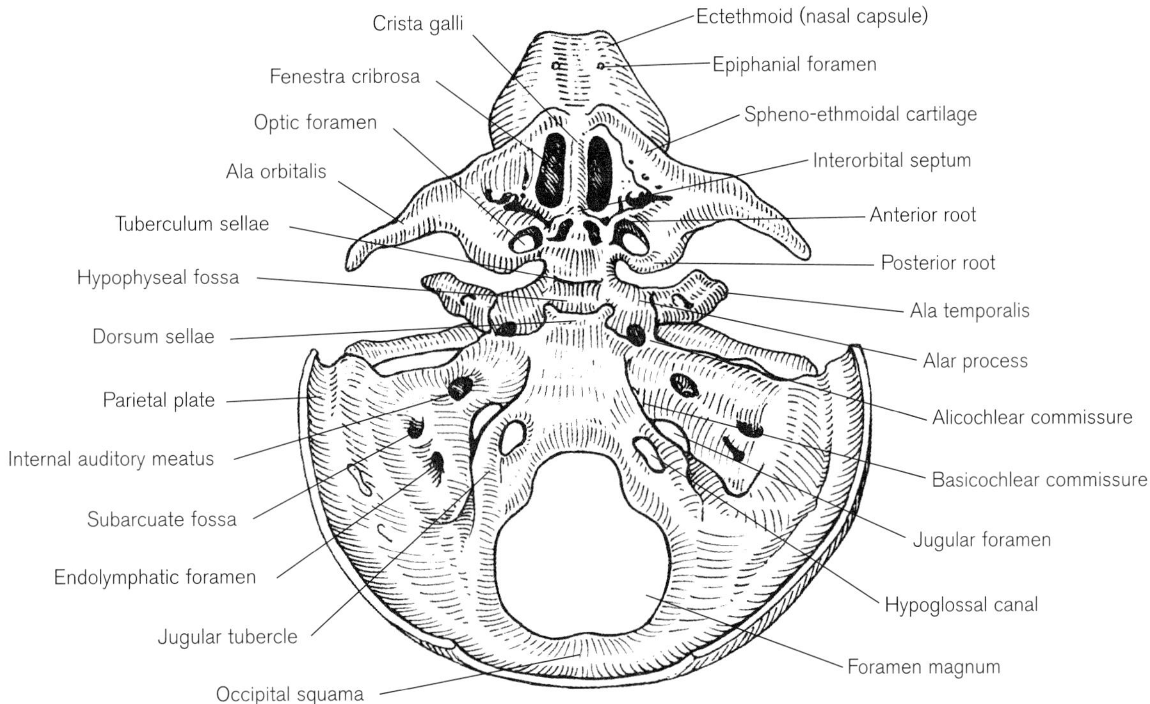

Figure 5.7 The chondrocranium from above.

ment of the different parts of the brain (Sperber, 1989). Growth of the different segments of the fetal skull is detailed by Ford (1956).

For descriptive purposes, during the embryonic period, the chondrocranium can be conveniently divided from posterior to anterior as occipital, otic, sphenoidal (orbitotemporal) and ethmoidal areas (Figs. 5.6–5.8). In the **occipital** region, the paired parachordal cartilages join to form the basi-occipital part of the basal plate, which lies anterior to the foramen magnum. This is at first deeply notched anteriorly but later becomes more rounded in shape. On either side lie the ex-occipitals, which give rise to the lateral parts of the occipital bone. They develop jugular tubercles, which separate the hypoglossal canals from the jugular fossae. The ex-occipitals are continued superiorly into the occipital plates (squamae), which at first are not united in the mid-dorsal line so that the foramen magnum is incomplete posteriorly. Initially, a thin band of cartilage, the tectum posterius (synoticum) joins the occipital plates, but later the whole inferoposterior occipital region is formed by the cartilaginous occipital plate. In detailed studies of quail-chick chimeras, Couly *et al.* (1993) found that the first five somites contribute to the occipital bone but in the human embryo, only four somites are involved in the occipital region (O'Rahilly and Müller, 1984a; Müller and O'Rahilly, 1986). The differences between avian and human embryos are discussed by Müller and O'Rahilly (1994).

The **otic capsules** lie lateral to the basal plate and are joined to it by basicochlear commissures. Each may be divided into a cochlear part, mostly formed from median paraxial mesoderm with contributions from neural crest, and a canalicular part, which is derived mainly from the first cranial somite. The internal auditory meatus, the endolymphatic foramen and the subarcuate fossa are obvious and the internal carotid artery and the VIIth (facial) cranial nerve are exposed on the rostral surface. Joined to the canalicular parts of the otic capsules by capsuloparietal commissures are two areas of cartilage called parietal (mastoid/nuchal) plates. They are incomplete superiorly, but joined posteriorly to the occipital plate and so partially cover the posterolateral part of the occipital area.

In the **sphenoidal region** the basisphenoid (postsphenoid) cartilage is continuous posteriorly with the basi-occipital and has the dorsum sellae protruding superiorly. On either side of the hypophyseal fossa is the alar process, over which the internal carotid artery runs in an anterior direction. The alar processes join the bases of the greater wings (alae temporales) to the body and are themselves connected posteriorly, via the alicochlear commissures, to the otic capsules. Anterior to the postsphenoid in the midline is the interorbital septum, which forms the presphenoid part of the body between the tuberculum sellae and the limbus sphenoidalis. It is connected to a lesser wing (ala orbitalis) on each side by two roots, a pre-optic (anterior/ventral) and a postoptic (posterior/dorsal/metopic) root, between which lies the optic foramen. The maxillary nerve runs forward to a cleft between the greater and

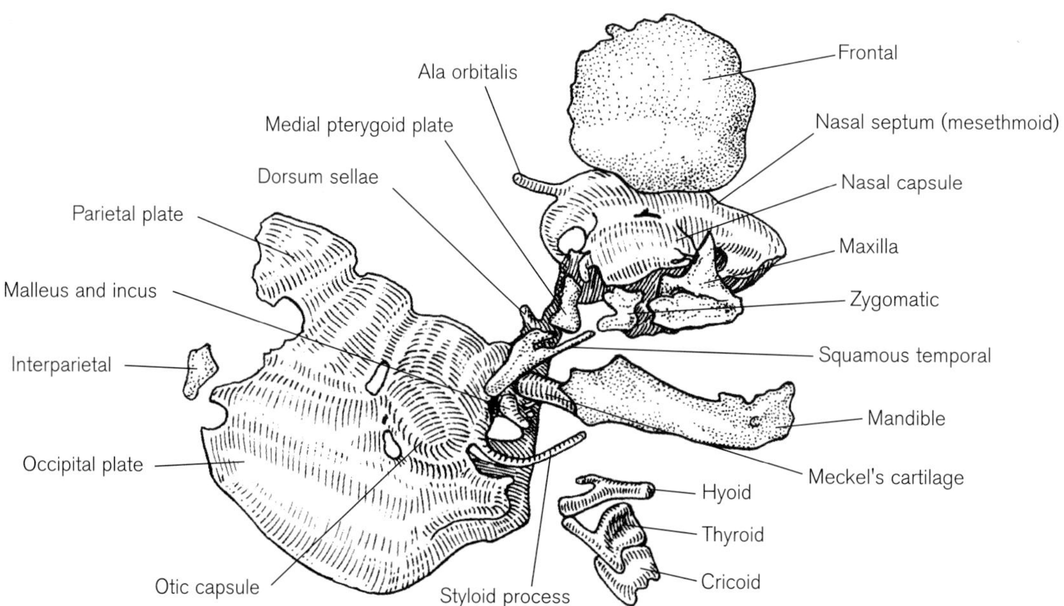

Figure 5.8 Chondrocranium with membrane bones from the right side.

lesser sphenoidal wings. At first this is wide open, but later becomes filled in medially as the foramen rotundum forms, and laterally as the rest of the wing develops in membrane. Some authorities consider that both the presphenoid part of the hypophyseal cartilage and the alae orbitales are derived from the trabeculae cranii of ancestral forms, but homologies are far from clear.

The **ethmoidal region** consists of a midline (mesethmoid) cartilage in the nasal septum from which the prominent crista galli protrudes superiorly. On either side are the nasal capsules consisting of small para-septal cartilages and ectethmoid cartilages from which the ethmoidal labyrinths develop. At first, they are incomplete, having side walls with a developing middle concha but almost no floor except the inturned edges where the inferior concha forms. Superiorly the anterior half has a roof, but posteriorly are the open fenestrae cribrosae. Epiphanial foramina in the roof allow passage of the anterior ethmoidal nerves. The posterior end of the nasal capsules are joined to the orbital wings of the sphenoid by spheno-ethmoidal cartilages, which support the developing frontal lobes of the brain.

Ossification of the chondrocranium begins posteriorly before chondrification is complete in the whole mass anteriorly. At the beginning of the second month the first ossification centres appear in the tectum posterius part of the occipital squama as the supra-occipital bone begins to ossify. Details of ossification in the cranial base are given under descriptions of individual bones.

The **vault** of the skull appears laterally at the end of the first fetal month, as curved plates of mesenchyme, which gradually spread both downwards to meet the forming cartilaginous base and upwards to meet each other over the top of the developing brain. This membranous **neurocranium** (desmocranium) is mainly derived from neural crest (Couly *et al.*, 1993). Most of the vault bones ossify directly in this mesenchyme, which requires the presence of the underlying brain in order to form bone. The induction of osteogenesis is lost in anencephalic fetuses, which do not form bony calvariae (Romero *et al.*, 1988). The mesenchyme of the sides of the vault is temporarily connected superiorly by three incomplete bands of cartilage called tecta (Fawcett, 1910a, 1923) but these ill-defined cartilaginous remnants soon disappear. By the end of the embryonic period, (Fig. 5.8) ossification can be seen posteriorly in the interparietal part of the occipital, laterally in the squamous temporal, medial pterygoid plate, zygomatic and anteriorly in the maxilla and the frontal bones. The goniale, which develops into the anterior process of the malleus, is represented by a small spicule of bone close to the end of Meckel's cartilage. The parietal bones and tympanic parts of the temporal bones start ossification during the fetal period (O'Rahilly and Gardner, 1972) and details of their later development can be found under descriptions of individual bones.

Neural crest cells are also thought to form the pia and arachnoid mater (leptomeninges), while most of the dura mater (pachymeninx) has, in addition to neural crest, contributions from prechordal plate and paraxial mesoderm. Details of the development of the human meninges can be found in O'Rahilly and Müller (1986). The internal attachments of the dura mater and their relationship to the suture systems of the skull are thought to take part in counteracting the force of the expanding brain. They are thus responsible in part for the final shape of the neurocranium (Moss, 1959; Smith and Töndury, 1978). This region has a very rapid rate of growth, concurrent with the precocious development of the brain and reaches 25% of its growth by birth, 50% by 6 months of age, 75% by 2 years and almost completes its growth by 10 years (Sperber, 1989). The circumference of the head almost doubles from midfetal life to birth and the biparietal diameter (BPD), as measured by ultrasound, is one of the common parameters by which normal development is monitored during pregnancy (Romero *et al.*, 1988).

The basic organization of the **face** begins at the end of the fourth week, when five swellings appear around the stomodeum. The mandibular (first pharyngeal) arch gives rise to bilateral maxillary and mandibular processes above and below the stomodeum and a median frontonasal process develops in the forehead area over the anterior end of the forebrain (Fig. 5.9a). During the fifth week, nasal placodes appear on the frontonasal process and the mesenchyme on either side of these ectodermal thickenings forms the medial and lateral nasal folds (processes). The placode invaginates beneath the surface to become the nasal pit. By a process of differential growth, the medial folds meet together to form the intermaxillary segment (Fig. 5.9b), which forms the bridge and centre of the nose, the philtrum of the upper lip and the primary palate (premaxillary area; Fig. 5.10a, b). The lateral nasal folds join with the maxillary processes to form the sides of the nose and the cheek area (Fig. 5.9c). Deep to the surface, the maxillary processes form palatal shelves (Fig. 5.10), which at first hang down beside the tongue. They rotate to a horizontal position and join with each other to complete the posterior growth of the secondary palate. A downgrowth from the base of the skull fuses in the midline of the palate (Wood and Kraus, 1962; Andersen and Matthiessen, 1967; Luke, 1976). In this way the primitive pharyngeal cavity is separated by the palate and nasal septum into

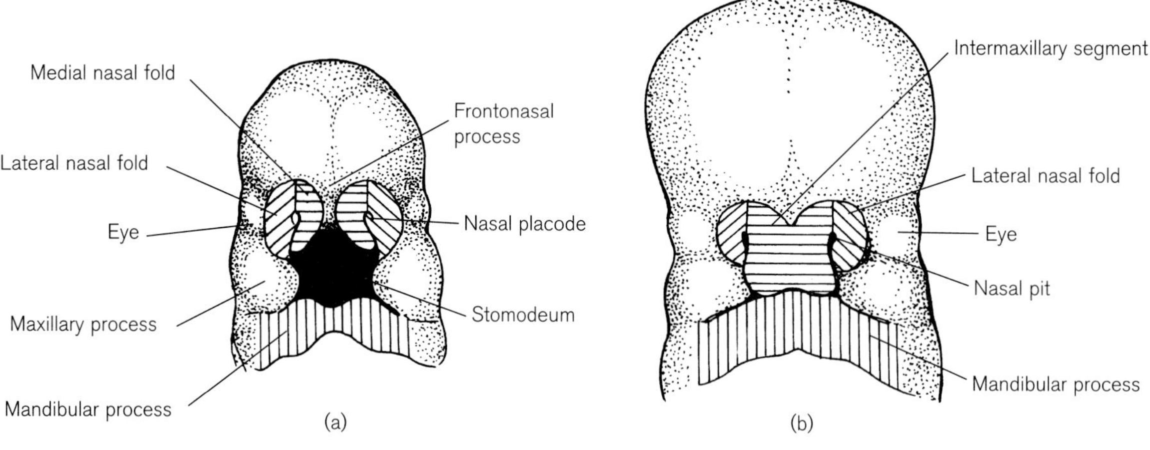

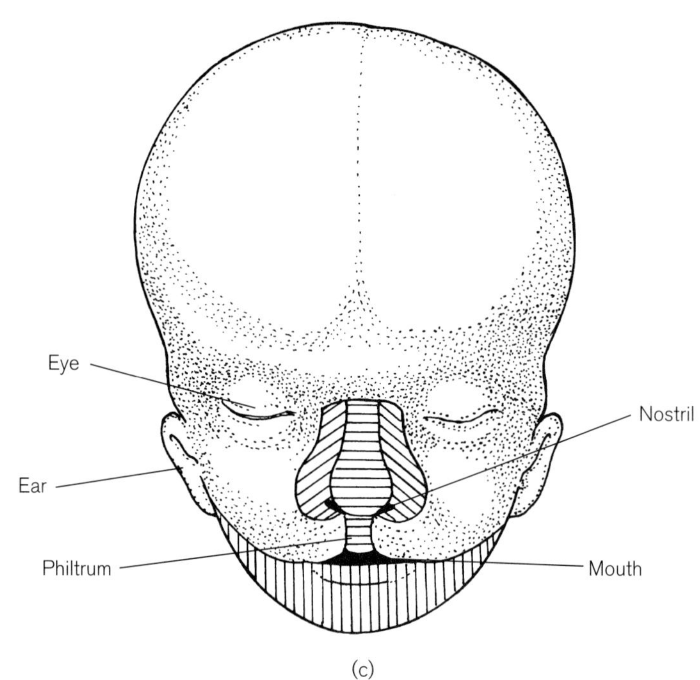

Figure 5.9 Formation of the face: (a) 5 weeks; (b) 7–8 weeks; (c) 10 weeks.

bilateral nasal cavities above and an oral cavity below (Fig. 5.10c). The transition of the palatal shelves from a vertical to a horizontal position takes place over a relatively short period of time between 7 and 8 weeks. However, the shelves remain vertical slightly longer in females, which could account for the greater incidence of cleft palate in girls (Burdi and Silvey, 1969a, b). The initiation of tooth development in each jaw begins during the sixth week (see section XV). The basic morphology of the facial and palatal region is laid down between 4 and 10 weeks. Details of major growth changes taking place during this time have been studied by Diewert (1985).

Most of the superficial facial bones develop in membrane from migrating cell populations that are derived mainly from neural crest but ossification entails a complex interaction between this mesenchyme and the overlying epithelium of the facial region. Early ossification centres for the maxillae and zygomatic bones can be seen in the side wall of the nasal capsule and those for the palatines and bilateral plates of the vomer lie in the posterior part of the nasal

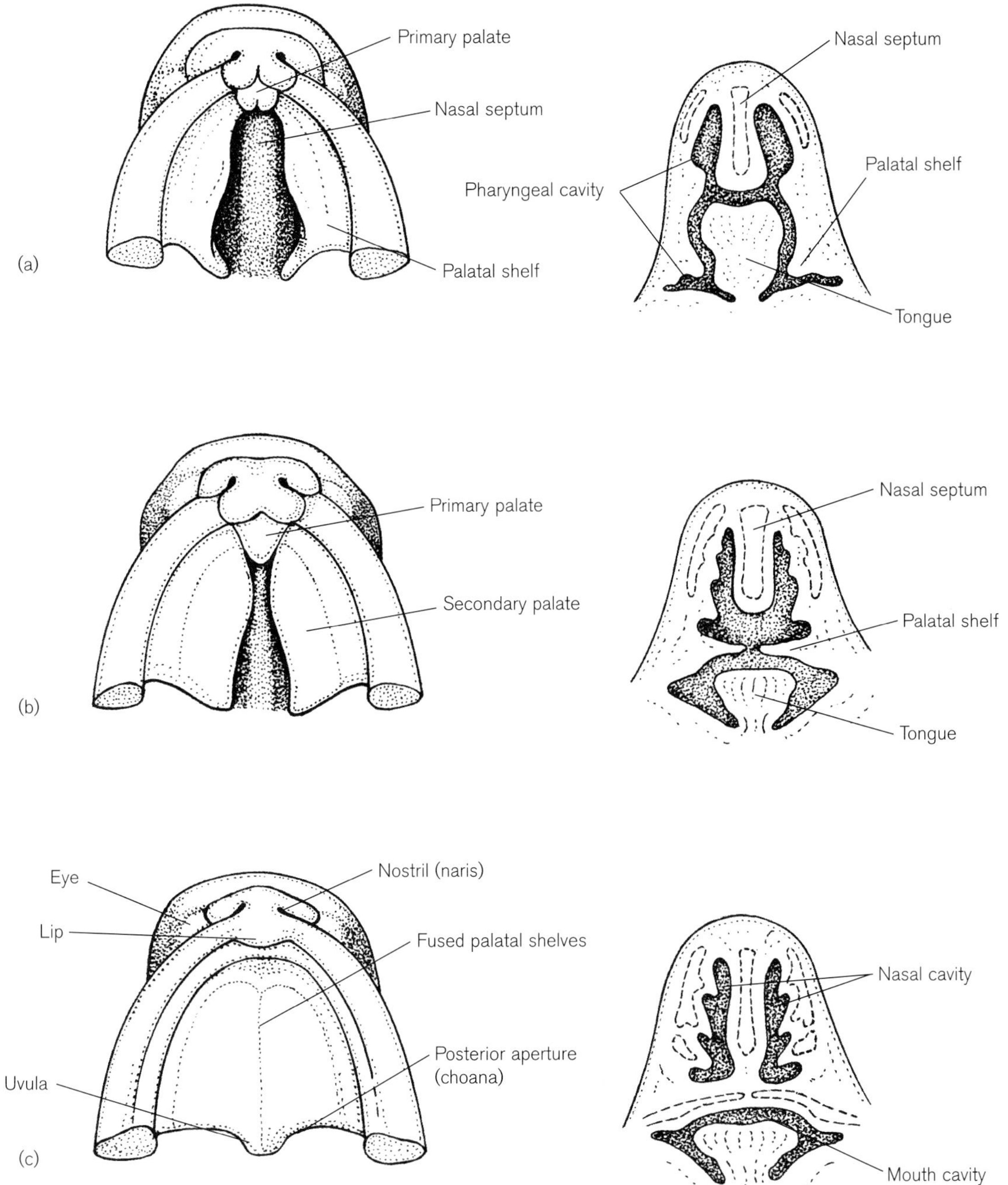

Figure 5.10 Formation of the palate: (a) 7 weeks; (b) 8 weeks; (c) 10 weeks. Left row – looking into roof of the mouth; right row – coronal sections through nose and mouth.

cavity. The nasal and lacrimal bones start to ossify slightly later in the fetal period. Details are given under development of individual bones.

The growth of the vault and eyes in their contained orbits follow the rapid pattern of neural growth, while the rest of the facial complex is primarily related to the development of the dentition and muscles of mastication. This results in a skull in the fetus, infant and young child that is very different in proportions from that seen later in adolescence and adult life, hence the large head and eyes and relatively small face of infants and young children (Figs. 5.11–5.14). At birth, the face is 55–60% of the breadth, 40–45% of the height and 30–35% of the depth of the adult value (Krogman, 1951). Calvarial to facial proportions are about 8:1 at birth, 4:1 at 5 years and about 2.5:1 in adult life (Sperber, 1989).

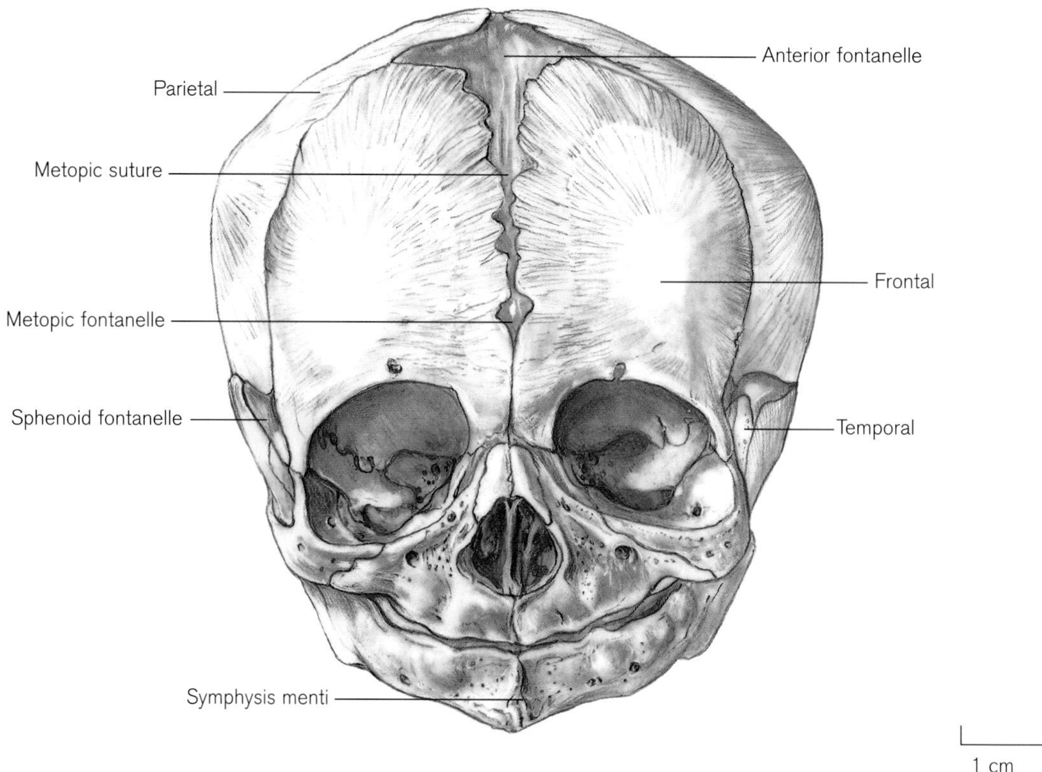

Figure 5.11 Anterior view of fetal skull and mandible.

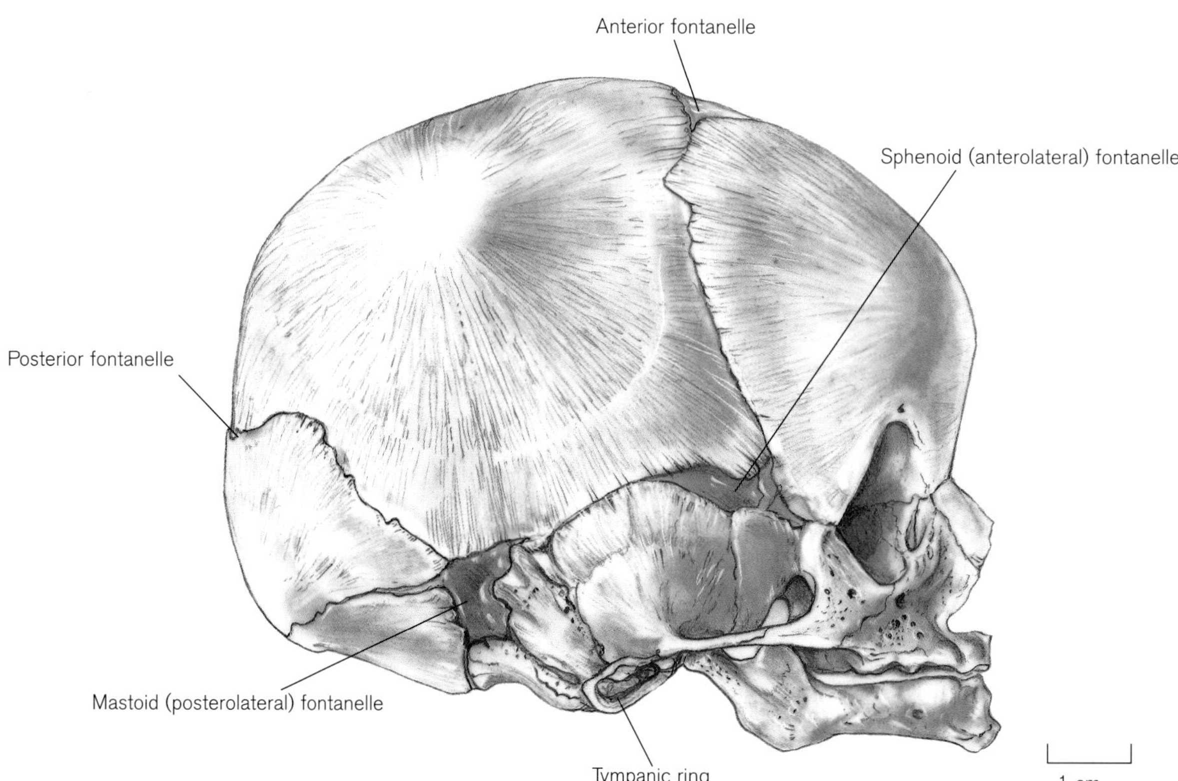

Figure 5.12 Lateral view of fetal skull and mandible.

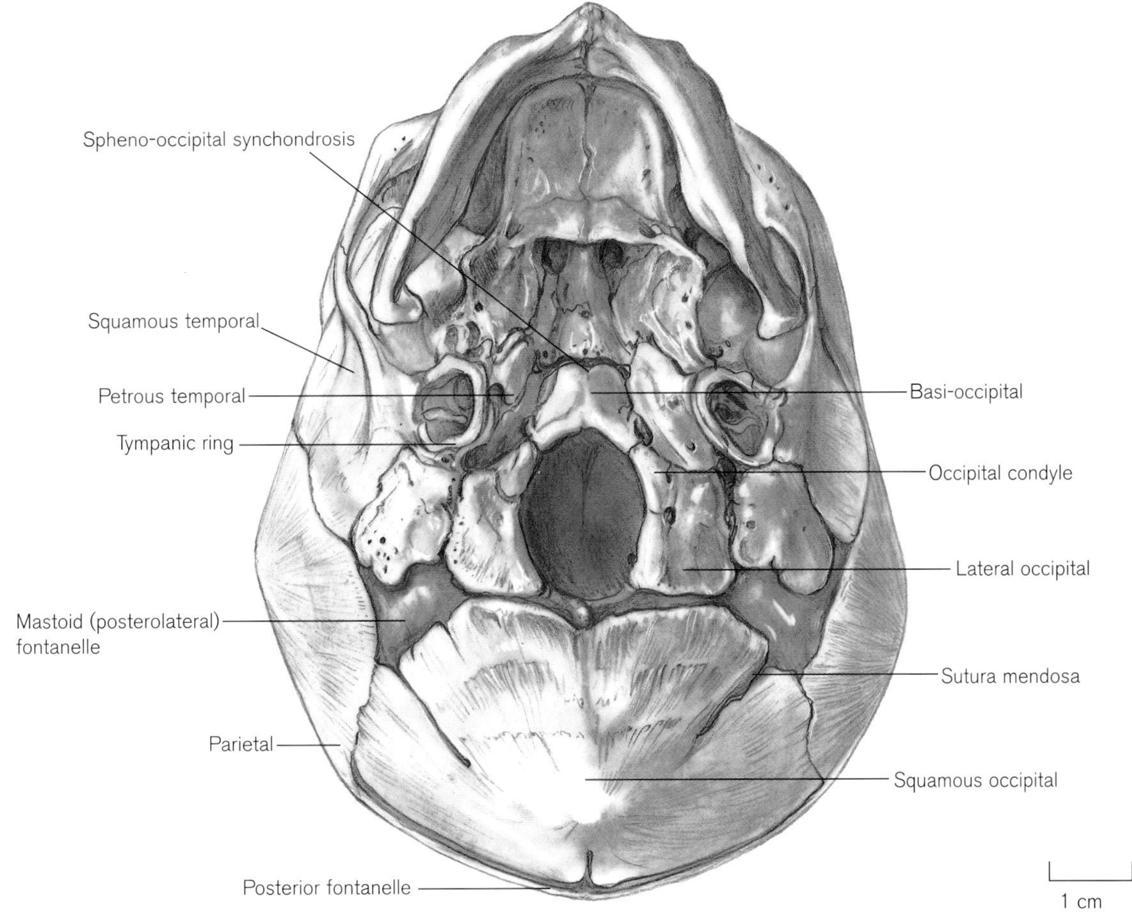

Figure 5.13 Basal view of fetal skull and mandible.

The **pharyngeal arches** are transitory structures, which form in the lateral walls and floor of the pharynx of all mammalian embryos. In mammals, they develop into a variety of structures in the head and neck, in contrast to aquatic forms, where the pharyngeal wall is perforated to form gill slits (for discussion, see O'Rahilly and Tucker, 1973). In the human embryo they develop in a craniocaudal sequence between 22 and 29 days. The first three are fairly prominent but the rest of the series, especially the fifth, are rudimentary and short-lived. It appears from experimental evidence in avian models that the mesoderm giving rise to the skeletal elements in the first three arches is of neural crest origin, while that in the fourth and sixth arches is derived from the lateral plate (Noden, 1988). Some of the structures that arise from the branchial arches develop in cartilage, which subsequently ossifies and others are formed directly in mesenchyme.

During the embryonic period (Fig. 5.8) Meckel's cartilages are represented by elongated cartilaginous rods, which extend inferiorly from the otic capsules to converge at an angle in the floor of the mouth. The upper end of each rod, forms the malleus and incus, which at this stage are still attached to the cartilage, but which later become separated by mesenchyme. On the lateral side of Meckel's cartilage the mandible is well ossified in membrane. The second arch cartilage is represented by the stapes and the styloid process of the temporal bone. At this stage, the stapes is disc-shaped, with a small central foramen. The styloid process is attached to the otic capsule above and projects downward from the base of the skull. Derivatives of subsequent branchial arches are represented by the cartilaginous anlagen of the hyoid bone and laryngeal cartilages, which lie below Meckel's cartilage.

There is a vast literature on the growth and development of the skull as a whole that lies beyond the scope of this text. Much of it is in dental and orthodontic papers, and further information, including details of the main planes and osteometric landmarks used in radiological cephalometric analysis, can be found in other texts (Knussmann, 1988; Sperber, 1989; Enlow and Hans, 1996).

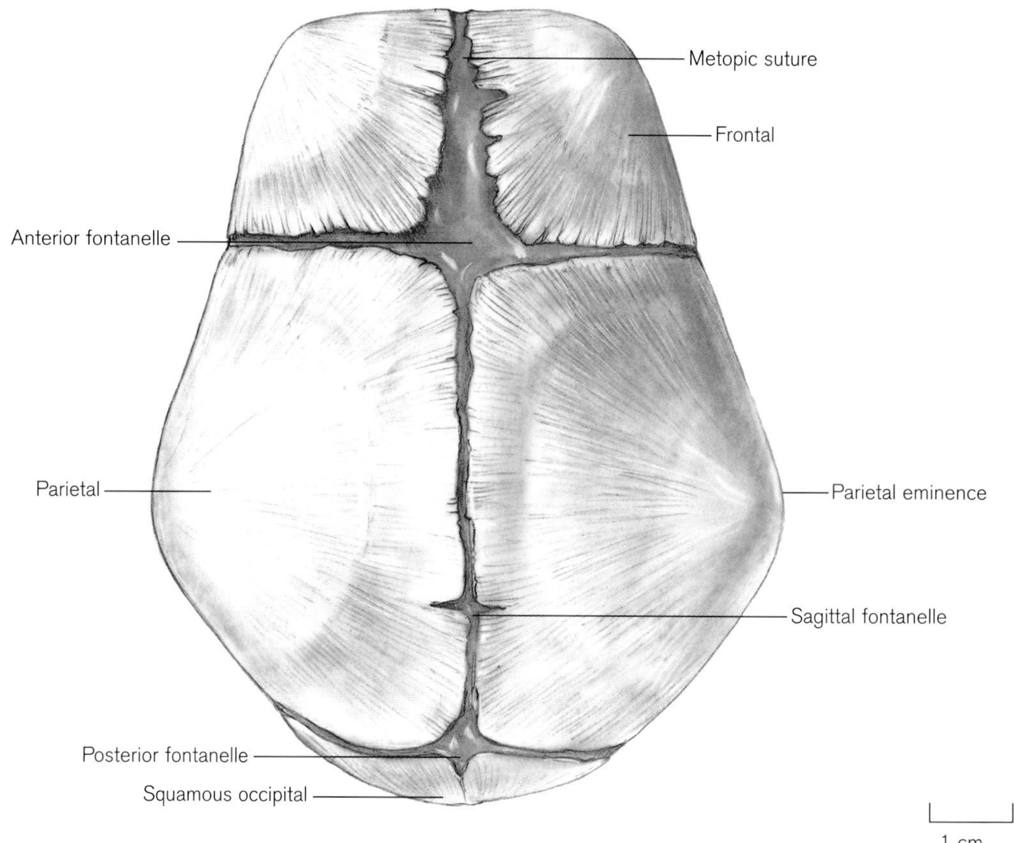

Figure 5.14 Superior view of fetal skull.

I. THE OCCIPITAL

The adult occipital

The adult occipital[1] forms part of the base of the skull and the posterior wall of the cranial cavity. It articulates with the parietals superolaterally, the petromastoid parts of the temporals inferiorly and laterally and the sphenoid anteriorly (Figs. 5.1–5.4). The bone consists of four parts: the squamous (tabular) part, two lateral parts and a basal part arranged around the foramen magnum.

The **squamous part** of the occipital is a diamond-shaped tabular bone, which is convex externally. The lower part of the bone faces inferiorly towards the neck and forms, in its central part, the posterior margin of the foramen magnum to which the posterior atlanto-occipital membrane is attached. On either side, the bone is fused with the lateral (ex-) occipitals and more posteriorly articulates at thick, smooth sutures with the petrous and mastoid parts of the temporal bones (Figs. 5.1–5.3). The upper part of the bone faces posteriorly and extends upwards from the lateral angles between the parietal bones with which it articulates at the deeply serrated lambdoid suture (Figs. 5.3 and 5.4). This is the most common site to find Inca (epactal) bones and accessory ossicles, so-called Wormian[2] bones (see below).

From the **external** protuberance, just below the centre of the bone, two lines curve laterally on either side (Fig. 5.15a). The upper ones, or highest nuchal lines, are faint and provide attachment for the galea[3] aponeurotica of the occipitofrontalis muscle, the posterior belly of which lies on the smooth surface of the bone above them. The lower lines are the superior

[1] *Occipio* (Latin meaning I 'begin'). Possibly derived from the fact that the back of the head is the first part of the baby to appear in a normal delivery.

[2] Ole Worm (1588–1654) was Professor of Greek, Philosophy and Anatomy at Copenhagen University.

[3] *Galea* (Latin meaning 'helmet') made of leather. May come from *galèe* (Greek meaning 'cat') as cat skins were used as head coverings. The term '*Galea aponeurotica*' was first used by Santorini (1681–1737), Professor of Anatomy and Medicine in Venice in about 1700.

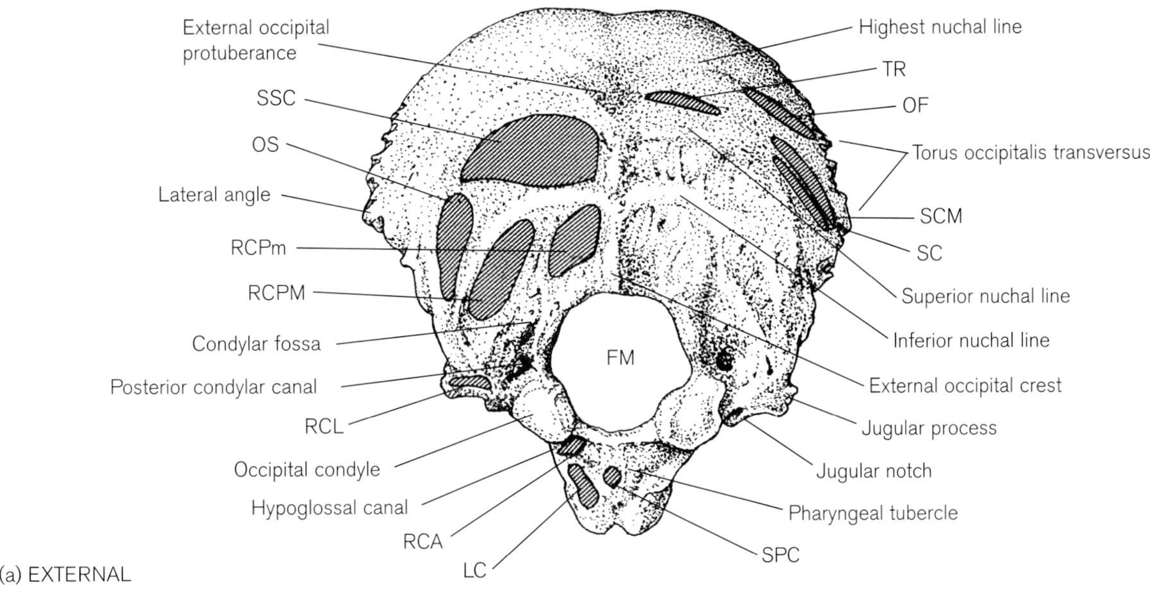

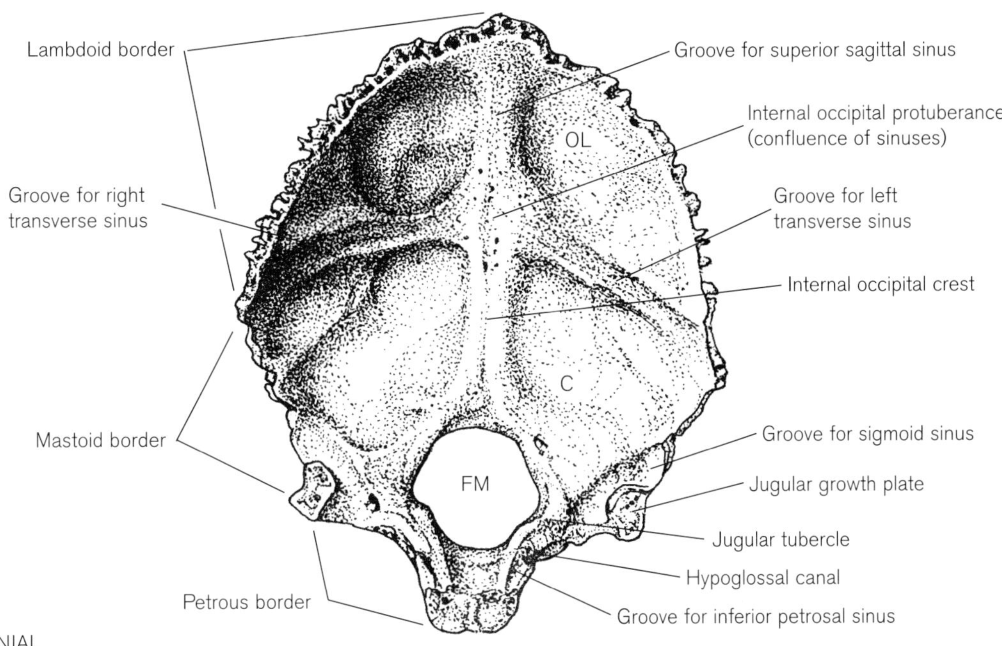

Figure 5.15 Adult occipital.

OF	Occipitofrontalis	RCPm	Rectus capitis posterior minor
TR	Trapezius	RCPM	Rectus capitis posterior major
SCM	Sternocleidomastoid	RCL	Rectus capitis lateralis
SC	Splenius capitis	RCA	Rectus capitis anterior
SSC	Semispinalis capitis	LC	Longus capitis
OS	Obliquus superior	OL	Occipital lobe of cerebral hemisphere
FM	Foramen magnum	C	Cerebellar hemisphere
SPC	Superior pharyngeal constrictor		

nuchal lines, which are roughened for the attachment of trapezius medially and sternocleidomastoid and splenius capitis laterally. About halfway from the external occipital protuberance to the foramen magnum, the inferior nuchal lines radiate laterally. On either side, between the superior and inferior lines lie the attachments of semispinalis capitis and obliquus superior muscles, while the rectus capitis posterior major and minor muscles are attached below the inferior line. The rectus capitis posterior major muscle is attached to the area of the bone that was originally part of the lateral occipital but, in the adult skull, no visible suture line remains. These muscles have both a postural role and rotate and extend the head on the neck. In the median plane, the external occipital crest runs down to the foramen magnum and provides attachment for the ligamentum nuchae.

The **intracranial surface** of the squama is concave and divided into four depressions (Fig. 5.15b). The sulcus for the superior sagittal sinus runs upwards in a groove from the internal occipital protuberance. A sharp ridge, the internal occipital crest, to which the falx cerebelli is attached, passes downward from the protuberance to the foramen magnum. Often there are well-developed occipital sinuses in the lower part of the posterior fossa, but their morphology can be very variable. Das and Hasan (1970) found that they are clearly marked in about 60% of skulls and they classified and illustrated five different types. They may be single or double in the midline, or continue round the posterior margin of the foramen magnum. They always appear to communicate with either the superior sagittal sinus or the confluence of sinuses. Running horizontally are grooves for the right and left transverse sinuses. Above, the bone has two triangular, ridged hollows to accommodate the gyri of the occipital lobes of the cerebral hemispheres. Below, there are two smooth quadrangular hollows to which the cerebellar hemispheres are related. The internal occipital protuberance is the site of the confluence of venous sinuses (torcular Herophili), which has a variable pattern (Woodhall, 1936, 1939; Hayner, 1949; Browning, 1953). The most common arrangement is dominance of the right transverse sinus, but there are other patterns. Frequently, the sinuses are unequal in size or, in rare cases, absent (Waltner, 1944). Woodhall (1936) found a close correlation between the arrangement of sinuses and their radiological appearance but Hayner (1949) and Browning (1953) reported that markings on the bone did not provide adequate data from which the pattern of sinuses could be deduced.

In the normal occipital bone there is either an occasional small foramen (the inio-endinial canal) in the region of the protuberance that transmits an occipital emissary vein that joins the confluence of sinuses with the occipital veins, or an internal or external vascular orifice (O'Rahilly, 1952).

The two **lateral (condylar) parts** of the occipital bone lie on either side of the foramen magnum and bear the occipital condyles on their inferior surfaces. The articular surfaces are convex both anteroposteriorly and transversely, with their long axes running anteromedially. They may be oval, kidney-shaped or have surfaces bisected by a strip of non-articular cartilage. They are not always symmetrical. Usually, the facets of the atlas vertebra, with which they articulate, show the same reciprocal division as the occipital articular surfaces (Singh, 1965; Reinhard and Rösing, 1985). This can be useful when faced with commingled remains and may enable a skull to be matched with an atlas, and thus sometimes the rest of the vertebral column. On the medial side of each condyle is a small tubercle to which is attached the alar ligament of the dens of the axis. Directly behind each condyle is a condylar fossa, which accommodates the posterior margin of the atlas when the head is fully extended. A posterior condylar canal is often found in the fossa and, when present, transmits a sigmoid emissary vein (Reinhard and Rösing, 1985). Above and lateral to each condyle is the hypoglossal (anterior condylar) canal, through which passes the XIIth (hypoglossal) cranial nerve and a meningeal branch of the ascending pharyngeal artery. The canal is often partially or fully divided and this may be present from an early fetal age (Lillie, 1917; Dodo, 1980; Hauser and De Stefano, 1985; Reinhard and Rösing, 1985). The canal's detailed normal and abnormal radiological anatomy has been studied by Kirdani (1967) and Valvassori and Kirdani (1967) and Berlis *et al.* (1992) have made direct and CT measurements. The intracranial side of the hypoglossal canal is raised to form the jugular tubercle, behind which is a groove accommodating the IXth (glossopharyngeal), Xth (vagus) and XIth (accessory) cranial nerves as they pass towards the jugular foramen.

A quadrangular area of bone, the jugular process, extends from the posterior half of each condyle and articulates laterally with the jugular surface of the mastoid part of the temporal bone (Fig. 5.1). The posterior part of this articulation is a normal cranial suture, but anteriorly there is a small triangular or quadrilateral area, the cartilaginous jugular growth plate, which may persist until early in the fourth decade (see below). The inferior surface is roughened for the attachment of the rectus capitis lateralis muscle. The intracranial surface of this area is curved to form a hook-like process that overhangs a deep groove containing the terminal part of the sigmoid venous sinus. Posteriorly, the jugular process merges with the squamous part of the occipital. The anterior border of the process forms the curved jugular notch which, with the petrous temporal bone, completes the jugular foramen. The anteromedial part of this (pars nervosa) transmits the inferior petrosal sinus and glossopharyngeal, vagus and accessory cranial nerves, while the posterolateral part (pars vascularis) accommodates the superior bulb of the internal jugular vein. The posterior condylar canal opens here. This important cranial venous drainage area was examined in a large series of adult skulls by Solter and Paljan (1973). They noted that the shape and dimensions varied widely, that the depth of the jugular fossa increases with age and that many dehiscences occur. These increase with age and may communicate with either the hypoglossal canal or with the middle or internal parts of the ear. Doubt has been cast by Glassman and Bass (1986) and Glassman and Dana (1992) on suggestions that the bilateral size asymmetry of the foramen could be related to handedness. In a significant proportion of skulls the jugular foramen is divided by an intrajugular process of bone from either (or both) the occipital or temporal sides (Toldt, 1919; Frazer, 1948; Ferner and Staubesand, 1983). A study of the incidence of this trait in both fetal and adult Japanese skulls and in adult skulls from nine other populations was reported by Dodo (1986a, b). Sawyer and Kiely (1987) and Sawyer *et al.* (1990) also studied bridging in East Asian and pre-Columbian Chilean populations. Correlations of the appearance in dried skulls and radiographs are reported by Di Chiro *et al.* (1964) and Shapiro (1972a).

The **basilar part** of the occipital bone forms part of the posterior region of the base of the skull and is a thick quadrilateral plate of bone which, in the adult, is fused anteriorly with the body of the sphenoid bone (Figs. 5.1 and 5.2). Posteriorly, it forms the curved anterior boundary of the foramen magnum to which is attached the anterior atlanto-occipital membrane and the apical ligament of the dens of the axis. Internal to this, the membrana tectoria passes to its attachment on the upper surface of the bone. Laterally, the basilar part of the bone articulates on either side with the petromastoid parts of the temporal bones (Figs. 5.1 and 5.2). The inferior surface is roughened for the attachment of the longus capitis and rectus capitis anterior muscles and in its centre it bears a small elevation, the pharyngeal tubercle, to which is attached the raphé of the superior pharyngeal constrictor. Immediately anterior to the tubercle there may be a depression, the fossa pharyngea (fovea bursa/mediobasal bursa), the incidence of which varies in different populations. Its anatomical significance is obscure (Collins, 1928). Together with the sphenoid bone, the intracranial surface forms the smooth, curved clivus[4] that supports the medulla oblongata and lower pons of the brainstem. On either side lie the grooves for the inferior petrosal venous sinuses.

The lambdoid suture is often the site for anomalous bones, commonly small accessory ossicles (Wormian bones) and less commonly, so-called Inca bones, which are larger. Descriptions and illustrations can be found in Hepburn (1907), Misra (1960), Kolte and Mysorekar (1966), Shapiro and Robinson (1976a), Srivastava (1977), Singh *et al.* (1979), Pal *et al.* (1984), Reinhard and Rösing (1985), Saxena *et al.* (1986), Pal (1987) and Gopinathan (1992). They have been regarded either as normal variants or as non-metric traits (Berry and Berry, 1967; Ossenberg, 1976; Saunders, 1989) and there appears to be no agreement on their aetiology. Bennett (1965) found that there was a positive correlation between their occurrence and the length of the basi-occiput in three different populations and concluded that their formation was not under direct genetic control, but represented secondary sutural characteristics, which are brought about by stress. The fact that Wormian bones are very common in hydrocephalic skulls, where normal ossification is thought to be prevented by liquid pressure, appeared to add weight to this view. Also, Ossenberg (1970) found that there was an increased frequency of posterior Wormian bones in skulls that had been deformed by the pressure of cradle-boards and bandages. However, El-Najjar and Dawson (1977) concluded that there is a genetic predisposition for these to form and they were not the result of deformation. Gottlieb (1978) reported that in deformed skulls there was an increase in sutural complexity in the upper part of the lambdoid suture and, if Wormian bones were present, then there was an increase in their numbers compared to normal skulls. Anomalous foramina are relatively rare, and when present, are usually associated with either meningo-encephalocoeles or dermoid cysts. They rarely occur above the occipital protuberance, sometimes at the protuberance, but more commonly between the protuberance and the foramen magnum. The defect may extend to become continuous with the foramen magnum and/or below as cervical spina bifida (O'Rahilly, 1952). Occasionally there is a small midline foramen in the centre of the basi-occiput, anterior to the pharyngeal tubercle. It leads to a canal, the canalis basilaris chordae (Huber, 1912; Schultz, 1918a), which exits intracranially in front of the foramen magnum. It normally closes during the third lunar month and is thought to be the remains of the path taken during fetal life by the notochord (chorda dorsalis) as

[4] *Clivus* (Latin meaning 'slope, gradient') – the name given to the road in Rome that led from the forum up the Capitoline Hill.

it emerges from the developing vertebral column to enter the cranial base (see also Chapter 5 – Introduction). Remnants of fetal notochordal tissue can give rise to a chordoma, a slow growing neoplasm (Salisbury and Isaacson, 1985; see also Chapter 6).

A variety of anomalies occur around the foramen magnum as the occipitovertebral border is an embryologically unstable area (see also Chapter 6). Barnes (1994) has reviewed these in some detail and divides them into two groups according to whether there has been a cranial or caudal shift at the occipitocervical junction. Cranial shifting is said to produce a precondylar tubercle or process at the anterior border of the foramen magnum (Marshall, 1955; Broman, 1957; Lombardi, 1961; Reinhard and Rösing, 1985; Lakhtakia *et al.*, 1991; Vasudeva and Choudhry, 1996), transverse basilar clefts (Limson, 1932; Kruyff, 1967; Johnson and Israel, 1979; Lang, 1995), bipartite condylar facets (Singh, 1965; Tillmann and Lorenz, 1978) and divided hypoglossal canals (Lillie, 1917; Dodo, 1980; Hauser and De Stefano, 1985). Caudal shifting may include occipitalization of the atlas (Shapiro and Robinson, 1976b; Black and Scheuer, 1996a), basilar impression/platybasia (Peyton and Peterson, 1942; Hadley, 1948) and the presence of paracondylar and epitransverse processes (Lombardi, 1961; Shapiro and Robinson, 1976b; Anderson, 1996). The biometry and sexual dimorphism of the bone have been investigated by Olivier (1975) and Routal *et al.* (1984).

Ossification

Ossification of the occipital arises from a number of centres that join during fetal life to form the four principal components of the bone (Fig. 5.16). The **squama occipitalis** (pars squama/tabular part) is subdivided into a **pars interparietalis** and a **pars supra-occipitalis**, which fuse in the central part of the **sutura mendosa** during fetal life. The interparietal part, which alone merits the name of squama, forms the posterior wall of the cranial cavity and extends upwards between the two parietal bones from the highest nuchal line into the triangular space at the lambdoid suture. The supra-occipital part forms the most posterior part of the skull base, defines the centre of the posterior border of the foramen magnum and articulates anteriorly with the lateral occipitals at the **sutura intra-occipitalis posterior**. The two **partes laterales/condylares** (lateral/ex-occipitals) form the lateral boundaries of the foramen magnum and articulate anteriorly with the **pars basilaris** (basi-occipital) at the **sutura intra-occipitalis anterior**. The basilar part forms the anterior margin of the foramen magnum and articulates anteriorly with the sphenoid at the **spheno-occipital synchondrosis**. All four main parts of the bone articulate with the temporal bone.

Ossification in the **squamous** part of the occipital bone is visible between 8 and 10 weeks of intra-uterine life (Noback, 1944; Noback and Robertson, 1951). Ossification centres can be seen by alizarin staining or by examination of histological sections before they are visible radiographically (O'Rahilly and Gardner, 1972). At stage 23 (eighth week) two small areas of bone representing the supra-occipital and interparietal portions can be seen: a small area of periosteal bone in the tectum posterior on the outer aspect of the chondrocranium and above it, on each side of the median plane, an intramembranous centre (O'Rahilly and Gardner, 1972; Müller and O'Rahilly, 1980). In studies of the developing fetal cranium by Kjær and colleagues, the sequence of appearance of the ossification centres was shown to be very consistent (Bach-Petersen and Kjær, 1993; Kjær *et al.*, 1993).

Most of the supra-occipital part is preformed in cartilage and ossification starts at the end of the embryonic period proper from either a single centre (Macklin, 1921; Noback, 1944) or a pair of centres (Mall, 1906; Müller and O'Rahilly, 1980), which rapidly fuse to form a solid plate of bone at the posterior border of the skull (Frazer, 1948; Fazekas and Kósa, 1978; Matsumura *et al.*, 1993, 1994). The interparietal part ossifies from several intramembranous centres. The detailed observations of Srivastava (1992) and Matsumura *et al.* (1993) agree fundamentally but, unfortunately, different terms have been used for the same parts of the developing bone. Early in the ninth week a small pair of centres appear in the membrane above the ossifying supra-occipital. These fuse with each other and then join with the supra-occipitals to form that part of the adult bone which lies between the superior and highest nuchal lines and is called the **torus occipitalis transversus** (Fig. 5.15a). This small, membranously formed area is called the 'intermediate segment' by Srivastava (1992) and the 'primary interparietal' by Matsumura *et al.* (1993). Srivastava considers that this part, and the endochondrally ossified part to which it fuses, constitute the supra-occipital. However, further studies by Matsumura *et al.* (1994) indicate that this division of bone forming either endochondrally or intramembranously is an over-simplification. They observed that the supra-occipital part is indeed originally formed from cartilage and the part that forms immediately superior to it appears in membrane. However, the first formed supra-occipital bone becomes covered on both the internal and external surfaces with fine periosteal

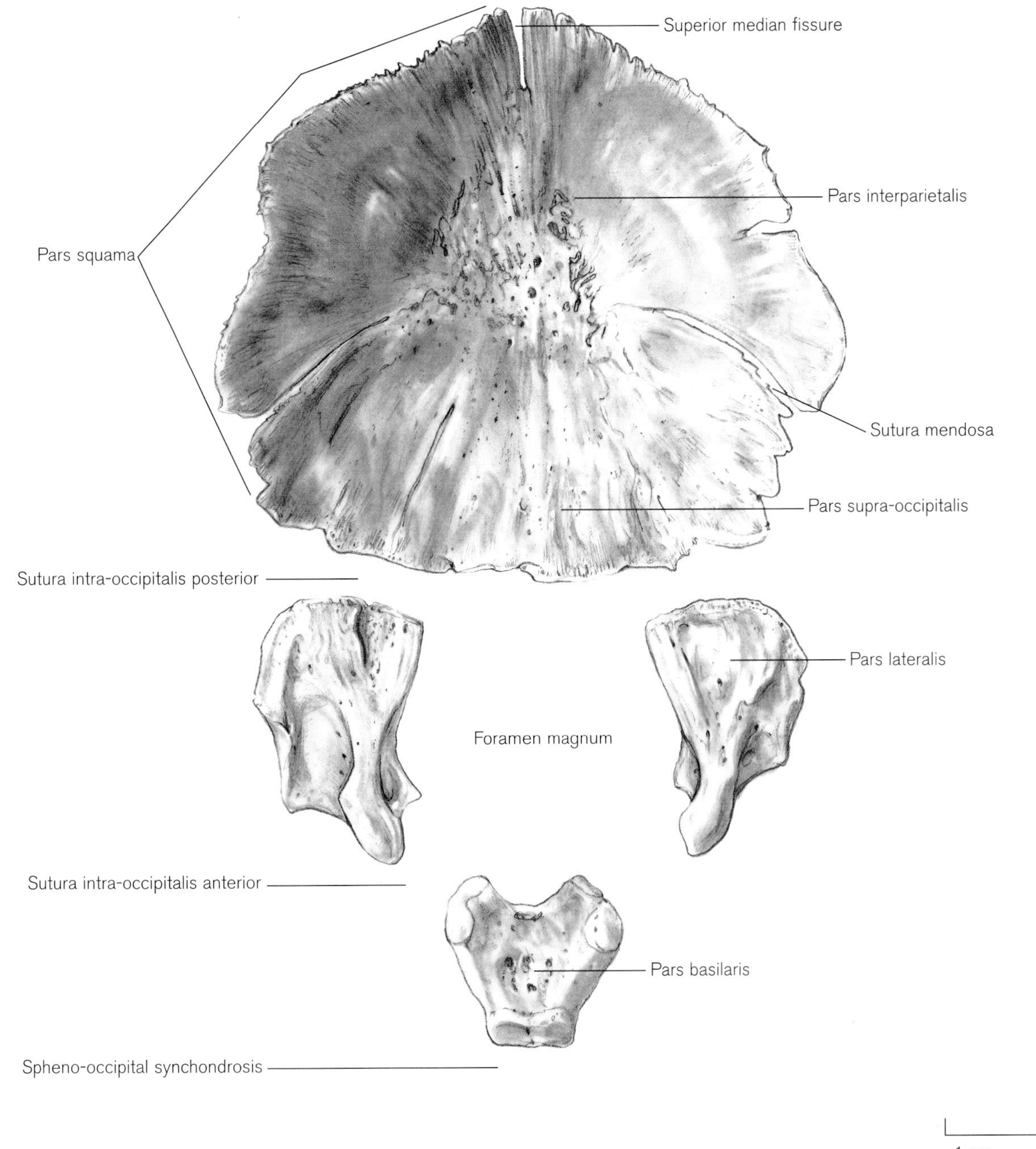

Figure 5.16 Intracranial view of the perinatal occipital.

cancellous bone, which appears to spread from the membrane-formed bone above (a similar process occurring in the maxilla). From the fifth fetal month, the supra-occipital bone is a three-layered structure consisting of a solid core of rough, spongy bone between two layers of trabecular meshwork. These appearances were originally described by Zawisch (1957) and have also been confirmed by Niida *et al.* (1992).

The true **interparietal** part of the bone, above the highest nuchal line, is formed from a variable number of ossification centres, which develop in the membrane above the supra-occipital during the third and fourth intra-uterine months. Srivastava (1992) describes a lateral plate on either side, each formed from medial and lateral centres and, above this, two medial plates composed of superior and inferior centres. Matsumura *et al.* (1993) call the medial and lateral plates 'secondary interparietals' and observed that the medial centres always appeared before the lateral ones. The use of the terms primary and secondary interparietal centres is misleading as both are in truth primary ossification centres. There is much variation in the pattern of fusion of these centres, causing this part of the skull to be subject to numerous anomalies (see above). However, as most of the descriptions are of adult specimens, it is not possible to deduce their true embryological origins.

Rambaud and Renault (1864), Augier (1931) and O'Rahilly and Meyer (1956) describe an inconstant 'pre-interparietal' centre and Matsumura *et al.* (1993) describe fetal skulls with occasional further ossification centres, which they also call pre-interparietals, which appear anterior to the main part of the interparietal bone. They view them as a group of separated bones that form in the triangular territory of the central lambdoid region, whose bases are situated higher than the highest nuchal line and distinct anatomically from the small sutural bones that sometimes form in this location. Srivastava (1992) considers that the term 'pre-interparietal' is a misnomer to be avoided and maintains that all the bones developing in the region of the lambdoid suture are sutural or Wormian bones with their own separate ossification centres.

Between 3.5 and 5 lunar months, the supra-occipital and interparietal parts of the bone start to fuse together in the middle of the bone, but there is sometimes a small aperture in the centre between the two parts (the inio-endinial canal) to accommodate a vascular channel between the occipital veins and the confluence of sinuses (O'Rahilly, 1952; O'Rahilly and Meyer, 1956). Fusion is incomplete laterally and this is called the lateral 'fissure' by Srivastava (1992) and the lateral 'incisure' by Niida *et al.* (1992), but is much more commonly known as the **sutura mendosa**. Niida *et al.* considered that lateral fusion is prevented by the existence of the **tectum synoticum posterior**, one of the three roof elements of the chondrocranium existing in the territory of the interparietal from about 10–16 fetal weeks (Fawcett, 1923; Jarvik, 1980), which interferes with the extension of the bone trabeculae in this area. It also represents the future site of the posterolateral fontanelle.

Noback (1944) and Moss *et al.* (1956) reported that the cartilaginous part of the squama has a different growth rate from the interparietal part. The latter, together with the other bones of the vault, has a rapid growth rate up to 12–13 fetal weeks, which is related to the early precocious growth of the cerebral hemispheres. The supra-occipital part is related to the different growth rate of the cerebellar hemispheres, which start to enlarge at about the end of the third lunar month. Confirming this, Fazekas and Kósa (1978) reported that from the fifth to the tenth lunar months the maximum width of the squama is in the interparietal part above the sutura mendosa, but by the perinatal period the longitudinal and transverse measurements are very similar. These proportions have also been confirmed in Japanese fetuses by Ohtsuki (1977), who measured the thickness of the occipital squama from 4 fetal months until birth.

By the perinatal period the pars squama has adopted a shallow, bowl-shaped appearance, which is composed of an inferior, thicker supra-occipital portion set at an angle to the thinner, fan-shaped interparietal part (Fig. 5.16). At the junction is the prominent external occipital protuberance on the convex (external) surface in the median plane. There is usually a median fissure of variable length at the superior angle of the interparietal part, which is continuous with the posterior fontanelle (Figs. 5.13 and 5.14). From here, the bone slopes down to the sutura mendosa, which may extend up to half way across the bone medially and is continuous laterally with the mastoid (posterolateral) fontanelle (Figs. 5.12 and 5.13). In the early fetal and perinatal stages the interparietal part is extremely thin with fragile, feathery borders. Later, these thicken and become finely serrated. The lateral borders of the supra-occipital are also serrated and become continuous with the inferior border, which is thickened on either side of the midline, where it will eventually fuse with the lateral occipitals.

There is an occasional midline ossicle or process in the posterior margin of the foramen magnum (Fig. 5.17). This structure was recognized by early anatomists and was originally described by Kerckring (1717) and illustrated by Albinus (1737). Kerckring observed that it appeared in the fourth or fifth fetal month and fused with the supra-occipital before birth. Sometimes, instead of a separate ossicle, this is represented by a projecting tongue of bone, called the manubrium squamae occipitalis by Virchow or the opisthial process (O'Rahilly and Meyer, 1956) but is more commonly known as the process of Kerckring. It is described and illustrated by Schultz (1917), Toldt (1919), Limson (1932), Redfield (1970) and Shapiro and Robinson (1976c, 1980) amongst others. Caffey (1953) believed that it could still be visualized as late as the first few months of life if a Towne projection radiograph of the skull was taken. Matsumura *et al.* (1994) indicated that this ossicle is sometimes formed when the inner surface of the newly formed supra-occipital is covered with periosteal bone from above, but its aetiology remains uncertain.

Schultz (1917) and Caffey (1953) describe other ossicles that develop laterally in the cartilaginous plate

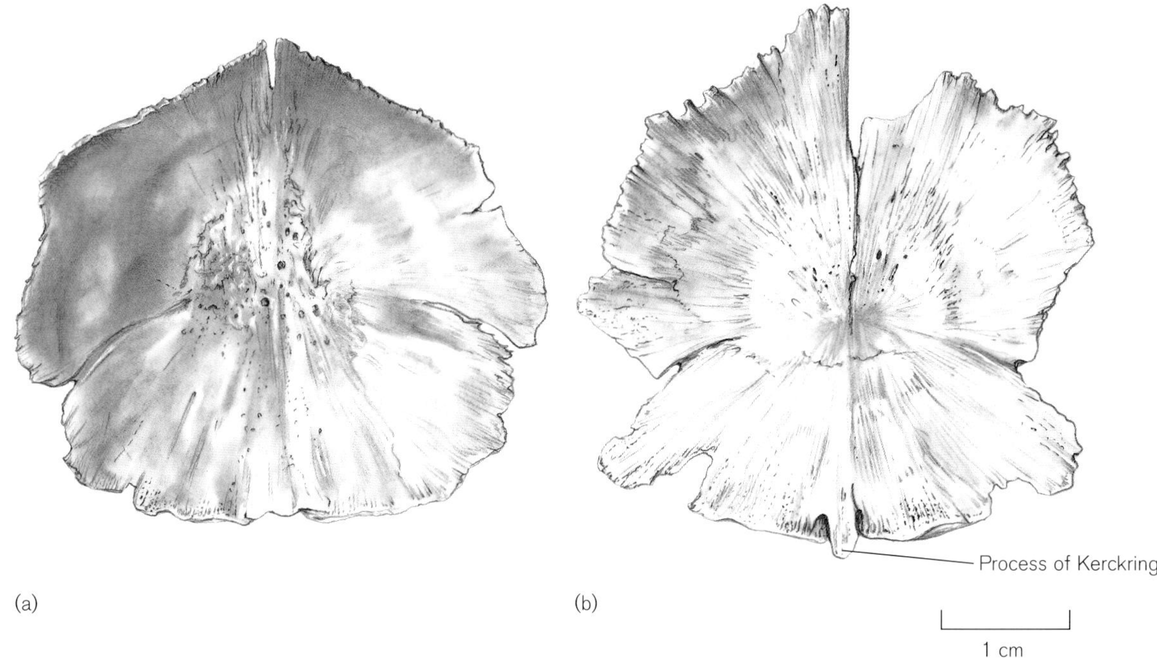

Figure 5.17 Perinatal pars squama. (a) Straight lower border, slightly thickened in the centre; (b) a damaged archaeological specimen with a process of Kerckring.

between the supra-occipital and the pars lateralis. They vary in number and size and fuse by the end of the first year with the lower edge of the supra-occipital, but never with the pars lateralis.

Vascular and neural markings begin to show on the intracranial surface of the bone in the perinatal period and details have been described by Vignaud-Pasquier *et al.* (1964). Radiographs of children's skulls normally show patchy areas of diminished density called digital impressions or convolutional rarefactions, which are most prominent in the posterior and lower lateral calvarial bones. Davidoff (1936) and Macauly (1951), scoring their appearance in different age groups, found that they rarely appeared before 18 months of age but then increased rapidly up to 4 years, reaching a plateau between 7 and 9 years. Although the aetiology is still unknown, they occur maximally during a period of very active growth of the brain and calvaria and are thought in some way to reflect the adaptation of the two tissues to one another. Contrary to previous suggestions, it is now considered unlikely that they are due to increased intracranial pressure (Du Boulay, 1956).

The centres for the **partes laterales** start to ossify endochondrally on either side of the foramen magnum between 8 and 9 fetal weeks. Noback (1944), Bach-Petersen and Kjær (1993) and Kjær *et al.* (1993) reported the onset of ossification as arising above the hypoglossal canal, but Zawisch (1957) described two perichondral centres for each bone, the posterior being the larger. Ossification spreads to form quadrilateral plates whose long axes run anteroposteriorly. During the early fetal period, two limbs, which will eventually enclose the hypoglossal nerve, begin to develop from the anteromedial corner of the bone. The posterior condylar canal is present from an early fetal stage, immediately posterior to the occipital condyle.

The neonatal pars lateralis (Fig. 5.18) has a thickened medial border, which forms the lateral boundary of the foramen magnum. It meets the wedge-shaped posterior border, which fuses postnatally with the supra-occipital, at a right angle. This ends laterally at a rounded angle, which at this stage is open to the mastoid (posterolateral) fontanelle. The lateral border articulates with the mastoid part of the temporal bone (Fig. 5.13). The anterolateral corner has a rounded profile and forms the occipital border of the jugular foramen. It may have one or more spicules of bone along its length, meeting reciprocal processes from the petrous temporal bone, which divide the foramen into one or more compartments (Dodo, 1986a). During the first year, the bone posterior to the foramen extends laterally to form the quadrangular jugular process.

At the anteromedial angle, the jugular (upper) and condylar (lower) limbs project from the bone. The upper limb bears the jugular tubercle on its intracranial surface, while the inferior surface of the lower

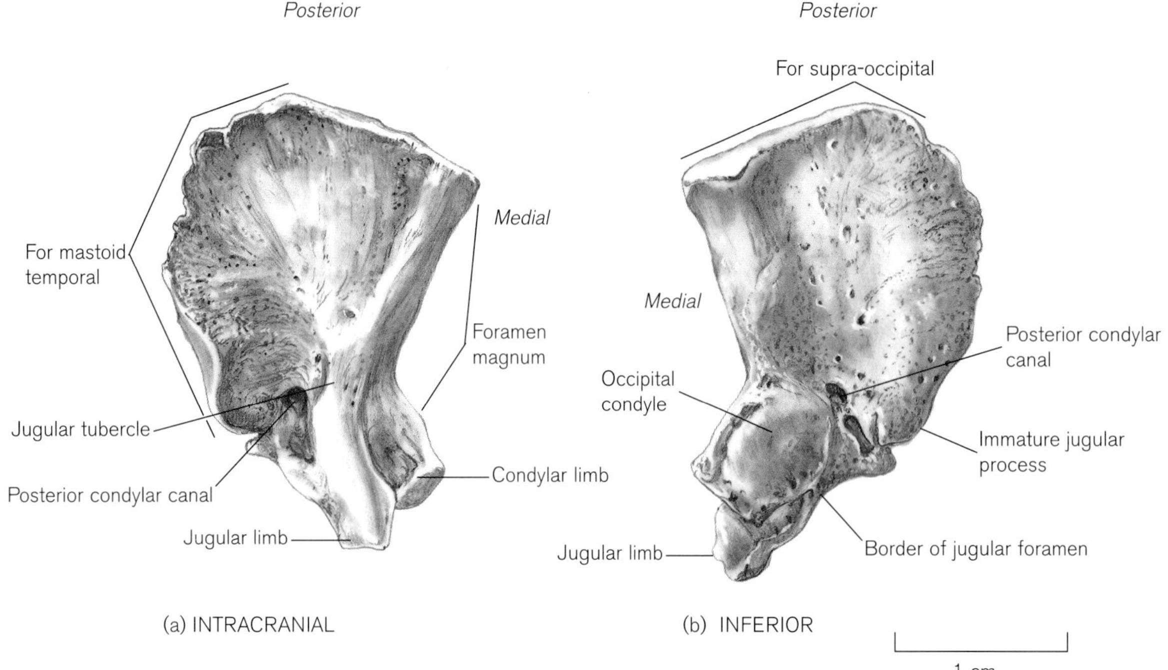

Figure 5.18 Right perinatal pars lateralis.

limb forms the posterior two-thirds of the occipital condyle. At first, the rounded ends of the two limbs articulate with reciprocal surfaces of the dual facet on the posterolateral border of the pars basilaris (see below), thus forming the hypoglossal canal. Between the ages of 1 and 3 years, the condylar limb develops a hooked extension which grows towards, and eventually fuses with the jugular limb, thus excluding the pars basilaris from the canal. The hypoglossal canal then lies entirely within the territory of the pars lateralis (Fig. 5.19).

The ossification centre for the **pars basilaris** appears in the basal plate anterior to the foramen magnum between the eleventh and twelfth weeks of fetal life (Macklin, 1921; Noback, 1944; Noback and Robertson, 1951; Fazekas and Kósa, 1978). Kjær (1990a, b), Kjær *et al.* (1993) and Kyrkanides *et al.* (1993) observed the centre in their radiographic series between 11 and 13 weeks. They divided the early development from 12 to 21 weeks into five maturity stages, which correlated closely with age, crown–rump length and the length of the humerus.

This part of the occipital bone becomes recognizable from an early fetal period and with advancing age, its characteristic features are intensified. At first, the bone is spindle-shaped, but around the beginning of the fourth month it becomes more triangular. The base, facing the foramen magnum is V-shaped, but during the next 2 weeks, it assumes a U-shaped curve and the basilar contributions to the occipital condyles become more obvious at the tips of the inferior surface. At the same time, the sides become parallel and the bone adopts a more quadrilateral shape. By the seventh fetal month, the lateral margins are angulat-

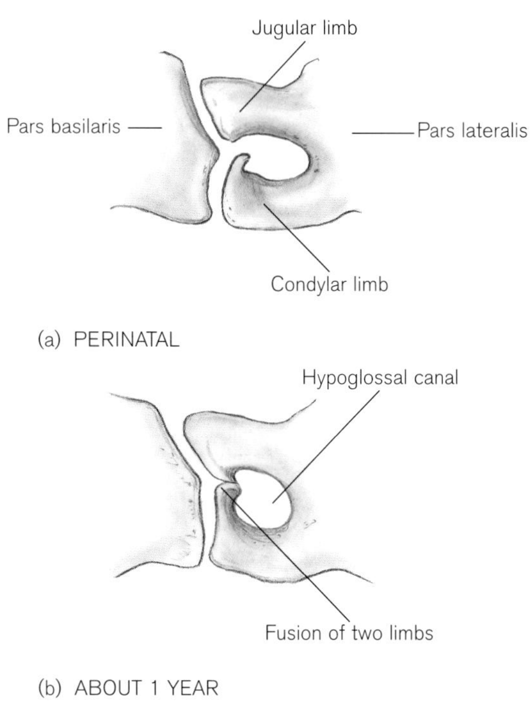

Figure 5.19 Formation of the hypoglossal canal.

ed outwards at about the midpoint and the bone becomes trapezoid in shape.

The perinatal pars basilaris is a robust bone (Fig. 5.20). The inferior surface is flattened and the intracranial surface is slightly concave from side to side and pitted with nutrient foramina. The anterior surface, which forms one side of the spheno-occipital synchondrosis, is D-shaped, with the straight edge on the intracranial surface. The posterior border, contributing to the foramen magnum, is thickened and forms a semi-lunar curve, each horn of which bears one-third of an occipital condyle inferiorly. This border reaches adult size at about the age of 2 years. The lateral border is divided into two parts. Anterior to the angle, it articulates with the petrous temporal bone, while posteriorly, there are two distinct facets that articulate with the jugular and condylar limbs of the pars lateralis (see above). The pharyngeal tubercle on the inferior surface cannot usually be identified until the second or third year of life.

The changing proportions throughout the development of the pars basilaris and the fact that it tends to survive inhumation intact have been used as a means of ageing immature skeletons. However, the exact osteological landmarks used for taking measurements are not always clearly defined. Redfield (1970), in a useful and carefully observed study, included both the pars basilaris and the partes laterales to identify seven developmental stages as an aid to ageing and described, but did not illustrate, the measurements. Fazekas and Kósa (1978) reported dimensions of all parts of the bone and illustrated measurements with photographs. However, the landmarks on both the pars basilaris and lateralis are not the same as those of Redfield (Fig. 5.21). The differences in the measurements are described and evaluated by Scheuer and MacLaughlin-Black (1994). In essence, if only the pars basilaris is available, the sagittal length is greater than the width in individuals less than 28 fetal weeks. If the maximum length is less than the width, then the

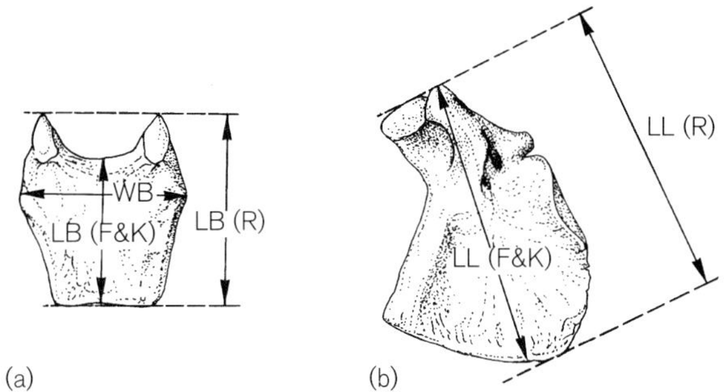

Figure 5.21 Measurements of the (a) pars basilaris and (b) pars lateralis.

LB (R)	Redfield's maximum length of pars basilaris
LB (F & K)	Fazekas & Kósa's mid-sagittal length of pars basilaris
WB	Width of pars basilaris
LL (R)	Redfield's length of pars lateralis
LL (F & K)	Fazekas & Kósa's length of pars lateralis

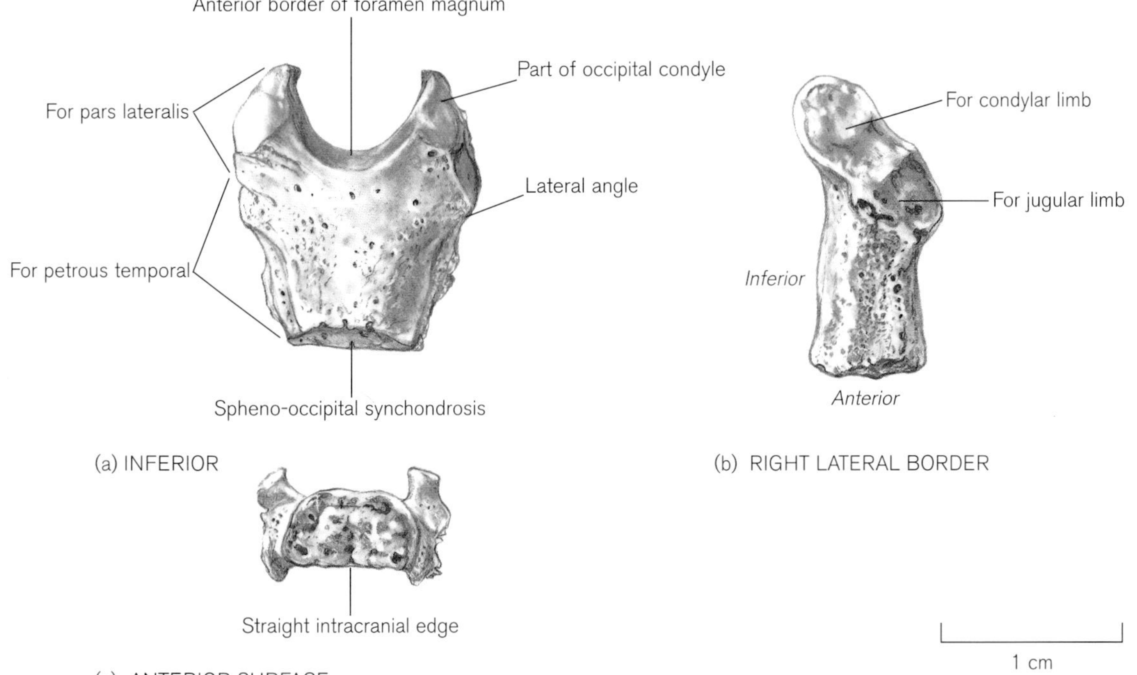

Figure 5.20 Perinatal pars basilaris.

individual is more than 5 months postpartum. If, however, both the pars basilaris and the pars lateralis are available, and they are of approximately the same length, then the fetus is less than 7 months *in utero*. In the perinatal period, the pars lateralis has a faster growth rate and is longer than the pars basilaris. The latter is itself either longer than wide or square in shape. After this time, the pars lateralis is always longer than the basilaris, but the latter always has a greater width than length.

Fusion of the individual parts of the occipital bone starts in the perinatal period and continues until the age of 5–6 years. The lateral sections of the sutura mendosa, which extend about half way to the median plane, start to close from about 4 months postpartum (Redfield, 1970) and are normally virtually closed but not necessarily obliterated, by the end of the first year of life (Molleson and Cox, 1993). Fazekas and Kósa, (1978) state that they can persist until the age of 3 or 4 years. Reinhard and Rösing (1985) report that the suture may remain in 25%, 10% and 1% of skulls at the age of 4 years, 5–6 years and 11–15 years, respectively and Keats (1992) shows a 17 year old male skull with persistent mendosal sutures. Abnormalities in the normal pattern of fusion of the ossification centres of the interparietal part of the bone can produce many varieties of Inca bones (see above).

The lateral occipitals fuse with the supra-occipital part of the squama between the first and third years at the **sutura** (synchondrosis) **intra-occipitalis posterior**. This is often referred to as the 'innominate synchondrosis' in the clinical literature (Caffey, 1953; Shapiro and Robinson, 1976c). Molleson and Cox (1993) reported that in a small skeletal sample of infants and children of documented age, the suture fused between 2 and 4 years. Redfield (1970), examining bones of estimated age at death, found that the suture was fused and obliterated in about half of the specimens by the fifth year, which is later than all other accounts. Exceptionally, traces of the suture may remain into adult life (Smith, 1912). Fusion starts where the partes laterales meet the mastoid parts of the temporal bones and proceeds medially. The last part to fuse is at the posterior border of the foramen magnum, where the open sutures on each side may leave a tongue of bone between them (Fig. 5.22). This must be distinguished from the process of Kerckring (see above) which is a much earlier structure (Fig. 5.17).

Complete fusion of the lateral occipitals with the basi-occipital at the **sutura** (synchondrosis) **intra-occipitalis anterior** takes place between the ages of 5 and 7 years but can start as early as 3–4 years of age (Tillmann and Lorenz, 1978). Moss (1958) remarked that the hyaline cartilage between the bones of both the anterior and posterior intra-occipitalis synchondroses are reduced to sutural dimensions well before

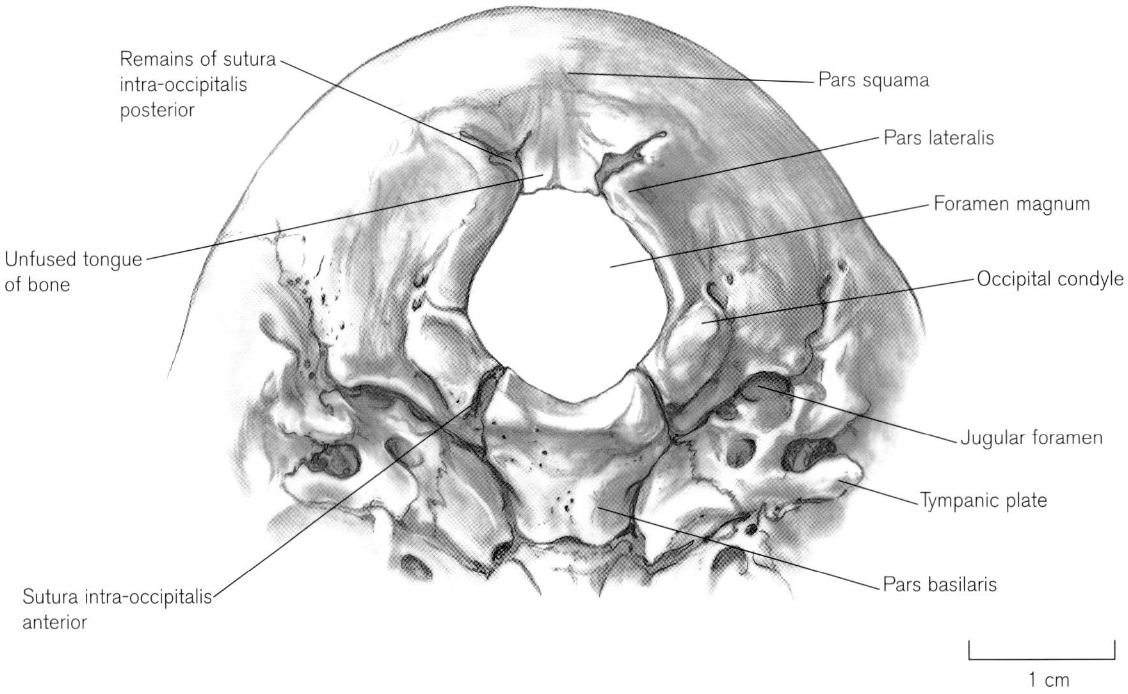

Figure 5.22 The sutura intra-occipitalis posterior. Drawn from a skull of dental age 18 months. Fusion is almost complete except for a small tongue of bone at the posterior border of the foramen magnum. The sutura intra-occipitalis anterior is still open.

final fusion takes place and this may account for the wide range of times reported. Fusion starts internally and proceeds outwards, often leaving a small gap across the occipital condyles. Redfield (1970) distinguished this from the 'dimple or fossa', which lies over the hypoglossal canal and noted that few condyles younger than 12 years of age are smooth. Tillmann and Lorenz (1978) also commented on a strip of unossified cartilage that sometimes divides condyles even into adult life, but rejected a developmental cause in favour of a still unknown mechanical explanation. This final fusion of the parts of the occipital bone halts any further growth in size of the foramen magnum, other than an increase in robusticity of its margins by subperiosteal deposition and this is necessarily mirrored by a concurrent completion of the atlas (see Chapter 6). It reflects the well-documented precocious maturation of the human central nervous system.

Most standard anatomical texts overestimate the age range of closure of the spheno-occipital synchondrosis (Fig. 5.13) at between 18 and 25 years (Frazer, 1948; Grant, 1948; Williams *et al.*, 1995). Ford (1958) and Scott (1958), in reviewing growth of the cranial base, also state that closure occurs between 17 and 25 years of age. Irwin (1960), in a tomographic study, found that the synchondrosis was complete by 18 years but did not distinguish between the sexes. Large series were reviewed by Powell and Brodie (1963), Konie (1964), Melsen (1969, 1972), Ingervall and Thilander (1972) and Sahni *et al.* (1998) (Table 5.1). They all report closure times during adolescence, with females being on average 2 years in advance of males. Melsen (1969), in observations on dry skulls of unknown age, notes that fusion occurs after the eruption of the permanent canines, premolars and second molar teeth and Konie (1964) found that the closure age coincided with skeletal age as estimated from hand–wrist X-rays (Greulich and Pyle, 1959). It seems likely that the slight discrepancies observed may be due to differences in methodology, but the closure of the synchondrosis almost certainly occurs during the adolescent rather than the young adult period. Closure occurs first on the intracranial surface and proceeds towards the base of the skull.

It appears that the fusion times of both the intra-occipital and the spheno-occipital synchondroses are related to significant maturational events. The posterior intra-occipital fusion occurs at between 2 and 4 years of age, when the deciduous dentition has erupted into the mouth and is nearing completion. The anterior fusion is usually complete by the age of 6 years, when the period of rapid brain growth has reached its peak and the permanent molars are starting to erupt. Spheno-occipital fusion occurs at the end of the adolescent growth spurt and when the permanent dentition (except the third molars) is nearing completion (see Appendix 1; Bogin, 1997).

A small area between the occipital and temporal bones does not fuse until early adult life. This is the cartilaginous jugular growth plate (jugular synchondrosis/petro-exoccipital articulation), a small triangular or quadrangular area, situated just posterolateral to the jugular foramen in the occipitotemporal suture (Figs. 5.1 and 5.2). Maat and Mastwijk (1995) found that, in a Dutch series, fusion did not begin until after the age of 22 years and that bilateral fusion was complete at 34 years. Hershkovitz *et al.* (1997) reported on a larger series (Hamann-Todd collection – Black and White American populations) and found that a small proportion (7–10%) underwent complete union before 20 years of age while 5–9% remained open after 50 years. It was concluded that the chance of finding individuals above the age of 40 years with a completely open suture was less than 13% and this area might be useful in assigning age in the young adult. The authors' 'anatomical perspective' in dividing the petro-occipital articulation into three regions is somewhat misleading. Only part of the petro-exoccipital articulation is the jugular growth plate. The rest of the suture between the exoccipital and the whole of the suture with the supra-occipital as far as the lateral angle is not 'petro-' at all, but in fact the occipitomastoid suture.

Table 5.1 Time of closure of the spheno-occipital synchondrosis

	Age (yrs)		Numbers		
	Female	Male	Female	Male	Method
Powell and Brodie (1963)	11–14	13–16	193	205	Radiographic
Konie (1964)	10.5–13.5	12.5–16	162	152	Radiographic
Melsen (1972)	12–16	13–18	44	56	Histological
Ingervall and Thilander (1972)	>13.75*	>16	21	32	Histological
Sahni (1998)	13–17	15–19	34	50	Direct inspection
			27	46	CT scans

*Never open.

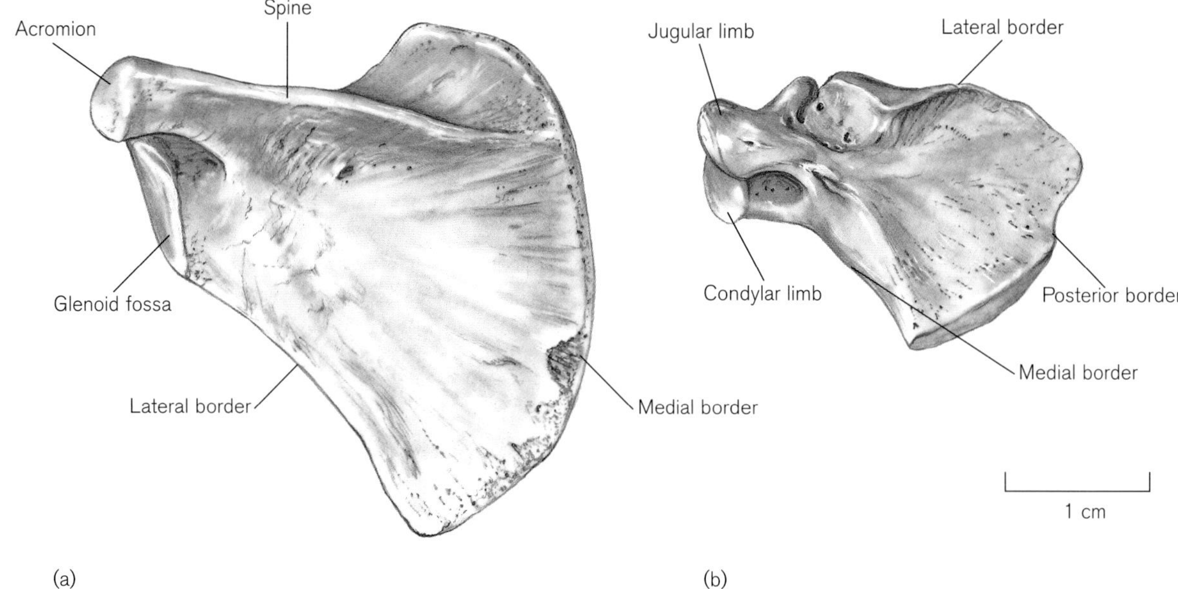

Figure 5.23 (a) Dorsal view of the perinatal left scapula; (b) intracranial view of right pars lateralis from the same skeleton. Note the superficial similarity.

Practical notes

Sideing/orientation of the juvenile occipital

Pars lateralis – identification is possible by midfetal life. Sideing depends on identifying the condylar and jugular limbs of the hypoglossal canal, which extend anteromedially. The greater part of the occipital condyle lies on the inferior surface of the condylar limb (Fig. 5.18).

Pars basilaris – the bone is identifiable by mid-fetal life, although it differs from its neonatal appearance in being longer and not so angled laterally. By 7 fetal months it is readily identifiable. The inferior surface is fairly flat and parts of the occipital condyles can usually be seen at the tips of the posterior curve. The intracranial surface is slightly concave (Fig. 5.20).

Bones of a similar morphology

Pars squama – fragments of the squama are probably indistinguishable from fragments of other vault bones or scapula unless a characteristic part such as the process of Kerckring is present. The lower part of the supra-occipital part of the bone tends to be more robust than other vault bones.

Pars lateralis – at the perinatal stage, a single pars lateralis viewed from the intracranial surface is very similar in shape to the dorsal surface of the scapula of the opposite side, as the jugular limb extends from the bone in a manner very like the scapular spine (Fig. 5.23). However, in any one individual the scapula is larger overall and the blade is more extensive than the body of the pars lateralis, which has the occipital condyle on its inferior surface (see Chapter 8 – Scapula).

Pars basilaris – an isolated pars basilaris is similar in shape to the manubrium sterni but at the perinatal stage of development the basilaris is a substantial, solid bone, while the manubrium is barely more than a thin disc (see Chapter 7 – Sternum). From the perinatal stage until the pars basilaris fuses with the rest of the occipital the manubrium is always smaller and thinner and has less well-defined borders.

Morphological summary

Fetal

8–10 wks	Ossification centres for supra-occipital, interparietal and pars lateralis appear in that order	
By mth 5	Supra-occipital and interparietal parts of squama fused	
By mth 7	Pars basilaris develops lateral angle	
By mth 8	Pars lateralis longer than pars basilaris	
Birth	Represented by:	pars basilaris two partes laterales pars squama
By mth 6	Pars basilaris width always greater than length	
During yr 1	Median sagittal suture and remains of sutura mendosa close Jugular process develops on pars lateralis Vascular and neural markings become apparent	
1–3 yrs	Fusion of partes laterales to squama	
2–4 yrs	Hypoglossal canal complete excluding pars basilaris	

5–7 yrs Fusion of pars basilaris and partes laterales
11–16 yrs (females) Fusion of spheno-occipital synchondrosis
13–18 yrs (males) Fusion of spheno-occipital synchondrosis
22–34 yrs Closure of jugular growth plate

Metrics

Fazekas and Kósa (1978) illustrated and tabulated measurements of the squamous, lateral and basilar parts of the bone during the fetal period (the length of the pars basilaris is the median sagittal length – Table 5.2). Moss *et al.* (1956) reported dimensions of the pars squama from 8 to 20 fetal weeks, but measurements

Table 5.2 Dimensions of the fetal occipital bone

	Pars squama			
	Height (mm)		Width (mm)	
Age (weeks)	Chord	Arc	Chord	Arc
12	7.5	7.5	12.0	12.0
14	10.6	10.6	14.4	14.4
16	15.0	15.7	18.6	19.6
18	18.8	19.9	22.5	23.8
20	23.7	24.7	27.5	29.4
22	27.3	28.9	31.2	34.2
24	28.7	32.1	32.9	39.0
26	32.8	36.0	36.5	40.9
28	35.4	40.8	39.6	45.9
30	39.0	44.4	43.0	49.0
32	42.5	47.7	47.6	55.9
34	49.4	59.2	50.0	60.5
36	50.3	61.3	51.6	63.1
38	53.5	63.8	56.3	67.0
40	55.2	68.8	59.3	70.5

Height: posterior border of foramen magnum to tip of squama; chord: direct distance; arc: distance on surface of bone.
Width: maximum distance across bone at right angles to height.

	Pars basilaris		Pars lateralis	
Age (weeks)	Length (mm)	Width (mm)	Length (mm)	Width (mm)
12	2.7	1.7	2.7	1.4
14	3.9	2.6	4.0	1.8
16	5.5	3.9	5.9	2.9
18	6.9	5.1	7.7	4.1
20	8.0	6.1	9.5	5.1
22	8.3	6.8	10.6	5.8
24	8.7	8.0	11.8	6.7
26	9.1	8.4	13.1	7.1
28	9.6	9.1	14.1	7.9
30	10.1	10.0	14.7	8.5
32	10.5	10.9	17.0	8.9
34	11.0	12.0	19.3	10.9
36	11.8	12.4	20.8	11.6
38	12.4	13.4	23.4	13.2
40	13.1	15.2	26.5	14.0

Pars basilaris: length: midsagittal distance from anterior border of foramen magnum to anterior border; width: maximum width at level of lateral angles.
Pars lateralis: length: maximum distance between anterior and posterior intra-occipital synchondroses; width: maximum distance between medial and lateral margins of the posterior intra-occipital synchondrosis.
Adapted from Fazekas and Kósa (1978).

were not defined. Kyrkanides *et al.* (1993) gave measurements of the pars basilaris related to other fetal parameters from 13.5 to 21 weeks (Table 5.3). Molleson and Cox (1993) published width and length measurements of the pars basilaris in the documented Spitalfields collection and commented on other aspects of the bone. Scheuer and MacLaughlin-Black (1994) gave data for the width, and both the sagittal and maximum length of the pars basilaris, in 46 documented juveniles from the St Bride's and Spitalfields collections (Table 5.4).

Table 5.3 Length of pars basilaris and humerus between 13.5 and 21 fetal weeks

Age (weeks)	Maximum length (mm)	Humeral length (mm)
13.5	3.4	12.0
16.5	6.3	19.5
17.2	8.0	27.9
21.1	10.7	32.4

Adapted from Kyrkanides *et al.* (1993).

Table 5.4 Dimensions of the pars basilaris in individuals of documented age at death

Documented age	*n*	Mean maximum width (mm) WB	Mean length (mm)	
			LB (F&K)	LB(R)
2 weeks	3	14.5	11.3	15.6
3 weeks	1	16.9	12.7	17.0
4 weeks	1	15.6	12.6	16.8
7 weeks	1	15.5	11.6	15.9
3 months	1	15.4	13.8	16.7
5 months	1	18.4	13.4	18.1
8 months	2	21.0	13.8	20.5
9 months	3	20.5	13.9	19.6
11 months	1	22.3	14.0	19.7
1 year	1	18.3	13.9	17.9
1 year 1 month	2	22.1	14.8	19.8
1 year 2 months	3	22.7	15.8	21.3
1 year 3 months	1	23.6	16.8	22.7
1 year 4 months	1	18.6	14.0	18.6
1 year 6 months	3	21.9	15.5	20.8
1 year 8 months	1	22.8	15.7	21.7
1 year 9 months	1	22.7	16.8	21.3
2 years 3 months	2	24.4	18.1	23.5
2 years 5 months	2	25.8	17.5	24.2
2 years 6 months	1	24.6	17.5	22.4
2 years 7 months	4	25.9	17.4	24.2
2 years 9 months	2	24.2	16.4	23.3
3 years 2 months	1	23.2	16.6	22.7
3 years 4 months	1	27.6	16.6	24.6
3 years 5 months	1	26.1	18.1	24.1
3 years 7 months	1	27.8	17.5	24.8
3 years 8 months	1	27.3	15.5	24.0
4 years 3 months	2	25.9	16.4	24.2
4 years 7 months	1	26.2	15.3	23.9

WB: maximum width; LB (F&K): length in median sagittal plane; LB(R): maximum length (see Fig. 5.21).
Adapted from Scheuer and MacLaughlin-Black (1994).

II. THE TEMPORAL

The adult temporal

The adult temporal[5] bones (Fig. 5.24) form part of the base of the skull and the lateral walls of the cranial cavity. They articulate with the occipital, parietals, greater wings and body of the sphenoid and the zygomatic bones (Figs. 5.1–5.3). Each bone is a compound structure composed of four main parts, the petromastoid, squamous, tympanic and the styloid process. As the ear also forms an integral part of the bone, it is essential to briefly consider its anatomy, especially with regard to its contained auditory ossicles. In addition, the VIIth (facial) and VIIIth (vestibulocochlear) cranial nerves and the internal carotid artery pass through the bone. Consequently, the temporal bone has attracted a vast clinical and surgical literature. However, the following account will attempt to describe only those features which are essential to follow the development of the bone. Further detail can be found in specialized texts (Proctor, 1989; Donaldson *et al.*, 1992).

The **petromastoid** part of the bone is situated in the base of the skull and forms both the posterior wall of the middle cranial fossa and the anterior wall of the posterior fossa. The **petrous**[6] part is a three-sided pyramid pointing anteromedially and filling in the space between the greater wing of the sphenoid anteriorly and the occipital bone posteriorly (Figs. 5.1 and 5.2). Its **base** is fused with the mastoid part on the outer surface of the skull and its apex limits the posterolateral boundary of the foramen lacerum. The **apex** carries the anterior opening of the **carotid canal**, which is often deficient superiorly. The petrous apex is usually diploic with contained marrow but can be pneumatized or sclerotic (Chole, 1985). Just superolateral to the apex, lie the double apertures of the **auditory** (pharyngotympanic/Eustachian) **tube** and the **canal for the tensor tympani** muscle. The **anterior** surface, facing the middle fossa, is smooth and joined at right angles to the squamous part of the bone at the petrosquamous suture (Fig. 5.24b). Just behind the apex is a hollow, lined with dura mater, the **trigeminal impression**, for the sensory (Gasserian) ganglion of the Vth (trigeminal) cranial nerve. Posteriorly is the raised **arcuate eminence**, chiefly caused by the superior (anterior) semicircular canal of the inner ear. Anterolaterally, the **tegmen tympani** forms the roof of the auditory tube, the middle ear cavity and the **mastoid antrum**. The **posterior** surface of the petrous pyramid faces the posterior cranial fossa and, on the ridge between it and the anterior surface, is attached the upper fixed margin of the tentorium cerebelli. Between the layers of dura mater the superior petrosal venous sinus runs backwards in a groove to drain into the **sigmoid sinus**. The anterior part of the base of the posterior surface articulates with the occipital bone, forming a groove for the inferior petrosal sinus, which empties into the jugular bulb lodged in the jugular foramen. Near the centre of the surface is the **internal acoustic meatus** (porus acousticus internus) through which pass the facial and vestibulocochlear nerves and the labyrinthine (internal auditory) vessels. The dimensions and shape of the meatus have been recorded from casts by Amjad *et al.* (1969), Papangelou (1972) and Faruqi and Hasan (1984) and its width and depth on histological sections by Olivares and Schuknecht (1979). The size and appearance on radiographs are detailed by Camp and Cilley (1939) and Valvassori and Pierce (1964). Bilateral asymmetry is of clinical significance in the diagnosis of acoustic neuromas. Behind the meatus, a slit in the bone conceals an aperture leading to the **aqueduct of the vestibule**. A second aperture, the **subarcuate fossa**, lies above and between the meatus and the opening of the aqueduct. Both are very variable in shape and size (Bast and Anson, 1950; Watzke and Bast, 1950; Donaldson *et al.*, 1992). The **inferior** surface of the petrous bone lies in the base of the skull (Fig. 5.24c). The apex has a roughened surface for the attachment of the levator veli palatini muscle and the cartilaginous part of the auditory tube. Behind is the circular opening of the carotid canal, while further posteriorly the bone forms the anterolateral border of the **jugular foramen** and the **jugular growth plate** (see occipital bone). At the anteromedial edge of the jugular fossa is a small triangular space for the inferior (petrosal) ganglion of the IXth (glossopharyngeal) cranial nerve. Next to it, is the cochlear canaliculus, through which the **perilymphatic** (periotic) **duct** opens into the subarachnoid space.

Currarino and Weinberg (1974) describe an anomalous pea-sized ossicle, which is visible on radiographs. It lies under the dura, or adheres to it, at the anterior superior tip of the petrous bone, medial to the position of the trigeminal ganglion. It is usually bilateral and may be observed at any age. Its incidence is not established and it has no clinical significance except in the differential diagnosis of anomalous calcifications of the region. A small, rounded mass of cartilage in just such a position in the fetal chondrocranium is described by Macklin (1914) as the 'supracochlear cartilage' and also recorded in seven embryos by Müller and

[5] *Tempus* (Latin meaning 'time'). The first area to show the ravages of time by greying of the hair at the temples.
[6] *Petros* (Greek meaning 'stone'), *petra* (Greek meaning 'rock'). Christ changed Simon's name to Peter as he would be the rock on which the Church was built.

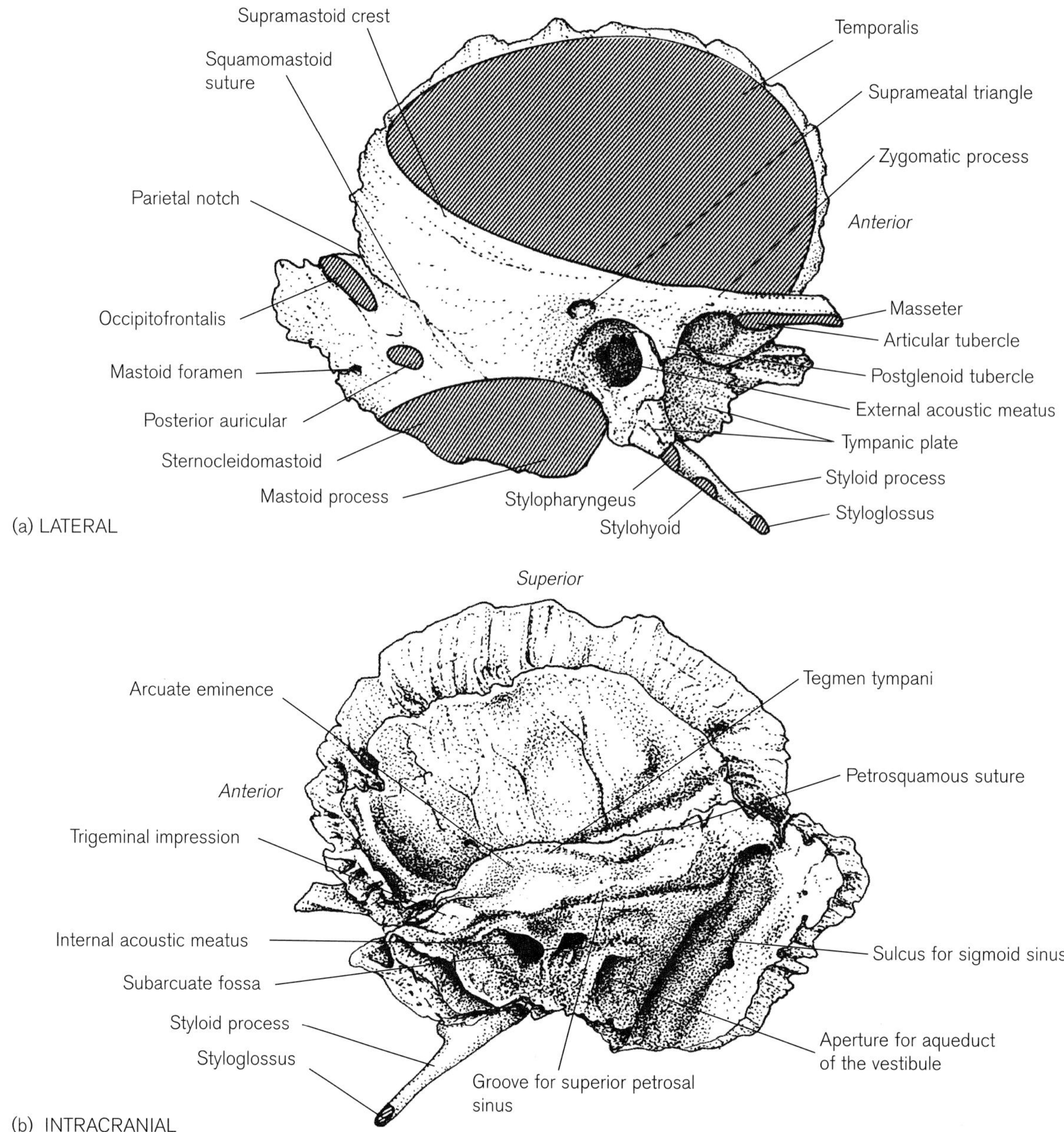

Figure 5.24 Right adult temporal.

O'Rahilly (1980). It seems likely that this osseous anomaly, called the 'os suprapetrosum of Meckel' could be this same unfused ossicle.

The **mastoid**[7] section of the bone is attached to the petrous part behind the external auditory meatus. It articulates with the squamous occipital bone between its lateral angle and the jugular process, and with the postero-inferior border of the parietal bone (Figs. 5.1 and 5.3). It fuses with the squamous part of the temporal bone at the **squamomastoid suture**, which can often be seen in adult skulls (Fig. 5.24a). At the superior end of the suture is the parietal notch, the location of sutural ossicles in certain populations (Laughlin and Jørgensen, 1956; Berry and Berry, 1967; Berry, 1975; Reinhard and Rösing, 1985). The outer surface is roughened for the attachment of the posterior belly of the occipitofrontalis and posterior auricular muscles. The mastoid foramen, transmitting a vein to the sigmoid sinus, is an inconstant feature. The conical **mastoid process** projects inferiorly and its external surface provides attachment for the sterno-

[7] *Mastos* (Greek meaning 'breast') The process is so named for its supposed likeness to the female breast.

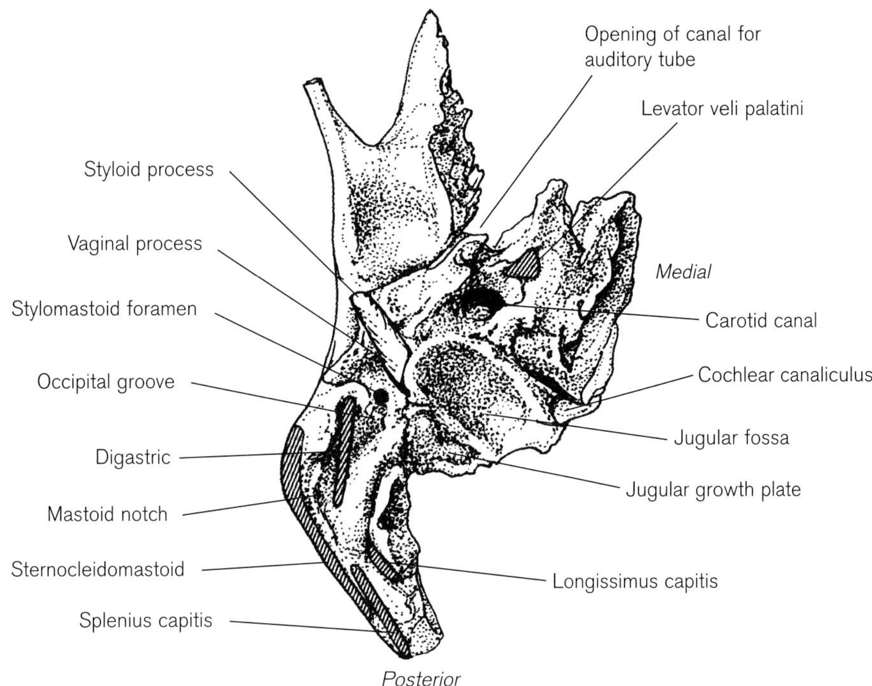

(c) INFERIOR

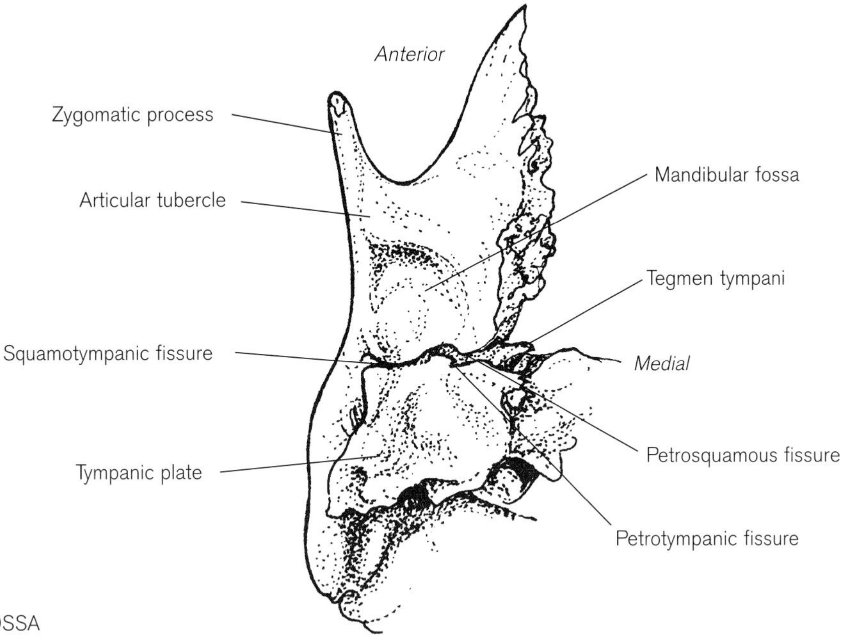

(d) MANDIBULAR FOSSA

Figure 5.24 *(Continued).*

cleidomastoid, splenius capitis and longissimus capitis muscles. Its size is sexually dimorphic, being larger in males. Immediately medial to the base of the process is a deep **mastoid notch** for the posterior belly of the digastric muscle and medial to this is an **occipital groove** for the occipital artery. The surface between the notch and groove may vary from a smooth, rounded ridge to an expanded, projecting process which, if conspicuous, is termed a paramastoid (juxtamastoid) process (Corner, 1896a; Taxman, 1963; Anderson, 1993; Barnes, 1994). The main feature of the inner surface of the mastoid part of the bone is the deep **sulcus for the sigmoid venous sinus**, which often has an opening for a mastoid vein. Pneumatization of the mastoid, extending into contiguous parts of the bone is very variable (Williams *et al.*, 1995). Turner and Porter (1922) identified cellular, or well-pneumatized and acellular mastoid processes, in a survey of 1000 crania from different population groups. 80% were of the first type and there appeared to be no sexual bias. The air cells are often separated from those of the adjoining squamous part by a thin septum of bone (Korner's septum). Middle ear disease has been diagnosed in archaeological material, either as a chronic condition (Gregg *et al.*, 1965) or when the tympanic cavity has perforated into the cranial cavity, which may lead to meningitis or chronic osteomyelitis (Ortner and Putschar, 1985). The pattern of the mastoid sinus cells has been used for identification in forensic cases (Rhine and Sperry, 1991). Kalmey and Rathbun (1996) report that discriminant function analysis of the measurements of the petrous part of the bone will achieve up to 74% accuracy in sex determination.

The **squamous** part of the temporal bone consists of a flat, vertical plate, forming part of the temporal fossa and lateral wall of the cranial cavity, and the **zygomatic process**, which projects anteriorly (Fig. 5.24a). The lateral surface of the squama is smooth and covered by the temporalis muscle, part of whose lower fascia is attached to the **supramastoid crest (crista supramastoidea)**, and sometimes the middle temporal artery grooves the bone vertically from the root of the zygomatic process. The inner, cerebral surface forms the wall of the middle cranial fossa and is marked, both by the sulci and gyri of the temporal lobe of the cerebral hemisphere and by branches of the middle meningeal vessels (Chandler and Derezinski, 1935). The bone's thinness in this area makes it liable to fracture, with consequent rupture of the vessels leading to extradural haematoma. Trephining may then be necessary to reduce cerebral compression. The superior border of the bone forms a semicircular curve, bevelled within, which articulates with the inferior border of the parietal bone at the squamosal suture (Fig. 5.3). Anteriorly, it usually articulates with the posterior border of the greater wing of the sphenoid and occasionally with the frontal bone. A frontotemporal articulation occurred in 1.5% of over 8000 skulls from American collections (Collins, 1926) and in 7.7% of Australian aboriginal skulls (Murphy, 1956), but it can be as high as 10% (Berry and Berry, 1967) depending on the population. There may also be a single or multiple epipteric bones (pterion ossicles) at this site, whose occurrence varies from 6% to 18%. They are regarded as non-metric variants (Berry and Berry, 1967; Reinhard and Rösing, 1985). They may later fuse to either the temporal or frontal bones (Collins, 1930), so that incidence figures would depend on the ages of the skulls examined. Posteriorly, the squamous bone is fused to the mastoid (see above). A depressed area above the **external acoustic meatus**, the **suprameatal triangle** (vascular spot), is the surface marking for the mastoid antrum and occasionally bears a suprameatal spine. More anteriorly (Fig. 5.24d) is the articular surface of the temporomandibular joint, the **mandibular fossa** and the root of the zygomatic process. Superiorly, the surface forms a smooth curve whose surface articulates with the disc of the joint, while posteriorly it projects downwards as the **postglenoid tubercle**. Here it articulates laterally for a short distance with the tympanic plate at the **squamotympanic** (Glaserian) **fissure**. More medially, the edge of the tegmen tympani can be seen between the two parts of the bone and splits the fissure into a petrosquamous suture anteriorly and a petrotympanic fissure posteriorly, with the latter providing an exit for the chorda tympani nerve into the infratemporal fossa. In front of the articular fossa is the **articular tubercle**, onto the surface of which the disc of the temporomandibular joint glides when the mouth is fully open. The **zygomatic** process projects horizontally and anteriorly in front of the external meatus and provides attachment on its upper surface for the superior temporal fascia and on its medial and inferior surfaces for fibres of the masseter muscle. Anteriorly, the process articulates at a serrated suture with the temporal process of the zygomatic bone. The area around its root is said to display sexual dimorphism as the supramastoid crest extends further posteriorly in males than in females (Keen, 1950; WEA, 1980). Schulter (1976) reported measurements for 25 different parameters of the bone in three different populations.

The **tympanic**[8] part of the temporal bone is a roughly quadrilateral plate lying below the squamous part and anterior to the mastoid process. Its posterior surface is drawn out into a scroll-like formation that forms the anterior, inferior and most of the posterior walls of the bony **external acoustic meatus**. It is fused to the squamous part, both anteriorly to the postglenoid tubercle and posteriorly to the mastoid process. The inner end of the meatus is grooved by the **tympanic sulcus** for the attachment of the tympanic membrane and the outer end is roughened to receive the cartilaginous part of the meatus. The quadrilateral surface faces antero-inferiorly and forms the posterior, non-articular part of the mandibular fossa. The inferior border of the plate is sharp and spread out posteriorly as the **vaginal process**, which encloses the base of the styloid process like a sleeve. Immediately behind it is the **stylomastoid**

[8] *Tympanum* (Latin meaning 'drum'). Fallopius first used the term.

foramen, which transmits the motor division of the facial nerve and the stylomastoid artery.

The tympanic plate may be perforated by a **foramen of Huschke**. The presence of the foramen is a normal stage during development (see below) but is considered a non-metric variable if it persists after the age of 5 years (Reinhard and Rösing, 1985). It shows a varying incidence in different populations (Krogman, 1932; Wood-Jones, 1933; Wunderly and Wood-Jones, 1933; Laughlin and Jørgensen, 1956; Anderson, 1960).

Reports of aural exostoses have been present in the anatomical, anthropological and medical literature for over 100 years (Field, 1878; Turner, 1879; Hrdlička, 1935; Gregg and Bass, 1970; Gregg and McGrew, 1970). Typically, they are bony masses arising from the walls of the auditory canal. Their aetiology is uncertain, but as there appeared to be large differences in incidence in various populations (Stewart, 1933; van Gilse, 1938; Roche, 1964a), an hereditary factor was thought to play a part. Irritation of the canal by physical means such as deformation with head binding, or by chemical factors (Jackson, 1909) were discussed in the early medical literature. Van Gilse (1938) first suggested that irritant stimulation by cold water might be a factor in their formation in individuals involved in aquatic sports or working activities involving swimming and diving. This was followed by many supportive clinical surveys (Adams, 1951; Harrison, 1951; Seftel, 1977). Fowler and Osmun (1942) produced bony growths in the meatuses of guinea pigs by irrigating them with cold water. A review of the historical, anthropological and clinical literature can be found in DiBartolomeo (1979). More recently, Kennedy (1986) surveyed the frequencies of exostoses by latitude among populations that exploit marine and fresh water resources and found a strong positive correlation between aquatic activity and aural exostoses. Further evidence of behaviour-induced exostoses has been reported from imperial Rome (Manzi *et al.*, 1991) and prehistoric Chile (Standen, 1996; Standen *et al.*, 1997). The aetiology has been recently reviewed by Hutchinson *et al.* (1997). As occurrence of some types of exostoses, or auditory tori, have been viewed as discrete non-metric traits (Berry and Berry, 1967), it would be misleading to use them in estimates of population distances based on discrete variables, if they have a behavioural rather than a genetic origin.

The **styloid process**[9] projects inferiorly and forwards from the underside of the temporal bone between the petrous part and the tympanic plate. Its tip is connected to the superior horn of the hyoid bone by the stylohyoid ligament. Both the bony process and the ligament give rise to the stylopharyngeus, stylohyoid and styloglossus muscles. Davis *et al.* (1956) dissected 350 craniofacial halves and found the process to be absent, sometimes bilaterally, in 36% of cases. From radiographs, Kaufman *et al.* (1970) reported a wide variation in length around a mean of 29 mm. Lengelé and Dehm (1988, 1989), in a gross and microradiographic study, measured the styloid on macerated skulls and concluded that short processes were generally invisible on radiographs, as they were hidden by the vaginal process. They recorded a bimodal distribution in the length of styloids: a group with short processes of less than 20 mm, and a larger group with long processes whose median was 27 mm. There appeared to be no correlation with either age or sex.

There is a well-documented clinical condition known as styloid chain ossification, styloid syndrome or Eagle's syndrome (Eagle, 1937). It may present as a solid pillar of bone as far as the hyoid, or as a chain of ossified articulated segments. It has been reported both in individuals from past populations (Sawyer *et al.*, 1980) and extensively in the anatomical, dental and radiological literature (Dwight, 1907a; Eagle, 1948; Steinmann, 1970; Gossman and Tarsitano, 1977; Mueller *et al.*, 1983; Lykaki and Papadopoulos, 1988; Genez *et al.*, 1989 and Kiely *et al.*, 1995). It occurs in about 4% of patients, rarely under the age of 30 years and is not sexually dimorphic. It may be asymptomatic, or give rise to dysphagia, or to pain in the ear, throat or temporomandibular joint. Eagle (1948) suggested that pain could sometimes be due to impingement of the calcified ligament on the carotid artery. Steinmann (1970), whose patient regrew a process 14 years after removal, concluded that the condition had a genetic basis, and that the second arch structures, originally formed in cartilage, may always retain their potential to ossify. Camarda *et al.* (1989a, b) have reviewed the extensive literature and, in a review of 150 children and adolescents, reported a significant number of both elongated styloid processes and stylohyoid ligament ossifications.

The ear

The **inner ear** includes the membranous labyrinth containing the peripheral receptors for hearing and balance, enclosed within the osseous labyrinth, a system of interconnecting cavities in the petrous part of the bone. The space between the bone and the membranous labyrinth is filled with **perilymph**, a fluid akin to cerebrospinal fluid.

[9] *Stylos* (Greek meaning 'pen'). *Stylus* (Latin) meaning a pointed iron or bone implement used by the Romans to mark wax tablets.

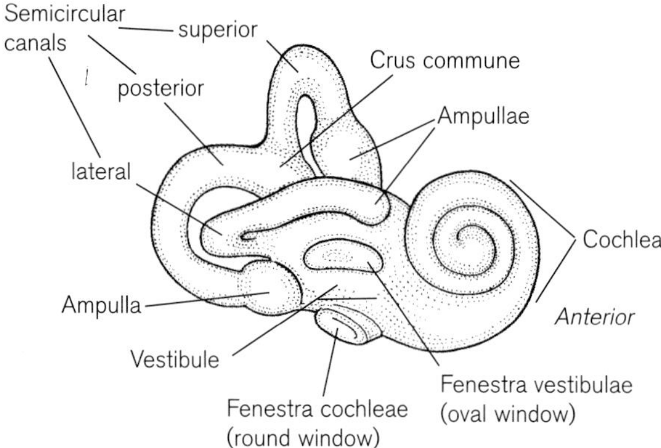

Figure 5.25 Right osseous labyrinth from the lateral side.

The **osseous labyrinth** (Fig. 5.25) consists of the **cochlea**, separated from the **semicircular canals** by a middle section, the **vestibule**. The cochlea is a hollow tube that spirals two-and-a-half turns around a central pillar, the modiolus. Projecting from the modiolus is a bony ledge, the **spiral lamina**, which partially divides the canal into a lower passage, the **scala tympani** and an upper passage, the **scala vestibuli**, which are continuous at the apex, the **helicotrema**. At the base of the cochlea the scala tympani is separated from the middle ear by the secondary tympanic membrane at the **fenestra cochleae** (round window). Near this is the **cochlear canaliculus** (aquaeductus cochleae/perilymphatic/periotic duct), which opens into the subarachnoid space at the apex of the jugular fossa. Also from the vestibule, a narrow duct, the **aqueduct of the vestibule**, opens onto the posterior surface of the petrous bone. The vestibule is also separated from the middle ear at the **fenestra vestibuli** (oval window), occupied by the footplate of the stapes. The three **semicircular canals**, lateral, posterior and superior, open into the vestibule by five apertures, the last two sharing a common entrance, the crus commune. Each canal has an expanded end, the ampulla. The **membranous labyrinth** (Fig. 5.26), lies within the osseous labyrinth and is a closed system of extremely small intercommunicating sacs and ducts containing a fluid called **endolymph** and Anson and Bast (1958) calculated that its volume displaces only 0.2 ml of water. Posteriorly, the **semicircular ducts** occupy the semicircular canals and open into the **utricle**[10] which, in turn is connected to the **saccule.**[11] The utricle and saccule, which lie within the vestibule of the bony labyrinth, and the semicircular canals contain the neural endings responsible for the detection of movement of the head and hence balance and orientation. From the utricle and the saccule a Y-shaped duct leads to the **endolymphatic duct and sac**. This duct lies in the bony vestibular aqueduct and the sac protrudes to lie in a hollow on the posterior surface of the petrous bone between the two layers of dura. Attached anteriorly to the saccule is the blind-ending, spiral **cochlear duct**, which follows around the spiral lamina between the scala tympani and the scala vestibuli. It is completely closed off from the scala tympani by the basilar membrane attached to the projecting edge of the spiral lamina, and from the scala vestibuli by Reissner's membrane. It contains the **organ of Corti**, the highly specialized sensory cells that respond to sound.

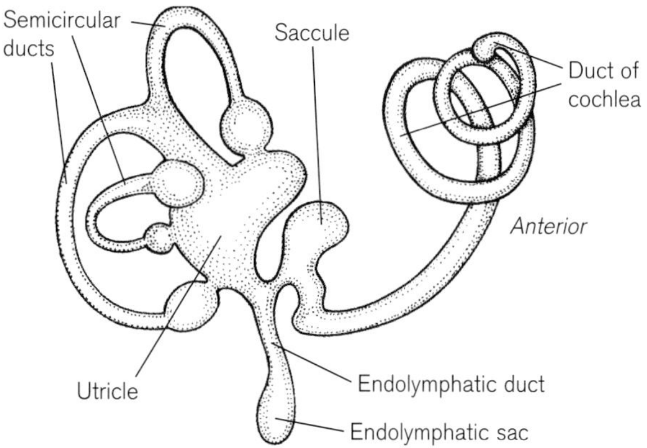

Figure 5.26 Right membranous labyrinth from the lateral side.

The **middle ear** (tympanic cavity/tympanum; Fig. 5.27) lies between the inner ear and the external auditory meatus and is responsible for the mechanical transmission of sound waves from the exterior, via a chain of three **auditory ossicles** (see below). It is a slim, air-filled cavity, slightly wider above than below, with a roof, floor and medial, lateral, anterior and posterior walls. The **roof** is formed from part of the tegmen tympani, which separates the cavity from the middle cranial fossa. The **floor** forms part of the **jugular plate** and is related to the bulb of the internal jugular vein, the carotid canal and the base of the styloid process. It is often extremely thin and may be deficient or contain air cells. Hence, in fractures of the skull there may be bleeding from the ear. The greater part of the **lateral wall** is taken up by the **tympanic membrane**, fixed in the sulcus of the **tympanic ring**, (annulus tympanicus), which is deficient superiorly at the **tympanic notch** (incisura tympanica). From the edges of the incisure the anterior and posterior malleolar folds subtend the pars flaccida of the membrane. At the centre of the membrane is the umbo, where the

[10] Literally 'a little womb', a diminutive of *uterus* (Latin).

[11] *Sacculus* (Latin meaning a 'small bag').

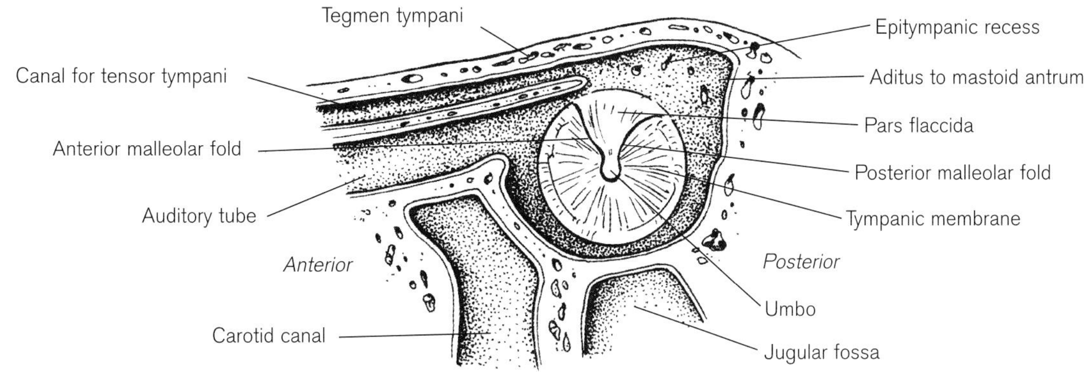

(a) LATERAL WALL

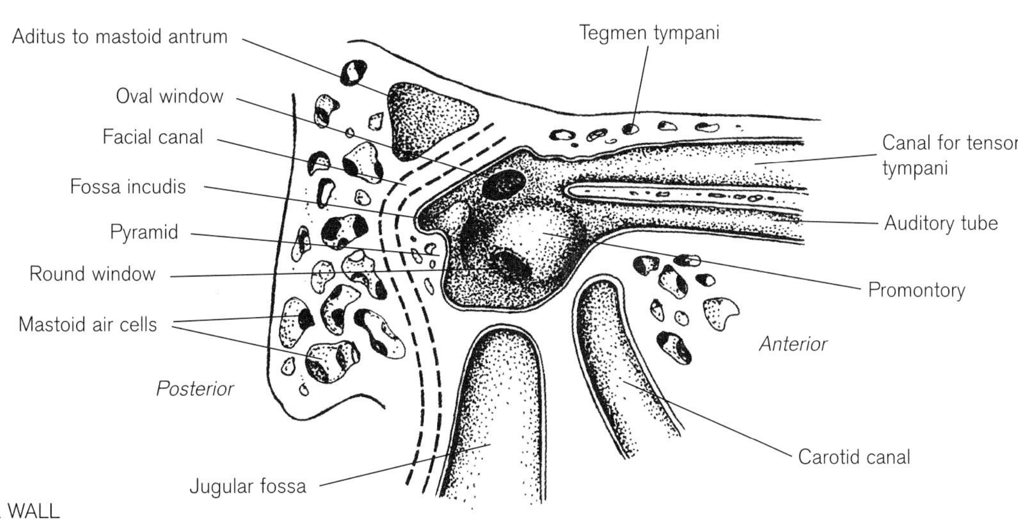

(b) MEDIAL WALL

Figure 5.27 Right middle ear.

handle of the malleus is attached. Above the membrane, a section of the squamous part of the bone, the **scutum**, forms the lateral wall of the **epitympanic recess**. This leads anteriorly into the double canal for the auditory tube and the tensor tympani muscle and posteriorly into the **aditus to the mastoid antrum**. The **medial wall** is the lateral wall of the inner ear. Inferiorly, the **promontory** is related to the basal turn of the cochlea. Posterosuperior to this is the oval window to which the footplate of the stapes is attached by the annular ligament. The oval window is overshadowed by the prominence of the **facial canal**, which runs from the geniculum to the posterior wall. This often bulges out so that the footplate is obscured (Hough, 1958). A little below and posterior to the oval window is a depression leading to the round window. It is separated from the oval window by an extension of bone, the **subiculum**, from the posterior end of the promontory. Posteriorly is a protrusion formed by the lateral semicircular canal. High on the **posterior wall** the aditus leads into the **mastoid antrum** and the air cells of the mastoid part of the bone. The facial canal lies in the medial wall of the aditus as it turns downward to run in the posterior wall of the tympanum. Dehiscences, or deficiencies, in the bony wall of the canal are common (Guild, 1949; Hough, 1958; Fowler, 1961; Beddard and Saunders, 1962), especially in the horizontal segment (Baxter, 1971). The vertical segment is related to mastoid air cells. At the anterior end of the facial canal is the **processus cochleariformis**, a curved projection of bone housing the tendon of the tensor tympani muscle as it turns through a right angle to insert into the upper end of the handle of the malleus. Beneath the aditus is the **fossa incudis**, which accommodates the short crus of the incus, and lower still is the prominence of the **pyramid** for the attachment of the tendon of the stapedius muscle. On the lateral side of the pyramid the chorda tympani nerve enters the middle ear via the posterior canaliculus. It crosses from posterior to anterior across the tympanic membrane between the mucosal and fibrous layers and passes medial to the upper part of the handle of the malleus. It leaves by the anterior canaliculus to enter the infratemporal fossa through the petrotympanic fissure. The **anterior wall** of the middle ear receives the openings of the canal for the tensor tympani muscle, and below it, the **auditory tube** which connects the middle ear with the nasopharynx. The thin floor, often covered with air cells, separates the cavity from the carotid canal and jugular bulb.

The middle ear cavity is crossed by a chain of three **auditory ossicles**, the **malleus** (hammer), the **incus** (anvil) and the **stapes** (stirrup), which stretch from the tympanic membrane laterally to the oval window medially. They articulate with each other via synovial joints and are attached by ligaments and folds of mucous membrane to surrounding structures. The system acts as a bent lever to amplify and convert vibrations in air at the tympanic membrane to pressure changes in the perilymph in the vestibule of the inner ear.

The ossicles have long been a source of interest and fascination to anatomists and anthropologists and, in spite of their very small size, they retain a remarkable survival rate following inhumation. It is always worth investigating the external auditory meatus of a buried skull for the presence of one or more ossicles. Basic measurements and variability were recorded by Urbantschitsch (1876) and Heron (1923). Botella Lopez and de Linares von Schmiterlow (1975) described Bronze Age ossicles from Granada, which were said to be of the gracile Mediterranean type. Masali (1964) reported that there appeared to be less variability in size and weight in a collection of Egyptian dynastic origin than in European populations. Arensburg *et al.* (1981), in a study of ossicles from three populations, stress that metric variation is extremely minor, even in prehistoric and historic populations separated by thousands of years. This consistency makes ossicular morphology useless as a taxon parameter, but when morphological variation occurs, it is extremely significant. Neanderthal and other prehistoric ossicles are described by Arensburg and Nathan (1972), Arensburg *et al.* (1977), Heim (1982), Arensburg and Tillier (1983) and Arensburg *et al.* (1996). A fossil malleus seen on radiographic examination of the left temporal bone of Kabwe (Rhodesian) man was reported by Price and Molleson (1974) and a fossilized right incus of *Australopithecus robustus* has been described by Rak and Clarke (1979).

The **malleus** (Fig. 5.28a) consists of a **head** (caput), a **neck** (collum), a **handle** (manubrium), a **lateral process** (processus lateralis) and an **anterior process** (processus anterior). The oval head lies in the **epitympanic recess** and is attached to the roof by the superior malleolar ligament. On its posteromedial surface it bears a saddle-shaped articular surface, covered with hyaline cartilage, the lower half of which is drawn out into the so-called **spur** (cog-tooth). This articulates with a reciprocal surface on the incus at the incudomalleolar joint, which is said to contain an interarticular disc (Wolff and Bellucci, 1956). The head is connected by the narrowed neck to the tapering handle, which points posteromedially away from the head. The handle is covered with cartilage on its lateral surface and attached by a fold of mucous membrane to the tympanic membrane, drawing it inwards towards the cavity and its tip marks a central depression, the **umbo** (Fig. 5.27a). The tensor tympani muscle is attached to the upper part of the manubrium of the malleus. Two processes are attached at the junction of the neck and the manubrium. The short, thick lateral process, which appears to be a continuation of the manubrium, points towards the tympanic membrane to which it is attached by the anterior and posterior malleolar folds enclosing the **pars flaccida** of the membrane. The slender anterior process is variable in length and anchored by dense fibres of the anterior ligament that pass forwards through the petrotympanic fissure to the sphenoid bone.

The **incus** (Fig. 5.28b), toothlike in form, consists of a **body** (corpus), a **short process** (crus breve) and a **long process** (crus longum), to whose tip is attached a **lenticular process** (processus lenticularis). The body, located in the epitympanic recess, is laterally compressed, bearing on its free, anterior surface a reciprocal articular surface for that of the malleus (see above). The short process, the tip covered in cartilage, points directly backwards and is attached to the **fossa incudis** on the posterior wall of the recess by the posterior ligament. A notch in the inferior border is not mentioned in the common texts, but is described by Urbantschitsch (1876), and illustrated as a common variation by Heron (1923), Lempert and Wolff (1945), Arensburg and Nathan (1971) and Botella Lopez and de Linares von Schmiterlow (1975). Wolff and Bellucci (1956) describe the notch as being filled with dense fibrous tissue, which is joined to atypical cartilage in its roof. The posterior ligament has medial and lateral expansions extending from the notch into the corresponding side of the fossa incudis. The notch is occasionally extended across the width of the crus, making the tip a separate ossicle, which is sometimes seen as a cartilaginous mass in the embryo. The long

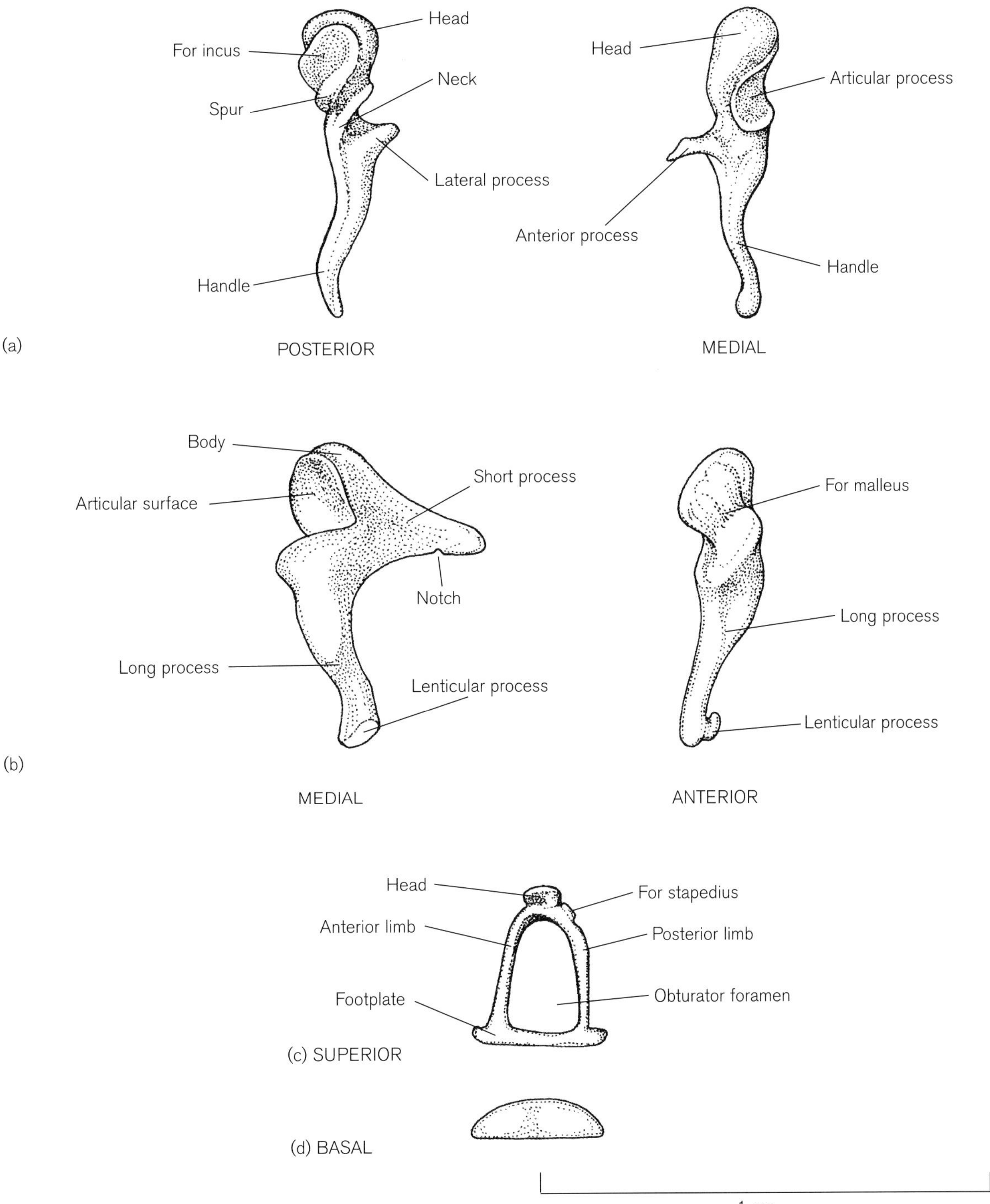

Figure 5.28 Right ear ossicles: (a) malleus; (b) incus; (c) stapes; (d) stapes footplate.

process lies parallel and posteromedial to the handle of the malleus. At its tip is the hook-like lenticular process, which is directed medially and articulates with the head of the stapes at the incudostapedial joint. There is said to be a minute intra-articular disc about 38 μm thick in some specimens (Wolff and Bellucci, 1956).

Anomalies illustrated by Donaldson *et al.* (1992) include the incus represented only by the long crus or lenticular process, and lacking both, or either, of the crura. Resorption of the long and lenticular processes is common in middle ear disease (Pollock, 1959; Ghorayeb and Graham, 1978) but Richany *et al.*

(1954) attribute this to normal remodelling that occurs throughout life. However, Frootko *et al.* (1984) and Lannigan *et al.* (1995) report resorption of the surface in normal ears and believe that it is positively correlated with age and also more obvious in males. They dismiss the possibility that its tenuous blood supply is a cause (Lannigan *et al.*, 1993) and suggest that it is possibly a biomechanical response to excessive noise.

The **stapes** (Fig. 5.28c) lies in a horizontal plane across the medial part of the tympanic cavity and consists of a **head** (caput), an **anterior limb** (crus anterius), a **posterior limb** (crus posterius) and a base or **footplate** (basis stapedis; Fig. 5.28d). It is extremely fragile and the most variable of the ossicles in form, an important factor to surgeons, as it is commonly removed in surgery for otosclerosis. There appears to be no correlation between weight and length, although wider bones are in general heavier (Dass *et al.*, 1966a). The head points laterally and has a small, cartilage-covered facet of variable shape that articulates with the lenticular process of the incus. The stapedius muscle, which arises from the pyramid, is attached by a tendon to a small spine (Hough, 1958) at the junction of the head and posterior crus. The two limbs, which are grooved on their inner surfaces, curve away from the head to attach to the footplate. The anterior limb is generally finer and slightly less curved than the posterior limb. The footplate is an almost oval disc whose vestibular surface and rim are covered with hyaline cartilage. It is fixed in the oval window at the stapediovestibular joint by the annular ligament. This contains elastin and consists of extensive fibres, which can stretch into the fissula ante-fenestram (Wolff and Bellucci, 1956). The superior surface of the footplate is convex and the inferior surface can be straight, concave or convex (Dass *et al.*, 1966b). The footplate sometimes consists only of a layer of cartilage and can be as thin as 50 μm (Anson and Bast, 1958). The footplate and bases of the crura are often joined by a complete or incomplete plate of bone, the **crista stapedis**, which alters the regular shape of the enclosed **obturator foramen** and occasionally even obliterates it. Its occurrence has been recorded and illustrated by Dass *et al.* (1966b), Galindo and Galindo, (1975) and Bruintjes *et al.* (1997). Donaldson *et al.* (1992) illustrate other, more extreme variations including partial, or complete absence of the whole ossicle. Anson *et al.* (1960) relate these anomalies to the extensive remodelling that occurs during development.

Fixation of the footplate of the stapes in the oval window (stapes ankylosis) can occur at any period of life. It may be congenital, caused by middle ear infection in children or due to otosclerosis in adults. Otosclerosis of the labyrinthine capsule is a common cause of deafness and is an inherited, non-infectious disease, which is more common in females and varies according to the population. It has not been found in native Americans (Holzhueter *et al.* 1965; Birkby and Gregg, 1975) but prevalence in white Caucasoids seems to have been constant at about 1% for many centuries. Ziemann-Becker *et al.* (1994) observed it in a skull from the Early Bronze Age of Austria, Sakalinskas and Jankauskas (1991) reported it in Lithuanian skulls from the fifth to sixth centuries and Dalby *et al.* (1993) observed the same prevalence in British material from the fourth to the seventeenth century.

Early development

The development of the ear and the surrounding temporal bone is a complex process involving the interaction of several different embryonic tissues (Fig. 5.29). A neurectodermal placode, with additions from neural crest, gives rise to the membranous labyrinth at an early embryonic stage. The surrounding otic capsule, which forms the major part of the petromastoid part of the bone, develops endochondrally from paraxial mesoderm with mesenchyme derived from the neural crest. Mesenchyme also gives rise, by intramembranous ossification, to the squamous and tympanic parts of the bone. In contrast, both the styloid process and the auditory ossicles develop endochondrally from pharyngeal arch tissue and the external and middle ear spaces arise from associated grooves and pouches.

Because of this complex development from different embryological components, congenital atresia may affect one part of the ear and leave another part unaffected or modifications may occur in associated structures, including the sigmoid sinus and the facial nerve. Clinical accounts (Altmann, 1955; Gill, 1969; De La Cruz *et al.*, 1985) suggest that the most frequent malformations involve the outer and middle ear only. Males are affected more than females and there is a bias towards unilateral involvement of the right ear. Anatomical and archaeological cases have been described by Greig (1927a) and Hodges *et al.* (1990).

The first signs of **ear** development are evident during the third week of embryonic life as dorsolateral thickenings on either side of the head at the level of the myelencephalon region of the hindbrain. These ectodermal placodes develop into the **membranous labyrinth** of the internal ear. The specialized cells of the placode originate in the neural folds but, unlike the cells of the neural tube, they stay in the surface ecto-

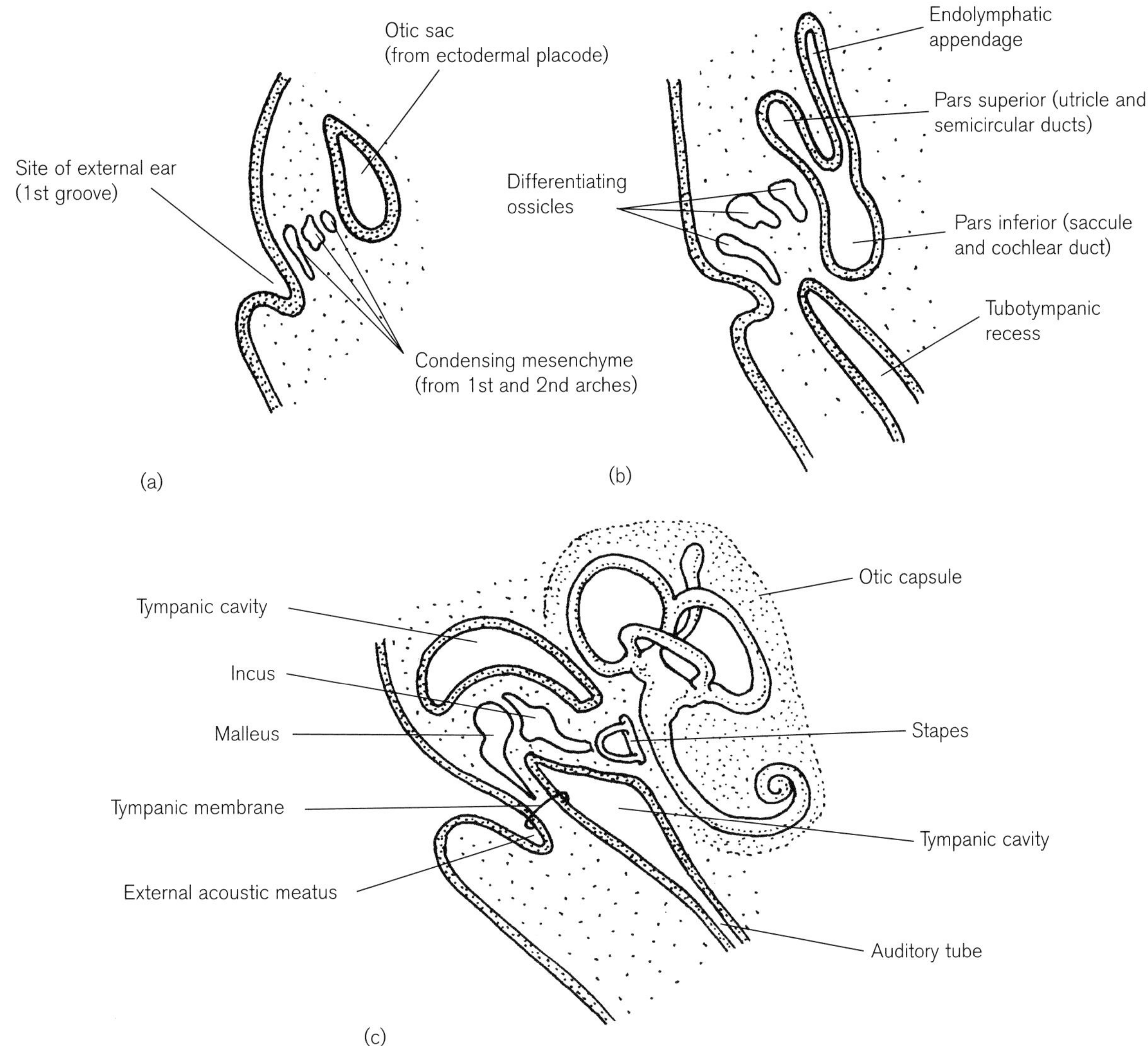

Figure 5.29 Embryology of the ear: (a) 3 weeks; (b) 5–7 weeks; (c) eighth month.

derm after closure of the tube. They give rise to most of the membranous labyrinth and the acoustic ganglion and also have a contribution from neural crest tissue, which migrates to form part of the vestibular ganglion. Details of cell derivations in the chick embryo may be found in D'Amico-Martell (1982), D'Amico-Martell and Noden (1983) and Mayordomo *et al.* (1998) and it is assumed that, in the human embryo, the derivation of the tissues is the same as indicated in chick-quail chimera transplant experiments. Each placode sinks below the surface, forming an **otic**/auditory **vesicle** the mouth of which closes off to form an **otic sac** which, for a time, is attached to the surface ectoderm by a stalk (Fig. 5.29a). Between the fifth and seventh weeks a fold separates off part of the vesicle, which will develop into the **endolymphatic appendage**. Further folds separate the remainder into two parts: a dorsal part (pars superior/vestibularis) forming the utricle and semicircular ducts and a ventral part (pars inferior/cochlearis), differentiating slightly later, forming the saccule and cochlear duct (Fig. 5.29b). The membranous labyrinth is fully differentiated by the week 25 of life. Further details may be found in Bast *et al.* (1947) and Streeter (1942, 1945, 1948, 1951) and the precise sequence of events in staged human embryos may be followed in O'Rahilly (1983).

Between 4 and 5 weeks, the primordia of the **tympanic cavity** and **auditory tube** develop from the **tubotympanic recess**. This is a diverticulum from the primitive pharynx derived from the first, and possibly second pharyngeal pouches. The exact derivation of the tissues is in some doubt and is discussed in detail by Frazer (1910a, 1914, 1922) and Kanagasuntheram (1967). The first pharyngeal groove, which will form the **external auditory meatus**, extends medially from the external surface towards the recess, leaving an area of mesenchyme between the two spaces in which the auditory ossicles develop from pharyngeal arch tissue.

By 8–9 weeks, the mesenchyme surrounding the developing otic vesicles condenses to form the cartilaginous **otic capsules**, which at this stage form prominent lateral bulges in the base of the chondrocranium. They are each divided into an anterior **cochlear** part and a posterior **canalicular** part separated by a sulcus (Lewis, 1920). They are connected to the cartilaginous basi-occipital by the basicochlear and capsulo-occipital commissures and to the temporal wings of the sphenoid by the alicochlear commissures (Müller and O'Rahilly, 1980). In the canalicular part, which develops first (Lewis, 1920) the subarcuate fossa, endolymphatic foramen and eminences of the semicircular canals soon become obvious. The cochlear part displays a wide internal auditory meatus, divided around the divisions of the VIIth and VIIIth cranial nerves. The opening for the duct of the cochlea can be seen in the posterior part of the sulcus and inferiorly the base of the stapes is in the fossa ovalis. At this stage, neither the internal carotid artery nor the facial nerve is incorporated in the capsule for any distance. The artery lies in a groove beneath the cochlear part and the nerve passes straight through the internal meatus and exits at the facial foramen in the anterior sulcus. A little later, a small projection, the mastoid process, develops posteriorly and the shelf of the tegmen tympani begins to project from the capsule (Macklin, 1914, 1921).

While the cartilaginous otic capsule is developing it is, at the same time, being resorbed to make way for the perilymphatic (periotic) fluid-filled spaces around the membranous labyrinth. These start in the region of the vestibule and spread to the cochlear duct, where they form the scala tympani and the scala vestibuli. The last part of the capsule to be transformed is around the semicircular ducts and their ampullae. By about 11 weeks, the spaces eventually form a continuous gap, the **periotic cistern**, between the membranous and bony labyrinths, which is filled with perilymph. Further details may be found in Streeter (1918).

The **auditory ossicles** are at first embedded in mesenchyme (see above) but, as the tympanic cavity enlarges, its mucous membrane covers the ossicles and acts as mesenteries, partially separating tympanic spaces (Proctor, 1964). The epithelium of the cleft, the intervening mesenchyme and the epithelium of the pouch, each contribute a layer to the trilaminar tympanic membrane. Between 5 and 6 weeks, the blastemal mass attached to the ends of the **first and second arches** is grooved and partially separated by the facial nerve. One side will develop into the **malleus** and **incus** and the other will become the **stapes** (Anson *et al.*, 1960). By 8 weeks the three blastemal ossicles are separated by joint cavities and are becoming cartilaginous. The head, body and manubrium of the malleus are recognizable, although it is still associated with the end of Meckel's cartilage. The body and crura of the incus are likewise obvious and the short crus is in contact with the otic capsule. At this stage, the stapes has an annular shape and is fused to the otic capsule, which will provide part of its footplate. The goniale, the primordium of the anterior process of the malleus is visible (Macklin, 1921; Müller and O'Rahilly, 1980) and is the only ossicular structure to form in membrane. The long-held classical view of the single mesenchymal origin for each of the ossicles has been modified by the detailed studies of Hanson *et al.* (1962). The head of the malleus and the body and short crus of the incus are derived from first arch tissue. The manubrium and long crus of the incus, as well as the head and crura of the stapes arise from the second arch. Additional to pharyngeal arch tissue, are the independent membranous anterior process of the malleus and part of the footplate of the stapes that develop from the otic capsule. Between 9 and 15 fetal weeks, the cartilaginous ossicles acquire their recognizable adult morphology and size (Richany *et al.*, 1954) and by the second half of fetal life, the main morphology of the ear is in place (Fig. 5.29c).

The **styloid** part of the temporal bone develops from the cartilage of the second pharyngeal arch. At 8 or 9 weeks the cranial end of the arch becomes attached to the otic capsule and the anlage of the styloid extends inferiorly and medially from the base of the chondrocranium (Macklin, 1921; Müller and O'Rahilly, 1980).

At about 10 weeks, the **tympanic ring** is represented only by a small nodule of cells surrounded with a little osseous matrix in the angle between the handle of the malleus and Meckel's cartilage (Macklin, 1921).

Ossification

The ossification of the temporal bone is unique in two ways. First, the osseous labyrinth, the auditory ossicles and the tympanic ring reach full adult proportions by fetal midterm and there is therefore no subsequent postnatal increase in size. Second, unlike other bones, the capsular part of the petrous part of the temporal does not undergo remodelling, and the first formed endochondral bone is retained throughout life. Interestingly, the otic capsule portion of the petrous temporal is one of the few bones that is spared from pathological change in Paget's disease, whose chief characteristic is a distortion of the normal remodelling process (Ortner and Putschar, 1985). In contrast to the otic capsule, the mastoid, squamous and tympanic parts of the bone change greatly in shape and proportion during postnatal life.

Ossification of the **pars petrosa** (petrous part of the temporal) proceeds first by the formation of the bony labyrinth immediately surrounding the otic capsule and then by extensions from this, which contribute to the extracapsular part of the bone. Ossification of the **otic capsule** is endochondral, except for the modiolus and spiral lamina of the cochlea, the external ostium of the vestibular aqueduct and part of the tympanic wall of the lateral semicircular canal, which form in membrane. Ossification begins only when the cartilaginous capsule, with its contained membranous labyrinth, has reached adult proportions. At this point, apart from the endolymphatic duct and sac, further growth of all the internal structures ceases. The first formed endochondral bone is not replaced by Haversian bone but keeps its primitive, relatively avascular structure. There are conflicting accounts of the number of ossification centres that contribute to the formation of the otic capsule. A careful reading of the definitive work by Bast (1930) makes it clear that, in the human embryo, there may be up to 14 separate centres, the first of which appears at 16 weeks in the outer part of the capsule overlying the first turn of the cochlea. Once begun, the process is very rapid and the greater part of the capsule is ossified by fetal week 23. Bast starts his account with an extensive historical review of previous observations, beginning with Kerckring in 1670. There is considerable variation in the order of appearance and it should be borne in mind that some of the centres may be of the inconstant, accessory variety. Ossification centres appear to arise in groups, in relation to nerve terminations, the internal acoustic meatus and the semicircular canals. Each centre is trilaminar, consisting of an inner layer surrounding the labyrinthine spaces, a middle layer made up of scattered islands of calcifying cartilage (globuli ossei), which lie in marrow spaces and an outer periosteal layer. Vascular osteogenic buds lay down endochondral bone and further bone (called endochondrial bone by Bast) is formed on the surface of the remaining cartilage. Fusion between the centres takes place without intermediate zones of epiphyseal growth so that no suture lines can be seen. Ossification takes place rapidly around the immediate area of the cochlear part of the membranous labyrinth but it is slower in the canalicular area. Spoor (1993) reported that there were no changes in size of the bony labyrinth as seen on CT scans after the ossification of the otic capsule at approximately fetal week 24. Bonaldi *et al.* (1997) measured the region of the round window and its fossula from 4 months fetal life to adults and found that, although there were very minor differences in shape of the window itself, adult dimensions are reached during fetal development. There is a burst of activity in the perinatal period, when the capsule finally attains its petrous character. Terms such as opisthotic, prootic, pterotic and epi-otic have been used by some authors (Sutton, 1883; Frazer, 1948) to name individual centres in an attempt to homologize these with individual bones in other vertebrates, but this does little to add to the understanding of the development in the human embryo and in fact probably confuses it further.

Several channels of communication still exist between the interior of the bony labyrinth and external structures. The internal acoustic meatus carries the facial and vestibulocochlear nerves and labyrinthine vessels to the internal ear and the subarcuate fossa transmits the subarcuate artery to the periotic bone. The relations and homologies of the subarcuate fossa in other primates are discussed by Gannon *et al.*, (1988). The vestibular aqueduct and the cochlear canaliculus transmit the endolymphatic duct and the periotic duct respectively, the latter communicating with the subarachnoid space in the posterior cranial fossa. There are also two areas of fibrous connective tissue: the fissula ante fenestram and the inconstant fissula post fenestram, which connect the vestibular region with the tympanic cavity. They are thought to be preferential sites for development of otosclerotic bone in the adult (Kenna, 1996).

The petrous bone first becomes recognizable in midfetal life (Fig. 5.30). It is irregularly shaped, with a rounded **anterior cochlear** end and a more expanded **posterior canalicular** end. Medially, the **internal acoustic meatus** lies anterior to the larger and wider **subarcuate fossa**. Above this, the uncovered curves of the anterior and posterior semicircular canals lie at right angles to each other. The superior surface is smooth and bears opposite to the internal meatus, the **facial foramen** for the exit of the facial nerve into the tympanic cavity. Beneath this, the lateral surface forms the irregular medial wall of the future middle ear. In its centre is the oval window above, which is a minute aperture leading to a groove, the partially formed **facial canal**, which bends postero-inferiorly over the oval window. Just inferior and posterior to the oval window is the fossula of the **fenestra cochleae**, in which the round window can be seen facing backwards. The inferior surface is slightly grooved anteriorly where the internal carotid artery passes under it but there is, as yet, no carotid canal. Posteriorly is

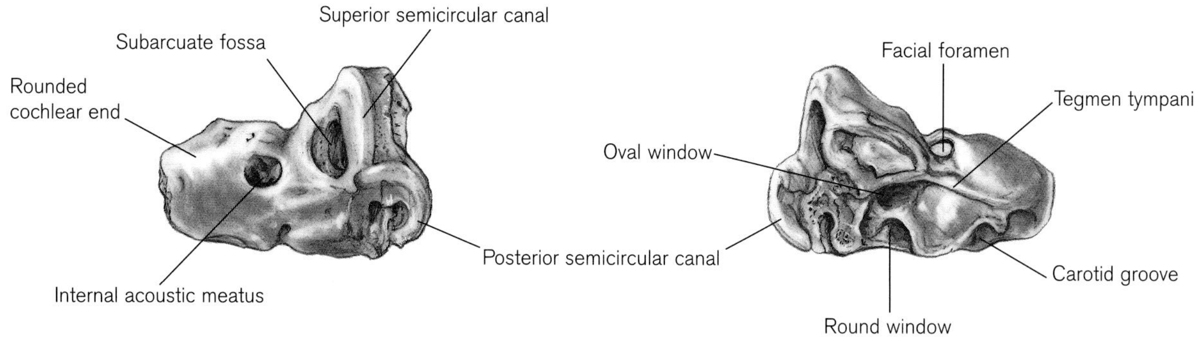

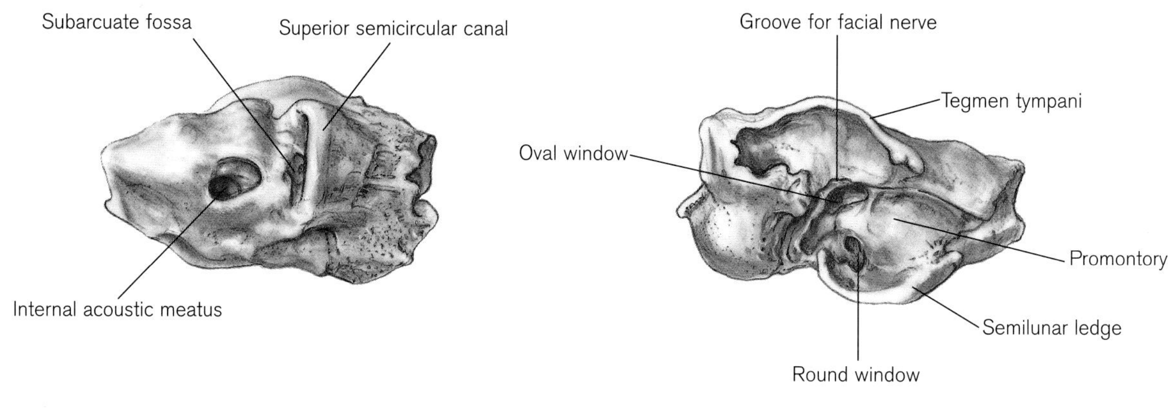

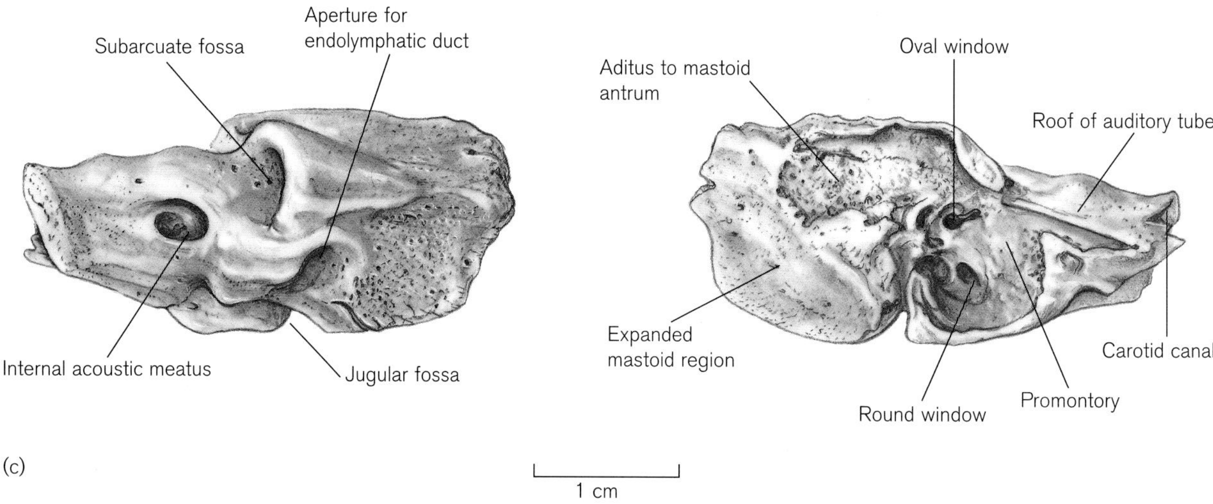

Figure 5.30 Ossification of the right pars petrosa: (a) midfetal life; (b) about 7 months; (c) late fetal life. Left row – medial side, anterior is to the left; right row – lateral side, anterior is to the right.

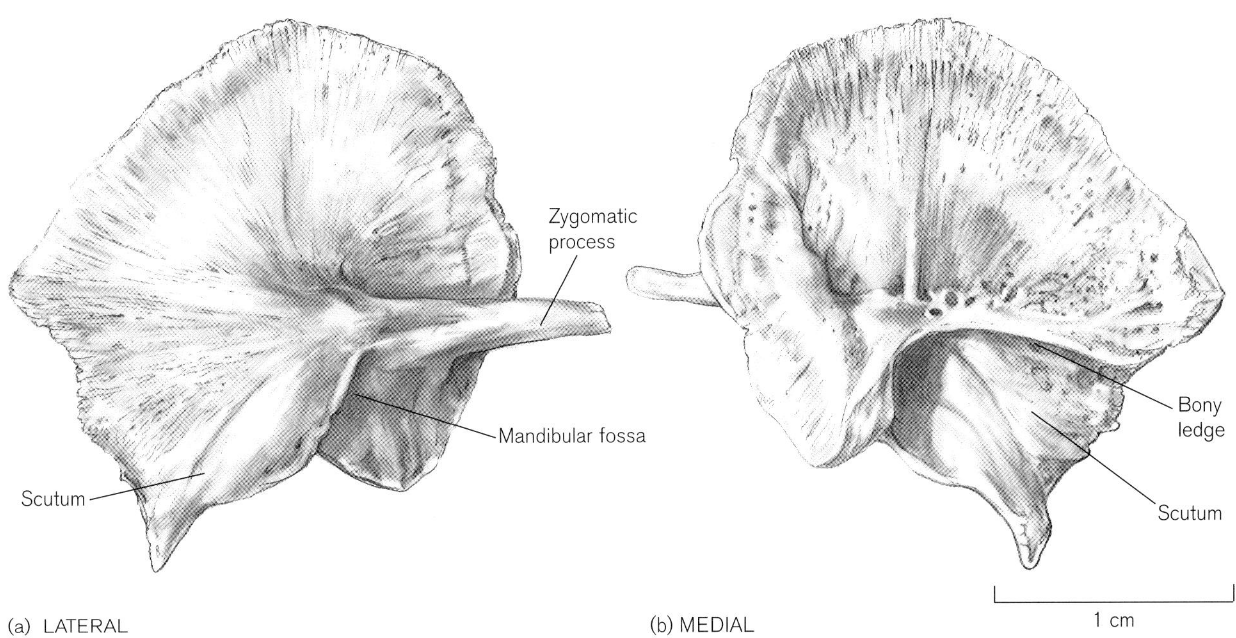

Figure 5.31 Right perinatal pars squama.

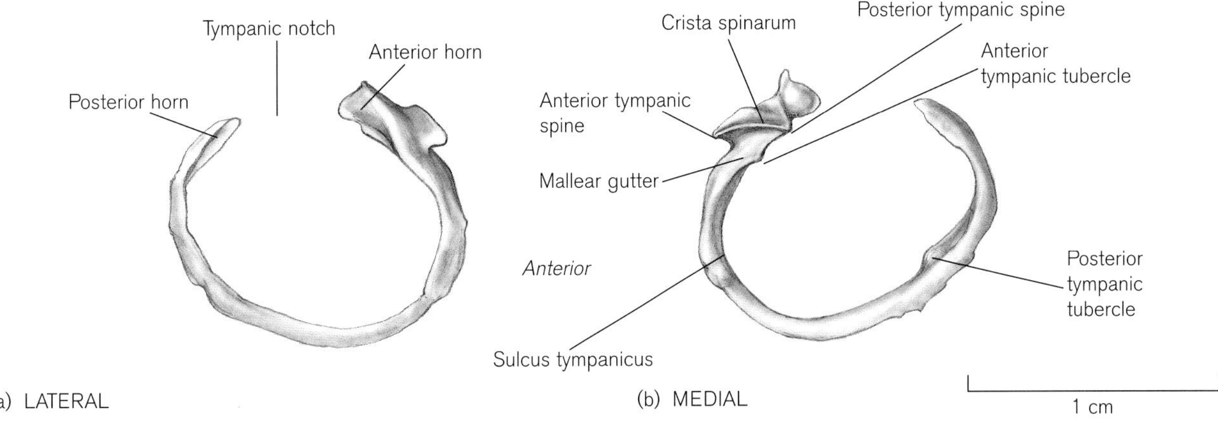

Figure 5.32 Right perinatal tympanic ring.

the smooth jugular part of the bone. The last part of the canalicular part to ossify is the region of the posterior and lateral canals and the lateral aspect of the superior canal, as they continue to grow for some time after the rest of the internal ear has reached maximum size (Bast, 1930). This whole area spreads posteriorly towards the future mastoid part of the bone.

In the second half of intra-uterine life, the ossification of most of the **extra-capsular** areas of the petrous bone takes place by extension from the outer periosteal layer of the capsule. The facial foramen becomes covered by a plate of bone, which is continued laterally as the **tegmen tympani**. It starts to ossify by fetal week 23 (Kenna, 1996) and eventually forms the roof of the middle ear, the antrum and part of the wall of the auditory tube. The **canal for the facial nerve** is formed partly by extension from the otic capsule with contributions from the second pharyngeal arch. At first the nerve lies in a groove on the lateral wall of the canalicular part of the capsule but by 26 weeks, together with the stapedius muscle and blood vessels, it is partially enclosed in a bony sulcus. The promontory may be seen at this stage as a bulge in the wall between the oval and round windows. The inferior edge of the lateral surface of the bone forms a **semilunar ledge**, which will eventually support the inferior part of the tympanic ring. Between 24 and 29 fetal weeks, a further petrosal ledge, the **jugular plate** extends laterally and begins to form part of the floor of the middle ear (Spector and Ge, 1981).

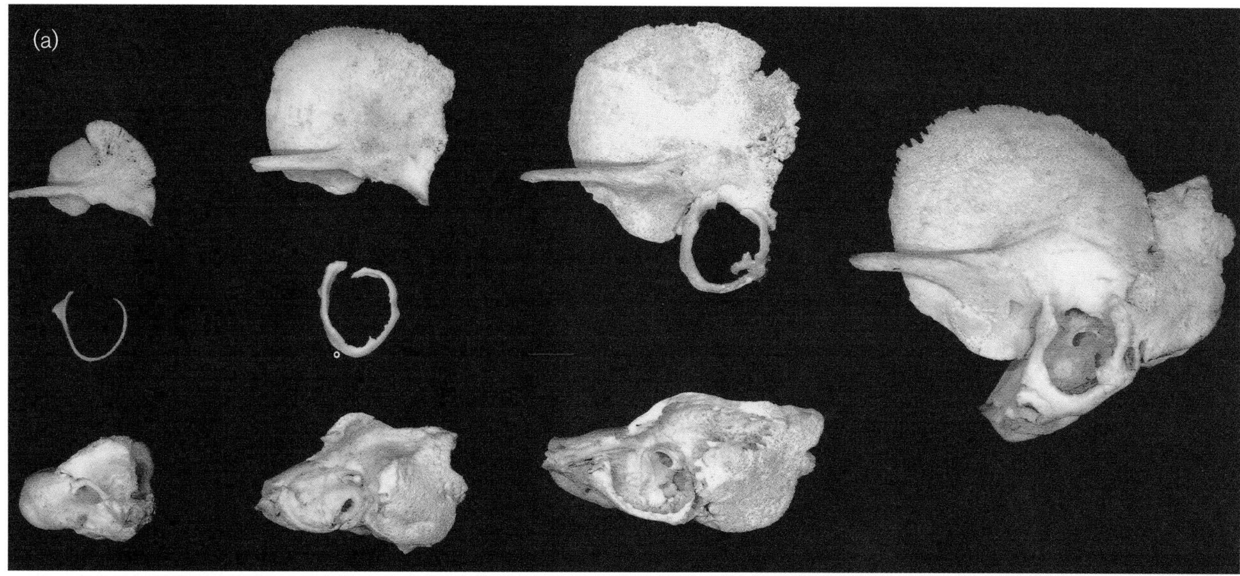

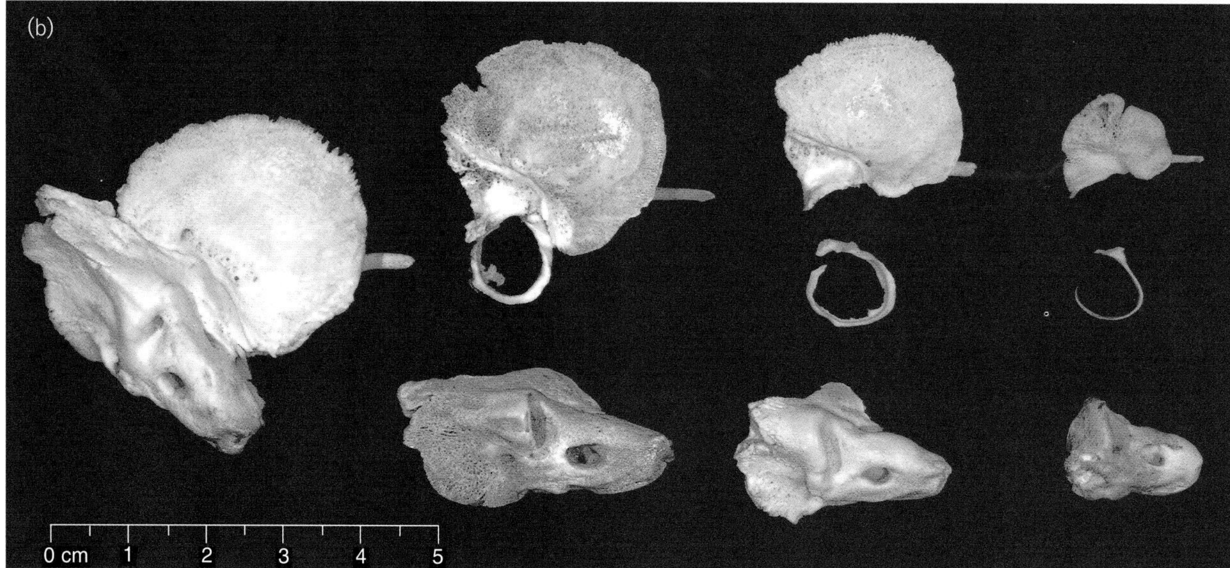

Figure 5.33 Development of the three parts of the temporal bone. (a) Lateral view, from left to right – fifth fetal month, eighth fetal month (note the stapes in the oval window), at birth, about 6 months postnatal. (b) Medial view of same specimens. (For other details see the text.)

During late fetal life, the arcuate fossa and the internal auditory meatus are about equal in size (Figs. 5.30 and 5.33) and the aperture of the **endolymphatic duct** can be seen inferior to them. The extracapsular parts of the bone expand further and a tongue of bone curves inferiorly from the anterior part of the semilunar ledge to form the entrance of the **carotid canal**. Behind this is the forming **jugular fossa** and the expanding mastoid part of the bone. The bony section of the **auditory tube** can be seen as a definite groove leading anteriorly from the middle ear.

The **tympanic cavity** is complete by fetal week 30 and the **epitympanum** by week 34. The facial canal is gradually enclosed by the end of the first year of life (Anson *et al.*, 1963), although up to 25% of canals may have dehiscences (Sataloff, 1990). Although pneumatization of the extracapsular parts of the bone starts at about 35 weeks, it does not accelerate until after birth, when air replaces amniotic fluid in the middle ear. It proceeds throughout infancy and early childhood (Bast and Forester, 1939) and may even continue at the petrous apex into early adult life (Shambaugh, 1967). Three principal groups of air cells, opening into the antrum, main cavity and the auditory tube are formed in the fetus and undergo postnatal growth until puberty (Ars, 1989).

The **squamous** part of the temporal bone starts to ossify in membrane in the seventh or eighth week of intra-uterine life (Noback and Robertson, 1951; Anson *et al.*, 1955; O'Rahilly and Gardner, 1972; Müller and O'Rahilly, 1980). Bach-Petersen and Kjær (1993) identified it radiographically at 9–10 weeks. Most accounts describe a single centre at the base of the zygomatic process from which ossification spreads. However, Augier (1931) described and illustrated a zygomatico-squamosal centre and a second squamomastoid centre posterior to it. Fazekas and Kósa (1978) described three independent centres, which unite by the third lunar month, the first being near the base of the zygomatic process, the second for the main part of the squama and a third posterior part, the last two centres being separated by a deep fissure until the eighth month. The bone in the ninth week is described by Macklin (1914, 1921) as a thin, narrow plate just lateral to the upper parts of the malleus and incus terminating in a pointed zygomatic process above the root of which there is a small foramen. The squama itself is short supero-inferiorly and the edges are serrated both behind and in front.

By mid-fetal life, the squamous temporal is recognizable as it has assumed more adult proportions (Figs. 5.31 and 5.33). The **squama** is a delicate, almost flat semicircular plate with finely serrated edges. About one-third of the way along the lower border, the **zygomatic process** projects anteriorly from a thickened root, below which is a small curved plate, which will become the **mandibular fossa**. Postero-inferior to the root of the zygomatic process is the **scutum**, a triangular extension with a sharp inferior angle, which later becomes pneumatized. On the medial surface, the scutum is delimited superiorly by a ledge of bone, which fuses with the tegmen tympani postnatally (see below).

A detailed histological account of the development of the **tympanic** part of the temporal bone can be found in Anson *et al.* (1955) and Ars (1989). At about 9 weeks, the first ossification centre is seen between the first and second pharyngeal arches, anterior to the cartilaginous anlage of the incus. It is posterior to the mandible and inferior to the squamous plate, both of which have already started to ossify. About a week later, the centre, which will become the anterior horn, is joined by intermediate mesenchymal tissue to four or more other centres arranged in a C-shape. Two weeks later the ossification centres fuse to form an incomplete ring that has expanded to twice its original size, with its anterior part now adjacent to the ossified anterior process of the malleus (goniale). The ring appears radiologically at about 12–13 weeks (Bach-Petersen and Kjær, 1993). By 19 weeks the diameter of the ring has increased by 3.5 times and the **tympanic sulcus** has begun to form on the inner surface, although the tympanic membrane is still not lodged within it.

The tympanic ring (Figs. 5.32 and 5.33) is usually recognizable in isolation from about halfway through fetal life. It is deficient at the upper **tympanic incisure** (notch of Rivinus), which is framed by **anterior** and **posterior horns**. Medially, just below the larger anterior horn, is a transverse groove, the **mallear gutter**, which accommodates the anterior process of the malleus. The groove is delimited above by a ridge (**crista spinarum**), whose ends form **anterior** and **posterior tympanic spines**. The lower, inner end of the mallear gutter protrudes as the **anterior tympanic tubercle**. The **posterior tympanic tubercle** lies about half way down the posterior limb of the ring. The inner surface of the ring is grooved by the **sulcus tympanicus** for the attachment of the tympanic membrane. By 35 weeks, it has attained almost full adult dimensions and there is a localized fusion of the posterior segment to the squamous part of the bone (Anson *et al.*, 1955). At term, the ring is slightly more robust and is usually fused to the squamous part of the temporal at its open ends (Fig. 5.33), the anterior being attached postero-inferior to the root of the zygomatic process and the posterior fusing to the pointed end of the scutum. Here, there is a sharp projection at the petrotympanic fissure, where the chorda tympani leaves the middle ear cavity (iter chordae anterius). At this stage it is still possible to look through the ring into the tympanic cavity of a dry skull and see the auditory ossicles and the oval and round windows.

The **styloid process** ossifies endochondrally from the second pharyngeal arch. The centre for the base of the process, usually called the tympanohyal, appears in the perinatal period (Augier, 1931), followed by several more centres for the main part of the process (stylohyal) during the third and fourth years of life (Rambaud and Renault, 1864).

In summary, at birth, the petrous part of the bone is well ossified. The pointed anterior end has, as yet, an incomplete carotid canal. On the medial side the internal acoustic meatus and the subarcuate fossa are about equal in size and the aqueduct of the vestibule is usually somewhat smaller. From the superior surface, the tegmen tympani projects laterally over the open wall of the middle ear cavity, which is delimited below by the semilunar ledge. The structures of the medial wall of the middle ear, including the oval and round windows, are obvious. Posteriorly, there is a small mastoid portion of the bone. The squamotympanic section of the bone consists of a delicate squama, separated by a ridge of bone on the medial side from a partially pneumatized scutum. The tympanic ring is attached below the root of the zygomatic process by its anterior and posterior ends (Fig. 5.33).

Postnatal growth and fusion

In the perinatal period, the combined squamotympanic part of the bone fuses to the petromastoid part along various segments (Fig. 5.33). First, the ledge on the medial surface of the squamous bone fuses to the reciprocal lateral edge of the tegmen tympani, forming the internal petrosquamous suture (Fig. 5.24b). The scutum, which becomes increasingly pneumatized during this period, thus becomes the lateral wall of the epitympanic recess of the middle ear. Second, the external petrosquamous (squamomastoid) suture is formed where the posterior border of the squamous part fuses with the mastoid part of the bone. This suture often remains evident, even in adult skulls. Gradually the squamous part extends inferiorly, covering the anterior part of the petromastoid and contributing to the tip of the rapidly growing mastoid process. Even after pneumatization, the air cells from the two parts may be divided by a septum of bone (Korner's septum). Finally, the lower part of the tympanic ring fuses with the semilunar ledge at the lower border of the tympanic cavity.

During the first year of life, the anterior and posterior tympanic tubercles enlarge, grow towards each other across the ring and eventually fuse to form a second opening, the foramen of Huschke, below the original meatus (Fig. 5.34). During the same period the

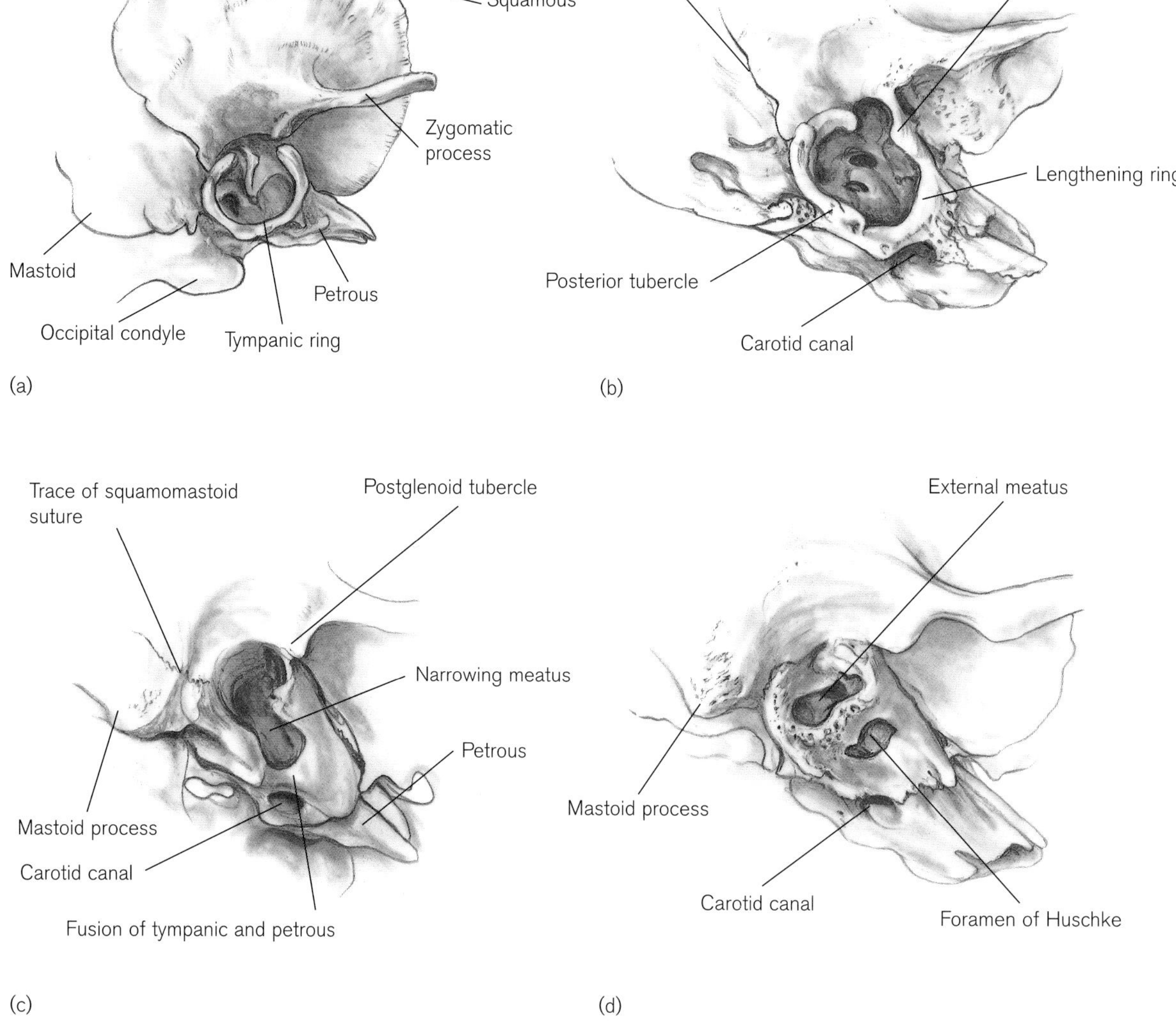

Figure 5.34 Formation of the foramen of Huschke. Drawn from skulls with dental ages of (a) birth; (b) 6 months; (c) 1 year; (d) 2.5 years.

tympanic plate grows laterally, gradually converting the ring into the bony external auditory meatus. Anderson (1960) reported that the anterior tubercle made the major contribution to the formation of the foramen and the posterior tubercle showed an inferior direction of growth. Later still, fingers of bone grow in from the edges of the foramen of Huschke, which gradually closes at about the age of 5 years (Reinhard and Rösing, 1985; Ars, 1989), although the opening may persist as a permanent feature in a significant proportion of adult skulls, depending on the population (see adult). Weaver (1979) and Curran and Weaver (1982) described a method for ageing the infant and child temporal bone using stages based on the growth of the tympanic plate. The first stage is described as 'tympanic ring not developed' and the second 'tympanic ring incomplete'. The stages are misleading as the ring is, in fact, fully developed by midfetal life and is never, despite its name, a complete ring at any age. Unfortunately, the method has been quoted and illustrated in many other texts, including Krogman and Işcan (1986).

The bony meatus continues to grow laterally, displacing the ring from the external osseous opening and this causes a considerable change in orientation of the plane of the tympanic membrane. At term it is almost horizontal but by 4–5 years of age it has acquired its more vertical adult position (Eby and Nadol, 1986; Ars, 1989). The growth of the plate also extends posteriorly and inferiorly to enclose the base of the styloid process in its vaginal sheath and a tongue of bone encloses the anterior border of the carotid canal. This eventually fuses with the petrous base (Fig. 5.24c) but can be seen as a separate entity in some skulls until puberty. On the inferior surface of the petrous bone, an edge of the tegmen tympani protrudes between the growing tympanic plate and the glenoid fossa, thus splitting the squamotympanic fissure into a petrotympanic part posteriorly and a petrosquamous part anteriorly (Fig. 5.24d).

Recent advances in technology and surgery have made cochlear implantation possible in profoundly deaf young children. In order to attach wires onto the skull surface, it has been necessary to record accurate measurements of those parts of the bone that show significant postnatal growth. Eby and Nadol (1986), in a radiological and histological study, found that a very slight increase in width of the tympanic cavity occurred in the first 6 months of life. Mastoid width and depth increased rapidly up to the age of 7 years with no apparent sexual dimorphism. Mastoid length, on the other hand, showed two periods of growth, the first occuring before 7 years and the second phase between 9 and 15 years in females and 11 and 19 years in males. Dahm *et al.* (1993) recorded a doubling in depth of the external auditory canal from birth to adulthood, with most of this occuring in the first 6 months of life. They confirmed the growth in all directions of the mastoid process and noted that the digastric ridge was only visible in bones older than 6 months of age. Simms and Neely (1989) measured the growth of the lateral part of the temporal bone, including the squama, from birth to adult life and found that there was very rapid growth increase in dimensions from birth to 4 years, after which growth slowed dramatically but continued until age 20.

Both the time and pattern of fusion of parts of the styloid process are very variable. Normally the base and various sections of the stylohyal part fuse to form a styloid process in late puberty or early adult life. Common variations include non-fusion throughout life or fusion together with the ossified ligament (ceratohyal) and superior horns (basihyal) of the hyoid bone. Lengelé and Dehm (1988), who recorded short and long types of hyoid bones, concluded that the short ones were the result of ossification of the tympanohyal alone, whereas those of the long group were the result of fusion of the tympano- and stylohyal segments (see adult bone).

The fusion of the petrous temporal to the lateral occipital at the jugular growth plate (petro-exoccipital synchondrosis/jugular synchondrosis) is described under 'Occipital bone'.

Ossification of the auditory ossicles

Ossification of the **auditory ossicles** begins at 16 weeks *in utero* and each bone has a different pattern of ossification and remodelling. Cartilage is retained on their articular surfaces and on the manubrium of the malleus, the short crus of the incus and the stapedial base.

Between 16 and 17 weeks the ossification centre for the **malleus** appears as a plaque of periosteal bone at the head, near its junction with Meckel's cartilage. It spreads rapidly forming a shell around the ossicle, except for the manubrium, which retains a cartilaginous covering around an endochondral bony centre until the perinatal period (Richany *et al.*, 1954). The anterior process (goniale), which was formed in membrane, finally fuses with the main part of the ossicle at about 19 weeks (Anson *et al.*, 1960). At the same time, the malleus loses its proximity to Meckel's cartilage, which is starting to undergo de-organization, although the anterior ligament of the malleus is thought to be a remaining part.

The ossification centre of the **incus** appears slightly before that of the malleus, at about 16 weeks, as a thin layer of perichondral bone on the anterior part of the long crus, which spreads rapidly to completely invest the surface of the ossicle. The main bulk of the ossicle then becomes converted into dense endochondral bone by late fetal life (Richany *et al.*, 1954). The incus, unlike the other two ossicles, is subject to remodelling, particularly in the long crus, at any time during life, although Lannigan *et al.* (1995) report that it often results in resorption without regrowth.

Ossification of the **stapes** starts about 2 weeks later than in the incus and malleus and takes a very different course. The other two ossicles keep the relative shape, size and bulk of their original cartilage anlage. The stapes undergoes such extensive resorption and remodelling that the final bone is actually less bulky than the fetal model. Richany *et al.* (1954) described a single perichondral centre that appears on the obturator surface of the base of the stapes at about 18 weeks of fetal life but Dass and Makhni (1966) described, and illustrated (with alizarin staining and histological sections), three centres appearing at about the same age. These fuse to form a U-shaped ossified area, which gradually spreads up the crura towards the head until the whole ossicle is converted to bone at about 24 weeks. As soon as a shell of bone has covered the whole surface, resorption begins and it loses most of its bulk, so that at 6 fetal months the stapes has acquired its relatively gracile adult structure. Both crura are converted to three-sided pillars of bone that open towards the obturator foramen (Richany *et al.*, 1954). The base and the head are also hollow on their obturator surfaces, but are bilaminar, consisting of a layer of cartilage and endochondral bone (Anson *et al.*, 1948). Dass *et al.* (1969) describe resorption continuing into postnatal life.

Practical notes

Sideing the juvenile temporal

Pars petrosa (Figs. 5.30 and 5.33) – the perinatal bone can be recognized at about midfetal life and the descriptions can be found in the main text. Sideing of the perinatal bone depends on identifying the middle ear cavity, which lies laterally and the intracranial surface, which is medial. On the lateral surface, the smooth mastoid part of the bone lies posterior to the semicircular ledge to which the tympanic ring may be fused. On the intracranial surface, the anteriorly pointing subarcuate fossa lies above the oval internal auditory meatus.

Pars squama (Figs. 5.31 and 5.33) – this part of the bone assumes adult morphology by midfetal life. Sideing depends on identifying either the zygomatic process, which points anteriorly from the lateral surface, or the triangular pneumatized scutum, with a straight anterior border lying below the ledge (see Fig. 5.31). Fragments of the rest of the squama are probably indistinguishable from other calvarial fragments. An isolated zygomatic process could be mistaken for an incomplete posterior arch of the atlas (see Chapter 6 – Fig. 6.34).

Pars tympani (Figs. 5.32 and 5.33) – the tympanic ring assumes its characteristic shape by midfetal life. It is difficult to side until late fetal life when the sulcus for the tympanic membrane has developed on the medial side. At the superior tympanic incisure the anterior horn is more robust than the posterior horn, which tapers off to a point. By birth, the ring is usually partly fused to the pars squama.

Sideing the auditory ossicles

Malleus (Fig. 5.28a)	Place with the head pointing superiorly and the manubrium inferiorly. Turn so that the slender anterior process is pointing downwards and the articular surface for the incus is visible on the head. The short lateral process points to the side from which the bone comes.
Incus (Fig. 5.28b)	Place with the short crus pointing horizontal and the long crus pointing inferiorly. Turn so that the lenticular process is pointing upwards and the superior half of the articular surface for the malleus is visible. The short crus points to the side from which the bone comes.
Stapes (Figs. 5.28c and 5.28d)	Place with the head pointing superiorly and the footplate pointing inferiorly. Turn so that the footplate has its flat surface below and its rounded surface uppermost. The more curved and slightly more robust posterior crus is on the side from which the bone comes. It is sometimes difficult to side a stapes, as many of the features are not at all well defined.

Morphological summary

Fetal

Wks 3–25	Development of membranous labyrinth
Wks 6–16	Cartilaginous anlagen of ossicles developing
Wk 7–8	Ossification centres for pars squama and goniale appear
Wk 9	First ossification centre for pars tympani appears
Wks 9–15	Development of cartilaginous otic capsule
Wk 12	Centres for tympanic ring joined together
Wk 16	First ossification centre for otic capsule appears. Ossification centre for incus appears
Wks 16–17	Ossification centre for malleus appears
Wk 18	Ossification centre(s) for stapes appear(s)

Wk 19	Goniale fuses to malleus
Wk 30	Tympanic cavity complete except for lateral wall
Wk 35	Epitympanum complete Pneumatization of petromastoid starts Posterior segment of ring fuses to squamous part
Birth	Bone usually represented by two parts: petromastoid and squamotympanic
During yr 1	Petromastoid and squamotympanic parts fuse. Anterior and posterior tympanic tubercles commence growth
1–5 yrs	Growth of tympanic plate and formation of foramen of Huschke. Mastoid process forming

Table 5.5 Dimensions of the fetal temporal bone

	Pars squama		
Age (weeks)	Height (mm)	Width (mm)	Length (mm)
12	2.8	2.8	7.0
14	3.6	3.6	9.3
16	6.7	10.1	11.5
18	9.0	12.4	15.0
20	10.6	14.0	17.4
22	11.8	15.4	18.8
24	13.0	16.9	20.5
26	14.3	18.6	21.0
28	16.0	20.2	22.2
30	17.7	21.5	23.6
32	19.8	24.1	26.5
34	22.4	26.1	28.3
36	22.9	26.9	29.6
38	24.1	29.9	31.6
40	25.4	32.6	34.2

Height: maximum distance from centre of tympanic notch to superior border of bone.
Width: maximum distance across bone parallel to length measurement.
Length: postero-inferior point on bone to anterior end of zygomatic process.

	Pars petrosa		Tympanic ring
Age (weeks)	Length (mm)	Width (mm)	diameter (mm)
14	–	–	4.0
16	10.5	5.3	5.7
18	12.3	5.7	7.5
20	14.4	8.7	8.0
22	17.3	9.7	8.5
24	18.8	10.2	9.0
26	19.9	10.6	9.5
28	21.4	10.9	9.9
30	22.5	13.1	10.5
32	27.7	13.5	10.8
34	29.7	15.4	11.5
36	33.0	16.1	11.8
38	35.1	17.0	12.0
40	38.1	17.5	12.5

Pars petrosa: length: maximum anteroposterior distance across bone; width: maximum distance at right angles to length across arcuate eminence.
Tympanic ring: diameter: maximum distance across ring at level of anterior tympanic tubercle.
Adapted from Fazekas and Kósa (1978).

Metrics

Measurements of the petrous, squamous and tympanic parts of the bone during fetal life are recorded by Fazekas and Kósa (1978, Table 5.5). Anson *et al.* (1955) record the increase in diameter of the tympanic ring from 9 fetal weeks to 1 year postnatal but do not state their osteological landmarks. Moss *et al.* (1956) recorded length and height of the pars squama from 8 to 20 fetal weeks but again, landmarks are not defined. Eby and Nadol (1986) and Dahm *et al.* (1993) recorded measurements for many different parameters of the bone from infancy to adult life. They are clinically, rather than dry bone, related and the relevant texts should be consulted for details. Schulter (1976) gave figures for 25 variables of the adult bone in three different populations. Spoor (1993) recorded different measurements and indices of the labyrinth as seen on CT scans from 24 fetal weeks to adult life and compared them with previous figures.

III. THE SPHENOID

The adult sphenoid

The sphenoid[12] (Fig. 5.35) lies in the centre of the skull and this is the key to an appreciation of its anatomy. It articulates with the ethmoid, frontal, zygomatics, parietals, squamous and petrous temporals, vomer and occipital (Figs. 5.1–5.3). It consists of a central body, lying in the skull base; two lesser wings contributing to the anterior cranial fossa and the orbits; two greater wings, which lie in the middle cranial fossa and form part of the lateral walls of the cranial cavity and two pairs of pterygoid plates extending vertically beneath the skull base.

[12] *Sphenoid* and *eidos* (Greek meaning 'wedge, shape'). *Wespenbein* (German meaning 'wasp bone') referring to its resemblance to a flying insect!

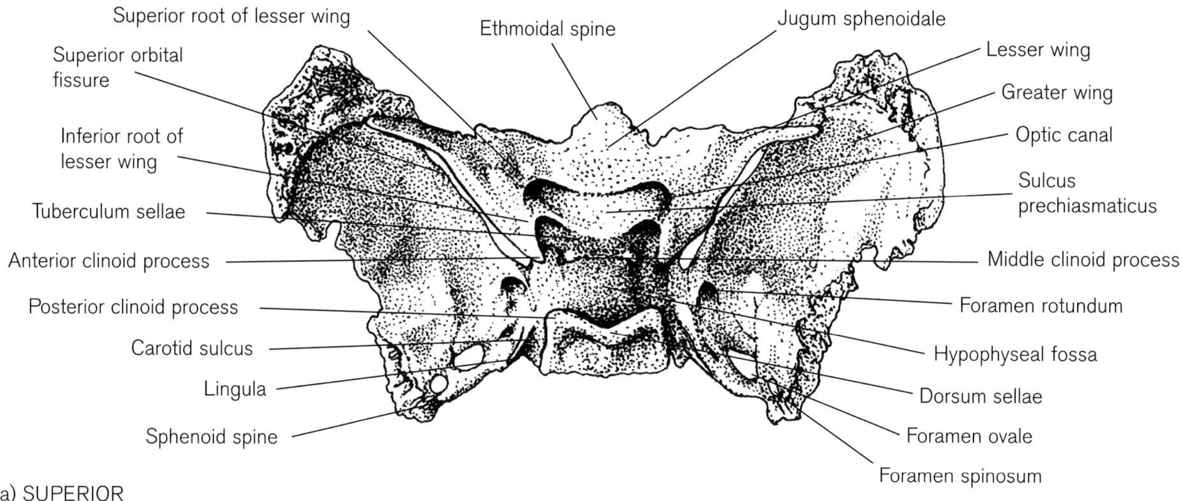

(a) SUPERIOR

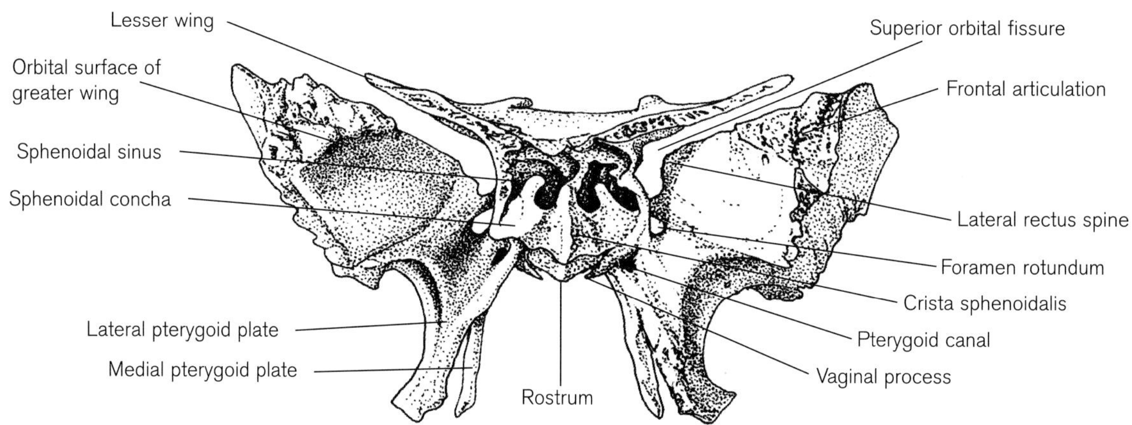

(b) ANTERO-INFERIOR

Figure 5.35 Adult sphenoid.

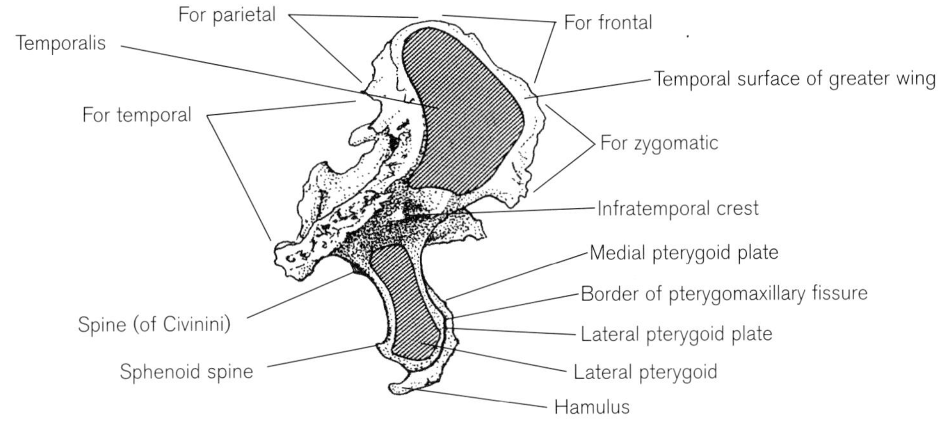

(c) RIGHT LATERAL

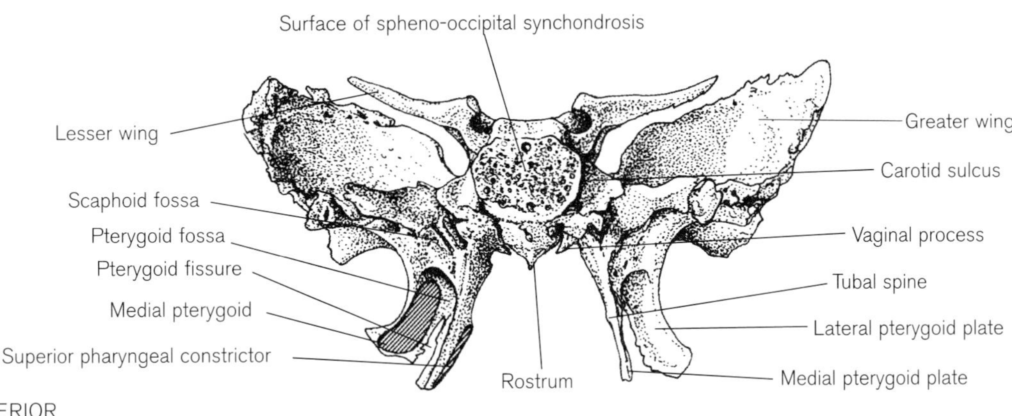

(d) POSTERIOR

Figure 5.35 *(Continued).*

The **corpus** (body) of the sphenoid is cuboidal. The front of the **superior** surface lies in the anterior cranial fossa where it forms a smooth bridge, the **jugum** (planum) **sphenoidale**, which normally articulates with the ethmoid bone, sometimes via an anteriorly pointing ethmoidal spine. In a minority of cases, retro-ethmoidal processes of the frontal bone meet and intervene between the cribriform plate and the jugum (see ethmoid bone). The jugum is continuous with a triangular lesser wing on either side the posterior corner of which forms an **anterior clinoid**[13] **process** overhanging the middle cranial fossa (Fig. 5.2). The free posterior edge of the jugum as seen on a lateral radiograph is known as the limbus sphenoidale. Posterior to the jugum is a groove, the **sulcus prechiasmaticus**, leading laterally on either side into the **optic canals**. Contrary to what may be expected, the optic chiasma does not usually occupy the sulcus, but tends to lie somewhat posterior to it (Lawrence, 1894; Schaeffer, 1924). The relative widths of the jugum and the sulcus depend on the variable posterior growth of the presellar part of the bone, with a wide jugum associated with a narrow sulcus and vice versa (Schaeffer, 1924; Kier, 1968). Posterior to the sulcus the superior surface forms the raised central portion of the middle cranial fossa known as the **sella turcica**, because of its supposed likeness to a Turkish saddle. The anterosuperior margin of the sella, (the pommel of the saddle) is the raised **tuberculum sellae** (olivary prominence) whose lateral ends commonly bear the small **middle clinoid processes**. The posterior part of the saddle forms a raised ridge, the **dorsum sellae**, the lateral ends of which form the pointed **posterior clinoid processes**. The anterior and posterior processes form attachments for the free and fixed borders

[13] *Kline* (Greek meaning 'bed'). The area of the sella with its clinoid processes and covered with the diaphragma sellae has a fancied resemblance to a canopied, four-poster bed. Hence clinical medicine – practised at the bedside.

of the tentorium cerebelli, respectively. The free edge of the dorsum often shows grooves, which are occupied by vessels and nerves (Bisaria, 1984).

A common anomaly reported by Augier (1931), Keyes (1935), Kier (1966) and Saunders and Popovich (1978) is bony bridging between the different clinoid processes. The most common form is fusion between the anterior and middle clinoid process, forming the clinocarotid (caroticoclinoid) canal through which the internal carotid artery passes upwards at the anterior end of the cavernous sinus. Less common is fusion between the anterior and posterior clinoid processes. The incidence of the various types of bridging were reported by Keyes (1935) in 4000 skulls of Black and White Americans, and Ossenberg (1970, 1976) in Native American populations. Some authorities (Shapiro and Janzen, 1960) believe that bridging is the result of ossification of either the clinocarotid ligament or a fold of dura. Ossification of this type is usually recognized as an age-related phenomenon, but as clinoid bridging is commonly reported in fetuses and infants, this seems an unlikely explanation. Augier's suggestion that it represents an abnormality at a much earlier stage in the development of the chondrocranium appears more likely. Evidence from a familial study by Saunders and Popovich (1978) suggests that there may be a mechanism of polygenic inheritance.

The seat of the saddle is the deep **fossa hypophysialis**, which is covered by the diaphragma sellae, a layer of dura pierced by the stalk of the pituitary gland. An occasional foramen in the floor of the sella turcica can lead back into a canal through the septum of the sinus, which can end in the vomer (Cave, 1931), or pass straight through the bone (Arey, 1950) to emerge on the base of the skull. Bowdler (1971) reported that these so-called craniopharyngeal canals are seen as vertical transradiant regions on X-rays of some neonatal and infant skulls, but are rare in the adult. At one time they were thought to represent the remains of the hypophyseal recess (of Rathké), which forms part of the developing pituitary gland. Arey (1950) and Lowman *et al.* (1966) made detailed studies of dry skulls and sections of early embryos and confirmed that the remains of Rathké's pouch disappear at 8–9 weeks of fetal life and that the canals provide a channel for vessels concerned with the ossification of the body of the bone. They would therefore be comparable with the basivertebral veins, which serve the same purpose as those seen associated with the body of a vertebra (see Chapter 6). Currarino *et al.* (1985) described a second type of canal, the large craniopharyngeal canal. It occupies most of the floor of the sella, tapers inferiorly and is prone to be associated with craniofacial abnormalities such as meningo-encephalocoeles. Pruett (1928) recorded the dimensions of the sella in dry bone and Di Chiro and Nelson (1962) and Oon (1963) calculated the volume from radiographs. Bruneton *et al.* (1979) reported on the appearance of normal variants of the structures immediately surrounding the sella. Lang (1977) illustrated a long, narrow process, the sella spine, protruding from the floor of posterior part of the sella in an adult male skull.

From the dorsum sellae the sphenoid slopes steeply backwards to fuse at its **posterior** surface with the occipital bone forming the clivus, which supports the pons and medulla oblongata. On either side of the body lies the cavernous venous sinus, through which the internal carotid artery runs forwards from the foramen lacerum. The bone is sometimes marked by a **carotid sulcus** at the posterior end of which there is a small sharp projection, the **lingula**. This, together with the posterior border of the greater wing and the apex of the petrous temporal bone, forms the bony boundaries of the **foramen lacerum**. The **inferior** surface of the body, which lies in the roof of the nasopharynx, bears a thick, wedge-shaped bar that articulates with the alae of the vomer. The centre of the **anterior** surface has a sharp crest, the **crista sphenoidalis**, which runs down from the ethmoidal spine to a sharp projection, the **rostrum**, which articulates with the vertical plate of the ethmoid, forming part of the nasal septum. On either side of the spine are the **sphenoidal conchae** (ossicula Bertini), curved plates of bone that are nearly always damaged when the skull is disarticulated. They cover the posterior surfaces of the lateral masses of the ethmoid and articulate with the orbital processes of the palatine bones. In their upper portions, they bear the foramina through which the air sinuses drain into the spheno-ethmoidal recess of the nasal cavity.

The **sphenoidal air sinuses** are extremely variable in shape and size. The right and left sides are separated by an intersphenoidal septum, which is normally in the midline anteriorly but often deviates posteriorly. Early anatomical studies (Cope, 1917; Congdon, 1920; van Alyea, 1941; Peele, 1957) classified the different patterns of sinus shape and related them to the ossification centres of the bone and also recorded variations in the walls caused by related structures. Later clinical and radiological studies (Hammer and Rådberg, 1961; Etter, 1963; Elwany *et al.*, 1983) were concerned with the effects that these variations might have on trans-sphenoidal hypophysectomy. The sinuses can be limited to the presphenoid area (conchal); extend back into the basisphenoid or occipitosphenoid; or laterally into the greater wings and pterygoid plates (Wigh, 1951).

The **alae minores** (lesser wings) of the sphenoid are triangular plates attached on either side of the jugum. The **anterior** border of each wing articulates with the posterior border of the orbital plate of the frontal bone lateral to the cribriform plate, and may also articulate with the greater wing towards its tip (Fig. 5.2). The **lateral** border passes posteromedially, forming the upper edge of the superior orbital fissure, and ends in the anterior clinoid process. The wing is attached at its **medial** border by two roots, which enclose the **optic canal** through which pass the optic nerve and the ophthalmic artery. The **superior root**, joining the jugum, is broad and flat. The **inferior root** (metopic root/posterior strut), which attaches at the lateral side of the prechiasmatic sulcus, is narrower and thinner. The intracranial entrance of the optic canal has its long diameter in the horizontal plane, whereas the orbital opening has the larger diameter in the vertical plane (Wolff, 1976). Detailed measurements of the size and angulation of the canals have been made by Lang (1995) and Berlis *et al.* (1992).

Anomalies and variations of the lesser wings include a variety of supernumerary ossicles and also abnormalities of the optic canal and superior orbital fissure. Duplication of the optic canal is comparatively rare but has been reported by White (1923), Augier (1931), Keyes (1935) and Warwick (1951). Kier (1966) made detailed observations of the development of the optic canal and believed that the previous descriptions probably referred only to the intracranial, rather than the orbital, opening of the canal. Both this condition and other anomalies, such as spurs of bone in the opening and the 'keyhole' and grooved optic floor anomalies, can be explained by malformation during development of the posterior root of the lesser wing (see below). Duplicated cranial openings appear to have a much higher incidence in certain populations (Kier, 1966), suggesting a possible genetic basis. The superior orbital fissure lies between the greater and lesser wings and may be divided into a medial, broad segment and a narrow, lateral segment. Subdivision of the medial end has been reported by Warwick (1951), Lang (1977) and Bisaria *et al.*, (1996a) and variations in the shape of the lateral end have been detailed by Ray (1955). Augier (1931) described and illustrated small bones along the suture of the anterior surface of the lesser wing, which he named ali-spheno-frontal or spheno-ethmoido-frontal ossicles, depending on their position relative to other bones.

The **alae majores** (greater wings) are continuous with the carotid sulcus at the sides of the body. Each wing extends laterally and superiorly and forms the anterior wall and floor of the lateral part of the middle cranial fossa and most of the lateral wall of each orbit. The **cranial surface** supports the anterior temporal pole of the cerebral hemisphere and is grooved by cerebral gyri and branches of the middle meningeal vessels. Around the medial surface of the greater wing is arranged the 'crescent of foramina' (Grant, 1948; Fig. 5.36). The greater and lesser wings form the margins of the **superior orbital fissure**, which transmits the ophthalmic division of the Vth (trigeminal), and the IIIrd (oculomotor), IVth (trochlear) and VIth (abducens) cranial nerves, which pass forwards from the cranial cavity into the orbit. The ophthalmic veins pass backwards through the fissure from the orbit to drain into the cavernous sinus. Below the medial end of the fissure the **foramen rotundum** transmits the

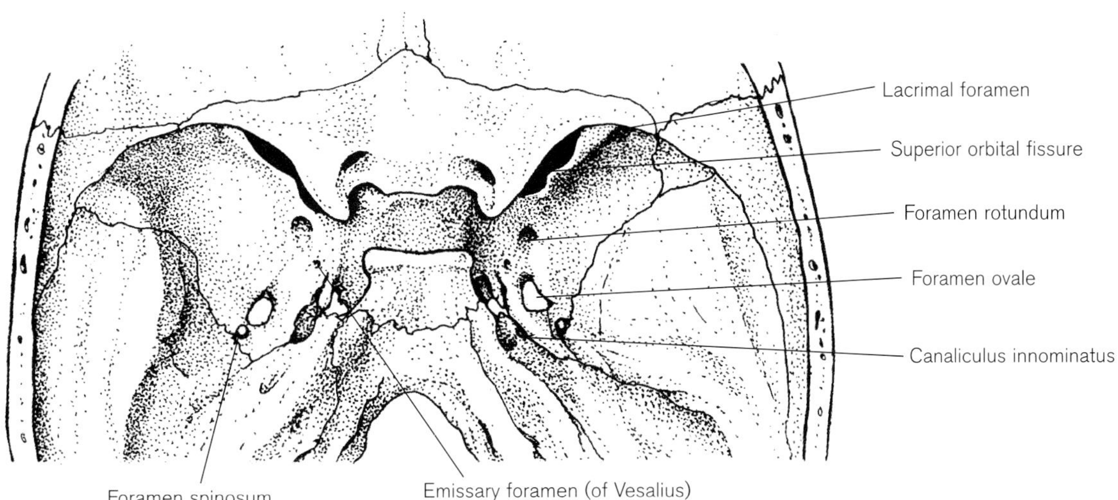

Figure 5.36 Crescent of foramina in the greater wing of the sphenoid.

maxillary nerve into the pterygopalatine fossa. The **foramen ovale** lies near the posterior border of the wing and carries the mandibular nerve, the accessory meningeal artery, and sometimes, the lesser petrosal nerve to the infratemporal fossa. Just posterior and lateral to this, the **foramen spinosum** transmits the middle meningeal vessels and a meningeal branch of the mandibular nerve, the nervus spinosus.

It is not uncommon to find variations in the arrangement of the normal crescent of foramina. Ginsberg *et al.* (1994) described openings in relation to the foramen rotundum that led to the infratemporal fossa, which they proposed calling the inferior and lateral rotundal canals. The foramen ovale and foramen spinosum may be conjoined and either, or both, may be incomplete and open posteriorly to the petrosphenoid suture (Greig, 1929; Augier, 1931; Berry and Berry, 1967; Ossenberg, 1970, 1976; Reinhard and Rösing, 1985; Ginsberg *et al.*, 1994). In addition, there may be a small meningo-orbital (lacrimal) foramen (of Hyrtl) lateral to the apex of the superior orbital fissure which, when present, can carry a communicating branch between the orbital and middle meningeal vessels (Royle, 1973; Santo Neto *et al.*, 1984; Mysorekar and Nandedkar, 1987). The small sphenoidal emissary foramen (of Vesalius) may lie anterior and medial to the foramen ovale. It opens near the scaphoid fossa and can transmit a vein, which joins the cavernous sinus with the pterygoid plexus. Boyd (1930) recorded this in 14% of skulls but more recent radiological observations (Lanzieri *et al.*, 1988; Ginsberg *et al.*, 1994) found it to be more common (60%) than previously reported. A further minute occasional foramen, the innominate canal (of Arnold) may lie between the foramen ovale and the foramen spinosum. It then transmits the lesser petrosal nerve, which otherwise passes through the foramen ovale. Chandler and Derezinski (1935) correlated the variations of the course of the middle meningeal artery with these inconstant foramina in dry and cadaveric skulls and Ginsberg *et al.* (1994) have reviewed the CT appearance and prevalence of the canals of the greater wing. Rak *et al.* (1996) have recently compared the arrangement of the foramina in the African great apes, early hominids and modern man. Much of the variability in the pattern of grooves and foramina results from the different routes taken by emissary veins of the middle meningeal plexus to reach the pterygoid plexus (James *et al.*, 1980).

The anterior part of the greater wing is thickened to form a triangular articular surface, which is only visible in the disarticulated skull. It divides the extracranial part of the wing into triangular orbital and quadrangular temporal surfaces set roughly at right angles to each other. The upper border of the **orbital surface** articulates with the frontal bone laterally, and medially forms the lower edge of the superior orbital fissure. Here, near its medial end, it normally bears the lateral rectus spine, to which is attached the common tendinous ring and possibly fibres of the lateral rectus muscle. Its variation in shape has been recorded by Bisaria *et al.* (1996b). The inferior border of the orbital surface forms the upper edge of the inferior orbital fissure, while the lateral border articulates with the zygomatic bone. The **temporal surface** of the greater wing articulates at its anterior border with the zygomatic and frontal bones, and with the squamous temporal at its posterior border. In the great majority of skulls, the superior border meets the parietal bone (Fig. 5.3), but the pattern of articulation in this region (the pterion) is variable and can be the site of anomalous epipteric bones (see Squamous temporal bone). The upper part of the surface gives origin to fibres of the temporalis muscle down to the level of a sharp, irregular, transverse ridge, the **crista infratemporalis**. Below this, the surface provides attachment for the upper fibres of the lateral pterygoid muscle and forms the upper part of the posterior edge of the pterygomaxillary fissure. The posterolateral corner of the greater wing bears the sharp **sphenoid spine**, to which is attached the sphenomandibular ligament. The undersurface of this part of the wing, where it borders on the petrous temporal bone, gives attachment to part of the cartilaginous auditory tube.

The **pterygoid processes**, (Greek meaning, 'wing') each consisting of a medial and a lateral lamina (plate), hang vertically from the base of the bone at the junction of the body and greater wings. The **medial plates** are almost parallel with each other, but the lateral plates diverge so that they lie at right angles to each other. The anterior borders of each medial and lateral plate are fused together above and diverge below to enclose the **pterygoid fissure**, whose margins articulate with the palatine bone. Posteriorly, the plates lie further apart and the space between them, the **pterygoid fossa**, gives rise to fibres of both the medial and lateral pterygoid muscles. Just above this fossa, at the junction of the medial plate and the body, is the smaller **scaphoid fossa**, to which part of the tensor veli palatini muscle is attached. Above and medial to the fossa is the posterior opening of the **pterygoid** (Vidian) **canal**, only visible in the disarticulated skull, which leads anteriorly through the bone to transmit nerves and vessels into the pterygopalatine fossa.

The lateral surface of the **lateral plate** forms part of the wall of the infratemporal fossa. Its anterior border forms the lower part of the posterior boundary of the **pterygomaxillary fissure**. Its posterior border is free, bearing near its root a small spine (of Civinini). The **medial** pterygoid plate forms the lateral boundary of the posterior naris, where it opens into the nasopharynx. The lower part of its posterior border gives attachment to the superior constrictor muscle of the pharynx and the upper part gives support to the pharyngeal end of the auditory tube, the two parts being separated by a small **tubal spine**. The cartilaginous part of the tube extends from its bony exit in the temporal bone and lies in the groove between the petrous bone and the greater wing of the sphenoid. The lower end of the posterior border is prolonged into the **pterygoid hamulus**, around which the tendon of the tensor veli palatini muscle turns to pass into the soft palate. The upper edge of the plate curves medially to form the **vaginal process** below the body, which articulates with the vomer.

The inferior surface of the greater wing and the pterygoid plates may develop two anomalous bony struts resulting from the ossification of the pterygospinous and the pterygo-alar bars. Their development is described by James *et al.* (1980) and their incidence in the adult is reported by Chouké (1946, 1947), Ossenberg (1970, 1976) and Shaw (1993). The pterygospinous bar passes medial to the foramen spinosum from the spine of Civinini on the lateral plate to the sphenoid spine and transects the foramen ovale. The branches of the mandibular nerve and the pterygoid vessels thus have to pass through the resulting foramen to reach the medial pterygoid muscle. The pterygo-alar bar connects the under surface of the greater wing, lateral to the foramen spinosum, to the root of the lateral pterygoid plate. It encloses a space originally rejoicing in the name of the porus crotophitico-buccinatorius (Hyrtl, 1862) but later, renamed the pterygo-alar foramen (canal) by Chouké (1947). He reported its incidence at about 7% in 6000 skulls. The presence of this anomaly in patients who need injections for trigeminal neuralgia, can cause difficulty in reaching the trigeminal sensory ganglion (Chouké, 1949; Chouké and Hodes, 1951; Shaw, 1993). Both these inconstant foramina and the bony bars are described and illustrated radiologically by Priman and Etter (1959), Shapiro and Robinson (1967) and Shaw (1993). Augier (1931) and Lang (1977) described occasional other bars of bone between the greater sphenoidal wing and the apex of the petrous temporal bone, which can impede the passage of cranial nerves passing forward from the brainstem to their anterior skull exits.

Ossification

The sphenoid bone ossifies from a large number of centres and accounts in the literature vary as to their exact number. Most of the centres fuse during prenatal life and again the pattern is variable. However, it is convenient to divide them into five main groups: those for the body, the lesser wings, the greater wings, the pterygoid plates and the sphenoidal conchae.

The **body** is formed endochondrally from anterior (basi/presphenoid) centres and posterior (basi/postsphenoid) centres. Fusion between the two groups of centres at the synchondrosis intrasphenoidalis takes place at the tuberculum sellae, which is at the junction of the prechordal and chordal regions of the skull base (see Introduction to the skull). Centres for the **presphenoid** part of the body appear at 12–14 fetal weeks and usually consist of bilateral single, or double, centre(s) medial to the optic foramen (Augier, 1931; Kier, 1966). Kodama (1976a) distinguished a constant pair of main centres, a pair of anterior accessory centres and a 'corporal deep centre' composed of two parts. Occasionally, there may be a pair of posterior accessory centres and a middle centre. By about 24 weeks, the main centres have fused together to form the medial wall of the optic foramen. Formation of the interoptic region, which will become the jugum, is variable and may be formed either by extension of the presphenoid centres or by the formation of a median, unpaired rostral centre at about 19–20 weeks. This lower part of the body, which will eventually form the crest, rostrum and ethmoid spine, derives from the corporal deep centre (Kodama, 1976a). The anterior wall of the sella turcica at his stage is still cartilaginous and gradually ossifies in the last trimester by the posterior and medial growth of the presphenoid centres. These extend from the superior to the inferior surface of the body, but may still not be fully ossified until the end of the first year of life (Kier, 1968). The **postsphenoid** centres for the body form in the base of the sella turcica, and are normally paired (Kodama, 1976b) but again, there may be an additional median centre. They appear at about 13 fetal weeks and are usually united by 16 weeks (Noback, 1944; Arey, 1950). Sasaki and Kodama (1976) distinguished pairs of medial basisphenoid and lateral basisphenoid centres, which showed distinct individual differences in size and pattern of fusion. Kjær (1990b, c), in a series of 145 fetuses, also identified different patterns of ossification. There were single and double ossification centres for the postsphenoid, with the single pattern being the more common. The most lateral part of the body, which will form the carotid sulcus and lingula, develops from a separate endochondral centre in the cartilaginous alar processes (see 'Early development of skull'). They join with the main postsphenoid centres some time after the fourth month.

The presphenoid part of body (Figs. 5.37a) is a Y-shaped bone with the single stem facing anteriorly and two limbs pointing posteriorly. The superior surface is relatively smooth and the inferior surface bears a blunt finger-like projection pointing antero-inferiorly. Each posterior limb has three surfaces: the supero-anterior and superoposterior are set at right angles and are articular for the lesser wings. The infero-posterior surfaces of both sides are approximately at right angles and form the upper boundaries of the cruciform space between the pre- and postsphenoid parts of the body. The postsphenoid part of body (Figs. 5.37b, c) becomes recognizable by about the fifth month of fetal life. It is a roughly quadrilateral bone, about twice as wide as it is long with two lateral alar projections extending postero-inferiorly. The centre of the superior surface is concave anteroposteriorly, forming the shallow hypophyseal fossa from which the blunt alar processes slope away laterally. The anterior and posterior surfaces of the body may be divided by deep central fissures, indicating the dual origin from two ossification centres. Later, the alar processes become separated inferiorly from the main part of the body by the carotid sulcus. They develop sharp projections pointing anteriorly, which articulate with the presphenoid part of the body and the posterior processes become the lingulae. Covell (1927) recorded the size of the sella turcica during fetal life and reported that the dimensions at birth were 0.89, 0.54 and 0.29 cm for the transverse, AP and vertical diameters, respectively.

The ossification centres for the **lesser wings** (alipresphenoid) are formed in the orbitosphenoid (ala orbitalis) cartilages at about 12 fetal weeks. This region has been described in detail by Fileti (1927), Kier (1966) and Kier and Rothman (1976) in studies on the development of the optic canal. Between 12 and 16 weeks two centres form in the cartilage on the superior and lateral sides of the cartilaginous optic foramen, which rapidly fuse together. They may appear before, or at the same time as, the presphenoid centres for the body. By 16 weeks, the optic foramen is almost surrounded by bone. A small linear process, the antero-inferior segment of the optic strut (posterior root/crus posterior) extends from the lesser wing and fuses with the postsphenoid centre of the body to form the inferolateral border of the optic foramen. At this stage, the foramen resembles a keyhole with the ophthalmic artery occupying the inferior, narrower part and the optic nerve above it in the wider part. The optic canal, as opposed to the foramen, starts to form during the fifth month of fetal life with the formation of a second, or posterosuperior strut, which joins the lesser wing to the presphenoid centre of the body. Normally at this time, the ophthalmic artery takes up a more superior position above the second strut and becomes incorporated into the dural sheath of the optic nerve. So for a relatively short time, the optic strut is composed of the two segments enclosing a transitory foramen between them which, on its closure, forms the cranial opening of the optic canal. There are three developmental malformations that may be associated with this stage of development. The 'figure of 8' anomaly occurs when the second strut develops above, instead of below, the ophthalmic artery and so it, and the optic nerve, occupy separate foramina at the cranial entrance to the canal. It would appear to be this arrangement that is described in the literature as a duplicated optic canal. The 'keyhole' anomaly occurs when the second strut does not develop at all, or is very rudimentary, so causing absence of the posterior wall of the canal. The orbital opening then retains its primitive fetal arrangement, with the artery lying in the narrow part below the nerve. There is also a very rare condition, reported by Le Double (1903), which occurs when neither of the struts is formed and the optic canal and superior orbital fissure remain confluent. The 'metopic foramen', described by Augier (1931), as transmitting an aberrant ophthalmic vein, was interpreted by Kier as the transitory foramen in the unfused optic strut.

The lesser wing (Figs. 5.37d) becomes recognizable about halfway through fetal life as a small flat piece of bone shaped like an arrow-head, with the tip of the wing pointing laterally. The superior root, called the anterior crus by Kodama (1976c) is slightly flatter and wider than the inferior root (posterior crus). Later, the difference between the two roots becomes more obvious and the upper root develops a posteromedial projection, which will articulate with the presphenoid part of the body.

Both endochondral and intramembranous ossification centres contribute to the formation of the **greater wings**. The intramembranous centre for each wing appears lateral to the cartilaginous foramen rotundum at about 9–10 fetal weeks and gradually expands to form the major part of the wing. At about 13 weeks, the cartilage in the region where the maxillary nerve branches from the trigeminal ganglion starts to ossify 'like a bent forefinger' to form the endochondral centre for the medial part of the wing (Fawcett, 1910b) and when this joins the lateral intramembranous centre, the foramen rotundum is complete. The inconstant foramen of Vesalius marks the junction of

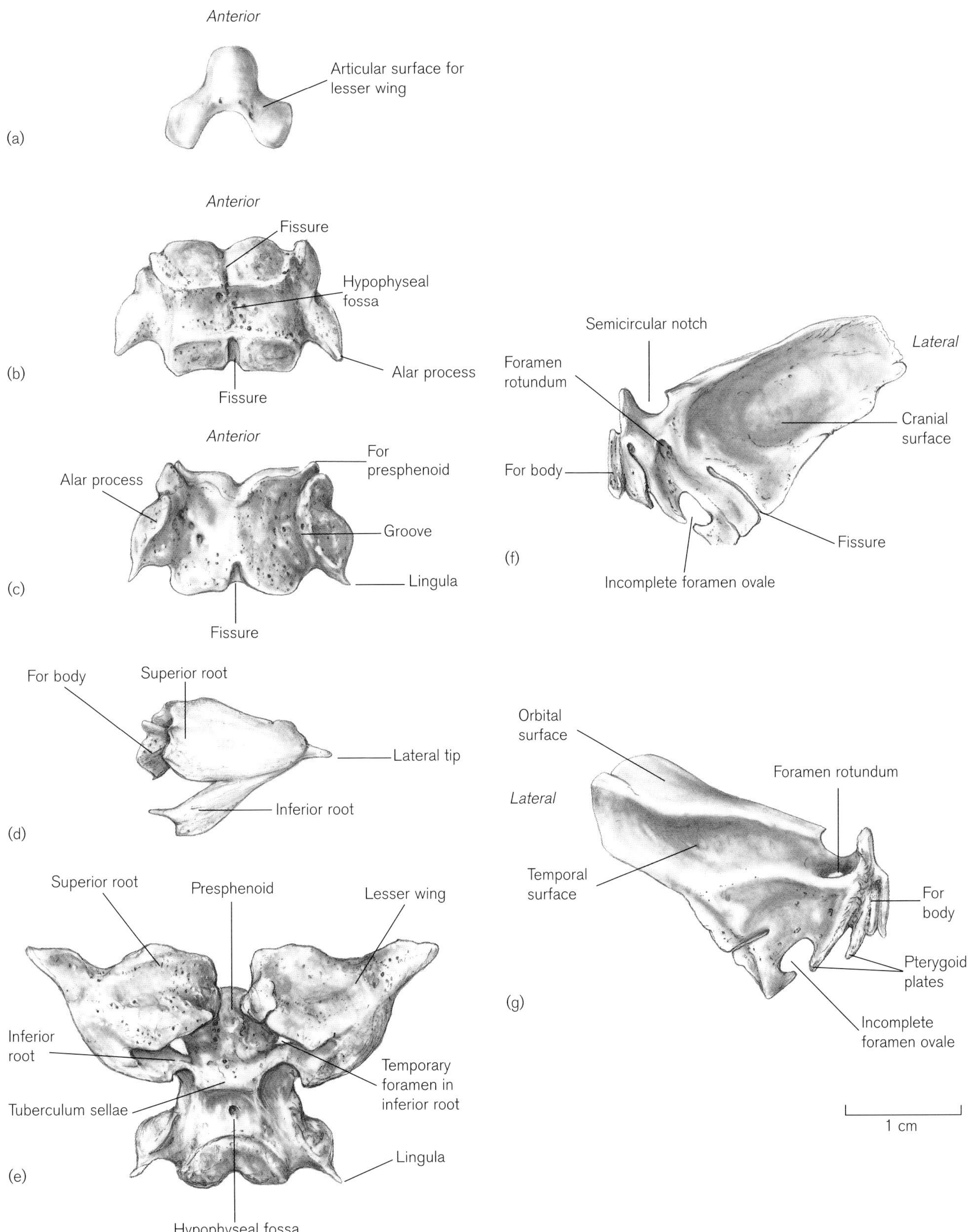

Figure 5.37 Fetal and perinatal sphenoid: (a) presphenoid, superior; (b) postsphenoid superior; (c) postsphenoid, inferior; (d) right lesser wing; (e) lesser wings fused to body; (f) right greater wing, superior; (g) right greater wing, inferior.

the endochondral and membranous portions of the wing so that the foramen ovale, being lateral to this, is entirely within the membranous part. Its margins are represented by a medial process and a lateral tongue of bone, which normally fuse behind the mandibular nerve to complete the foramen. This usually takes place either late in fetal life or during the first year (Augier, 1931), but occasionally fusion may never take place and the foramen ovale remains open to the petrosphenoid suture. The foramen spinosum is normally complete by the second year (Frazer, 1948). The posterior limitations of both the foramen ovale and the foramen spinosum are variable (Kier and Rothman, 1976; Sasaki and Kodama, 1976). James *et al.* (1980) interpret the inconstant pattern of grooves and foramina to be caused by the variable nature of the emissary middle meningeal veins passing to the pterygoid plexus. Braga *et al.* (1998) have suggested that the variations in positions of the two foramina in the great apes, fossil hominids and modern humans can aid in phylogenetic studies of human ancestry.

The intramembranous centre for the **medial pterygoid plate** can be seen medial to the developing tensor veli palatini muscle at about 9–10 fetal weeks, but the **hamulus** develops separately in cartilage at about the third month and rapidly ossifies. The **lateral plate** also ossifies in membrane during the early part of the third month (Fawcett, 1905a). Both the medial and lateral plates become fused to the undersurface of the greater wing between the sixth and eighth fetal months.

The morphology of the greater wing and pterygoid plates (Figs. 5.37f, g) becomes recognizable about halfway through fetal life. The wing can be divided into a posteromedial third and an anterolateral two-thirds by a line running through the foramen rotundum anteriorly and a fissure running for a variable distance into the bone towards it from the posterior surface. Medially, there is a complex surface for articulation with the alar process on the lateral surface of the body. The incomplete foramen ovale can be seen on the posterior surface of the bone, but the foramen spinosum has not yet formed. The lateral two-thirds of the wing has three surfaces. The anterior surface is relatively thicker than the other two and turns up at right angles to form part of the lateral wall of the orbit. Its upper border just above the opening of the foramen rotundum forms a semicircular notch at the medial end of the superior orbital fissure. The gently concave upper (cranial) surface tapers down to the thin, serrated lateral and posterolateral border and the inferior surface is reciprocally convex. At its medial end, the lateral and medial pterygoid plates project downwards. They are closer together anteriorly than posteriorly and the lateral plate extends further posteriorly.

The **sphenoidal conchae** develop from ossification centres, which appear on the medial part of the cartilaginous cupola of the nasal capsule, the future ethmoidal bone, between 4 and 6 lunar months (Schaeffer, 1910a; van Gilse, 1927). Further lower centres are added during the perinatal period and growth continues after birth.

The order in which the different parts of the bone **fuse** together is variable, but the lesser wings always fuse with the presphenoid part of the body in about midfetal life as the optic foramina are forming (Fig. 5.38). The time of fusion of the pre- and postsphenoid parts of the body is variable and, almost certainly, that given in some standard accounts is too early. Augier (1931) stated that it can occur as early as 17 weeks *in utero*, or be delayed until after birth. Ortiz and Brodie (1949) described the appearance on radiographs of unfused pre- and postsphenoidal centres in almost one-third of 139 newborn infants. Shopfner *et al.* (1968) recorded the incidence of a sphenoidal cleft from 750 radiographs and found that it was present in 64% of infants of less than 1 month in age and then progressively decreased to 3% at 3 years. The cleft had a histological structure similar to that of the spheno-occipital synchondrosis. It is difficult to distinguish between these descriptions and those of the craniopharyngeal canal (see adult bone). Also, the late fusion of the two parts of the body does not correspond with Kier's description of the formation of the optic canal, which has the posterior root joining the postsphenoid part of the body at the time of the formation of the optic foramen. Sprinz and Kaufman (1987) described and illustrated the appearance of the lesser wings and the body in a series of perinatal Egyptian crania. The lateral side of the pre- and postsphenoid parts of the body were fused, leaving a space that was commonly triangular or funnel-shaped in the centre, which they called the sphenoidal canal and interpreted as the remaining central, unfused area. They also distinguished this canal from the craniopharyngeal canal which, when present, occurs more posteriorly. Certainly their photographs and descriptions are the most commonly observed appearance in the perinatal period. A similarly shaped foramen is often seen at the junction of the body and dens of the incompletely fused axis vertebra (Chapter 6).

In summary (Fig. 5.38, (1–6)), at **birth** the bone is usually represented by three parts (4): the body with attached lesser wings and two separate greater wings, each with attached pterygoid plates (centre column). The fusion of the two parts of the body may be delayed until

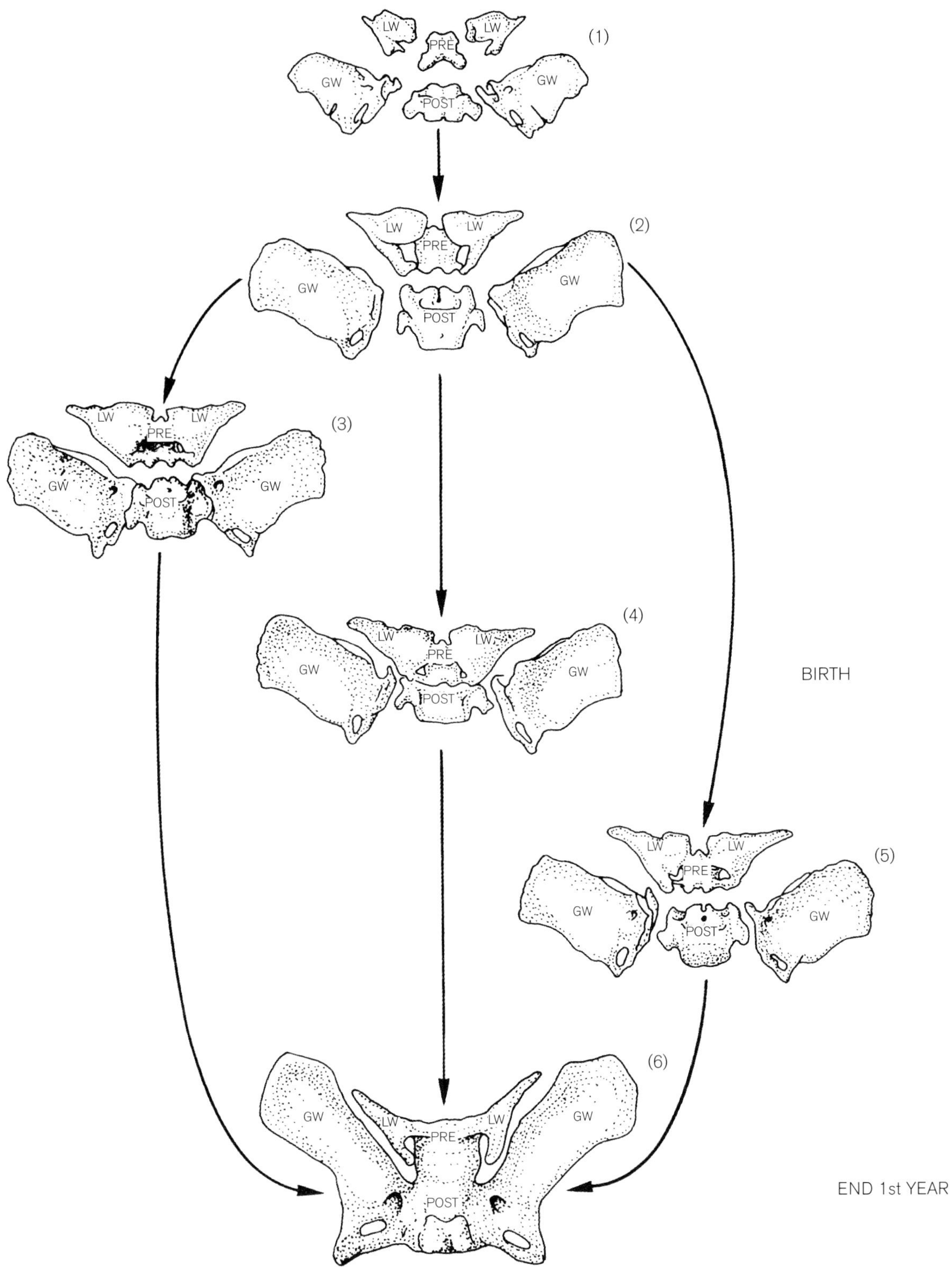

Figure 5.38 Fusion of sphenoid. Centre column usual order of fusion; right and left columns are possible variations.

PRE	Presphenoid part of body	LW	Lesser wing
POST	Postsphenoid part of body	GW	Greater wing

after birth (5) (right column) or, the other less common order of fusion is that the greater wings fuse to the post-sphenoid part of the body before birth (3) (left column). However, by the end of the first year of life, all parts of the bone have usually consolidated into a single structure (6). Variations in the order of fusion are illustrated in Fig. 5.38. In the Spitalfields juvenile crania, Molleson and Cox (1993) found that fusion had already occurred between the body and the greater wings by the fifth postnatal month. The jugum is undeveloped in the perinatal period, as the lesser wings are separated by a cleft, which is filled in by bone during the first year. The anteroposterior growth of the jugum is variable (Figs. 5.39 and 5.40) and is reflected in the reciprocity of the widths of the jugum and sulcus (see adult bone). The posterior margin of the jugum and the limbus sphenoidale may remain separate from the underlying presphenoid for several years leaving a cleft between them. By adulthood, the two structures fuse (Kier, 1968).

Van Alyea (1941), Fujioka and Young (1978) and Wolf *et al.* (1993) recorded the appearance of the sphenoidal sinus from radiographs. Pneumatization is first seen at about 6 months of age and is an extension from the nasal cavity into the conchal area, which gradually spreads into the presphenoid part of the body. It can extend into the basisphenoid by 4 years and is present in 50% of individuals by 8 years and 95% by 12 years. Van Gilse (1927), in a study of the sinus in different species, called this anterior conchal part, which is intimately connected with the nasal capsule, the palaio-sinus, as it is the only one present in certain animals. In the human sphenoid, after the fusion of the nasal capsule and the sphenoid body, pneumatization spreads posteriorly into the basisphenoid. This was named the neo-sinus. According to Vidić (1968a), the dorsum sellae and the posterior clinoid processes are pneumatized in about 20% of individuals between the ages of 12 and 20 years. The sphenoidal conchae gradually become attached to the ethmoid bone by resorption of intervening cartilage. The time of fusion is very variable as it may begin as early as 4 years of age, or be delayed until puberty (Lang, 1995).

Postnatal growth of the sella has been recorded by Acheson and Archer (1959), Latham (1972), Underwood *et al.* (1976) and Chilton *et al.* (1983). As the distance between the sella and the foramen caecum of the ethmoid (Fig. 5.2) remains constant after

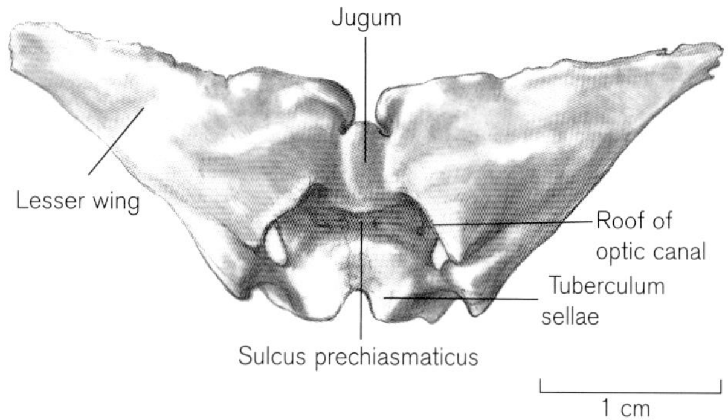

Figure 5.39 Immature jugum sphenoidale.

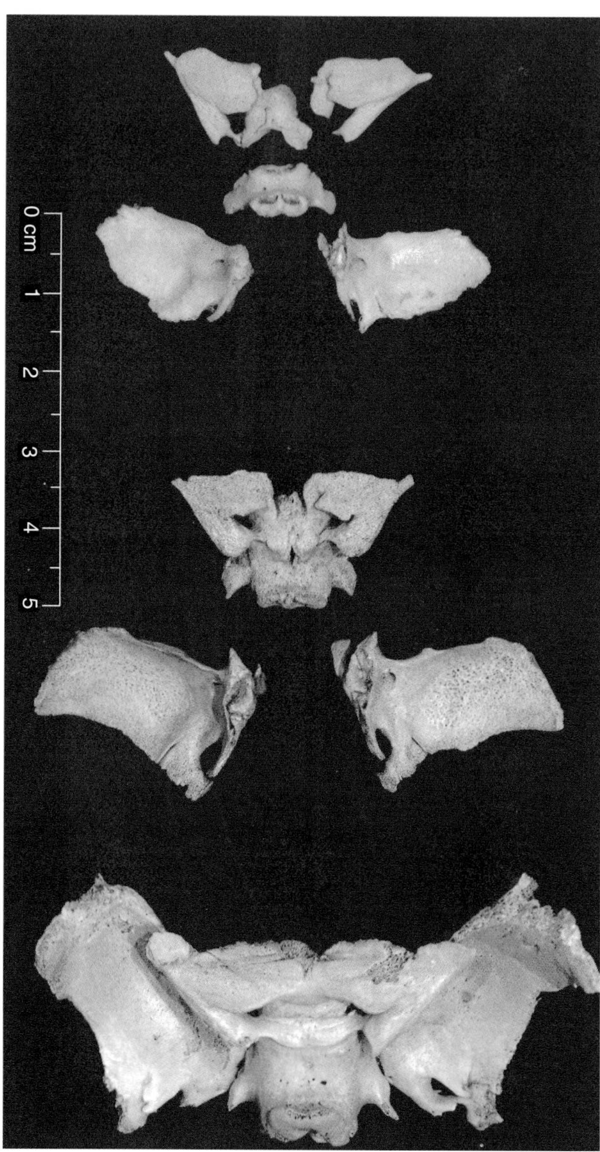

Figure 5.40 Development of the sphenoid. Top – fetal, the presphenoid and postsphenoid parts of the body are separate, the right lesser wing is still unfused to the body; middle – birth, body and lesser wings are fused; bottom – about 6 months *postpartum*, the jugum is still immature, the foramen ovale is open posteriorly and the dorsum sellae is not yet ossified.

about the seventh year, there is probably little growth at the spheno-ethmoidal suture after the end of the first decade (Scott, 1958). Latham (1972) reported histological evidence of bone resorption in the posterior wall of the fossa for at least the first 10 years of life. This resulted in the upward and backward movement of the sella point, which would not have been obvious by measurements taken on radiographs alone.

Knott (1974) used the increase in distance between the centres of the right and left foramen rotundum, as recorded from radiographs, as one of the parameters in a longitudinal study of cranial growth. Increase in size in individuals between the ages of 6 and 26 years ranged from 3.2 mm to 8.3 mm. The spheno-occipital synchondrosis at birth is wide and extends superiorly to include the region of the dorsum sellae and posterior clinoid processes (Moss-Salentijn, 1975). This remains largely cartilaginous for at least 5 years after birth (Latham, 1966, 1972) and there are still small areas of cartilage up to the age of puberty (Ingervall and Thilander, 1972). It ossifies by extension from the posterior part of the body (Augier, 1931). The age of closure of the spheno-occipital synchondrosis is discussed under the section on the occipital bone.

Practical notes

Sideing/orientation of the juvenile sphenoid (Fig. 5.37)

Body – recognition of this part of the bone will depend on the state of fusion (see text) but by late fetal life the pre- and postsphenoid parts are normally fused together and the hypophyseal fossa has assumed its characteristic shape.

Lesser wing – this part of the bone becomes recognizable by mid-fetal life, as it resembles an arrowhead with the superior root anterior and flatter than the narrower posterior root. Both lesser wings are usually fused to the body before birth and form a characteristic shaped bone.

Greater wing – this is usually recognizable by mid-fetal life. Sideing depends on recognizing the concave intracranial surface with the obvious foramen rotundum pointing anteriorly and a posterior fissure in the bone. The pterygoid plates are attached inferiorly. Both wings normally fuse to the body soon after birth.

Table 5.6 Dimensions of the fetal sphenoid bone

	Body		Lesser wing		Greater wing	
Age (weeks)	Length (mm)	Width (mm)	Length (mm)	Width (mm)	Length (mm)	Width (mm)
12	–	–	–	–	5.0	1.5
14	–	–	–	–	5.1	2.3
16	2.7	4.5	4.7	4.0	10.3	5.7
18	3.7	5.5	5.9	4.8	13.1	7.0
20	5.1	9.6	6.3	5.2	15.3	8.5
22	5.9	10.6	7.9	6.0	17.1	9.2
24	6.1	11.7	9.0	6.4	19.0	10.1
26	7.4	12.2	10.6	7.0	19.7	10.5
28	7.9	12.5	12.5	7.6	21.6	11.7
30	8.1	13.5	13.7	8.2	22.0	12.6
32	8.6	14.5	14.7	8.5	24.5	13.7
34	9.1	15.0	15.1	9.3	25.4	14.8
36	9.5	16.0	15.8	10.3	26.4	15.4
38	10.9	17.2	17.1	11.0	28.7	16.1
40	11.7	17.9	19.4	12.4	31.0	17.4

Body: length: midline distance between the synchondrosis intrasphenoidalis and spheno-occipitalis;
width: maximum transverse distance in the mid-hypophyseal fossa.
Lesser wing: length: lateral tip of lesser wing to midline of synchondrosis intrasphenoidalis (lateral tip of lesser wing to medial end of lesser wing in younger fetuses);
width: maximum distance of lesser wing across optic canal.
Greater wing: length: maximum distance between medial pterygoid plate and lateral tip of greater wing;
width: maximum distance between sphenoidal spine and anterior end of pterygoid plate.
Adapted from Fazekas and Kósa (1978).

Morphological summary

Fetal	
Wks 9–10	Medial pterygoid plate and lateral part of greater wing commence ossification in membrane
Wks 12–14	Endochondral centres for postsphenoid part of body appear Endochondral centres for lesser wings appear
Early mth 3	Lateral pterygoid plate commences ossification in membrane Endochondral centre for hamulus appears
Wk 13	Endochondral centre for medial part of greater wing appears
Mths 4–6	First ossification centres for sphenoidal conchae appear
Mth 5	Ossification centre for lingula appears Lesser wings usually fused to body
By mth 8	Pterygoid plates fused to greater wings Pre- and postsphenoid parts of body usually fused together
Birth	Usually represented by body with lesser wings and two separate greater wings with attached pterygoid plates
During yr 1	Greater wings fuse to body. Foramen ovale is completed. Sinus commences pneumatization
By yr 2	Foramen spinosum is completed
By yr 5	Dorsum sellae ossified
Yr 4 – puberty	Sphenoidal conchae fused to ethmoid

Metrics

Fazekas and Kósa (1978) recorded the dimensions of the body, the lesser and greater wings during fetal life (Table 5.6).

IV. THE PARIETAL

The adult parietal

The right and left parietal (Latin – *paries* meaning 'wall') bones form a large part of the side walls of the cranial cavity. They articulate with each other, the squamous occipital, the mastoid and squamous parts of the temporals, the greater wings of the sphenoid and the frontal (Figs. 5.3 and 5.4). In common with some other bones of the cranial vault, they are composed of an inner and outer table of compact bone sandwiching the cancellous, erythropoietic **diploë** between them.

Each bone (Fig. 5.41) is a curved quadrilateral with four borders, four angles and two surfaces. The **frontal** (anterior) border is deeply serrated and bevelled outwards medially and inwards laterally and forms half of the coronal suture with the frontal. The **sagittal** (superior) border is also serrated and articulates with the opposite parietal at the midline sagittal suture. The **occipital** (posterior) border is deeply serrated and bevelled internally and forms half of the lambdoid suture with the occipital. The **squamosal** (inferior) border is curved and consists of three sections. A short, anterior, protruding segment normally articulates with the greater wing of the sphenoid except occasionally, when the frontal meets the temporal, and thus excludes the parietal (see 'Temporal bone'). Posteriorly, the border articulates with the temporal bone: the squamous part overlaps the middle section, which curves gently upwards and the mastoid articulates with the thick, serrated posterior segment. Ossicles may exist in any of the sutures surrounding the bone, but are seen most frequently in the lambdoid suture (see 'Occipital and Temporal bones'). A suture within the parietal bone itself is quite rare, usually unilateral, and appears to be unrelated to age but is reported more frequently in males (Turner, 1891, 1901; Berry, 1909; O'Rahilly and Twohig, 1952; Shapiro, 1972b; Reinhard and Rösing, 1985; Anderson, 1995). It may be horizontal, vertical or oblique, the last cutting off one angle of the bone. A horizontal suture running between the coronal and lambdoid sutures is more common in man, as opposed to a vertical one seen more often in primates. A divided bone on one side is usually larger than the undivided one, due to increased growth perpendicular to the anomalous suture and this may cause asymmetry of the skull. The most likely aetiology of complete division is the failure of the two ossification centres to fuse (see 'Development'), whereas an angular subdivision would be difficult to distinguish from a Wormian bone (Shapiro, 1972b).

All four angles are situated at recognised anthropometric landmarks, are of a different shape, and are associated with blood vessels (Grant, 1948; Figs. 5.3 and 5.4). Each of the angles coincides with the previous site of a fetal fontanelle (Fig. 5.12). The **frontal** (anterosuperior) is a right angle and meets its opposite fellow and the frontal bone at the bregma. The **occipital** (posterosuperior) angle is slightly rounded and joins the occipital and the other parietal at the lambda. Both these superior angles are related to the superior sagittal venous sinus. The blunt **mastoid** (postero-inferior) angle lies at the asterion and is marked on its internal aspect by the transverse venous sinus. The **sphenoid** (antero-inferior) angle is acute,

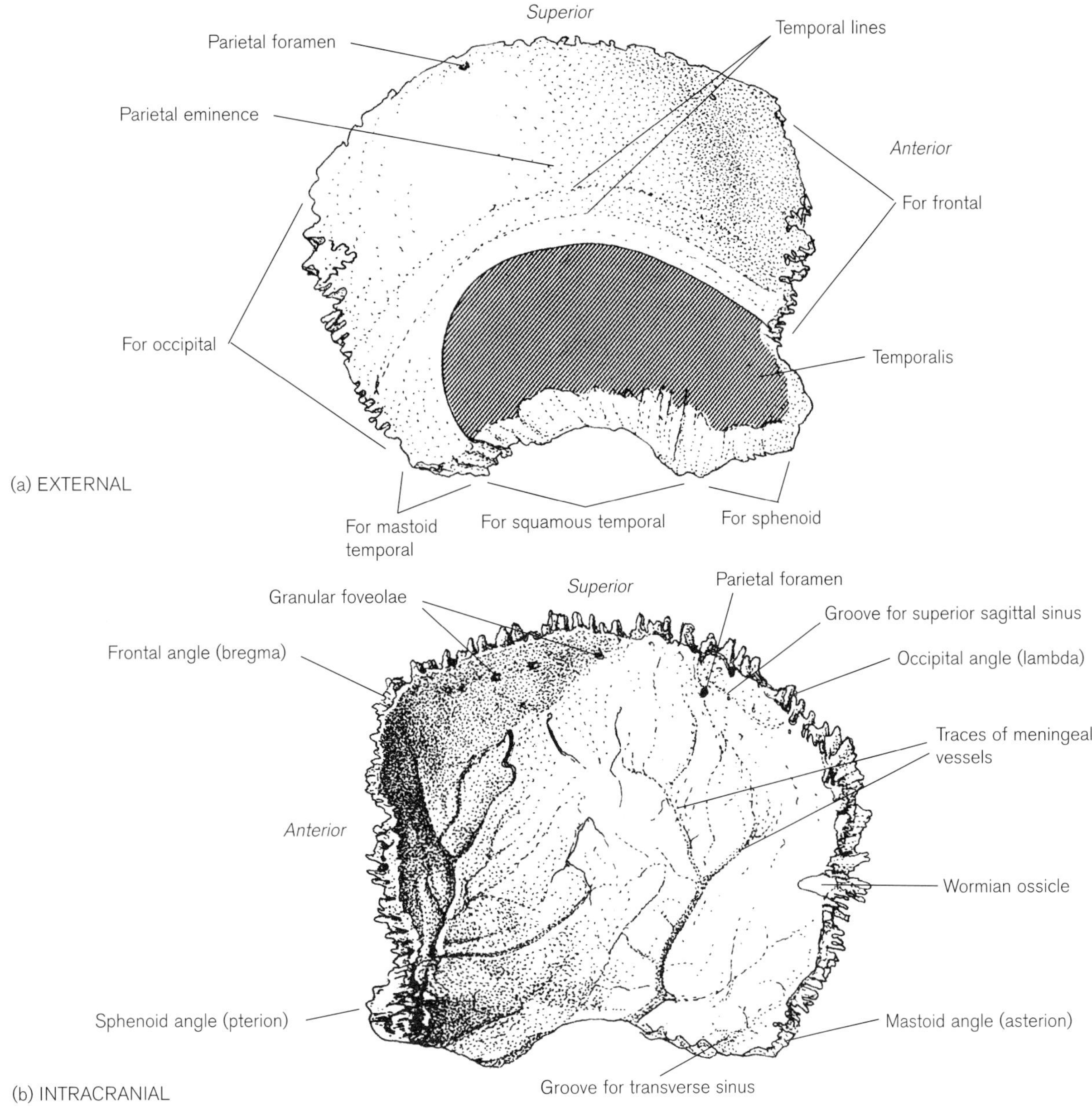

Figure 5.41 Right adult parietal.

situated at the pterion, and internally bears markings for the middle meningeal vessels.

The **external surface** (Fig. 5.41a) is markedly convex and has a **tuber parietale** (parietal eminence), which forms the most protruding part of the bone. Towards the posterior end of the sagittal suture there may be a **parietal foramen**, which when present, transmits a vessel connecting the superior sagittal sinus, the diploic veins and the surface veins of the scalp. The reported incidence of foramina varies from 20% (Boyd, 1930) to 60% (O'Rahilly and Twohig, 1952; Reinhard and Rösing, 1985) and they may be unilateral or multiple. The **pars obelica** is that part of the sagittal suture in the region of the foramina. It is often less serrated than the rest and may even be depressed. Greig (1926) noted that this grooving was more frequent in skulls that showed sagittal instead of parietal foramina. Shore (1938) described interparietal grooving both in a series of Egyptian skulls and in skulls from East Anglia. The grooves were sometimes limited to the region of the obelion (see 'Ossification'), or continued into the lambdoid suture. Curved **superior** and **inferior temporal lines**, often difficult to recognize (Corner, 1896b) and variable in their position (Riesenfeld, 1955), divide the surface of the bone into a smooth upper two-thirds covered by the **galea aponeurotica**, the intermediate tendon of the occipitofrontalis muscle, and a lower third, which is part of the temporal fossa. The temporal fascia is attached to the upper line and the lower line is the limit of attachment for its muscle fibres.

The concave **intracranial surface** of the parietal (Fig. 5.41b) is marked both by convolutions of the cerebral hemispheres and by blood vessels. Along the sagittal border, the bone is grooved to accommodate the dural attachment of the superior sagittal sinus. Within the groove there are **granular foveolae**, small depressions, which increase in number with age, for the **arachnoid granulations** (Pacchionian bodies) that are concerned with the circulation of cerebrospinal fluid. Barber *et al.* (1995) reported that the number of these pits correlate highly with age at death in both archaeological and modern postmortem material. The surface of the bone also shows grooves for the middle meningeal vessels which may, especially in the antero-inferior corner, pass through small tunnels in the bone. This arrangement could complicate treatment of epidural haematomas after fracture of the bone. Because veins are normally wider than arteries and in direct contact with the bone, Wood-Jones (1912) concluded that these vessel traces were primarily venous in nature, but Diamond (1992) argued that traces may be produced by either arteries or veins, depending on the relative dimensions of the two components at any particular point.

The region of the obelion (Fig. 5.4) is the site of many bony variants and developmental anomalies, which may be limited to the bone, but can also involve the scalp or central nervous system (Currarino, 1976). The remnants of the embryonic parietal notch sometimes remains as a fissure (incisura) and a small parietal fontanelle or parietal foramina of varying sizes may occur (see 'Ossification'). Most foramina do not exceed 1 mm in diameter but accounts of grossly enlarged foramina, up to the size of 3–4 cm, are commonplace in the anatomical literature (Turner, 1866; Greig, 1892, 1917, 1927b; Symmers, 1895; Paterson and Lovegrove, 1900; Cave, 1928; Stibbe, 1929; Boyd, 1930; Stallworthy, 1932). They can be unilateral or bilateral and are sometimes connected by a suture that crosses the sagittal suture at right angles. The aetiology of the condition is not clear but from clinical accounts (Greig, 1917; Goldsmith, 1922;[14] Alley, 1936; Irvine and Taylor, 1936; Pepper and Pendergrass, 1936; Travers and Wormley, 1938; O'Rahilly and Twohig, 1952; Fein and Brinker, 1972), it is obvious that there is some inherited factor as the anomaly has been traced through at least five generations in some families.

Symmetrical thinness (biparietal osteodystrophy) is the other extensively reported anomaly of the parietal bone (Shepherd, 1893; Smith,[15] 1907; Greig, 1926; Cave; 1927; Durward, 1929; Camp and Nash, 1944; Wilson, 1944, 1947; Steinbach and Obata, 1957; Bruyn and Bots, 1977). In spite of its name, areas of unilateral or bilateral thinness appear as flat patches or grooves in the bone, lying midway between the sagittal suture and the parietal prominence and anterior to the parietal foramina. The inner table of bone remains intact, but the outer table tapers off and leaves the affected area covered with dense connective tissue (Nashold and Netsky, 1959). The condition was previously described as 'senile atrophy' (Virchow, 1854) but Camp and Nash (1944) and Wilson (1944) maintained that it was neither age-related nor progressive. Clinical interest centres on possible increased susceptibility to skull fracture and difficulties with radiological differential diagnosis. An excellent historical review, including archaeological and clinical cases, may be found in Bruyn and Bots (1977), who concluded that the lesion occurs predominantly in females over the age of 60 years.

Terminology of these anomalies is obviously confusing. Nashold and Netsky (1959) suggest that small parietal foramina, which transmit emissary veins, are normal anatomical variants, whereas large foramina, which they prefer to call fenestrae, and patches of thinness, are true defects of ossification, differing from each other only in extent.

Many other types of foramina may be found in the parietal and other bones of the vault in archaeological specimens. The causes vary from developmental and pathological causes to traumatic intervention, such as trepanning (trephining) or military injuries. Reviews of the differential diagnosis of different foramina may be found in Kaplan *et al.* (1991) and Kaufman *et al.* (1997).

[14]Goldsmith calls this 'the Catlin mark'. The slightly sinister name is called by O'Rahilly and Twohig (1952) 'a perfect example of futile eponymous terminology'. It refers to the name of the family whose several members had this anomaly.

[15]Professor Sir Grafton Elliot Smith noted that these lesions were found on skulls of wealthy Egyptians between the fourth and nineteenth dynasties. They were accustomed to wearing wigs of enormous proportions and great weight, in accordance with their position in society. He put forward the unlikely suggestion that this was responsible for the bone thinning.

Ossification

There is no agreement on either the time of appearance or the number of ossification centres for the parietal bone. The major reason for this is the variety of methods used to study the intramembranous development of the bones of the cranial vault (see Chapter 2). Mall (1906), Noback (1944) and Noback and Robertson (1951) reported that, in alizarin-stained fetuses, the bone can be seen between 7 and 8 weeks of intra-uterine life. Hill (1939), first saw a centre of ossification in the fifth lunar month in a radiographic study, but it almost certainly starts to ossify before then. A single centre, corresponding to the site of the future parietal eminence is described by Rambaud and Renault (1864) and Pendergrass and Pepper (1939). However, Mall (1906), Augier (1931) and Frazer (1948) describe two centres, one above the other, which rapidly unite. Noback (1944) reported that eight out of nine fetuses showed evidence of ossification from two centres. Limson (1932) described a perinatal skull with a completely divided left parietal, in which each part possessed a distinct protuberance, suggesting development from separate centres. The early fusion of two centres is almost certainly the explanation of the hourglass-shaped bone described and illustrated by Mall (1906). Noback also stressed that the ossification centre is not necessarily coincident with the parietal eminence, which occurs at the region of greatest curvature and is thought to be a response to the mechanical stimulus of the growth of the underlying brain and dural tracts.

Moss *et al.* (1956) studied the rate of growth of the calvarial bones of the skull between 8 and 20 fetal weeks and recorded an interphase at about 12.5 weeks. This coincides with the time when the major portions of the fetal brain have attained their definitive topographical relations and the tentorium cerebelli has ceased its backward migration in relation to the overlying neurocranial capsule. The bones then assume a size and shape roughly proportional to their position in the adult skull. Silau *et al.* (1995) described the detailed radiographic appearance at the tuber, the sagittal suture and the anterior fontanelle, and the general shape of the bone between 14 and 21 fetal weeks. Ohtsuki (1977, 1980) measured various parameters of the fetal parietal bone from the fifth lunar month until birth and found a fairly constant rate of increase in area, whereas the increase in thickness shows some deceleration as term is approached.

The later development of the bone is described by Noback (1943, 1944), O'Rahilly and Twohig (1952) and Fazekas and Kósa (1978). At about 5 lunar months, the bone appears as a delicate, ellipsoidal membranous disc with a thickened central eminence from which a fine network of trabeculae radiate outwards. At first, the individual borders and angles are not identifiable, but after the sixth month, the margins of the bone begin to straighten out and the angles take on their characteristic shapes (Fig. 5.42). The frontal border is gently concave and finely serrated, ending laterally at the sphenoidal angle, which points acutely forwards. The sagittal border usually runs directly posteriorly from the rounded frontal angle for

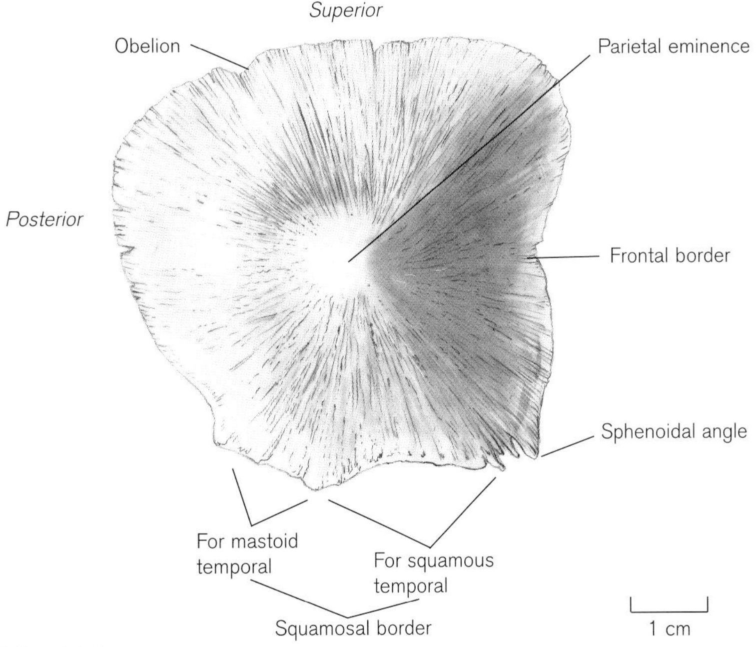

Figure 5.42 Right perinatal parietal.

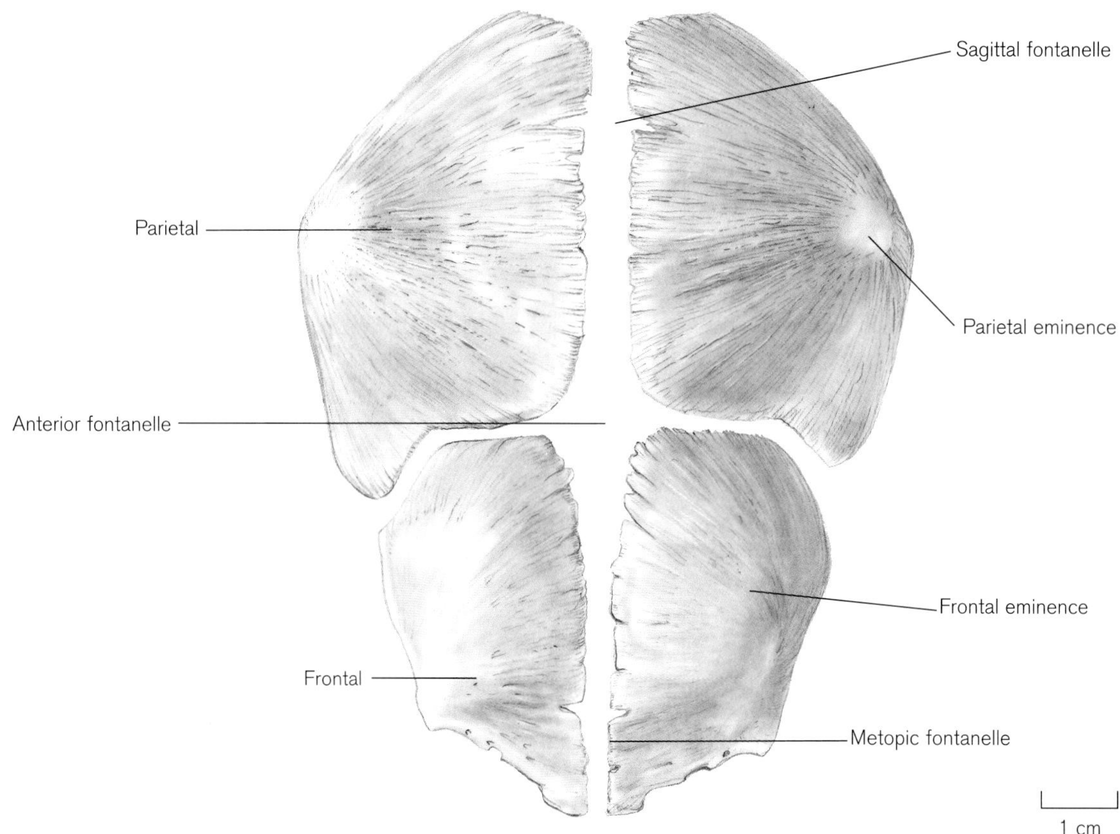

Figure 5.43 Perinatal parietals and frontals.

about two-thirds of its length. This is the position of the **obelion**, and there may be a slit in the bone (Fig. 5.43), after which the serrations on the border become more fringe-like as it slopes away towards the rounded occipital angle at the posterior fontanelle. The occipital border is also finely serrated and may contain one or two slits. The squamosal border is usually divided into two sections, a posterior blunt portion and an anterior curved part, to accommodate the mastoid and squamous parts of the temporal bone, respectively.

In the region of the future parietal foramina, there is often an unossified section between the foramen and the superior border of the bone, which, when joined across the median plane, forms the **sagittal fontanelle** (third fontanelle/fontanelle obélique/Gerdy's fontanelle). This cleft may disappear *in utero*, but is often present at birth, where it has been recorded in 50%–80% of perinatal skulls (Paterson and Lovegrove, 1900; Augier, 1931). Adair and Scammon (1927) recorded a 30% incidence during the first postnatal month and followed its progress in a series of healthy newborns. Its position was highly variable, but it rarely existed after the third postnatal trimester. There is evidence, however, of an increased incidence of the third fontanelle in babies born with Down's syndrome and other abnormalities (Chemke and Robinson, 1969; Tan, 1971).

The development of parietal foramina has been followed by consecutive radiographs in individual patients (Pendergrass and Pepper, 1939; Hollender, 1967; Murphy and Gooding, 1970; Fein and Brinker, 1972). At birth there is a large unossified midline defect, which is gradually filled in by tongue-like growths of bone from the centre. Some unknown factor, regarded as an erratic hereditary defect of ossification, causes the bone formation to cease, leaving bilateral foramina of varying sizes. Warkany and Weaver (1940) reviewed the anomaly in relation to other heredofamilial disorders.

Craniolacunia (lacunar skull/Lückenschädel) is an abnormality of the calvarial bones of the skull, which develops during fetal life and is present at birth. It differs from the normal digital impressions, which only appear after the first year (see 'Occipital'). Kerr (1933) and Doub and Danzer (1934) described the condition in the newborn and Maier (1934) claimed the first prenatal, radiological diagnosis. The bones of the cranial vault have large, rounded areas of decreased density outlined by a web-like pattern of thicker bone bars and ridges, while the cranial base remains normal. It nearly always occurs in conjunction with other malformations, commonly spina bifida, hydrocephalus and meningocoele (Vogt and Wyatt, 1941). Hartley and Burnett (1943a, b) illustrated the skeletal and radiological appearance of affected vault bones, some of which show actual perforations, which they termed craniofenestria. Early reports suggested increased intracranial pressure as the most likely aetiological factor, but this has not been substantiated, as it occurred in skulls of normal size. Hartley and Burnett (1944) suggested that some sort of dietary deficiency might be the cause, as the condition appeared more often in babies from mothers of a financially poorer class. It also occurred more frequently in those children who were conceived during the starvation winters of World War II in the Netherlands (van Waalwijk and Boet, 1949). The aetiology is still far from clear and Caffey (1993) classifies it as a probable dysplasia of the calvaria and its internal periosteum, which is almost always associated with meningocoele and with the Arnold-Chiari (Chiari II/Treacher-Collins/mandibulofacial dysostosis) malformation (Stovin *et al.*, 1960).

Ortiz and Brodie (1949) studied the postnatal growth of the bone from birth to 3 months of age and reported that, after recovery from moulding of the skull during labour, dolichocephalic and brachycephalic skull types could be distinguished at a very early period. In both types, the parietals rise markedly on a lateral view of the head radiograph. Growth of the bone was also measured by Young (1957) on radiographs of a longitudinal series of 20 boys from 1 month to 16 years. The parietal, as measured by the parietal arc from bregma to lambda, increased its maximum curvature rapidly until about the ninth postnatal month, after which growth slowed and the bone became progressively more flattened.

Practical notes

Sideing/orientation (Fig. 5.42)

It is unusual to recover a complete separate parietal, as most bones of the vault are damaged, but sideing will depend on the ability to distinguish the four borders and angles from each other. The sharp, protruding sphenoidal angle lies at the antero-inferior corner. There may be a parietal notch or foramen near the posterior end of the sagittal border and the squamosal (inferior) border becomes characteristically bevelled soon after birth.

Bones of a similar morphology

Small fragments of the parietal bone are probably indistinguishable from other vault fragments unless a characteristic marking is present. Structures to be aware of include venous sinus grooves with granular foveolae, grooves for meningeal vessels, a distinct parietal foramen near a serrated border, temporal lines and characteristic bevelling on the squamosal border.

Morphological summary

Fetal

Wks 7–8 — Two centres of ossification form which rapidly fuse

By mth 6 — Borders and angles become definitive. There may be a sagittal fontanelle

Birth — Single bone with prominent eminence. Sagittal fontanelle usually obliterated

Childhood — Gradually takes on the appearance of the adult bone as the eminence becomes less obvious.

Metrics

Fazekas and Kósa (1978) measured the increase in height and width of the dry parietal bone during fetal life (Table 5.7). Moss *et al.* (1956) reported the lengths of borders of the bone in alizarin-stained wet material between about 8 and 20 fetal weeks. Ohtsuki (1977, 1980) reported on increase in area and thickness of the dry bone from 5 months to term. Young

Table 5.7 Dimensions of the fetal parietal bone

	Height (mm)		Width (mm)	
Age (weeks)	Chord	Arc	Chord	Arc
12	10.0	10.0	14.0	14.0
14	12.3	12.3	16.0	16.0
16	22.1	26.1	25.3	26.7
18	28.4	31.6	30.7	32.6
20	33.8	38.0	36.9	37.0
22	36.6	44.4	39.7	43.0
24	38.1	49.1	43.0	49.6
26	41.6	50.7	46.0	51.6
28	45.2	58.2	50.4	55.9
30	48.8	61.6	56.0	61.7
32	52.5	66.9	58.5	64.8
34	56.0	73.9	63.3	71.6
36	57.1	78.4	66.9	78.6
38	63.5	84.4	70.5	79.5
40	65.7	86.8	72.4	82.0

Height: midsquamous border to midsagittal border across parietal eminence parallel to coronal suture; width: frontal to occipital borders across parietal eminence parallel to sagittal suture.
Adapted from Fazekas and Kósa (1978).

Table 5.8 Dimensions of the parietal bone as measured from radiographs from 1 month to adult

	Chord (mm)		Arc (mm)	
Age	Mean	Range	Mean	Range
1 month	94.3	84–109	107.1	95–135
3 months	104.3	94–119	120.2	104–149
6 months	111.1	104–130	127.2	117–159
9 months	114.7	107–135	131.2	122–165
1 year	119.6	112–139	135.8	124–170
2 years	127.8	118–146	143.0	129–179
3 years	128.1	117–147	143.8	127–179
4 years	129.8	122–150	146.1	134–182
6 years	130.5	119–146	146.0	129–177
8 years	130.4	119–147	146.5	129–179
10 years	131.9	119–149	147.9	130–179
12 years	132.2	120–148	147.9	130–177
14 years	132.4	119–149	148.3	129–178
16 years	130.6	120–149	146.6	129–179
Adult	130.1	123–150	145.6	121–177

Adapted from Young (1957).

(1957) measured the increase in the parietal cord and arc from lateral skull radiographs from 1 month to adult life (Table 5.8). Original texts should be consulted for type of preparation of material and osteological landmarks. The bones of the vault at the fetal and perinatal period are so thin that when disarticulated, they tend to deform and caution needs to be used when comparing measurements. As the bone increases in robusticity in early infancy, this becomes less of a problem.

V. THE FRONTAL

The adult frontal

The frontal (Latin – *frons* meaning 'forehead, brow') is an irregular, bowl-shaped bone, which articulates with the parietals, greater wings of the sphenoid, zygomatics, frontal processes of the maxillae, lacrimals, nasals and the cribriform plate of the ethmoid (Figs. 5.2–5.5). It is both calvarial and facial, forming part of the roof and side walls of the cranial cavity, the floor of the anterior cranial fossa, and the roofs of the orbits. These functionally different parts are reflected in its morphological form (Moss and Young, 1960).

The **external surface** of the **squama** (pars frontalis) forms the forehead and curved anterior part of the cranium, which is covered with the occipitofrontalis muscle and anteriorly, with part of the orbicularis oculi (Fig. 5.44a). It articulates posteriorly with both parietal bones along the deeply serrated coronal suture, which is bevelled internally in its central part, and externally at the lateral ends. The **bregma** is at the junction of the three bones and is the site of the former anterior fontanelle (see below). The area of greatest curvature of the bone, forming the rounded **tuber (eminentia) frontale**, lies above the centre of each orbital margin. The orbits, the thickened **supraciliary arches** (ridges/tori) above them and the **glabella**, the area between the arches, display sexual dimorphism (WEA, 1980; Krogman and Işcan, 1986). The orbital margins in the female tend to be sharper and less rounded than in the male, whilst both the supra-orbital ridges and the glabella are more strongly developed in the male. The forehead is said to be more paedomorphic in character in the female, being smoother, more vertical and displaying prominent frontal bosses. The medial third of the **supra-orbital margin**, marked by the **incisura/foramen supra-orbitalis**, for the supra-orbital vessels and nerve, is smooth, while the lateral two-thirds has a well-defined edge, ending in the articular **processus zygomaticus**. The two branches of the frontal nerve, and their accompanying vessels, which leave the orbit to supply the front of the scalp, mark the bone in a variety of ways. The larger branch, the supra-orbital nerve, usually passes over the margin in a notch, but this may be converted into a foramen. The passage of the smaller, more medial, supratrochlear branch may also mark the bone with a **frontal foramen** or incisure (Reinhard and Rösing, 1985; Chung *et al.*, 1995). Either or both nerves and vessels may make grooves on the external surface of the bone. Dixon (1904) described the incidence of grooves in various populations and suggested that they could result from a growth differential between the superior orbital margin and the nerves (and/or vessels) that have to cross the margin at right angles. Ossenberg (1970, 1976) used these features as discrete traits in the estimation of population distances.

The **temporal surface** is at right angles to the facial surface of the bone and usually shows the anterior ends of the **temporal lines** (lineae temporales), which continue onto the parietal bone. Between the lateral end of the coronal suture and the zygomatic process is a thickened, triangular articular surface for the greater wing of the sphenoid. This region is the pterion and occasionally there may be a frontotemporal articulation, an additional ossicle or epipteric bone at the inferior end of the suture (see 'Temporal bone').

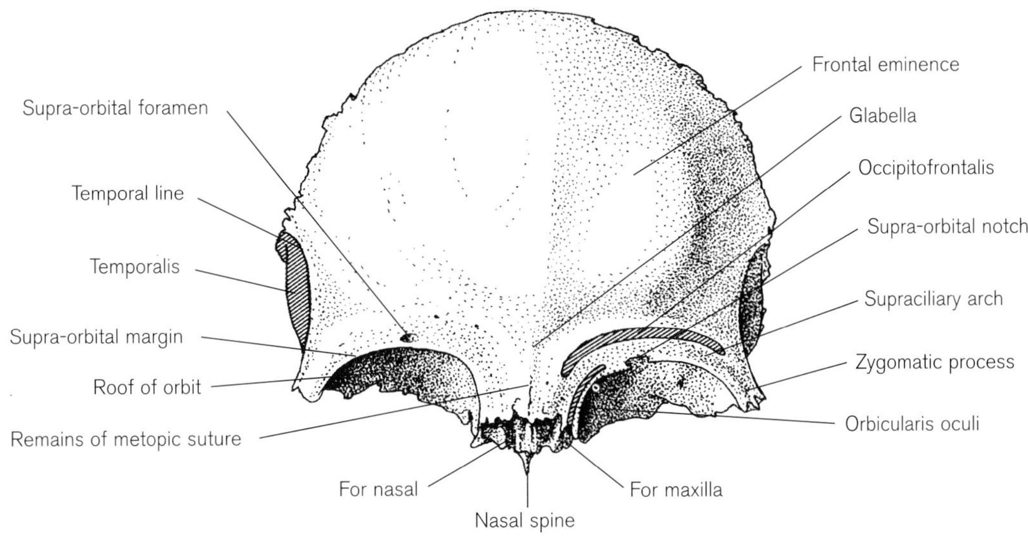

(a) ANTERIOR

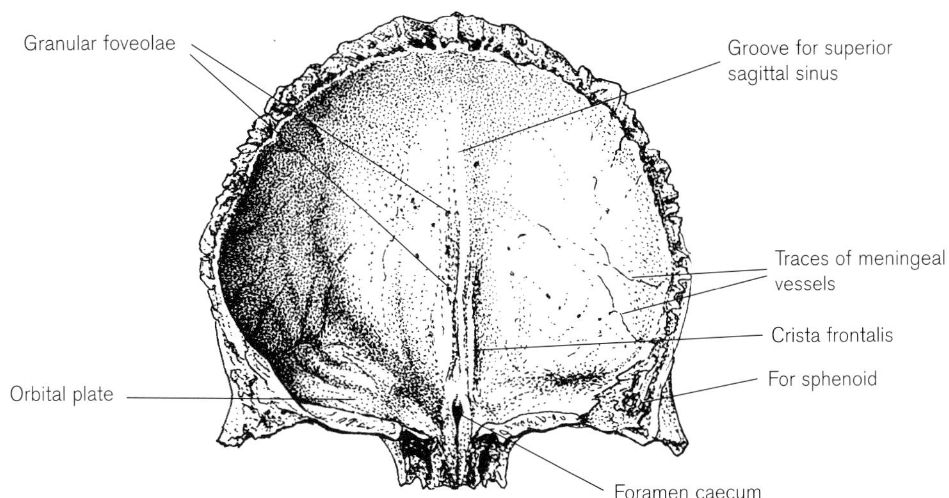

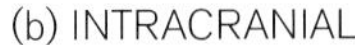
(b) INTRACRANIAL

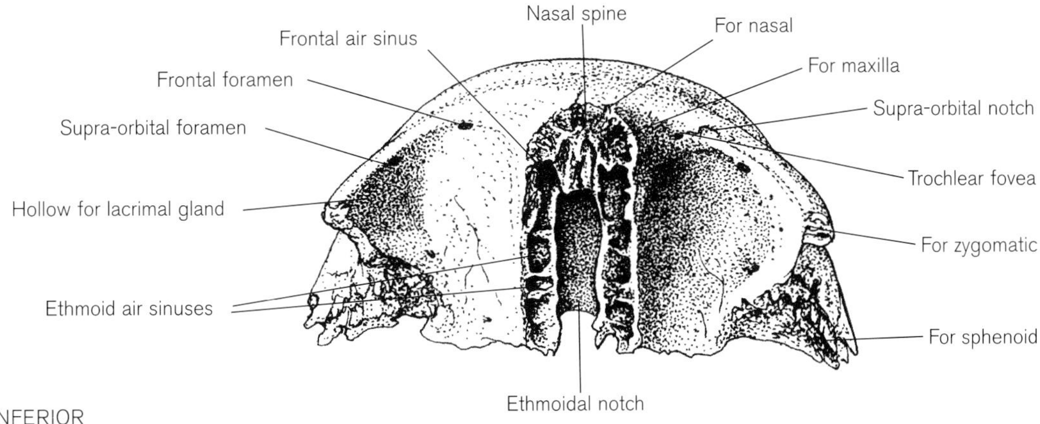

(c) INFERIOR

Figure 5.44 Adult frontal.

The **intracranial surface** of the squama (Fig. 5.44b) shows traces of anterior branches of middle meningeal vessels laterally. In the centre, it is marked by a groove for the superior sagittal sinus, which continues antero-inferiorly into a crest, the **crista frontalis**. The margins of the sulcus and the crest form the anterior attachment of the falx[16] cerebri. The groove often contains small depressions, the **granular foveolae**, caused by the arachnoid granulations, which are concerned with the circulation of cerebrospinal fluid (see also parietal bone). Most anatomical texts state that the **foramen caecum** at the anterior end contains a vein connecting the upper part of the nasal cavity to the superior sagittal sinus. However, Kaplan *et al.* (1973) in a series of 200 autopsies, from age 7 months *in utero* to over 50 years of age, found no sign of a venous channel. They described, and Lang (1989) illustrated, the foramen filled with a plug of periosteal dura.[17]

The **partes orbitales** (orbital plates) are triangular laminae, set at right angles to the vertical part of the squama, which form the floor of the anterior cranial fossa and roofs of the orbits (Fig. 5.44c). The posterior borders of the plates articulate with the lesser and greater wings of the sphenoid (Fig. 5.2). The orbital surface is smooth and near the medial, anterior edge there is usually either a **trochlear spine** or **fovea**, to which is attached a fibrocartilaginous pulley for the superior oblique muscle of the eye. Ossenberg (1970) regarded these features as discontinuous morphological traits achieving stable frequencies at puberty, but they are described as normal structures in most anatomical texts. Rarely there is an osseous ring through which the tendon passes (Augier, 1931). The orbital surface is hollowed anterolaterally to accommodate the lacrimal gland. Lateral and inferolateral to the orbital plate, there are articular surfaces for the zygomatic and sphenoidal greater wings, respectively.

The superior surface of each plate bears marks of the frontal gyri of the cerebral hemispheres. Their medial parallel borders form the quadrangular **incisura ethmoidalis** (ethmoidal notch), occupied by the cribriform plate of the ethmoid (for variations, see 'Ethmoid bone'). The borders of the ethmoidal notch contain the upper parts of the ethmoidal air sinuses and there are usually two grooves that run across their medial edges. When the ethmoid bone is articulated at the notch, the sinuses are complete and the grooves are converted into the anterior and posterior ethmoidal canals for nerves and vessels travelling between the anterior cranial fossa and the nasal cavity. Downie *et al.* (1995) found that there was a middle ethmoidal foramen in 28% of skulls examined.

The openings of the **frontal air sinuses**, which are spaces of variable size and shape between the inner and outer tables of the bone, can be seen in the U-shaped anterior part of the ethmoidal notch. They are normally divided into right and left chambers by a septum, which is commonly midline in its lower part, but can deviate markedly in its upper segments and even divide the sinus spaces into three or more chambers. The sinuses may extend a considerable way between the inner and outer tables of the bone of the forehead and sometimes penetrate horizontally into the orbital plates, or even into the crista galli of the ethmoid (Augier, 1931). In a study of 250 skulls, Monteiro *et al.* (1957) distinguished that 4–8% of sinuses were large, 35–43% were medium and 49–61% were small or absent. Harris *et al.* (1987) reported that the male sinus was significantly larger in size and had more loculations than that of the female. Detailed measurements of sinus size can be found in Lang (1989). Once adult size and shape has been established, the frontal sinuses are unique to each individual and this may be used to advantage by forensic scientists for purposes of identification (Schuller, 1943; Ubelaker, 1984; Krogman and Işcan, 1986; Harris *et al.*, 1987; Yoshino *et al.* 1987; Kullman *et al.*, 1990). Absent or hypoplastic sinuses are characteristic of Down's syndrome (trisomy 21) or Apert's syndrome (acrocephalosyndactyly), but occasionally the condition appears to be unrelated to pathological conditions. Koertvelyessy (1972) investigated the relationship between frontal sinus area, as measured from radiographs, and wind chill equivalent temperatures in Eskimo crania. The conclusion was reached that, although populations from cold areas are characterized by smaller mean sinus surface areas than populations living in warmer climates, multiple factors, rather than simple adaptation to cold, are involved in determination of sinus size.

Anterior to the openings of the sinuses lies the **pars nasalis** (nasal part) of the bone, whose central part protrudes forwards as the **nasal spine**. On either side of the spine the bone forms the grooved, narrow roof of each side of the nasal cavity. The spine articulates with the crest of the nasal bones anteriorly and the perpendicular plate of the ethmoid posteriorly. The anterior border of the nasal part has bilateral, thickened articular surfaces for the nasal bones medially and the frontal processes of the maxillae laterally.

Developmental anomalies equivalent to those at the obelion in the parietal bone (see above) can occur in

[16] *Falx* (Latin meaning 'sickle'), referring to the shape of the median fold of dura between the right and left cerebral hemispheres.

[17] *Caecus* (Latin meaning 'blind, obscure'), so unlikely to be a passageway, and therefore it appears well named.

the frontal bone, but are less frequent. A **metopic**[18] **fontanelle** may lie between the two halves of the bone in the inferior third of the interfrontal suture at the level of the frontal bosses. It usually contains lateral emissary veins and, with age, adopts a more posterior location as the bone grows in height. Traces may remain as a median, or two lateral paramedian, frontal foramina, which may be connected by an orthometopic suture, which is sometimes reduced to a bony, star-shaped scar (Schultz, 1918b, 1929b; Augier, 1931).

A major anomaly of the frontal bone is the failure of the two halves to fuse in the midline during early childhood. The terminology of this condition, usually referred to as **metopism**, is confusing and its use in the literature has not been consistent. The remnant of any part of the suture remaining after the age of about 2 years is usually called a **sutura metopica persistens** (Reinhard and Rösing, 1985). Wood Jones (1953) described a complete suture as appearing typically dentate from the nasion to about 2 cm anterior to the bregma, the pars bregmatica, when it becomes more simple in structure. The partial metopic suture is typically complex in form in its supranasal section (Das *et al.*, 1973; Agarwal *et al.*, 1979; Ajmani *et al.*, 1983). The incidence of metopism and metopic suture varies in different populations (Bryce and Young, 1917; Limson, 1924; Jit and Shah, 1948; Woo, 1949a; Berry and Berry, 1967; Ossenberg, 1970; Das *et al.*, 1973; Berry, 1975; Agarwal *et al.*, 1979; Ajmani *et al.*, 1983) arguing for some sort of genetic basis and Torgersen (1950, 1951) followed its incidence in 16 Norwegian families. Its presence is not related either to skull shape or to cranial capacity, but is positively correlated with an increase in frontal curvature (Bolk, 1917; Schultz, 1929b; Woo, 1949a). All theories concerning metopism focus on reasons for the non-fusion of the two parts of the frontal bone and none are very convincing (Bolk, 1917; Bryce and Young, 1917; Ashley-Montagu, 1937; Hess, 1945). A more interesting question is why, in the vast majority of individuals, the interfrontal suture closes much earlier than the rest of the sagittal suture, rather than why the suture remains open in a minority of cases. Because of its morphology and position, the frontal bone plays a major part in connecting the facial and neurocranial skeleton. Ethmoid centres cease growth at about 2 years of age, so that the early fusion of the halves of the frontal could be a way of maintaining maximum stability in the region of the fronto-ethmoidal-nasal suture system. However, if there is premature fusion of the metopic suture (metopic synostosis), severe defects in the orbital region and compensatory expansion in other cranial areas occur (Kolar and Salter, 1997). It is obviously essential for increase in width to take place at the interfrontal suture until ethmoid centres have completed their growth. Both ethmoid and normal metopic fusion occur at about the time of completion of eruption of the deciduous dentition, when there are maximum masticatory forces on the facial skeleton. Experimental approaches, such as those of Hylander *et al.* (1991) and Ross and Hylander (1996), on the mechanical forces on the facial and anterior calvarial skeleton, may throw further light on the reasons for the early closure of the interfrontal suture. The mechanics at the cellular level (Hall, 1967; Manzanares *et al.*, 1988) also seem to suggest that the formation of chondroid tissue, which is involved in the closure of the interfrontal suture, is linked to the action of forces exerted in different directions on the sutural space.

Ossification

There has been much disagreement about both the number of centres and the manner in which the frontal bone ossifies. This was in part due to misinterpretation of the development of the somewhat complex structure at both ends of the supra-orbital ridges and also to the attempts of early zoologists and anatomists to homologize parts of the human frontal bone with pre- and postfrontal elements of premammalian skulls. A careful and definitive study was carried out by Inman and Saunders (1937), who reviewed the previous extensive literature and made observations on fetal and infant frontal bones from the sixth week of intra-uterine life to the tenth postnatal month.

Each half of the bone ossifies from a single centre, which appears in membrane between 6 and 7 weeks. At first, each centre has an oval-shaped form, whose long axis lies in the region of the supraciliary arch, which forms the lower part of the squama and the anterior portion of the orbital plate. Ossification spreads as a network of radiating trabeculae, at first more rapidly in the pars frontalis than in the pars orbitalis. The rapid expansion upwards has led to many accounts of the centre of ossification being in the region of the frontal eminence, but this does not appear to be the case (Inman and Saunders, 1937; Noback, 1943, 1944). This first burst of ossification gives rise only to that part of the supraciliary arch medial to the future supra-orbital notch. The lateral two-thirds of the arch and the zygomatic process develop later, between 10 and 12 weeks, thus separating the orbital cavity from the temporal fossa.

[18]*Meta* (Greek meaning 'between'); *ops* (Greek meaning 'eye'). Literally, 'between the eyes.'

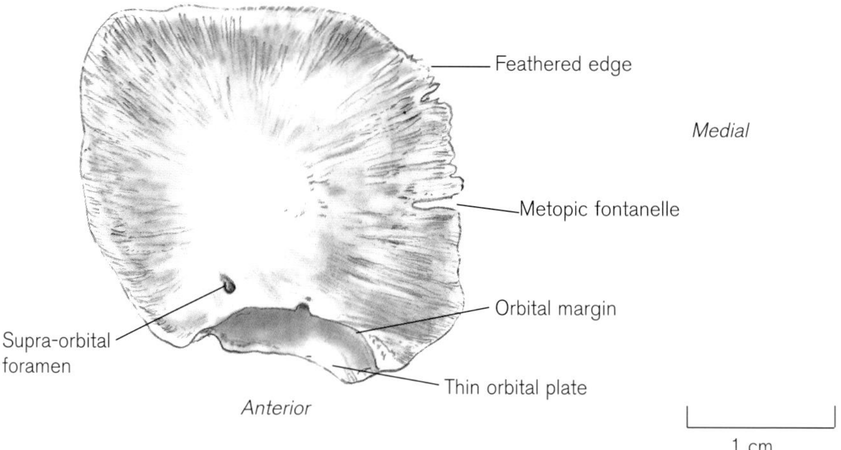

Figure 5.45 Right fetal frontal.

This process, which includes the formation of the linea temporalis and a fissure for the attachment of the membrane of the anterolateral fontanelle, tends to accentuate the appearance of a separate ossification centre. A similar process occurs at the medial end of the supraciliary ridge, where the orbital plate is slow to ossify and this is complete by about 13 weeks.

The bone becomes recognizable at the end of the first trimester of fetal life. It is a fragile, oval-shaped dome, whose long axis runs from anteromedial to posterolateral (Fig. 5.45). The anterior edge is thickened as the orbital margin, which may show a supra-orbital notch or foramen. The orbital plate is extremely slight and thin. As the bone develops, the frontal plate grows more rapidly and by about the fifth lunar month, the anteroposterior length is greater than its lateral width. Moss *et al.* (1956) measured four parameters of the prenatal frontal bone and found that, like the parietal, there is a definite interphase in rate of growth at between 12 and 13 weeks. Ohtsuki (1977) recorded developmental changes in thickness between 4 months and term.

In the last 2 months of fetal life, the bone is more substantial (Fig. 5.46a). The inferomedial angle of the bone, which will form the glabella, shows transverse striations and from here the medial border is fairly smooth for a short distance. About halfway between the frontal eminence and the medial border there may be a foramen, which is continuous with a groove or slit joining it to the medial border. This is the site of the metopic fontanelle (see below). More posteriorly, the medial edge of the bone is very finely serrated and then slopes away laterally to form the margin of the anterior fontanelle. There is a rounded posterior angle at the lateral edge of the fontanelle and from here the coronal margin is also serrated as far as the lateral end

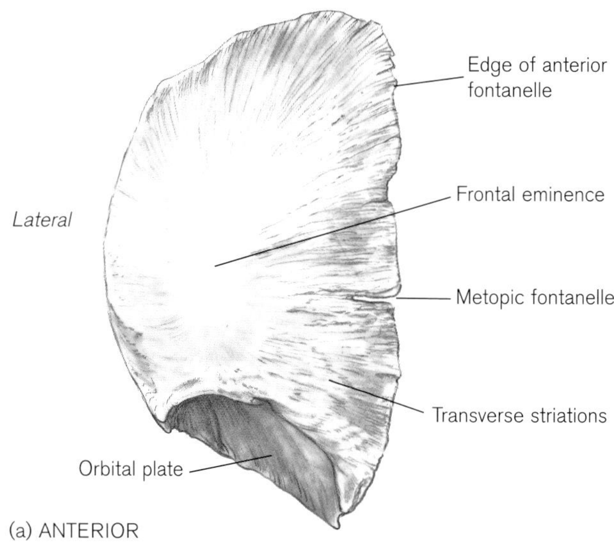

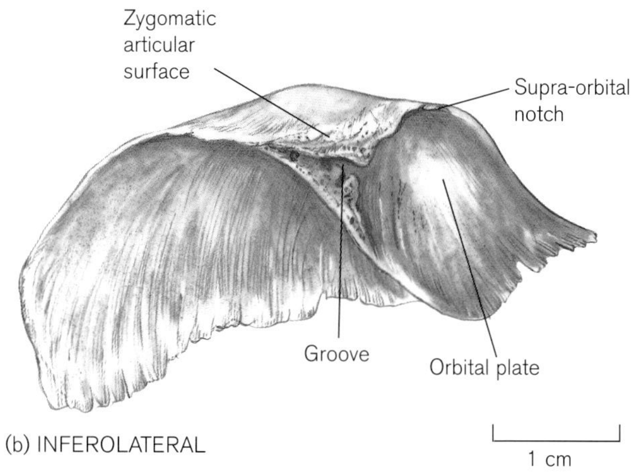

Figure 5.46 Right perinatal frontal.

of the supra-orbital ridge. Here, the bone is thickened for the zygomatic articulation, which, at this stage, is an elongated triangle containing a groove whose apex points posteriorly (Fig. 5.46b). The lateral edge of the supra-orbital margin is sharp and the medial third smooth as in the adult bone.

It is not clear whether there is a separate secondary centre for the nasal spine. Rambaud and Renault (1864) and Augier (1931) stated that this part of the bone develops from a double cartilaginous centre between 2 and 8 years of age. Inman and Saunders (1937) were unable to see a separate centre but noted that the nasal spine became obvious in radiographs at about 10 years of age. Both the thickened articulations for the maxilla and nasal bones and the undulations in the orbital plate become obvious in the perinatal period.

At birth, the frontal bone is composed of two symmetrical halves, which are separated from each other by the metopic suture (Figs. 5.11, 5.14 and 5.43). The anterosuperior angles meet the parietal bones at the diamond-shaped **anterior fontanelle**,[19] which is the largest of the fetal fontanelles. Dimensions are very variable (Popich and Smith, 1972; Duc and Largo, 1986), but tend to increase in the first month of life, as the shape of the vault settles after moulding in the birth canal. The size of the fontanelle does not appear to be significantly related to sex, head circumference or bone age, or be predictive of time of closure. 38 percent of fontanelles are closed by the end of the first year and 96% by 2 years. It is not uncommon for the fontanelle and its contiguous sutures to contain separate ossicles (Barclay-Smith, 1909; Willock, 1925; Girdany and Blank, 1965), which may be present at birth or develop later. They do not seem to interfere with normal growth and usually fuse with the surrounding bones before the fifth year of life. The frontal arm of the sagittal suture regularly reaches below the level of the frontal tuberosities, and in about 15% of infants it persists to birth or into postnatal life. In some cases, the entire frontal arm of the suture is open, but more usually the upper part closes and the lower open part is then known as the metopic fontanelle (Schultz, 1929b). A persistent metopic fontanelle (cranium bifidum occultam frontalis) is one of the signs of cranio-cleidodysostosis (Epstein and Epstein, 1967; Jarvis and Keats, 1974; see also Chapter 8).

[19] *Fontanelle* (French meaning 'little fountain'). Medieval surgeons attempted to cure brain and eye diseases by placing a cautery at the site of the anterior fontanelle. The wound remained open by application of an irritant so that poisonous substances could supposedly escape. The welling of blood from the site was supposed to have looked like water bubbling from a spring.

Closure of the metopic suture normally takes place during the first year (Molleson and Cox, 1993) but completion can last until the fourth year. It starts to close just above the nasal end. In a number of individuals, which varies with the population, the suture is retained in its entirety into adult life (see above), but many skulls show some sign of an irregular suture just above the junction with the nasal bones.

Postnatal growth was recorded by Young (1957) in boys aged from 1 month to 16 years and by Meredith (1959) in girls from 5 to 15 years. After a rapid increase in chord, arc and thickness measurements the bone becomes increasingly more arched until the third year, reflecting early brain enlargement. After this time, there is a deceleration of growth leading to a flattening of the bone. Adjustments also have to be made both to the growth of the frontal sinus and to the facial skeleton.

The sinus starts in fetal life, either as a mucosal evagination at the anterior end of the middle meatus of the nose or from anterior ethmoidal cells, but does not pneumatize the frontal bone until the postnatal period. Expansion begins at the age of 3.5 years (Lang, 1989; Wolf *et al.*, 1993), is level with the orbital roof between 6 and 8 years (Caffey, 1993) and then increases slowly until puberty. Dimensions in childhood are given by Peter *et al.* (1938) and Wolf *et al.* (1993). Brown *et al.* (1984) made detailed measurements from radiographs in 49 males and 47 females from the age of 2 years until over 20 years. Over half of the subjects had a sinus visible on first examination, but the mean age of appearance was 3.25 years in boys and 4.58 years in girls. This agrees with Maresh (1940), who gave an age range of 2–6 years. As expected, the main period of enlargement coincided with the pubertal growth spurt, the end of which was about 13 years in girls and 15 years in boys. Thus, the period of growth was shorter in girls and the mean final size was smaller than in boys. Lang (1989) reported that the sinus may go on increasing in size well into the fourth decade of life.

Practical notes

Sideing/orientation (Fig. 5.46)

It is unusual to recover a complete separate perinatal frontal as most bones of the vault are damaged. Sideing and orientation relies on recognizing the orbital margin, which is thickened and often survives inhumation. The sharp, projecting margin is on the lateral side and ends in the thickened, triangular articular surface for the zygomatic bone.

Table 5.9 Dimensions of the fetal frontal bone

	Length (mm)		Width (mm)	
Age (weeks)	Chord (mm)	Arc (mm)	Chord (mm)	Arc (mm)
12	7.0	7.0	11.5	11.5
14	10.1	10.1	13.8	13.8
16	21.5	21.6	17.9	18.8
18	24.5	26.5	21.3	23.2
20	28.7	30.3	24.4	26.3
22	30.5	31.8	26.1	27.5
24	32.8	36.4	29.1	32.6
26	35.0	40.0	31.0	33.7
28	37.8	42.9	33.0	37.4
30	40.8	46.5	34.6	38.5
32	43.7	49.6	37.8	41.2
34	46.9	54.0	39.7	45.0
36	50.4	58.0	41.3	49.2
38	53.1	61.8	43.6	52.0
40	54.8	64.5	45.2	54.1

Length: middle of superior margin of orbit to superior peak of bone across frontal eminence.
Width: width across frontal eminence at right angles to length (width at superior border of orbit in younger fetuses).
Adapted from Fazekas and Kósa (1978).

Bones of a similar morphology

Small fragments of the frontal bone are probably indistinguishable from other vault fragments unless a characteristic part of the bone is present. Only the frontal bone has orbital rims and orbital plates set at an angle to the rest of the bone. There may be traces of frontal air sinuses or the highly characteristic crista frontalis.

Morphological summary

Fetal

Wks 6–7	Primary centre of ossification appears
Wks 10–13	Zygomatic process and medial angular processes start ossifying
By mth 5	Anteroposterior longer than medio-lateral length
Birth	Represented by right and left halves
1–2 yrs	Anterior fontanelle closed
2–4 yrs	Metopic suture normally closed

Metrics

Fazekas and Kósa (1978) measured the dimensions of the dry frontal bone during fetal life (Table 5.9). Moss *et al.* (1956) reported the lengths of borders of the bone in alizarin-stained wet material between about 8 and 20 fetal weeks. Young (1957) measured the increase in the frontal arc and chord from lateral skull radiographs from one month to adult life (Table 5.10). Original texts should be consulted for type of preparation of material and osteological landmarks, as measurements are unlikely to be comparable. The frontal bones during the fetal and perinatal period are very thin and when disarticulated, tend to deform. The bone increases in robusticity in early infancy and, as with the parietal bone, this is then less of a problem.

Table 5.10 Dimensions of the frontal bone as measured from radiographs from 1 month to adult

	Chord (mm)		Arc (mm)	
Age	Mean	Range	Mean	Range
1 month	73.0	67–80	81.2	72–90
3 months	81.9	74–92	93.3	80–106
6 months	89.3	82–96	103.6	91–115
9 months	93.4	86–99	107.5	98–113
1 year	99.6	90–109	114.8	100–125
2 years	109.2	97–115	127.6	110–127
3 years	110.0	101–117	128.4	113–140
4 years	111.5	99–118	130.1	114–142
6 years	113.2	103–123	130.9	114–147
8 years	114.2	104–120	131.2	118–142
10 years	116.3	104–125	133.5	118–149
12 years	117.9	105–128	134.6	119–149
14 years	118.9	105–129	134.9	118–149
16 years	120.0	107–126	135.4	121–145
Adult	122.1	107–121	140.5	125–158

Adapted from Young (1957).

VI. THE NASAL BONE

The adult nasal bone

The right and left nasal bones (Fig. 5.47) form the bridge of the nose and articulate with each other, the frontal bone, perpendicular plate of the ethmoid, nasal septal cartilages and the frontal processes of the maxillae (Figs. 5.3, 5.5 and 5.52). Each bone resembles an elongated rhomboid in outline and can be very variable in shape and size (Martin and Saller, 1959; Lang and Baumeister, 1982). Einy *et al.* (1984) noted that, because of variations in nasal and glabellar contour, it was difficult to measure skull thickness at the nasion and proposed an accurate and easily reproducible alternative method of measurement.

The **external surface** is usually convex transversely and concavo-convex from above downwards. There is normally a vascular foramen in the middle third of the bone. The **internal (nasal) surface** is reciprocally concave and bears a longitudinal groove, the **sulcus ethmoidalis** for the anterior ethmoidal nerve. The **superior border** is thick and serrated and articulates with the central part of the pars nasalis of the ethmoidal notch of the frontal. The thin **lateral border** articulates with the medial edge of the frontal process of the maxilla. The **medial border** is thick in its upper part and bears an articular surface, which meets the bone of the opposite side at an angle. Together they form a pronounced **crest** on the internal surface, which rests on the nasal spine of the frontal bone above and the perpendicular plate of the ethmoid and/or the septal cartilage below. The **inferior border** is the most irregular, but commonly slopes upwards from lateral to medial and meets the lateral (superior) nasal cartilage. There is often a notch in the middle of the border, through which the external nasal nerve reaches the overlying skin.

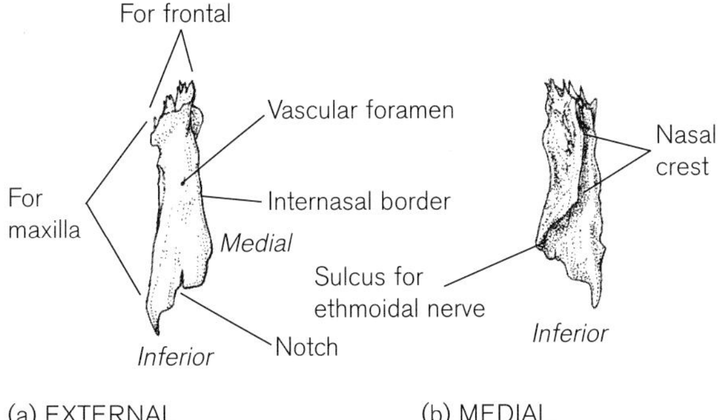

Figure 5.47 Right adult nasal.

Anomalies of the nasal bones may vary from unilateral or bilateral agenesis, through hypoplasia to hyperdevelopment (Duckworth, 1902; Wahby, 1903; Augier, 1931; Barnes, 1994). In their absence, the neighbouring frontal or maxillary bones may compensate by sending a process into the normal territory of the nasal. Each bone may occasionally be bi- or tripartite, with transverse or vertical sutures and there are sometimes small ossicles between the nasal and adjacent bones (Reinhard and Rösing, 1985).

The nasal (piriform) aperture, the space bounded by the nasal bones and the maxillae, exhibits some sexual dimorphism. It tends to be higher and narrower and have sharper margins in the male than in the female. The two nasal bones also meet in the midline at a more acute angle, producing the prominent male nose (Krogman and Işcan, 1986). The aperture also varies in height, width and shape in different populations (Macalister, 1898; Schultz, 1918c; Burkitt and Lightoller, 1923; Gower, 1923; Cameron, 1930; Krogman, 1932) and it was postulated that climatic factors acted by natural selection to produce global differences in size of the nasal aperture, as indicated by the nasal index (Thompson and Buxton, 1923; Davies, 1932). However, further studies on a large variety of skulls indicated that the difference shown in the nasal index (maximum breadth/height × 100) is too simple an explanation for this. Both nasal height and breadth are themselves correlated more directly to other parameters of the skull, such as prognathism and dental arch shape, which produce secondary changes in the nasal index (St Hoyme, 1965; Wolpoff, 1968; Glanville, 1969).

Ossification

The nasal bones develop in membrane in the dense mesenchyme overlying the cartilaginous nasal capsule. They are first visible histologically at 9–10 weeks (Macklin, 1914; Sandikcioglu *et al.*, 1994) and become recognizable in radiographs a little later (O'Rahilly and Meyer, 1956; Sandikcioglu *et al.*, 1994). Most accounts describe a single ossification centre for each bone, although there are reports, not well substantiated, of a second, medial endochondral centre (Augier, 1931; Frazer, 1948). Dedick and Caffey (1953) reported that in rare cases the nasal bones fail to mineralize and this may possibly be associated with conditions like Down's syndrome.

Limson (1932) commented on the variety in size and shape of fetal nasal bones and distinguished four distinct classes according to overall shape, the percentage frequencies being different in Black and White fetuses. Niida *et al.* (1991), using scanning electron

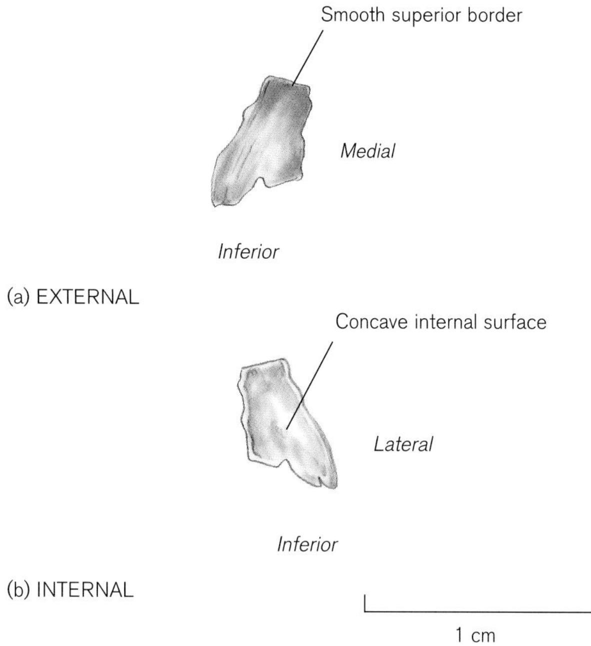

Figure 5.48 Right fetal nasal.

microscopy, distinguished three separate patterns of trabecular bone growth in Japanese fetuses. The most common was a concentric arrangement in the lower part and a vertical arrangement in the upper part of the bone. The patterns, already apparent in the fetus, were thought to be responsible for the variations that are common in the adult bone. Fazekas and Kósa (1978) measured the length and breadth of the dry bone throughout fetal life and Sandikcioglu *et al.* (1994) recorded the length from radiographs from about 3 to 7 lunar months. Although the measurements were not strictly comparable, both showed a relatively linear rate of growth in length.

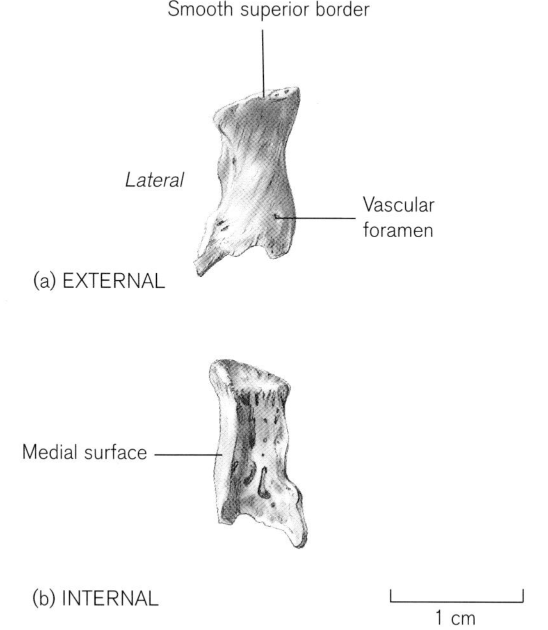

Figure 5.49 Right perinatal nasal.

Because of its extreme fragility, the nasal bone is probably not identifiable in isolation before the third trimester of fetal life. It can be recognized from its adult morphological shape, but differs in size and overall proportions (Fig. 5.48). An obvious articular surface on the medial border for the corresponding bone does not develop until late in fetal life. At birth, the bone is surprisingly robust. The borders are smooth and the vascular foramen can usually be seen in the lower half of the bone (Fig. 5.49). Its length is about twice the breadth across the lower part of the bone (Fazekas and Kósa, 1978; Lang, 1989) but its overall shape, even at this stage, is quite variable. After one year of age, the bone starts to increase in length in its lower part, so that by puberty it is about three times as long as it is wide.The serrated superior border develops after the age of 3 years at about the time that ossification is proceeding inferiorly in the perpendicular plate of the ethmoid. Enlow and Bang (1965), in a study of the maxilla and its neighbouring bones, observed that the outer and inner surfaces of the nasal bones show typical appositional and resorptive surfaces, respectively, as the bone grows in size and noted that there was much individual variation in size and shape. In young children, the nasofrontal and frontomaxillary sutures are both level with the roof of the nasal cavity, whereas in older children and adults the nasofrontal suture is somewhat higher (Fig. 5.50). This is caused by the overlapping nature of the suture so that as it develops, the nasion ascends on the frontal bone with age and becomes closer to the upper orbital margin in adults than in children. Because of this changing relationship, Scott (1956) warned that the nasion cannot be used as evidence of the growth and separation of the frontal and maxilla. It must be used with care as a fixed point when measurements are taken on radiographs.

Practical notes

Sideing/orientation of the perinatal nasal (Fig. 5.49)

The bone does not become recognizable in isolation until late fetal life as it is small and fairly fragile, but by birth it is more robust. It is narrower superiorly than inferiorly. The medial border is shorter than the lateral border and bears the thickened articular surface for the bone of the opposite side.

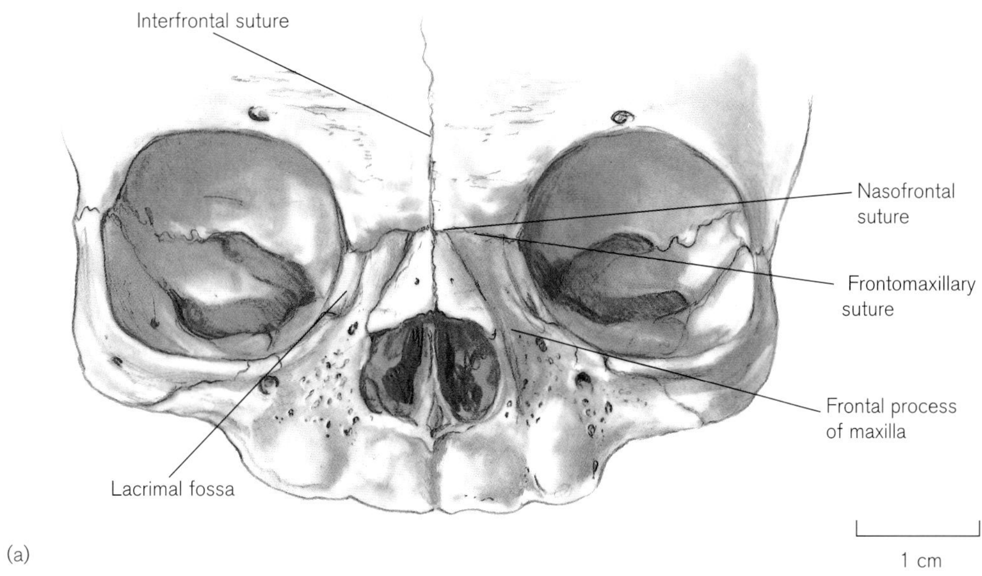

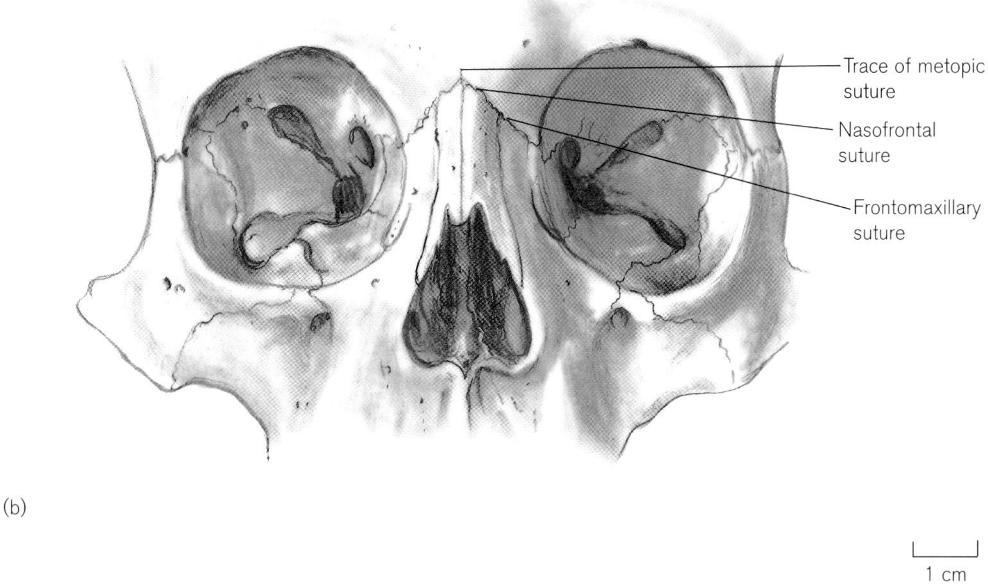

Figure 5.50 Frontonasal sutures. (a) Perinatal – frontonasal and frontomaxillary sutures at same level. Note triangular nasal bone. (b) Child of 8 years – frontonasal sutures superior to frontomaxillary sutures.

Morphological summary

Fetal

Wks 9–10	Intramembranous ossification centre appears for each bone
Mths 9–10	Medial articular border develops
Birth	Morphology similar to adult except: length to width proportion different, borders are smooth and vascular foramen is in lower half of the bone
About year 3	Superior border becomes serrated
Puberty	Adopts adult morphology and size

Metrics

Fazekas and Kósa (1978) reported the dimensions of the nasal bone during fetal life (Table 5.11). Lang (1989) measured size of the piriform aperture (Table 5.12) and the height and breadth across both nasal bones (Table 5.13) in the neonate, at 1 year, 5 years, 13 years and in adults.

Table 5.11 Dimensions of the fetal nasal bone life

Age (weeks)	Length (mm)	Width (mm)
16	4.5	2.5
18	5.1	3.0
20	5.9	2.9
22	6.1	3.9
24	6.8	4.0
26	7.3	4.2
28	7.9	4.2
30	8.7	4.3
32	9.6	5.2
34	10.6	5.3
36	11.6	5.9
38	11.8	6.6
40	12.3	7.4

Length: superior to inferior margin in midline.
Width: maximum distance across the inferior border.
Adapted from Fazekas and Kósa (1978).

Table 5.12 Dimensions of the piriform aperture from birth to adult life

	Height (mm)		Superior width (mm)		Inferior width (mm)	
	Mean	Range	Mean	Range	Mean	Range
Neonate	9.8	7–11	12.4	11–13.5	11.3	10–13
1 year	11.9	11–13	16.5	16–18	17.4	15–19
5 years	13.3	11–18	18.2	14–20	22.6	20–33
13 years	14.0	13–15	19.7	19–21	26.0	25–27
Adult	16.3	10–22	23.6	20–28	29.1	21–37

Height: maximum height from superior to inferior piriform aperture.
Superior width: width across aperture at level of inferior lateral border of nasal bones.
Inferior width: maximum width across aperture.
Adapted from Lang (1989).

Table 5.13 Dimensions of the nasal bones from birth to adult life

	Height (mm)		Breadth (mm)	
	Mean	Range	Mean	Range
Neonate	8.3	7.9–9	8.4	6–10
1 year	12.8	11–14	11.2	9–15
5 years	16.2	13–19	11.4	9–18
13 years	22.8	22–24	12.0	11–15
Adult	24.9	18–31	13.0	7–18

Height: highest point of internasal suture.
Breadth: distance across both nasal bones at point at which frontal process of maxilla meets lateral border of nasal bones.
Adapted from Lang (1989).

VII. THE ETHMOID

The adult ethmoid

The ethmoid[20] (Fig. 5.51) is a component of the nasal cavity and orbits and also lies in the anterior cranial fossa. It occupies the ethmoidal notch of the frontal bone and also articulates with the sphenoid, vomer, maxillae, lacrimal and nasal bones and the septal cartilage (Figs. 5.2, 5.3 and 5.52). It consists of a horizontal cribriform plate, a midline perpendicular plate and two lateral labyrinths.

The **lamina cribrosa** (cribriform plate) lies horizontally in the centre of the anterior cranial fossa, separating it from the roof of the nose. The upper part

[20]*Ethmos* (Greek meaning 'a sieve') referring to the holes in the cribriform plate, whose name is taken from *cribrum* (Latin meaning a 'sieve').

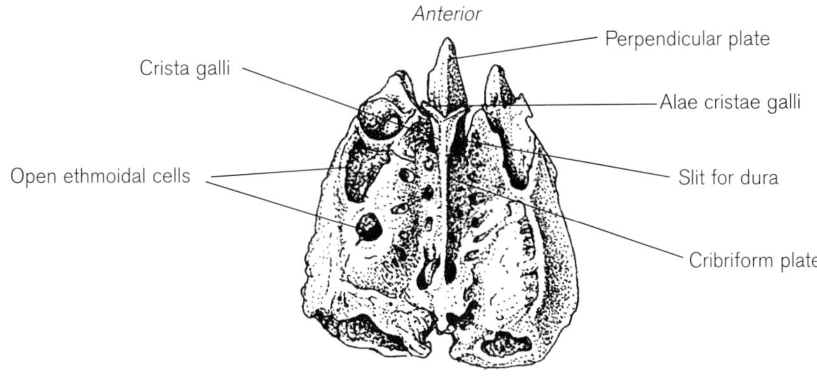

(a) SUPERIOR

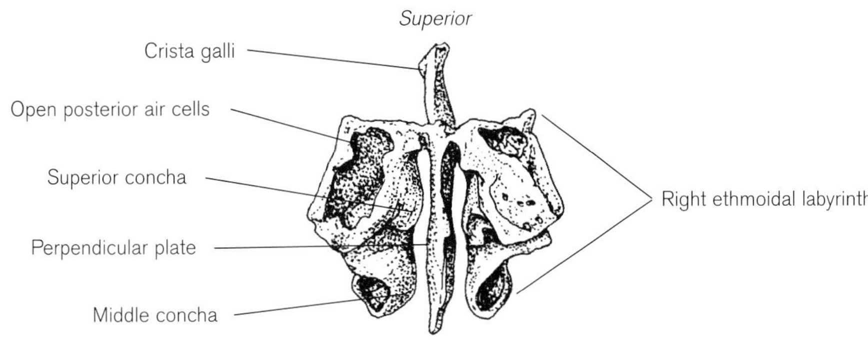

(b) POSTERIOR

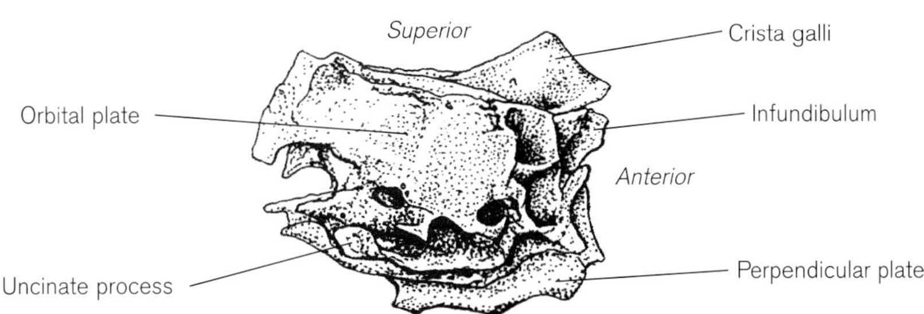

(c) LATERAL

Figure 5.51 Adult ethmoid.

of the perpendicular plate, the **crista galli** (cock's comb), appears above it in the centre and on either side it is perforated by small foramina, through which the olfactory cranial nerves pass from the olfactory mucosa into the cranial cavity. Kalmey *et al.* (1998) reported that the area of patent foramina in the posterior part of the cribriform plate decreases significantly with increasing age in both sexes. It was suggested that this could be associated with the supposed impairment of olfactory function in the elderly. At the anterior extremity on either side of the crista galli are foramina through which the anterior ethmoidal nerves and vessels pass to the nose after lying in grooves on the surface of the cribriform plate. An inconstant small slit may be seen in this region, which is said to anchor the dura mater.

The **lamina perpendicularis** (perpendicular plate) consists of the crista galli above and a large segment below the horizontal plate that forms part of the bony nasal septum (Fig. 5.52). The dural fold of the falx cerebri, which contains the superior sagittal venous sinus, is attached to the crista galli. The anterior border of the crista divides into two wings, the **alae cristae galli**, which fuse with the frontal bone and enclose the foramen caecum. The posterior border falls sharply back towards the cribriform plate. Moss (1963) distinguished two morphological types of cristae galli. Type 1 skulls had a thickened orbital roof, an inflated 'clubbed' crista galli, well-defined medial orbital margins and a so-called cryptocribriform plate, which was overshadowed laterally. By contrast, Type 2 skulls had a thin crista and medial orbital margins that blended with the sides of the cribriform plate so that it was easily visible. The prominent orbital margins were possibly the result of enlarged fronto-ethmoidal sinuses. Type 1 skulls were associated with relative depression of the petrous pyramid, indicating that the neurocranium was posteriorly rotated with respect to the splanchnocranium. It was thought that the more posterior attachment of the dura increased the tensile force exerted on the crista galli and expanded its bulk. Posteriorly, the cribriform plate usually articulates with either the ethmoidal spine or the jugum of the sphenoid bone. However, in a minority of cases, retro-ethmoidal processes of the orbital plates of the frontal bone join together behind the plate so that the ethmoid is cut off from the sphenoid and is surrounded by frontal articulations. Another minor variation is the presence of a non-cribriform area behind the perforated part of the plate (Murphy, 1955).

The section of the perpendicular plate below the cribriform plate is thin, flat and rhomboidal and covered with mucous membrane. It forms part of the nasal septum, separating the right and left cavities of the nose. The **posterior border** is fused to the crest and rostrum of the sphenoid above and articulates with the vomer below, while the **inferior border** joins the septal cartilage. The **anterior border** supports the frontal spine and articulates with the median crest of the nasal bones for a variable distance along its length. Details are given by Lang (1989).

The two **ethmoidal labyrinths** are delicate masses of bone attached on either side of the cribriform plate and articulate with the frontal above, the sphenoid behind and the orbital plate of the maxilla below. Each is composed of air cells (sinuses) separated by thin septa, many of which are completed by adjoining bones and which therefore appear open in the disarticulated skull. The lateral surface of the labyrinth, **orbital plate** (lamina papyracea/os

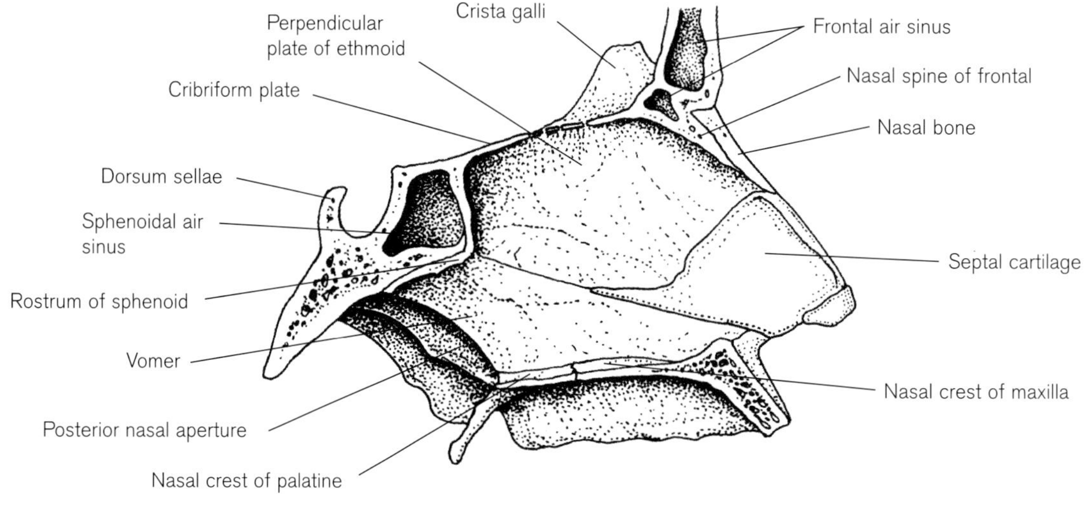

Figure 5.52 Components of the adult nasal septum.

planum) is extremely thin and outlines of the air cells may be seen through it in the medial wall of the orbit. Anteriorly, articulation with the lacrimal covers the infundibulum of the frontal sinus and the anterolateral air cells. The **medial surface** of each labyrinth, forming the lateral wall of the nasal cavity, normally bears the **superior** and **middle nasal conchae**[21] (turbinate bones). A common variation is the presence of a **supreme concha** above the superior concha and a 30% incidence rate has been reported by Swanson and Logan (1999). The middle concha covers the expanded **bulla ethmoidalis** and the groove beneath it, the **hiatus semilunaris**. A curved piece of bone, the **uncinate process**, which usually articulates with both the lacrimal and the inferior concha and partly covers the opening of the maxillary sinus, extends posteriorly under the bulla. Variations of the uncinate process have been described by Isobe *et al.* (1998). The ethmoidal sinuses are grouped into posterior, middle and anterior. The posterior sinuses are behind, above and medial to the middle group and open into the superior meatus. The middle and anterior groups are more extensive and open into the hiatus beneath the bulla, together with the infundibulum leading from the frontal sinus. Pneumatization may spread into the uncinate process (Schaeffer, 1910a).

Each part of the ethmoid bone shows minor anomalies. The crista galli is variable in form, may deviate laterally or be pneumatized (Lang, 1989). The perpendicular plate also commonly deviates and its articulation with the frontal and nasal bones is variable, depending partly on the size of the frontal spine. The orbital surface may be divided by sutures or show dehiscences. Its articulation with the lacrimal bone is also variable (Thomson, 1890). The conchae are variable in size, shape and number (Harris, 1926b; Augier, 1931; Lang, 1989).

[21] *Concha* (Latin meaning a 'shell') especially pearl-oyster or mussel.

Ossification

The first centres of ossification appear in the middle conchal region of the labyrinths of the ethmoid bone during the fifth lunar month (Vidić, 1971). In general, ossification spreads from inferior to superior and medial to lateral and there may be several centres for the main concha, the bulla and the uncinate process (Augier, 1931). The ethmoidal and frontal sinus systems begin as air cells, which bud out from the superior and middle meatuses to invaginate the ectethmoidal part of the nasal capsule (See 'Early development of skull'). Ossification extends into the superior concha and then slowly spreads into intercellular septa as far as the orbital laminae, which form as the external surfaces of ethmoidal cells, so that by about 6 lunar months, each labyrinth is almost completely ossified. At birth, the bone consists of the two bony labyrinths held together by the cartilaginous cribriform and perpendicular plates. In the perinatal period, an individual labyrinth may be identified by its characteristic morphology although it is rarely recovered, owing to its extremely fragile nature (Fig. 5.53). It is a slim rectangle, the medial side of which is 'wrinkled' bone and the lateral side is the smooth orbital plate. This forms a more or less continuous covering, except at the anterior end where open air cells are usually visible. The upper and middle conchae may be distinguished on the medial side.

The cribriform plate and the upper part of the perpendicular plate start to ossify quite rapidly during the first year of life, the external parts by spreading from the labyrinth and the internal parts from paramedian centres. From 4–8 months *postpartum* the internal and external sections unite, commencing in the posterior third. The crista galli ossifies either by extension from the internal part of the cribriform plate or from a separate centre of ossification and there may be an occasional centre for the tip (Augier, 1931). Growth in length and width of the cribriform plate

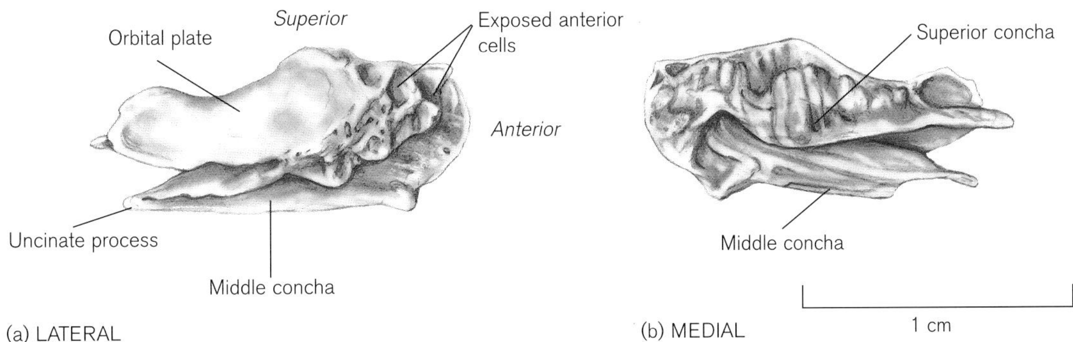

Figure 5.53 Right perinatal ethmoidal labyrinth.

ceases by the age of 2–3 years, when it fuses with the labyrinths (Ford, 1958; Scott, 1959). After this, the width of the labyrinths can only increase by surface deposition during further pneumatization on the orbital side (Scott, 1959). Measurements of the ethmoidal sinuses at birth and during childhood are given by Peter *et al.*, (1938) and Wolf *et al.* (1993). The most anterior group of air cells sometimes give rise to the frontal air sinuses (Schaeffer, 1916), which start to pneumatize the frontal bone in early childhood (see 'Frontal bone'). Ethmoidal air cells may also invade the sphenoid, maxilla and lacrimal bones.

The lower part of the perpendicular plate ossifies later and more slowly. An endochondral centre appears in the mesethmoid cartilage during the first year and bone gradually spreads in the cartilaginous septum towards the vomer (see 'Ossification of vomer'). At first, only the edge of the ossifying area is thickened and the rest of the plate is very thin and may be perforated (Cleland, 1862). Verwoerd *et al.* (1989) reported on the radiological appearances of the nasal septum from birth to 30 years of age. No ossification was visible in the upper part of the septum during the first year, but the alae of the vomer showed clearly. Ossification began in the upper, posterior part of the septum and gradually enlarged antero-inferiorly towards the vomer, the lower rim of the bony area becoming obvious. The age at which the ossification reached the vomer varied between 3 and 10 years of age. There was usually an unossified posterior part of the septum – the 'sphenoidal tail' – between the thickened rim of the perpendicular plate and the line of fusion of the vomerine alae. From 10 years of age until the late teens, there was a progressive expansion of ossification of the perpendicular plate at the expense of the cartilaginous septum and overlap was visible radiologically. Bony integration between the two structures took place between 20 and 30 years of age.

Practical notes

Sideing/orientation of the ethmoid (Fig. 5.53)

The ethmoidal labyrinth is usually ossified by the seventh month of fetal life and resembles the adult in its morphology. The smooth orbital plate lies laterally and the wrinkled conchal surface is medial with the free edge of the middle concha inferiorly. Air sinuses can usually be seen anteriorly on the superior surface. A whole ethmoid is not usually recognizable until some time after birth, as the perpendicular plate does not start to ossify until the first year of life.

Bones of similar morphology

Small fragments of any of the pneumatized bones could be mistaken for the ethmoidal labyrinth. Probably the only recognizable parts are the crista galli or a large part of the nasal septum in late juvenile life.

Morphological summary

Fetal	
Mth 5	Ossification centres appear in the cartilage of the conchal regions of the labyrinth
Birth	Represented by two labyrinths joined by cartilage
1–2 yrs	Cribriform plate and crista galli ossify and fuse with labyrinths
3–10 yrs	Ossified perpendicular plate reaches vomer and 'sphenoidal tail' usually visible posteriorly
10 yrs–puberty	Progressive expansion of ossification into nasal septum
20–30 yrs	Ethmoid and vomer fuse

VIII. INFERIOR NASAL CONCHA

The adult inferior nasal concha

Functionally, the inferior nasal concha should probably be viewed as a detached piece of the ethmoid bone. It lies below the ethmoidal labyrinth in the lateral wall of the nose and is covered with mucous membrane on both sides. It is a delicate plate of bone, boat-shaped in outline, with two surfaces, two ends and two borders (Fig. 5.54).

The **medial** (septal) **surface** is convex and roughened by ridges and grooves for nerves and vessels. The **lateral surface** is concave and smoother and lies across the inferior half of the opening of the maxillary sinus, thus reducing its size. The rounded **anterior end** and the pointed **posterior end** attach to the conchal crests of the frontal process of the maxilla and the perpendicular plate of the palatine bone, respectively. The **inferior border** is thickened and inrolled and curves upwards at both ends. The **superior border** bears three processes, which are variable in size and shape. Anteriorly, a **lacrimal process** articulates with the descending process of the lacrimal bone, forming part of the nasolacrimal canal; in the centre, a flat **maxillary process** projecting inferiorly articulates with the edge of the maxillary hiatus; and posteriorly there is an **ethmoidal process** which articulates, sometimes at several points, with the uncinate process of the ethmoidal labyrinth.

Abnormalities of the inferior concha can include agenesis, variations in size and shape of the superior border or it may appear as a bilobed, or trilobed struc-

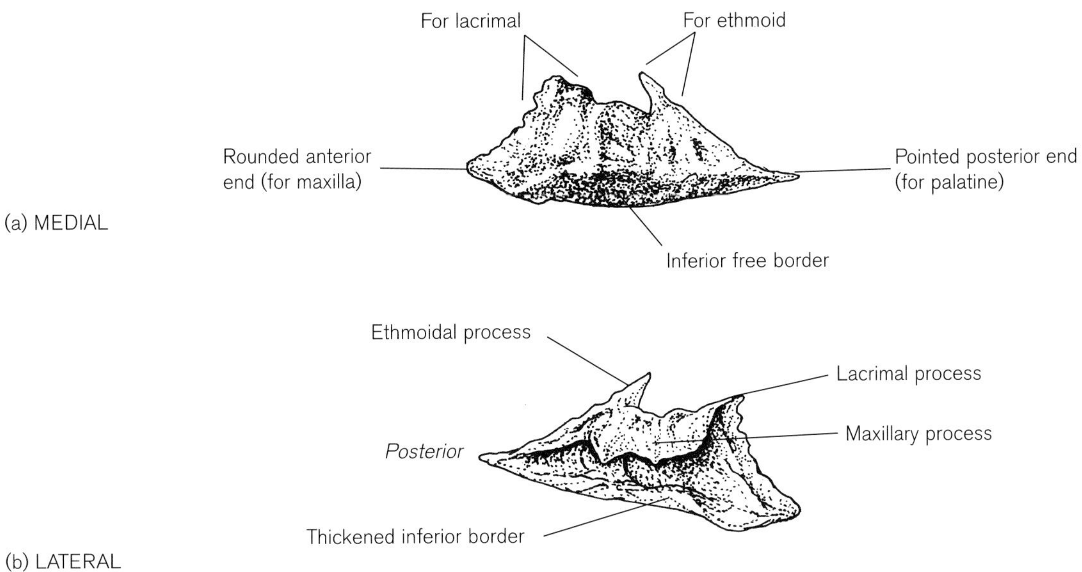

Figure 5.54 Right adult inferior concha.

ture. It may also fuse with the uncinate process of the ethmoid bone (Augier, 1931).

Ossification

The inferior concha develops endochondrally in the lateral wall of the nasal capsule. As with the other conchae, it is part of the ectethmoid cartilage (see 'Early development of skull'), which forms the incomplete floor (solum nasi) of the nasal region before the palatal shelves develop. It is the first part of the region to ossify and appears before any of the ethmoid centres. According to Augier (1931), a single ossification centre appears at about 16 weeks in the middle of the cartilaginous anlage and rapidly grows inferiorly towards the free edge. It loses continuity with the capsule during ossification and so develops into an independent bone. Limson (1932) describes a second bony plate, which appears at the inferior border of the first centre during the seventh month. During the later part of fetal life it spreads upwards as a corrugated mass of bone and covers the medial surface of the upper plate. The maxillary process appears first and is recognizable in the seventh month, while the ethmoidal and lacrimal processes do not develop until the eighth month. At birth, the bone has all the characters of the adult bone, except that it is more wrinkled and the processes of the superior border are less obvious (Fig. 5.55). It frequently fuses with the maxilla before middle life (Augier, 1931; Frazer, 1948).

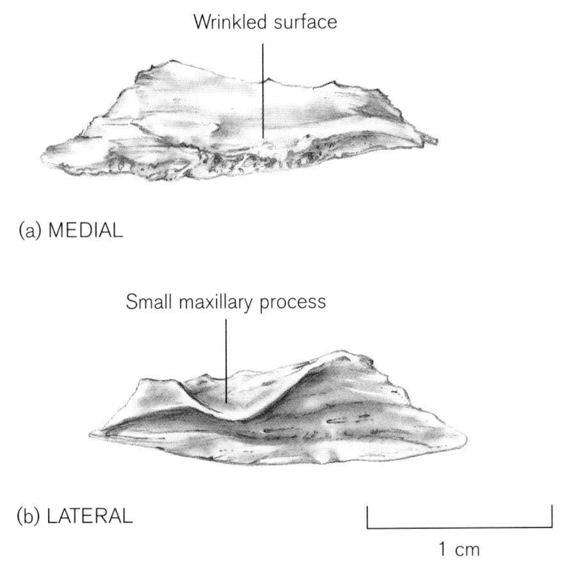

Figure 5.55 Right perinatal concha.

Practical notes

Sideing /orientation

Recovery of an isolated juvenile inferior concha would be a rare event, as it is a very fragile bone and correct sideing would depend on the completeness of the specimen. The medial surface is wrinkled and convex and the lateral surface is smoother and concave. The posterior end is more pointed than the anterior and the inferior border is thickened and curved under (Fig. 5.55).

Bones of a similar morphology

Parts of an inferior concha would be very difficult to distinguish from fragments of the labyrinths of the ethmoid bone.

Morphological summary

Fetal

Wk 16 Single intramembranous ossification centre appears
Mth 7 Maxillary process develops
Mth 8 Ethmoidal and lacrimal processes develop
Birth Adult morphology except more wrinkled and lacrimal, maxillary and ethmoid processes less well developed

Metrics

The length of the bone was recorded during fetal life by Fazekas and Kósa (1978, Table 5.14) and at birth, 1 year, 5 years, 13 years and in adults by Lang (1989, Table 5.15).

Table 5.14 Length of the fetal inferior nasal concha

Age (weeks)	Length (mm)
16	4.0
18	4.8
20	5.5
22	6.1
24	6.3
26	7.9
28	9.3
30	10.2
32	11.9
34	14.2
36	15.0
38	18.7
40	19.9

Length: maximum distance measured in the horizontal plane.
Adapted from Fazekas and Kósa (1978).

Table 5.15 Length of the inferior nasal concha from birth to adult life (mm)

	Mean	Range
Neonate	20.50	17.5–23.0
1 year	26.37	22.5–30.5
5 years	33.31	32.0–39.0
13 years	40.01	38.0–42.0
Adult	43.43	35.0–51.0

Adapted from Lang (1989).

IX. LACRIMAL

The adult lacrimal

The lacrimal (Latin – *lacrima*, meaning 'tear') is probably the most delicate of all the bones of the body and, despite its small size, quite variable in morphology. It lies at the anterior edge of the medial wall of the orbit and articulates with the frontal and ethmoidal bones and with the maxilla and the inferior nasal concha (Fig. 5.3). It has two surfaces and four borders (Fig. 5.56).

The **superficial** (lateral/orbital) **surface** is divided by the sharp, anteriorly curved **posterior lacrimal crest**, which ends in the **lacrimal hamulus**. The section posterior to the crest is translucent and lies anteriorly in the medial orbital wall. The part anterior to the crest forms the posteromedial wall of the nasolacrimal canal, which is completed by the frontal process of the maxilla. The lacrimal part of the orbicularis oculi is attached to the crest and the surface posterior to it. The **deep** (medial/nasal) **surface** completes the lateral wall of the ethmoidal labyrinth and covers some of the anterior ethmoidofrontal air cells and the infundibulum to form part of the lateral wall of the middle meatus of the nose. Most of the surface contains very thin patches, which are impressions of the sinus walls and the lower part has an articular area for the inferior nasal concha. The **posterior border** articulates with the orbital plate of the ethmoid and the small **superior border** meets the frontal bone. The **anterior border** articulates with the frontal process of the maxilla and the **inferior border**, behind the crest, meets its orbital plate. In front of the crest it is prolonged downwards and articulates with the lacrimal process of the inferior concha and the uncinate process of the ethmoid and so completes the wall of the nasolacrimal canal. Normally a lacrimal fossa, accommodating the lacrimal sac, is formed at the junction of the bone with the frontal bone and the maxilla, but its boundaries and shape are not always distinct. Its structural variability is described by Martin and Saller (1959) and Bisaria *et al.* (1989).

Anomalies of the lacrimal bone have been reported by Macalister (1884), Thomson (1890), Reid (1910), Flecker (1913) and Barnes (1994). If the lacrimal is absent or rudimentary, its place may be taken by the maxilla or ethmoid bones. The crest may vary in shape and angulation and the bone may be limited to that part behind the crest. The hamulus, present more commonly in males, normally articulates at the orbital margin with the maxilla, but it can meet an extended maxillary process of the zygomatic bone.

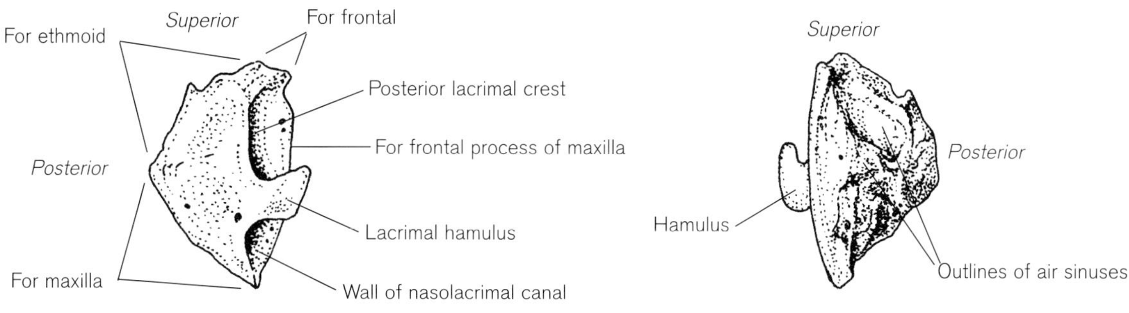

(a) SUPERFICIAL (b) DEEP

Figure 5.56 Right adult lacrimal.

Perilacrimal ossicles between it and neighbouring bones are common on all borders.

Post (1969) used the differences in size of the opening and length of the nasolacrimal canal to assess sex, age and racial affinity. Females had a more restricted entrance than males. After the fifth decade, there is an increase in size of the opening and a decrease in length in both sexes. In American Blacks the opening of the canal was larger and the length shorter than in Whites. This appears to correlate with an increased incidence of dacrocystitis (inflammation of the nasolacrimal canal) in those groups with a more restricted entrance and a longer canal.

Ossification

The lacrimal bone develops in membrane on the surface of the nasal capsule. It arises from a single ossification centre at about 10 fetal weeks (Macklin, 1921; Noback and Robertson, 1951) in a cleft in the chondrocranium between the posterior maxillary process and the posterior prominence, with the nasolacrimal duct lying immediately lateral to it (Macklin, 1921). The main part of the bone forms first, followed by the crista and then the hamulus, with the orbital part last. Rambaud and Renault (1864) describe two calcified tracks, which would explain the occasional bipartite bone. There is sometimes a separate inferior ossicle for the hamulus (Augier, 1931). In fetuses between 5 and 8 lunar months, the orbital part of the bone is very small compared to the facial part, but by birth the two parts have become nearly equal in size (Limson, 1932). The perinatal bone is long and slim supero-inferiorly, with the facial and orbital parts separated by the lacrimal crest (Fig. 5.57). It may not articulate with the orbital plate of the ethmoid until after birth. Peter *et al.* (1938) described two periods of growth in length of the nasolacrimal duct, which were related to the eruption of the deciduous dentition and the second permanent molars, first, from 7 months to 3 years and second between 12 and 14 years.

Practical notes

Sideing a perinatal lacrimal (Fig. 5.57)

It is unlikely that the lacrimal bone would be recovered in isolation, owing to its extremely fragile nature. The lacrimal crest lies on the lateral side and ends inferiorly in the lacrimal hamulus.

Bones of a similar morphology

Fragments of the orbital plate of the ethmoid have a similar structure to the lacrimal, which could only be identified if a characteristic part such as the crest or hamulus were preserved.

Morphological summary

Fetal

Wk 10 Single intramembranous ossification centre appears

Birth Long, slim bone with narrow section posterior to crest

2–3 yrs Adult morphology

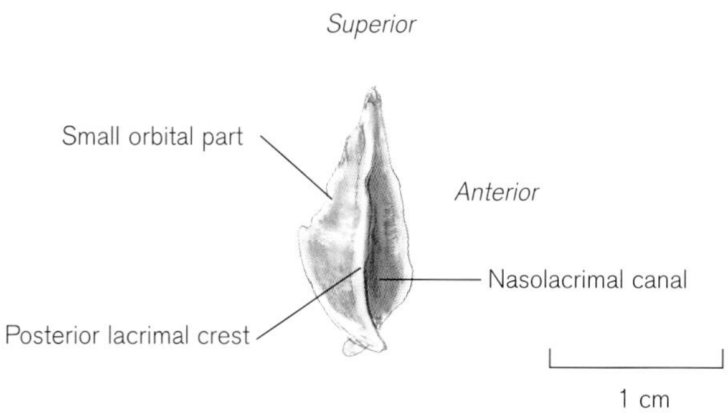

Figure 5.57 Right perinatal lacrimal.

X. THE VOMER

The adult vomer

The vomer[22] (Fig. 5.58) is a thin, trapezoid-shaped plate of bone that lies in the midline and forms part of the nasal septum. It articulates with the sphenoid, ethmoid, and palatine bones, and with the maxilla and septal cartilage (Figs. 5.1 and 5.52). It has two surfaces and four borders.

The **two surfaces**, forming part of the medial wall of each half of the nasal cavity, are both covered by mucous membrane and bear grooves for nasopalatine nerves and vessels. The **posterosuperior border** bears two thickened **alae** with a deep groove between them into which articulates the underside of the body and the rostrum of the sphenoid. The alae are overlapped by the vaginal processes of the medial pterygoid plates and the sphenoidal processes of the palatine bones. The long **anterosuperior** border articulates behind with the perpendicular plate of the ethmoid and in front with the nasal septal cartilage. There may be a band of cartilage between the ethmoid and vomer even into old age (Augier, 1931), but more usually the two bones fuse in early adult life (see above). The joint between the vomer and the septal cartilage is unusual in that it is the only freely moveable joint composed of non-cartilage-covered bone on one side and cartilage on the other. The perichondrium of the septum and the bone of the vomer are separated only by a fat pad (Fig. 5.59). This would appear to be a safety device to prevent dislocation of the septum, as pressure on the anterior border causes the cartilage to bend obliquely on itself in its long axis (Aymard, 1917). The **inferior border** rests on the median crest formed by the horizontal plates of the palatine bone and the maxilla. The **posterior border** forms a gently curving, free edge that forms a midline division between the posterior choanae. It is thin below and thickens above as it slopes towards the two alae.

Incomplete ossification may lead to perforations in the bone or to a narrow cavity between the two sides. Most of the variations in the shape of the vomer play a part in the clinical condition of deviated septum (Takahashi, 1987). Deviation is rarely seen in the newborn or before the age of 7 years and so may be related to the growth of the maxillae after the appearance of the deciduous dentition (Augier, 1931; Frazer, 1948). It appears to be more common in Whites and males. Rarely, the sphenoidal sinus may project inferiorly and pneumatize the vomer (Lang, 1989).

[22] *Vomer* (Latin meaning a 'ploughshare') or *vomere* (Latin meaning 'to vomit, throw up'), because the ploughshare threw up the earth on either side in a fanciful resemblance to vomiting.

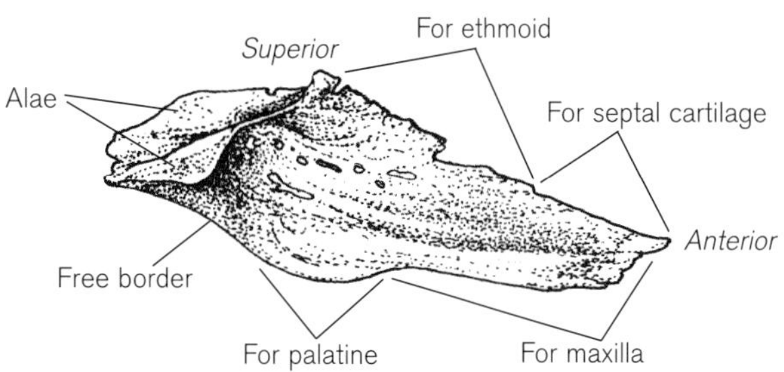

Figure 5.58 Adult vomer.

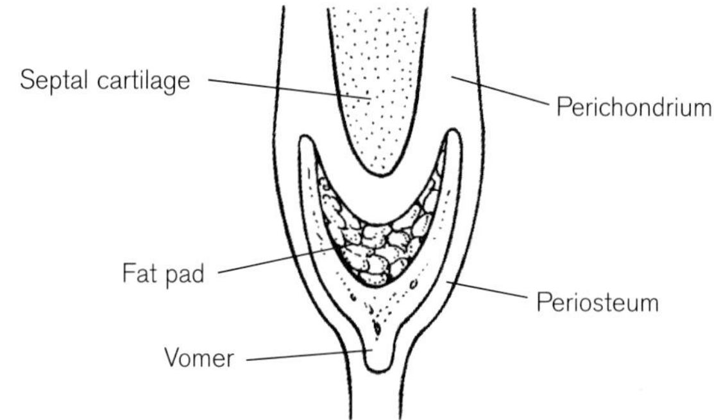

Figure 5.59 Chondrovomeral joint (redrawn after Scott, 1958).

Ossification

The vomer develops from two intramembranous ossification centres that appear in the mucoperichondrium at the lower border of the nasal septum during the ninth week of uterine life (Fawcett, 1911a; Macklin, 1914, 1921; Müller and O'Rahilly, 1980). Histologically, they appear as two slender strips of bone, widest in the middle and tapering off towards their ends. After about 2 weeks, they fuse at their lower borders beneath the septal cartilage to form a V- or U-shaped bone. Later still, this becomes Y-shaped in coronal section. The vomerine groove, which extends from the sphenoid posteriorly to the premaxillary area in front, supports the lower edge of the septal cartilage, the posterior part of which will ossify later as the perpendicular plate of the ethmoid. The vomer is visible radiographically at about 11 weeks (O'Rahilly and Meyer, 1956). Sandikcioglu *et al.* (1994), in a histological and radiological study, reported a concavity inferiorly at the site of fusion, which took place at a mean age of 17 fetal weeks. The bone assumed its Y-shape from between 19 and 23 weeks and, from the lateral aspect, looked fan-shaped, with bony trabeculae spreading radially from the base.

The vomer in the third trimester of fetal life is boat-shaped, consisting of two leaves of bone joined inferiorly into a single lamina with a flattened base (Fig. 5.60). Each leaf has a feathery free edge and is pointed and almost vertical anteriorly. Posteriorly, the two leaves open out to form a scoop-shaped end, which develops into the vomerine alae.

The involvement of the paraseptal (Jacobsonian) cartilages in the development of the vomer is complex and has remained a matter of some controversy. Fawcett (1911a) described the vomer invading and ossifying the posterior end of the anterior paraseptal cartilages, which he believed originated from the roof of the nasal capsule. Augier (1931) described the paraseptal cartilages ossifying independently into paraseptal ossicles, which then fused with the vomer later in the perinatal period or even after birth. Eloff (1952) agreed with Augier on the existence of independent paraseptal ossicles, but could not confirm Fawcett's finding of fusion with the vomer. More recently, Wang *et al.* (1988) attempted to elucidate the fate of the paraseptal cartilages, which they believed originated directly from the antero-inferior part of the septal cartilage as it grows down to meet the palatal shelves. They were unable to identify any separate paraseptal ossicles and agreed with Fawcett that the vomer invades the posterior end of the paraseptal cartilages, while the anterior end seemed to be resorbing. The time of ossification varied greatly from 14 to 32 weeks *in utero*. They were unable to identify any posterior paraseptal cartilages. Whatever the exact relationship of the paraseptal cartilages to the vomer, they obviously contribute to the development of the bone, so that although primarily of membranous origin, the vomer is ontogenetically a mixed bone with contributions from both membranous and cartilaginous elements. The role of the paraseptal cartilages and the surgical approaches to cartilaginous remnants were reviewed by Beck (1963).

The postnatal growth of the vomer is intimately connected with the growth of the nasal septum as a whole and the consequent increase in size of the facial skeleton (Scott, 1953, 1967). Takahashi (1987), in a study of septal deformity, gave a detailed account of the changes in the vomer and distinguished nine phases of development. The downward spread of ossification in the perpendicular plate of the ethmoid reaches the vomer during early childhood and contact between the two structures induces further ossification at the open edges of the vomerine groove. By the age of 10 years, the height of the posterior edge of the nasal septum is about 85% of its adult size (Scott, 1967). The superior left and right edges of the vomer fuse, converting the groove into a vomerine canal by the age of puberty. During adult life, the bone undergoes compaction and thinning and also increases in height. In early adult life, there is usually fusion with the perpendicular plate of the ethmoid (see above).

Practical notes

Orientation (Fig. 5.60)
The boat-shaped bone is composed of two laminae, which are fused inferiorly. They are more pointed and closer together anteriorly.

Bones of a similar morphology

The complete vomer is unlikely to be mistaken for any other bone as it has a characteristic shape. However, fragments would be indistinguishable from other delicate nasal and facial fragments.

Morphological summary

Fetal	
Wks 9–10	Two intramembranous ossification centres appear
Wks 11–12	Fusion at the lower edges of the two leaves of bone
Mths 3–5	Change from U-shaped to Y-shaped base
Birth	Boat-shaped bone composed of two laminae
3–10 yrs	Ossification of perpendicular plate of ethmoid towards vomer
10 yrs–puberty	Edges of vomerine groove fuse to form canal
20–30 yrs	Vomer normally fuses with perpendicular plate of ethmoid

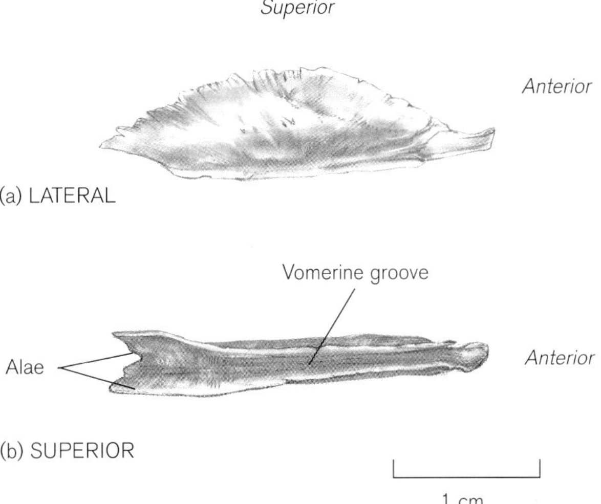

Figure 5.60 Perinatal vomer.

Metrics

Fazekas and Kósa (1978) recorded the increase in length of the vomer during fetal life (Table 5.16).

Table 5.16 Length of the fetal vomer

Age (weeks)	Length (mm)
12	4.0
14	5.6
16	9.9
18	12.0
20	14.1
22	15.9
24	17.5
26	18.2
28	20.1
30	21.3
32	23.1
34	23.8
36	28.3
38	28.7
40	30.6

Length: maximum length from anterior end to posterior end of alae.
Adapted from Fazekas and Kósa (1978).

XI. THE ZYGOMATIC

The adult zygomatic

The zygomatic[23] (malar[24] bone/jugal[25]) forms the prominence of the cheek and separates the orbit from the temporal fossa. It articulates with the maxilla, the greater wing of the sphenoid, and the zygomatic processes of the frontal and temporal bones (Figs. 5.1, 5.3 and 5.5). It is an irregular shape and has three surfaces, two processes and five borders (Fig. 5.61).

The **lateral** (external) **surface** may be flat, or have a pronounced malar **tubercle** in its centre. It usually has at least one foramen for the zygomaticofacial nerve and vessels, but this may be double or multiple. The **temporal surface** faces inferoposteriorly and is divided into two. The upper part is deeply concave and forms the anterior wall of the temporal and infratemporal fossae. It is also pierced by neurovascular foramina and provides attachment for the vertical, anterior fibres of the temporalis muscle. The lower part is a roughened triangular articular area for the maxilla. The **orbital surface** forms the anterolateral wall and part of the floor of the orbit and in 95% of bones bears a tubercle in its upper part, the **eminentia orbitalis**, first described by Whitnall (1911). It provides attachments for the check ligament of the lateral rectus muscle, the lateral extremity of the tendon of the levator palpebrae superioris muscle, the suspensory ligament of the eye and the lateral extremities of the tarsal plates. Zygomatico-orbital foramina allow the passage of branches of the zygomatic nerve from the orbit to the skin over the bone.

The stout **frontal process** extends superiorly from the junction of all three surfaces and articulates at a serrated end, with the zygomatic process of the frontal bone above and the greater wing of the sphenoid below. The **temporal process** extends posteriorly from the lateral and temporal surfaces to meet the zygomatic process of the squamous temporal bone and so complete the zygomatic arch.

The **anterosuperior** (orbital) **border** extends from the frontal to the maxillary articulation and forms the blunt inferolateral part of the circumference of the orbit. It normally extends along the inferior margin as far as the infra-orbital foramen. The **antero-inferior** (maxillary) **border** lies on the front of the face and forms one side of the maxillary articulation. The **posterosuperior border** is convex above where it forms the posterior border of the frontal process. Here there is a tuberosity, the **tuberculum marginale**, to which a strong band of temporal fascia is attached. Both the malar tuberosity and the tuberculum are more strongly developed in males (WEA, 1980). The border is concave below where it continues onto the superior border of the temporal process. The **postero-inferior** (masseteric) **border** forms the inferior border of the temporal process and is often roughened for the attachment of the masseter muscle. The **posteromedial border** is serrated in its upper half and articulates with the frontal bone and the greater wing of the sphenoid. Below this, there is usually a small non-articular section that forms the anterior end of the inferior orbital fissure and the border continues horizontally to articulate with the maxilla in the floor of the orbit.

The size and curvature of the bone varies greatly in different populations (Woo, 1937–8), being smaller and flatter in Caucasian skulls and larger and more curved in Mongoloid races. There are several anomalies of the zygomatic bone. The infra-orbital process can extend medially beyond its usual distance to articulate with the lacrimal bone and form

[23] *Zygoma* (Greek meaning 'yoke').
[24] *Mala* (Latin meaning 'cheek')
[25] *Lugum* (Latin meaning 'yoke') *iugare* (Latin meaning 'to bind together') – the bone binds the maxilla, frontal and temporal bones together.

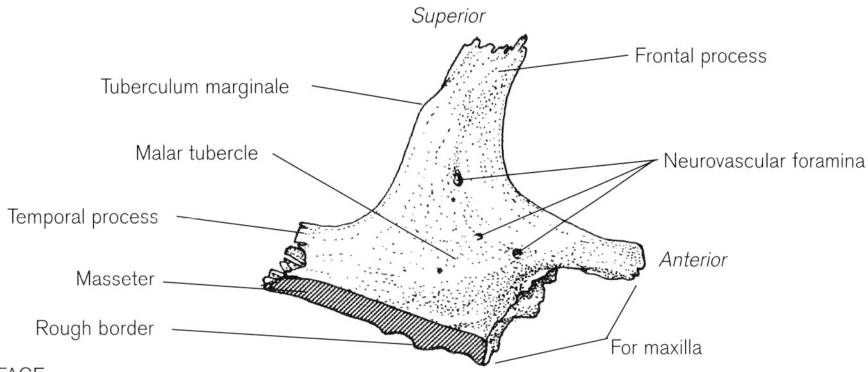

(a) LATERAL SURFACE

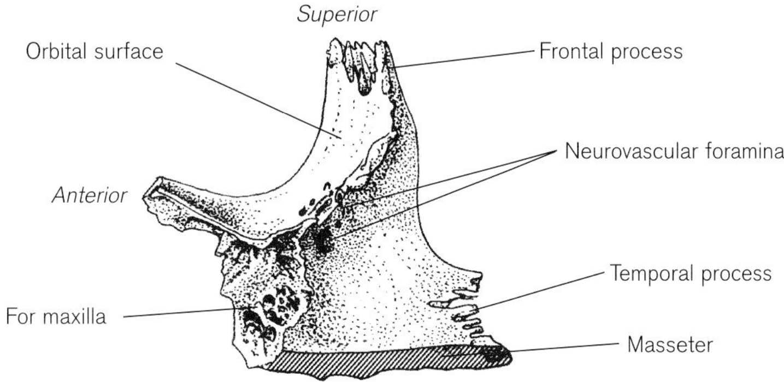

(b) TEMPORAL SURFACE

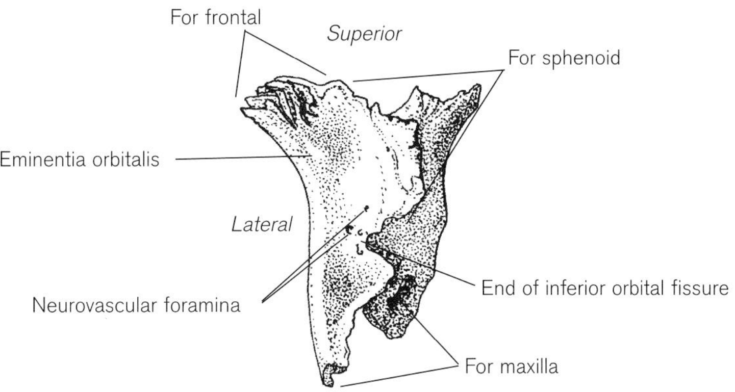

(c) ORBITAL SURFACE

Figure 5.61 Right adult zygomatic.

part of the nasolacrimal canal (Augier, 1931). The bone may be divided by anomalous sutures and may be bi-, or tripartite (Barclay-Smith, 1897; Hrdlička, 1902, 1904). This is extremely rare in Caucasian skulls (0.5–2%), but in certain Far Eastern populations it is much more common (e.g. Japan, 20%) and has earned the name 'os japonicum' (Reinhard and Rösing, 1985). Hanihara *et al.*, (1998) have reviewed the worldwide incidence of bipartite os zygomaticum. Another variation, often classified as os japonicum, is seen when the zygomatic process of the maxilla may meet that of the temporal bone without the zygomatic bone itself being divided, a condition known as 'arcus maxillotemporalis infrajugalis'. The trace of a suture, misnamed an 'os japonicum', is fairly common in other Asiatic and New World populations (Bhargava *et al.*, 1960; Ossenberg, 1970; Jeyasingh *et al.*, 1982). Perimalar ossicles may occasionally be found between the zygomatic and any of the bones with which it articulates. The number of neurovascular canals in the bone is very variable. The most common arrangement is a single foramen on the orbital surface, which divides into zygomaticotemporal and zygomaticofacial canals that exit on the lateral surface, but it is not uncommon for there to be double or supernumerary foramina.

Ossification

The single ossification centre for the bone develops in the mesenchyme below and lateral to the orbit during the eighth week of intra-uterine life (Noback and Robertson, 1951; O'Rahilly and Gardner, 1972) and evidence for two or three separate centres appears doubtful, at least in Europeans. The bone appears as a triangular squama, with the temporal process most advanced and the frontal process the last to form (Augier, 1931). By the ninth week it already bears a resemblance to the adult bone, being an incurved quadrilateral with four angles. The border between the cranial and ventral angles forms the part that will fuse with the maxilla (Macklin, 1914, 1921). At first the temporal process is the most obvious, but it does not complete the zygomatic arch until late in fetal life, or occasionally after birth. The ossification centre becomes apparent radiologically by about 11–12 weeks (O'Rahilly and Meyer, 1956; Bach-Petersen and Kjær, 1993).

By the end of the first half of fetal life, the zygomatic is sufficiently similar to the adult bone to be recognizable, although the proportions are somewhat modified. It is also comparatively large and robust and is therefore one of the most frequently recovered complete juvenile cranial bones. Perinatally, (Fig. 5.62) it is a gracile triradiate bone with slender frontal, temporal and maxillary processes, which project from a relatively small, curved body. The three surfaces have the same relationship to each other as in the adult bone, but the borders of the bone are different because the facial skeleton is relatively small at this stage. The inferior border bears a prominent notch about one-third of the way from the medial end, which marks the future angle between the antero-inferior and postero-inferior borders. The posteromedial border just touches the frontal bone and then articulates with the greater sphenoidal wing. There is a big non-articular area below this as the inferior orbital fissure is relatively large at this stage and the inferior part of the border articulates with the maxilla obliquely along the middle of the orbital floor.

During infancy and early childhood, the zygomatic develops to keep pace with the rapid growth of the maxilla, which increases in height and width to accommodate the deciduous dentition. This causes a change in position of the articulation with the maxilla and angulation at the notch on the inferior border. The infra-orbital zygomaticomaxillary suture shifts from the middle to the lateral side of the orbital floor and the antero-inferior and the postero-inferior borders become defined. By the time of completion of the eruption of the deciduous dentition, the bone has assumed adult proportions. Both the tuberculum marginale and the eminentia orbitalis become palpable during the second or third year of life. At about the same time, the ends of the frontal and temporal processes become serrated. As the development of a malar tubercle is a secondary sexual characteristic, it is not usually obvious much before puberty.

Practical notes

Sideing/orientation (Fig. 5.62)

The bone is recognizable in isolation from mid-fetal life and by the perinatal period is surprisingly large and robust, compared to other facial bones. Sideing depends on orientating the convex triradiate external surface correctly. The curved orbital surface lies anteromedially and the notched border is inferior. The concave temporal surface and the slender temporal process then point posteriorly.

Bones of a similar morphology

A complete zygomatic bone is readily recognizable, but fragments of one of its processes could be confused with pointed parts of other cranial bones, such as the zygomatic process of the temporal or lesser wing of sphenoid.

Morphological summary

Fetal

Wk 8	Single intramembranous ossification centre appears
Mth 6	Adopts recognizable adult morphology
Birth	Slender triradiate bone with notched inferior border
2–3 yrs	Adopts adult proportions with serrated frontal and temporal processes. Tuberculum marginale and eminentia orbitalis palpable

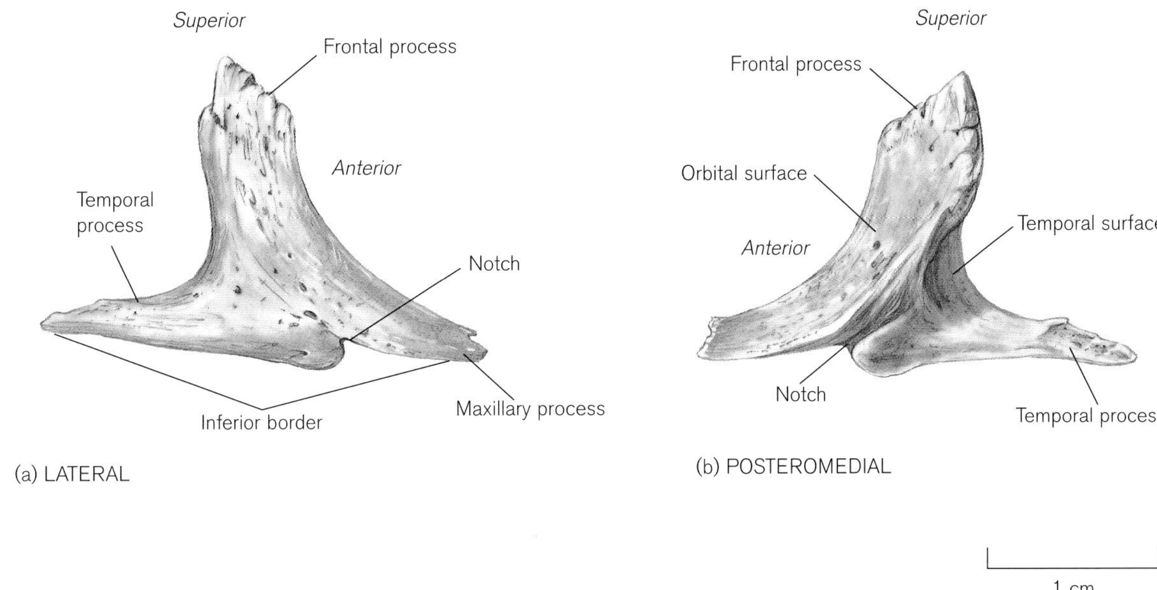

Figure 5.62 Right perinatal zygomatic.

Metrics

Fazekas and Kósa (1978) recorded the length and width of the bone during fetal life (Table 5.17). Moss *et al.* (1956) recorded length and height of the bone from 8 to 20 fetal weeks but landmarks are not defined.

Table 5.17 Dimensions of the fetal zygomatic bone

Age (weeks)	Length (mm)	Width (mm)
12	4.5	4.0
14	5.8	4.9
16	9.0	7.1
18	11.5	9.6
20	13.5	10.3
22	14.2	11.2
24	15.0	12.1
26	16.5	13.4
28	17.5	14.1
30	18.5	14.8
32	19.5	15.6
34	20.9	16.6
36	21.8	17.2
38	24.6	18.4
40	25.8	20.2

Length: medial end of infra-orbital border to posterior end of temporal process.
Width: medial end of infra-orbital border to superior end of frontal process.
Adapted from Fazekas and Kósa (1978).

XII. THE MAXILLA

The adult maxilla

The maxillae[26] (Fig. 5.63) form a large part of the visible surface of the lower face and nasal aperture. They also extend inwards to take part in the floor and lateral walls of the nasal cavity, the floors of the orbits and the anterior part of the roof of the oral cavity and they bear all the upper teeth. The right and left bones join with each other in the midline of the hard palate and articulate with the zygomatics, frontal, nasals, lacrimals, inferior conchae, ethmoid and palatine bones (Figs. 5.1, 5.3 and 5.5). Each maxilla consists of a body from which four processes extend.

The **body** is said to resemble a hollow, three-sided, pyramid, whose base forms part of the middle and inferior meatuses of the lateral wall of the nose. A large part of this **nasal surface** is open postero-superiorly as the **maxillary hiatus**, above which are parts of air cells covered in life by the ethmoid and lacrimal bones. Most of the surface below the hiatus is the smooth wall of the inferior meatus, but posteriorly there is a roughened articulation for the perpendicular process of the palatine bone. Anterior to the hiatus is a deep groove forming part of the nasolacrimal canal, which is completed by the inferior

[26] *Maxilla* (Latin meaning 'jaw'). Until comparatively recently, the upper and lower jaws were termed superior and inferior maxillae.

concha and the lacrimal bone. The anterior part of the concha rests on the **conchal crest**, which lies anterior to the groove at the base of the frontal process. The **anterior surface** actually faces anterolaterally and is limited medially by the nasal aperture and above by the medial half of the lower orbital rim. About 0.5 cm below the rim, there is normally a single large foramen for the passage of the infra-orbital nerve and vessels onto the face but multiple foramina have been reported (Riesenfeld, 1956; Reinhard and Rösing, 1985). The position of the foramen in relation to the supra-orbital notch/foramen in Korean skulls has been reported by Chung *et al.* (1995). Many of the muscles of facial expression take partial origin from this

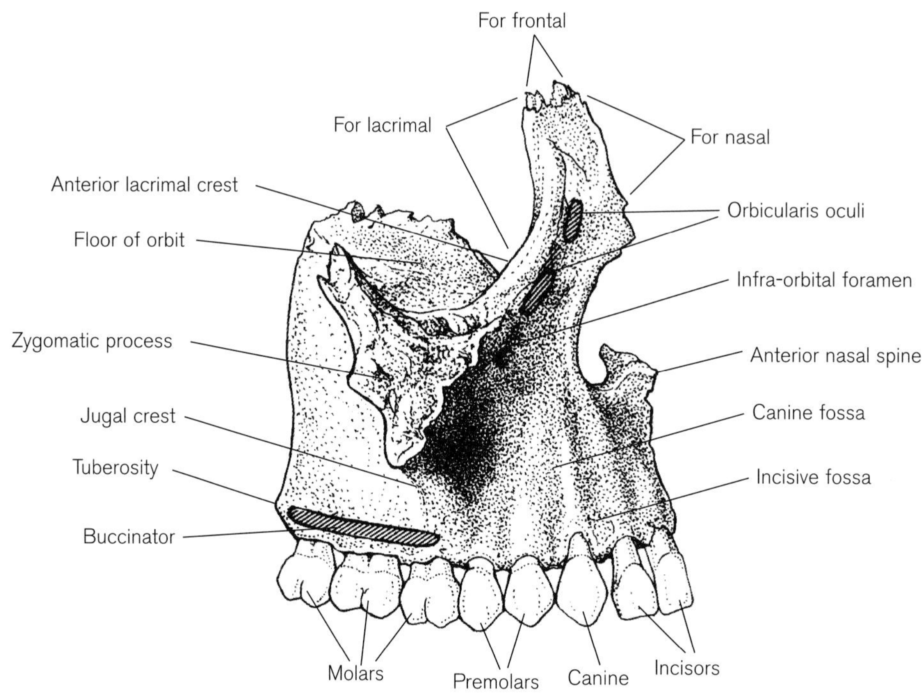

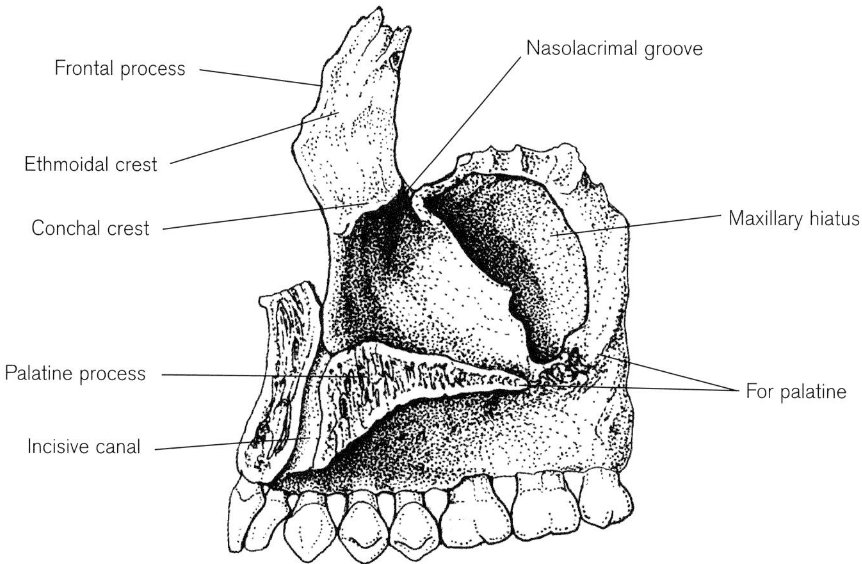

Figure 5.63 Right adult maxilla.

surface but rarely leave any impressions on the bone. It is marked by the teeth, especially the canine, which usually forms an elongated eminence reaching to the lower border of the nasal aperture. If this is sufficiently prominent there is an **incisive fossa** medial, and a **canine fossa**, lateral to the tooth. The **infratemporal surface** faces posterolaterally and is separated from the anterior surface by a rounded ridge, the zygomatico-alveolar (jugal) crest, which runs down from the zygomatic process at the level of the first molar tooth. The surface bulges posteriorly as the maxillary **tuberosity** and forms part of both the infratemporal fossa and more medially, with the palatine and sphenoid, the pterygopalatine fossa. The tuberosity is pierced in the centre by several foramina for superior alveolar nerves and vessels and roughened posteromedially, where it articulates with the palatine bone. The **orbital surface** is a thin, smooth, triangular plate that forms most of the floor of the orbit. The medial border articulates from before backward with the lacrimal, the orbital plate of the ethmoid and the orbital process of the palatine bone. The posterolateral border forms the medial edge of the inferior orbital fissure and the anterior border is the orbital margin, which is continuous with the frontal process medially. The infra-orbital nerve passes across the surface in a groove of variable length, which usually converts to a canal in the anterior part of the floor before opening onto the face via the foramen.

The **maxillary sinus** (antrum of Highmore) is the space enclosed by the base and walls of the body of the bone. Underwood (1910), Schaeffer (1910b, 1916), Wood Jones (1939), Anagnostopoulou *et al.* (1991) and Doig *et al.* (1998) have described its detailed anatomy and variations. It may be divided by septa and its apex can extend into the zygomatic process. Its floor is lower than that of the nasal cavity and often bears elevations caused by the roots of the second premolar and molar teeth. They are separated from the sinus space by a thin layer of bone, which may be deficient so that roots of the teeth are then covered only by sinusoidal mucosa and may project into the sinus. Because of the close proximity of the root apices, it is easy for infection from dental abscesses to spread into the sinus. Drainage is difficult because of the position of the opening high above the floor of the sinus. Prevalence of maxillary sinusitis in medieval populations has been studied by Lilley *et al.*, (1994), Boocock *et al.* (1995), Lewis *et al.* (1995) and Panhuysen *et al.* (1997). Shea (1977), in a study of populations from different geographical areas, reported a significant correlation between the mean maxillary sinus volume and the mean temperature of the coldest month of the year in the region inhabited. Indications are that mean maxillary sinus volume decreases in Eskimo populations from colder areas.

The **frontal process** is interposed between the nasal and lacrimal bones and articulates at its tip with the nasal part of the frontal bone via a serrated suture. Its outer surface bears the **anterior lacrimal crest**, to which is attached the medial palpebral ligament of the eye. Anterior to this are attachments for the lower parts of the orbicularis oculi muscle. Posterior to the crest, this bone, with the lacrimal bone, forms the **nasolacrimal groove**, which accommodates the nasolacrimal sac and duct. The inner surface of the frontal process lies in the lateral wall of the nose, where it articulates with the ethmoid. Its apical part may close some of the air cells, and just below, it meets the middle concha at the oblique **ethmoidal crest**.

The **zygomatic process** projects posteriorly from the junction of the anterior, infratemporal and orbital surfaces of the body. Its anterior border continues laterally from the anterior surface; its posterior border is concave and continuous with the infratemporal surface; its inferior border is sharp and continues into the ridge separating the anterior and posterolateral surfaces. The superolateral border forms a triangular, roughened surface for articulation with the zygomatic bone.

The **palatine process** projects horizontally and medially from the body to form the anterior two-thirds of the hard palate. Its smooth superior surface in the nasal floor is concave transversely. The inferior surface is ridged and grooved for palatine vessels and nerves and bears many vascular foramina. The medial surface of the process is rough for articulation in the midline of the palate, with the bone of the opposite side at the **intermaxillary** (sagittal) **suture**. This forms the nasal crest superiorly, which accommodates the vomer and septal cartilage. The crest ends in front at the **anterior nasal spine** and continues posteriorly onto the palatine bones. There are documented differences both in anterior nasal spine prominence and prognathism between Black and White populations (Schultz, 1918c; Mooney and Siegel, 1986), with the latter having a more prominent anterior nasal spine and less prognathism than the former. Behind the spine, between the two maxillae, are the openings of the **incisive canals**, which form a groove on the medial surface of each bone and transmit palatine arteries and nasopalatine nerves (Fig. 5.64). There are occasionally additional anterior and posterior incisive foraminal openings into the canal. Bellairs (1951), in a detailed study of the development of the region, observed a large blood vessel in the anterior canal and this was confirmed by Norberg (1963). These observations question the traditional textbook account that the nasopalatine (long sphenopalatine) nerves pass asymmetrically through the anterior and posterior median canaliculi. From the posterior edge of the incisive canal opening there may be an **incisive suture** extending anterolaterally to reach the alveolar process, usually between the lateral incisor and canine teeth. This delimits the 'os incisivum' or premaxillary part of the bone (see below). The posterior surface of the palatine process articulates at the squamous **palatomaxillary** (transverse palatine) suture, with the maxilla overlapping the horizontal plate of the palatine on the oral surface. At the lateral end of the suture the maxilla contributes to the lateral border of the **greater palatine foramen**, through which nerves and vessels travel from the sphenopalatine fossa to the surface of the palate (see 'Palatine bone').

The **alveolar process** extends from the inferior surface of the body and is composed of crypts for the eight permanent teeth: two incisors, one canine (cuspid), two premolars (bicuspids) and three molars. Its outer surface (labial or buccal plate) is a continuation of the anterior and infratemporal surfaces and may show fenestrae when large tooth roots pierce the bone. Its inner surface (lingual or palatal plate) extends from the anterior and lateral surfaces of the palatine process. Each tooth socket extends from its floor (fundus) to the rim (alveolar crest) and is divided from the neighbouring socket by a thin, interalveolar (interdental) septum. In multirooted cheek teeth there are interradicular septa. The alveolar sockets only persist in the presence of teeth, so that in the edentulous condition, resorption occurs and the process is much reduced in height and can be rounded or sharp in appearance. The buccinator muscle is attached to the outer alveolar surface as far forward as the first molar tooth.

The most common anomalies of the maxilla are caused by abnormalities at the blastemal stage of development. Failure of the normal morphogenesis of the frontonasal and medial nasal processes (see 'Introduction to the skull') result in different types of defects. These include cleft lip and palate, absence of the premaxillary region (Walker, 1917; Derry, 1938), various forms of facial clefting, and Binder's syndrome (hypoplasia of the median nasal prominence; Horswell *et al.*, 1987). Frontonasal process field defects seen in archaeological material have been reviewed by Barnes (1994). Information on clinical conditions can be found in Stricker *et al.* (1990).

Minor anomalies can occur at the ossification stage of development. The retention of the incisive suture on the palatal aspect has been used, together with other palatal sutures, for age determination, but there is wide variation in the time of obliteration (Mann *et al.* 1987, 1991a; Gruspier and Mullen, 1991). The remains of the incisive suture on the frontal process

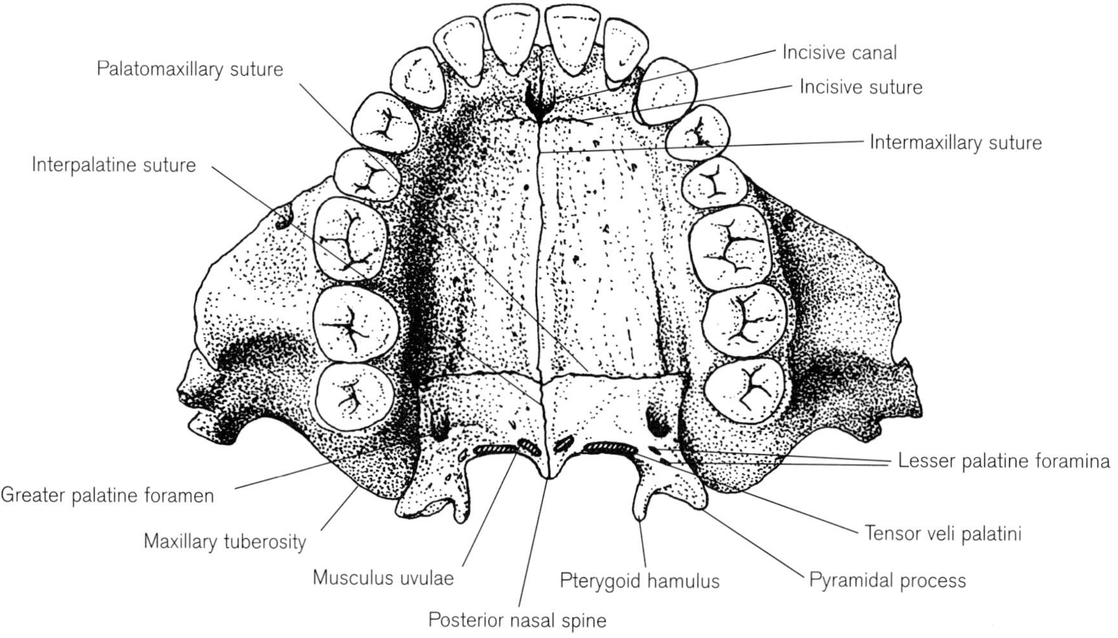

Figure 5.64 Adult hard palate.

(the sutura notha[27]) have been reported by Augier (1931). Partial or complete sutures in the palate delineating extra ossicles or complete supernumerary bones have been described and illustrated by Ashley-Montagu (1940) and Woo (1948), who named them 'anterior' or 'posterior medio-palatine bones' respectively, depending upon their position in the maxillary or palatine part of the hard palate.

The shape of the palate and nasal aperture varies depending on the ethnic origin of the population. Palate shape has been used in an attempt to identify racial groups in North American populations (Byers *et al.*, 1997). The nasal aperture also varies in height, width and shape in different populations (see 'Nasal bone').

Torus palatinus maxillaris is a bony protuberance situated along the midline palatal suture. Its appearance in the living, described by Miller and Roth (1940), varied from a slight uniform midline crest to a large prominence occupying two-thirds of the palate. It occurred in a surprisingly high 24% of 1024 routine American dental patients. It rarely appeared before the age of 5 years but on appearance, grew progressively and was twice as common in males as females. There is an extensive anthropological literature (Hooton, 1918; Hrdlička, 1940a; Woo, 1950; Witkop and Barros, 1963; Sawyer *et al.* 1979; Axelsson and Hedegaard, 1985; Reinhard and Rösing, 1985) describing a normal bilateral appearance, but unilateral occurrence has been reported. The exostosis is formed by hypertrophy of the spongy and compact layers of the oral surface of the bone, but the nasal layer remains unchanged (Vidić, 1968b). Familial studies have been reported by Krahl (1949), Kolas *et al.* (1953) and Suzuki and Sakai (1960). Torus maxillaris is a similar bony ridge running along the lingual side of the palate alongside the molar teeth (Woo, 1950; Berry and Berry, 1967). Both types of tori may need surgical removal as they can cause difficulties in fitting dentures. The prevalence of both types of tori has been used to identify and define population groups.

Ossification

Accounts of the ossification of the human maxilla have been bedevilled with disagreements about the supposed presence of a separate premaxilla (os incisivum), based on the partial separation of the adult bone by the incisive (premaxillary) suture (fissure) that is sometimes present on the palatal aspect in the adult. As stressed by Noback and Moss (1953) and Jacobson (1955), the argument has been further complicated by similar terms being used for both the mesenchymal processes and the ossification centres. Ossification centres are independent of, and secondary to, the fusion of the early mesenchymal facial processes and their boundaries do not coincide. Further confusion has been created by attempts to homologize the parts of the human maxilla with the separate premaxilla and maxilla that exist in other mammals, particularly primates. A full review of the literature from the time of Vesalius may be found in Ashley-Montagu (1935).[28]

No agreement exists on whether there are separate centres of ossification for the premaxillary and maxillary parts of the bone. Separate centres have been reported by Chase (1942), Woo (1949b), Noback and Moss (1953), Shepherd and McCarthy (1955), Kraus and Decker (1960) and Latham (1970). However, Fawcett (1911a), Jacobson (1955) and Wood *et al.*, (1967, 1969) stated categorically that there is no separate premaxillary ossification centre. Wood *et al.* (1969) described the whole bone developing from a lamina of osteoid tissue that may contain separate foci of calcification, which rapidly fuse together. They attribute the observations of supposed separate centres to misinterpretation of material; alizarin staining showing only actual calcification, but not the preliminary formation of osteoid tissue, and serial sections possibly being viewed at too high a level to see the continuous osteoid lamina at the base of the bone.

There is also controversy regarding the subsequent development of the maxilla and there are two main interpretations based on its developing appearance. The overgrowth theory (Callender, 1869; Vallois, 1930; Ashley-Montagu, 1935; Johnson, 1937; Wood Jones, 1947; Woo, 1949b) described the maxillary part gradually covering the premaxillary centre on the facial aspect, thus obliterating the incisive suture, which remains only on the palatal aspect. The other view (Felber, 1919; Chase, 1942; Noback and Moss, 1953; Kvinnsland, 1969a) is that the two parts of the bone fuse together at the incisive suture, which then becomes obliterated on the facial aspect but remains

[27] *Notha* (Latin meaning 'illegitimate, bastard,' i.e. spurious).

[28] In Ashley-Montagu's (1935) review of the literature, he states, 'Ever since the time of the publication of Vesalius' immortal *De Humani Corporis Fabrica* in the year 1543, the premaxillary bone has formed the subject of much contention, some of it extraordinarily vituperative, and some of it characterised by a vigour of expression which was apparently inversely proportional to the writer's understanding of his subject.' For example, 'Sylvius delivered himself in 1551 of an attack upon Vesalius so vitriolic that it probably remains unique and unparalleled in the annals of scientific literature. Of Vesalius himself, Sylvius is pleased to say, in no round terms, that he is a madman as well as a liar.'

open in the palate. Other studies adopted an intermediate position. Shepherd and McCarthy (1955) described a mixture of fusion and overgrowth with erosion of the premaxillary territory by the maxilla. Kraus and Decker (1960) described a secondary overgrowth of bone, the external trabecular network, which obliterated the incisive suture. The description of this type of development is similar to that described by Matsumura *et al.* (1994) in the supra-occipital (see above), where the endochondrally formed bone is overgrown by cancellous bone formed in the membranous interparietal above it. Wood *et al.* (1969, 1970) followed the course of ossification on the frontal aspect of the body and frontal process of the maxilla. They regarded the so-called 'incisive suture' not as a true suture, in that it never truly separates parts of the bone at any stage in its development, and preferred the term 'incisive fissure' for the feature, which undoubtedly exists at an early stage. However, as emphasized by O'Rahilly and Gardner (1972), the existence of a separate bony element does not depend on a separate centre of ossification and these differing accounts do not preclude the convenient use of the term 'premaxilla' for that part of the bone that lies in front of the incisive suture and bears the incisor teeth (Dixon, 1953).

The early development of the maxilla is described in detail by Fawcett (1911a), Dixon (1953) and Jacobson (1955). The first ossification centre is seen at Stage 19 (seventh week) in the membranous tissue covering the anterior part of the nasal capsule. At this stage, the tongue is high in the undivided pharyngeal cavity and the palatal shelves are still vertical (see above – 'Early development of the skull'). The centre is just above the part of the dental lamina that gives rise to the canine tooth and where the infra-orbital nerve gives off its anterior superior alveolar branch. The definitive parts of the maxilla spread rapidly from this centre. Dixon (1953) envisaged the bone as functionally subdivided into neural and alveolar areas. Outer and inner neural plates, which develop into the zygomatic (malar) process and the inner orbital margin respectively, form on either side of the anterior superior dental nerve, which runs forward to reach the incisor teeth. Under the nerve, the ossific tissue rejoins to form a subneural plate, which develops into the infra-orbital groove, in which the nerve lies in the floor of the orbit. About 2 weeks later, two further limbs extend superiorly and inferiorly from the centre to start formation of the frontal and alveolar processes. The latter eventually forms a gutter, which envelops the dental lamina. From the junction of the two processes, ossification spreads medially into the palatal shelves, which have by then reached a horizontal position. Small centres of secondary cartilage are present at both the upper end of the frontal process on the outer side of the lacrimal duct (the paranasal process of Mihalkovics) and at the alveolar border of the zygomatic process, but these quickly become converted to bone.

Descriptions of the radiographic appearance of the developing maxilla emphasize a maxillary centre at 7–8 weeks, followed by a premaxillary centre at 9–10 weeks (Kjær, 1990d). O'Rahilly and Meyer (1956) described and illustrated its structure at about 11–12 weeks. A gap can be seen between the palatine processes of the premaxillary and maxillary parts and there is a prominent anterior nasal spine. Njio and Kjær (1993) described the gross, radiological and histological appearance of both the incisive fissure and the maxillopalatine sutures. They concluded that the latter is likely to have a function in the anteroposterior growth of the bony palate, while the former is associated with accommodation of the increased volume of the tooth germs during the development of the dentition.

The prenatal maxilla towards the end of the embryonic period is described and illustrated in detail by Macklin (1914, 1921), Augier (1931) and Müller and O'Rahilly (1980). The main body of the bone is small, the nasal notch, the infra-orbital margin and all four processes are recognizable. The frontal process, triangular in shape, lies on the side wall of the ectethmoid part of the nasal capsule in front of the epiphanial foramen with the lacrimal bone above, and the paraseptal cartilage below it. Its derivation from the premaxillary and maxillary parts sometimes shows as a cleft. The zygomatic process points dorsolaterally but at this early stage, there is a wide interval between it and the zygomatic bone. The alveolar process is an irregular crescentic groove with rough edges, filled with developing tooth germs. At this stage, the palatine process is still not completely developed and is represented by a shelf of bone extending from the inner alveolar area towards the midline. It is divided into maxillary and premaxillary parts, but does not meet either the bone from the opposite side or the palatine bone posteriorly. The infra-orbital nerve lies in a groove in the bone of the orbital floor. Later, it usually becomes closed over in the anterior part of the orbital floor and emerges on the facial aspect through the infra-orbital foramen. Variations in the formation of the infra-orbital suture are described by Schwartz (1982) and Bollobás (1984a). Occasionally, the foramen remains open at the infra-orbital margin into adult life (Turner, 1885).

The maxillary sinus starts to develop between 10 and 12 fetal weeks as a small epithelial sac outpouching from the infundibulum of the middle meatus into the ectethmoid cartilage (Schaeffer, 1910b; Van Alyea, 1936). At first, it lies above the floor of the nose and medial and superior to the infra-orbital foramen, but these relationships change as pneumatization proceeds into the ossifying maxilla (see below).

The whole of the palatine process consists of a thin plate of bone until the late fetal period. After this, the medial surface anterior to the incisive canal increases in height as it becomes the interdental septum between the central incisor tooth germs. The growth of the whole alveolar process is complex and develops in close relationship to the developing deciduous and permanent tooth germs (Scott, 1959). A series of radiographs with corresponding dissections of fetal specimens from 3–10 lunar months shows the developing tooth germs *in situ* (Boller, 1964). Other details have been reported by Kraus (1960), Schwartz (1982) and Bollobás (1984b). In general, the alveolar crypts develop in an anteroposterior direction, with the lingual lamina in advance of the buccal lamina and the interalveolar septa being the last parts to complete each crypt. At 11 weeks of intra-uterine life, the crypts of the deciduous incisors start formation and septa spread between the tooth germs about 2 weeks later. The crypts of all the teeth from the central incisors to the first molars are complete by about 17–18 fetal weeks.

The perinatal maxilla (Fig. 5.65) has a very small body so that the tooth germs are close to the orbital floor. Although the air sinus is very small, its bony outline can be seen as a spindle-shaped depression in the lateral wall of the nose immediately lateral to the inferior concha. It is about 10 mm long, 3 mm wide and 4 mm high (Cullen and Vidić, 1972; Wolf *et al.*, 1993), and is usually circular or pyramidal in shape in the living and is radiographically identifiable. All the air sinuses contain amniotic fluid at birth and do not become fully aerated until about 10 days *postpartum* (Wasson, 1933). A prominent infra-orbital foramen is visible on the anterior surface and may still be open superiorly and continuous with the groove in the floor of the orbit. The frontal process is lanceolate in shape, with the anterior lacrimal crest prominent on the outer surface, although the oblique ethmoidal crest on the nasal aspect is only faintly marked. The slender zygomatic process extends posterolaterally from above the infra-orbital foramen and consists almost entirely of a triangular articular surface for the zygomatic bone. The palatine process is thin except for the medial border. Anteriorly, the premaxillary part of the bone displays racial differences. There is a less prominent anterior nasal spine and more alveolar prognathism in Black individuals compared to White (Limson, 1932). Between the central incisors there is a smooth interdental septum, behind which the incisive canal runs almost vertically. Posteriorly, the bone then becomes thinner as it forms the main part of the intermaxillary suture. The incisive fissure on the palatal surface extends from the incisive canal medially to a variable position at its lateral end. It may be continuous with a fissure on the nasal aspect of the frontal process or end in alveolar bone. According to Schwartz (1982), this may be between the crypts of the lateral incisor and canine, at the middle, or even posterior to the canine crypt. Detailed discussion of these variable positions appears to be based on assumptions about direct derivation of the premaxilla and maxilla from embryological mesenchymal processes. The calcified crowns of the deciduous teeth cause prominent bulges on the external border of the alveolar process and the inferior view of the maxilla is dominated by the curve formed by the alveolar crypts that envelop the palate. The first three dental crypts are triangular and arranged in a cuneiform pattern. The apices of the central incisor (i^1) and canine (c) face lingually, while the lateral incisor (i^2) fits between them, with its apex facing in a labial direction. The crypt of the first molar (m^1) is rectangular and that of the second deciduous molar (m^2) and first permanent molar (M^1) is still incomplete and continuous posteriorly with the infratemporal fossa (Fig. 5.65c). The infratemporal surface of the body only becomes identifiable late in fetal life as it lies postero-inferior to the orbital floor and superior to the alveolar process and both these structures are late to ossify fully posteriorly.

The alveolar bone in infants consists mainly of fine cancellous bone, which is constantly undergoing remodelling as the dentition forms. Van der Linden and Duterloo (1976) distinguish four stages that take place in bone of the alveolar socket immediately surrounding each developing tooth, each of which is related to a specific morphological stage of crown or root development. They illustrate the appearance of the crypts both before and after the removal of the deciduous and permanent tooth germs.

The maxillary tuberosity as such does not exist during childhood as its place is taken by the posterior extensions of the alveolar processes. After eruption of the second and third molars, the tuberosity then becomes closely related to the pyramidal process of the palatine bone (Scott, 1967).

Postnatal growth of the maxilla is rapid and related to different functional areas of the anterior part of the skull. The increase in size of the eyeballs and the nose both influence the development of the main part of the body. The growth of the nasal septum carries the maxilla downwards and forwards, more anterior-

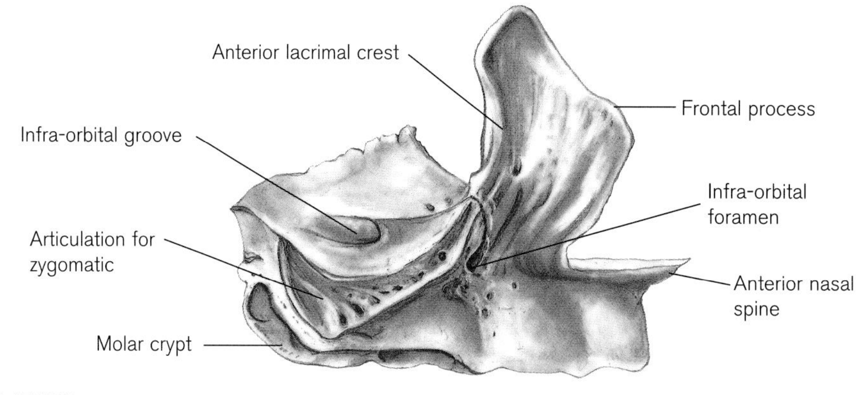

(a) LATERAL

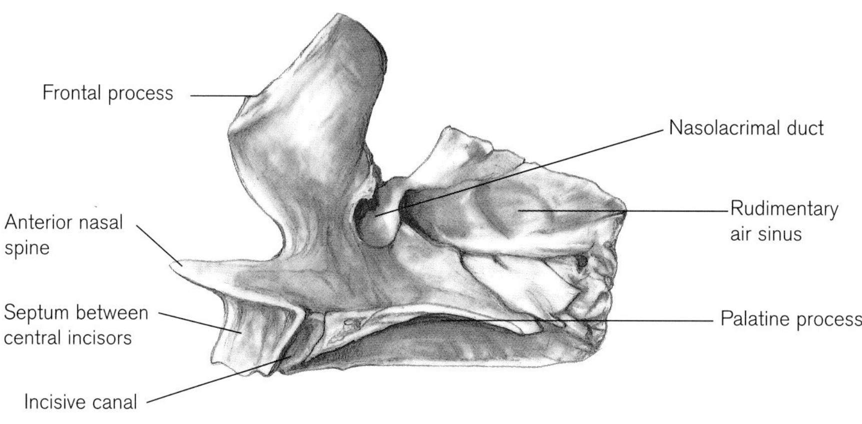

(b) MEDIAL

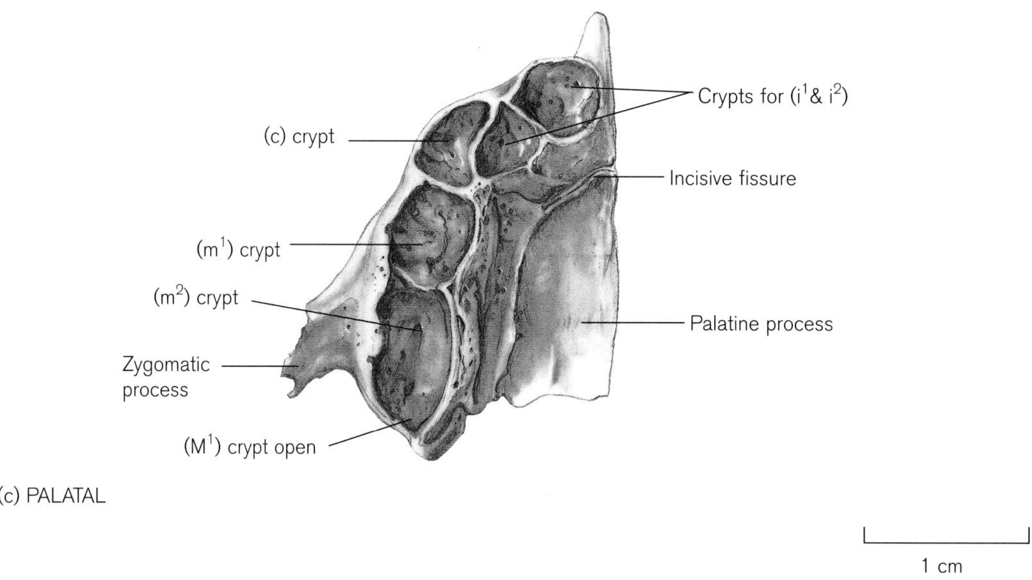

(c) PALATAL

Figure 5.65 Right perinatal maxilla.

ly in the first decade and more vertically in the second. Enlow and Bang (1965), described growth by sutural activity and cartilaginous expansion up to the age of about 7 years, after which overall apposition becomes the dominant mechanism of growth. This occurs mainly at the alveolar region, the facial surface and the posterior border (Scott, 1967). Björk and Skieller (1977) followed the growth of the maxilla from 4 years to adult life radiographically by using metallic implants in living patients.

The contained air sinus enlarges by resorption and deposition of bone surfaces. By 4 years of age, pneumatization has reached laterally to the infra-orbital foramen and inferiorly to the attachment of the inferior concha (Wolf *et al.* 1993). By 8 or 9 years, it has reached beyond the infra-orbital foramen and by 12 years has reached the same level as the floor of the nose inferiorly and as far as the molar teeth laterally (Van Alyea, 1936; Wolf *et al.* 1993). By puberty, its lower limit is usually below that of the nose, but the size and shape can be very variable (Schaeffer, 1910b). Dimensions of the sinus from birth to adulthood may be found in Peter (1938), Maresh (1940) and Lang (1989).

The other major influence on the growth of the maxilla is the need for space for the increasing number and size of teeth. As the eruption of the deciduous dentition nears completion, the calcified crowns of the permanent central and lateral incisor teeth can be seen through foramina in the palatal process behind the corresponding deciduous incisor teeth. These are the openings of the gubernacular canals, occupied by fibrous cords that connect the tooth follicles of the permanent teeth to the overlying mucous membrane. With the formation of each subsequent molar tooth, the posterior wall of the crypt of the tooth anterior to it is completed, leaving the newly formed crypt behind it open to the infratemporal fossa. Thus, at about 1 year of age, the crypt of the second deciduous molar (m^2) completes formation and that of the first permanent molar (M^1) is open posteriorly. At about 3 years of age, the second permanent molar (M^2) socket is open. In dry skulls, the maxillary tuberosity appears to remain partially unossified until the third molar (M^3) becomes properly surrounded by alveolar bone. However, Norberg (1960) distinguished a sutural line between the bone formed by the follicular sac of the second permanent molar and that of the maxilla proper. This would seem to concur with later observations on experimental animals that the alveolar bone is derived from the tooth germ and is therefore of a different origin from that of the main body of the maxilla with which it fuses (Ten Cate and Mills, 1972; Freeman *et al.*, 1975).

The time of closure of the incisive suture is very variable and is therefore not a good indicator for determination of age. Although the facial aspect of the suture closes in infancy, the internal aspect in the region of the incisive canal between the two maxillae is slow to fuse and about one-third remain unfused into the adolescent period (Behrents and Harris, 1991). The palatal aspect of the suture may close laterally as early as the perinatal period, where the palatal processes fuse with the alveolar bone (Schwartz, 1982), but the medial part often remains open into adult life. Mann *et al.* (1987) found that the earliest age at which total obliteration of the suture occurred was 25 years. Sejrsen *et al.* (1993) studied the suture and its enclosed premaxillary area in a series of medieval Danish skulls. They showed that the degree of closure of the suture was related to tooth maturation and took place soon after the crowns of the permanent incisors had reached their final width. The size of the premaxillary area appeared to be related to tooth spacing and was reduced in some cases of tooth agenesis. Both these observations and those of Njio and Kjær (1993) on the prenatal structure of the suture suggest that the function of the suture is likely to be directly related to the maturation of the anterior tooth germs, rather than general increase in size of the palate. Palatal growth as a whole is considered under the palatine bone.

Scott (1967) described three main periods of skull growth. During the first, which extends from late fetal life until about the third year, all the sutural systems are very active as the brain, eyeballs and tongue increase in size. By the end of the first year, the greater wings of the sphenoid unite with the body and the two parts of the frontal bone commence fusion. Within the next 2 years, the mesethmoid unites with the labyrinths and this limits growth of the craniofacial suture system. The second phase is from the third to the tenth year. Surface deposition generally replaces sutural growth as the main method of development, although there is still some enlargement at the lambdoid, coronal and circum-maxillary sutures and growth is still active at the spheno-occipital synchondrosis. The distance from the pituitary fossa to the spheno-ethmoidal suture reaches adult dimensions (Brodie, 1941), as does the distance from the fossa to the foramen caecum (Ford, 1958). By about 10 years, when the third period begins, adult dimensions have been reached by the cranial and orbital cavities, the upper nose and the petrous parts of the temporal bones. During this time, the spheno-occipital synchondrosis ceases to be a growth centre and growth slows in the nasal septum. Growth by bone deposition is still marked at the alveolar processes, the orbital margins and muscular processes, including the zygoma and the pterygoid plates. During all three phases, growth of the mandible continues to keep pace with that of the skull (see below).

There is a large amount of information in the dental and anatomical literature on the postnatal growth of the face in relation to the development and eruption of the dentition. Details of the growth of the face and its sutures are outwith the scope of this text and further details can be found in dental and orthodontic texts (Scott, 1954, 1956, 1957, 1967; Enlow and Hans, 1996).

Practical notes

Sideing /orientation (Fig. 5.65)

The maxilla does not ossify completely until late fetal life and is a relatively fragile bone, especially in the alveolar region. Sideing relies on orientating the bone so that the dental crypts lie inferiorly, the frontal process extends anterosuperiorly and the palatal process points medially.

Bones of a similar morphology

Fragments of damaged alveolar processes of the maxilla and mandible may appear similar, but the supporting bone in the mandible is narrow with compact and dense cortices. In the maxilla, the bone related to the alveolar process is the thin, flat nasal or orbital floor.

Morphological summary

Fetal

Wk 6	Intramembranous ossification centre appears
By wk 8	Body and four processes identifiable
Wks 10–12	Maxillary sinus starts to develop
Wk 11	Formation of crypts for deciduous dentition
Wks 14–16	Deciduous tooth germs start to form
Wks 17–18	All deciduous crypts completed
Birth	Main parts of bone present. Sinus rudimentary. Crowns of deciduous teeth in crypts. Calcification of first permanent molar commenced
Infancy and childhood	Gradual increase in size of body of bone. Increase in size of sinus. Eruption and replacement of deciduous teeth
By 12–14 yrs	All permanent teeth emerged except third molars (further details of teeth in section on dentition)

Metrics

Fazekas and Kósa (1978) recorded the measurements of the maxilla during fetal life (Table 5.18). Detailed measurements of the postnatal maxilla can be found in orthodontic texts (e.g. Enlow and Hans, 1996). Lang (1989) recorded the dimensions of the maxillary sinus from birth to 14 years (Table 5.19).

Table 5.18 Dimensions of the fetal maxilla

Age (weeks)	Length (mm)	Height (mm)	Width (mm)	Longest oblique length (mm)
12	4.2	3.1	–	6.0
14	6.3	5.6	5.6	9.3
16	8.9	8.9	9.8	14.0
18	10.6	10.0	11.6	15.3
20	12.6	12.3	13.0	18.8
22	13.5	13.4	14.2	20.0
24	15.1	14.1	15.4	21.6
26	15.9	15.6	15.9	22.3
28	17.3	17.1	17.7	23.3
30	17.8	18.2	18.7	23.8
32	19.4	19.6	20.0	26.0
34	20.0	20.9	21.2	28.2
36	22.0	21.9	22.3	28.9
38	24.1	24.1	24.2	32.1
40	24.1	24.5	25.1	34.3

Length: anterior nasal spine to posterior border of palatal process in sagittal plane.
Height: alveolar process to tip of frontal process in vertical plane.
Width: posterior border palatal process and lateral end of zygomatic process.
Longest oblique length: anterior nasal spine to lateral end of zygomatic process in oblique plane.

Adapted from Fazekas and Kósa (1978).

Table 5.19 Dimensions of the maxillary sinus from birth to 14 years

Age	Width (mm)		Height (mm)	
	Mean	Range	Mean	Range
0–12 months	12.0	7.0–17.0	12.5	8.0–17.0
13–18 months	13.0	7.0–19.0	13.5	10.0–19.0
19–24 months	16.0	9.0–20.0	16.0	10.0–22.0
3 years	18.0	14.0–29.0	18.0	12.0–24.0
4 years	19.5	14.0–27.0	19.5	14.0–27.0
5 years	20.5	14.0–27.0	20.0	14.0–27.0
6 years	21.5	15.0–31.0	22.0	14.0–29.0
7 years	22.5	17.0–31.0	23.0	19.0–29.0
8 years	23.0	18.0–31.0	24.0	19.0–30.0
9 years	25.0	18.0–31.0	26.5	20.0–30.0
10 years	27.0	19.0–31.0	27.0	19.0–33.0
11 years	28.0	20.0–32.0	29.0	21.0–33.0
12 years	28.0	21.0–34.0	29.0	22.0–35.0
13 years	28.0	22.0–34.0	30.0	26.0–35.0
14 years	28.5	22.0–35.0	30.0	27.0–38.0

Adapted from Lang (1989).

XIII. THE PALATINE

The adult palatine

The palatine bones contribute to the posterior part of the roof of the mouth and floor and lateral walls of the nose, the medial wall of the maxillary sinuses and the orbital floors. Each bone (Fig. 5.66) consists of horizontal and perpendicular plates (laminae) set at right angles to each other. Orbital and sphenoidal processes are attached to the superior border of the perpendicular plate and a pyramidal process extends posterolaterally from the junction of the two plates. The right and left bones join with each other in the midline of the palate and also articulate with the maxillae, inferior conchae, ethmoid and sphenoid bones (Figs. 5.1 and 5.64). Together with the vomer, the palatine bones form the skeleton of the posterior choanae, which lead from the nasal cavity into the nasopharynx.

The quadrilateral **horizontal plate** lies posterior to the maxilla and has a **nasal** (superior) surface and a **palatine** (inferior/oral) surface. The **anterior** border is serrated and overlapped on the oral side by the palatine process of the maxilla at the palatomaxillary (transpalatine) suture. The **medial** border is thick and also serrated and articulates with the bone of the opposite side at the **interpalatine** (sagittal) **suture** to form the posterior part of the nasal crest, which accommodates the vomer. The free **posterior** border is thin and concave and continues in life into the soft

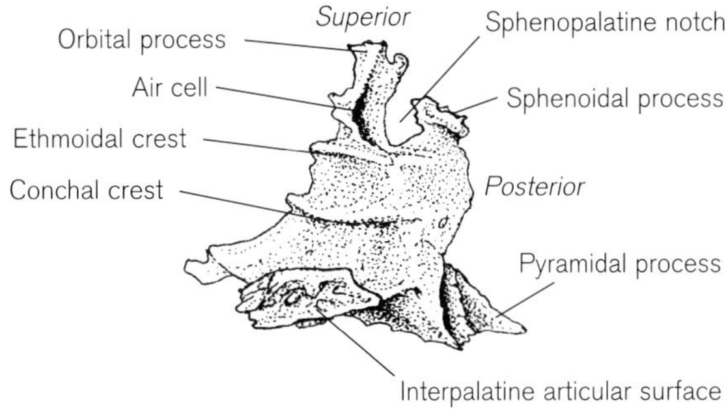

(a) MEDIAL

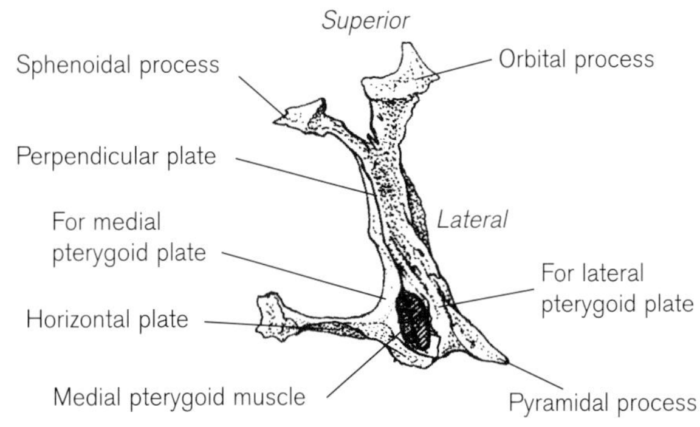

(b) POSTERIOR

Figure 5.66 Right adult palatine.

palate. Just anterior to it on the oral side, there may be a thickened palatine crest that provides attachment for the palatine aponeurosis. The medial end of both horizontal plates is extended posteriorly to form the posterior nasal spine (Fig. 5.64). The musculi uvulae are attached on either side and the tensor veli palatini laterally. The **lateral** border is continuous at right angles with the perpendicular plate.

The **perpendicular plate** extends upwards in the posterolateral wall of the nasal cavity, where it lies on the medial side of the maxilla anteriorly and articulates posteromedially with the medial pterygoid plate of the sphenoid. The **nasal** (medial) surface forms the posterior part of the three nasal meatuses separated by two crests. The conchal crest, for articulation with the posterior end of the inferior concha, is one-third of the way up the wall and separates the inferior from the middle meatus. The middle and superior meatuses lie on either side of the smaller ethmoidal crest for the middle concha. The **maxillary** (lateral) surface is irregular and has a smooth anterior part, which is attached to the maxilla and overlaps the posterior part of its antral opening. Behind this, and separated by a crest, is a narrow area forming the medial wall of the pterygopalatine fossa, which leads down into the deep groove carrying the palatine vessels and nerves from the fossa to exit on the surface of the palate at the **greater palatine foramen** (Fig. 5.64). The bone contributes to the anterior, medial and posterior borders of the foramen, which is completed by the maxilla. The exact location of the foramen is important clinically in injection procedures to anaesthetize the palatal region, but most anatomical descriptions are incomplete and inconsistent. Its direction of opening and position in relation to the molar teeth is variable, but the most common arrangement is for the opening to be vertical and medial to the third molar tooth. In a significant proportion of skulls there is a bony projection, similar to the mandibular lingula, extending from the posterior margin of the foramen (Westmoreland and Blanton, 1982; Ajmani, 1994).

From the superior surface of the perpendicular plate the orbital and sphenoidal processes extend laterally and medially, respectively. The **orbital process** is variable in size and forms a small part of the floor of the orbit and the inferior orbital fissure. It may contain air cells and usually articulates with the maxilla, the sphenoid and ethmoid, but can sometimes meet the frontal bone (Russell, 1939). The **sphenoidal process** is usually smaller and articulates with the medial pterygoid plate of the sphenoid and the vomerine ala. Between the two processes there is the deep sphenopalatine notch, which is converted to a foramen by the sphenoidal concha or by a large orbital process. It connects the pterygopalatine fossa to the superior meatus and transmits sphenopalatine vessels and posterior superior nasal nerves.

The **pyramidal process** (palatine tuberosity/tubercle) extends posterolaterally from the junction of the horizontal and perpendicular plates to lie in the angle between the medial and lateral pterygoid plates of the sphenoid. Its posterior surface has a small, smooth, triangular area between the two roughened articular surfaces for the pterygoid plates. This is the lower part of the pterygoid fossa and provides part of the attachment for the medial pterygoid muscle. The inferior surface bears a variable number of foramina for lesser palatine nerves and vessels.

Most of the reported anomalies of the palatine are minor in nature and consist of variations and dehiscences in the perpendicular plate, which are compensated for by neighbouring bones. The greater palatine canal may exist entirely within the territory of the palatine bone (Augier, 1931) and extra ossicles, 'posterior medio-palatine bones', are sometimes seen in the horizontal process (Woo, 1948).

Ossification

The ossification centre for the perpendicular plate of the palatine appears at about 7–8 weeks on the medial aspect of the nasal capsule between the primitive oropharyngeal cavity medially and a palatal nerve bundle laterally (Fawcett, 1906). At this stage of development, the mesenchymal palatal processes are hanging vertically beside the tongue, which is still high in the cavity. About a week later, as the palatal shelves take up a horizontal position, the ossification centres assume a boomerang-like shape as bone begins to spread into them. By about 10 weeks, the orbital and sphenoidal processes are visible as outgrowths from the perpendicular plate and are separated by a shallow notch. At first, the orbital process is directed upwards and forwards and is largely maxillary in surface, but later turns upwards and backwards and becomes mainly orbital. During fetal life there is a prominent groove for the medial pterygoid plate (Fawcett, 1906).

The palatine is recognizable in isolation from about mid-fetal life, when it assumes the main morphological features of the adult bone, although the relative proportions of its component parts are different. In the perinatal period (Fig. 5.67), the thin horizontal plate is almost square. The medial border is slightly thickened for the sagittal suture and the palatine crest may be seen running transversely across the oral surface. The perpendicular plate is about the same height as the width of the horizontal plate and is also very

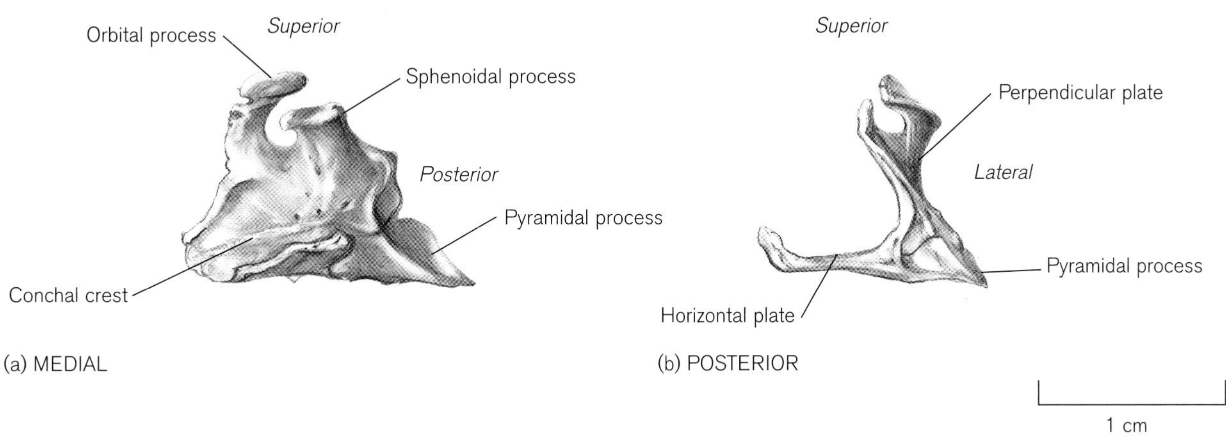

Figure 5.67 Right perinatal palatine.

thin. On its nasal surface, the conchal crest for articulation with the posterior end of the inferior concha is just above the junction of the two plates, reflecting the small height of the nasal cavity compared to the adult. The groove leading down to the greater palatine foramen is obvious on the maxillary surface. A notch separates the orbital and sphenoidal processes, which extend from the upper border, the former being the larger and turning laterally and the latter inclining medially. The pyramidal process, extending posterolaterally, is relatively larger than in the adult but bears the same recognizable morphology. Up to about the age of 3 years, the horizontal and perpendicular plates are roughly equal in size but, associated with the rapid increase in size of the face and nasal cavity during childhood, the perpendicular plate increases in height. By puberty, its height is about twice the width of the horizontal plate.

Growth of the palate

The palate is a septum dividing the first part of the alimentary and respiratory tracts. It extends from behind the mouth and nostrils anteriorly to the junction of the naso- and oropharynx posteriorly and is bounded laterally by the alveolar processes. The anterior four-fifths is composed of the bony (hard) palate and is composed of the palatal processes of the maxilla and the horizontal plates of the palatine bones, which meet in the midline at the continuous intermaxillary and interpalatine sutures. In the dry skull, the posterior border of the palate, together with the medial pterygoid plates and the inferior surface of the sphenoidal body, form the posterior choanae leading to the nasopharynx. The right and left sides are divided by the vomer. In the living, the muscular (soft) palate is attached to the posterior border of the hard palate and is composed of the aponeuroses and fibres of the tensor veli palatini, levator veli palatini and uvulae muscles.

Prenatal growth of the palate as a whole has been studied by Freiband (1937), Kraus (1960), Lebret (1962), Burdi (1965), Ewers (1968), Kvinnsland (1969a), Latham (1971) and Silau *et al.* (1994). Kraus (1960) distinguished eight morphological stages of development between 7 and 18 weeks. Only two of 151 specimens were reported to show separate premaxillary and maxillary ossification centres. Networks of bony trabeculae spread out into the palatine processes from the region of the canine tooth germ. At first, the maxillary and palatine components are separated from each other and from the opposite side, so that the developing plates of the vomer can be seen between them. By about 13 weeks, both maxillary processes reach the midline, but the bony palatine processes do not fuse until after 18 weeks. Increase in length is more rapid than that in width before 18 weeks. After this, length increases in a linear fashion, with the maxillary component contributing approximately two-thirds and the palatine component one-third (Silau *et al.*, 1994). Palatal width increases more rapidly as growth at the midpalatal suture and the buccal surfaces of the alveolar processes is very active and this leads to the typical broad, infantile palate (Ewers, 1968). At term, the length and width are approximately equal.

Postnatally, growth at the midpalatal suture slows and ceases between 2 and 4 years of age. Appositional growth at the alveolar margins continues to widen the palate, particularly posteriorly, until about the age of 7 years (Sperber, 1989). Increase in height appears to cease after 9 years of age (Knott and Johnson, 1970), but increase in length takes place up to adult life. Melsen (1975) found that until the age of 13–15 years, growth occurred at the transverse (palatomaxillary) suture and also by apposition at the tuberosity of the maxilla. After this, sutural growth appeared to cease, but appositional growth continued for some years. The morphology of the suture changed during the growth period from a broad, sinuous type in infants to a typical squamous suture in childhood, when the palatine overlapped the maxilla on the cranial side. Growth in width at the mid-palatal (sagittal) suture continued up to the age of 16 in girls and 18 in boys. Again, the nature of the suture changed from a simple Y-shaped structure enclosing the vomer seen in infancy, through an increasingly sinuous type in childhood to a densely interdigitated type by puberty. The nasal cavity increases in height throughout childhood, with bone apposition on the oral side and resorption on the nasal side. This is accompanied by an increase in depth of the palatal arch from an almost flat palate at birth to an arched palate at puberty, mainly caused by the alveolar bone around erupting teeth. Further details of palatal growth may be found in orthodontic texts (e.g. Lavelle, 1970; Foster *et al.*, 1977; Enlow and Hans, 1996).

Slavkin *et al.* (1966) measured the position of the greater palatine foramen posterior to the last molar tooth from birth to 18 years of age. As each tooth erupted, the position of the foramen moved posteriorly, due to sutural growth at the transverse palatine suture and appositional growth at the posterior palatine processes. Sejrsen *et al.* (1996) used a similar method to measure palatal growth in a series of medieval child and adult crania. They concluded that the growth increment between the incisive foramen and the transverse palatine suture was greater than that between the transverse suture and the greater palatine foramen. The distance between the greater palatine foramen and the posterior margin of the palate did not increase significantly with age, which argues against significant appositional growth at the posterior border. Growth in width appeared to continue into adult life. There are little data on the age at which palatal sutures start to close. Persson and Thilander (1977) investigated the intermaxillary and transverse palatine sutures on histological sections of autopsy material in the adolescent and young adult age ranges. They concluded that there was great variation between individuals and, although sutures may show obliteration during the juvenile period, any marked degree was rare until the third decade. Any closure that was observed seemed to be more rapid on the oral rather than the nasal side and in the posterior more often than the anterior part of the intermaxillary suture. Mann *et al.* (1987, 1991a) attempted to use obliteration of palatal sutures for estimating skeletal age in dry skulls, but concluded that it was only possible to place an individual within a very broad age category, as there was such a wide range in the age of closure.

Practical notes

Sideing /orientation (Fig. 5.67)

In spite of its seemingly fragile nature, an isolated palatine bone often survives intact, due to its central position and protection by surrounding bones. It is sometimes found still fused to the maxilla. The horizontal plate is rectangular and the perpendicular plate has two processes extending superiorly from it. The relatively robust pyramidal process extends posterolaterally from the side to which the bone belongs.

Bones of a similar morphology

There is no complete bone that looks similar. Fragments of the palatine are unlikely to be identified, except perhaps the pyramidal process, which bears some similarity to the pointed lateral end of the lesser wing of the sphenoid. However, the fine structure of each is characteristic.

Morphological summary

Fetal	
Wks 7–8	Ossification centre for perpendicular plate appears
Wk 10	Orbital and sphenoidal processes start to develop
Wk 18	Palatal processes fuse
Mid-fetal life	Has adopted adult morphology, but not proportions
Birth	Adult morphology except horizontal and perpendicular plates are of equal width and height. Orbital process does not contain air cells
From yr 3	Perpendicular plate starts to increase in height
Puberty	Adult morphology and proportions

Metrics

Fazekas and Kósa (1978) reported on the length of the perpendicular plate during fetal life (Table 5.20). Their illustration should be consulted, as it appears to show an oblique maximum distance from the superior border of the orbital process to the tip of the pyramidal process.

Table 5.20 Oblique height of the fetal palatine bone

Age (weeks)	Height (mm)
12	2.2
14	2.9
16	5.8
18	6.7
20	7.7
22	8.4
24	8.9
26	9.7
28	9.9
30	10.5
32	11.5
34	12.1
36	12.7
38	13.7
40	15.3

Height: described as 'length of perpendicular plate' but illustration shows oblique distance from tip of pyramidal process to maximum height of orbital process.

Adapted from Fazekas and Kósa (1978).

XIV. THE MANDIBLE

The adult mandible

The lower jaw is the only skeletal element of the head, apart from the ossicles of the middle ear, to enjoy independent movement. It articulates with the mandibular fossae of the squamous temporal bones at the synovial temporomandibular joints. The mandible[29] gives attachment to the muscles that form the floor of the mouth and the tongue, to the muscles of mastication and also bears all the lower teeth. Each half of the mandible consists of a horizontal body and a vertical ramus (Fig. 5.68).

The anterior end of the **body** meets its opposite fellow at the midline **symphysis menti**.[30] This is usually marked on the external surface as a vertical ridge dividing inferiorly to enclose a triangular area, the **mental protuberance** (chin), at the base of which is a **mental tubercle** on either side. A shallow depression, the **incisive fossa**, lies above the protuberance.

On the outer surface, an **oblique line**, part of which provides attachment for the buccinator muscle, extends posterolaterally from the tubercle to the anterior surface of the ramus. Above the line lies the **mental foramen** for the exit of the mental nerve and vessels. Gershenson *et al.* (1986) describe the opening as sometimes cribrotic or trabecular and their illustrations of the foramen resemble the morphology at the entrance of the internal auditory meatus. The traditional textbook account places the position of the foramen between the roots of the premolar teeth, in spite of many reports that it can be as far forward as the first premolar, or between the second premolar and the first molar tooth (Tebo and Telford, 1950; Miller, 1953; Ashley-Montagu, 1954; Gabriel, 1958; Azaz and Lustmann, 1973; Wang *et al.*, 1986). There is data to suggest that the position varies in different populations (Simonton, 1923; Murphy, 1957a; Green, 1987; Chung *et al.*, 1995) and Green and Darvell (1988) reported a significant correlation between tooth wear and anteroposterior position. In the tooth-bearing young adult, the height of the foramen lies about midway between the base of the bone and the alveolar border and its relationship to the lower border remains constant, even in the edentulous state. As alveolar bone is resorbed, the foramen comes to lie much nearer to the top of the bone, or resorption may even reach below the level of the foramen, leaving the inferior alveolar nerve exposed on the bone and soft tissue (Gabriel, 1958). The direction of the opening alters during development (see below), but in the adult it has a sharp border, except in the posterosuperior quadrant, where the nerve emerges (Warwick, 1950). Occurrence of multiple foramina varies between 2% and 30%, depending on the population (Ashley-Montagu, 1954; Riesenfeld, 1956; Murphy, 1957a; Azaz and Lustmann, 1973; Reinhard and Rösing, 1985; Gershenson *et al.*, 1986). Serman (1989) described a variation in which two foramina faced anteriorly and posteriorly, respectively. After giving off the mental nerve, the incisive branch re-entered the bone through the anterior foramen and for the distance between the two foramina there was no mandibular canal within the bone.

On the inner surface, just lateral to the lower end of the symphysis, is an oval hollow, the **digastric fossa**, for the attachment of the anterior belly of the digastric muscle. Above this, and close to the symphysis, is a small projection, the **mental spine**, sometimes divided into upper and lower sections (genial[31] tubercles), to which are attached the genioglossus and

[29] *Mandere* (meaning 'to chew, masticate'). Mandible is a relatively new term for the lower jaw. Many of the older texts refer to the bone as the inferior maxilla (Latin meaning 'jaw') although the Nomina Term is now Mandibula.

[30] *Mentum* (Latin meaning 'chin').

[31] *Geneion* (Greek meaning 'chin').

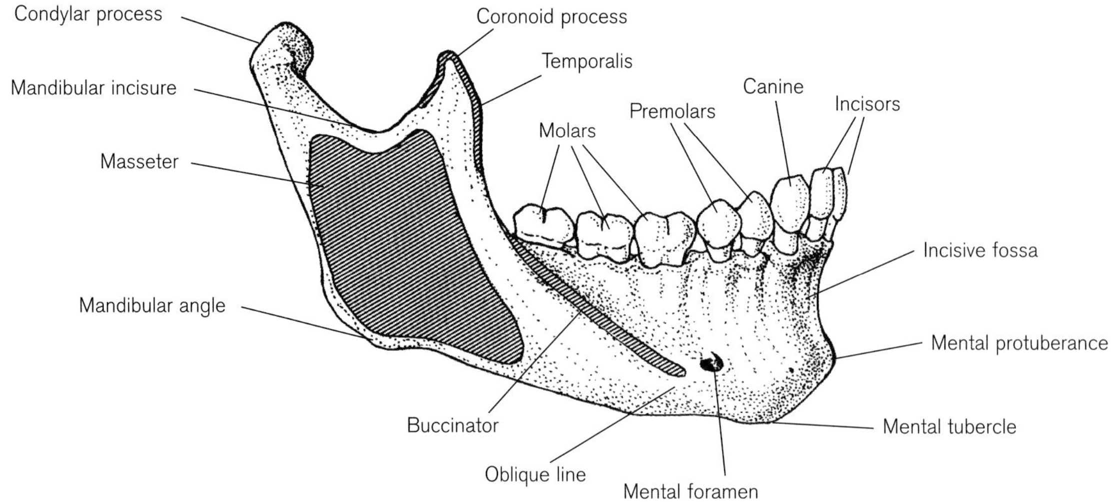

(a) LATERAL

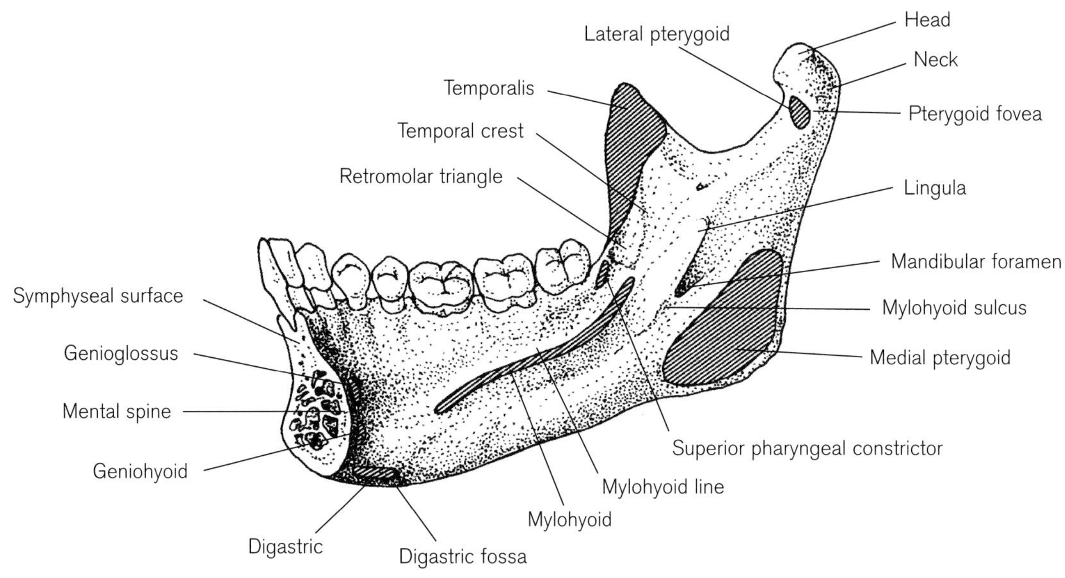

(b) MEDIAL

Figure 5.68 Right adult hemi-mandible.

geniohyoid muscles. Greyling *et al.* (1997) have given a detailed description of the area of the genial tubercles and reviewed the literature. Above the tubercles, a midline (lingual) foramen is present in over 80% of mandibles. Shiller and Wiswell (1954) and Sutton (1974) traced nerves from the incisive plexus to this foramen, but McDonnell *et al.* (1994) reported that it contained an artery formed by anastomosis of the right and left sublingual vessels. From the digastric fossa, an oblique ridge, the **mylohyoid line**, passes upwards and backwards. It provides attachment for the mylohyoid muscle, forming the floor of the mouth, and divides the surface into an anterior (buccal) and a posterior (cervical) area. Above and below the line are two hollows, in which the lingual and submandibular salivary glands lie in relation to the bone. The lower border of the body (splenium) is thick and rounded, while the upper border forms the alveolar process. Like that of the maxilla, it is composed of sockets for the eight permanent teeth: two incisors, one canine, two premolars and three molars. Each crypt has a buccal and lingual plate and is divided from the next by an interalveolar (interdental) septum.

The **ramus** extends superiorly as a flat, quadrilateral plate behind the body and its posterior border is continuous with the lower border of the body at the **mandibular** (gonial) **angle** (see below). Especially in males, the lower part of the outer surface is often roughened with ridges for the masseter muscle, while the corresponding inner surface provides attachment for the medial pterygoid muscle. The superior border of the ramus is formed from two processes separated by a deep notch, the **mandibular incisure** (coronoid/sigmoid notch), which provides a passage for structures to pass from the infratemporal fossa to the oral cavity. Posteriorly, the **condylar process** consists of a narrow **neck** from which arises a transverse **head** whose anteroposterior dimension is about half that of its mediolateral width. The long axis of the condyle is not at right angles to the ramus, but diverges so that the medial end is slightly posterior to the lateral end. The size and shape of the condyle varies considerably and may be asymmetrical (Costa, 1986). There is a relatively rare anomaly in which the mandibular head is divided in an anteroposterior plane, producing a double-headed condyle. It is described in both dry skulls and living patients by Hrdlička (1941), Schier (1948), Stadnicki (1971) and Forman and Smith (1984). Blackwood (1957) postulated that this could be a developmental abnormality where the connective tissue septa that are normally present during the growth of the condylar cartilage up to 2 years of age persist, and so possibly impair normal ossification.

The anterior surface of the neck has a **pterygoid fovea** for the attachment of part of the tendon of the lateral pterygoid muscle. Anterior to the incisure, the **coronoid process** is a slim triangular extension of bone, to which is attached the temporalis muscle. From the tip of the process a ridge of bone, the **temporal crest**, runs down the anteromedial surface and the lower part of both this line and the anterior border of the ramus delimit an area behind the molar teeth called the **retromolar triangle**. In this region, the pterygomandibular ligament extends from the sphenoid and has attached to it, and to the adjoining bone, the superior constrictor muscle of the pharynx posteriorly and the buccinator muscle anteriorly, the muscles being separated by a raphé. About halfway up the inner surface of the ramus is the large **mandibular foramen**, which is the entrance to the **mandibular canal**. Before they enter the canal, the inferior alveolar nerve and vessels give off mylohyoid branches, which lie in the **mylohyoid sulcus**, which extends antero-inferiorly from the foramen. A bony projection, the **lingula**, lies anteromedial to the foramen and is the site of attachment of the sphenomandibular ligament. The position of the mandibular foramen and the lingula has been the subject of much attention (Fawcett, 1895; Harrower, 1928; Morant, 1936; Cleaver, 1937-8; Miller, 1953; Gabriel, 1958) as its exact location is important for the administration of dental anaesthesia. However, as the width of the ramus and its angle with the body varies, it is not possible to define its position exactly. Most accounts place it at the junction of the lower third and the upper two-thirds of a line joining the tip of the coronoid process to the mandibular angle, and this usually passes just posterior to the midpoint of the width of the ramus.

Mylohyoid bridging, occurring between 16% and 60% depending on the population, is a hyperostotic variant where the mylohyoid groove (sulcus) becomes variably ossified (Ossenberg, 1974, 1976; Sawyer *et al.*, 1978; Arensburg and Nathan, 1979; Lundy, 1980; Kaul and Pathak, 1984; Reinhard and Rösing, 1985). The groove, beginning antero-inferior to the mandibular foramen and containing the neurovascular bundle, is normally closed over to become a connective tissue canal, which is a prolongation of the sphenomandibular ligament attached to the lingula. Either or both parts of this tissue may become partially or completely transformed into bone, forming bridges or an elongated canal, which may extend above the foramen. This has been regarded as a genetic marker and Ossenberg (1974) has suggested that it is a remnant of Meckel's cartilage that has undergone hyperostosis. The clinical importance of mylohyoid bridging again centres on possible interference with administration of dental anaesthesia.

The mandibular canal runs forward from the foramen into the body of the bone and, beneath the level of the premolar or canine teeth, divides into mental and incisive branches. The mental nerve runs upwards, backwards and laterally to emerge at the foramen and the incisive nerve travels forward to the midline and normally supplies the incisor and canine teeth. The level of the canal within the bone is very variable (Starkie and Stewart, 1931; Gabriel, 1958; Carter and Keen, 1971) and has been reviewed in over 3000 radiographs by Nortjé *et al.* (1977). It may be so high that the roots of the molar teeth penetrate it, lie within 2 mm of the lower border of the mandible or, in a minority of cases, it can be duplicated. There appears to be no correlation between the frequency of a double canal and multiple mental foramina (Gershenson *et al.*, 1986).

There are numerous reports of accessory foramina on the lingual surface of the mandible. These are commonly seen at the level of the premolar teeth (Shiller and Wiswell, 1954; Sutton, 1974) and in the retromolar region (Schejtman *et al.*, 1967; Carter and

Keen, 1971; Azaz and Lustmann, 1973; Ossenberg, 1987). The latter can be up to 0.5 mm in diameter and often contain a recurrent branch of the inferior alveolar nerve that ends either on the temporalis tendon or buccinator muscle, or sends accessory branches to the third molar tooth. A similar, but distinct and rare variant, the temporal crest canal, was described by Ossenberg (1986), where a tunnel ran horizontally across the temporal crest midway between the third molar crypt and the tip of the coronoid process. Again, the importance of these posterior canals is that they probably provide an alternative route for pain fibres that may not be reached by routine inferior alveolar nerve block.

The gonial angle can vary from 100° to 140° and the mean angle is highest in Caucasians, nearly as high in Chinese, Eskimos and Blacks and lowest in Australians and American Indians (Hrdlička, 1940b, c; Zivanovic, 1970). In all racial groups, the mean angle in females is 3–5° higher than in males, but the wide range of variation makes this trait of little or no value for racial classification (Jensen and Palling, 1954; Zivanovic, 1970). Mandibles with a broad, well-marked ramus tend to have a smaller gonial angle, than ones with a slender ramus. Symons (1951) distinguishes between the gonial angle and 'true angle of the mandible', the latter being the angle between a line from the middle of the condyle to the mandibular foramen and the occlusal surfaces of the second and third molar teeth. This angle is much less variable than the gonial angle which is altered by 'filling in' of alveolar bone to maintain the true angle.

As in the maxilla, tori are extensively reported in the anthropological literature. Torus mandibularis is a single or multiple bony exostosis, on the lingual side of the mandible below the mylohyoid line, usually in the premolar segment, although it may extend more anteriorly. Like the torus palatinus, this varies in occurrence and degree of expression. In general, incidence appears to be higher in populations from the northern hemisphere such as Inuit, Aleuts and Icelanders (Hooton, 1918; Hrdlička, 1940a; Mayhall *et al.*, 1970; Mayhall and Mayhall, 1971; Axelsson and Hedegård, 1981; Reinhard and Rösing, 1985), although it has also been reported in modern Khoisan and pre-Columbian Peruvians (Drennan, 1937; Sawyer *et al.*, 1979). Muller and Mayhall (1971) found that the presence of torus is strongly affected by age amongst Eskimos and Aleuts, but they also stress that these incidence figures may be biased, depending on whether observations are carried out on living or skeletal populations. Tori are easier to see in skeletal material, but skeletal collections are often deficient in juvenile material. Diet and other environmental factors have been suggested to explain the development of torus, but familial studies have indicated that a genetic component may be involved (Krahl, 1949; Kolas *et al.*, 1953; Suzuki and Sakai, 1960; Johnson *et al.*, 1965; Axelsson and Hedegård, 1981). Recently, a Finnish study of individuals with Turner syndrome gives some support to the suggestion that the sex chromosome may have an influence on the occurrence, expression and timing of development of torus formation (Alvesalo *et al.*, 1996).

There are many studies using the mandible for sex determination and ascribing racial affinity. The value of early mathematical analyses is debatable, as although they show the expected quantitative differences in size between the sexes, the material on which they are based appears to be of undocumented sex (Martin, 1936; Morant, 1936). Differences in racial characteristics exhibited by the mandible are described by Houghton (1977, 1978) and Angel and Kelley (1986) and reviewed by St Hoyme and Işcan (1989). It is generally accepted that the male mandible has a greater body height, a more prominent chin and robust lower border and a less obtuse gonial angle (Hrdlička 1940c; WEA, 1980). Giles (1964) reported an accuracy of 85% in sex prediction using documented American Black and White mandibles and suggested that sexual dimorphism outweighed racial differences. However, Calcagno (1981), using discriminant function analysis, showed that removal of the size factor and formulating new functions or altering sectioning points was not successful and population specificity restricts their use. This problem has again been highlighted by Maat *et al.* (1997) using non-metric features of the mandible, in a population from the Low Countries. The large size of Dutch females resulted in a high degree of mismatching between pelvis and mandible. Morphology of the ramus alone may be a better discriminator of sex as Hunter and Garn (1972) found that from late adolescence onwards there was a disproportionate difference in ramal size in males and females compared to other facial components. More recently, Loth and Henneberg (1996, 1998), using dry bones, described a flexure in the posterior border of the ramus at the occlusal level in male mandibles, which is absent in females. They reported that this resulted in an overall accuracy of over 94% for assessment of sex. The method has been criticized on slightly dubious grounds by Koski (1996), who used lateral radiographs and only examined females. An accuracy of 94% in females and 90% in males was achieved using the method on an Indonesian population (Indrayana *et al.*, 1998).

It is a common observation that mandibles with loss of alveolar bone, and consequent adoption of a more obtuse gonial angle, belong to elderly individuals. In the great majority of cases this is so, but as both changes are secondary to the edentulous condition, direct correlation of this morphology with age should be viewed with caution. Although there is great individual variation in bone density, there appears to be reduction in cross-sectional girth of the mandible following tooth loss but, unlike postcranial sites, there is an increase in bone density with age. Highest densities were found at the midline, inferiorly at the mental foramen and buccally at the level of the third molar (Kingsmill and Boyde, 1998a, b).

Ossification

The mandible is the second bone in the body (after the clavicle) to commence ossification. A centre for each half of the bone appears at stage 18 (seventh week of intrauterine life) lateral to Meckel's cartilage in the ventral part of the first pharyngeal arch (Mall, 1906; Noback and Robertson, 1951; Dixon, 1958; O'Rahilly and Gardner, 1972). Before ossification can begin, the ectomesenchyme within the lower jaw must react with the epithelium of the mandibular arch and there is evidence that the presence of the trigeminal nerve is also essential for the induction of ossification (Sperber, 1989). Similarly, Jacobsen *et al.* (1991) described an archaeological adult mandible in which there was unilateral absence of the mandibular canal and foramen, and teeth from the second premolar to the second molar. They suggest that the nerve was also absent and that this observation suggests interaction between nerve tissue and tooth formation at an early stage of development.

Detailed descriptions of the initial stages of mandibular ossification are given by Fawcett (1905b, c, 1930) and Low (1905, 1909). The centre is first seen as a delicate lamella on the lateral aspect of Meckel's cartilage between the lateral incisor and canine tooth germs. The inferior alveolar nerve lies between the bone and Meckel's cartilage and gives off its mental branch, which at first lies in a notch on the superior border of the bone. Ossification spreads rapidly until there is a sheet of bone from the midline to the auriculotemporal nerve posteriorly. From this lateral plate, the bone spreads beneath the nerve and a medial plate forms between the nerve and the cartilage so that vertical sections appear V-shaped around the nerve, and then Y-shaped as the base of the bone (splenium) thickens. The terms medial and lateral alveolar plates (walls) were considered inappropriate by Symons (1951) as the tooth germs are well above the bone at this stage. True alveolar bone on either side of the developing teeth is formed above the level of the bone that bridges over the nerve.

The coronoid process differentiates topographically within the temporal muscle mass in the seventh week and by 8 weeks unites with the main part of the ramus (Spyropoulos, 1977). Kvinnsland (1969b) noted a difference in degree of ossification between the medial and lateral walls, which were distinct as far back as the angle. At 10 weeks, the medial wall, in close relation to Meckel's cartilage, was more active, whereas the lateral wall, continuous with the coronoid and condylar regions, was less well ossified. The angle at this stage was very obtuse, so that the condylar process was nearly in direct line with the body. By 12 weeks, the angle and the coronoid and condylar processes were well ossified and the mental foramen was visible on the lateral wall.

The lower jaw at the end of the embryonic period is described and illustrated by Macklin (1914, 1921), Augier (1931) and Müller and O'Rahilly (1980). Meckel's cartilage appears as a long rod of mature cartilage, which is continuous posteriorly with the malleus and is enlarged and flattened anteriorly, where it meets its fellow of the opposite side at a wide angle in the midline. The cartilage is covered laterally for three-quarters of its length by a plate of bone, whose lower border runs parallel with it. In the centre is the large mental foramen. Posteriorly, the upper end is notched and separated from the zygomatic process of the temporal bone in the region of the future condyle and, anterior to this, a thin projecting spur shows the position of the future coronoid process. The lateral surface of the body is a rounded, vertical ridge and the medial wall is serrated, with the gutter between them occupied by developing tooth germs. In front of the mental foramen, spicules of bone pass from one alveolar wall to the other to cover in the mental and incisive nerve canals.

At about week 10, the anterior end of the perichondrium of Meckel's cartilage from the mental foramen to the symphysis shows signs of incipient ossification and this section of the cartilage becomes incorporated into the bone. Kjær (1975, 1997) reported that, before this ossification began, the two halves of Meckel's cartilage were fused at a 'rostral connection' across the midline for a short time and then separated. Although this has been described and named the 'rostral process' in the rat (Bhaskar, 1953; Bhaskar *et al.*, 1953) and the mouse (Frommer and Margolies, 1971), it is the only report of midline fusion in the human embryo. More posteriorly, from the mental foramen to the lingula, the cartilage disappears completely by 24 weeks (Friant, 1960; Sperber, 1989). The extreme posterior end becomes converted into the malleus, incus, anterior ligament of the malleus and the sphenomandibular ligament (Bossy and Gaillard, 1963).

Between 12 and 14 weeks, secondary cartilages develop in the region of the condyle and coronoid processes, and a small number of cartilaginous nodules can be seen at the symphysis. Goret-Nicaise and Dhem (1982) studied the histological and microradiographic structure of the symphyseal region and maintain that the tissue in both the extremities of the hemi mandibles and in the ossicles (ossicula mentalia) differs from both bone and calcified cartilage, suggesting that it be designated chondroid tissue. The condylar cartilage develops in the cellular blastema covering the dorsal extension of the bony mandible and soon becomes a 'carrot-shaped wedge' that passes down the ramus to end at the base of the coronoid process (Fawcett, 1905c; Charles, 1925). About two weeks later, the temporomandibular joint is clearly defined and the posterior end becomes covered by articular hyaline cartilage (Symons, 1952; Blackwood, 1965). At first, the cone-shaped mass of the condylar cartilage reaches well forwards, but by the fourth lunar month, it starts to be replaced by bone. By 5 months, all that remains is a narrow strip of cartilage immediately beneath the condyle (Symons, 1951). The coronoid cartilage becomes rapidly converted to bone and all traces of the cartilage have usually disappeared by the sixth lunar month. The ossicles at the symphysis ossify about the seventh prenatal month and fuse with the anterior part of the body during the first year of life. The condylar cartilage, however, continues to act as the main growth centre until the beginning of the third decade of life (Rushton, 1944; Blackwood, 1965). At about 5 lunar months, early woven bone starts to be replaced by lamellar bone. It is suggested that this replacement of woven bone by mature Haversian systems at such an early stage of ontogeny is related to the fact that the mandible is subjected to intense activity from sucking and swallowing (Goret-Nicaise and Dhem, 1984).

The shape of the dental arch and the proportionate growth of the prenatal maxilla and mandible have been much studied (Burdi, 1965, 1968; Scott, 1967; Lavelle and Moore, 1970). At 6 weeks, the mandible is further advanced than the maxilla but 2 weeks later, the maxilla has overtaken it in size. By 11 weeks, they are equal in size, then again the maxilla becomes larger between 13 and 20 weeks. At birth, they are about equal with the mandible retrognathic to the maxilla. The rapid postnatal growth of the mandible should lead to a normal occlusion, but inadequate or overgrowth can result in abnormal occlusal positions (Sperber, 1989). A series of radiographs with corresponding dissections of fetal specimens from 3–10 lunar months shows the developing tooth germs *in situ* (Boller, 1964).

The perinatal mandible (Fig. 5.69) consists of a body and a ramus of about half its length that extends posteriorly in an almost straight line, so that the head of the condyle is at the same level as the superior surface of the body. The outer surface of the body is flattened anteriorly but becomes rounded just above the base, at the level of the canine and first molar crypts by the bulging tooth germs contained within it. The mental foramen lies about two-thirds of the way from the base of the bone with its entrance pointing anteriorly. The mylohyoid line and mental spines can be seen on the inner surface. The angle between the body and ramus is obtuse, measuring about 135–145°. The articular surface of the condyle points posteriorly and between it and the thin pointed coronoid process there is a wide, shallow notch. The prominent mandibular foramen, with a well-formed lingula, lies in the centre of the inner surface of the ramus. The crypts for the two incisor tooth germs (i_1 and i_2) are rounded or oval and the mesial wall of the central incisor crypt forms the U-shaped symphyseal surface. The inferior edge of the surface curves away so that there is a gap between the two sides when the two halves of the mandible are articulated together. The canine crypt (c) is triangular in shape, with its base on the labial side and its apex pointing lingually. The crypt for the first deciduous molar (m_1) is square and behind it is a long, rectangular crypt that extends into the ramus. This is imperfectly divided by an incomplete interdental septum at its base and contains the tooth germ of the second deciduous molar (m_2) and the forming crown of the first permanent molar (M_1). The detailed appearance of the alveolar bone and crypts during the development of the deciduous dentition is described and illustrated by van der Linden and Duterloo (1976).

Postnatally, the mandible undergoes more variation in shape and greater increase in size than any other facial bone. It has to grow in harmony both with development of the deciduous and permanent dentition, with changes of size and shape of the maxilla and with increase in width of the cranial base. Growth at the symphysis is limited, as the right and left halves of the body join at the midline during the first year of life. Fusion starts on the outer and inferior surfaces and proceeds towards the inner and superior surfaces. Using archaeological populations, Becker (1986) suggested a fusion date between 7 and 8 months and Molleson and Cox (1993) found that in the Spitalfields collection the two halves of the mandible were always separate before 3 months of age, but that most had fused by 6 months.

As early as 1878 Humphry, carrying out experimental work on the pig, forecast most of the results of subsequent studies of mandibular growth. Growth has since been studied in archaeological specimens

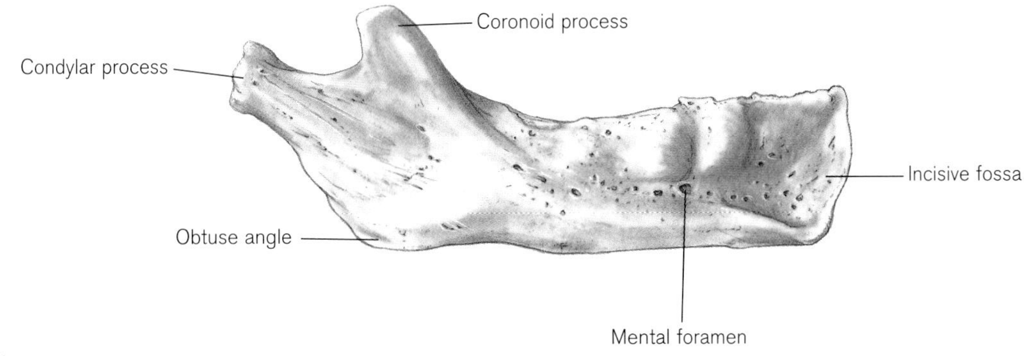

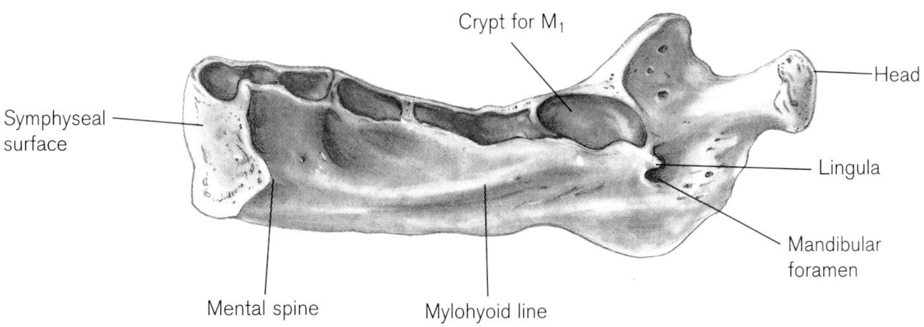

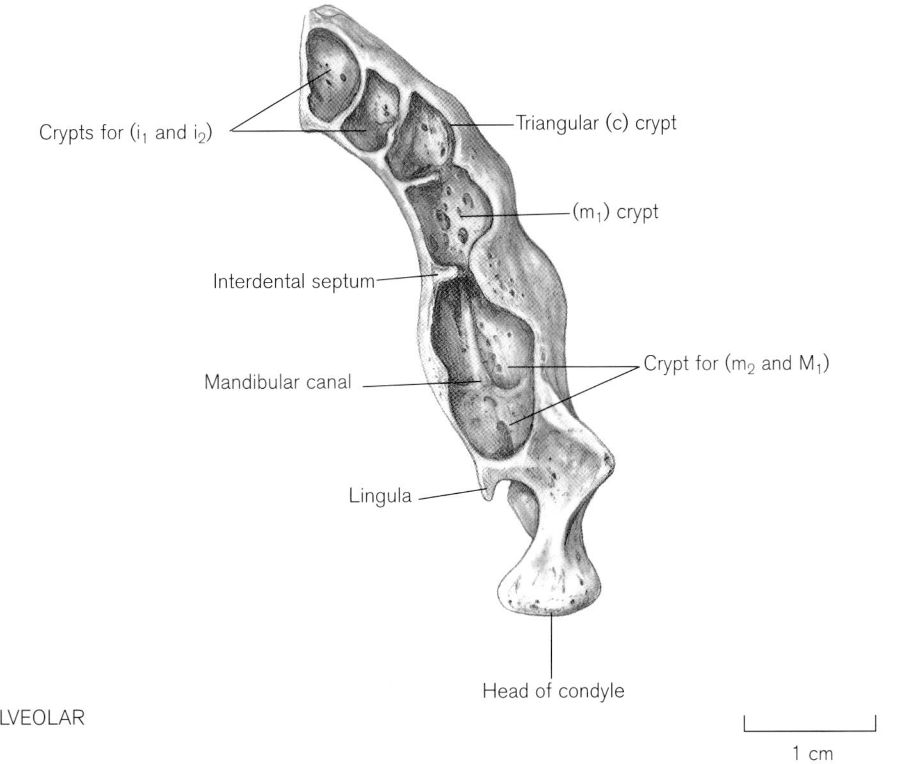

Figure 5.69 Right perinatal hemi-mandible.

(Murphy, 1957b), in living patients via the implant method (Björk, 1963), by histological examination of ground sections of dry bone (Enlow and Harris, 1964) and by Fourier analysis (Ferrario *et al.*, 1996).

The condyle plays a major role in the development of the lower jaw and its role is reviewed by Scott (1967) and Meikle (1973). It causes a downward and forward movement of the mandible from the cranial base. At first, there is an increase in length of the body because of the almost straight line formed by the body and ramus. The angle at birth is between 135° and 150°, but soon afterwards it decreases and this becomes most obvious at about the time of the completion of the deciduous dentition, when it is between 130° and 140° (Jensen and Palling, 1954).

Alveolar bone is deposited at the superior surface of the body as the deciduous dentition develops but, once the occlusal plane is established, it maintains a stable relationship with the lower border of the body (Brodie, 1941). The concomitant decrease in the mandibular angle, together with a rapid growth in height of the ramus, results in the condyle reaching a higher level than the occlusal plane of the teeth. The angle measures between 120° and 130° after the eruption of the second permanent molars (Jensen and Palling, 1954). To maintain constant relationships during progressive increases in size, bone deposition occurs on the posterior border of the ramus and resorption on the anterior border. In this way, the ramus is backwardly displaced and the posterior part of the body is lengthened, making further space for developing teeth. As in the maxilla, each succeeding crypt occupies the same position relative to the surrounding structures, in this case, the mandibular canal and the anterior border of the ramus (Symons, 1951).

To keep pace with increase in width of the cranial base, there is an overall widening of the mandibular body by resorption and deposition, with consequent increase in bigonial breadth. A similar mechanism occurs at the mandibular notch and in the neck to further define their shape. The mental foramen lies below a line between the canine and first deciduous molar until the completion of eruption of the deciduous dentition. It subsequently moves posteriorly relative to the dentition, first lying under the first molar and then between the first and second molars. The foramen also changes its position vertically as the alveolar process increases in depth. At birth, it points anteriorly and upwards but there is a change during childhood, so that in the adult the neurovascular bundle occupies a posteriorly placed groove (Warwick, 1950). This is possibly brought about by differential rates of growth in the bone and periosteum as the body grows in length.

The chin alters considerably during childhood. Its depth increases rapidly after the eruption of the incisor teeth (Fig. 5.70) to make space for the developing roots, but the triangular mental area is variable in shape in different individuals. Brodie (1941) reported a rapid growth until the age of about 4 years, after which growth slowed. Meredith (1957) found that the concavity of the chin changed from very shallow at 4 years of age to a distinctly concave shape at 14 years. The crowns of the permanent incisors (I_1 and I_2) can be seen through the openings of the gubernacular canals on the lingual surface of the symphyseal region behind the deciduous teeth between 3 and 4 years of age.

Most sexual dimorphism starts to appear in the skeleton at puberty but, as nearly all the increase in craniofacial growth takes place before this time, it would seem reasonable to expect differences in growth between boys and girls in the craniofacial bones in childhood. There have been many studies in this area (Newman and Meredith, 1956; Hunter and Garn, 1972; Walker and Kowalski, 1972; Baughan and

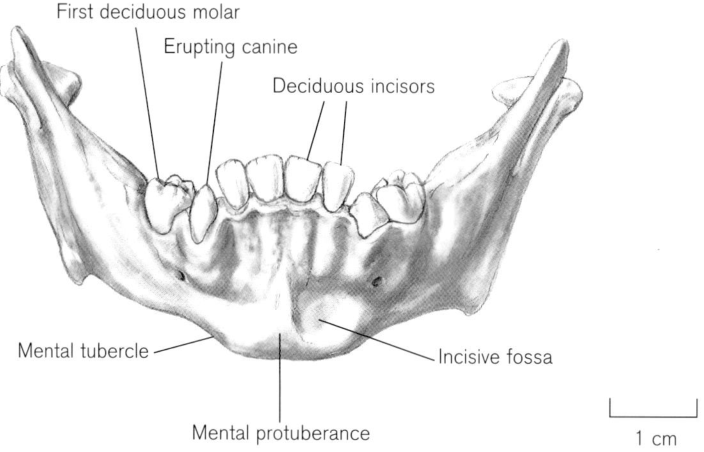

Figure 5.70 Formation of the chin. Mandible of a child of dental age about 1 year.

Demirjian, 1978; Buschang *et al.*, 1983, 1986; Schutkowski, 1993; Humphrey, 1998), which suggest that sexual dimorphism in both the face and mandible does exist from quite an early age. However, its manifestation is complex, and dimorphism does not usually reach a sufficiently high level to allow useful positive determination of sex until after the skeletal changes that take place at puberty. Molleson *et al.* (1998) found that the mandibular angle and the shape of the chin proved useful in determination of sex in juvenile skulls, but indicated that this needs to be tested on larger samples of known sex.

Practical notes

Sideing/orientation (Fig. 5.69)

The mandible is identifiable in isolation by mid-fetal life. The two halves remain separate until the first or second year of life. To side a complete half mandible, the coronoid and condylar processes extend posterosuperiorly and the anterior end of the body curves medially.

Bones of a similar morphology

Fragments of the alveolar area may appear similar to those of the maxilla, but the bone of the body beneath the crypts of the mandible is thick and rounded. The bone related to the crypts of the maxilla is part of the thin nasal or orbital floor. The condyle bears similarities to the acromial end of a scapular spine, the acetabular end of a perinatal pubis and to the pedicle end of vertebral half arches.

Morphological summary

Fetal

Wk 6	Intramembranous ossification centre develops lateral to Meckel's cartilage
Wk 7	Coronoid process differentiating
Wk 8	Coronoid fuses with main mass
About wk 10	Condylar and coronoid processes recognizable. Anterior part of Meckel's cartilage starting to ossify
Wks 12–14	Secondary cartilages for condyle, coronoid and symphysis appear
Wks 14–16	Deciduous tooth germs start to form
Birth	Mandible consists of separate right and left halves
During yr 1	Fusion at symphysis
Infancy and childhood	Increase in size and shape of bone Eruption and replacement of teeth
By 12–14 yrs	All permanent teeth emerged except third molars

Metrics

Fazekas and Kósa (1978) recorded the measurements of the mandible during fetal life (Table 5.21). Moss *et al.* (1956) recorded length and height of the bone from 8 to 20 fetal weeks, but landmarks were not defined. Detailed measurements of the postnatal mandible can be found in orthodontic texts (e.g. Enlow and Hans, 1996).

Table 5.21 Dimensions of the fetal mandible

Age (weeks)	Body length (mm)	Width (mm)	Longest length (mm)
12	8.0	–	10.7
14	9.6	3.2	12.6
16	13.0	6.5	17.9
18	14.2	6.9	21.4
20	17.6	8.0	25.6
22	19.2	9.0	27.3
24	21.5	10.2	30.1
26	22.6	10.9	31.9
28	24.2	11.3	34.0
30	26.0	13.0	35.9
32	27.7	14.1	39.0
34	30.0	15.1	40.2
36	31.7	16.4	42.7
38	34.7	17.0	47.5
40	36.5	18.0	49.7

Body length: from tuberculum mentale to mandibular angle.
Width: posterior border of condyle to tip of coronoid process.
Longest length: from tuberculum mentale to posterior border of condyle.
Adapted from Fazekas and Kósa (1978).

XV. THE TEETH

Teeth are the only skeletal structures of the living body that are in part visible to the naked eye. Their composition, anatomy and development are also quite different from the rest of the skeleton and in addition, they tend to be more resistant than bone to the effects of inhumation. As a result, the study of teeth forms a large and important part of the investigations of palaeontologists, anthropologists, skeletal biologists and forensic scientists. In common with many mammals, humans are diphyodont; that is, they have two generations of teeth: the deciduous, or 'milk', teeth and the permanent teeth. Deciduous teeth begin to form at about 6 weeks *in utero* and the last permanent tooth does not reach completion until early adult life, so that the development and maturation of both sets cover almost the whole of the juvenile life-span. In fact, they have proved to be one of the most accurate indicators of age at death, especially in immature individuals. No text on the juvenile skeleton would be complete without some reference to dental development and its relation to age determination (see also Chapter 2). However, there are many excellent texts detailing the gross and microscopic anatomy of tooth development and therefore in this section, no attempt is made to cover the morphology and development of the dentition in the same detail as with the bones of the skeleton in the rest of the text. Only those features of dental anatomy, terminology and development that may enable the reader to more readily appreciate the literature on estimation of age from the dentition will be reviewed.

Terminology

Teeth are arranged in both the upper and lower jaws in the form of a dental arch (arcade), or so-called catenary curve (like a chain suspended from two points). Both halves of each jaw contain the same number of teeth and for descriptive purposes are called the right and left, upper and lower quadrants. The deciduous and the permanent dentition both contain two incisors and a canine tooth in each quadrant and these are commonly referred to as anterior teeth. Behind them are the cheek, or posterior teeth, which consist of two molars in the deciduous series. These are replaced by premolars in the permanent dentition, and the arcade is normally completed posteriorly by a further three permanent molars. There are therefore 20 deciduous and 32 permanent teeth. In summary, the dental formulae for the deciduous dentition is:

$i\,\frac{2}{2}\;c\,\frac{1}{1}\;m\,\frac{2}{2}$, often individually named di1, di2, dc, dm1, dm2

and that for the permanent dentition is:

$$I\,\frac{2}{2}\;C\,\frac{1}{1}\;PM\,\frac{2}{2}\;M\,\frac{3}{3}$$

often individually named I1,I2, C, PM1, PM2, M1, M2, M3.

Figures given a super- or subscript position in relation to the letter designate a maxillary or mandibular tooth, respectively. For example, a right mandibular first deciduous molar will be Rdm_1 and a left maxillary second premolar will be LPM^2. Terminology can appear somewhat confusing, as clinical dentistry has several systems of shorthand to identify tooth position and these differ from that used by both zoologists and palaeontologists. For example, the latter often refer to the premolars as PM3 and PM4 as they are the remaining pair of a series of four premolars found in many mammals.

The two most common systems in clinical use are the Zsigmondy and the FDI (Fédération Dentaire International, 1971). The Zsigmondy system, in common use by clinicians, assigns letters a–e to the deciduous teeth and numbers 1–8 to the permanent teeth in each quadrant and the mouth is displayed diagrammatically, as if the observer is facing the patient (Fig. 5.71a). Thus d⌉ is a mandibular right first deciduous molar and ⌊5 is a maxillary left second premolar. The FDI system assigns two digits to each tooth, the first of which designates the appropriate quadrant and the second, the number of the tooth. The quadrants are numbered:

1 – permanent right upper	5 – deciduous right upper
2 – permanent left upper	6 – deciduous left upper
3 – permanent left lower	7 – deciduous left lower
4 – permanent right lower	8 – deciduous right lower

Thus, the same two teeth in the FDI system would be numbered as 84 (mandibular right first deciduous molar) and 25 (upper left maxillary second premolar – Fig. 5.71b). The FDI system appears to be less straightforward than the Zsigmondy system, but was developed for the purpose of entering individual teeth into a computer database.

Each tooth has four surfaces: labial, buccal, palatal and lingual, named according to their position relative to the midline of the mouth and to the lips, cheeks, palate and tongue, respectively. In a clinical situation, the positions of cusps of the premolar and molar teeth are similarly designated but again, zoologists and palaeontologists use a different terminology. This again derives from comparative mammalian dental anatomy, the corresponding terms

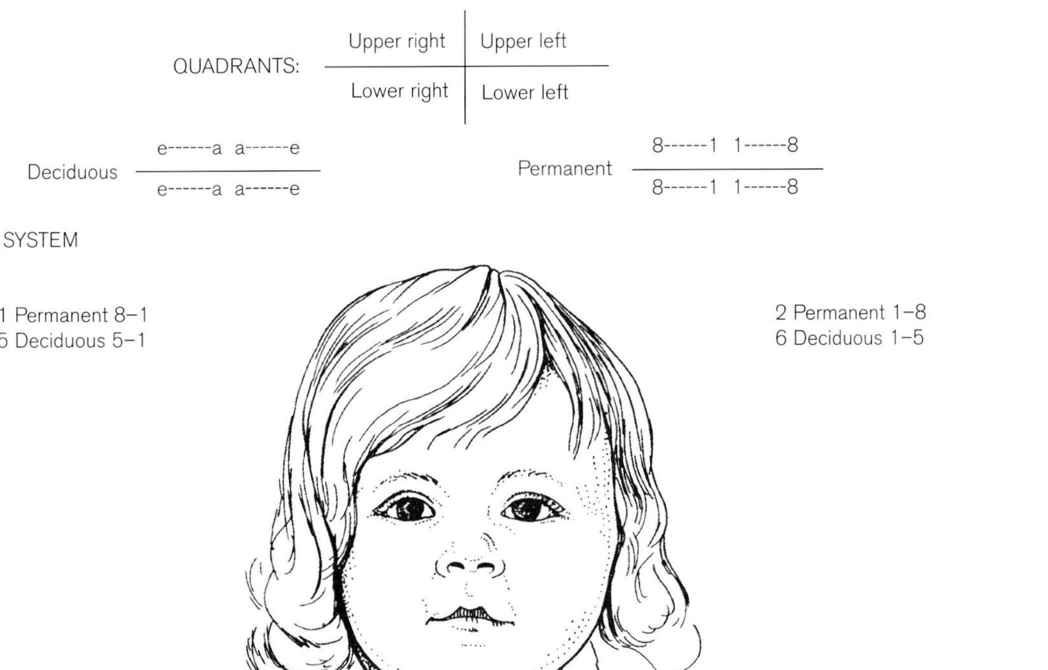

Figure 5.71 Terminology of tooth position. (a) Zsigmondy system; (b) FDI system.

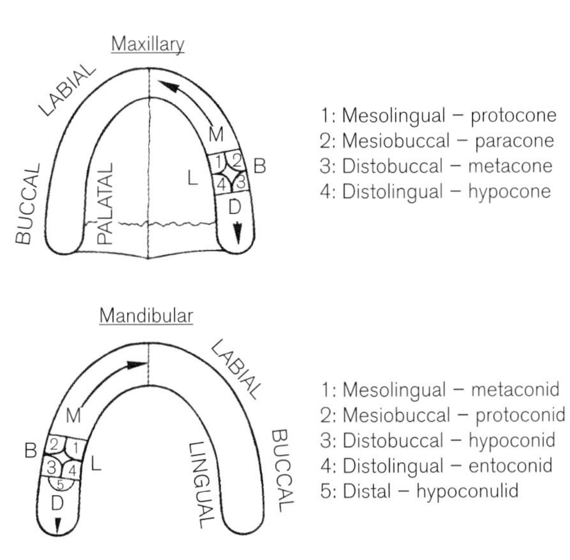

Figure 5.72 Dental arcades and molar cusp terminology. B buccal, D distal, L lingual, M mesial.

being given in Fig. 5.72. Equivalent teeth in the maxilla and mandible are termed isomeres, whereas those in the opposite right and left quadrants are called antimeres.

The mature tooth

The human tooth is composed of three types of hard tissue: dentine, enamel and cementum, each of which is different in composition from bone. The major part of both the crown and root of each tooth consists of dentine, which is covered by enamel on the crown and by a thin layer of cementum around the root. The junction between enamel and cementum occurs at the neck, or cervix. The innermost section of each tooth is occupied by the pulp chamber and root canal, composed of loose connective tissue containing nerves and blood vessels, which gain access to the pulp through the apex of the root. Each tooth is anchored by fibres of the periodontal ligament, which run from the cementum of the root to the alveolar bone of the jaw (Fig. 5.73). Covering the alveolar bone and attached around the tooth is the gum, or gingiva. Details of the gross anatomy and light and electron microscopy of the tissues of the tooth may be found in Berkovitz *et al.* (1978), Bhaskar (1980), Aiello and Dean (1990), Hillson (1996) and Ten Cate (1998).

It is important to recognize the normal appearance of developing teeth on an X-ray as one of the most commonly used methods of ageing relies on devel-

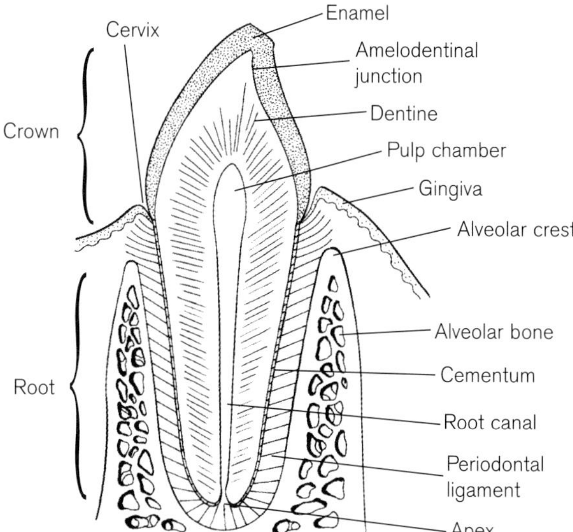

Figure 5.73 Section through a mandibular tooth to show tissues.

opmental stages as seen on radiographs (Fig. 5.74). X-rays also provide information on unerupted teeth that is not available when the jaw is viewed with the naked eye. Enamel is the most radiopaque tissue of the tooth and so the crown, or developing crown of a tooth can be distinguished as the whitest part. Dentine and cementum contain less radiopaque material than enamel and therefore appear greyer, but they are not easily distinguished from one another as their density is similar and in addition, cementum is extremely thin. The soft tissues of the pulp cavity and the periodontal ligament are radiolucent and appear dark in radiographs. Two parts of the supporting alveolar bone stand out on radiographs: the lamina dura, the layer of compact bone that lines the tooth socket and the alveolar crest, which is the gingival margin of the alveolus. The appearance of the crest depends on the space between the teeth, often producing points between the anterior teeth and flat crests between the cheek teeth. In a healthy erupted tooth, the alveolar crest is just below the level of the cervical margin of the tooth.

Each tooth develops within the alveolar bone of the jaw from a soft tissue tooth germ that is subsequently mineralized. The crown and part of the root is formed before eruption commences. Eruption is the movement by which a tooth advances from the alveolar crypt to its functional occlusal position in the mouth and can be regarded as a potentially lifelong process. Depending on the tooth, between one-third and three-quarters of the root is formed by the time of emergence into the mouth (Gleiser & Hunt, 1955; Grøn, 1962) and the remainder of root growth, including the closure of its apex, continues after emergence has occurred. A tooth may be stimulated to overerupt at any time in response to local conditions, such as the loss of an antagonist (Fanning, 1962), or to compensate for attrition, so that different fractions of the crown and root are visible in the mouth during the life history of a single tooth. Any part of the tooth visible in the mouth is termed the clinical crown and this obviously comprises less than the anatomical crown during emergence. In fully emerged teeth, the cementum/enamel junction (CEJ) is just subgingival. Only with gingival recession and/or continuous emergence to compensate for attrition, does the CEJ become visible intra-orally in life. However, in certain pathological conditions, such as periodontal disease (and therefore often in old age), where there is continued loss of attachment of the periodontal ligament from the alveolar crest, the visible part of the tooth above the gingival margin sometimes consists of the anatomical crown plus part of the upper section of the root covered with cementum, hence the term 'long in the tooth'. In this case, the clinical crown

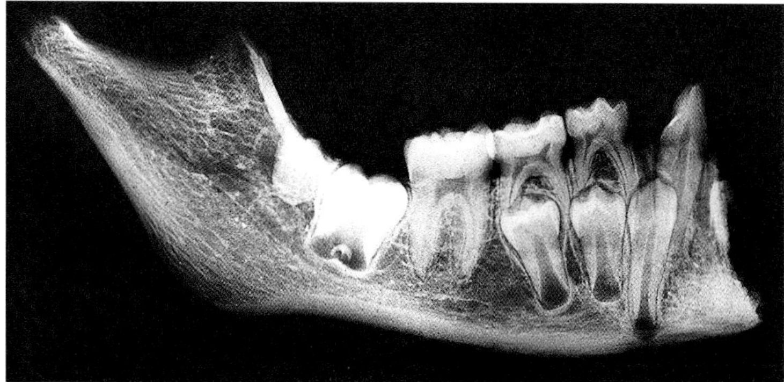

Figure 5.74 Radiograph of part of a hemi-mandible from a Romano–British archaeological specimen from Peterborough. The deciduous canine, first and second molars and the first permanent molar are in occlusion. Unerupted teeth visible are the permanent canine, both premolars, the partially complete second permanent molar and part of the crown of the third molar.

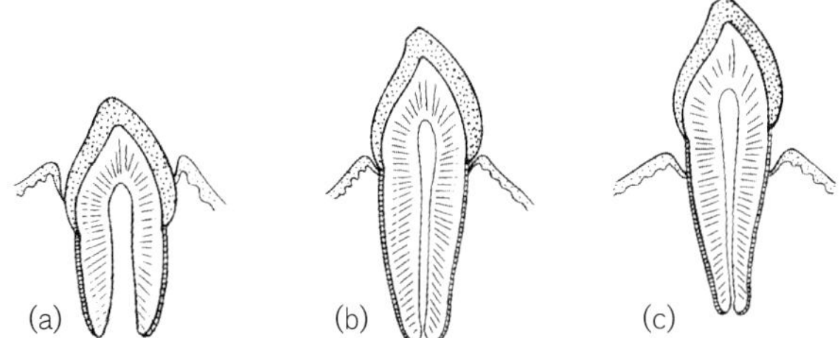

Figure 5.75 Anatomical and clinical crowns. (a) Emerging tooth, clinical < anatomical crown; (b) healthy tooth in occlusion, anatomical = clinical crown; (c) over-erupted tooth clinical > anatomical crown. Tissues as in Fig. 5.73.

comprises more than the anatomical crown (Fig. 5.75). In skeletal material where gingival tissues are absent, the anatomical crown is always at, or above, the level of the crestal alveolar bone, even in juvenile specimens where a tooth is fully erupted.

There are many texts with excellent descriptions and illustrations of the detailed morphology of the deciduous and permanent dentition and the reader is directed to these for the identification of individual teeth (Berkovitz *et al.*, 1978; Van Beek, 1983; Brown, 1985; Hillson, 1996). White (1991), Hillson (1996) and Whittaker[32] also give diagnostic criteria for categorizing tooth type, distinguishing deciduous and permanent teeth and then identifying each individual tooth in the upper or lower jaws. Metrical and non-metrical variations are also described by Hillson (1996). Photographs of the *in situ* state of the dentition from late fetal life to adulthood may be found in van der Linden and Duterloo (1976).

General chronology of tooth development

Although the development of the dentition is a continuous process that extends from embryonic to early adult life, it may be divided into a number of stages that are visibly active in the mouth as bouts of tooth emergence separated by apparently more quiescent periods. Within the jaws, however, there is continuous growth throughout most of embryonic and fetal life and postnatally until 18–20 years. By birth, all the teeth of the deciduous dentition and the first permanent molars have started to mineralize. By the age of about 3 years the deciduous dentition has emerged into the mouth and completed root formation. During the first year, the permanent first molar and anterior teeth begin formation and between the ages of 2 and 4 years, mineralization in the premolars and second molars is initiated. The third molars commence formation between 6 and 12 years of age.

The emergence of all the permanent teeth, except the third molars, takes place in two stages, between the ages of about 6 and 8 years and again between 10 and 12 years, separated by two relatively inactive periods. In the first active stage, the first permanent molar appears behind the second deciduous molar. At the same time, the deciduous incisors are shed and replaced by their permanent successors. The usual emergence order is the mandibular central incisor, followed by the maxillary central and the mandibular lateral incisors about a year later. The maxillary laterals are normally the last incisors to appear. There is then a quiescent period of 1.5–2 years before the second visibly active stage commences. This involves shedding deciduous canines and molars and their replacement by permanent canines and premolars, together with the emergence of the second permanent molars. Thus, the first active period begins with the emergence of the first molars at about 6 years and the second period ends at about 12 years with the emergence of the second molars.

Third molars in humans appear late in development and are said to be more variable in their development, size, shape and presence. They usually commence formation between 6 and 12 years, complete their crowns in 4 years and emerge and complete development during adolescence or early adulthood. Garn *et al.* (1962) compared the variability in timing to other posterior teeth and found it no different from the general biological trend that variability increases directly with mean age of attainment. Stewart (1934a) compared their emergence to other skeletal markers and found it was variable in relation to the closure of both long bone epiphyses and the spheno-occipital synchondrosis. Agenesis appears to vary in different populations from about 2% to 35% (Chagula, 1960; Thompson *et al.*, 1974; Bermúdez de Castro, 1989) and is not sexually dimorphic (Garn *et al.*, 1962; Levesque *et al.*, 1981). It also has a close association with other missing teeth (Thompson *et al.*, 1974) and Garn *et al.* (1961a) found it to be associated with relatively late emergence of second molars. In a large French Canadian sample, crown mineralization began at 9.8 years and was complete about 5 years later, with females being in advance of males, as with the development of other molar teeth. However, further developmental emergence and root

[32]Five excellent audiovisual tapes demonstrating tooth morphology (I – Introduction, II – Incisors and canines, III – Premolars, IV – Molars, and V – Deciduous teeth) by D.K. Whittaker are available for study by appointment in the Odontology Museum of the Royal College of Surgeons of England, Lincoln's Inn Fields, London WC2A 3PN, UK.

completion was faster in males, apex closure occurring about 1.5 years earlier in males (Levesque *et al.*, 1981).

The total time taken for an individual tooth to develop is considerable, lasting from 2–3 years for the deciduous teeth and up to 8–12 years for the permanent teeth. In general, anterior tooth crowns take 4–5 years and molar tooth crowns 3–4 years. This means that roots take approximately 6–7 years to grow. Normal emergence is correlated between antimeres and isomeres rather than neighbouring teeth (Garn and Smith, 1980), but if there is early loss of deciduous predecessors, or malocclusion, there may be delayed emergence (Fanning, 1961, 1962; Maj *et al.*, 1964; Anderson and Popovich, 1981).

Sex differences exist in developmental timing of the deciduous dentition. Boys are in advance of girls in the prenatal stages (Burdi *et al.*, 1970a; Garn and Burdi, 1971). There is also a sequence precedence, established very early in development, for tooth formation and emergence, with the anterior teeth more commonly having a mandibular precedence and the posterior teeth tending to a maxillary precedence (Burdi *et al.*, 1970b, 1975).

There is a large volume of literature on emergence times of both the deciduous and permanent teeth from all parts of the world and reports vary greatly in the size of the samples and in the methodology of recording. Some accounts failed to find differences in timing of emergence or sequencing of the deciduous teeth between the sexes (Friedlander and Bailit, 1969; Brook and Barker, 1972; Bambach *et al.*, 1973; Saleemi *et al.*, 1994) but Robinow *et al.* (1942), Meredith (1946) and MacKay and Martin (1952) reported that males were in advance of females in emergence timing. However Tanguay *et al.* (1986) pointed out that in young children, although this was true relative to chronological age, there was no significant difference between the length/height of an individual child and the time of tooth emergence. They suggested that clinical standards might be more accurate and efficient if scaled relative to height, as reflecting general physical development, rather than age. McGregor *et al.* (1968) also found that young children who are tall or heavy for their chronological age tended to have more teeth in the mouth than those who were smaller and lighter and there is some evidence that emergence was delayed in a severely undernourished population (Ulijaszek, 1996). In both these studies, children with a delayed dentition were systematically assessed as younger than their chronological age. Evidence on difference in timing between populations is equivocal, but reported differences appear to be small and it is difficult to isolate the effects of socio-economic status with its consequent nutritional effects. Shedding, or exfoliation, of the deciduous teeth begins at about the same time in boys as in girls, but sex differences increase with age, girls being in advance of boys (Fanning, 1961; Haavikko, 1973; Nyström *et al.*, 1986a).

There is more general agreement about the development of the permanent dentition as differences are more apparent. There is evidence from sibling studies that there is a genetic component in the sequence of development (Garn *et al.*, 1956; Garn and Lewis, 1957; Barrett *et al.*, 1964; Garn and Burdi, 1971; Kent *et al.*, 1978; Garn and Smith, 1980; Smith and Garn, 1987). Sex differences in both mineralization and emergence are usually in reverse of those for the deciduous dentition, girls being in advance of boys by about 6 months (MacKay and Martin, 1952; Garn *et al.*, 1958; Friedlander and Bailit, 1969; Helm, 1969; Helm and Seidler, 1974; Thompson *et al.*, 1975; Anderson *et al.*, 1976; Brown, 1978; Demirjian and Levesque, 1980; Levesque *et al.*, 1981; Jaswal, 1983). The difference is most marked in the emergence times for the canine teeth (Steggerda and Hill, 1942; Moss and Moss-Salentijn, 1977). Studies on tooth crown size in individuals with sex chromosome anomalies and their normal male and female relatives have demonstrated that genes on the X and Y chromosomes have differential effects on growth. This would explain the expression of sexual dimorphism of size, shape and number of teeth and differences in the proportions of enamel and dentine (Alvesalo, 1997).

Indications for differences in timing between populations are stronger than in the deciduous dentition (Brown, 1978; Blankenstein *et al.*, 1990) and some studies have taken into account socio-economic levels (Garn *et al.*, 1973c; De Melo e Freitas and Salzano, 1975). There is also evidence for difference in sequencing between populations (Dahlberg and Menegaz-Bock, 1958) and it is possible that sequencing could be affected by seasonality (Nonaka *et al.*, 1990). As with the deciduous dentition, some studies suggest that emergence of the permanent teeth is also related to general somatic development (Maj *et al.*, 1964; Helm, 1969). Filipsson (1975) and Moorrees and Kent (1978) developed methods based on the number of emerged teeth in living children. Factors affecting growth and emergence are discussed in more detail by Liversidge *et al.* (1998).

Age may be estimated using tooth emergence, but is not as accurate as some other methods (see below). In the living child, a tooth is normally recorded as having emerged if any part of the crown has broken through the gum. In a skull, emergence is usually defined as the appearance of the tip of the tooth, or

Table 5.22 Times of emergence (mths) of the deciduous dentition

		Mean	Range ± 1 SD
Maxilla	i^1	10	8–12
	i^2	11	9–13
	c	19	16–22
	m^1	16	13–19 (boys)
			14–18 (girls)
	m^2	29	25–33
Mandible	i_1	8	6–10
	i_2	13	10–16
	c	20	17–23
	m_1	16	14–18
	m_2	27	23–31 (boys)
			24–30 (girls)

Adapted from Lysell *et al.* (1962).

its cusps, at the same level as the alveolar crest. In either case, it is not usually possible to know the exact time of the event, as it may have happened at an unknown time before the examination of the child or skull. However, there are some occasions when the use of tooth emergence times is the only possible option, for example, in some fieldwork or forensic situations, where radiography is not practicable and speed and expense are paramount. Tables 5.22 and 5.23 give ages of emergence of the deciduous and permanent dentition. Because of the wide age range of each stage of third molar development, it is not a very useful estimator of age at death in a forensic situation, where accuracy is all important. Developmental standards can be found in Johanson (1971) and Nortjé (1983). Regression formulae and probabilities that an individual has reached the medicolegally important age of 18 years are given by Mincer *et al.* (1993).

Early development of the teeth

The first indications of dental development are visible in the early embryonic period before even the nose and mouth cavities are completely separated by formation of the secondary palate (Chapters 4 and 5). At about 28 days, an island of ectodermal epithelial thickening appears on each side of the maxillary processes and on the dorsolateral aspects of the mandibular arch. Additional thickenings appear about a week later on the lateral borders of the frontonasal process (see Fig. 5.9). The maxillary and frontonasal islands coalesce and the mandibular thickenings join in the midline. They form continuous arch-shaped plates, the **primary epithelial bands** in both the upper and lower jaws from which the vestibular and dental laminae develop (Nery *et al.*, 1970). On the labial side, apoptosis of the central cells of the **vestibular lamina** results

Table 5.23 Ages (yrs) for alveolar and clinical emergence of permanent teeth

		Boys				Girls			
		Maxillary		Mandibular		Maxillary		Mandibular	
Tooth	Stage	Median	± SD	Median	± SD	Median	± SD	Median	± SD
I1	alv	6.2	0.86	5.9	0.74	6.1	0.35	5.8	0.43
	clin	6.9	0.86	6.3	0.70	6.7	0.66	6.2	0.55
I2	alv	7.3	1.29	6.9	0.78	7.0	0.90	6.5	0.55
	clin	8.3	1.25	7.3	0.70	7.8	0.86	6.8	0.70
C	alv	11.2	1.21	9.8	1.09	9.3	1.25	8.8	0.63
	clin	12.1	1.41	10.4	1.17	10.6	1.45	9.2	1.06
PM1	alv	9.8	1.41	9.6	1.29	9.0	1.09	9.1	0.90
	clin	10.2	1.41	10.3	1.80	9.6	1.37	9.6	1.48
PM2	alv	11.1	1.60	10.3	1.72	9.5	1.37	9.2	1.64
	clin	11.4	1.48	11.1	1.72	10.2	1.60	10.1	0.67
M1	alv	5.3	0.74	5.3	0.35	5.3	0.47	5.0	0.39
	clin	6.4	0.63	6.3	0.55	6.4	0.55	6.3	0.55
M2	alv	11.4	1.09	10.8	1.02	10.3	0.90	9.9	1.06
	clin	12.8	1.25	12.2	1.41	12.4	1.17	11.4	1.41
M3	alv	17.7	1.52	18.1	2.15	17.2	2.46	17.7	2.34

Alv: alveolar emergence; clin: clinical emergence.
Table from Liversidge *et al.* (1998) with cross-sectional data from Haavikko (1970).

in the formation of a sulcus, the **oral vestibule**, which will separate the lips and cheeks from the tooth-bearing alveolar bone.

From each **dental lamina** ten swellings, the **enamel organs**, are budded off, which subsequently produce the enamel crowns of the teeth. Beneath each epithelial component is an aggregation of mesenchymal tissue, the **dental papilla**, derived from neural crest cells, which have migrated from the caudal mesencephalic and rostral metencephalic regions of the neural tube. The dentine, cementum and pulp of each tooth are derived from the dental papilla. The study of tooth development has provided much insight into induction mechanisms and tissue interactions (Lumsden and Buchanan, 1986; Mina and Kollar, 1987; Lumsden, 1988; Linde, 1998). By the tenth week the components derived from these two tissues become surrounded by a capsular **dental follicle** and each unit, or **tooth germ**, develops into a deciduous tooth. For descriptive purposes bud, cap and bell stages are distinguished before the late bell stage, when mineralization begins (Fig. 5.76). As with bone, the production of both enamel and dentine involve the deposition of an organic matrix, which is subsequently mineralized. Dentine is formed first, followed closely by enamel, with the two tissues being laid down between the original two components of the tooth germ. **Ameloblast** cells from the inner layer of the original epithelial enamel organ produce enamel and also induce the outer layer of the mesenchymal papilla to differentiate into **odontoblasts**, which form dentine. A layer of epithelial cells, known as Hertwig's **epithelial root sheath**, covers the future root and in the cheek teeth some of these cells invaginate to produce multi-rooted teeth. Cells of the dental follicle are involved in the production of **cementum**, the **periodontal ligament** and part of the surrounding alveolar bone. Permanent teeth that have deciduous predecessors develop as downgrowths from the dental lamina on the palatal or lingual side of their respective deciduous tooth germs. The permanent molars arise from an extension of the dental lamina posterior to the deciduous molars. Details of dental histodifferentiation may be found in Ten Cate (1998).

Mineralization

Mineralization of the tooth germ can be viewed as the equivalent of the ossification stage of bone formation. As with studies of ossification, prenatal observations are from entirely different source material than those obtained postnatally. Similarly, detection of mineralization depends on the technique used and reported timing is also affected by the inaccuracies incurred in the estimation of fetal age (see Chapter 2). Postnatal observations of mineralization are nearly all from cross-sectional and longitudinal radiological studies of living populations, some of the latter employing the same children that took part in the long-term skeletal growth studies discussed in Chapter 2.

Prenatal dental development has been studied histologically by serial sectioning, dissection and alizarin staining of fetal tooth germs and by radiology.

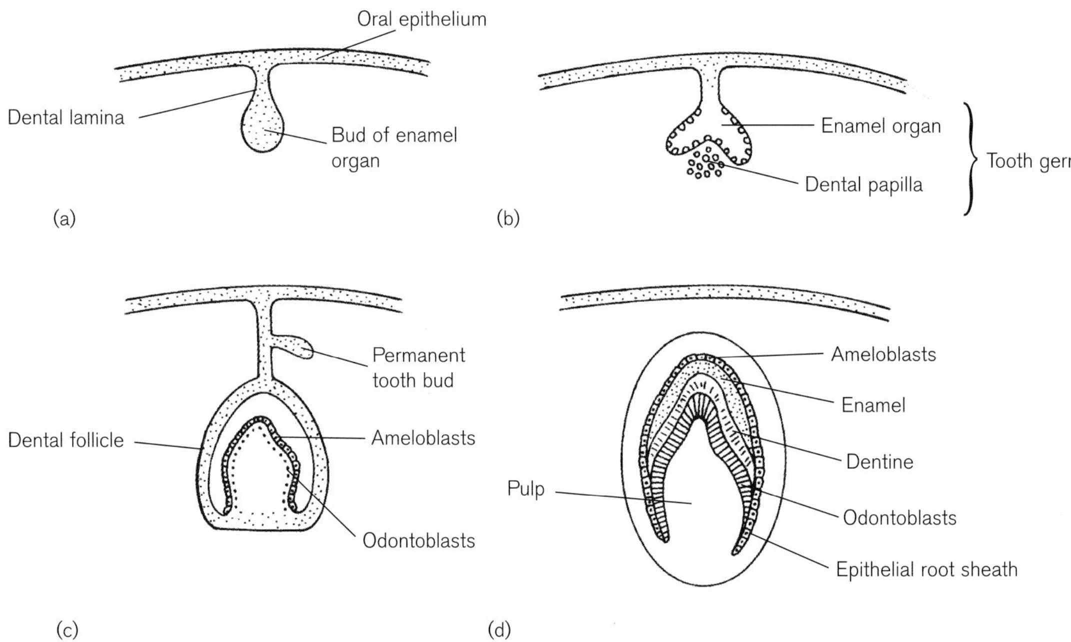

Figure 5.76 Tooth development: (a) bud stage; (b) cap stage; (c) bell stage; (d) late bell stage.

Some authors (Logan and Kronfeld, 1933; Kronfeld, 1935; Garn *et al.*, 1959; Nolla, 1960) reported that there are discrepancies in recorded timing of developmental stages, albeit smaller than in the ossification process, depending on whether the tooth germs are dissected or examined radiologically. Mineralization can be detected histologically up to 6 months before it can be seen on radiographs, as initially both enamel and dentine are not very radiopaque (Hess *et al.*, 1932). As a result, mineralization times from radiographs are usually shorter than the actual times taken for full crown and root formation.

Kraus (1959a) and Kraus and Jordan (1965), using dissection and staining techniques, demonstrated that initial mineralization began earlier than had previously been reported using other methods. Calcification proceeded faster mesiodistally than vertically and between 13–18 weeks *in utero* showed a sigmoid type of growth curve (Kraus, 1959b). Formation times of crown soft tissue, initiation of mineralization and maturation of enamel observed by all three techniques were reported by Nomata (1964). Lunt and Law (1974) reviewed previous studies on times of initial mineralization and produced a modified chronology table, which agrees with later histological work by Sunderland *et al.* (1987). Lunt and Law's (1974) timing appears to be about 2 weeks in advance of the times given by Sunderland *et al.* (1987), but is an example of the difference incurred in recording fetal age from fertilization or from LMP (see Chapter 2).

The sequence of prenatal mineralization in the deciduous teeth starts with the central incisor followed by the first molar, lateral incisor, canine and second molar. The maxillary central incisors and first molars are usually seen before those in the mandible. The lateral incisor appears first in the maxilla, but subsequent development is ahead in the mandible. Sunderland *et al.* (1987) reported mineralization in the mandibular canine before that in the maxilla, but it occurred simultaneously in the maxillary and mandibular second molars. Both Turner (1963) and Kraus and Jordan (1965) are in agreement that the sequence of calcification in the molar cusps of both the maxillary and mandibular teeth is mesiobuccal, mesiolingual, distobuccal, distolingual, with the distal cusp of the mandibular molar being the last to form.

Metrical studies of fetal molar tooth germs from 12 weeks to term have been reported by Butler (1967a, b; 1968) who concluded that the initial growth of the tooth germ and its subsequent calcification are independent processes. Kjær (1980) studied the development of the mandible and its anterior deciduous teeth and found that up to about 19 fetal weeks, the development of the lateral incisor was in advance of that of the central incisor. It was suggested that the envelopment of Meckel's cartilage by bone at the site of the canine tooth germ influenced the lateral incisor germ first. However, Deutsch *et al.* (1984) found that from 20 fetal weeks, the crown height of both the mandibular and maxillary anterior teeth proceeded in order of central incisor, lateral incisor and canine. Using gravimetric methods, Stack (1964, 1967, 1971) demonstrated that during the last trimester, fetal age is linearly related to the square root of the weight of mineralized tissue in the deciduous anterior teeth and Deutsch *et al.* (1981, 1984) confirmed that both the weight and crown height of the anterior teeth were correlated with fetal age. Initiation of mineralization, as visualized by alizarin staining, takes place in the first permanent molars between 28 and 32 fetal weeks, the mandibular germs being slightly in advance of those of the maxilla (Christensen and Kraus, 1965).

The mineralization status of the deciduous teeth and first permanent molars has been tested against other methods for the estimation of gestational age. Luke *et al.* (1978) tested the Kraus and Jordan (1965) stages of molar calcification and Stack's (1964) gravimetric method on fetuses whose LMP ages and crown–rump lengths were reliably known. Although the mean error produced by each method was similar, the correlation coefficients between actual and estimated ages were higher with the gravimetric method. They concluded that between 24 and 42 weeks of gestation, dental methods were more reliable in the estimation of gestational age than crown-rump length. Although there is a close correlation between tooth germ weight and fetal age, its use in age at death estimation is limited in most forensic and archaeological situations where there has been prolonged inhumation. Large changes in weight, presumably caused by chemical processes during diagenesis, render the gravimetric method hugely inaccurate (Scheuer, unpublished data).

Kuhns *et al.* (1972) correlated radiographic tooth mineralization with chest radiographs and knee ossification in premature infants and again found dental age correlated better with gestational age than did skeletal age. Lemons *et al.* (1972) attempted the estimation of age in small-for-dates babies from 2 weeks before the expected date of delivery, by correlating mineralization of the teeth with the appearance of the distal femoral epiphysis. They also confirmed that fetal age could be determined with greater accuracy from dental rather than skeletal development, but the method had a limited use as tooth germs could only be visualized sufficiently clearly if the fetus was in breech position with the head well clear of the pelvis.

At birth, the deciduous incisors have about 60–80% of their crowns complete and the incisal edges are usually elaborated into three small cuspules, or mamelons, which wear flat soon after emergence. In spite of this initial shape, there is no evidence that mineralization proceeds from more than a single centre as had been previously suggested, the lobed appearance being merely a function of depressions in the amelodentinal junction (Kraus, 1959a). Canine crowns are a simple conical shape and approximately 30% formed by birth. The first deciduous molars have a complete occlusal cap of mineralized tissue, the maxillary tooth being more fully calcified than the other molars. The mandibular

Table 5.24 Chronology of the deciduous dentition

Beginning of mineralization (number of weeks postfertilization)

Tooth	Fiftieth percentile	Range
di1	15	13–17
di2	17	14–19
dc	19	17–20
dm1	16	14–17
dm2	19	18–20

From Sunderland *et al.* (1987).

Age of crown completion (yrs)

	MFH Mean	MFH ±2SD	K & S	LDM Latest age or range
di 1	–	–	0.1–0.2	0.1
di 2	–	–	0.2	0.4
dc	–	–	0.7	0.7–1.4
Females	0.7	0.4–1.0	–	–
Males	0.7	0.4–1.0	–	–
dm 1	–	–	0.5	0.4–0.8
Females	0.3	0.1–0.5	–	–
Males	0.4	0.2–0.7	–	–
dm 2	–	–	0.8–0.9	0.7–1.4
Females	0.7	0.4–1.0	–	–
Males	0.7	0.4–1.0	–	–

Age of root completion (yrs)

	MFH Mean	MFH ±2SD	K & S	LDM Latest age or range
di 1	–	–	1.5	1.1–1.6
di 2	–	–	1.5–2.0	1.5
dc	–	–	3.25	2.6–2.9
Females	3.0	2.3–3.8	–	–
Males	3.1	2.4–3.8	–	–
dm 1	–	–	2.25	2.6
Females	1.8	1.3–2.3	–	–
Males	2.0	1.5–2.5	–	–
dm 2	–	–	3.0	3.0
Females	2.8	2.2–3.6	–	–
Males	3.1	2.4–3.9	–	–

MFH: data of Moorrees, Fanning and Hunt (1963a) from Smith (1991a).
K & S: data of Kronfeld and Schour (1939) from Smith (1991a).
LDM: Liversidge, Dean and Molleson (1993).

molars lack the characteristic pattern of grooves and pits, which only develop with later postnatal deposition of enamel (Kraus and Jordan, 1965). The crown of the second molar tooth normally has calcified cusps continuous with a large central area of uncalcified occlusal surface (Kraus and Jordan, 1965). Calcification may be present on as many as four cusp tips of first permanent molars at birth (Christensen and Kraus, 1965). In archaeological specimens, the fragile ring of mineralized tissue in the second deciduous molars rarely remains intact and it is often difficult to recover the tiny calcified cusps of the first permanent molars. Most maxillary and mandibular incisors reach maximum crown size between birth and 3 postnatal months but the canines can take up to 14 months to reach maximum size. The first permanent molars grow more slowly, but finally attain a total weight that is 2–2.5 times that of the deciduous molars (Stack, 1968). Postnatal changes in the size, morphology and weight of the deciduous dentition have been detailed by Deutsch *et al.* (1985). The accuracy of these standards tested on a crypt sample of known age between birth and 1 year was found to be high and accuracy during the first postnatal year was highest for deciduous molar tooth length (Liversidge *et al.*, 1993; Liversidge, 1994). Age of formation standards for individual teeth reported by Liversidge (1995a) fall within the range of previously published standards. Mays *et al.* (1995) also found that there was a highly significant relationship between permanent molar crown height and dental age amongst juveniles from an archaeological population of unknown age. Details of the appearance of the enamel matrix in decalcified sections from birth to 2.5 years, useful for age estimation in a forensic context, have been reported by Calonius *et al.* (1970).

The literature on the prenatal development of the teeth is complex and historical reviews may be found in Garn *et al.* (1959), Lunt and Law (1974) and Smith (1991a). Many of the early studies give no clear indication of methods, ageing or sample size. However, it seems unlikely that there will be many new studies on the very early developmental stages because of the rarity of fetal tissue. Also, in the UK at least, radiographic studies *per se* are unlikely to be ethically approved as radiographs of young children are only taken if treatment is needed (Liversidge and Molleson, 1999). Information on the initiation of mineralization and the completion of crown and root formation of the deciduous teeth taken from Smith (1991a) and Liversidge *et al.* (1993) is shown in Table 5.24.

The majority of postnatal studies of mineralization have been radiological surveys of varying sizes. Starting with the classic study of the life history of the permanent mandibular first molar by Gleiser and Hunt (1955), defined stages of crown and root development were assessed from panoramic or lateral radiographs to construct chronological time scales of normal tooth growth. Most employed 11–14 stages, but the number varied in different studies as stages were either interpolated or omitted. Crown stages start with first evidence of mineralization and then coalescence of the cusps, followed by complete cusp outline, then half, three-quarters and completion of the crown. This is followed by root initiation, and usually by fractions of root completion with an added cleft formation stage in multi-rooted teeth. Some surveys used additional stages for closure of the root apex. Accepted standard stages are shown in Fig. 5.77 and their abbreviations in Table 5.25. The majority of studies included all the mandibular permanent teeth, but some omitted the third molars and there is very little information on maxillary teeth, owing to the practical difficulties in their radiographic visualization.

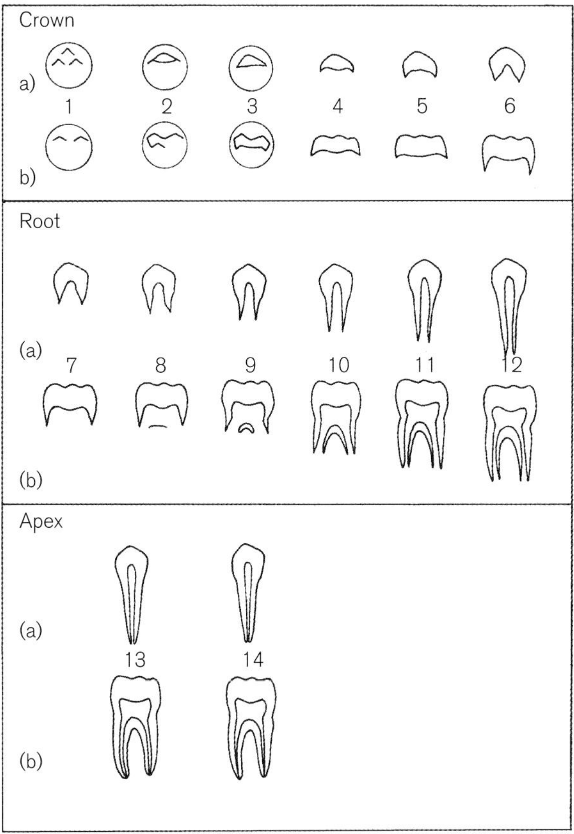

Figure 5.77 Stages of mineralization in the development of the crown, root and apex of permanent teeth as defined by Moorrees *et al.* (1963b). (a) Single-rooted teeth; (b) mandibular molars. Abbreviations in Table 5.25.

Table 5.25 Standard abbreviations of tooth formation stages

1	C_i	Initial cusp formation
2	C_{co}	Coalescence of cusps
3	C_{oc}	Cusp outline complete
4	$Cr_{1/2}$	Crown half complete
5	$Cr_{3/4}$	Crown three-quarters complete
6	Cr_c	Crown complete
7	R_i	Initial root formation
8	Cl_i	Initial cleft formation
9	$R_{1/4}$	Root length quarter
10	$R_{1/2}$	Root length half
11	$R_{3/4}$	Root length three-quarters
12	R_c	Root length complete
13	$A_{1/2}$	Apex half closed
14	A_c	Apical closure complete

From Moorrees *et al.* (1963b).

Chronologies using stages of mineralization were reported by Demisch and Wartmann (1956), Garn *et al.* (1958, 1959), Nolla (1960), Fanning (1961), Moorrees *et al.* (1963a, b), Haataja (1965), Wolanski (1966), Haavikko (1970, 1974), Fanning and Brown (1971), Liliequist and Lundberg (1971), Anderson *et al.* (1976) and Nyström *et al.* (1977). A variety of teeth, or combinations of teeth, were employed and nearly all the children studied were either from European-derived populations of North America, or from Scandinavia. Most were used to produce age-of-attainment schedules; that is, the proportion of children who had reached a particular developmental stage was plotted against the midpoint of each age group.

The most commonly used method in estimation of age in archaeological material is that of Moorrees *et al.* (1963a, b) but accounts of its accuracy vary in different studies. In general, the times for M1 crown completion and incisor and M1 root formation are too low. In a cemetery sample of ten individuals of known age tested by Saunders *et al.* (1993b), it proved to be more accurate for age prediction than the method of Anderson *et al.* (1976). Even so, the authors advise the omission of the Moorrees' maxillary incisor standards because these have a biasing effect on the estimation, as they include values only from the age of 4 years.

In growth-related studies of older archaeological populations, accuracy cannot be tested, as the individuals are of unknown age. However, tooth formation standards have been applied in an attempt to compare differences between populations. This has identified methodological problems such as systematic and patterned differences in tooth formation timing, which have complicated their use (Owsley and Jantz, 1983).

Another type of mineralization study was developed by Demirjian *et al.* (1973) to estimate dental maturity in children of known age, using subjects of French Canadian origin. The number of stages was reduced to eight and each tooth was assigned a score depending on its state of development. Weighted scores were then added to produce a total maturity score, which was plotted against age. This was the same principle as that used to estimate skeletal maturity from wrist bone age (Tanner *et al.*, 1983). It was modified by Demirjian and Goldstein (1976), and used by Prahl-Andersen and Roede (1979), Demirjian and Levesque (1980), Levesque *et al.* (1981) and Nyström *et al.* (1986b). The Demirjian *et al.* (1973) method or its modification (Demirjian and Goldstein, 1976) has been tested on Black, White and Latino children of known age by Loevy (1983) and by Nyström *et al.* (1986b) on Swedish children. Both studies reported more advanced maturity scores than for the original French Canadian sample. Although the Swedish authors found the eight-stage system easy to use, with little intra-observer error, they recommended that maturity standards should be based on studies made on the same population for which they are used. Although this system was developed to assess dental maturity, it has also been used for estimation of age by Hägg and Matsson (1985) and Staaf *et al.* (1991) on Scandinavian children, by Davis and Hägg (1994) on Chinese children and by Koshy and Tandon (1998) on South Indian children. Not surprisingly, it did not correlate well with the samples tested, although it was more accurate in the younger than older age groups. This is a common finding, as variability increases with age when environmental influences have a cumulative effect (Garn *et al.*, 1959; Haavikko, 1970; Anderson *et al.*, 1976). Its use would be very limited on fragmentary remains.

All radiographic studies vary somewhat, depending on the number of formation stages used, the time interval between examinations and the intra- and interobserver error (Pöyry *et al.*, 1986). Training and experience in the reading of dental radiographs is essential in order to recognize fractions of crown and root development. It is obviously easier to assess these in longitudinal studies, where successive radiographs of the same individual are available. In cross-sectional studies, evaluation has to be made by comparing each tooth with more mature neighbouring teeth and this is inevitably less accurate.

Smith's (1991a) review chapter on tooth formation stages in the assessment of age is essential reading. She stresses that data collected for various tooth chronologies have been subjected to different statistical procedures and many studies are not comparable with each other as the underlying variables are fundamentally different. As a result, it is likely that some of the conclusions that claim population, and other differences are more likely to be due to the use of statistical treatments, or to sampling effects, rather than real differences between samples. There are also many gaps in the present knowledge of tooth development stages. The majority of samples are truncated in the early age ranges, owing to scarcity of very young children and the problems incurred in radiographing them. There is no single study that provides a chronology for all the deciduous teeth. Ages are usually available for mandibular teeth only, as there is very little information on maxillary teeth, owing to the practical difficulties of visualizing them. There is also sparse information on both deciduous and permanent incisors mainly due to the difficulty of visualizing anterior teeth. Some samples have an uneven distribution of ages, or do not give variances and there is also very little information other than from white, European-derived populations. Most clinical studies are expressed as either age-of-attainment of a growth stage, or produced for maturity assessments, but few chronologies are suitable for age prediction. Smith (1991a) re-worked the data of Moorrees *et al.* (1963b) so that each tooth may be assessed independently, making it more suitable for use with archaeological or fragmented remains (Table 5.26). The mean of the ages attributed to any available teeth can then be designated as the dental age. As most of this type of material is likely to be of unknown sex, the average of the male and female estimates would be

Table 5.26 Estimation of age (yrs) from the permanent mandibular dentition

Stage	I1	I2	C	PM1	PM2	M1	M2	M3
Female								
C_i	–	–	0.6	2.0	3.3	0.2	3.6	9.9
C_{co}	–	–	1.0	2.5	3.9	0.5	4.0	10.4
C_{oc}	–	–	1.6	3.2	4.5	0.9	4.5	11.0
$Cr_{1/2}$	–	–	3.5	4.0	5.1	1.3	5.1	11.5
$Cr_{3/4}$	–	–	4.3	4.7	5.8	1.8	5.8	12.0
Cr_c	–	–	4.4	5.4	6.5	2.4	6.6	12.6
R_i	–	–	5.0	6.1	7.2	3.1	7.3	13.2
Cl_i	–	–	–	–	–	4.0	8.4	14.1
$R_{1/4}$	4.8	5.0	6.2	7.4	8.2	4.8	9.5	15.2
$R_{1/2}$	5.4	5.6	7.7	8.7	9.4	5.4	10.3	16.2
$R_{2/3}$	5.9	6.2	–	–	–	–	–	–
$R_{3/4}$	6.4	7.0	8.6	9.6	10.3	5.8	11.0	16.9
R_c	7.0	7.9	9.4	10.5	11.3	6.5	11.8	17.7
$A_{1/2}$	7.5	8.3	10.6	11.6	12.8	7.9	13.5	19.5
A_c	–	–	–	–	–	–	–	–
Male								
C_i	–	–	0.6	2.1	3.2	0.1	3.8	9.5
C_{co}	–	–	1.0	2.6	3.9	0.4	4.3	10.0
C_{oc}	–	–	1.7	3.3	4.5	0.8	4.9	10.6
$Cr_{1/2}$	–	–	2.5	4.1	5.0	1.3	5.4	11.3
$Cr_{3/4}$	–	–	3.4	4.9	5.8	1.9	6.1	11.8
Cr_c	–	–	4.4	5.6	6.6	2.5	6.8	12.4
R_i	–	–	5.2	6.4	7.3	3.2	7.6	13.2
Cl_i	–	–	–	–	–	4.1	8.7	14.1
$R_{1/4}$	–	5.8	6.9	7.8	8.6	4.9	9.8	14.8
$R_{1/2}$	5.6	6.6	8.8	9.3	10.1	5.5	10.6	15.6
$R_{2/3}$	6.2	7.2	–	–	–	–	–	–
$R_{3/4}$	6.7	7.7	9.9	10.2	11.2	6.1	11.4	16.4
R_c	7.3	8.3	11.0	11.2	12.2	7.0	12.3	17.5
$A_{1/2}$	7.9	8.9	12.4	12.7	13.5	8.5	13.9	19.1
A_c	–	–	–	–	–	–	–	–

From Moorrees *et al.* (1963b) modified by Smith, B.H. (1991).

Table 5.27 Estimation of age (yrs) from tooth length of the deciduous dentition

di1	−0.653 + 0.144 × length ± 0.19
di2	−0.581 + 0.153 × length ± 0.17
dc	−0.648 + 0.209 × length ± 0.22
dm1	−0.814 + 0.222 × length ± 0.25
dm2	−0.904 + 0.292 × length ± 0.26

Tooth length (mm) = distance from cusp-tip or mid-incisal edge to developing edge of crown or root in the midline; only appropriate if root is incomplete, i.e. tooth still growing.
From Liversidge *et al.* (1998).

appropriate. Two tests of accuracy of age estimation on individuals of known age using these revised data are contradictory. Saunders *et al.* (1993b) found no substantial difference between age-of-attainment and the age-of-prediction tables, whereas Liversidge (1994) found the age-of-prediction tables to be significantly more accurate.

Other methods of age estimation

Tooth length

There have been a few studies on living children, which have produced reference charts based on tooth length alone in relation to age (Israel and Lewis, 1971; Ledley *et al.*, 1971; Carels *et al.*, 1991) and they appear to give good information for maturity assessment. Results from measurements of tooth length in the Spitalfields archaeological collection of known age at death individuals indicate that the age of crown completion is later than that reported in radiographic studies (Liversidge, 1995b). This is partly due to the condition known as 'burnout', where the last formed enamel in the cervical region is not seen at all on dental X-rays. There is also difficulty in visualization of the whole of the curving cementum/enamel junction in a two-dimensional radiograph. The enamel contour extends on the buccal and lingual surfaces 2–4 mm more towards the root than on the mesial and distal surfaces. Also, enamel on the buccal and lingual surfaces can occur up to 2 years after initial root formation begins on the approximal surfaces (Liversidge *et al.*, 1998). Recent histological studies (see below) agree with this. Regression equations to estimate age from the lengths of all the deciduous teeth and from the anterior teeth and first permanent molar are from Liversidge *et al.* (1998, Tables 5.27 and 5.28). Liversidge and Molleson (1999) extended these data for permanent teeth and gave updated regression equations that included earliest and latest age for when they are appropriate as well as dispersion, but they still remain to be tested.

Tables and charts

Many skeletal studies use estimated ages derived from the mean stage of development of the dentition as a whole, compared to a chart or atlas. The most commonly used are by Schour and Massler (1941), van der Linden and Duterloo (1976) and Ubelaker (1978). The last, although originally adapted for Native Americans, has been widely used with many different samples and is recommended by the WEA (1980, Fig. 5.78). Comparing an individual with a set stage in an atlas is easy and rapid but, as with skeletal atlases, difficulties occur with matching. Dentally, this happens when numbers of teeth, or sequencing between the two, do not match. However, accuracy of age estimation on a large sample of known age juveniles below the age of 5.4 years from the Spitalfields crypt was found to be higher using the Schour and Massler atlas than by other methods (Liversidge, 1994).

Another method in common use is the chart developed by Gustafson and Koch (1974), which includes both deciduous and permanent teeth. It was compiled from the accumulated data of about 20 different studies, regardless of histological or radiological

Table 5.28 Estimation of age (yrs) from tooth lengths of some permanent teeth

		Max t/l
I1	0.237 − 0.018 × length + 0.042 × (length)^2 ± 0.21	<11.3
I^2	− 0.173 + 0.538 × length + 0.003 × (length)^2 ± 0.14	<9.9
I$_2$	0.921 − 0.281 × length + 0.075 × (length)^2 ± 0.12	<9.8
C	− 0.163 + 0.294 × length + 0.028 × (length)^2 ± 0.25	<9.8
M1	− 0.942 + 0.441 × length + 0.010 × (length)^2 ± 0.25	<11.5

Length: maximum tooth length in mm; max t/l: maximum tooth length on which data based.
From Liversidge *et al.* (1998).

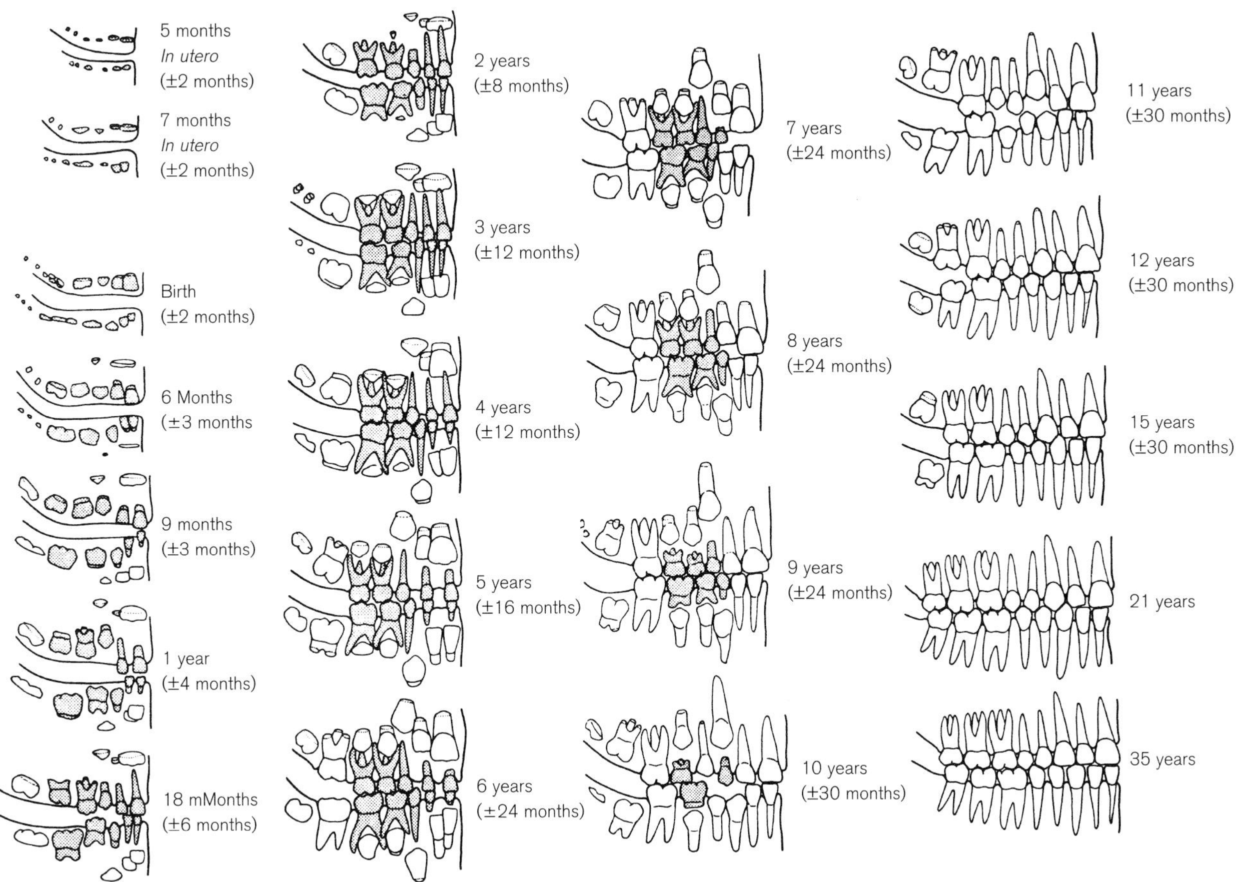

Figure 5.78 Chart of development of the teeth from 5 months *in utero* to 35 years. From WEA (1980) after Ubelaker (1978).

observations, or of the application of different statistical methods. It is based on four recognizable stages of development: initiation of mineralization, crown completion, tooth emergence and root completion. These are drawn as triangles on the chart, the base representing the range and the apex the mean. Age is estimated by placing a ruler across the available teeth and adjusting to 'best fit'. The authors tested it on a sample of 41 children of known age and found that an individual could be aged with an accuracy of ±2 months and that the 95% confidence interval for a single estimation was ±4.79 months. It has been tested independently on children of known age by Crossner and Mansfield (1983), who found it to be reliable irrespective of sex or race. Hägg and Matsson (1985) found that it was more accurate for males than for females, but that its precision (intra- and interobserver variability) was low, presumably because of the difficulty of its application. Reported overall accuracy for a known age crypt sample between birth and 5 years was 0.1 ± 0.37 years (Liversidge, 1994).

Dental microstructure

All the dental hard tissues show incremental lines that occur during the laying-down of their organic matrix and subsequent mineralization and there is a considerable volume of literature concerned with age estimation that makes use of this process. A long-established method for ageing in adults using cementum apposition, secondary dentine formation and other associated criteria was established by Gustafson (1950) and modified by Johanson (1971) and Maples and Rice (1979). It was recently compared with other methods against a known modern population by Lucy *et al.* (1994) and Lucy and Pollard (1995) have offered an alternative statistical analysis of Gustafson's data. Further techniques have been tested by Charles *et al.* (1986) and Condon *et al.* (1986). Their use in archaeological skeletal remains is hampered by the damage and possible diagenesis that occurs to cementum and dentine and the majority of the methods are only applicable in the young adult and adult age ranges.

Incremental lines in enamel provide a much more accurate method of age determination and their use in the estimation of age at death of a child from an archaeological site was first reported by Boyde (1963). The method is based on the recognition of two types of lines visible in enamel. Cross-striations occur along the length of the enamel prisms and it is generally accepted that they result from a circadian rhythm inherent in the rate of enamel matrix secretion by ameloblasts (for a review, see FitzGerald, 1998). Fairly regular numbers of cross-striations appear between darker and coarser lines, the striae of Retzius, which form with a periodicity of 7–8 days, although there are variations (Huda and Bowman, 1994; FitzGerald *et al.*, 1996; Hillson, 1996). Enamel is first laid down appositionally over the cusps and then secreted over the sides of the teeth, where the striae pass from the amelodentine junction to the surface. Here the overlapping layers, or imbricational enamel, are recognized as perikymata. The method has since been extended to estimate age in juvenile fossil hominids (Bromage and Dean, 1985; Dean *et al.*, 1986, 1993) and Dean and Beynon (1991) have used cross-striation counts, perikymata counts and root formation times to calculate the age of an unknown child from the Spitalfields archaeological collection. They found that incremental markings in the enamel were internally consistent between three different teeth of the same individual. Also, the estimates of average rate of root growth of the three teeth are consistent with each other and with the known chronological age of the child. Huda and Bowman (1995) have since used this technique to identify individual juvenile skulls in a sample of commingled remains between 1 and 4 years of age, by correlating them with information on their respective coffin plates. The advantage of this procedure is that it provides a much more accurate age at death estimate than can be obtained with previous mineralization standards. It is also an absolute method of age determination without reference to the growth standards of a particular population. Its disadvantages are that it is destructive of valuable or rare material, requires the facilities of a hard tissue laboratory, experience in technique and in addition, is both expensive and very time consuming. For these reasons, it is unlikely to become routinely used for the ageing of juveniles in samples of skeletal remains, although it could well be applied to an occasional forensic case.

The neonatal line, described independently by Rushton (1933) and Schour (1936), is a pronounced incremental line formed at birth or very soon afterwards. It can be seen on all teeth that start mineralization before birth, that is, all the deciduous teeth and usually at least the mesiobuccal cusp of the first permanent molar. Enamel prisms change direction as they cross the neonatal line and on the postnatal side, they appear to be less tightly packed (Whittaker and Richards, 1978). The visualization of the line could be of significance for medicolegal reasons, where it is important to determine if an infant was liveborn or stillborn. In practice, the neonatal line can be visualized by light microscopy if the child has survived for about 3 weeks after birth, or by electron microscopy, within a day or two after birth (Whittaker and MacDonald, 1989). Change in the normal location of the line in relation to the cervix of the tooth or a double neonatal line may indicate that the child has suffered premature birth or prolonged neonatal disruption of health (Skinner and Dupras, 1993; Huda and Bowman, 1995).

Chemical methods

There have been several attempts to estimate age at death from the teeth by measurement of biochemical norms. For instance, the calcium/phosphorus ratio in peritubular dentine increases significantly with age (Kósa *et al.*, 1990) and the rate of racemization of D and L enantiomers of aspartic acid residues in the collagen of dentine is accurately time dependent (Whittaker, 1992). Problems such as diagenesis caused by soil organisms have complicated the use of chemical methods thus far, but they provide a potentially interesting field for further investigation.

Conclusions

Detailed reviews of the principles and methods involved in the estimation of juvenile age from dentition can be found in Smith (1991a) and Liversidge *et al.* (1998). Recommendations include:

- Ideally, growth standards should be appropriate for the sample being aged with regards to sex, historic time and regional group. However, with many archaeological samples there are unknown variables and insufficient data for comparison.
- As many teeth as possible should be aged separately and a mean taken to give an age interval for a specific confidence and to state which interval this is.
- Because of the difficulty in assessing crown and root fractions in cross-sectional data, when ageing by developmental standards, the use of tooth lengths is recommended.
- In infancy and early childhood, the atlas of Schour and Massler (1941) or the chart of Gustafson and Koch (1974) is recommended.

- For older age groups, selection of the least variable mandibular teeth (Haavikko, 1974) may lead to greater accuracy. These are:

< 10 yrs. M_1, M_2, PM_1, I_1

> 10 yrs. M_2, PM_1, C

XVI. THE HYOID

The adult hyoid

The hyoid bone forms part of the rather insubstantial skeleton of the anterior part of the neck. It does not normally articulate directly with other skeletal structures, but is suspended by muscles and ligaments from the base of the skull and the mandible above, and connected to the larynx and sternum below. It gives attachment to muscles of the tongue, pharyngeal wall and anterior neck from the mandible to the thoracic inlet.

The hyoid consists of a central body, two greater and two lesser horns (Fig. 5.79) The **body** has superior, inferior and lateral borders and anterior and posterior surfaces. The superior border is sharp with a slight notch in the midline, on either side of which the surface is convex upwards. The inferior border is thicker and rougher and situated in a more anterior plane than the upper border. The upper parts of the lateral borders are either articulated or synostosed to the greater horns, while their lower sections slope downwards and inwards to meet the lower border. The anterior surface is either quadrilateral or hexagonal, depending on the slope of the lateral borders. It may be divided by a thick bar of bone into a narrow upper section facing anterosuperiorly and a lower section facing anteriorly, set at an obtuse angle to each other. The bar of bone, which has a slight downwards convexity, is occasionally separated from the main part of the body so that a thread can be passed behind it (Parsons, 1909). There may be a median vertical ridge on either or both sections of the surface. The posterior surface of the body is concave supero-inferiorly and laterally and usually pierced by several vascular foramina. Parsons (1909) reported the ranges and means of the dimensions of the body of 81 adult hyoid bones.

The **cornua majora** (greater horns) are attached to the upper part of the lateral border of the body. Each is a horizontally flattened bar, which tapers until about 5 mm from the end, when it expands into a tubercle. The lateral surface is roughened for muscle

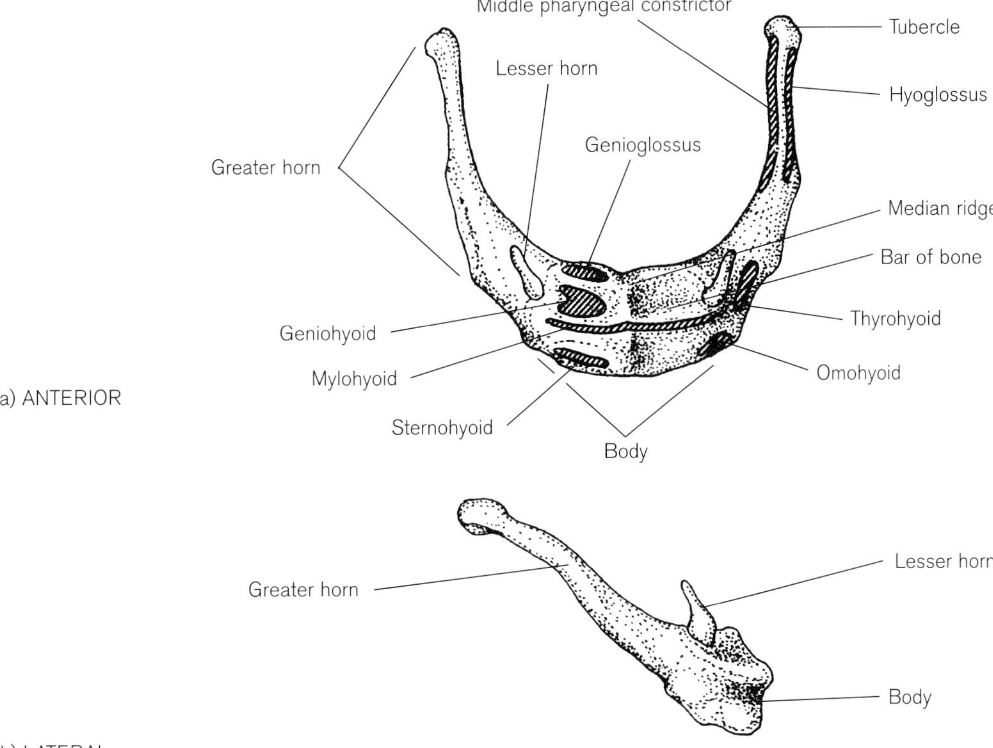

Figure 5.79 Adult hyoid.

attachment and may be everted, especially in the male. The attachment to the body is either by a strip of cartilage or through synostosis. The **cornua minora** (lesser horns) are small pyramidal cartilages or bones that jut outwards and upwards from the body at the point of attachment of the greater horns. They are usually attached to the body by fibrous tissue and sometimes to the greater horns by synovial joints.

The geniohyoid and genioglossus muscles arise from the upper part of the body of the hyoid and pass to the mandible and the tongue and the mylohyoid muscle, forming the floor of the mouth, is attached to the lower anterior surface of the body. The sternohyoid and omohyoid muscles pass from the lower part of the body to the sternum and scapula, respectively. The middle constrictor muscles of the pharynx and the hyoglossus muscles attach along the length of the greater horn and the stylohyoid and thyrohyoid muscles and the thyrohyoid membrane arise from the anterior segment of the greater horn. The inferior end of the stylohyoid ligament and the intermediate tendon of the digastric muscle are attached to the lesser horn.

The size, shape and symmetry of the hyoid is very variable and Papadopoulos *et al.* (1989) attempted to classify different types, but there appeared to be no significant relationship between a particular type and age or sex. Hypertrophy of the horns of the bone can cause occasional puzzling clinical symptoms. They may come into contact with the mandible (Morrissey and Alun-Jones, 1989) or even the cervical vertebrae (Hilali *et al.*, 1997) and possibly require excision. A well-preserved fossil hyoid from the Kabara Cave (Middle Palaeolithic of Israel) was almost identical in size and shape to the present-day bone, arguing that the morphological basis for speech was present some 60 000 years BP (Arensburg *et al.*, 1989).

Early development

The hyoid develops from the second and probably the third pharyngeal arches. The upper part of the second (Reichert's) cartilage, the tympanohyal and stylohyal form the vaginal process and the styloid process of the temporal bone (see above), but the origins of the named parts of the skeletal elements below this vary in different texts (Dwight, 1907a; Augier, 1931; Frazer, 1948). The segment below the styloid process (cerato-/epihyal) normally persists in the adult as the stylohyoid ligament, which is connected to the lesser horn at its inferior end. The lesser horn is either included in the ceratohyal, or called apohyal (Augier, 1931) or hypohyal (Dwight, 1907a). Part, or whole, of the ceratohyal may become ossified as a stylohyoid chain (see 'Temporal bone').

The second and third bars meet at their ventral ends to form the body of the hyoid, while the dorsal ends project posteriorly to form the lesser and greater horns. A cartilaginous centre appears in the body at about 5 weeks of intra-uterine life and by the seventh week the hyoid body and both horns have chondrified and the greater horns may be attached directly to the superior horns of the thyroid cartilage of the larynx (Frazer, 1910b; Müller *et al.*, 1981).

Macklin (1921) and Müller and O'Rahilly (1980) described the appearance of the hyoid cartilage at the end of the embryonic period. It resembles its adult form, but the body is slightly V-shaped with a notch or groove in the lower surface which, at this stage, is continuous with the upper edge of the thyroid cartilage of the larynx. The lesser horns are connected to the body by a zone of densely packed cells, while the greater horns are still separated by mesenchymal tissue. Koebke (1978) described the later prenatal development of the relationships between the horns and the body. Between 5 and 6 fetal months, there is either a joint cavity or a cartilaginous connection between the greater horns and the body, while the lesser horn is attached directly to the greater horn but separated from the body by a strip of fibrous tissue. Tompsett and Donaldson (1951) reported that the body of the hyoid appeared as a radio-opacity in 75% of 500 newborn infants, but care must be taken to distinguish it from the anterior arch of the atlas, which was ossified in 20%.

Ossification

Ossification has been reported in the body and greater horns as early as 30 fetal weeks (Reed, 1993), but may not be present until the first few months of life (Parsons, 1909). At first, the centre in the body occupies that part above the curved bar which is continuous above with the lesser horns (Fig. 5.80), but by the end of the first year, ossification has invaded the rest of the body. Parsons suggested that the body above the bar and the lesser horns are derived from the second arch, and that the rest of the body and the greater horns develop from the third arch. In a radiographic study of 86 juveniles from birth to 15 years, Reed (1993) found that after the age of 4 months, ossification had always begun in the body of the hyoid. Initially, the body appeared crescentic, changing to triangular in early childhood and then square in early adolescence. In the older age groups, the width of the body was significantly wider in boys than in girls. Ossification was first seen in the medial end of the greater cornua after the age of 6 months and this gradually extended posteriorly throughout childhood and ado-

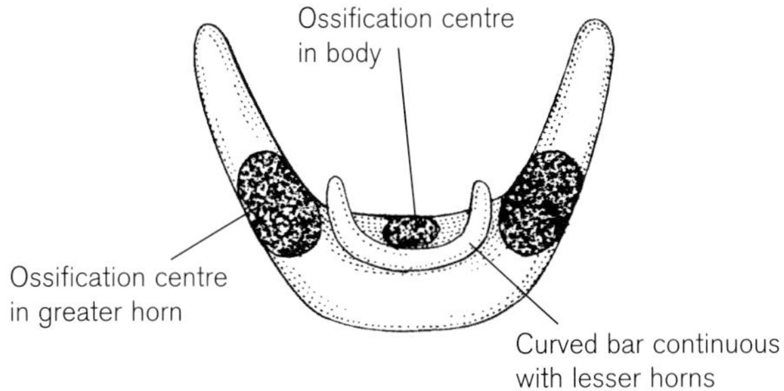

Figure 5.80 Perinatal hyoid (redrawn after Parsons, 1909).

lescence. The lesser horns, and the distal ends of the greater horns do not usually complete ossification until puberty, but may remain unossified throughout life.

Normally, both the greater and lesser horns eventually fuse with the body, but timing is very variable. Evans and Knight (1981) found both fusion of the greater horns and the body at 18 years and also non-fusion in the eighth and ninth decade. O'Halloran and Lundy (1987), in a review of 300 autopsy cases, reported that fusion did not usually occur until the third decade. Incidence of fusion generally increased with age and reached a plateau in the sixth or seventh decades, with approximately 70% of joints in males and 60% of joints in females fused by the age of 60 years. Bilateral fusion was found to be more common in men than women in all age groups. These findings are of interest to the forensic pathologist, as fracture of the hyoid bone is a well recognized indicator of strangulation, although only one-third of such victims actually have a fractured hyoid (Ubelaker, 1992). Pollanen *et al.* (1995) reported that fractures occurred at vulnerable angles of curvature and were usually restricted to the middle and posterior segments of the greater horn. Pollanen and Chiasson (1996) found that fractured hyoids occurred in older victims of strangulation (39 ± 14 years) when compared to victims with unfractured hyoids (30 ± 10 years). This age-dependency correlated with either the degree of ossification or fusion of the synchondroses, unfused hyoids being more flexible than fused ones. Indeed, hyoid fracture is rare in infants and children but becomes increasingly likely in adults with advancing age (Ubelaker, 1992).

Practical notes

Sideing/orientation (Fig. 5.79)

In a complete hyoid, the body faces anteriorly and the greater horns extend superoposteriorly. An isolated body is convex anteriorly and the smaller, biconcave section of the anterior surface faces superiorly. Isolated greater horns are difficult to side if not well marked. The wider anterior end can usually be distinguished from the tubercle at the posterior end and the lower surface tends to be smoother than the upper surface, which has muscle markings.

Bones of a similar morphology

The body of the hyoid bone is similar to an unfused anterior arch of atlas (see Chapter 6), both having a concave posterior surface. An isolated anterior arch of the atlas has a tubercle in the middle of its anterior surface, while a hyoid body is usually divided into two horizontal sections set at an angle to each other. If the two bones from the same individual are compared, the atlas is more robust and about twice the size of the hyoid. Isolated fragments of the greater horn may look like ossified horns of the laryngeal thyroid cartilage.

Morphological summary

Fetal	
Wk 5	Cartilaginous centre for body appears
Wk 7	Body, greater and lesser horns chondrified
Birth	Ossification centres may be present in the upper part of the body and ventral ends of greater horns
By yr 2	Body usually completely ossified
Puberty	Body and most of greater horns ossified
Throughout adult life	Complete ossification of bone and usually fusion of some elements

XVII. THE LARYNX

The adult larynx

The larynx developed primarily as an organ to guard the upper end of the respiratory tract and only secondarily took on the function of vocalization (Negus, 1929, 1949). It is composed of cartilages, ligamentous membranes and muscles and lies opposite the third to sixth cervical vertebrae in the anterior part of the neck, between the hyoid bone above and the trachea below. The principal cartilages are the single thyroid, cricoid and epiglottic cartilages and the paired arytenoids (Fig. 5.81). There are also small bilateral triticeal cartilages that lie in the edge of the thyrohyoid membrane between the hyoid bone and the larynx. The epiglottis, together with small paired corniculate and cuneiform cartilages, are composed of fibro-elastic cartilage, which has little tendency to ossify. This description will therefore be confined to the thyroid,

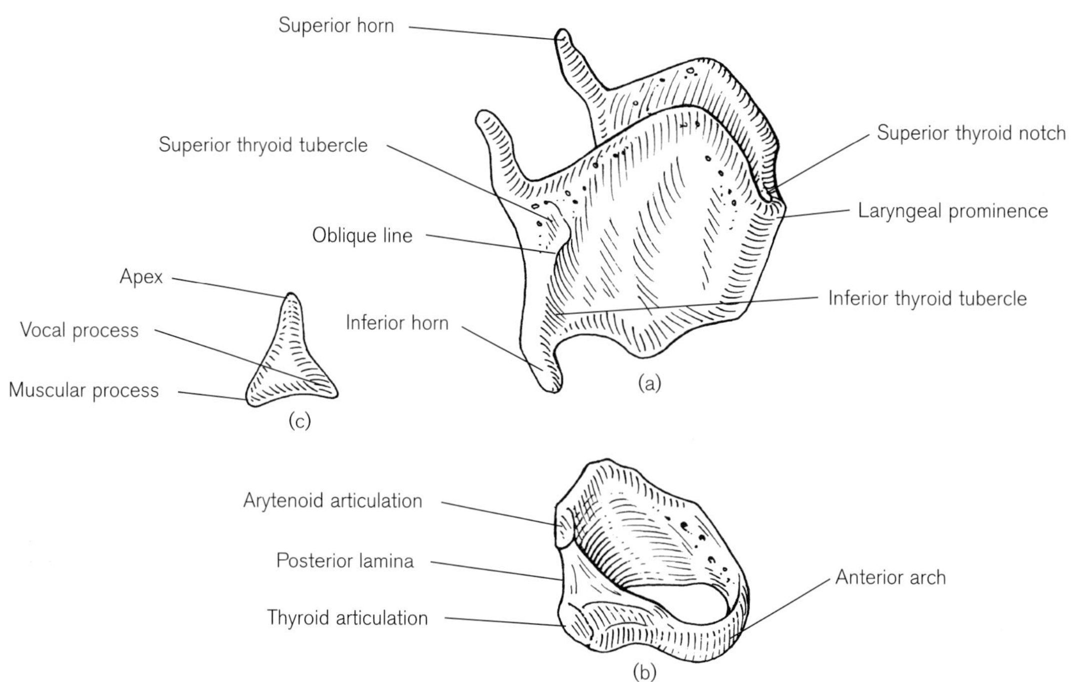

Figure 5.81 Laryngeal cartilages: (a) thyroid; (b) cricoid; (c) arytenoid.

cricoid and arytenoids, as they are composed of hyaline cartilage and commonly calcify, or ossify, even within the young adult time period.

The **thyroid cartilage** (Greek meaning 'shield-shaped') consists of two quadrilateral laminae whose anterior borders are joined at an angle in their lower two-thirds. The upper end of the junction forms the **laryngeal prominence** (Adam's apple), which lies subcutaneously in the anterior surface of the neck. This is usually visible in the male due to the more acute angle of the laminae and often only palpable in the female, where the angle is more obtuse. Ajmani *et al.* (1980) recorded mean angles of 78° and 106° for males and females, respectively. The space between the upper thirds of the anterior borders forms the **superior thyroid incisure** (notch). The superior border of each lamina has an inverted V-shape and is joined by the thyrohyoid membrane to the body and greater horn of the hyoid bone. The posterior borders of the laminae diverge and are prolonged into **superior** and **inferior cornua** (horns). The borders are thickened for the attachment of muscles of the pharynx. The inferior border of each lamina is straight anteriorly, curves concavely down to the inferior horn posteriorly and provides attachment for the cricothyroid membrane and muscle. Towards the posterior margin of the external surface of each lamina an **oblique line** curves from the **superior** to the **inferior thyroid tubercle** and the sternothyroid, thyrohyoid and part of the inferior constrictor muscle of the pharynx take origin here.

The **cricoid cartilage** (Greek meaning 'ring-shaped') is a complete circle around the respiratory passage and consists of a posterior quadrilateral lamina, which slopes down to a narrow anterior arch. Its horizontal lower border is attached to the trachea by the cricotracheal membrane. The upper border of the arch slopes steeply backwards to the lamina, which lies between the open posterior borders of the thyroid laminae. The lateral surface articulates at a synovial joint, with the inferior horn of the thyroid cartilage allowing the thyroid to rotate up and down on the cricoid, rather like the visor of a helmet (Grant, 1948). The posterior surface of the lamina has a median raised ridge, on either side of which are two hollows that accommodate the crico-arytenoideus posterior muscles.

The paired **arytenoid cartilages** (Greek meaning 'cup-shaped vessel, pitcher') are pyramid-shaped and sit on top of the sloping shoulders of the posterior lamina of the cricoid. The base of each is concave and forms one of the surfaces of a synovial joint with the cricoid (Sellars and Keen, 1978). Each cartilage has a blunt **muscular process** laterally, a sharp **vocal process** extending anteriorly and an **apex** that points superiorly. Detailed measurements of the laryngeal cartilages, for precise positioning in clinical practice, have been recorded by Ajmani *et al.*,

(1980) and Ajmani (1990) in Indians and Nigerians, respectively and in Europeans (Eckel *et al.*, 1994).

Early development

Classic studies of the development of the larynx were made early in the twentieth century by Soulié and Bardier (1907) and Frazer (1910b), but it was not until much later that development was followed in staged human embryos (Tucker and O'Rahilly, 1972; O'Rahilly and Tucker, 1973; Tucker and Tucker, 1975; Müller *et al.*, 1981; O'Rahilly and Müller, 1984b; Müller *et al.*, 1985). The respiratory and alimentary systems develop from the foregut, which is itself a diverticulum of the yolk sac. At about 20 days (Stage 9), when the embryo has one to three somite pairs and the first pharyngeal arch is beginning to form, the first sign of the respiratory primordium is a median groove in the floor of the pharynx. About a week later (Stage 12) both the gut and respiratory tubes elongate from the groove and a tracheo-oesophageal septum starts to form, which separates the two systems. By 32–33 days (Stages 14 and 15), the hypobranchial eminence, in the floor of the pharynx between the fourth pair of pharyngeal arches, and bilateral mesenchymal arytenoid swellings mark the site of the laryngeal inlet. It is not at all clear which pharyngeal arches give rise to the larynx, as the number of arches beyond the fourth, and particularly the actual existence of the fifth arch in the human embryo, is in some doubt. With the present state of knowledge it does not seem possible to assign various laryngeal components to specific arches (O'Rahilly and Tucker, 1973).

Chondrification of the thyroid, cricoid and arytenoid cartilages starts at the beginning of the eighth week (Stage 20). Bilateral centres appear in the laminae of the thyroid cartilage and about a week later, they become joined cranially and caudally, leaving the mesenchymal thyroid copula in the centre. This chondrifies separately and by 12 weeks has joined the laminae. Bilateral centres for the cricoid arch and the arytenoids appear at the same time as those for the thyroid cartilage (Doménech-Mateu and Sañudo, 1990). The shape of the cartilages at the end of the embryonic period have been described in some detail by Macklin (1921), Hast (1970), Müller and O'Rahilly (1980) and Müller *et al.* (1981). The thyroid cartilage is composed of two laminae, which may still be unfused in the midline, so there is no laryngeal prominence or thyroid notch. It is directly joined to the hyoid bone as the upper edges are continuous with the body of the hyoid cartilage. The superior horns are a direct prolongation of the greater horns of the hyoid. Both superior and inferior thyroid tubercles and an oblique line are present on each lamina and there is a foramen where chondrification is incomplete near the posterior border. The cricoid cartilage has already adopted its signet-ring form but the right and left halves of the posterior lamina are set at an angle, causing the lumen to be triangular, rather than circular. Tucker *et al.* (1977) comment on this shape in relation to intubation injuries in the infant larynx and Too-Chung and Green (1974) reported that the different rate of growth of sagittal and coronal diameters in the juvenile cricoid compensates for this early inequality. The arytenoid cartilages are composed of young cartilage and have distinct muscular and vocal processes. They are still joined to the cricoid by mesenchymal condensations, as the crico-arytenoid joints are as yet undeveloped and there are no corniculate or cuneiform cartilages at this stage. The epiglottis is composed of mesenchyme and fibro-elastic cartilage does not appear until the fifth lunar month (Tucker and Tucker, 1975). León *et al.* (1997) have investigated the incidence of the foramen thyroideum in embryos, fetuses and adults. It occurred in 57% of prenatal larynges, but only 31% of adults and in the latter the foramen is always traversed by a nerve or vessel. They proposed that it represents a failure of the complete fusion of the fourth and sixth arches which, when present, may be invaded by neurovascular elements. If this does not occur, then the lamina chondrifies completely and the foramen disappears.

By the end of the second trimester, the laryngeal cartilages have adopted their neonatal form, which is morphologically similar to that of the adult. The hyoid and thyroid horns become separated by the thyrohyoid membrane and the former connection between them is sometimes represented by small triticeal cartilaginous nodules. The fetal larynx is higher in the neck with respect to the vertebral column compared to its postnatal position, the tip of the epiglottis to the lower border of the cricoid cartilage reaching from C1 to C3/4 (Roche and Barkla, 1965; Müller and O'Rahilly, 1980; Magriples and Laitman, 1987). At birth, the larynx lies between C2 and superior C4 and there is then a marked descent between birth and 3 years as the lower rim of the cricoid cartilage reaches the C4/5 level. This has important clinical consequences during intubation of infants and small children because, as the larynx descends, so a greater number of vertebrae can be flexed and access to the upper respiratory tract becomes easier (Westhorpe, 1987). There is little change after this period until puberty when, with the growth of the thyroid cartilage, the larynx approaches the adult position.

The larynx also begins to display sexual dimorphism towards the end of the pubertal growth spurt (Sinclair,

1978). In the male, the size of the thyroid laminae is larger and the angle between them is more acute, allowing a greater length for the vocal cords and thus a deeper voice. Kahane (1978) found that, although there appeared to be no sexual dimorphism in the prepubertal larynx, females were closer to their adult counterparts than males and therefore had less growth per unit time to reach maturity. At puberty, the differential growth of the cartilages caused an increase in vocal fold length in males that was more than twice that in females. Harjeet and Jit (1992) reported that sexual dimorphism occurred in Indian subjects between the ages of 13 and 15 years in both sexes, but that increase in size in males continued until the age of 40 years.

Ossification

Calcification of the laryngeal and tracheal cartilages has been reported in infancy (Nabarro, 1952; Russo and Coin, 1958; Goldbloom and Scott Dunbar, 1960), but this is very rare and must be regarded as pathological. Later calcification and ossification of the laryngeal cartilages have been much studied (Taylor, 1935; Roncallo, 1948; O'Bannon and Grunow, 1954; Keen and Wainwright, 1958; Yoshikawa, 1958; King, 1963; Hately *et al.*, 1965; Cerný, 1983; Harrison and Denny, 1983; Jurik, 1984; Curtis *et al.*, 1985; Pryke, 1990, 1991; Turk and Hogg, 1993). It is well known that ossification occurs towards the end of the second decade and this possibly begins slightly later in females than in males. Details of different studies vary, but two principles appear to be established. First, ossification, especially in the thyroid cartilage, and to a lesser extent in the cricoid cartilage, follows a progressive pattern. Second, although the pattern is very similar in different individuals, its timing is highly variable and appears not to be sex-related. Evidence that there may be a genetic basis for the timing and pattern of ossification comes from studies of identical twins (Vastine and Vastine, 1952). The same pattern of ossification was seen in the hyoid and laryngeal cartilages in five pairs of twins ranging in age from 13 to 64 years.

Keen and Wainwright (1958) divided the ossification process into five, four and two stages, for the thyroid, cricoid and arytenoid cartilages, respectively. In the thyroid cartilage, ossification begins near the postero-inferior border of the lamina and then extends into the inferior horn and along the whole inferior border (Fig. 5.82a). It then extends upwards in the posterior border of the lamina towards the superior horn, before spreading into the main part. Often an anterior midline tongue forms (Fig. 5.82b), and it is common for there to be one or two 'windows' of unossified, or less ossified, material in the centre of each lamina (Fig. 5.82c). Eventually, the whole cartilage may ossify to produce an 'os thyroideum' (Fig. 5.82d). In the cricoid cartilage ossification starts at the superior edge of the posterior lamina and then spreads down the sloping lateral sides towards the anterior arch, which is always the last part to complete its ossification (Fig. 5.82e, f). In the arytenoid cartilages, there is often ossification in the main body and muscular processes but it is rarely seen in the vocal processes (Fig. 5.82g). Calcification precedes endochondral ossification and fatty and cellular marrow may be seen in both the thyroid and cricoid (Keen and Wainwright, 1958; Pryke, 1990). Partially calcified or ossified laryngeal cartilages may be mistaken for a foreign body in a cervical radiograph (O'Bannon and Grunow, 1954; Zoller and Bowie,[33] 1957; Hately *et al.*, 1965; Morreels *et al.*, 1967). The variability of the triticeal cartilages and their ossification has been reviewed by Grossman (1945) and Watanabe *et al.* (1982).

In summary, although most studies have demonstrated a gradual increase in ossification in both sexes with advancing age, there is no correlation between actual age and the degree of ossification. Nor is there a substantial difference in pattern between the sexes and it is therefore an unsuitable parameter with which to attempt ageing and sexing of skeletal remains. It is unfortunate that Krogman and Işcan (1986) quote an age-related pattern (Cerný, 1983) that appears to have been tested on only five individuals.

There is some reported sexual dimorphism in the bony texture of the thyroid cartilage, in that the ossification appears more homogeneous and hazy in the male, and more irregular and dense in the female. It is interesting that the same difference between trabecular and sclerotic type of calcification is also found in the costal cartilages (see Chapter 7). Arytenoid cartilages are more likely to be ossified in females than in males. Hately *et al.* (1965) found that between the ages of 21 and 80 years, 48% of female arytenoids were ossified, against only 8% in males and Jurik (1984) reported that arytenoid ossification was dense and homogeneous in 74% of females and 19% of males.

[33]A patient came into the Accident and Emergency Department complaining that he had swallowed a turkey bone. After oesophagoscopy, he was told that there was no sign of a turkey bone but a large piece of oyster shell had been removed. 'Oh yes' replied the patient 'the turkey *was* stuffed with oysters.'

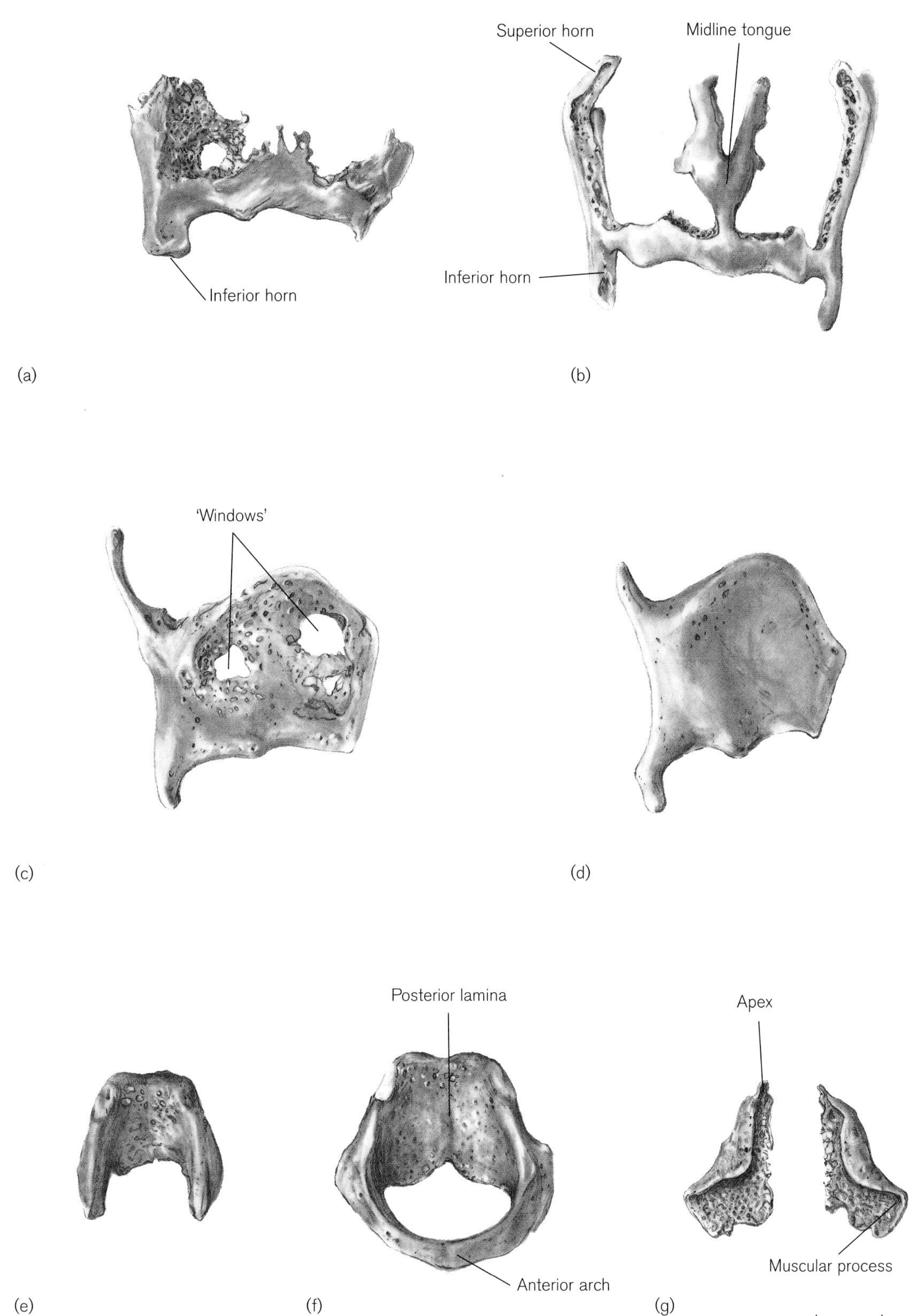

Figure 5.82 Ossification of laryngeal cartilages. (a) Thyroid, male age 55 years; (b) thyroid, male age 81 years; (c) thyroid, male age 42 years; (d) thyroid, male age 41 years; (e) cricoid, female age 51 years; (f) cricoid, male unknown age; (g) arytenoids, female 43 years.

Tracheal rings may become ossified in the adult. Although original sources of information are difficult to locate, standard anatomical texts suggest that this may occur after 40 years in the male and 60 years in the female (Schäfer and Symington, 1898; Ellis, 1992).

Practical notes

Sideing/orientation (Fig. 5.81)

The laminae of the thyroid cartilage (or 'os thyroideum') are joined **anteriorly** and open **posteriorly** and the thyroid notch is **superior**. The **superior** horns are thinner and longer than the **inferior** horns.

The **posterior** lamina of the cricoid cartilage (or 'os cricoideum') is quadrilateral in shape and the **lateral** borders slope down to a narrow **anterior** arch.

Bones of a similar morphology

Small fragments of ossified laryngeal cartilages are probably not recognizable in isolation and horns of the thyroid cartilage have a similar morphology to hyoid greater horns.

Morphological summary

Fetal	
Wk 8	Cartilaginous centres for the thyroid, cricoid and arytenoids appear
By mth 6	Cartilages adopt adult morphology
Birth	Adult morphology but larynx position high in the neck
By yr 3	Larynx descends to childhood position
Puberty	Larynx adopts adult position. Sexual dimorphism begins
By end of 2nd decade	Ossification usually begins in thyroid and cricoid cartilages

CHAPTER SIX

The Vertebral Column

The metameric segmentation of the central axis of the skeleton is the primitive phylogenetic phenomenon from which the subphylum vertebrata derives its name. Interestingly, the word spine, the term that is more favoured by clinicians, seems to have been adopted from the realms of the Roman circus.[1]

The vertebral column extends in the midline from the base of the skull above to the pelvis below and then beyond as the rudimentary tail (Fig. 6.1). It is made up of a number of individual components (vertebrae) that articulate above and below with each other, thus forming a segmented structure.

One of the major influences on the eventual morphology of the 'back bone' is the form of locomotion adopted by the animal. As such, the shape and construction of the human vertebral column bears testament to the virtually unique specializations and constraints imposed by habitual bipedal locomotion (Gadow, 1933). Although the adult vertebral column represents some two-fifths of total standing height, only three-quarters of its length is derived from the bony vertebrae. The remaining quarter of the column is comprised of intervening fibrocartilaginous intervertebral discs. Only a small degree of movement occurs between any two individual vertebrae, but the cumulative effect of this, results in a column of considerable flexibility that has neither sacrificed its stability nor its strength. In fact, the term vertebra is derived from the Latin '*verto*' meaning 'I turn' (Holden, 1882).

[1]The Roman racecourse was divided down the middle by a length of wall whose ends marked the turning points for the chariots. This central wall, which divided the two straight stretches of the course, was adorned with statues and altars to the appropriate Gods and was in fact termed the 'spina'. This was applied to the vertebral column in early anatomical nomenclature in reference to the way the spinous processes projected outwards and appeared to separate the region of the back into two straight portions (Field and Harrison, 1957).

The column as a whole subserves four major functions:

- it is the means whereby body weight is transferred from the upper regions to the pelvic girdle and then to the ground via the lower limbs,
- it provides a large site of attachment for the muscles of posture and locomotion,
- it offers a protective canal for the spinal cord and its covering meninges, and
- it is an important site of haemopoietic activity.

The adult vertebral column

Although somewhat variable, there are normally said to be 33 vertebrae in the adult column, of which 24 are true or presacral and a further nine which are false vertebrae (Danforth, 1930; Allbrook, 1955; Kaufman, 1977). The true vertebrae are to be found in the region of the neck (cervical – of which there are seven), in the chest (thoracic – of which there are 12) and in the small of the back (lumbar – of which there are five). The nine false vertebrae occur in two parts in the adult, with the upper five fusing to form the sacrum, which is the central axis of the pelvic girdle, and the remaining four fusing to form the diminutive coccyx (rudimentary tail). In the adult, the thoracic segment constitutes approximately half the length of the entire free column, the lumbar column approximately one-third and the cervical region approximately one-fifth or one-sixth (Crelin, 1973). It is interesting to note that the proportions are significantly different in the newborn, with the cervical segment constituting approximately one-quarter of the free column, the thoracic region approximately a half and the lumbar around one-quarter (Crelin, 1973). The newborn free column (first cervical to fifth lumbar vertebra) is approximately 19–20 cm at birth and is equal to about 40% of the total body length.

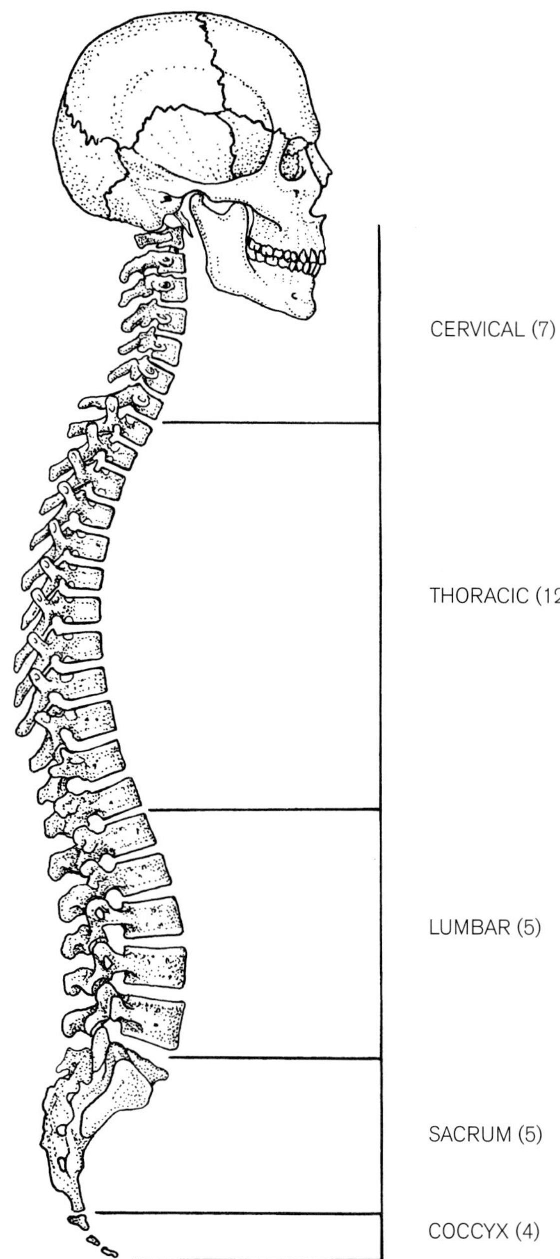

Figure 6.1 Lateral view of the adult vertebral column.

Not only do these different segments develop in response to the functional demands of the column as a whole, but they are also greatly influenced by more localized regional requirements. Therefore, the morphology of an individual vertebra reflects a compromise between these two requirements, and as such the differences that are subsequently manifested permit ready regional identification. For example, there are paired costal elements associated with virtually every individual vertebra, yet their form is widely different in each region of the column and in fact, Cave (1975) went so far as to propose that 'the regional status of a vertebra is determined by the ontogenetic fate of its costal element'. Whilst this is perhaps somewhat of an oversimplification, there is some degree of truth in the statement. The transition from one region to another can be quite sudden or indeed more gradual in nature. It has been suggested that gradual changes in morphology between adjacent regions may be under the influence of *Hox* genes (Kostic and Capecchi, 1994). It has been proposed that whilst in some structures morphological change is loosely controlled and numerous variations may ensue, in other features the structural elements are more rigidly restricted and so exhibit fewer forms of morphological variability (Shinohara, 1997). Aubin *et al.* (1998) found that correct expression of the *Hoxa* 5 gene was critical for the normal development of the C3–T2 region of the vertebral column. Le Mouellic *et al.* (1992) found that a disruption of the *Hox c*-8 gene resulted in a transformation of the first lumbar vertebra into a thoracic vertebra including paired ribs.

The **cervical** column extends from the base of the skull above to the articulations with the first thoracic vertebra below at the root of the neck. This is the most mobile region of the column and is the site of attachment for the strong vertebral muscles of the neck, which contribute to the maintenance of the erect position of the head. In addition, the cervical column houses the region of the spinal cord, which carries the greatest proportion of white matter. Thus, damage to the cord in this region can lead to widespread neurological disruption and even death. The first and second cervical vertebrae have been extensively modified to permit the movements of nodding and rotation of the head on the neck. They are strikingly different in appearance from the remainder of the presacral vertebrae and, as such, are perhaps the easiest to identify. Cave (1937) labelled the first and second cervical vertebrae as 'handmaidens to the cranium' as their function and morphology are so closely linked with that of the skull. He proposed that the third cervical vertebra should be named the 'vertebra critica' as it represents a critical site of union between the mobile cervicocranium above and the more stable column proper, below. He found a high incidence of fusion between the second and third cervical vertebrae and interpreted this as an attempt to form a cervical sacrum not only to secure cervicocranial stability but also to facilitate uninterrupted transmission of cranial weight.

The **thoracic** column articulates with the last cervical vertebra above and the first lumbar vertebra below. It is specialized for articulation with the ribs laterally and is generally considered to be one of the least mobile regions of the presacral column (Kapandji, 1974). Not only are the thoracic vertebrae responsible for transferring body weight in a caudal direction from the cervical region above, but they also relay the upper lateral body weight (upper limbs and thorax) to the lumbar vertebrae below (Pal and Routal, 1987; Routal and Pal, 1990). In older texts, these vertebrae are often referred to as 'dorsal' vertebrae.

The **lumbar** column extends from the last thoracic vertebra above to the first sacral vertebra below at the lumbosacral angle. It is specialized for substantial weight transfer, being responsible for relaying all the upper body weight to the sacrum from where it is eventually transferred to the lower limbs. It also offers a large surface area for the muscles that are essential for maintenance of the upright posture of the trunk.

In the adult, the terminal region of the spinal cord (conus medullaris) rarely descends below the level of the second lumbar vertebra, although the meninges may extend as far as the second sacral vertebra (Fig. 6.2). Using MRI images, MacDonald *et al.* (1999) reported that the termination of the spinal cord may range between the middle third of the eleventh thoracic vertebra to the middle third of the third lumbar vertebra, with the median occuring at the middle third of the first lumbar vertebra. Similarly, they found that the termination of the dural sac can range from the upper border of the first sacral vertebra to the upper border of the fourth sacral vertebra, with the median occurring at the middle third of the second sacral vertebra. These results showed terminations that were slightly higher than those reported previously and suggested that this may have arisen due to the previous use of cadaveric material, which tends to display tissue shrinkage (Choi *et al.*, 1996). The importance of this variation in the practice of spinal and sacral anaesthesia is obvious. It is, however, generally accepted that a needle inserted between the third and fourth lumbar vertebrae (lumbar puncture) will allow the safe removal of cerebrospinal fluid from the subarachnoid space with minimal risk of neurological damage. The vertebral column grows at a faster rate than the spinal cord, such that the adult vertebral column is 22 times longer than that of the fetus, whilst the adult spinal cord is only 12 times longer than that of the fetus (Reimann and Anson, 1944). This explains why the adult cord terminates at such a relatively high vertebral level. At 20 weeks of intra-uterine life, the cord extends as far as L4 and by term it lies between L2 and L3 and interestingly, maldevelopments of the vertebral column tend to be associated with a lower terminal level of the spinal cord (Barson, 1970; O'Rahilly *et al.*, 1980). The cord is said to reach its adult location, between L1 and L2, by 2 months *postpartum*.

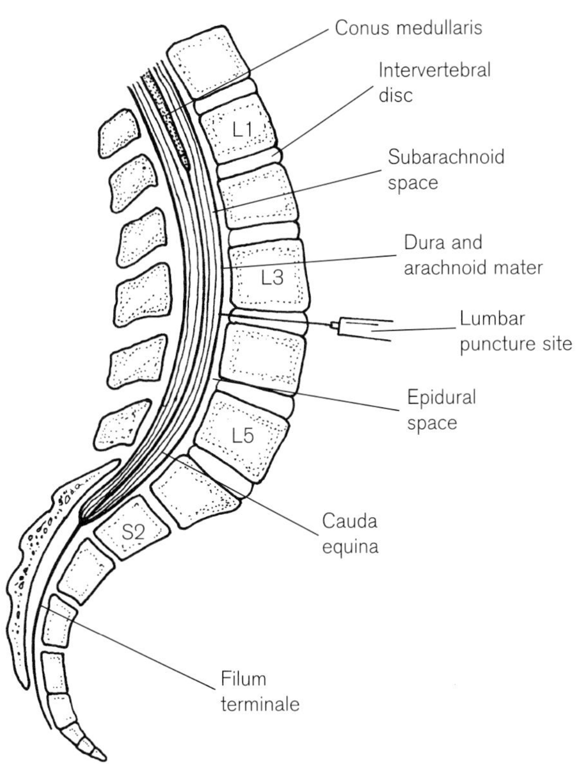

Figure 6.2 Sagittal section through the lower vertebral column showing the termination of the spinal cord and meninges.

The **sacral** vertebrae are fused in the adult and the sacrum articulates laterally with the innominates to form the pelvic girdle. It is wedge-shaped, being broader above than below as only the upper segments are involved in weight transfer to the sacro-iliac joints. The large surface area of the sacrum provides attachment for muscles of posture as well as for the muscles and ligaments of the gluteal region, whilst the sacral canal offers protection to the cauda equina. In midwifery, caudal or sacral anaesthesia can be performed to anaesthetize the sacral nerves which supply the bladder, cervix, vagina and rectum. A needle is inserted through the lower part of the sacral canal but cannot be advanced beyond the third sacral level for fear of perforating the meninges (Ellis and Feldman, 1993). For this reason, variations in the shape of the sacral canal are of significant clinical importance (Trotter and Lanier, 1945; Trotter, 1947).

The **coccygeal** column is a vestigial structure showing considerable variation in both morphology and number of components. It is the site of attachment of muscles of the internal pelvis and for ligaments and muscles of the gluteal region. It houses the lowest spinal nerve roots and the filum terminale. With advancing age the coccygeal elements generally fuse and the first may eventually fuse to the last sacral vertebra (Oldale, 1990).

The human vertebral column shows considerable numerical stability when compared to the degree of variation seen in many other primates (Bardeen, 1900; Brash, 1915; Willis, 1923a; Schultz, 1930; Mitchell, 1938; Hill, 1939), but transitional vertebrae do occur in the overlap zone between any two regions. The most common site for this, is at the lumbosacral articulation where the last lumbar vertebra may become sacralized and, conversely, the first sacral vertebra may become lumbarized (Bardeen, 1904, 1905; Todd, 1922; Lanier, 1939; Bernstein and Peterson, 1966; Castellvi *et al.*, 1984; Jonsson *et al.*, 1989; Barnes, 1994). It has been reported that the addition of a vertebra into the presacral region (25 vertebrae) is more likely in the male whilst the reduction by one vertebra (23 presacral) is more common in the female (Bernstein and Peterson, 1966). Therefore, the number of vertebrae in both the lumbar and sacral regions may vary from the common pattern, although this is usually by only plus or minus one vertebra. Although less common, variation is also found in the upper extremity of the column, either by increasing the number of vertebrae through the presence of an occipital vertebra or reducing the number by assimilation of the atlas with the occipital bone (Gladstone and Erichsen Powell, 1915; McRae and Barnum, 1953; Lombardi, 1961; Black and Scheuer, 1996a). Numerical variation is also encountered at the other extremity of the column, where it is not uncommon for the first coccygeal segment to fuse to the last sacral vertebra (Bardeen, 1905; Barnes, 1994).

The vertebral column is not a straight pillar of bone but consists of several curved segments which act like independent springs and so bestow considerable flexibility and resilience to the structure as a whole (Singer *et al.*, 1990). The curvatures are described as either primary or secondary, with the former being concave anteriorly and the latter convex anteriorly. In the fetus, the vertebral column is flexed in a 'C' shape with the concavity facing anteriorly, and this shape is fundamentally maintained until birth (Fig. 6.3). Crelin (1973) noted that the vertebral column of the neonate is so flexible that when dissected free it can easily be bent (flexed or extended) into a perfect half circle. It is generally held that once the child starts to hold its head up independently, around 2–3 months *postpartum*, a compensatory secondary curve, which is convex anteriorly, develops in the cervical region. However, Bagnall *et al.* (1977a) found the cervical curve to be present in the 10-week fetus and considered that it may arise in direct response to the well-documented reflex

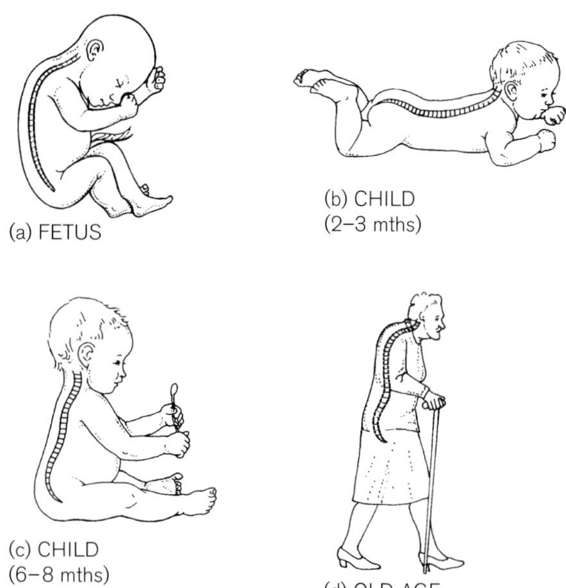

Figure 6.3 Changes in the curvatures of the vertebral column with advancing age.

movements of the fetal head *in utero*. Once the child begins to sit up unaided, around 6–8 months *postpartum*, a further secondary compensatory curve, which is also convex anteriorly, is said to develop in the lumbar region. It is generally recognized that the primary curves are maintained through the shape of the bony vertebrae whilst the secondary curves arise from a modification in shape of the intervertebral discs. With age, discs may degenerate and the integrity of the secondary curves become impaired. The column may then revert to its original primary curves, thereby partly explaining the curved shape of the vertebral column in the elderly (Oda *et al.*, 1988). Given the developmental and functional origin of the secondary curves, it is perhaps not surprising to note that over 80% of all back pain occurs in the compensatory regions of the neck and lumbar region (Woolf and Dixon, 1988).

The typical vertebra

Although the morphology of each vertebra is a product of both localized factors and general requirements that are placed on the column as a whole, there is a basic pattern that can be identified in all adult vertebrae throughout the length of the column (Fig. 6.4). When viewed from above, the typical vertebra has an anterior **body** and a posterior **vertebral** (neural) **arch**, which forms the boundaries of the **vertebral** (spinal) **canal**. The vertebral arch is formed from paired anterior **pedicles** and posterior **laminae** and

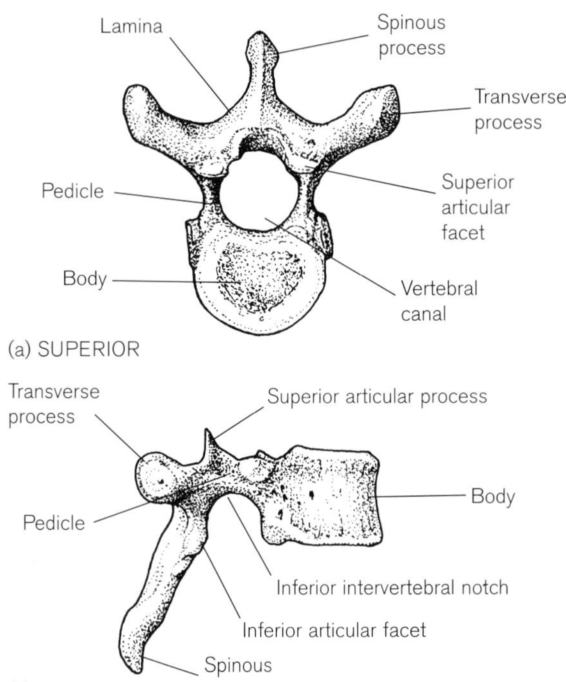

Figure 6.4 A typical adult vertebra.

seven processes that extend outwards from this arch – a single **spinous process**, paired lateral **transverse processes** and paired **superior and inferior articular processes**.

The main function of the **body** of a vertebra is to transmit weight from the inferior surface of the vertebral body above to the superior surface of the body below. As with all bone architecture, the cancellous struts and plates are aligned along the paths of principal stress (trajectories) and so adhere to Wolff's law (Wolff, 1870; Pal *et al.*, 1988). The internal architecture of the vertebral body shows this close relationship between form and function particularly well (Amstutz and Sissons, 1969). Bony trabeculae within the body are aligned in such a way that the majority run in a vertical direction (Fig. 6.5), indicating that the predominant force is compressive in nature (Francois and Dhem, 1974; Keller *et al.*, 1989; Smit, 1996). However, under axial compression the intervertebral disc introduces a horizontal tensile stress near the end plates, which results in the presence of horizontal trabecular struts in this location (Horst and Brinckmann, 1981; Smit, 1996). It is interesting to note that with age-related degradation of the nucleus pulposus there is a concomitant resorption in the horizontal struts at the end plates (Smit, 1996).

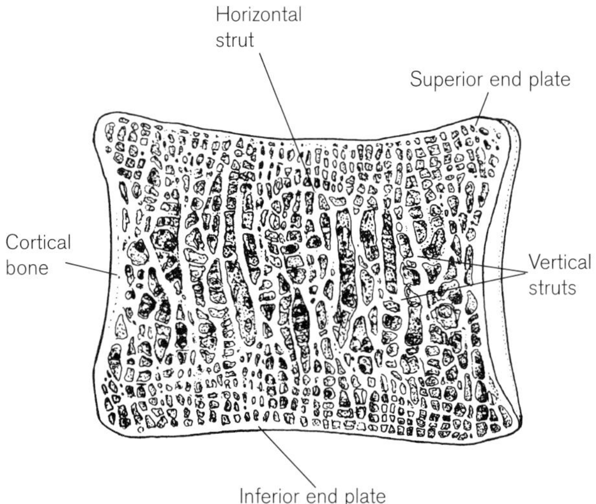

Figure 6.5 The cancellous architecture of an adult lumbar vertebral body.

As an individual column is descended, the bodies increase in both width and height to accommodate the proportional increase in body weight that passes through them. Therefore, the lumbar vertebrae have the largest bodies and the cervical vertebrae, the smallest.

However, sexual dimorphism in vertebral body size is more complicated as it does not only reflect differences in the transfer of absolute body weight. It has been shown that the horizontal vertebral growth is also dependent in part on mechanical influences such as muscle activity (Feik and Storey, 1983). It has also been shown that between 9 and 13 years, growth in the length of the female column exceeds that found in the male (Taylor and Twomey, 1984). This differential growth pattern ultimately leads to the female possessing a more slender vertebral column, which is more likely to buckle in the coronal plane than the relatively shorter, wider vertebral column of the male. It has been suggested that this might be a contributory factor in the greater prevalence of scoliosis among adolescent females (Miles, 1944; Taylor and Twomey, 1984; Oldale, 1990).

The essentially flat superior and inferior surfaces of the body are the site of attachment of the **intervertebral discs** that separate adjacent vertebrae. These act both as shock absorbers to dissipate the forces placed on the column during locomotion and to facilitate changes in the vertebral position; for example during alterations in posture. This is a secondary cartilaginous joint, with a layer of hyaline cartilage covering the superior and inferior surfaces of the bodies, which are further separated by a fibrocartilaginous disc. The disc is composed of an outer **annulus fibrosus** and an inner **nucleus pulposus** and is a remnant of the embryological notochord (see Chapter 4 and below).

The functions of the **neural arch** are to provide sites for muscle attachment and offer a protective bony canal for the spinal cord and its coverings. The primary function of the **pedicles** is to transfer lateral weight from the transverse processes to the midline vertebral body. They tend to be attached towards the superior poles of the bodies, resulting in two notches of uneven depth when two vertebrae are articulated and viewed from the side (Fig. 6.4b). The inferior notch is deeper than the superior notch, and when two vertebrae articulate an **intervertebral foramen** is formed for the transmission of the roots of the spinal nerves and the vascular structures supplying the spinal cord.

An articular pillar of paired **superior** and **inferior articular processes** lies behind the pedicles. The superior articular process of one vertebra articulates with the inferior articular process of the vertebra above via a synovial joint. The superior articular facet is more ventrally placed, with its articular surface facing posteriorly, while the inferior facet is more dorsally placed, with the articular surface facing anteriorly. The superior articular facets are more closely related to the pedicles while the inferior facets occur on the inner surface of the laminae of the neural arches. While it has always been accepted that body weight is transferred anteriorly through the body of a vertebra there is considerable evidence to suggest that in the thoracic region in particular, the articular facets may also be involved (Adams and Hutton, 1980; Pal and Routal, 1986). Pal and Routal (1987) and Routal and Pal (1990) have suggested that lateral body weight can be transferred via the transverse process and costotransverse ligaments through the synovial articular facets to the body of the vertebra below.

The **transverse processes,** the **laminae** and the **spinous process** all provide extensive sites of attachment for ligaments and deep postural muscles.

Regional characteristics of vertebrae

Cervical column

A typical cervical vertebra is to be found in the middle of the segment, for example, C3–C6 (Fig. 6.6). C1 the atlas, C2 the axis and C7 are atypical and will be considered separately.

The **typical cervical vertebra** has a relatively small body, which is wider in the transverse than in the anteroposterior plane. Its superior surface is concave transversely and slightly convex in the anteroposterior direction. The lateral aspects of the superior surface are elevated into two lateral lips, or **uncinate processes**, which are the sites of two small synovial joints, unco-vertebral joints (of Luschka). These joints are reported to be absent at birth but develop around 6 years of age to allow the intervertebral disc to maintain rotational function in harmony with the intervertebral joints (Boreadis and Gershon-Cohen, 1956; Penning, 1988). Osteoarthritic change is common in these joints with advancing age and this can lead to a narrowing of the intervertebral foramen, with subsequent irritation of the roots of the cervical spinal nerves (Cave *et al.*, 1955).

The inferior surface of the cervical body is concave anteroposteriorly and slightly convex in the transverse plane. The body is shallow in height and the antero-inferior border projects downwards so that it interlocks with the body of the vertebra below when the two are articulated.

The bodies are raised in the midline anteriorly for the attachment of the anterior longitudinal ligament, while there are two muscular hollows lateral to it for the attachment of the anterior deep muscles of the neck. This ligamentous area is narrower in the upper cervical vertebrae, becoming wider as the column is descended, indicating that the ligament is broader below and more cord-like above.

The transverse process contains a **foramen transversarium** for the passage of the vertebral artery and its associated venous and postganglionic sympathetic plexuses. In some instances, the foramen may be divided by a spicule of bone into a larger anterior compartment for the vertebral artery and a smaller posterior compartment for the venous and sympathetic plexuses and most commonly occurs in C6 and C7 (Francis, 1955a; Sawhney and Bahl, 1989; Vanezis, 1989). The foramina transversaria increase in size from C7 to C1 and are generally larger on the left to accommodate the larger size of the left vertebral artery (Francis, 1955b; Taitz *et al.*, 1978). The pedicles form the posteromedial limit of the foramen and are rounded and situated near the middle of the height of the body so that the superior and inferior vertebral notches are of almost equal depth. The pillar of bone associated with the superior articular facet forms the posterior boundary of the foramen transversarium, whilst the true transverse process (posterior bar) forms the posterolateral boundary and terminates in the **posterior tubercle**. The costal process of a typical cervical vertebra is represented by the anterior bar, which terminates in the **anterior tubercle** and is connected to the posterior tubercle by an **intertubercular lamina** of bone forming a shallow neural groove for the passage of the anterior (ventral) roots of the spinal nerves. Therefore, the costal element, which is the homologue

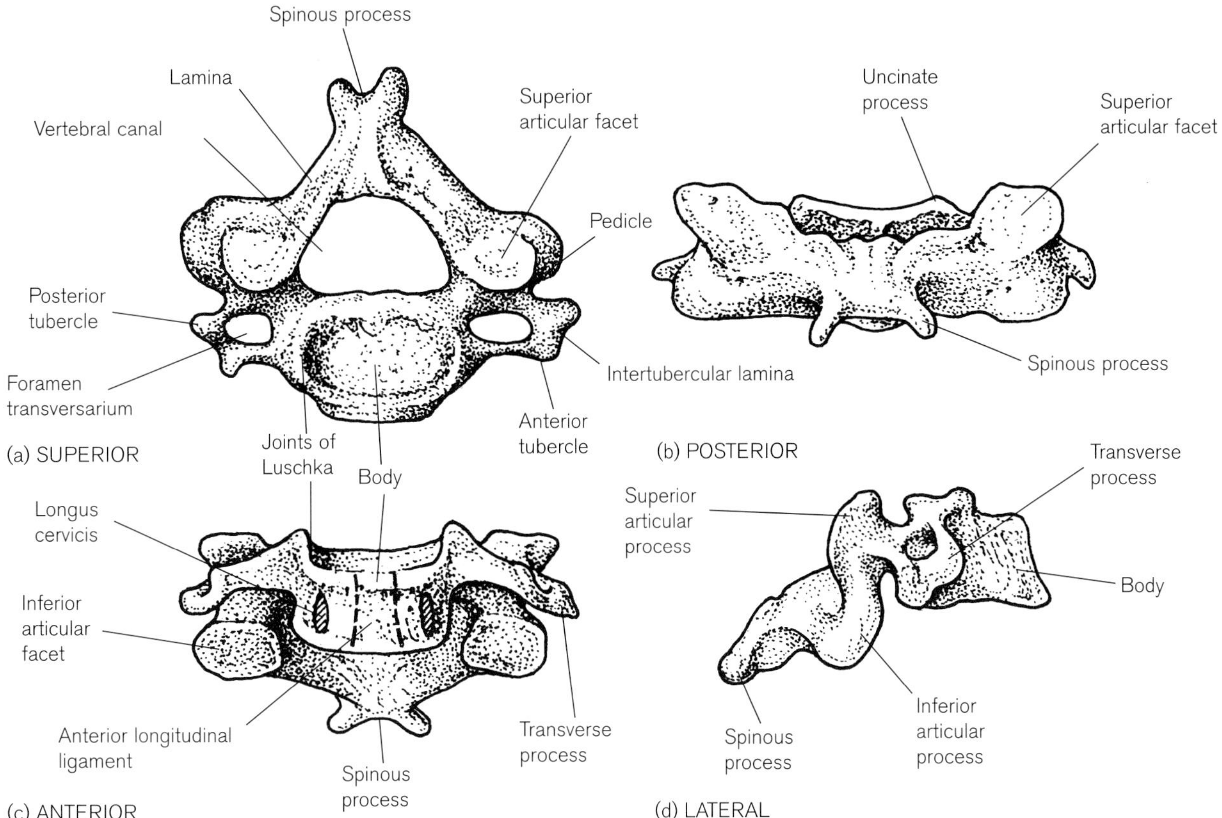

Figure 6.6 A typical adult cervical vertebra.

of the thoracic rib, forms the entire transverse element apart from the posterior bar, which in fact represents the true transverse process (Fig. 6.7). The anterior bar and tubercle are said to be homologous with the head of the rib, while the intertubercular lamina is equivalent to the neck of the rib. The posterior tubercle is homologous with the tubercle of the rib and in the cervical region there is no equivalent to the rib shaft unless a cervical rib develops (Honeij, 1920; Cave, 1975). Accessory articulations arising from the anterior tubercles have been reported and this intercostal articulation is thought to be homologous with pattern of fusion of the lateral masses of the sacrum (Cave, 1934; Stewart, 1934b).

Within each neural groove, the roots of the spinal nerve pass behind the position of the vertebral artery as it traverses the foramen transversarium (Fig. 6.8). Only the anterior ramus of each spinal nerve crosses the groove as the posterior (dorsal) ramus passes around the articular pillar to gain access to the muscles and skin of the back. The superior and inferior articular facets are to be found at the junction between the pedicles and the laminae. They form a cylindrical column of bone, sliced obliquely so that the superior facets face superiorly and posteriorly whilst the inferior facets face more or less anteriorly, with a slight downwards inclination. Throughout the cervical column there is little variation in the angle of inclination of these facets (Francis, 1955a) but when alterations

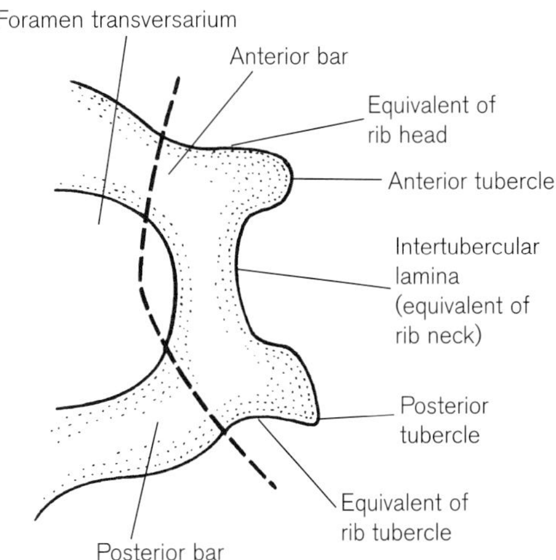

Figure 6.7 Developmental origins of the transverse process of a typical adult cervical vertebra.

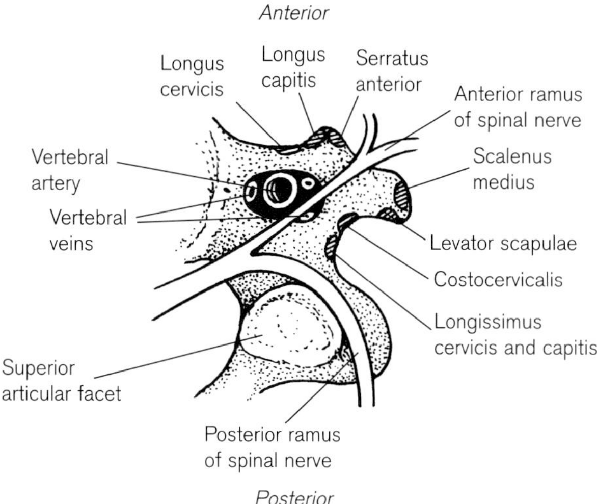

Figure 6.8 The immediate soft tissue relations of the lateral aspect of the adult fourth cervical vertebra.

do arise they can often result in abnormal loads and stresses, which can result in pain and particularly headaches (Morton, 1950; Overton and Grosman, 1952).

The **laminae** are flat and long, increase in depth from C3 downwards and terminate in a bifid spinous process, which may be single in C6. Pal and Routal (1996) reported that the laminae of C2 and C7 are load-bearing whilst the intervening laminae are not and minimal loading is found in C5. Therefore, they cautioned against surgical laminectomy of either C2 or C7 to minimize instability and subsequent neck deformity.

The **vertebral canal** is somewhat triangular in cross-section and increases in size from C2 to C5. This corresponds with the thickest part of the cervical enlargement of the cord, which provides the innervation to the thoracic diaphragm (C3–C5) and to the upper limb via the brachial plexus (spinal nerves C5–T1). The relative size of the vertebral canal decreases below the level of C5 (Yousefzadeh *et al.*, 1982).

Other than the general increase in body size dimensions relative to increasing weight transmission as the column is descended (Murone, 1974; Gilad and Nissan, 1985), there are some minor morphological modifications in the typical cervical vertebrae that may aid in the identification of individual members (Frazer, 1948). The superior articular facets of C3 and C4 are fairly round in shape, while the superior facets of C5–C7 are more elliptical. The costal process of C3 lies at a higher level than the true transverse process of that vertebra, thus forming a sloping lateral mass that is higher in front than behind. The intertubercular lamina of C3 is very narrow and the neural groove is shallow, with the anterior tubercle often being poorly defined. In addition, a faint groove can often be seen around the lateral aspect of the articular pillar, which is formed by the passage of the posterior ramus of the third cervical spinal nerve. In C4 the costal and transverse elements occur at the same level and the neural groove is deeper than that of C3 above. The anterior tubercle sits higher than the posterior tubercle in C4. In C5 the intertubercular lamina is virtually horizontal and the groove is wider and deeper, corresponding to the comparatively greater size of the roots of the C5 spinal nerve. In C6 the groove is wide and has a large anterior tubercle, the carotid (Chassaignac's) tubercle, against which the common carotid artery can be compressed. This serves to modify the blood flow to the head, neck and brain and unconsciousness will result if the artery is occluded for more than a few seconds. Herrera and Puchades-Orts (1998) reported on several characteristics which they considered to be restricted to C6. These included the presence of a sharp incisure on the lamina interposed between the superior and inferior articular facets (reportedly caused by the passage of the dorsal ramus of the sixth cervical nerve). In addition, they reported on the presence of a muscular tubercle located in the dorsocaudal region of the interarticular portion that is not present in children (Sato and Nakazawa, 1982).

The **atlas** (first cervical vertebra) is atypical both in function and morphology.[2] It is readily identifiable, as it is essentially a ring of bone that does not possess a body. As such, the weight of the head is transmitted through the occipital condyles to the upper articular facets of the atlas and then through its inferior articular facets to the axis below (Hinck *et al.*, 1962). The atlas has robust **anterior** and **posterior arches** that are united by thick **lateral masses** that carry the upper and lower articular facets (Fig. 6.9).

The anterior arch is shorter than the posterior arch and its ventral surface has a prominent tubercle, which

[2]This term is derived from the Greek 'atlao' meaning 'to endure or sustain'. The name was given to the Greek god who had to endure the weight of the world on his shoulders when he was turned to stone for refusing refuge to Perseus after he vanquished the Gorgons. The image of Atlas supporting the globe was adopted by ancient cartographers and so the term 'atlas' has come to mean a collection of maps, or subsequently any collection of informative illustrations (Skinner, 1961). The vertebral atlas therefore supports the weight of the globe of the head. Pollux applied the term to the seventh cervical vertebra as it carries the weight of the head and neck, but this was never adopted into general usage.

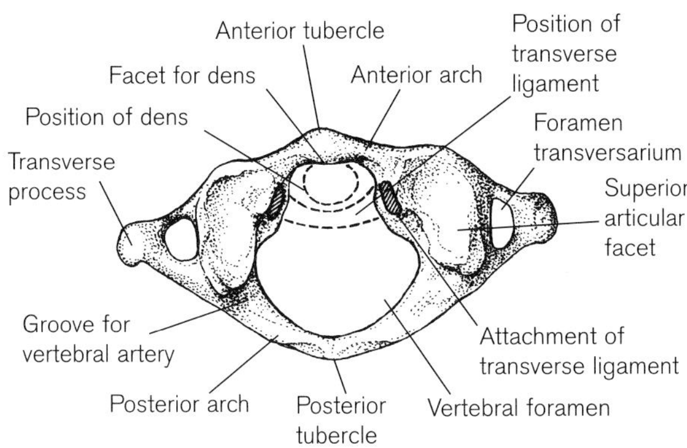

Figure 6.9 The superior surface of the adult atlas.

points downwards and is the site of attachment of the anterior longitudinal ligament. On the posterior surface of the anterior arch is a smooth round articular facet for the synovial articulation with the odontoid process (dens) of the axis.

The posterior arch is longer than the anterior arch and has a small tubercle on its posterior surface that is homologous with the spinous process and is the site of attachment of the ligamentum nuchae. The superior surface of the posterior arch is grooved by the passage of the vertebral artery as it passes from the foramen transversarium towards the foramen magnum. It is accompanied in this position by the first cervical (suboccipital) spinal nerve (Fig. 6.10). Ossification in the oblique posterior atlanto-occipital ligament can give rise to a small spicule of bone that passes from the edge of the superior facet over the vertebral artery to the posteromedial region of the vertebral groove. This bony bridge is well documented in the literature and is most commonly known as the posterior bridge, although it is also referred to as the posterior ponticle, ponticulus posticus, Kimmerle's anomaly, retro-articular canal, the spiculum or the posterior glenoid process. This converts the vertebral groove into a foramen, which is called either the foramen arcuale or the foramen retro-articulare superior (Ossenfort, 1926; Selby *et al.*, 1955; Pyo and Lowman, 1959; Saunders and Popovich, 1978). The incidence of this anomaly varies in different populations but is reported to be between 9% and 16% (Pyo and Lowman, 1959; Taitz and Nathan, 1986; Mitchell, 1998). It has been reported in children as young as 6 years of age and so is not necessarily an age-related phenomenon (Kendrick and Biggs, 1963). Distinct from this posterior bridge is a lateral bridge (ponticulus lateralis), which passes from the lateral mass to the posterior root of the transverse process. Lateral bridging is less common than posterior bridging and is not so well documented (Taitz and Nathan, 1986). It is clear that these bony bridges can compromise blood flow in the vertebral artery and so lead to cerebrovascular insufficiencies, with potential subsequent neurological complications (Bradshaw and McQuaid, 1963; Parkin *et al.*, 1978). However, there is now some controversy over whether or not mechanical obstruction of the vertebral artery flow does contribute significantly to vertebrobasilar insufficiency. The retrotransverse foramen (canaliculus venosus or posterolateral foramen) is a third anomaly of this region and is characterized by a small foramen found in the dorsal aspect of the transverse process. In life, it is said to be traversed by an anastomotic vein that connects the atlanto-occipital and atlanto-axoidial venous sinuses (Le Minor, 1997). Interestingly, this characteristic is restricted to man alone and is not found in any other primate (autapomorphic trait). It occurs in approximately 14% of humans and is more common on the left. Le Minor (1997) suggested that its presence is related to the development of upright posture and locomotion and results from regional modifications to the venous circulation.

In the absence of a body, the weight-bearing function of the atlas is borne by the massive lateral masses with their superior and inferior articular facets (Marino, 1995). The superior facets are kidney-shaped, although these articular surfaces can show quite considerable variation in shape (Pate, 1936; Singh, 1965; Barnes, 1994). In general though, they are deeply concave, being reciprocal in shape to the

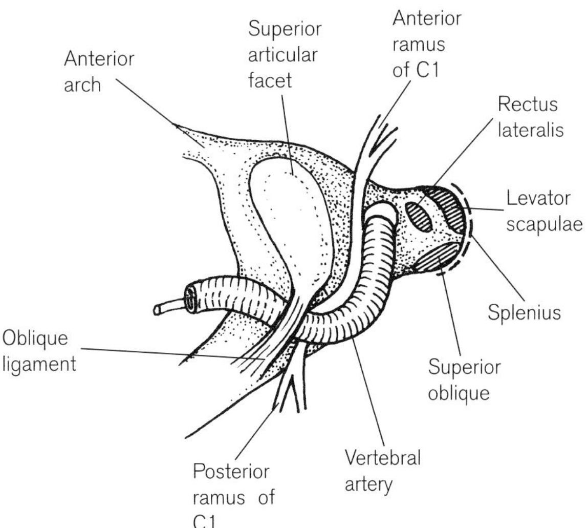

Figure 6.10 The immediate soft tissue relations of the lateral aspect of the adult atlas.

convex occipital condyles of the skull above (see Chapter 5). The shape of this synovial joint allows extensive forward and backward nodding of the head, as well as a considerable degree of lateral flexion. Variation in the shape of the atlantal articular facets (e.g. if double) can prove to be extremely valuable when attempting to associate a vertebral column with a particular skull. Rotation of the head in relation to the neck occurs at the atlanto-axial articulation between the facet on the posterior surface of the anterior arch and the anterior surface of the dens. The inferior articular process of the lateral mass is more rounded in shape and flat for articulation with the superior facet of the axis. This joint does not provide a clear indication of association as the joint surfaces differ markedly in their morphology. For this reason, it is often easier to associate a skull with its atlas than it is to correctly match the atlas with the axis of the same individual. The inferior articular facet of the atlas is virtually circular in shape and is flattened or slightly concave, facing medially and slightly backwards.

The lateral masses project into the vertebral canal forming two spaces of unequal size. The anterior compartment is smaller and is occupied by the dens, held in position by the transverse component of the cruciform ligament, which attaches to small tubercles on the inner surface of the lateral masses. The larger posterior compartment of the vertebral canal, behind the transverse ligament, houses the transitional zone between the lower limits of the medulla oblongata and the first cervical segment of the spinal cord (Doherty and Heggeness, 1994).

The transverse processes of the atlas are particularly long and are the sites of attachment for the muscles involved in rotation of the head. The apex of the transverse process is homologous with the posterior tubercles of the other cervical vertebrae and can be palpated in the living in the gap between the mastoid process and the angle of the mandible. The remainder of the transverse process of C1 is the equivalent of the posterior root and intertubercular lamina only, with the remainder of the costal process being essentially absent, although a small tubercle may be found on the anterior surface of the anterior arch, lateral to the anterior tubercle.

The **axis** (second cervical vertebra) is the pivot or axis upon which the atlas, but not the head, turns. The axis may be referred to as the 'epistropheus', which is derived from the Greek term meaning 'to turn upon'.[3]

The axis is readily identifiable due to the projecting **dens** (odontoid process) (Fig. 6.11) which bears an articular facet on its anterior aspect for articulation with the posterior surface of the anterior arch of the atlas. The two bones also articulate via superior and inferior facets. C2 articulates with C3 via the secondary cartilaginous articulation of the bodies and by the synovial joints at the inferior articular facets. Thus, by the inferior surface of the axis the typical pattern of intervertebral articulation is established.

The true body of the axis is said to lie below the level of the dens, which is generally considered to represent the displaced body of the atlas. The apex of the dens is attached to the occipital bone by apical ligaments and the slightly flattened postero-lateral surfaces are the site of attachment of the alar ligaments, which also pass superiorly to the occipital bone (Dvorak and Panjabi, 1987). The dens is waisted inferiorly by the passage of the transverse component of the cruciform ligament, which helps to keep it securely in place. Quick death from hanging results when the transverse ligament snaps and the dens crushes the lower medulla oblongata and the adjacent spinal cord. However, in most cases of judicial hanging it is uncommon for either the transverse ligament or the odontoid process to be damaged. The classic 'hangman's fracture' passes through the neural arch of C2 anterior to the position of the inferior articular facet and may in fact traverse the foramen transversarium (Marshall, 1888; Robertson, 1935; Duff, 1954; Elliott *et al.*, 1972).

The anterior aspect of the true body of the axis is hollowed out laterally for the attachment of the longus colli muscles, whilst the inferior border is characteristically pulled downwards and articulates with the concave superior surface of the body of C3. Unlike the remainder of the cervical vertebrae, the superior and inferior articular facets of the axis do not form a vertical articular pillar. The superior facets are large, virtually horizontal, slightly convex and ovoid in shape for articulation with the atlas, while the inferior facets are much smaller, more vertically inclined and displaced more posteriorly. The superior articular facet does not morphologically mirror the shape and orientation of the inferior atlantal facet as the concavity of the latter crosses the convexity of the former. The

[3]Another term used to denote the second cervical vertebra was 'astragalus', which is derived from the Greek meaning 'a die'. In Homer's Iliad and Odyssey, the word was used in connection with the second cervical vertebrae of sheep, from which the arches were removed and the remainder then fashioned into six-sided dice. The Romans however, made their dice from the tali of horses with the name being derived from the Latin 'taxillus' which means a small die. It is via this connection with the production of dice, that the older name for the talus was also 'astragalus' and it may still be referred to in this way in some clinical communications (Skinner, 1961).

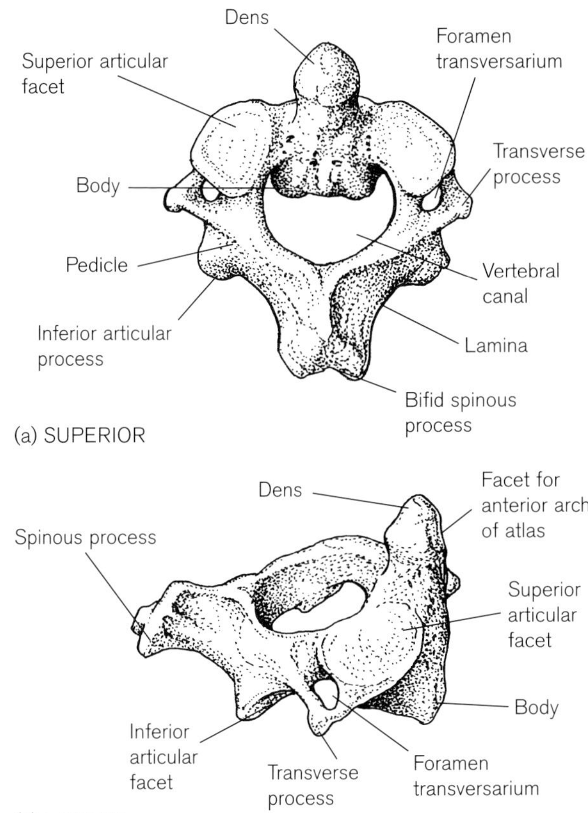

Figure 6.11 The superior surface of the adult axis.

pedicles are stout with deep inferior vertebral notches. The laminae are particularly robust, fusing in a powerful bifid spinous process for the attachment of the muscles that extend, retract and rotate the head. The transverse processes are small with a single tubercle, which is homologous with the posterior tubercle, although an anterior tubercle may be found at the junction between the root of the transverse process with the body. Each foramen transversarium is directed superolaterally as the vertebral artery deviates laterally (by about 45°) at this point to be in the correct position to pass through the corresponding foramen in the atlas. Therefore, unlike any of the other cervical vertebrae, the foramen transversarium of the axis is not a simple short foramen but is in fact an angulated canal with one opening facing inferiorly and the other laterally. The roof of this canal may show evidence of erosion due to the marked tortuosity of the artery. These erosions are thought to be caused by so-called 'reserve loops' of the vertebral artery, required to enable the artery to follow the movements of the head and neck without being overstretched (Hadley, 1958; Krayenbuhl and Yasargil, 1968; Lindsey *et al.*, 1985; Taitz and Arensburg, 1989). The anterior ramus of the second cervical spinal nerve passes lateral to the position of the vertebral artery and so excess tortuosity can lead to nerve compression (Fig. 6.12).

The **vertebra prominens** (seventh cervical vertebra) is characteristic because of its particularly long spinous process that is visible under the skin, although in reality, the spinous process of T1 may prove to be more prominent. C7 is a transitional vertebra that combines the characteristics of both the cervical vertebrae above and the thoracic column below. Like the cervicals, it usually possesses a foramen transversarium in the lateral mass, although the vertebral artery does not in fact pass through it, as the artery first enters through the foramen of C6. As such, the foramen transversarium of C7 is usually smaller than in the other cervical vertebrae and may be bipartite or indeed absent. In some instances, the costal element of C7 may be separate from the transverse process and so form a cervical rib (Fig. 6.13). These are usually asymptomatic but they can lead to both neurological and circulatory disruption in the upper limb (Black and Scheuer, 1997). The spinous process of C7 is generally not bifid but ends in a single tubercle.

Thoracic column

As in the cervical column, the typical thoracic vertebrae occur in the middle of the segment (T2–T9) and the atypical members are located at the extremities of the region (T1 and T10–T12).

The **typical thoracic vertebrae** are characterized by the presence of articular facets on the bodies and transverse processes for articulation with the heads and tubercles of the ribs, respectively. The description of a typical vertebra, as given above, closely applies

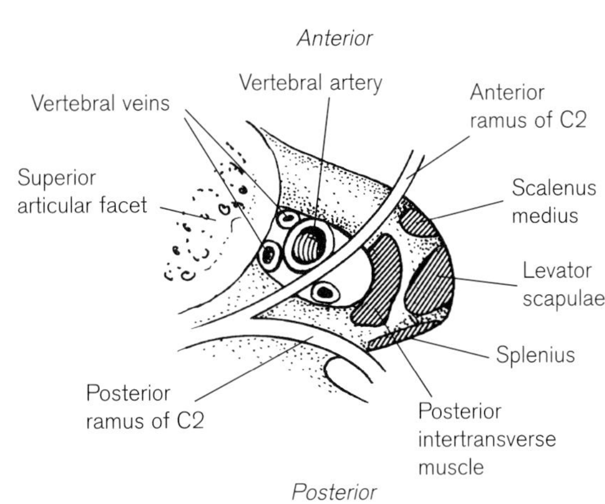

Figure 6.12 The immediate soft tissue relations of the lateral aspect of the adult axis.

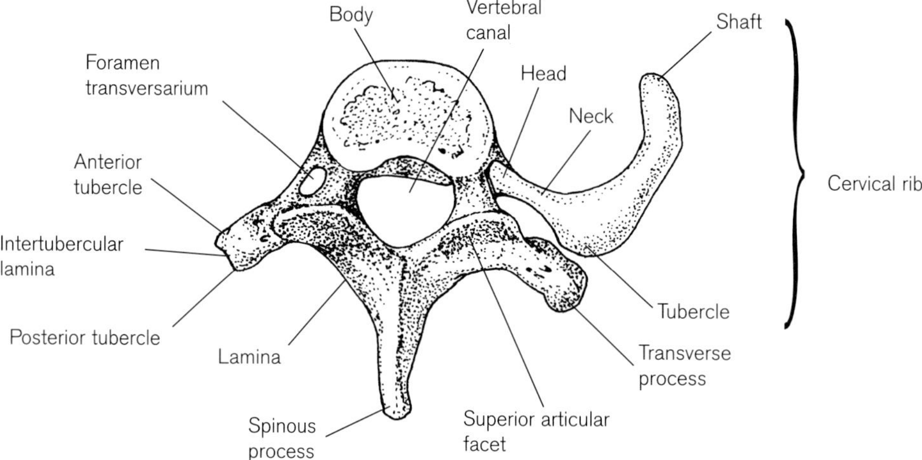

Figure 6.13 The superior surface of the adult seventh cervical vertebra showing a cervical rib on the right side.

to most of the thoracic vertebrae. The bodies are said to be somewhat heart-shaped when viewed from above and have a large costal demi-facet on the lateral side of the body at the level of the superior border and a smaller costal demi-facet in the same lateral location but on the inferior border (Fig. 6.14). The superior demi-facet is the site of the synovial articulation with the lower facet on the head of the rib of the corresponding number, e.g. the second rib articulates with the superior demi-facet on T2. The inferior demi-facet is generally smaller and articulates with the upper facet on the head of the rib that is one number lower in the series, e.g. the inferior demi-facet of T2 articulates with the head of the third rib.

The inferior vertebral notches are deep, while the superior notches are shallower so that the intervertebral foramen is predominantly formed by the inferior boundaries of the vertebra above. The transverse processes are directed backwards and laterally, each carrying a costal facet on its ventral aspect for articulation with the tubercle of the rib of the same number. The costal processes, which were fairly rudimentary in the cervical region, are particularly well developed in the thoracic region as the thoracic ribs (see Chapter 7).

The superior and inferior intervertebral articular facets are located in the position described above for typical vertebrae, and form a strong longitudinal articular pillar of bone. The spinous processes are generally long, slender, point downwards and end in a single tubercle, although the lower vertebrae adopt a more lumbar morphology. The vertebral canal is somewhat circular in shape and small in comparison with the cervical region.

Other than the atypical thoracic vertebrae, it is often quite difficult to identify single members of the thoracic vertebrae, but there are some characteristics which offer sufficient information to allow each vertebra to be placed within at least one or two vertebrae of its true anatomical position.

The shape of the thoracic vertebral bodies change as the column is descended and often this is the clearest indication of the location of a single vertebra within the thoracic segment. The bodies of T1–3 are wider in the transverse than in the anteroposterior plane, mimicking the typical cervical body shape. This is most obvious in T1 and less so by T3, which is said to have the smallest body in the thoracic segment. By T4, the anteroposterior diameter of the body exceeds the transverse diameter, thereby forming the so-called 'typical' thoracic body shape. From T4 downwards, the bodies increase in all dimensions.

The bodies of the middle thoracic vertebrae may come into direct contact with the descending thoracic aorta. This can leave a flattened impression on the left sides of the bodies of T5–T7, resulting in a slightly asymmetrical outline. Aneurysms of the descending aorta, usually as a result of arteriosclerosis, may erode the cortical surface of a number of vertebral bodies in this location. When this occurs, it presents as deeply scalloped resorption defects on several adjacent vertebral bodies with relatively intact vertebral endplates (Kelley, 1979a; Ortner and Putschar, 1985).

A difference is also found in the size, shape and direction of the articular facets on the transverse processes, depending upon whether the vertebra articulates with a vertebrosternal or a vertebrochondral rib (see Chapter 7). In T1–T7 (vertebrosternal) the articular facets on the transverse processes are well marked, large, concave and located on the ventral surface of the transverse process in a more vertical orientation. In T8–T10 (vertebrochondral) the facets

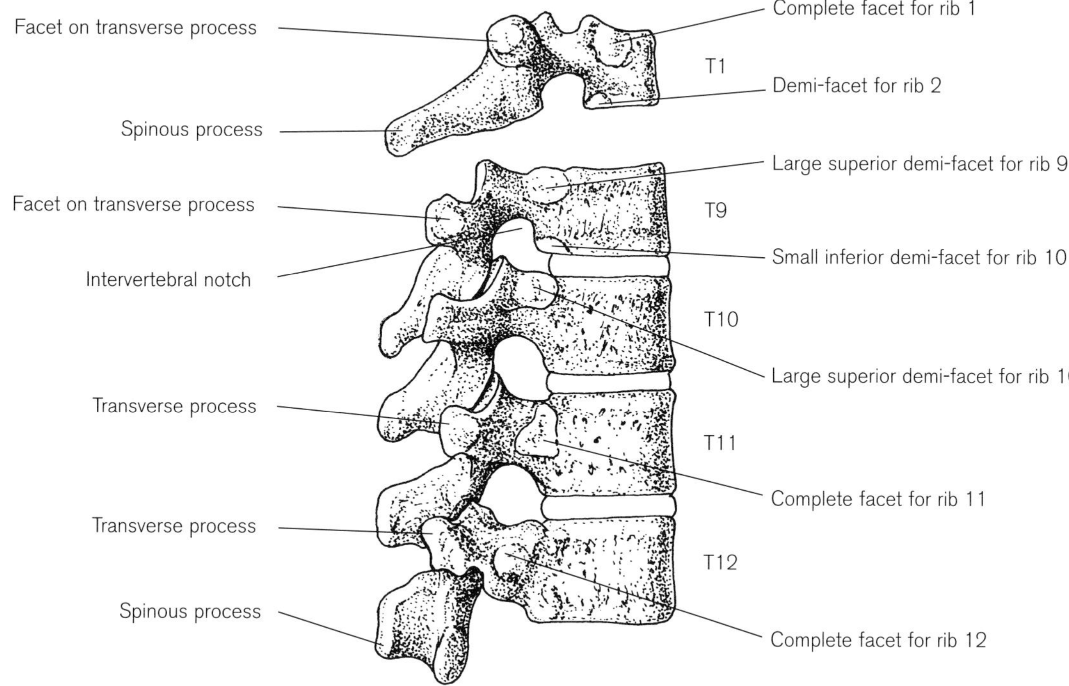

Figure 6.14 Lateral view of adult thoracic vertebrae to show the positions of the costal facets on T1 and T9–T12.

are smaller, flatter and tend to lie on the upper aspect of the process and to face more superiorly. From T10 to T12, the transverse processes markedly reduce in size.

The **first thoracic vertebra** is similar in its morphology to C7. Its body is shaped more like a cervical vertebra, with the superior surface being somewhat concave from side to side and wider in the transverse than in the anteroposterior direction. The vertebral canal is more cervical than typically thoracic in shape, as it contains the final stages of the cervical enlargement of the cord. Unlike the cervical vertebrae, there is no foramen transversarium in the transverse process. The upper costal facet on the body for articulation with the first rib is complete and a small demi-facet is present on the lower border for the upper facet of the head of the second rib. T1 also possesses an upward-facing articular shelf on the lamina, in association with the superior articular facet. This shelf projects backwards and is at virtually right angles to the lower margin of the superior articular facet, acting as a stop to limit the downward displacement of the inferior articular surface of C7. These so-called 'butting facets' are reported to permit a more even downward transmission of forces rising from muscles attached to the cervical transverse processes and during excessive vertical compression, their impingement clearly supports some of the compressive forces and thus gives relief to the vertebral bodies (Davis and Rowland, 1965; Keats and Johnstone, 1982). This shelf can be seen to a lesser extent on T2.

The **ninth thoracic vertebra** may only have a costal demi-facet on the superior part of the body and be devoid of one below, although there is always a corresponding articular facet present on the transverse process for the tubercle of the ninth rib. The **tenth thoracic vertebra** has a whole costal articular facet above but does not possess an inferior one. A small articular facet may be present on the transverse process for the tenth rib. The **eleventh** and **twelfth thoracic vertebrae** are essentially transitional in shape between the thoracic and the lumbar column (Shinohara, 1997). They are more robust and both have a single facet on the body for articulation with the rib of the corresponding number. The position of this facet migrates posteriorly from the sides of the bodies to occupy a position on the pedicles. The change in morphology of the superior and inferior articular facets from an essentially thoracic to a more lumbar form tends to occur around the level of the eleventh vertebra. In a vertebra which is occupying this transitional position, the superior facets may face posterolaterally (as for the typical thoracic vertebrae), while the inferior facets adopt the lumbar form by being convex in the transverse plane and facing anterolaterally. This demarcation is said to mark the site of the change from an essentially rotational to a non-rotational function (Davis, 1955). The transverse processes are reduced in length and no longer articulate with the ribs (Cave, 1936). The spinous processes are also reduced in size and are more horizontally aligned. The vertebral canal begins to widen again in the lower thoracic region to accommodate the lumbar spinal enlargement for the innervation of the lower limbs.

Lumbar column

These vertebrae are distinguished by their size and the lack of both foramina transversaria and costal articular facets. The bodies are large and kidney-shaped and the pedicles are short and stout (Zindrick *et al.*, 1987; Amonoo-Kuofi, 1995), indicating the importance of weight transfer as a function in this region of the column (Fig. 6.15).

The transverse processes are slender and the small **accessory** and **mamillary processes** found behind them are in fact said to be the true transverse process. There is, however, some debate on the true origin of the lumbar transverse process and this will be considered in the section on ossification of this region.

The articular processes are vertically orientated and curved transversely so that the lower pair are convex and look forwards and laterally and are placed closer together than the upper pair, which are concave, wider apart and curve to look inwards and backwards. This vertical positioning of the articular facets is peculiar to man and is not seen in any quadruped (Cotteril *et al.*, 1986). In fact, it is not present even in the human neonate but is reported to develop once the child starts to walk (Lanz and Wachsmut, 1982) and so this particular joint orientation may well be an indication of an adaptation to bipedal locomotion (Haher *et al.*, 1994).

The laminae are deep and short and the spinous processes are thick and square. The vertebral canal is triangular in shape and, below the level of L2, carries only the cauda equina and the filum terminale with the associated meninges, blood vessels, connective tissue and cerebrospinal fluid (Schatzker and Pennal, 1968).

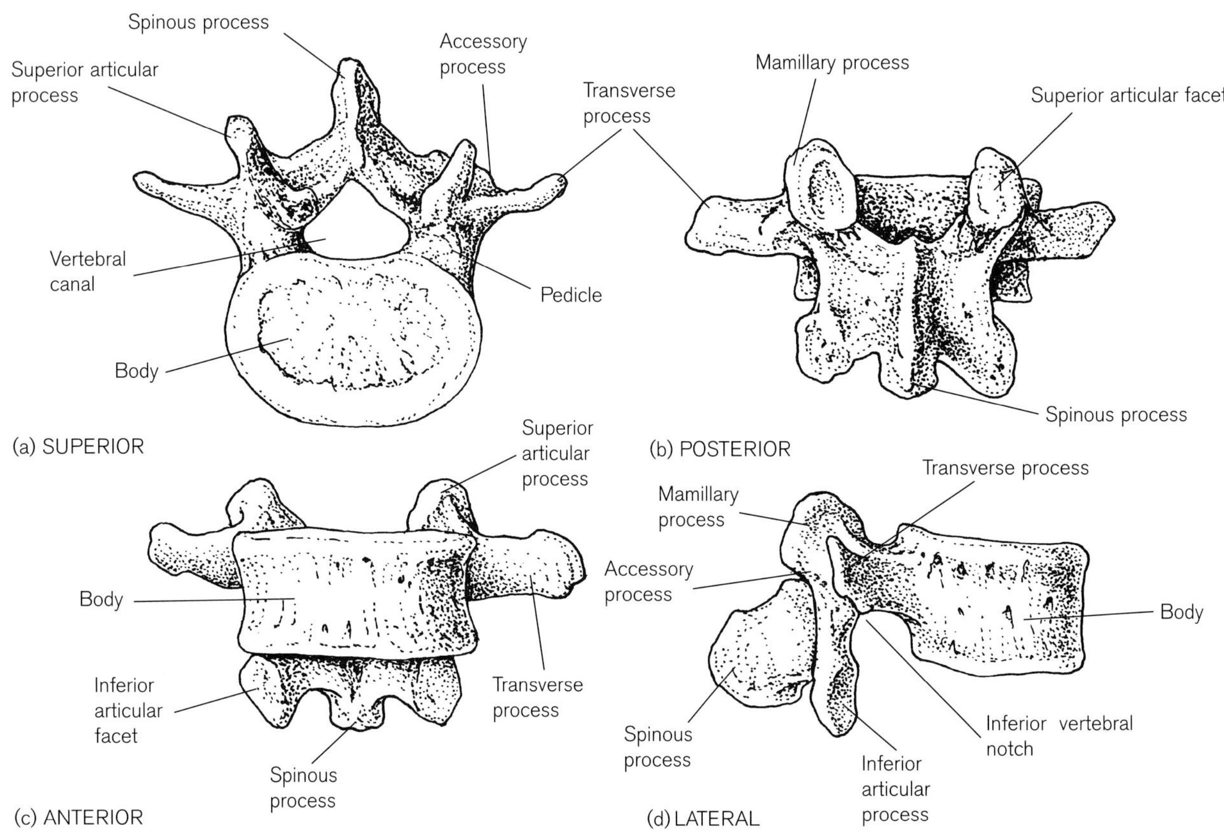

Figure 6.15 A typical adult lumbar vertebra.

Only the last lumbar vertebra has sufficiently individual characteristics to permit ready identification when presented in isolation; however, there are subtle differences in the other vertebrae of this segment. The bodies increase in width from above to below, as do the pedicles. The vertical height of the anterior aspect of the body is shorter than the posterior height in the upper two vertebrae but longer in the lower three bones of this segment. The transverse processes increase in length from L1 to L3 and then reduce in length towards L5. Fawcett (1932) noted that when the lumbar vertebrae are examined from behind, a four-sided figure can be constructed if the articular facets are taken to represent the angles of the geometric shape. In L1 and L2 the vertebral shape is trapezoid in form, with the superior margin being longer than the inferior margin so that the lateral sides pass obliquely downwards and medially. L3 is essentially a parallelogram in shape with long vertical sides and superior and inferior margins of equal length. L4 is virtually square in shape and L5 is represented by an elongated parallelogram with short vertical sides. However, L5 can be identified in isolation as its overall morphology is significantly different from the other vertebrae in this segment. The lower articular facets of L5 articulate with the upper sacral facets, which are widely separated (Brown, 1937). Thus, in the last lumbar vertebra the distance between the two superior articular facets and that between the two inferior articular facets are approximately equal, leading to a splayed appearance of the lower region of this vertebra (Fawcett, 1932). In addition, the anterior vertical height of the body is generally greater than its equivalent posterior height so that the body of this vertebra is somewhat wedge-shaped. The fifth lumbar vertebra might become included into the sacrum and so become sacralized, or alternatively the first sacral segment might remain separate from the rest of the sacrum and become lumbarized. The last lumbar and first sacral vertebrae are therefore transitional in nature (Willis, 1923b; Shore, 1930; Mitchell, 1938; Young and Ince, 1940; Wigh and Anthony, 1981; Castellvi *et al.*, 1984; Elster, 1989; Barnes, 1994). The lumbosacral region of the column is the site of many varied pathological conditions (Willis, 1923b; Brailsford, 1929; Stewart, 1956; Nathan, 1959; Reilly *et al.*, 1978; Wigh, 1982; Merbs, 1989; Barnes, 1994). It is not uncommon for such anatomical variants to result in low back pain with consequent sciatic radiation (Willis, 1929; Badgley, 1941; Willis, 1941).

Sacrum

The term 'sacrum' is said to be derived from the Latin 'sacer' meaning holy or sacred, but its relevance to the naming of the bone is uncertain.[4] In the adult, the five (or six) vertebrae below the lumbar segment fuse together to form the sacrum, which is the central axis of the pelvic girdle (Fig. 6.16). This bony mass articulates superiorly with the last lumbar vertebra at the lumbosacral angle, laterally with the innominates at the sacro-iliac joints and inferiorly with the first coccygeal segment (Brown, 1937). The lateral masses that pass outwards from the region of the promontory towards the sacro-iliac articulation are called the wings (alae) of the sacrum.[5]

The sacrum is a wedge-shaped bone that is wider above at its base and narrower below at its apex. The wider areas, i.e. S1–S2 are involved in weight transfer but below this level, the influence of body weight diminishes and so the vertebrae reduce in size (Pal, 1989). The sacrum is concave anteriorly and convex posteriorly, both from above to below and also from side to side. The incidence of a flat ventral surface is reported to be as high as 20% in females and this may give rise to prolonged labour, necessitating operative delivery due to parturition arrest in the midpelvis (Posner *et al.*, 1955). On the ventral aspect, it is clear that the central part is formed from the fusion of the bodies of the sacral vertebrae and four transverse lines of fusion generally persist even into old age. Lateral to this are four **anterior sacral foramina**, which are the remnants of the anterior boundaries of the intervertebral foramina for the passage of the anterior rami of the sacral spinal nerves. These foramina are not simply single canals but are in fact a complex network of interconnecting 'Y'-shaped canals that run at approximately 45° to the coronal plane (Jackson and Burke, 1984). The rounded bars of bone between adjacent foramina are said to be the remnants of the heads and necks of ribs and are therefore costal in origin. Lateral to the foramina are the **lateral masses** which are marked by neural grooves leading from the foramina and are also said to be costal in origin, although there is some debate over the truth of this statement – see below (O'Rahilly *et al.*, 1990a). The lateral surfaces of the upper two (or three) lateral masses articulate with the auricular surface of the innominate forming the synovial sacro-iliac joint (Flander and

[4]Suggestions have included the fact that the sacrum is resistant to decay and so would form the basis of resurrection and that perhaps it was considered divine through its protective role for the sacred organs of reproduction (Field and Harrison, 1957).

[5]It is interesting that 'ala' actually relates to any side compartment or structure and it is the word from which 'axilla' may be derived (Skinner, 1961).

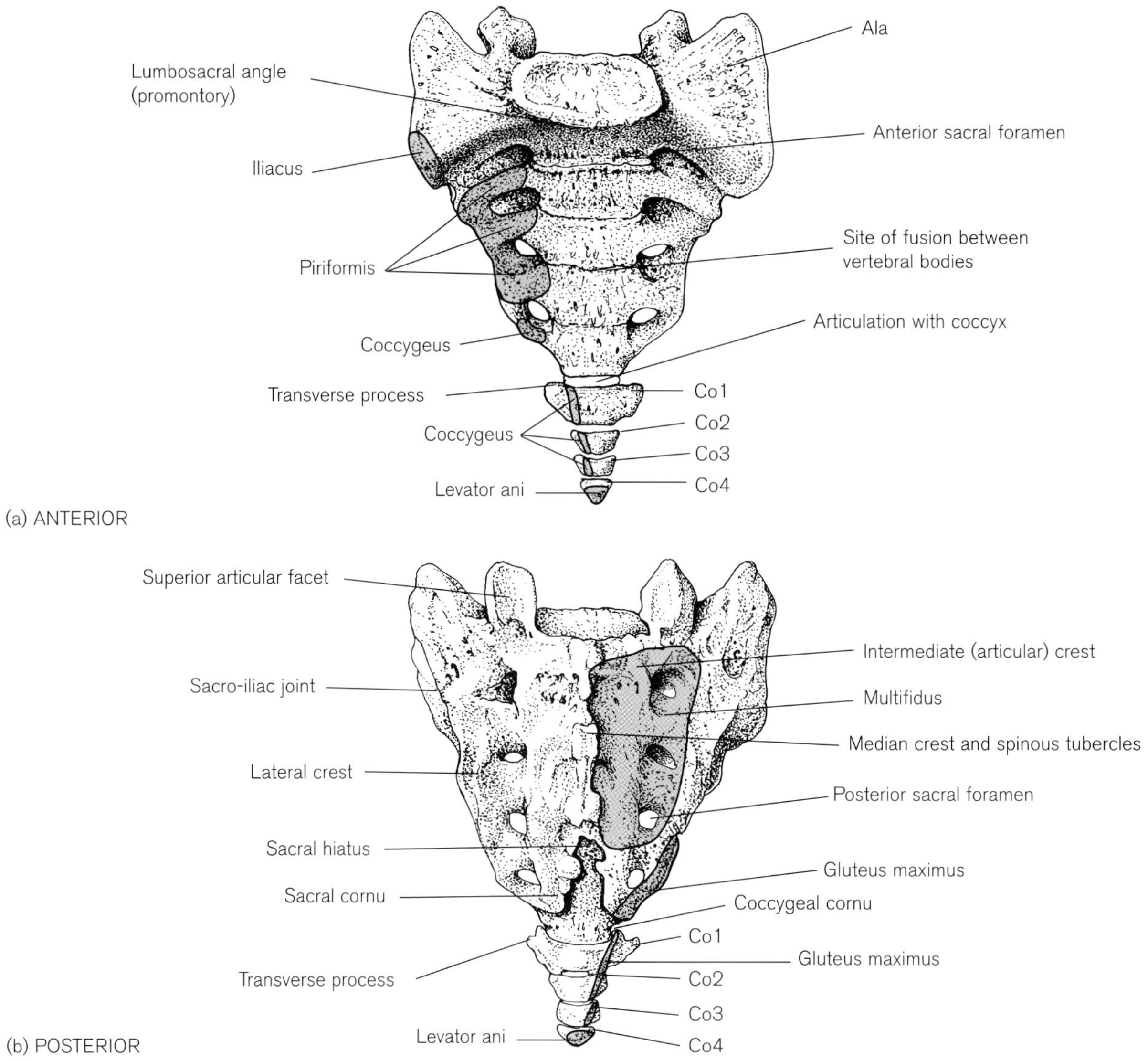

Figure 6.16 The adult sacrum and coccyx.

Corruccini, 1980). Despite the position of the joint in relation to body weight transfer, it is not actively weight-bearing, as all the forces are transmitted through the associated ligaments (Last, 1973) and this is borne out by the lack of sexual dimorphism exhibited by this joint (Ali and MacLaughlin, 1991). In addition to the sacro-iliac joint, a number of small accessory articulations can occur between the sacrum and the ilium (Derry, 1910; Trotter, 1937, 1940; Stewart, 1938; Hadley, 1952), with the most common site for these being at the level of the posterior second sacral foramen. They are generally asymptomatic, more common in males, positively correlated with increasing age, possibly the site of initiation for synostosis, but otherwise of unknown function and aetiology.

Bellamy *et al.* (1983) proposed that the more weight and forces that are transmitted through the lower limbs, the more segments of the sacral column will participate in the sacro-iliac articulation. Occasionally, and more frequently in the male, the third sacral segment may be incorporated into the sacro-iliac joint (Brothwell, 1981; Ali and MacLaughlin, 1991).

The convex posterior surface of the sacrum represents the fused neural arches of the individual vertebrae, with the **midline sacral crest** and spinous tubercles representing the fused spinous processes. Lateral to this is the **intermediate (articular) crest**, which is formed from the fusion of the synovial articular pillar. Lateral to this are the four **posterior sacral foramina**, which are the remnants of

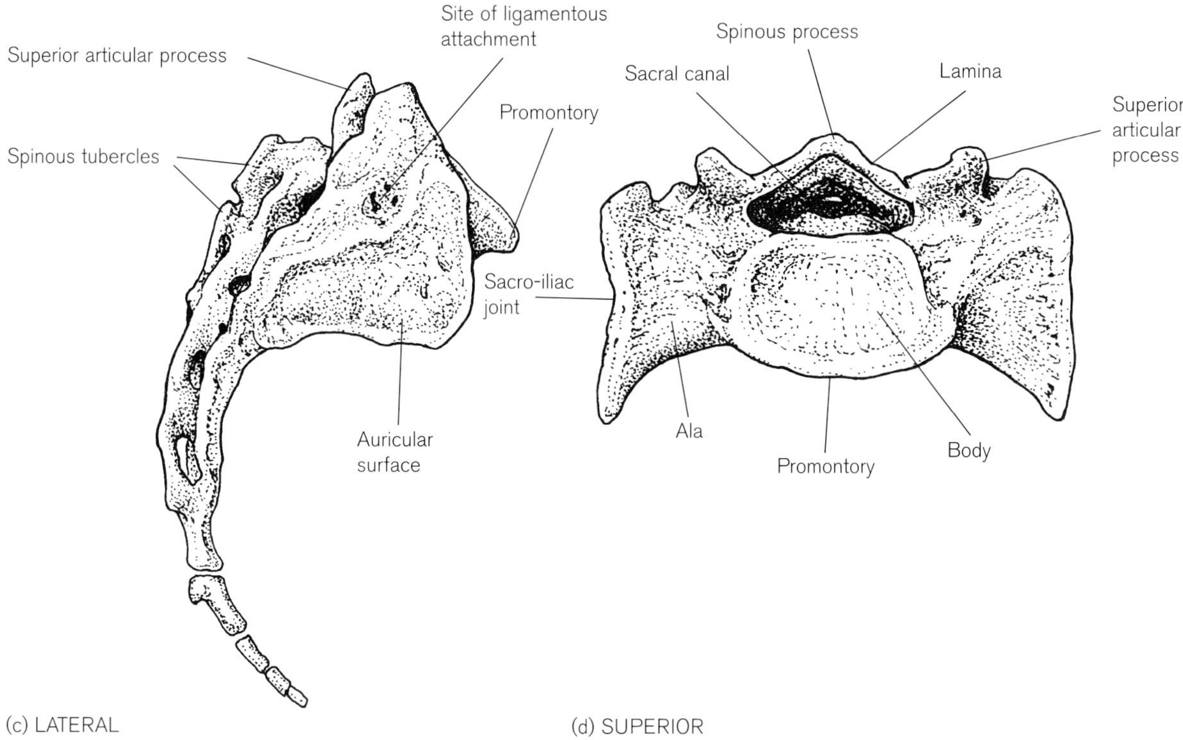

Figure 6.16 *(Continued).*

the posterior boundaries of the intervertebral foramina for the passage of the posterior rami of the sacral spinal nerves. Lateral to these is the **lateral sacral crest**, which is formed from the fusion of the transverse processes.

In the lower part of the sacrum the laminae fail to meet and fuse in the midline, leaving a **sacral hiatus** bounded by the **cornua** of the sacrum. The sacral canal is triangular in cross-section and transmits the cauda equina, with the meninges terminating at the level of the second sacral segment. Thus, the lower regions of the sacral vertebral canal contain only the roots of the spinal nerves passing to the appropriate sacral foramina and the filum terminale which attaches to the coccyx.

Coccyx

The term 'coccyx' comes from the Greek 'kokkyx' meaning 'cuckoo', due to its resemblance to the cuckoo's bill (Holden, 1882).[6] This small region of the column is comprised of the fused final four or five coccygeal vertebrae that make up the rudimentary tail. The first segment usually carries vestiges of the transverse processes and upper articular facets (cornua), which are attached to the corresponding sacral cornua by ligaments (Fig. 6.16). The upper surface of the superior coccygeal segment articulates with the apex of the sacrum and with age this joint may synostose. Sacrococcygeal fusion is more common in the male and whilst it is generally considered to be indicative of advancing age, it can be found in individuals as young as 30 years of age (Oldale, 1990). The coccyx is the site of attachment for muscles of both the floor of the pelvis and the gluteal region. The anterior surface of the coccyx is found in the pelvic floor and the posterior surface is in the buttock beneath the skin of the natal cleft.

Fractures of the coccyx are not uncommon and generally arise as a result of a fall onto the gluteal region. This is probably one of the most painful of fractures, due to the abundance of nerve fibres in the region. Coccygeal dislocation at the sacrococcygeal junction is rare and this also tends to arise following a fall or a slip (Bergkamp and Verhaar, 1995).

Extremely rare 'chevron' bones have been reported in relation to the first coccygeal segment in particular (Harrison, 1901; Schultz, 1941a). These are described as bony arches, which articulate or may synostose with the ventral surface of the body of the upper coccygeal

[6]Another more colourful derivation has been suggested, in that in the breaking of wind 'per anum', the sound echoes from the coccyx and produces a noise like the cry of a cuckoo! Thus the old name for the coccyx was the 'whistle bone' (Field and Harrison, 1957).

segments. They are reported to ossify from two separate centres of ossification, which may eventually fuse in the midline. It is thought that they represent rudiments of a mechanism designed to increase the surface area for muscle attachments in animals with large tails. It is also thought that they have an accessory role in protecting the caudal vessels that run in the bony canals formed from a series of these arches – hence their other name of 'haemal arches'.

Early development of the vertebral column

The earliest stages of the development of the column are considered in Chapter 4 but a discussion on the development of the vertebral column would not be complete without mention of *Hox* genes, which have revolutionized the understanding of the developmental processes (Burke *et al.*, 1995). A *Hox* axial code has been identified that appears to specify developmental position along the craniocaudal axis (Kessel and Gruss, 1991). It is believed that each *Hox* gene represents an overlapping domain and as such provides specific positional information. Kessel and Gruss (1991) suggested that each individual vertebra might be based upon a unique *Hox* code and so its ultimate form will be dependent upon the successful expression of that code (Johnson and O'Higgins, 1996). However, despite the fact that the *Hox* code is believed to be highly conserved in most mammal groups, it is interesting to speculate upon which factors influence not only the interspecies but also the intraspecies variations in vertebral morphology (Johnson *et al.*, 1999). It is clear that this rapidly expanding field of research will continue to dominate the field of vertebrate development.

In the fourth week of intra-uterine life, the sclerotome develops a central cavity that becomes populated by diffuse core cells. It then ruptures on the medial side and cells from its ventromedial wall, along with core cells, migrate towards the notochord anteriorly and the developing neural tube posteriorly (Fig. 6.17). A defect in the growth and migration of the sclerotome at this time results in a blanket condition known as caudal regression, which manifests as a deficiency in the development of the caudal region of the embryo. This can range from very minor coccygeal defects, which are asymptomatic, to sirenomelia where there is extensive agenesis of the caudal viscera and a fusion of the developing lower limb buds, resulting in a mermaid-like appearance (Blumel *et al.*, 1958; Duhamel, 1961; Frantz and Aitken, 1967; Banta and Nichols, 1969; Kallen and Winberg, 1974; Mills, 1982). This condition, which has an extensive array of clinical appearances, is of essentially unknown aetiology.

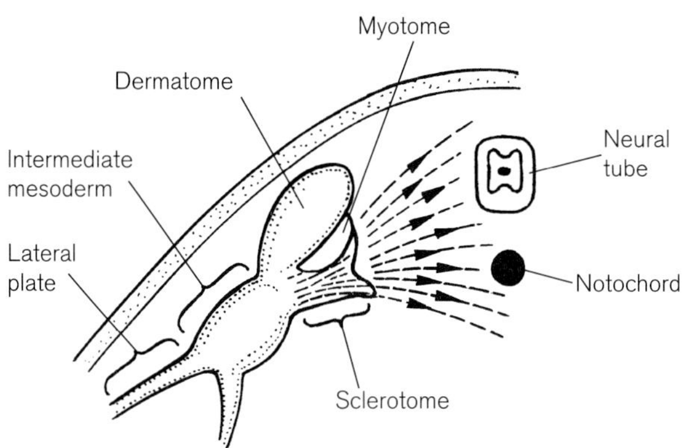

Figure 6.17 Diagrammatic representation of the embryonic migration of the cells of the sclerotome.

The ventral portion of the migrating sclerotome surrounds the notochord so that by the end of the fourth week it has become encased in a continuous investment of mesenchyme. This region will go on to develop into the vertebral centrum. The dorsal region of the sclerotome surrounds the neural tube and forms the precursor of the neural arch. Grafting experiments have shown that the normal development of the centrum depends upon the proximity of the notochord (or more precisely perhaps, the perinotochordal cellular sheath – Müller and O'Rahilly, 1994) and following ablation, the centrum fails to develop. Similarly, for normal development of the neural arches to occur, an inductive signal is necessary from the neural tube (Campbell *et al.*, 1986; Jacobson and Sater, 1988; Gurdon *et al.*, 1989). If a defect occurs in the early development of the neural tube then failure to close (spinal dysraphism) may result. This neurological failure most commonly occurs at the cranial and caudal neuropores and therefore most developmental defects of the posterior part of the column arise in the cranial and caudal regions. Failure of closure of the cranial neuropore can lead to anencephaly, which is incompatible with fetal survival. Failure of closure of the caudal neuropore can lead to partial or complete sacral agenesis. Providing the S1 and preferably S2 components develop, then the individual may only experience neurological disruption in the lower limbs, although incontinence and impotence are also possible consequences. If sacral agenesis is complete, then the individual will experience more pronounced lower limb dysfunction in association with the inability to walk or stand due to the loss of the bony connections to the innominates and therefore the means to transfer body weight to the ground (Hotson and Carty, 1982).

Following a neural tube defect, it appears that the inductive signal is either absent or insufficient to initiate normal development of the neural arches and spina bifida will result. This is a developmental abnormality involving failure of the laminae of one or more neural arches to fuse in the midline. It is important to make the distinction between spina bifida and cleft vertebrae as only the former involves a neural tube defect. Cleft vertebrae are a result of non-union of the bony elements and are not indicative of a serious congenital defect (Barnes, 1994). True spina bifida will result in the edges of the affected bone being displaced outwards due to the bulging of the underlying neurological tissues. The most innocuous form of this defect is spina bifida occulta where only a few vertebrae are affected and there is no herniation of either the spinal cord or the meninges. This most commonly occurs in the lumbosacral region, is often asymptomatic and has a reported incidence of 3–18% in the general population (Shore, 1931; Saluja, 1988; Waldron, 1993). A tuft of hair, a dimple or a small pigmented area on the adjacent skin frequently indicates the underlying location of this defect. Spina bifida cystica occurs where gross deficiencies of the vertebral arch exist or when several vertebrae are affected so that the meninges may protrude through the defect, resulting in a meningocoele. In some cases, the spinal cord itself may protrude beyond the limits of the spinal canal, resulting in the formation of a myelomeningocoele and consequent neurological disturbances may ensue. Recent clinical research has indicated that there are strong genetic and nutritional components to the incidence of spina bifida abnormalities. It has been shown that maternal diets low in either folic acid or selenium, severely impair zinc metabolism, which is a necessary element for normal neural tube development (Zimmerman and Lozzio, 1989; Shelby, 1992). Dietary supplements of folic acid are now regularly recommended to all women who are attempting to conceive in an effort to reduce the relatively high incidence of spina bifida, particularly in older mothers. In the USA, folic acid is now routinely added to grain products such as cereals and breads.

The pattern for the future development of the vertebral column is set during the third and fourth weeks of intra-uterine life. The complexity of the embryology of the axial skeleton leaves it open to many potential developmental abnormalities and it is important to realize that these can occur at any stage from the somite development through to the eventual ossification of the cartilage anlage (Peyton and Peterson, 1942; Hadley, 1948; Spillane *et al.*, 1957; Gunderson *et al.*, 1967; Kruyff, 1967; Tsou *et al.*, 1980; Barnes, 1994).

The traditional theory states that during migration, each segmental sclerotome splits into a smaller, more loosely arranged cranial and a larger, more densely organized caudal part, which will eventually resegment (Tanaka and Uhthoff, 1981; Bagnall *et al.*, 1988). The caudal part of one sclerotome fuses with the cranial part of the sclerotome segment below, to form an intersegmental structure, which will go on to develop into the vertebral column (Fig. 6.18). It is noteworthy that although the future vertebral bodies reputedly develop from the recombination of the sclerotome, the neural arches, pedicles and costal elements develop almost entirely from the more dense caudal part of each segmental sclerotome (Verbout, 1985; Selleck and Stern, 1991). This may explain why, in the typical adult vertebra, the pedicles that originally arise from the caudal portion of the sclerotome are generally attached towards the upper pole of the vertebra. The surrounding structures, e.g. the muscles, nerves and blood vessels, maintain their original segmental pattern (Fig. 6.18).

The seven cervical vertebrae are formed from eight cervical somites. The cranial portion of the first vertebral somite fuses with the caudal portion of the fourth occipital somite, which is then incorporated into the formation of the base of the skull (Fig. 6.19). This explains why there are eight pairs of cervical spinal nerves and only seven cervical vertebrae. Similarly, it explains why in the cervical region, the spinal nerves exit from the column above the vertebra of the corresponding number, whereas in the remaining regions of the column they exit below the vertebra of the corresponding number. The segmental spinal nerves are then free to exit from the vertebral canal in the space between two adjacent vertebrae to supply their appropriate segmental dermatome and myotome (Fig. 6.19).

This resegmentation theory has been widely accepted as the mechanism for formation of the vertebral column, but several authors have suggested an alternative mechanism that is very convincing given the detailed embryological specimens that are illustrated in the Uhthoff text in particular (Baur, 1969; Verbout, 1976; Dalgleish, 1985; O'Rahilly and Benson, 1985; Müller and O'Rahilly, 1986; Uhthoff 1990a). They suggested that the resegmentation theory was in error as it represented an incomplete and therefore incorrect extrapolation of information that was only seen in the earlier embryological stages. The differentiation between the more densely packed caudal section of a sclerotome and its less densely packed cranial segment can be identified in early embryological sections when the sclerotome occupies a more lateral position prior to the process of medial migration. However, once the cells have reached the midline, the

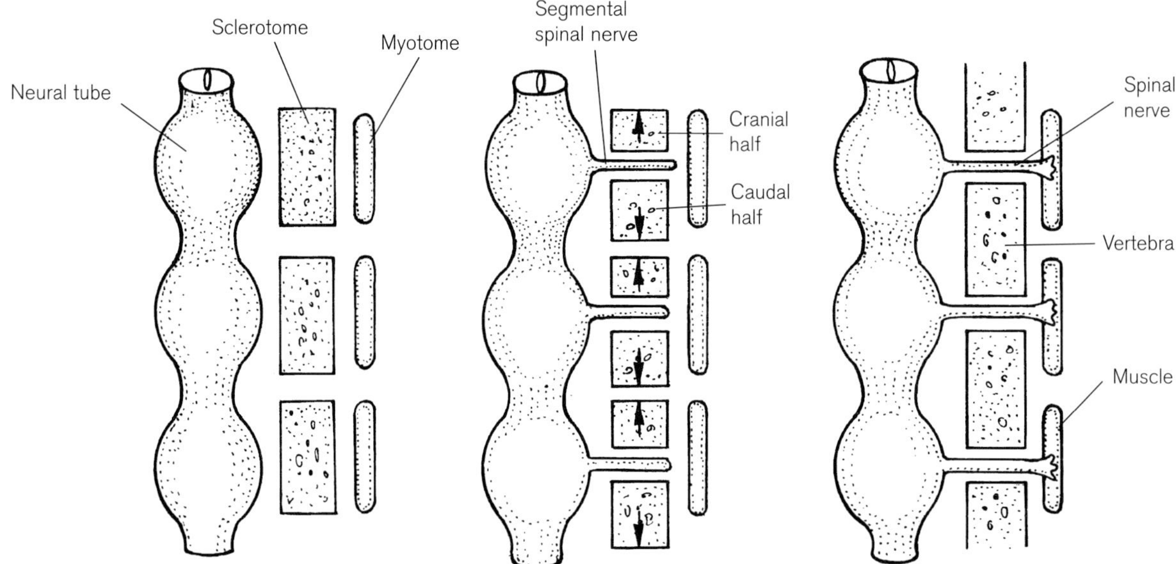

Figure 6.18 Diagrammatic representation of the embryonic recombination of the sclerotome.

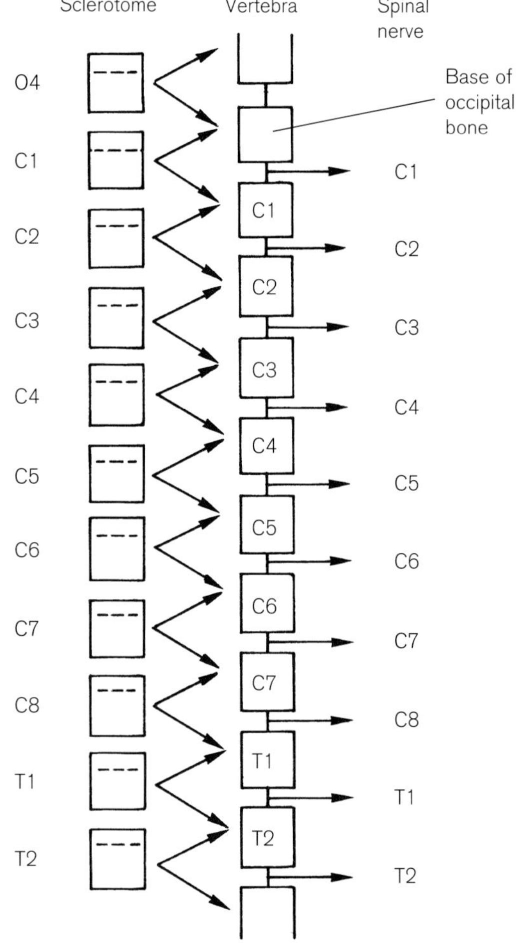

Figure 6.19 Embryonic differentiation of the upper regions of the vertebral column (redrawn after Larsen, 1993).

differentiation is non-existent and proponents of the resegmentation theory accepted that the observed changes were temporal rather than spatial, and this is where Uhthoff (1990a) believed that the error had been made. He strongly proposed that the changes were not only temporal but also spatial and that extrapolation of the situation that could be observed when the migrating cells were in the lateral position were incorrectly superimposed on the final definitive vertebral anlage in the midline. Thus, no account had been taken of any medial to lateral drift alterations in the relative positions of the migrating cells. In summary, they considered that while the vertebral column is indeed formed via a segmental process, there is unlikely to be any true resegmentation of the structure. In agreement with Dalgleish (1985), Müller and O'Rahilly (1994) stated that the centra develop from the perinotochordal territory and not from the sclerotome halves. Rather, they may develop from chondrific centres that originate in the somite-derived tissue surrounding the notochord – the perichordal tube.

The notochord and developing neural tube are enclosed within a mesenchymal template by the twenty-eighth intra-uterine day and this represents the blastemal stage of vertebral development (Fig. 6.20). Small lateral mesenchymal condensations (costal processes) arise in association with the lateral surface of the neural arch of all developing vertebrae at this stage. However, it is only in the thoracic region that these will separate from the developing vertebral mass and elongate into ribs, although all costal processes

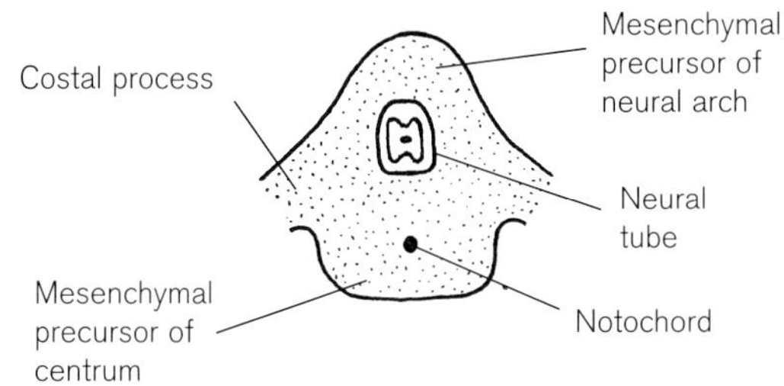

Figure 6.20 Blastemal stage of the developing vertebra – approximately 28 days gestation.

retain the potential to develop independently in any region of the column. This is often seen in the cases of cervical ribs, which generally occur in association with C7 but can also be found less frequently associated with C6 and C5 (Struthers, 1875). Lumbar ribs are less common but when they do arise it is usually in association with the first lumbar vertebra.

During the sixth week of intra-uterine life, up to six chondrification centres may appear in the mesenchymal template (Fig. 6.21). Typically, there is one centre for each lateral half of the centrum, but these probably fuse together shortly after formation to form a single centre. In this region, the notochord becomes increasingly restricted and retrogresses until it eventually disappears. However, in the space between developing vertebrae, the notochord expands, forming the nucleus pulposus of the future intervertebral disc (Peacock, 1951, 1952) (Fig. 6.22). If one of these chondrification centres fails to develop, then the pathological conditions of either hemi- or butterfly vertebrae may arise, which manifest as a congenital scoliosis (Hollinshead, 1965; Parke, 1975; Ogden, 1979; Müller *et al.*, 1986).

After the sixth month of fetal life, the notochordal cells within the nucleus pulposus undergo mucoid degeneration and are replaced by cells from the inner aspect of the annulus fibrosus. This degeneration continues until the second decade of life, by which time all the true notochordal cells have disappeared. Persistence of notochordal tissue results in 'notochordal remnants' that may subsequently develop into a chordoma, a slow-growing neoplasm most frequently located in either the basi-occiput (see Chapter 5) or in the lumbosacral region. In addition, failure of proper retrogression of the notochord may facilitate the formation of Schmorl's nodes by creating a defect in the cartilaginous end-plate through which intervertebral disc material may prolapse into the vertebral body (Saluja *et al.*, 1986). It is believed that these nodes may give rise to congenitally weak spots in the cartilaginous end-plates, which may lead to other vertebral orthopaedic conditions and may in fact be the first indicators of degenerative disc disease (Ortner and Putschar, 1985; Taylor and Twomey, 1986; McFadden and Taylor, 1989). Other authors believe that Schmorl's nodes may develop as a post-traumatic condition (Kornberg, 1988), or indeed as a result of vascular channel regression, resulting in weak spots or scars into which the disc can herniate (Harris and MacNab, 1954; Chandraraj *et al.*, 1998).

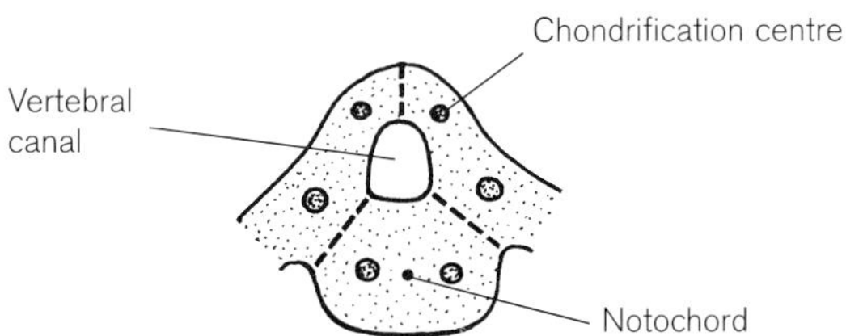

Figure 6.21 Appearance and position of the vertebral chondrification centres – approximately 40 days' gestation.

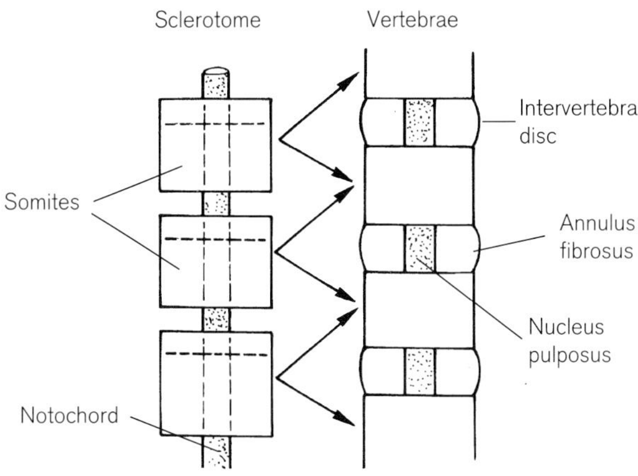

Figure 6.22 The embryological fate of the notochord (redrawn after Larsen, 1993).

Each half of the cartilaginous neural arch develops from a single centre, which commences chondrification at around 6 fetal weeks (Fig 6.21). These will eventually spread into the regions of the transverse and articular processes and anteriorly into the pedicles. A further two chondrification centres appear at the junctions between the centrum and the neural arch and by lateral extension form the costal elements in the thoracic region and contribute to the transverse processes in the other regions of the column (Maat *et al.*, 1996). By expansion of all the chondrification centres, a solid cartilaginous vertebral unit is formed when the fusion finally occurs at the spinous process in the fourth fetal month. Defects in this normal sequence of events can result in posterior arch anomalies, which can occur on either an isolated basis or may be related to defects in adjacent bone formation. For example, the 'absent pedicle complex' results from a failure of development and formation of the more ventral part of the chondrification centre of the neural arch at 6 fetal weeks (Schwartz *et al.*, 1982).

When ossification does commence at around 10 weeks, thoracic ribs will separate from the neural arches through the development of costovertebral joints while in the cervical, lumbar and sacral regions the costal processes will maintain continuity with the transverse processes in particular (Tsou *et al.*, 1980). The type of vertebra (cervical, thoracic, etc.) is established very early on in development and so it is perhaps not surprising to find that if a portion of thoracic somites is transplanted into the cervical region, ribs will still develop in this location (Kieny *et al.*, 1972; Goldstein and Kalcheim, 1992)

More detailed information on the embryonic and fetal development of the vertebral column can be found in Wyburn (1944), Sensenig (1949), Verbout (1985), Töndury and Theiler (1990) and Christ and Wilting (1992).

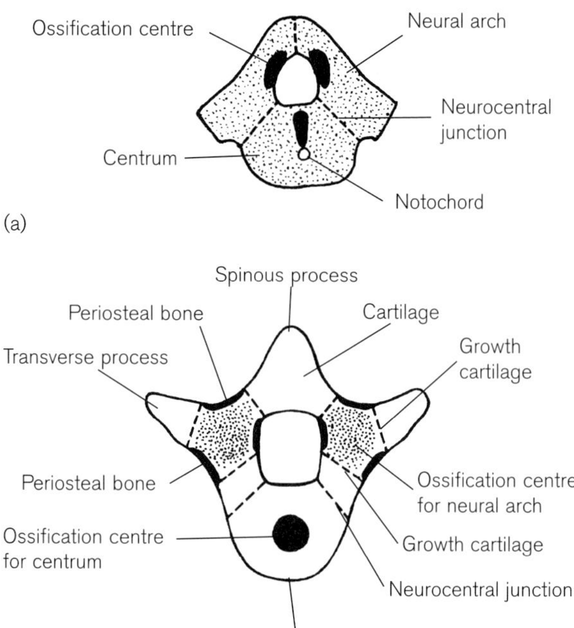

Figure 6.23 Early stage of vertebral development showing the position of the centres of ossification. (a) Approximately 11–12 fetal weeks and (b) 13–14 fetal weeks (redrawn after Chandraraj and Briggs, 1991).

Ossification

Primary centres

The ossification of the cartilaginous anlage begins at the end of the second embryonic month. While it is agreed that a single ossification centre develops for each half of the neural arch, the situation is more contentious regarding the development of the centrum. Some authors have stated that there is a single ossification centre (Fawcett, 1907; Birkner, 1978; Ogden, 1979; Richenbacher *et al.*, 1982; Williams *et al.*, 1995), while others maintain that there are two centres, one anterior and one posterior, that fuse shortly after formation (Frazer, 1948; Cohen *et al.*, 1956; Hollinshead, 1965; Last, 1973; Fazekas and Kósa, 1978). However, Tanaka and Uhthoff (1983) have shown that when two ossification centres do arise, they are always connected by a bony bridge, which carries a blood vessel. Therefore, it can be said that each typical vertebra is formed from at least three and in some instances possibly four separate primary centres of ossification (Fig. 6.23). While there are regional and individual bone variations in the patterns and timings of ossification, there are some basic principles that apply to the centra and the neural arches in general.

Centra

The ossification of the centrum is initiated dorsal to the position of the notochord within the cartilaginous anlage and so represents true endochondral ossification (Fig. 6.23). This primary centre first appears in the lower thoracic and upper lumbar regions (T10–L1) between the ninth and tenth fetal weeks (Fig. 6.24). Ossification in the centra then continues in a bi-directional pattern, appearing at successively higher and lower levels, reaching the fifth lumbar vertebra by the end of the third month and the second cervical vertebra certainly by the end of the fourth fetal month.

The morphology and development of the juvenile centrum is heavily influenced by its profuse vascular supply (Fig. 6.25) (Ratcliffe, 1981, 1982). According to Skawina *et al.* (1997) ossification commences in the region of the notochord remnants and they suggested that the notochordal cells contained some angiogenic inhibiting factor that delayed vascular penetration into this region. As a result, a vertebral centrum from the first trimester of pregnancy shows an axial avascular area around the notochord region, resulting in a ring-shaped area of ossification. They proposed that if the vascular penetration into this area was abnormally delayed then it could give rise to congenital malformations, such as a persistent notochordal canal or even cleft

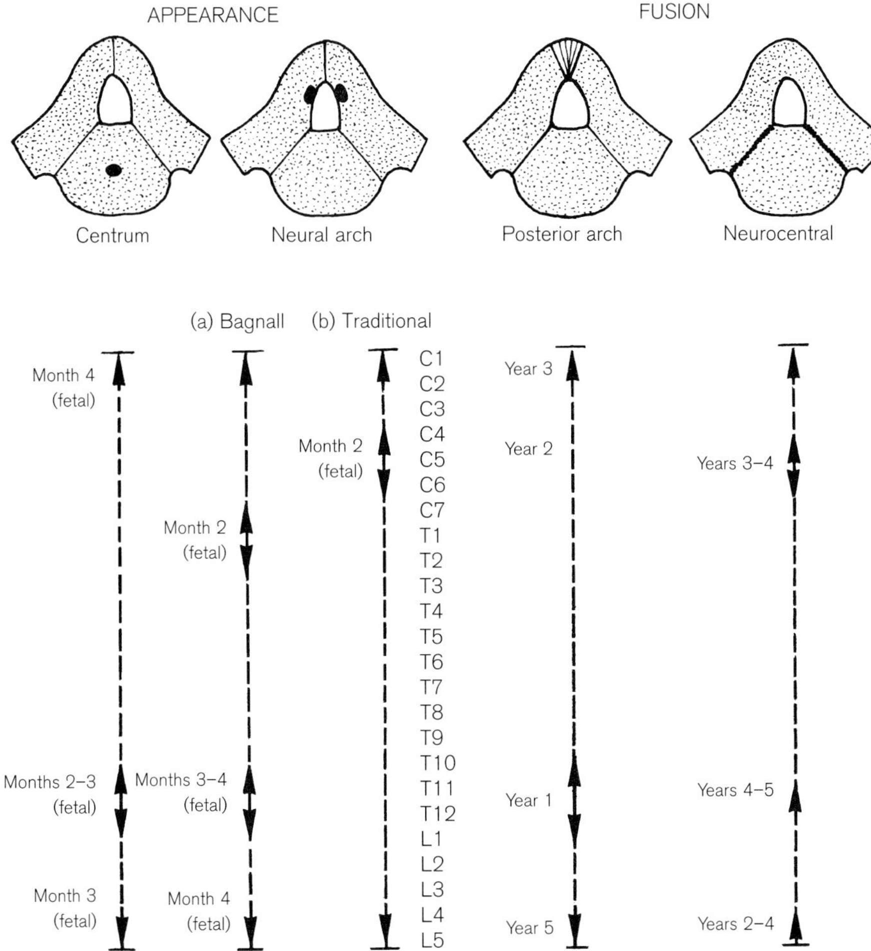

Figure 6.24 General pattern for the appearance and fusion of the primary centres of ossification in the presacral vertebrae.

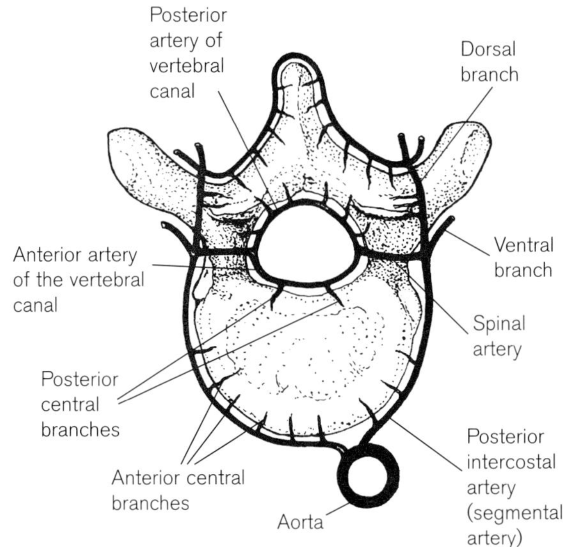

Figure 6.25 The arterial supply of a typical adult vertebra.

vertebral bodies (Hensinger and MacEwan, 1975). The notochord essentially disappears by the end of the first trimester, when the blood vessels then advance centrifugally to increase the size of the centre and centripetally to invade the previously avascular region. Each centre is normally supplied by paired (i.e. segmental) posterior (nutrient) arteries and they are accompanied by a venous network (Willis, 1949; Ferguson, 1950; Crock *et al.*, 1973). Ratcliffe (1982) noted that the arterial supply to the centrum undergoes fundamental changes throughout growth. He noted that the extensive intra-osseous arterial anastomotic networks found in the centra of the infant and young child started to reduce in number around 7 years of age and continued to do so until approximately 15 years. By adolescence, he found that the blood supply of the vertebral body was zoned into isolated regional compartments and felt that this might go some way towards explaining the distribution of angiogenic-related osseous pathological conditions.

In general terms, however, the vertebral bodies receive their arterial supply from a rich arborescent dorsal plexus that runs the length of the column and is fed by segmental arteries (Harris and Jones, 1956; Guida *et al.*, 1969; Brookes and Revell, 1998). Each segmental artery gives off a number of anterior central branches that penetrate the anterior and lateral surfaces of the centrum (Rothman and Simeone, 1975). The anterior central branches are largest on the anterior aspect of the centrum, where they penetrate into the core of the bone in the embryological segmental position. These prominent vascular channels are obvious in the middle of the anterior surface of the juvenile centrum (Fig. 6.26a), although they will eventually reduce in size as a layer of compact bone is laid down on this surface and by puberty there is little evidence of the anterior vascular foramina. These vascular channels are most prominent on the anterior surfaces of the thoracic vertebrae, possibly due to the size of the posterior intercostal arteries. At the level of the transverse process, the segmental artery bifurcates into a ventral and a dorsal branch. The dorsal branch gives off the spinal artery, which passes medially across the pedicle before bifurcating into the anterior and posterior arteries of the vertebral canal. The anterior artery courses along the posterior surface of the centrum and sends perforating posterior central arteries into the dorsal surface of the centrum. Unlike the anterior channels, these posterior vascular foramina tend to persist even into adulthood as so-called basivertebral foramina, which transmit the basivertebral veins to the anterior internal vertebral veins (Fig. 6.26b). As the anterior and posterior central perforating arteries pass across the superior and inferior surfaces of the centrum they form vascular radiating channels, which produce the characteristic billowed appearance of both the juvenile centrum and later the vertebral body (Donisch and Trapp, 1971) (Fig. 6.26c). It is only when the annular epiphyses of the body have fused that these furrows are no longer visible. It is important to remember at this stage that the adult vertebral body is derived from the juvenile centrum plus a small portion of the neural arch on each side. Thus, the adult vertebral body equates to more than the juvenile centrum and so in developmental terms it is incorrect to use the term 'vertebral body' as the term 'centrum' is more appropriate (MacLaughlin and Oldale, 1992).

Agenesis of the centrum is rare and can result either from a failure in the ventral part of the migrating

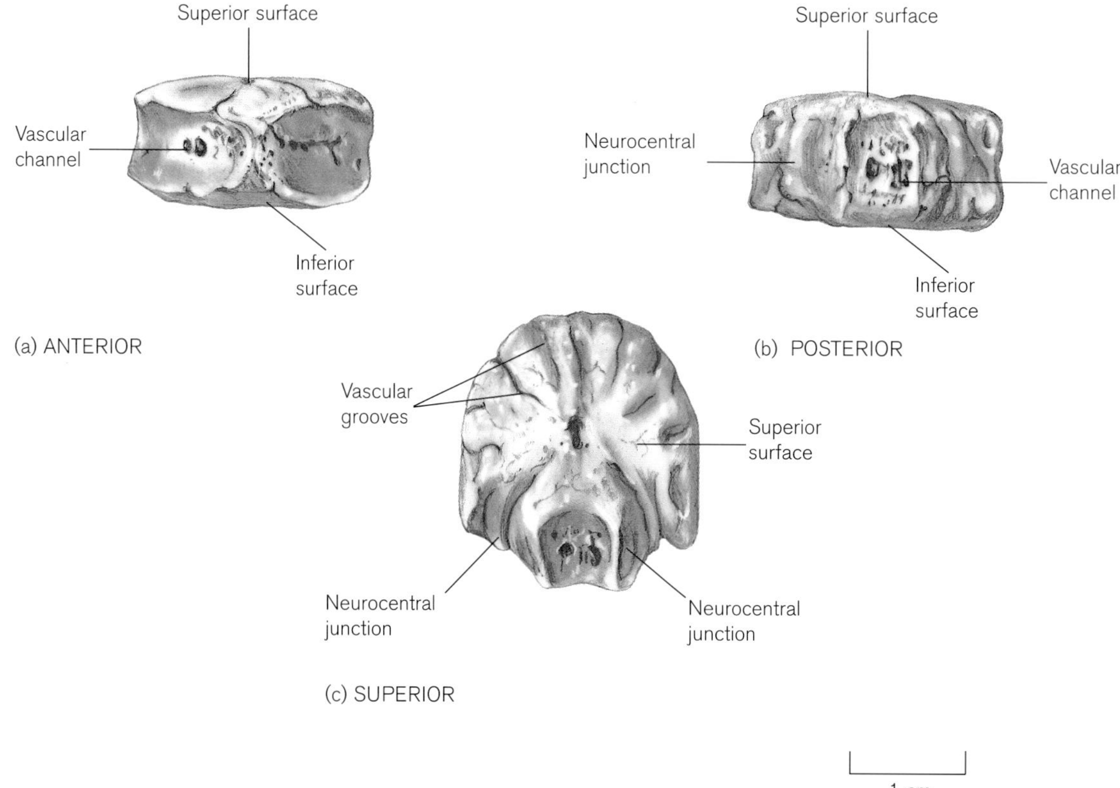

Figure 6.26 A typical juvenile vertebral centrum (T8 from a child of approximately 4 years).

sclerotome, the failure of chondrification or ossification centres to appear or indeed through a failure in the vascular supply (Tsou *et al.*, 1980). In this condition, the neural arch elements develop normally and the pedicles may in fact fuse anterior to the spinal cord, resulting in a congenital kyphosis (Tsou *et al.*, 1980). If untreated, aplasia of the centrum leads to rapidly progressive spinal deformity and neurological defects (Lorenzo *et al.*, 1983).

Neural arches

Ossification of the neural arches commences on the inner surface of each hemi-arch (Fig. 6.23b) as a perichondral lamella from which osteogenesis extends into the cartilage anlage (Richenbacher *et al.*, 1982). Technically therefore, the neural arches initially form via intramembranous ossification. Periosteal lamellar bone is first observed on the internal surface of an arch around week 12. By week 13, periosteal bone appears on the external surface, as the zone of hypertrophying cartilage has extended across the arch. Periosteal vessels then invade the calcifying mass and introduce osteogenic cells, which begin to lay down spicules of bone. The ossification centre eventually resembles a curved growth zone with three separate growth cartilages – one for the region of the pedicle, one for the lamina/spinous process and one for the transverse process (Fig. 6.23b). Ossification and subsequent growth of the neural arch therefore occurs centripetally (Chandraraj and Briggs, 1991).

This peripheral initiation of ossification supports the theory by Bagnall *et al.* (1977b) that the stimulus for the commencement of ossification in the neural arches is the attachment of muscles involved in early fetal reflexes. They proposed that these neurological reflexes initiated muscle contraction, thereby stimulating bone development on the perichondral surface of the cartilage template at the site of the muscle attachment. They found that primary centres of ossification for the neural arches first appeared in the lower cervical and upper thoracic regions in the second fetal month and then spread upwards and downwards in a fairly orderly fashion towards the mid-thoracic region (Fig. 6.24). Bagnall *et al.* (1977b) proposed that this initiation of ossification was concomitant with the head jerk reflex (gasp reflex) seen in the fetus around week 10. By the twelfth week, a second group of centres appeared in the lower thoracic and upper lumbar regions, spreading up towards the mid-thoracic and down to the lower lumbar and sacral regions in a fairly ordered sequence, with the neural arches of L5 being the last to develop towards the end of the fourth month. Bagnall *et al.* (1977b) proposed that the initiation for this second group of ossification centres arose again from muscle contraction associated with reflex movements in the fetal lower limbs. Thus, they suggested that both the initiation and the mode of ossification differed between the centra and the neural arches and that they therefore developed independently of each other, explaining why there is no apparent integrated pattern of timing of ossification (Fig. 6.24). Hill (1992) reported that early embryonic and fetal movements are vital to align the trabeculae within bones.

The more widely held and traditional view of ossification in the neural arches (Fig. 6.24), is that it commences in the cervical region in the second fetal month and is essentially monodirectional in a craniocaudal sequence (Mall, 1906; Fawcett, 1907; Hodges, 1933; Frazer, 1948; Noback and Robertson, 1951; Fazekas and Kósa, 1978; Ogden, 1979; Budorick *et al.*, 1991; Bareggi *et al.*, 1993; Williams *et al.*, 1995). A third theory is that neural arch ossification appears at three distinct locations and then each progresses independently in a cranial and caudal direction. Ford *et al.* (1982) stated that the first group to appear was in the lower cervical and upper thoracic regions, followed by a second group in the upper cervical region and finally by a third group in the lower thoracic and upper lumbar region.

In an attempt to get away from this controversy of different developmental sequences, Bareggi *et al.* (1994b) simply correlated the total number of centres present in a column and related this to fetal crown–rump measurements. They found that this offered a simple and reliable method for establishing the maturity of a fetus.

Regardless of which of the developmental sequence theories is accepted, it is clear that all three primary vertebral centres are present in all presacral vertebrae certainly by the end of the fourth fetal month, if not earlier (Budorick *et al.*, 1991). It is also true that in the cervical region, the ossification centres for the neural arches are present before the centra, whereas in the lower thoracic and upper lumbar regions, the centra may appear before the neural arches. In the upper to mid-thoracic regions the primary ossification centres for the centra and neural arches probably appear concurrently (Fig. 6.24). Thus, in regional terms the maturation of the centra parallels the maturation of the notochord, while the pattern of maturation in the vertebral arches parallels that of the somites and therefore the peripheral nervous system (Sperber, 1989; Kjaer *et al.*, 1993).

During the first year of postnatal life, the neural arches commence fusion posteriorly at the spinous process (Fig. 6.24). This occurs initially in the lower thoracic and upper lumbar regions in the latter part of the first year and progresses in a systematic cranial and caudal direction so that the cervical arches may not fuse until the beginning of the second year and the lowest lumbar may not fuse until the end of the fifth year. Therefore, in any individual below the age of 6 years some degree of non-fusion of the primary elements of the presacral vertebrae should be expected. The histological make-up of this junction is not, however, simply a plug of mesenchyme or cartilage, but is in fact a true growth plate which plays an integral part in the overall co-ordinated increase in size of the developing vertebra (Maat *et al.*, 1996).

Spondylolysis is defined as a separation in the neural arch, excluding that which can occur in the midline as a result of failure of the laminae to unite at the spinous process (Merbs, 1996). Such separation usually occurs through the isthmus separating the superior from the inferior articular facets (pars interarticularis). This is a uniquely human condition as its incidence is closely related to the development of the lumbar curvature (Letts *et al.*, 1986).

Fusion between the primary centres of the neural arches and the centra occurs ventral to the pedicles at the neurocentral junction between 2 and 5 years of age. The adult vertebral body is formed from the centrum and the paired anterior extensions (boutons) of the pedicles. It is important to remember that the head of the costal process only ever articulates with the lateral surfaces of these boutons and never directly with the centrum (Fig. 6.27). Histologically, the growth plate at the neurocentral junction (epiphysis arcus vertebrae) clearly displays growth columns on both sides and therefore is responsible for contributing not only to growth in the neural arch but also in the centrum (Maat *et al.*, 1996). Even when the neurocentral junctions have begun to fuse, their position remains clearly marked externally by a crescentic impression whose concavity is directed dorsolaterally on both the cranial and caudal aspects of the body. Thus, the pedicular bouton of the neural arch element forms a wedge that extends across the full height of the future vertebral body, with its upper and lower boundaries being limited by the cranial and caudal annular epiphyses respectively. The morphology of this wedge has been likened, appropriately, to a carpenter's dovetail joint (Maat *et al.*, 1996). Evidence of the neurocentral junction is maintained throughout adult life and persists as a permanent bilateral plate of bone inside the dorsolateral region of every adult vertebral body that is not obliterated by age-related remodelling. The persistence of this dense plate of bone makes this region of a vertebra extremely suitable for the strategic positioning of pedicular screws in spinal surgery (Maat *et al.*, 1996). It is also interesting to note that vertebral fracture lines seem to avoid the region of the neurocentral junction in the adult and this probably explains the typical pattern seen in traumatic burst fractures of a vertebra (Panjabi *et al.*, 1994).

Neurocentral fusion tends to occur first in the lumbar region, followed closely by the cervical segment, with the thoracic vertebrae generally being the last to

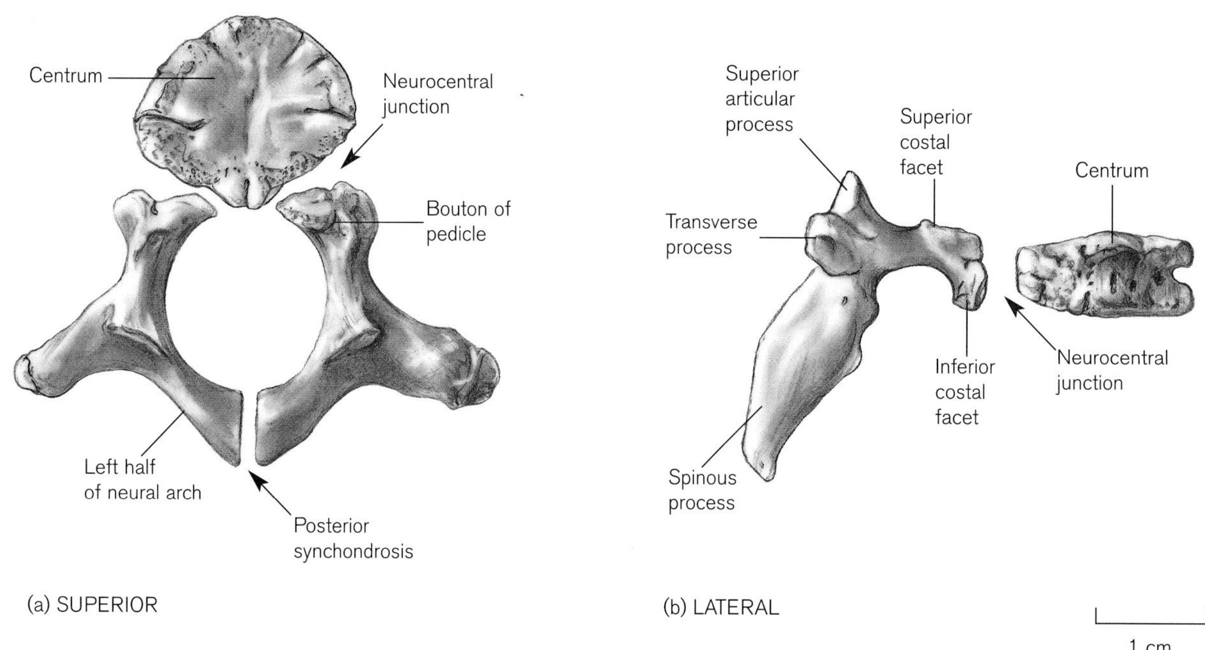

Figure 6.27 A typical thoracic vertebra from a child of approximately 1.5 years.

close. It is perhaps for this reason that the crescentic impressions of this junction are most clearly seen in the thoracic region of the juvenile column. It is likely that all neurocentral junctions will be closed by the fifth and certainly by the sixth year.

Premature osseous fusion, either anteriorly at the neurocentral junctions or posteriorly at the spinous process, would preclude further canal widening and thus impair proper diametric increase of the canal. Improperly timed fusion may be the mechanism of spinal stenosis in conditions such as achondroplasia (Ogden, 1979).

Cervical vertebrae

The embryological development of the first two cervical vertebrae is complicated and sufficiently different from that of the more typical vertebrae to require some further detailed discussion (Fig. 6.28).

The caudal part of the fourth occipital somite fuses with the cranial part of the first cervical somite to form what is known in zoological terms as the proatlas. In some lower vertebrates this remains a separate bone located between the occipital bone above and the first cervical vertebra below, but in man it is assimilated into the occipital condyles and the apex (ossiculum terminale) of the odontoid process of the axis (Shapiro and Robinson, 1976b; Müller and O'Rahilly, 1994). The caudal part of the first cervical sclerotome segment forms the lateral masses and anterior and posterior arches of the atlas (O'Rahilly *et al.*, 1983). The remainder of the dens develops from the fusion of the caudal part of the first cervical somite with the cranial part of the second cervical somite. The true centrum of the axis and its neural arch is then formed from the fusion of the caudal part of the second cervical somite with the cranial part of the third cervical somite. Müller and O'Rahilly (1994), identified three complete centra that develop in the region of the atlanto-axial region, although they are related to only 2.5 sclerotomes and two neural arches. They concluded that these three centra, which they termed the 'xyz' complex, belong ontogenetically to the axis so that the atlas does not appear to possess a central element.

David *et al.* (1998) reported that chondrification commenced in the lateral masses of the atlas around day 45, by which time the embryonic centrum of C1 had already become detached. The anterior tubercle of C1 develops from a separate chondrification centre around 50–53 days, which coincided with chondrification of the anterior arch. The intervertebral foramina of C1 and C2 are simply grooves by day 45 but have converted into foramina by day 58. At day 45, the odontoid process is simply represented by the embryonic centra of C1 and C2, but by day 58 it is well developed and extends above the level of C1 and actually reaches into the foramen magnum, thereby forming the so-called 'third occipital condyle' (Müller and O'Rahilly, 1980; O'Rahilly *et al.*, 1983).

There is some evidence that, in phylogenetic terms, the craniovertebral junction moves caudally, as vertebrae are assimilated into the posterior segment of the skull. This is therefore a phylogenetically inconstant region of the column and, given the complexity of its embryological derivation, it is not surprising that a relatively high incidence of congenital and acquired

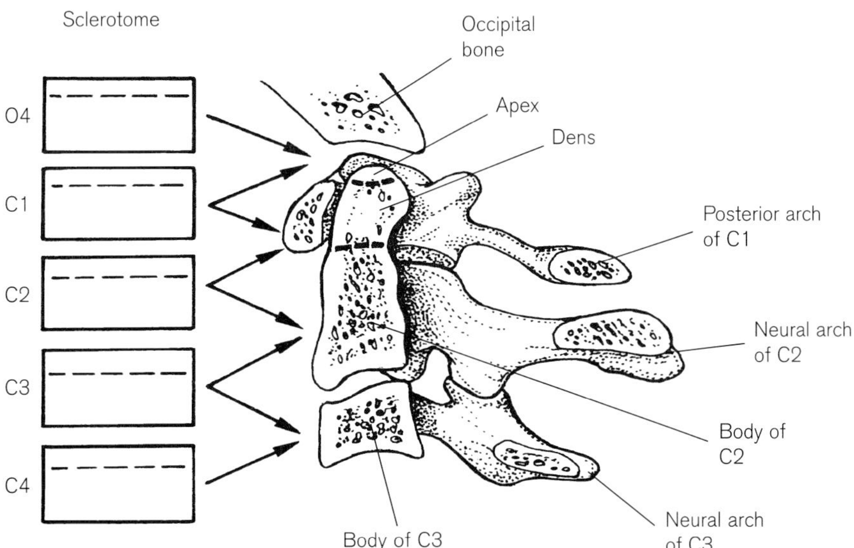

Figure 6.28 Embryological differentiation of the upper cervical vertebrae.

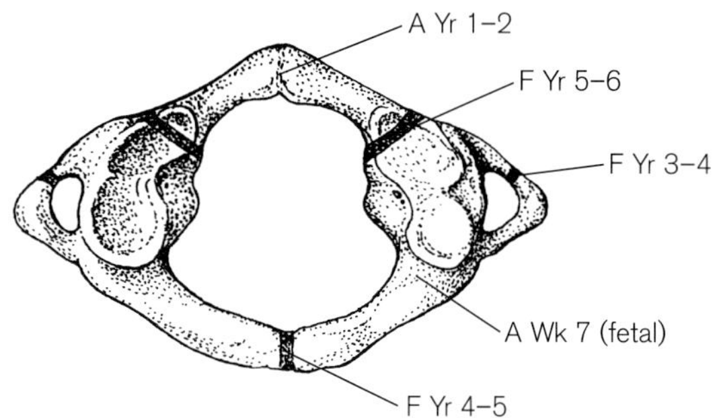

Figure 6.29 Times of appearance (A) and fusion (F) of the primary centres of ossification in the atlas.

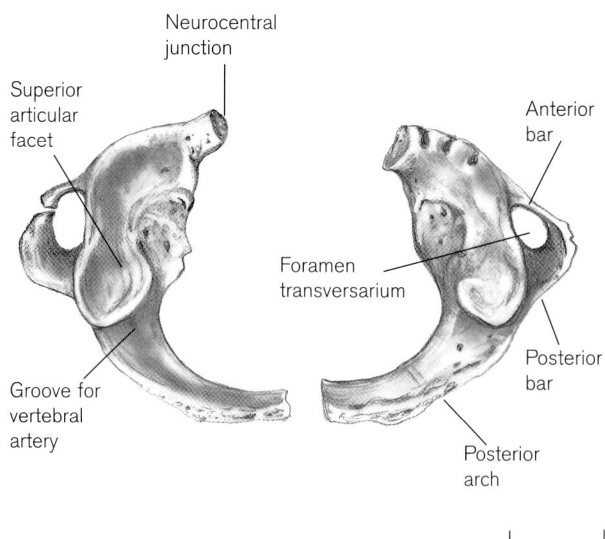

Figure 6.31 Superior surface of the atlas showing the formation of the transverse process in a boy aged 3 years 4 months.

abnormalities are seen in this region (Peyton and Peterson, 1942; Hadley, 1948; Spillane *et al.*, 1957; Kruyff, 1967; Ozonoff, 1979; Yochum and Rowe, 1987).

It is generally recognized that the **atlas** ossifies from three primary centres of ossification (Fig. 6.29) and is recognizable in isolation from the fourth fetal month onwards. A centre appears for each of the lateral masses, posterior to the articular pillar, in the seventh week of intra-uterine life. These centres increase in size and form the majority of the upper and all of the lower synovial articular facets (Castellana and Kósa, 1999). Ossification spreads backwards from these primary centres to form the two halves of the posterior arch and laterally to form the thick posterior bar of the transverse process (Fig. 6.30). At birth, the atlas is represented by two bony masses, which display larger concave articular facets anteriorly on their upper surface and smaller flatter articular facets on their lower surface. A relatively large nutrient foramen can usually be found on the inferior surface at the junction between the limits of the inferior articular facet and the transverse process. The groove for the vertebral artery is present behind the superior articular facet and the posterior arches are curved towards the midline. The anterior bar is not present at this stage and the superior articular facet may look somewhat foreshortened (at the neurocentral junction), as the remainder of the surface will form from the anterior centre of ossification. At this stage, the transverse process is only represented by a thick posterior bar, but this will eventually fuse with a thinner anterior bar, which develops from the ventrolateral aspect of the articular pillar between the third and fourth years (Fig. 6.31). It is clear that the posterior tubercle is formed from the thick posterior bar, as fusion with the anterior bar, to complete the foramen transversarium, occurs anterior to the posterior tubercle. Thus, in the

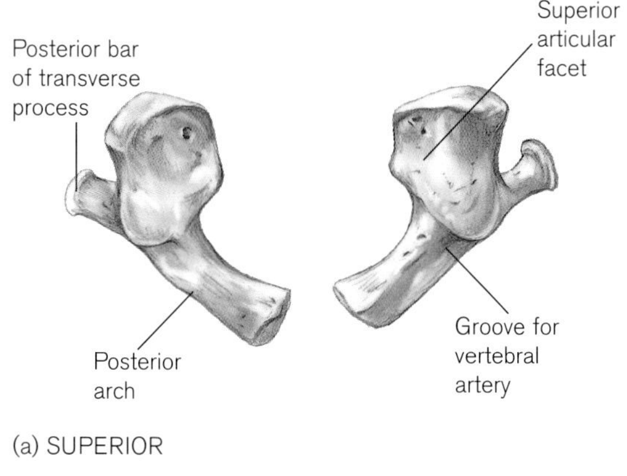

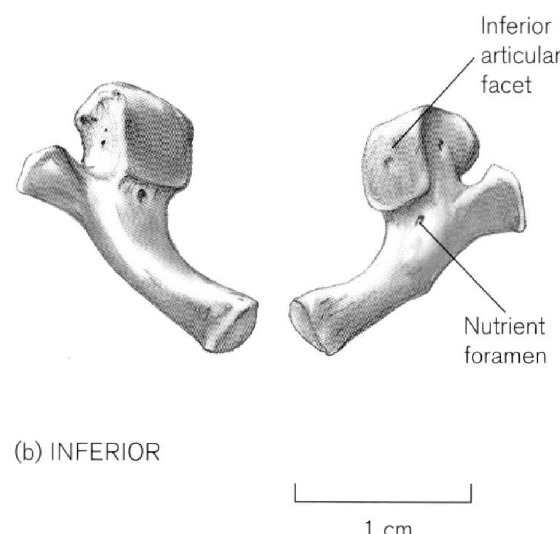

Figure 6.30 The morphology of the perinatal atlas.

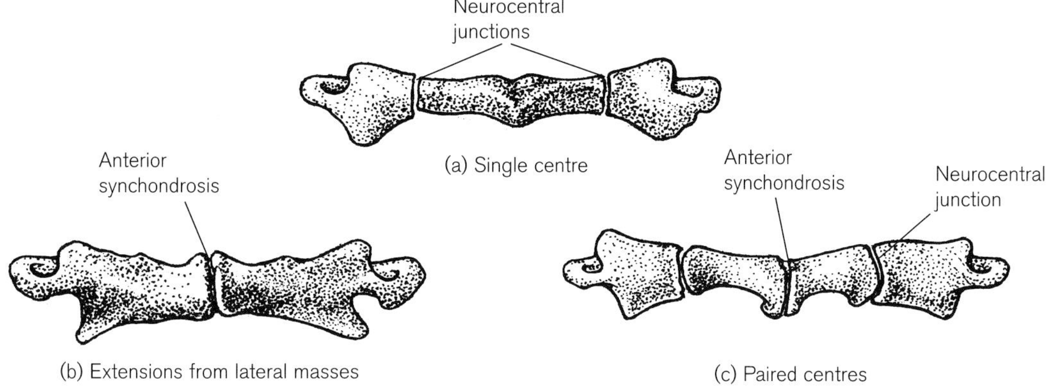

Figure 6.32 Variation in the mode of development of the anterior arch of the atlas.

atlas, the posterior tubercle represents the end of the true transverse process. The foramina transversaria are therefore formed by the fusion of the anterior and posterior bars as they pass around the position of the vertebral artery. The foramina are usually near to completion by years 3–4. Occasionally, the foramen transversarium of the atlas may be absent or sufficiently rudimentary to obviously exclude the passage of the vertebral artery (Vasudeva and Kumar, 1995). Since the presence of the vertebral vessels are an important factor in the genesis of the foramen, a variation in its course will influence the presence/absence and indeed the form, of the foramen transversarium. Therefore, if the foramen is not going to develop, this will be apparent by 3 years of age, if not earlier.

The morphology of the atlas remains virtually unchanged for the first year following birth, with the major growth emphasis being placed on an increase in overall size. In the first or second year, ossification commences in the cartilaginous mass of the anterior arch either as a single centre, paired centres, multifocal nodules or from ossification bars that spread directly from the lateral masses (Fig. 6.32), although the most common form is said to arise from a single separate centre (Fig. 6.33). As a result, the pattern of fusion in the anterior arch will depend upon the manner in which it originally ossified. A separate anterior arch of the atlas is probably identifiable at 3–4 years of age. It appears as a short bar of bone that has a downward-projecting tubercle on its anterior surface and a smooth articular facet on its posterior surface for articulation with ventral aspect of the dens (Fig. 6.33).

The posterior arch usually fuses in the fourth or even fifth year, although it is not unusual for it to remain open even in the adult (Fig. 6.34). The anterior (effectively neurocentral) junctions may not close until the fifth or sixth year at the earliest (Fig. 6.29). The line of union between the anterior arch and a lateral mass passes across the anterior portions of the superior articular facet, thereby mimicking the pattern of fusion seen in the occipital condyles – see Chapter 5.

Endochondral growth occurs prior to fusion at all junctions, ensuring an overall integrated expansion of the vertebral canal as the three ossified units grow away from each other. C1 reaches close to its final adult size by 4–6 years of age, after which there is little increase in the width of the vertebral canal, only a growth in the overall robusticity of its bony limits to facilitate increased muscle mass attachment (Tulsi, 1971; Ogden, 1984b). This early limitation on the size of the vertebral canal is a clear indication of the well-documented precocious maturation of the human central nervous system (Tanner, 1978).

There are several abnormalities seen in the developing first cervical vertebra. The occipito-atlanto-axial

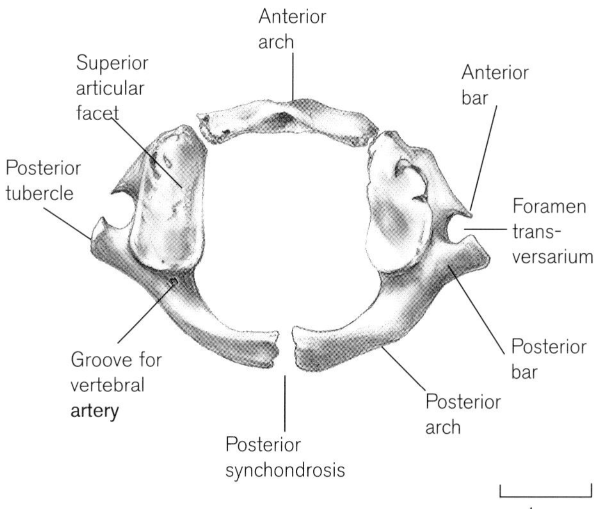

Figure 6.33 The three primary centres of ossification for the atlas in a child aged between 2 and 3 years.

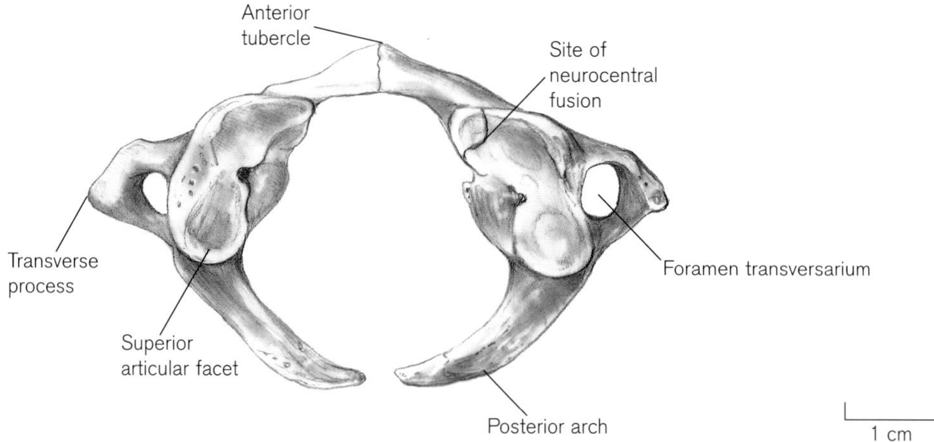

Figure 6.34 Spina bifida atlantis in a girl aged 8 years 7 months.

region is both a phylogenetically and ontogenetically inconstant region of the axial skeleton. Its embryological development is complex and gives rise to a high incidence of congenital and acquired abnormalities (Wilson *et al.*, 1940; Wade, 1941; Skeletal Dysplasia Group, 1989). Occipitalization or assimilation of the atlas occurs as a result of the maldevelopment of the craniovertebral junction from an incomplete segmentation of the first cervical sclerotome segment during the early embryonic period. The fusion between the occipital bone and the atlas may be localized or extensive and it can be uni- or bilateral (Griffith, 1896; Green, 1930; Nayak, 1931; Pate, 1936; Motwani, 1937; Stratemeier and Jensen, 1980; Kalla *et al.*, 1989). In the majority of cases, the fusion is localized to the region of the atlanto-occipital joint (McRae and Barnum, 1953; Black and Scheuer, 1996a). Around 10% of cases of assimilation of the atlas are asymptomatic, but it can present as weakness or ataxia of the lower limbs, numbness or pain in the extremities and a dull ache in the upper neck and occipital region (Smith, 1908a; McRae and Barnum, 1953; Malhotra and Leeds, 1984). These symptoms are thought to arise following the abnormally high position of the dens in relation to the medulla oblongata. Incomplete incorporation or failure of segmentation of the last occipital and C1 sclerotomes leads to a spectrum of fusional anomalies and accessory structures, many of which are asymptomatic (MacAlister, 1893a; Gladstone and Wakeley, 1924; Peyton and Peterson, 1942; Hadley, 1948; McRae, 1953; Spillane *et al.*, 1957; Lombardi, 1961; Keats, 1967; Kruyff, 1967; Nicholson and Sherr, 1968; Dalinka *et al.*, 1972).

A caudal shift in the position of the atlanto-occipital demarcation, causing an assimilation of the atlas into the occipital bone, is more common than a cranial shift, which results in an occipital vertebra – see Chapter 5. However, this phenomenon of cranial – caudal border shifting is not clearly understood, but it is thought that the cause may lie more with the neural arch components of these transitional vertebrae, rather than the centra. As the neural arches develop from the more dense caudal part of the sclerotome, it may be that the formation of the sclerotomic fissure is responsible for the delay in proper segmentation between two adjacent regions.

Non-union of the posterior arch (spina bifida atlantis) is not an uncommon anomaly (Fig. 6.34). It has a reported incidence of around 1% and is generally asymptomatic (Motateanu *et al.*, 1991).

The **axis** ossifies from five primary centres of ossification (Fig. 6.35) – one for each half of the neural arch, one for the true centrum of the axis, and one for each half of the body of the dens. In keeping with the

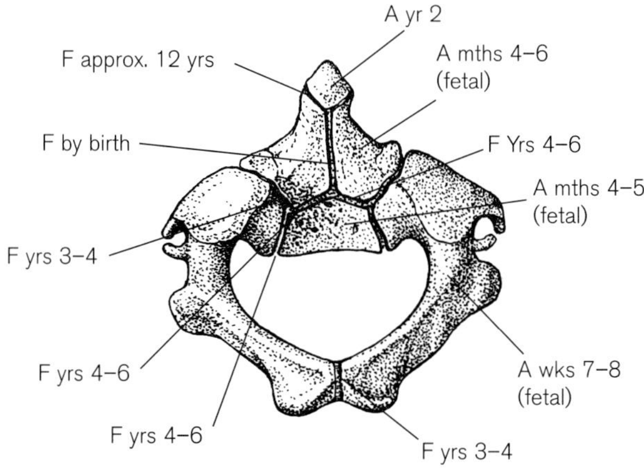

Figure 6.35 Times of appearance (A) and fusion (F) of the primary ossification centres of the axis.

prevailing pattern of ossification in the cervical region, the centres of ossification for the neural arches appear before the centra (between 7 and 8 weeks of intra-uterine life). In each half, the ossification centre appears posterior to the articular pillar and a nutrient foramen generally persists in this region on the inferior surface, posterior to the inferior articular facet. Ossification spreads backwards into the laminae and anteriorly to the neurocentral junction. As with the atlas, the first part of the foramen transversarium to form is the posterior boundary and this is represented in the perinatal axis by a small, laterally projecting spicule of bone, which is considerably more gracile than that seen in the atlas (Fig. 6.36). As with the atlas, the posterior tubercle is present at an early stage of development and is therefore unlikely to be costal in origin. Even from an early age, the neural arches are robust compared with the other cervical arches and end in a slightly bulbous terminal area that is deflected laterally to form the precursor of the bifid spinous process seen in the adult. Only the lateral two-thirds of the superior articular facet is formed from the neural arch component, as the remainder will be formed when the odontoid process fuses at the dentoneural synchondrosis (note the similarities between the pattern of formation of the superior articular process of C1 above and that of the occipital bone in Chapter 5).

The true centrum of the axis commences ossification from a single centre between the fourth and fifth months of intra-uterine life (Wollin, 1963; Sherk and Nicholson, 1969). Around the same time, two laterally placed ossification centres appear in the odontoid process, which rapidly coalesce so that the intradental

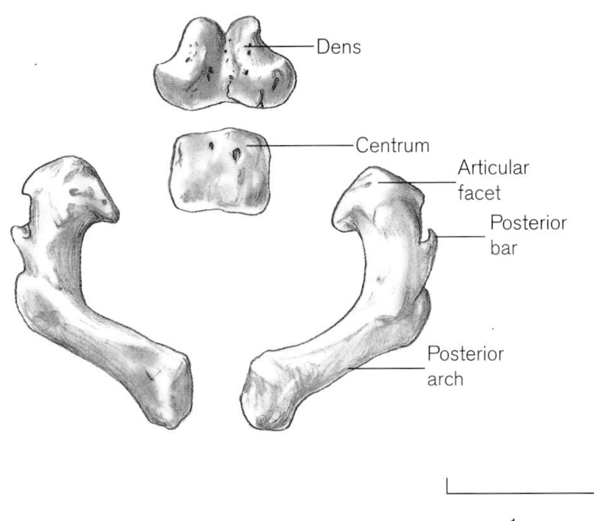

Figure 6.36 The morphology of the perinatal axis.

synchondrosis fuses, certainly by the time of birth and possibly as early as 7 or 8 months *in utero*, to form the characteristic forked appearance of the upper aspect of the juvenile dens (Freiberger *et al.*, 1965; Kline, 1966; Michaels *et al.*, 1969; Rezaian, 1974; Juhl and Seerup, 1983; Ogden, 1984c).

Although the components of the axis can be identified in isolation from approximately 4–5 fetal months, the centres for the centrum and the dens are only clearly recognizable towards the end of fetal life and realistically around the time of birth. The perinatal dens is slightly pyramidal in shape with a broader base that passes up towards a forked apex (Fig. 6.36). The axial centrum is very similar in morphology to all other cervical centra (see below) except that it has a horizontal superior surface that is the same size as the horizontal inferior surface and is therefore not wedge-shaped (see below). In addition, it is the largest of the cervical centra in all dimensions. Therefore, the perinatal axis presents as four separate bones, each of which is theoretically identifiable in isolation.

A longitudinal midline (intradental) sulcus is found on the posterior surface of the dens and this persists certainly until 3 or 4 years of age, when it begins to fill in, initially from below, concomitant with the period of development for the ossiculum terminale (see below). A posteriorly tilted dens can be detected, particularly on radiographs, and it is thought that this arises due to unco-ordinated growth on the anterior and posterior aspects of the dens (Swischuk *et al.*, 1979; Kattan and Pais, 1982).

The posterior synchondrosis between the neural arches, fuses between 3 and 4 years of age, and, at approximately the same time, the dens is fusing laterally to the neural arches at the dentoneural synchondrosis (Fig. 6.37). This fusion line passes across the superior articular facet, so that the medial one-third of the facet is formed by the dens and the lateral two-thirds by the neural arch (keeping in continuity with the location seen in both C1 and the occipital bone). The inferior articular facet is formed entirely from the neural arch component. This fusion of the anterior and posterior elements effectively halts any further substantial growth in the dimensions of the vertebral canal, apart from minor areas of continual subperiosteal remodelling. As with the atlas, this precocious fusion again clearly displays the early maturation of the central nervous system. Therefore, between 3 and 4 years of age, the axis may be represented by only two bony components (Fig. 6.37). The larger element is formed from the fusion of the neural arches with the dens and the smaller element represents the true centrum of the axis. At this stage, the transverse processes, and therefore the foramina

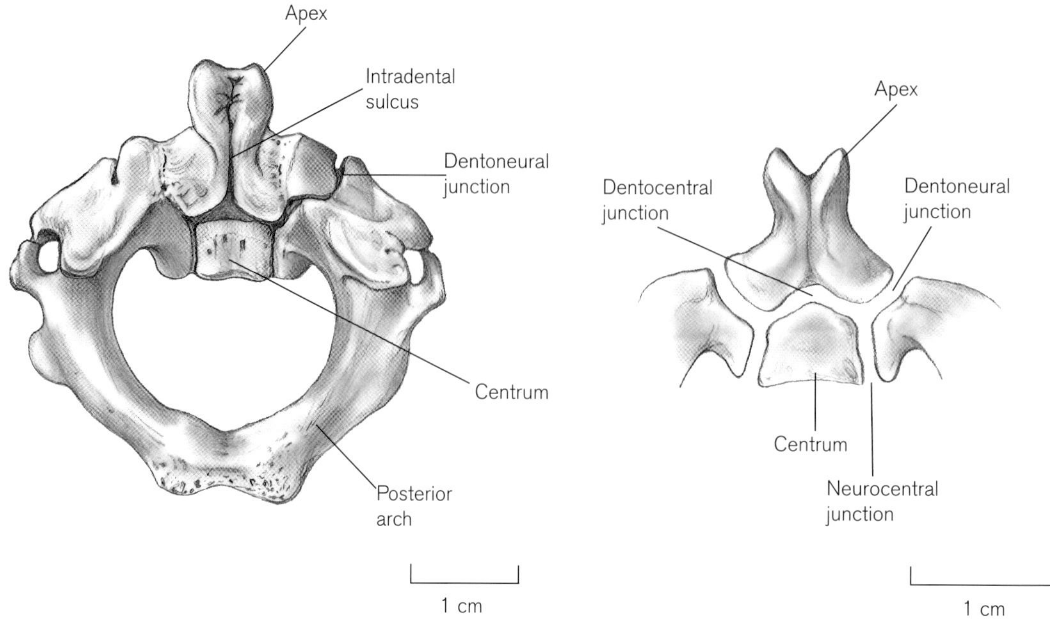

Figure 6.37 The axis in a boy aged 3 years 4 months.

transversaria, will be near to completion. The posterior bar of the transverse process extends anterolaterally from the laminar section of the neural arch element, while the more slender anterior bar is formed from a posterolateral outgrowth from the superior articular region. Between the ages of 3 and 5 years, the foramina transversaria will be completed by fusion of the anterior and posterior bars (Fig. 6.37). In this way, the medial boundary of the foramen transversarium of the axis is formed directly by the lateral border of the superior articular facet.

The dentocentral junction and the paired neurocentral junctions fuse between 4 and 6 years of age (Fig. 6.37) (Fullenlove, 1954; Rezaian, 1974; Dyck, 1978). All lines of fusion will usually disappear by 9–10 years, although a small horizontal crevice may remain for quite some time in the region of the posterior dentocentral junction, as this is generally the last region to complete fusion (Fullenlove, 1954). It is thought that this might prove to be a site of potential weakness if there is trauma to this region.

At approximately 2 years of age, a small ossific nodule (ossiculum terminale) appears in the cartilage plug (chondrum terminale) that fills the apical cleft (Gwinn and Smith, 1962; Freiberger *et al.*, 1965; Dyck, 1978). This nodule increases in size and eventually fuses with the 'v'-shaped apex of the dens at around 12 years of age (Fig. 6.35). Therefore, a forked apex to the axis is usually indicative of an age younger than 12 years. However, the ossiculum may persist as a separate ossicle in one in every 200 cases (Todd and D'Errico, 1926), when it is clinically known as 'ossiculum terminale persistens Bergmen' (Yochum and Rowe, 1987) and is generally asymptomatic. A separate bone in this situation may arise following trauma that involved stress on the apical ligament of the dens. A detailed understanding of the timing of appearance and fusion of axial elements is critical in clinical evaluations, as it is not uncommon for normal variations to be misdiagnosed as fracture sites (Cattell and Filtzer, 1965).

Odontoid abnormalities can result in biomechanical atlanto-axial instability, which can of course be fatal, so perhaps it is not surprising that there is a considerable amount of clinical research into developmental abnormalities and the effects of trauma in this region (Burke and Harris, 1989).

The traditional view of the odontoid process is that it represents the displaced centrum for the first cervical vertebra (MacAlister, 1868; Moreno *et al.*, 1982). However, this is certainly too simplistic a viewpoint (Ganguly and Roy, 1964; Cone *et al.*, 1981; Ogden *et al.*, 1986). Jenkins (1969) found that a dens of some form or another is present in all mammals except the Cetacea. He proposed that the dens evolved as an addition to the atlas body as a means of replacing the midline atlanto-axial articular surfaces, which were lost when the mammalian atlanto-axial joint became specialized for rotational movement.

Fractures of the odontoid generally arise from impact trauma, such as severe falls or automobile accidents (Sherk *et al.*, 1978; Kaplan *et al.*, 1990). The odontoid peg rarely fractures in children under 7 years, and trauma in this age group is more likely to result in damage to the dentocentral growth plate. It is thought that if damage is not treated, then it can result in resorption of the dens, leading to either a hypoplastic dens or indeed total agenesis, which is rare (Gwinn and Smith, 1962; Fielding, 1965; Freiberger *et al.*, 1965; Yochum and Rowe, 1987; Anderson, 1988a). An odontoid fracture in a child older than 7 years frequently manifests below the level of the upper articular facet, in the position of the most recently fused dentocentral synchondrosis. This is a site of potential weakness for a considerable number of years even after fusion as the dentocentral cartilaginous disc first ossifies peripherally, leaving a cartilaginous centre that may persist even into adulthood (Williams *et al.*, 1995). This is considered to support the view that the dens is truly the displaced body of C1, as this peripheral form of fusion at the dentocentral junction is consistent with the type of fusion that occurs between the annular epiphyses of, for example, two adjacent sacral bodies. However, as will be discussed later, there is some debate as to whether or not the annular rings are indeed epiphyseal in nature.

Stillwell and Fielding (1978) and Fielding *et al.* (1980) believed that following a fracture in the dentocentral region, there may be some compromise to the blood supply at the base of the dens and a clinical condition known as 'os odontoideum' could result (Wollin, 1963). This manifests as persistent neck discomfort with pain that can be transferred to the upper limbs and between the shoulder blades, a resistance to cervical extension and in extreme cases, transient paraplegia or tetraplegia. Radiologically, this presents as a separate ossicle in the normal position of the dens that is not attached to the vertebral body of C2. This can result in extreme atlanto-axial instability with significant risk for spinal cord injury unless a halo-cast is employed. Traction of the skull in this situation is to be avoided as it can increase the instability and does not permit close juxtaposition of the odontoid fragment to the main body of the bone (Ryan and Taylor, 1984). It is thought that the dystopic position of the fragment occurs following an upward pull on the tip by the alar ligaments (Spierings and Braakman, 1984). Schuller *et al.* (1991) considered that os odontoideum could be either congenital or traumatic in origin, with the evidence for congenital aetiology arising from the identification of this condition in only a single individual suffering from Klippel-Feil syndrome (Sherk and Dawoud, 1981).

A traumatic aetiology with subsequent non-union is the more widely accepted theory (Fielding and Griffin, 1974; Hawkins *et al.*, 1976; Hukuda *et al.*, 1980). The dentocentral synchondrosis prevents vascularization of the dens by direct extension of vessels from the centrum of C2. Thus, the arterial supply to the dens is achieved via arteries that enter either in the region of the apex or from small arteries that lie just medial to the facet joints (Schiff and Parke, 1973). There is also evidence of a large contribution from the ascending pharyngeal artery (Haffajee, 1997). Thus, following a fracture at the base of the dens, the dentocentral growth plate may be damaged but the dens itself will survive as it has its own independent blood supply, although the inferior portion may be resorbed. The presence of an os odontoideum in identical twins in the absence of trauma, suggests that there may even be a genetic component to this condition (Kirlew *et al.*, 1993).

A rare congenital condition arises when the odontoid process fails to separate from the anterior arch of the atlas and becomes fused in what would be considered to be the location of the atlantal vertebral body (Hunter, 1924; Cave, 1930; Olbrantz and Bohrer, 1984). Less than 10 cases of this type have been reported in the clinical literature and the patient obviously experiences restricted rotational movement of the head, especially when the lower cervical vertebrae are fixed in position. This condition arises when normal resegmentation and failure of sclerocoele formation occurs in the caudal half of the first and cranial half of the second cervical somites, resulting in an abnormality of the synovial joint formation.

The **third** to **seventh cervical vertebrae** develop in accordance with the general ossification pattern for any typical vertebra, as given above. Each is formed from three centres of ossification, which are all recognizable from mid-fetal life (Fig. 6.38). The neural arches are the first to show evidence of ossification, appearing at the end of the second fetal month and they are characterized by the presence of the developing foramen transversarium, which will not be complete until 3–4 years of age. The centra commence ossification a little later, appearing in C7 at the beginning of the third month and finally reaching C3 certainly by the beginning of the fourth fetal month (Noback, 1944; Noback and Robertson, 1951). They have a flat inferior surface, which may even tend towards being slightly convex, while the superior surface is flat posteriorly but slopes downwards anteriorly (Fig. 6.38). Thus, the superior surface has a smaller horizontal area than the inferior surface and the whole structure is wedge-shaped anteriorly (note the different appearance of the C2 centrum). At birth each

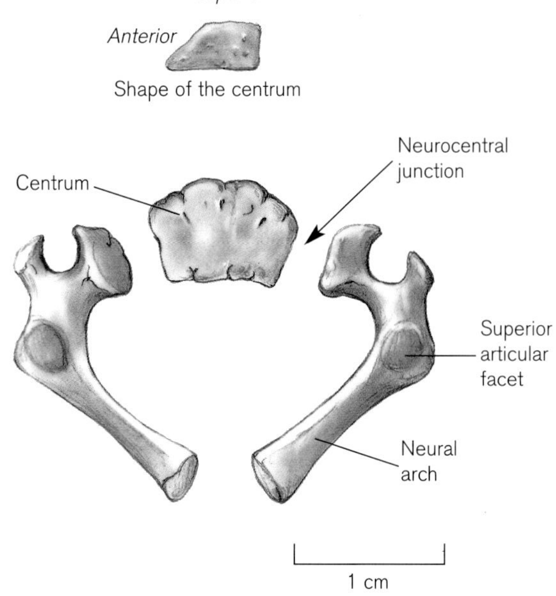

Figure 6.38 The morphology of a typical perinatal cervical vertebra.

cervical vertebra is represented by three separate bony elements (Fig 6.38).

All cervical laminae unite posteriorly within the second year and neurocentral fusion is complete in the cervical segment between the ages of 3 and 4 years (Fig. 6.39). It is only once neurocentral fusion takes place that the synovial uncovertebral joints of Luschka can form on the sloping and elevated articular sides of the neural element of the vertebral body. Therefore,

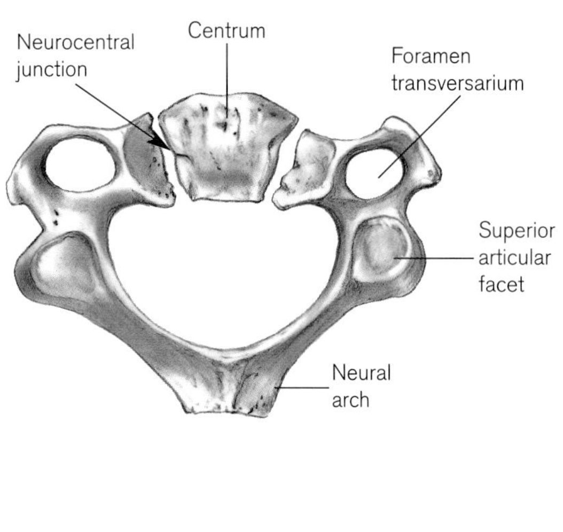

Figure 6.39 A typical cervical vertebra in a boy aged 3 years 4 months.

in the second year each cervical vertebra may be represented by two bony elements (Fig. 6.39) but by the end of the fourth year, fusion will have occurred and each vertebra will be represented by a single bony element and so close to adult morphology is achieved.

The costal processes of C7 (and sometimes C5 and C6 – Applbaum *et al.*, 1983) develop independent of the transverse processes and ossify from centres that appear around the sixth fetal month (Meyer, 1978). These centres remain independent from the vertebral column until around 4–10 years, when they generally fuse with the transverse process of the last cervical vertebra. However, there is a differential rate of growth between the costal process and the transverse process of C7 such that at an early age, the costal element may extend lateral to the transverse process (Keating and Amberg, 1954) but as the time for fusion approaches, the transverse process catches up and they become of equal length. This differential growth rate and the late fusion of the two processes have frequently resulted in clinical misdiagnoses of a cervical rib in children (Southam and Bythell, 1924; Davis and King, 1938; Weston, 1956). A true cervical rib cannot therefore be correctly diagnosed until the child is in excess of 10 years of age (Black and Scheuer, 1997). This rather late fusion may explain the phenomenon of cervical ribs being apparently more frequent in incidence in radiographs of the new born than is reflected in the incidence in the adult population as a whole (Keating and Amberg, 1954). A cervical rib may possess a definite head, neck and tubercle and the shaft can vary quite considerably in size (Turner, 1869; Dwight, 1887; Barclay-Smith, 1911; Todd, 1912). Only one-third of cases will present with clinical symptoms and the degree of development of the shaft generally dictates whether or not the rib will remain asymptomatic. Cervical ribs are generally bilateral, although symptoms are more frequently expressed on the right- than on the left-hand side (probably because of the position of the brachiocephalic trunk) and they are reported to be more common in females (Adson and Coffey, 1927). Symptoms do not generally appear until late adolescence or early adulthood, as the growth of the rib is not completed until 25 years of age. The lower trunk of the brachial plexus and the subclavian vessels are likely to be affected by the presence of a cervical rib, although it may not be discovered until the patient starts to complain of nervous or vascular disruptions. These symptoms generally include pain in the forearm and hand, muscle wastage along the C8 distribution, cyanosis, paraesthesia of the forearm and fingers, weakened radial and ulnar pulses, etc. (Kammerer, 1901; Tachdjian, 1972; Ozonoff, 1979).

Although the aetiology of cervical ribs is unknown, there is some evidence for a familial predisposition towards the condition (Southam and Bythell, 1924; Denninger, 1931; Gladstone and Wakeley, 1932a; Davis and King, 1938; Green, 1939; Purves and Wedin, 1950; Keating and Amberg, 1954; Weston, 1956; Cave, 1975).

It is generally recognized in the surgical literature that when cervical ribs are well developed, the symptoms are more commonly vascular than neurological (Ross, 1959). This is believed to result from the superior displacement of the brachial plexus by one segment (prefixed plexus) so that there is limited neurological compression on the lower cervical spinal nerves. However, arterial compression with a concomitant poststenotic dilatation is much more common in this situation, due to the position of the cervical rib in relation to the subclavian artery.

Smaller cervical ribs tend to be attached to the first thoracic rib by a fibrous band that fuses with the scalene tubercle on the superior surface of the latter rib. The presence of this restrictive band generally causes compression on the lower trunk of the brachial plexus, but rarely causes any vascular complications (Ross, 1959). Larger cervical ribs can either articulate with the cartilage of the first thoracic rib or in rare cases extend as far anteriorly as the manubrium. In this location, the subclavian artery is forced to pass over the site of the articulation, where it may be further compressed by the attachments of the scalenus anterior muscle (Patterson, 1935). Symptoms are most effectively alleviated by resection of the cervical rib and the first reported operation for this procedure was in St Bartholemew's Hospital, London in 1861 (Coote, 1861). Tenotomy of the scalenus anterior muscle has also been undertaken, but in the case of larger cervical ribs, with limited success (Davis and King, 1938).

Interestingly, some texts state that the presence of cervical ribs is atavistic, as there is an evolutionary trend towards the reduction in the total number of ribs (Tredgold, 1897; Jones, 1913). The evidence for this seems to rest on the fact that animals that develop limb buds require greater mobility in the region of the girdles and that the presence of cervical ribs in this location would be intrusive. In more recently evolved mammal groups, the limb buds tend to cover several vertebral segments and nerves from these segments grow outward at approximately right angles to the vertebral column and into the developing buds. As the column grows in length and the position of the root of the limb buds remains static, the nerves are forced to adopt an oblique course to reach the developing limbs. It is here that a conflict is said to arise between the nerves and the developing ribs. Large nerve trunks that press on comparatively small ribs will impede their growth and stunt them so that they ultimately merge with the transverse processes of the vertebrae. Therefore, the degree of development of the cervical rib depends on the nature of the obstruction in its path and if the brachial plexus is prefixed (i.e. comes off one segment higher), then it is free to develop and grow as it would in more primitive animal groups (Davis and King, 1938). In this way there are few neurological complications, but due to the involvement of the subclavian artery more anteriorly, vascular symptoms may arise. If this is true, then it is difficult to interpret the finding that cervical ribs are more common in man than in any of the apes (Aiello and Dean, 1990).

Elongated anterior tubercles at the C5–6 levels have been found concomitant with a narrowing of the disc space and deformity of the vertebral bodies and it has been suggested that elongation of the anterior tubercles may be indicative of incomplete segmentation of this specific region of the column. This hypertrophy of the costal element of the cervical vertebra has been likened to the development of cervical ribs and although the incidence of this condition is not common, it is sufficiently important to note in clinical situations as it can be misdiagnosed as a pathological finding such as osteochondroma, avulsion fracture or paravertebral calcification (Lapayowker, 1960; Applbaum *et al.*, 1983).

All **thoracic vertebrae** develop in accordance with the general ossification pattern for any typical vertebra, as given above. The centres of ossification are present in each of the three primary elements by the end of the third month of intra-uterine life and are identifiable by the end of the fourth fetal month. The centres for the neural arches of the first two thoracic vertebrae are first to appear in week 8 and by the end of week 10 an ossification centre is present in each half arch of the thoracic segment (O'Rahilly *et al.*, 1990b). The ossification centres for the centra appear during week 9 in the mid- to lower thoracic region and by the end of week 10, each centrum of the thoracic segment will show ossification. Thus, in the upper regions of the thoracic column, the ossification centres for the neural arches are the first to appear, while in the mid- to lower thoracic levels ossification commences in the centra prior to that in the arches (Flecker, 1932a; Noback, 1944; Noback and Robertson, 1951; Birkner, 1978). The costal elements elongate and extend around the thoracic region as ribs and these will be considered in detail in Chapter 7. It is sufficient to say at this stage that the costal elements of the thoracic segment commence ossification in the eighth to ninth fetal weeks and their development progresses independent of that in the vertebrae. At birth, each thoracic vertebra is represented by three bony masses (Fig. 6.27).

The laminae unite posteriorly within the first and often into the second year of life, with the lower thoracic usually the first to show union. Neurocentral fusion commences in the lower thoracic region in the third and fourth years and will be completed in most of the thoracic segment by the fifth and certainly the entire segment by the sixth year. Neurocentral fusion occurs anterior to the site of articulation with the ribs, as the ribs always remain associated with the neural arch component of the vertebrae and never articulate directly with the centrum (Fig. 6.27). A rare condition of persistent neurocentral synchondrosis has been reported (March, 1944). Therefore, in years 1–2, each thoracic vertebra will be represented by two bony masses and it is only from around the age of 6 years that each is represented by only a single bony structure.

The **lumbar vertebrae** develop in accordance with the general ossification pattern (Fig. 6.24) for any typical vertebra as given above, although there are reports of some rare developmental anomalies (Roche and Rowe, 1951; Stelling, 1981).

Ossification commences in the centra of the upper lumbar vertebrae in weeks 9–10 and reaches L5 by the end of the third fetal month. Ossification commences in the neural arches of the upper lumbar vertebrae in the eleventh week and reaches L5 in the fourth fetal month. Thus, it is a general rule that, in the lumbar segment of the column, the centra develop in advance of the neural arches. As with all the other presacral vertebra, the lumbar vertebrae are readily identifiable from the end of the fourth fetal month. At birth, each lumbar vertebra is represented by three bony masses.

It is reported that the synovial articular facets do not adopt their characteristic vertical position until the child starts to walk at approximately 1 year (Lanz and Wachsmut, 1982). The laminae unite towards the end of the first year in L1–L4, but fusion may not occur in L5 until the fifth year of life, if at all, as spina bifida in the last lumbar segment is not uncommon. Neurocentral fusion commences between the second and third years for L5 and fusion is generally completed in the lumbar segment by the fourth year.

There is considerable disagreement as to the ultimate fate of the true transverse process and the costal elements of the lumbar vertebrae and the degree of involvement of the accessory and mamillary processes (Jones, 1912). Fazekas and Kósa (1978) and Ogden (1979) both considered that the lumbar 'transverse process' is formed from the fusion of the true transverse process with the costal element. The former authors stated that the accessory and mamillary processes only develop around 6–8 years of age as muscle mass starts to increase. Frazer (1948) also concluded that the processes were sites of muscle attachment, with the accessory process representing the true transverse process, being the site of attachment of the longissimus thoracis muscle. He concluded that the mamillary process was a site of attachment for the multifidus muscle and that the 'transverse process' was predominantly costal in origin. Last (1973) agreed that the 'transverse process' was costal in origin, but stated that the true transverse process was represented by a small mass of bone that is grooved by the posterior ramus of the lumbar spinal nerve and that the mamillary and accessory processes belonged to this true process. Whatever the actual origin of the lumbar transverse process, it does not start to develop and become visibly detectable until the end of the first and the beginning of the second year of life.

Lumbar ribs are most commonly associated with the first lumbar vertebra (Lanier, 1944), are less frequent than cervical ribs, generally bilateral, more common in females and can result in considerable discomfort in the region of the lower back (Decker, 1915; Steiner, 1943).

The ossification pattern in the **sacrum** is complex as it develops from approximately 21 separate primary centres of ossification (Fig. 6.40). Each of the five sacral segments is represented by the usual three primary centres seen in all other vertebrae, but in addition, the first to third, and sometimes fourth, sacral segments also incorporate paired lateral (costal) elements. These form the ventral aspect of the alae or wings of the sacrum and are the site of articulation with the auricular surface of the innominate bone at the sacro-iliac joint (Fig. 6.40b). Sacra from individuals younger that 4 fetal months are said to be straight, with the natural concavity of the bone not developing until after this age. The sacrum is said to alter shape again when the individual starts to adopt upright posture and commence walking as the promontory is forced downwards and forwards, thereby also altering the shape of the pelvic inlet (Morton, 1942a).

In the third month of fetal life, ossification centres appear in the first and second sacral centra (Francis, 1951). By the fourth month, ossification is evident in the centra of the third and fourth sacral segments and in the neural arches of S1–3. By the fifth month, ossification occurs in the centrum of S5 and in the neural arches of S4–5. The paired costal elements of S1–3 appear between fetal months 6 and 8. Thus, all primary centres are generally present by birth, although some may be represented by no more than

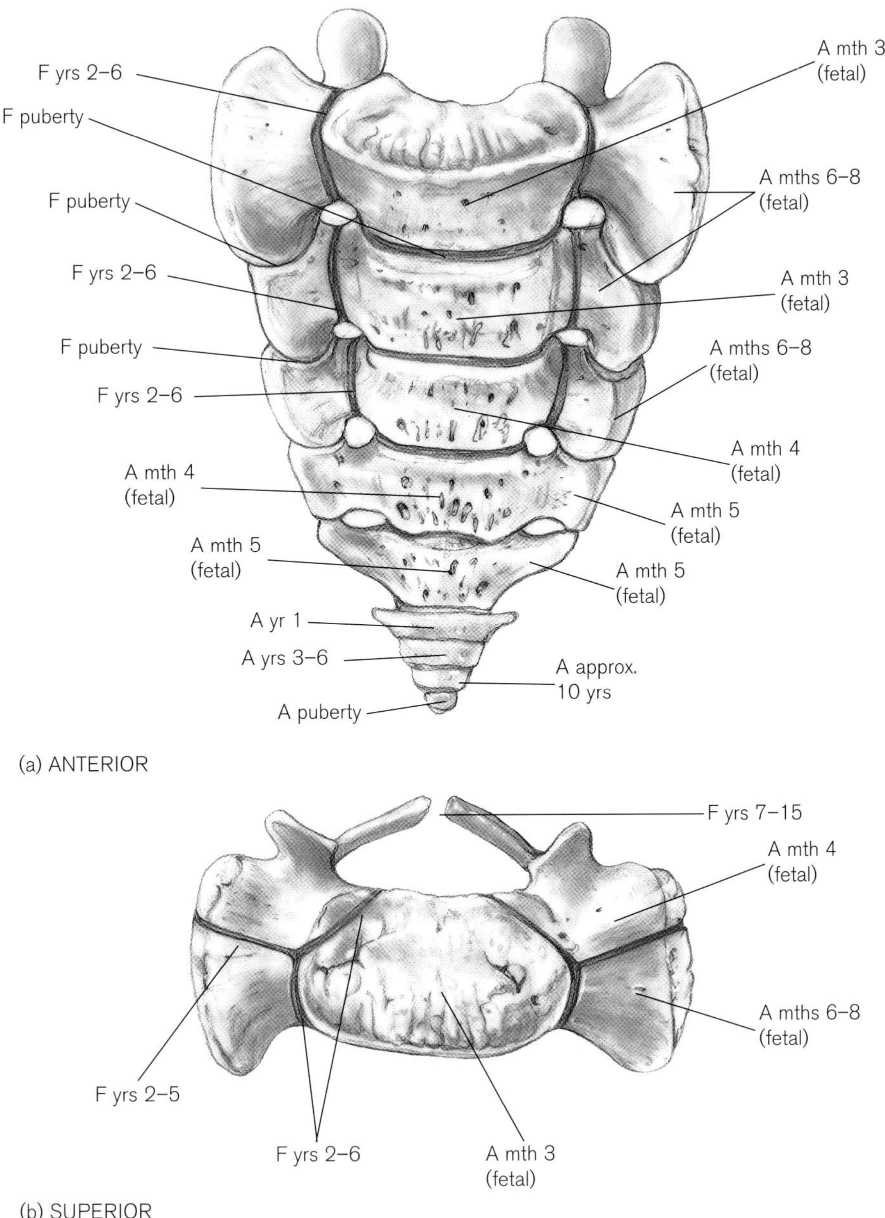

Figure 6.40 The times of appearance (A) and fusion (F) for the primary ossification centres of the sacrum and coccyx.

a small ossific nodule. Therefore, each element of the sacrum only becomes recognizable in isolation within the first year of life (Fig. 6.41). At this stage, the laminae of S1 are gracile and short in comparison to the bulk of the remainder of the neural arch. The superior articular facets are much larger than the inferior facets, which lie at the lateral extent of the inferior border of the lamina. The remainder of the neural element is square in shape and has a billowed articular surface on its medial aspect for articulation with the centrum. On its anterior aspect is another billowed surface for articulation with the lateral element, which forms the ala or wing of the sacrum. The inferolateral border bears a small oval facet that abuts onto an identical facet on the superolateral aspect of the neural arch of the second element. The morphology of the second sacral neural arch is very similar to that of the first, although considerably reduced in size. By the time the third and fourth sacral neural arches are reached there is frequently no articulation with a lateral element and the laminae are considerably reduced in size.

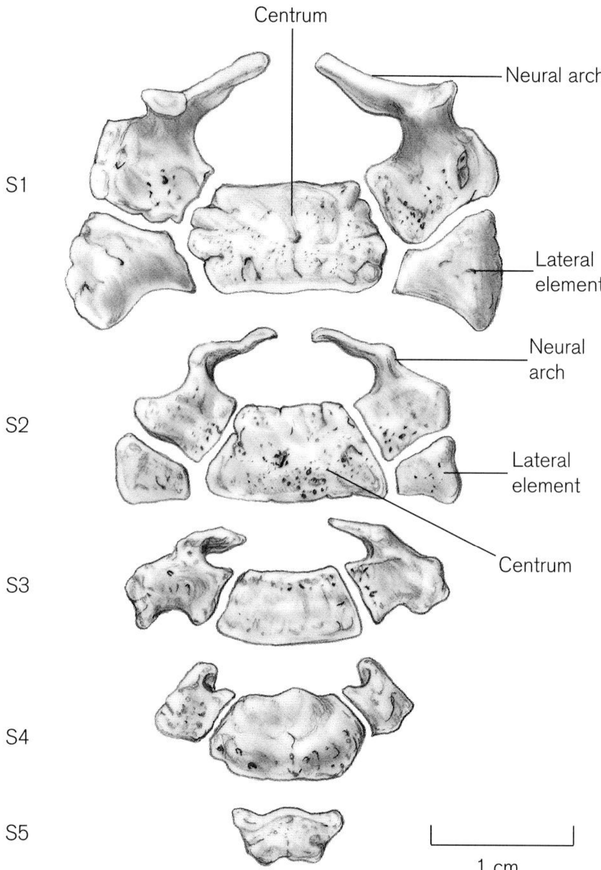

Figure 6.41 The sacral segments from a child of approximately 1 year.

The sacral centra are identifiable by their increased height and also by the concave shape of the anterior surface. The centra are wider anteriorly than posteriorly and the upper two centra show paired billowed articular surfaces on their lateral borders (Fig 6.41). Of these two surfaces, the anterior one is for articulation with the lateral/costal element and the posterior one is for articulation with the neural element. Although the centra decrease in size from above to below, the superior surface is noticeably larger than the inferior surface.

The lateral (costal) elements can only be identified with any certainty in the first two segments (Fig 6.41). If they arise at other sacral levels they often appear as little more than small spherical nodules of bone. The lateral elements are pyramidal in shape, with their apices facing medially for articulation with the centrum and their bases facing laterally to form the auricular surface of the sacro-iliac joints. The anterior surface is concave forming the identifiable curvature of the sacral alae and the inferior surface is also concave, forming the upper margin of the sacral foramen (Fig. 6.40). The posterior surface is billowed for articulation with the anterior aspect of the neural element.

The sacro-iliac joint forms in the second month of fetal life (see Chapter 10) and is not completed until the seventh fetal month (Schunke, 1938). At birth, the sacro–iliac joint resembles that of quadrupeds, being straight and parallel to the vertebral column (Abitbol, 1989). Due to the mechanical forces induced by growth, posture and locomotion, the joint curves in a caudodorsal direction to adopt the classical adult morphology (Bellamy *et al.*, 1983). At birth the surface area of the joint is said to be 1.5 cm^2, 7 cm^2 at puberty and 17.5 cm^2 in adulthood (Brooke, 1924).

Each half neural arch unites with its costal element in years 2–5, before uniting with the centrum slightly later in years 2–6. Therefore, by 6 years of age, all primary centres have fused in each sacral segment except posteriorly at the spinous processes (Fig. 6.42). The laminae fuse posteriorly between 7 and 15 years of age and each sacral segment remains separate until puberty, when the lateral elements commence fusion and secondary centres appear (Fawcett, 1907; Cleaves, 1937; Flecker, 1942; Frazer, 1948; Noback and Robertson, 1951; Birkner, 1978; Fazekas and Kósa, 1978).

O'Rahilly *et al.* (1990a) proposed that the lateral elements of the sacrum were not costal in origin, as the costal and transverse processes fused more posteriorly. They suggested that in fact the alar regions of the sacrum were new developments of bone and were restricted only to the sacrum. This is borne out to some extent by the fact that the alae of the sacrum articulate with the centra, which is a situation that does not arise in any other region of the column.

There is very little information available regarding the ossification of the **coccyx**. The consensus of opinion proposes that each coccygeal segment arises from a single centre of ossification although separate centres may be present for the cornua of the first segment (Fig. 6.40). The ossification centre for the first coccygeal body appears either towards the end of fetal life or certainly within the first year of life concomitant with the centres for the cornua (Francis, 1951). The centre for the second body appears between years 3 and 6, that for the third body around 10 years of age and that for the fourth body around puberty (Frazer, 1948; Birkner, 1978; Fazekas and Kósa, 1978; Williams *et al.*, 1995). It has been reported that the appearance of the ossification centres is later in females than in males (Frazer, 1948).

The centres for the coccyx appear as indistinct ossific nodules but it is only as puberty is approached that they will begin to adopt the final recognizable adult form.

Secondary centres

It is generally held that the typical vertebra possesses five epiphyses or secondary centres of ossification.

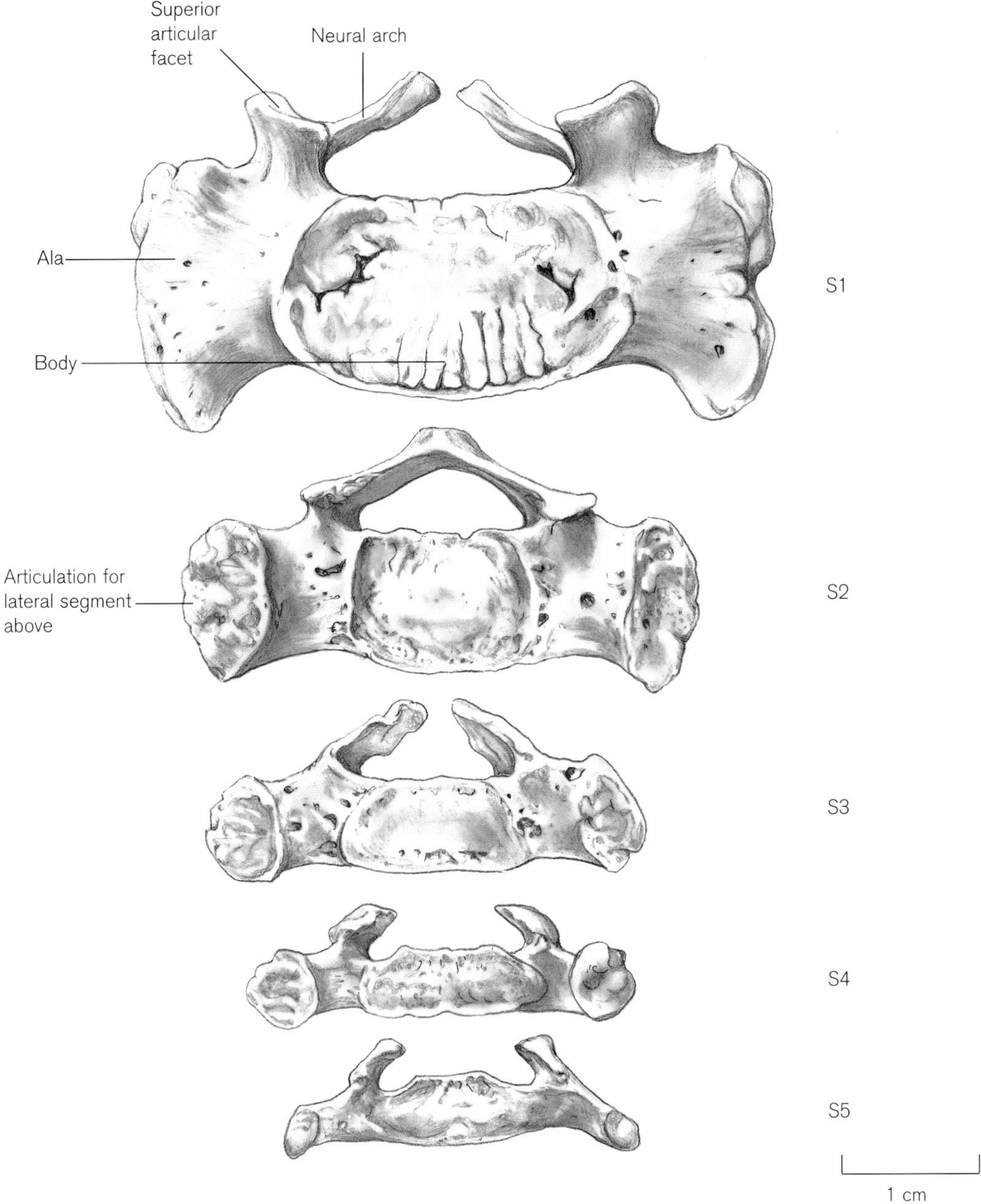

Figure 6.42 The sacral segments from a child aged between 7 and 8 years.

These occur at the tips of the transverse and spinous processes and as annular rings that cover the periphery of the superior and inferior surfaces of the vertebral bodies. Most texts concur that the secondary centres appear at the beginning of puberty (12–16 years) and finally fuse at the end of puberty (18+ years), and certainly by 24 years of age.

Hindman and Poole (1970) reported that the ossified **annular epiphyses** (which, being deficient posteriorly, are more akin to horseshoe than ring-shaped) can be detected on radiographs as early as 2–6.5 years. Both Bick and Copel (1950) and Gooding and Neuhauser (1965) have confirmed this early age of radiographic appearance, with calcification present by 6 years of age and ossification by 13 years. In fact, there is some debate as to whether or not these rings ought to be called 'epiphyses' as they may simply represent initial calcification and ultimate ossification in the vertebral end plate. They do not cover the entire surface of the vertebral body but are located only around the periphery, as their main function may be to serve as anchor points for the annulus fibrosus of the intervertebral disc (Lewin, 1929; Haas, 1939; Birkner, 1978). In most quadrupeds however, these rings cover the entire area of the endplate and display characteristic histological growth columns that clearly take an active part in the increase in height of the vertebral body (Töndury and Theiler, 1990). In a very convincing histological study of growth in the vertebral body, Bick and Copel (1950, 1951) showed that the annular rings do not take part in the active metaphyseal surface of a developing human vertebral body and so only fuse with the vertebral surface when it has completed growth in the later pubertal period. Schmorl (cited in Bick and Copel, 1950) used the term 'randleiste', meaning 'rim moulding', to describe the annular rings, and if indeed they are not epiphyseal in nature, then perhaps it is perfectly normal for them to be present in younger individuals. Interestingly, Bick and Copel found a higher frequency of early calcification of these rings in females and suggested that it may be hormonally induced. What is clear, is that the appearance of ossification in the annular rings may not be a reliable indicator of the age of skeletal material, but perhaps the age at which they fuse to the vertebral body may be considered to be more meaningful.

There is an alarming paucity of detailed information concerning secondary vertebral centres of ossification and most texts offer no more than a basic outline of the times and patterns of development and fusion. Needless to say, each region displays its own pattern of epiphyseal development and within that, certain individual vertebrae are of specific interest. From our experience, the appearance and fusion of these centres cannot be used to identify a specific age at death, but their presence does indicate a time around puberty which is in itself an extremely variable event in terms of onset, duration and cessation (Sinclair, 1978).

It is generally stated that the **typical cervical vertebra** has six epiphyses, one for the tip of each transverse process, a ring for both the superior and inferior surfaces of the body (if indeed these are epiphyses – see above) and one for each terminal ending of the bifid spinous process. Avulsion fractures of the superior rings often occur after extreme flexion of the cervical column, while avulsion of the inferior rings often follows extremes of extension (Jonsson *et al.*, 1991). It is debatable whether or not epiphyses exist for the transverse processes of C3–7 as, developmentally, they do not represent the true transverse processes but are in fact costal in origin. If epiphyses do exist they are likely to be restricted to the posterior tubercles and to be highly transitory in nature. The epiphyses for the spinous processes are small, flake-like structures that probably do not exist as separate entities but fuse directly with the process as it forms. The spinous process for C7 is different in this respect, first because it is not bifid in nature and second because the epiphysis is considerably larger and more readily identifiable than in any of the other cervical vertebrae.

The annular rings first start to fuse to the bodies in the upper cervical region and then fuse in a progressively caudal direction. The rings lie around the periphery of the body and pass upward to cover the uncinate processes. Buikstra *et al.* (1984) examined the pattern of annular epiphyseal union in 32 black females from the Terry collection. They noted that at any given age, the more cranially placed vertebrae tend to be at a more advanced stage of maturation than their more caudal counterparts. They found that union had commenced in their 17–19 year age group and that it was complete by 25 years.

The **atlas** is reported to show epiphyses at the tips of the transverse processes, but these are likely to be small, fugacious, flake-like structures, which are associated with the posterior aspect of the process.

The **axis** usually possesses five secondary ossification centres, although this rises to six if the ossiculum terminale is considered to be epiphyseal in nature. There are two flake-like epiphyses for the transverse

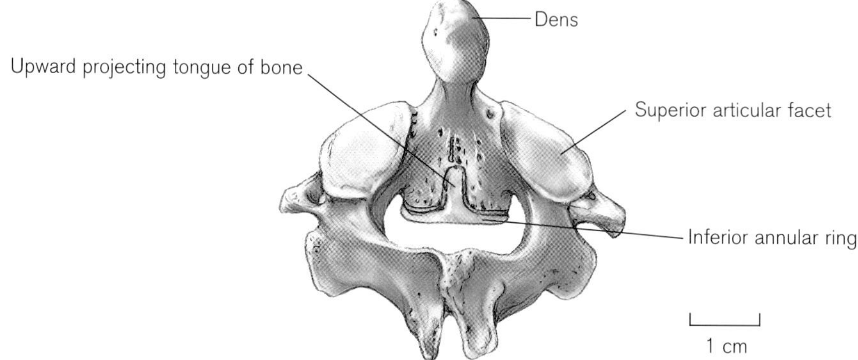

Figure 6.43 Prolongation of the inferior annular ring onto the posterior surface of the body of the axis in a female aged between 16 and 18 years.

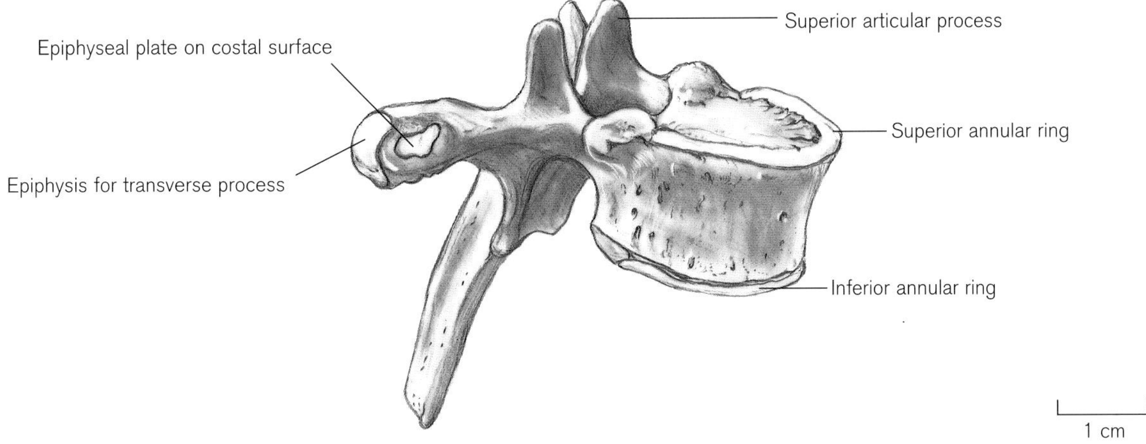

Figure 6.44 The epiphyses of the thoracic transverse process (T6) in a female aged between 16 and 18 years.

processes that probably do not exist as separate structures but fuse to the process as they form. In addition, there are two distinct plate-like epiphyses for the bifid spinous process. The inferior annular ring is the first to commence fusion in the cervical column. It can display an interesting phenomenon whereby a tongue of bone passes upwards from the posterior border of the annular ring on the posterior surface of the dens to terminate in the region of the dentocentral junction (Fig. 6.43). This does not occur on all axes but does seem to arise concomitant with a notched posterior border of the inferior surface of the axial body. To our knowledge this has not previously been reported and its phylogenetic and ontogenetic origins are uncertain.

Most reports state that each **typical thoracic vertebra** possesses five epiphyses – two annular rings, two for the tips of the transverse processes and one for the spinous process. However, in the upper regions of the column, separate epiphyseal flakes can exist for the costal articular surfaces of the transverse processes (Fig. 6.44). These are thin plates of bone and are likely to fuse as they form and never manifest as separate centres. They cover the medial costal articular surface, while the epiphysis of the lateral area that extends out onto the tip of the transverse process, arises from a separate, more clearly defined epiphysis (Fig. 6.44).

In the first seven thoracic vertebrae, the annular epiphyses commence fusion in the region of the costal demi-facet and send thin, scale-like prolongations to cover these articular surfaces (Fig 6.45a) (Dixon, 1920). In the lower thoracic vertebrae separate flakes will arise for the articular surfaces with the heads of the ribs, independent of the annular ring, as they are topographically removed from it (Fig. 6.45b). The

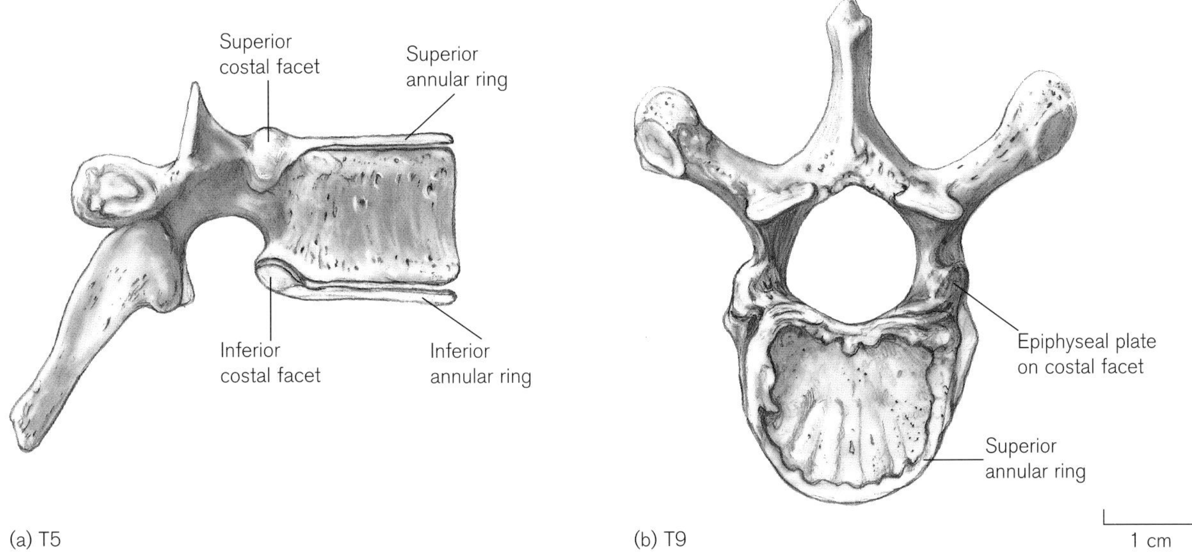

Figure 6.45 The annular epiphyses of the upper and lower thoracic region in a female aged between 16 and 18 years.

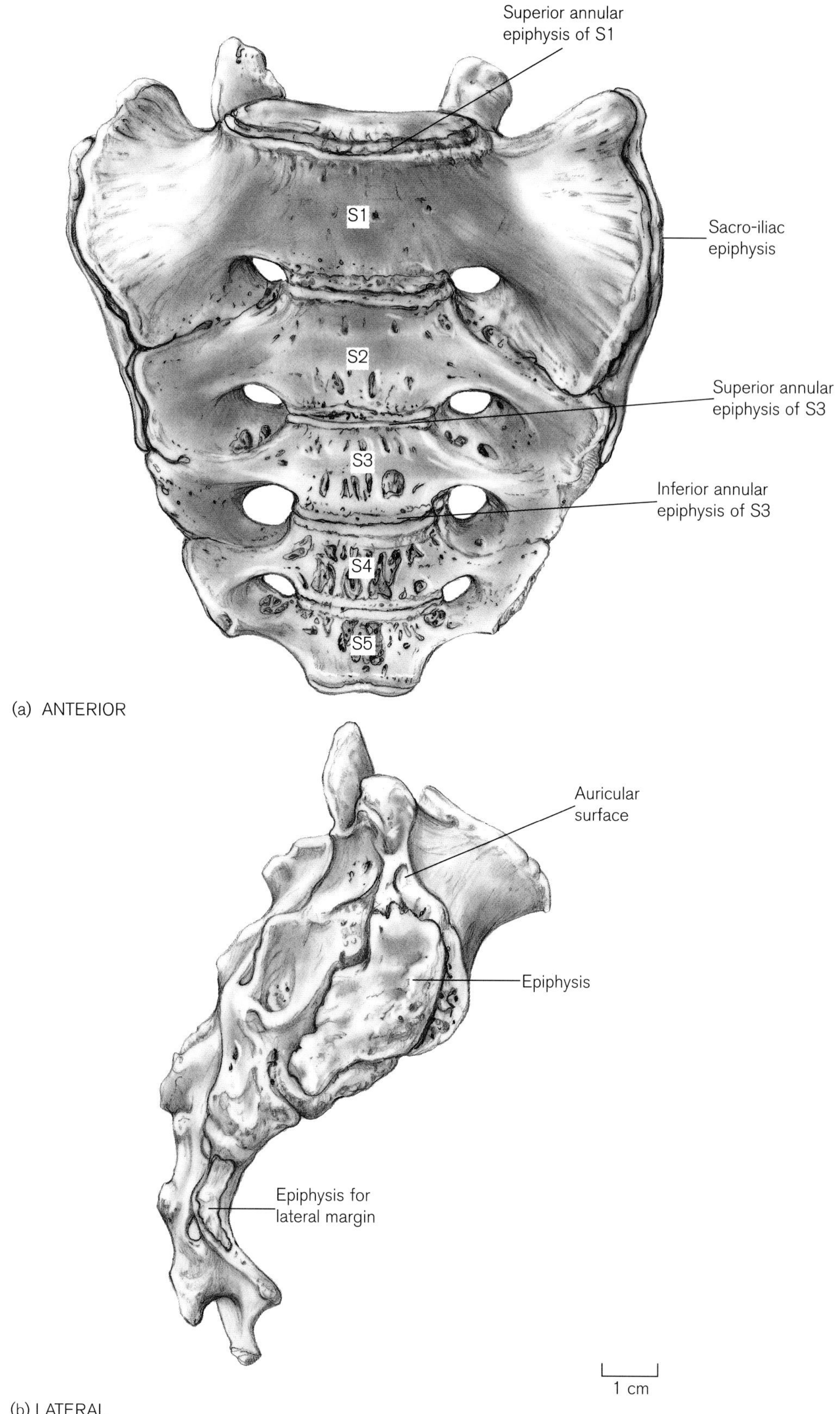

Figure 6.46 The constant epiphyses of the sacrum.

annular rings first begin to fuse at the extremities of the thoracic segment and then progressively towards the middle, so that the annular rings of T5–6 are often the last to fuse. It is only once annular fusion is complete that the crescentic depressions indicating the position of the neurocentral junctions are finally covered.

Albert and Maples (1995) examined the pattern and charted stages of union of ring epiphyses in thoracic and upper lumbar vertebrae from 55 cadavers. They identified three stages of union and separated each into an early and a late phase, thereby effectively using a six-stage process. They found that there was no evidence of epiphyseal union prior to 14 years in females and 16 years 4 months in males. The youngest female to show complete union in any vertebra was 18 years and the youngest male was 18 years 9 months. The youngest female to show complete union in all the vertebrae was 25 years and the youngest male was 24 years 2 months. Although they could not confirm any clear pattern to the sequence of union from T1 to L2, they did suggest that union might commence in the T8–12 region in advance of the T2–7 region. However, they could not uphold the finding of McKern and Stewart (1957), who suggested that T4 and T5 were always the last to complete union. Further, Albert and Maples (1995) could not identify any differences regarding the sequence of union between the superior and inferior ring epiphyses.

Only Last (1973) reported the presence of two secondary epiphyses for the mamillary processes of the last thoracic vertebra which appear in the early twenties.

Each **lumbar vertebra** is reported to have seven secondary centres of ossification – one for each mamillary process and transverse process, two annular rings and one for the spinous process. The centres for the mamillary processes are said to be the first to appear and those for the transverse and spinous processes are the last, with those for L5 appearing before those for L1. The ring epiphyses for L5 also appear and fuse before those for L1. The posterior aspect of the ring epiphyses in this region are susceptible to stress-related factors (Abel, 1985).

The number of secondary centres of ossification in the **sacrum** is not constant and it is likely that it varies between any two individuals. There are 14 constant centres (Fig. 6.46) representing ten annular rings for the five sacral bodies, two auricular epiphyses for the sacro-iliac joints and two epiphyses for the lateral margins of the sacrum below the level of the sacro-iliac joint (Fawcett, 1907; Frazer, 1948). In addition there are a number of variable elements including small, flake-like epiphyses in the position of the fused spinous processes on the median sacral crest and on the transverse processes, which are represented by the lateral sacral crest. In addition, small epiphyseal nodules can occur anywhere at the junctions between any two individual sacral vertebrae.

The lateral (costal) elements of the primary sacral centres start to fuse with each other around 12 years of age. This first occurs in the lower regions of the sacrum, with the lateral masses of S1 and S2 being the last to fuse. At this stage, the annular epiphyses have formed and they too commence fusion in a caudocranial direction (Johnston, 1961). As a general rule, if spaces can be detected between the sacral vertebral bodies, then the individual is younger than 20 years of age. If the space only occurs between S1 and S2, then the individual is likely to be younger than 27 years of age, and complete union is often not seen until 25+ years (McKern and Stewart, 1957). Spondylolysis in the sacrum is rare, as it tends to occur as a result of a stress-related fracture produced by the movement of the affected vertebra relative to the vertebra below. As the sacrum is a fixed bone, spondylolysis in this region must occur before fusion of the vertebral bodies, when there is still movement possible between adjacent, bones, i.e. in the case of S1 around the time of puberty or before (Merbs, 1996).

The epiphysis of the sacro-iliac joint generally develops from a number of ossific islands, which eventually coalesce to form a lamina of bone that covers the articular surface and projects into the demarcation lines between lateral costal elements (Fig. 6.46a). This epiphysis appears around 15–16 years of age and fuses by 18+ years (Rogers and Cleaves, 1935; Bollow *et al.*, 1997). It is probable that the epiphyses for the lateral margin follow a similar time schedule for appearance and fusion.

There do not appear to be any constant epiphyseal structures associated with the **coccyx**. However, when the coccyx becomes incorporated into the sacrum, vestiges of annular rings may occur.

Practical notes

Identification of juvenile vertebrae

Cervical vertebrae

The juvenile atlas and axis are both readily identifiable at birth and may in fact be recognizable from as early as the fourth fetal month. Similarly, the remainder of the cervical vertebrae are well-developed at birth. Their neural arches bear the characteristic foramina transversaria and the laminae are long and slender (Fig. 6.38). The centra are identifiable as they have a flat horizontal inferior surface and a superior surface that is flat posteriorly but slopes anteriorly so that they are

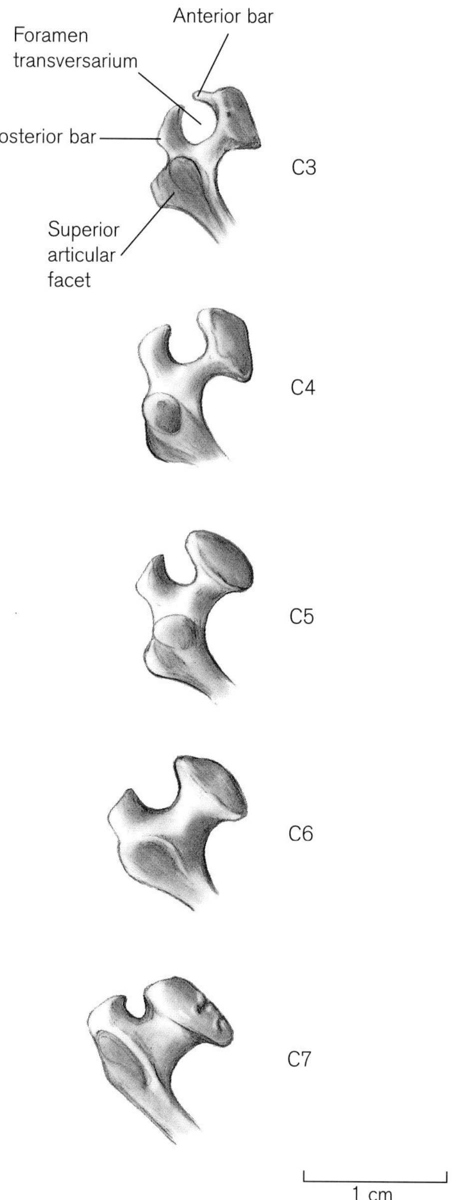

Figure 6.47 Changes in the shape of the posterior bar and foramen transversarium in the perinatal cervical neural arches.

wedge-shaped. Identification of individual centra is not possible, other than by following the premise that they increase in size as the segment is descended. However, the neural arches can be identified and this relies on the fact that as the segment is descended, the true transverse element (posterior bar) adopts a more lateral position relative to the superior articular facet (Fig. 6.47). In addition, the posterior bar increases in robusticity and becomes more square in shape in the lower cervical region. Once neurocentral fusion has occurred, identification of individual vertebrae follow the guidelines given above for the adult.

Thoracic vertebrae

Thoracic centra can be separated from cervical centra as they are more round in shape and of an even height, although the T1 centrum is essentially cervical in shape (Fig. 6.48). By T10, the transverse width of the centrum exceeds the anteroposterior dimensions and by T12, the centrum is clearly lumbar in shape, being more robust and wider in its transverse dimensions. Other than the extremes of the segment, individual identification of centra is extremely difficult and relies on all centra of the segment being present so that they can be ranked according to size and small shape alterations. Further, we have been unable to detect any differences that would allow the superior and inferior surfaces of a young juvenile centrum to be identified.

Identification of individual half thoracic arches is extremely difficult and in our opinion, only upper, middle and lower regions can be separated with any

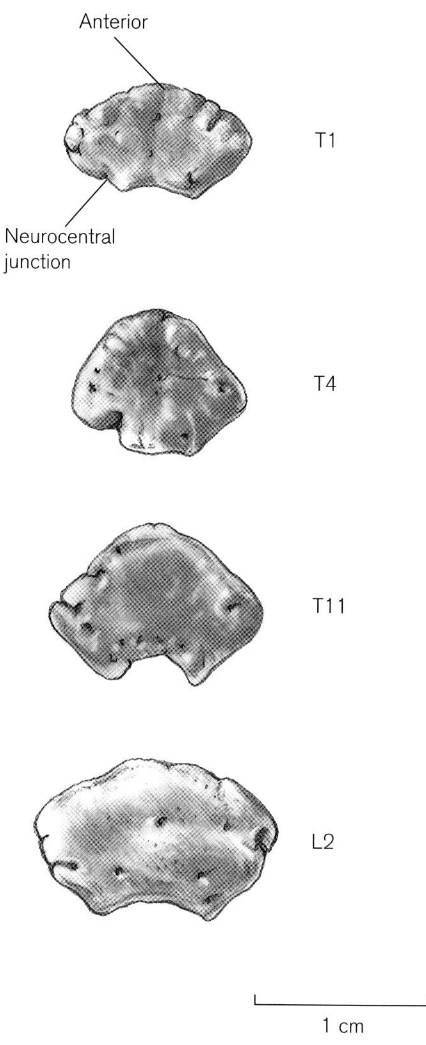

Figure 6.48 Variation in the shape of the perinatal thoracic and lumbar centra.

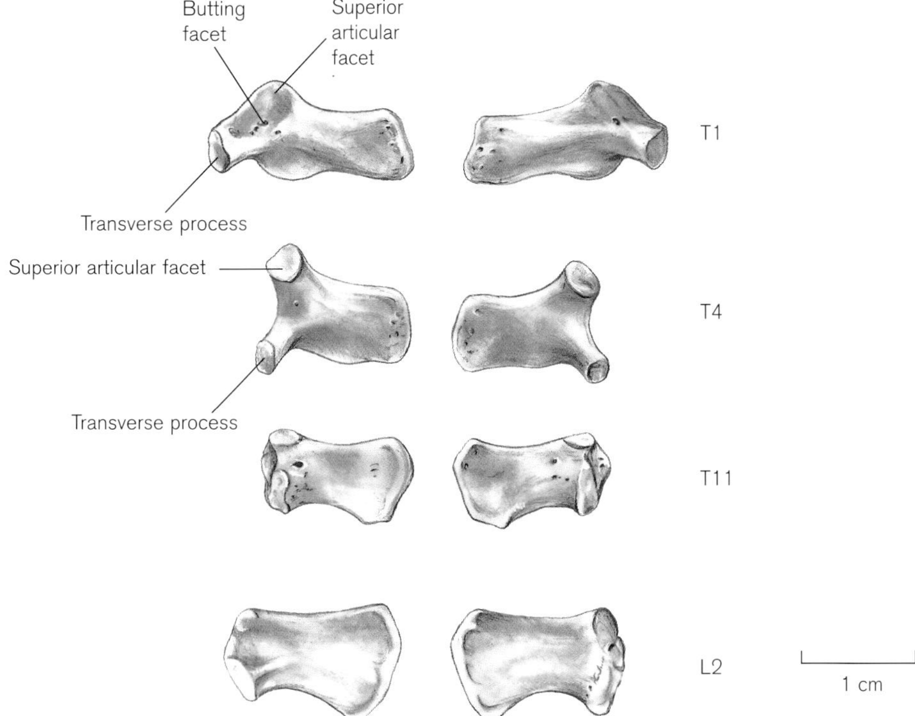

Figure 6.49 Variation in the shape of the perinatal thoracic and lumbar half neural arches.

degree of certainty (Fig. 6.49). The morphology of T1, and to a lesser extent T2, are sufficiently different from the middle, more typical, thoracic vertebrae that they can be identified with relative ease. T1 has the longest and most slender laminae of the thoracic segment and possess a well-developed butting facet associated with the superior articular facet (see above). Further, the inferior articular facets of T1 and T2 are to be found in the angle that is formed between the transverse process and the pedicle.

The middle thoracic segment comprises T3–10. These are the typical thoracic neural arches, which if viewed from above, are roughly T-shaped, with the cross bar being represented by the transverse process and the pedicle and the leg of the T being represented by the lamina. As the thoracic segment is descended, a number of changes gradually occur that allow an individual half arch to be roughly placed – the transverse processes become more robust, reduce in size and come to be more horizontally placed; the laminae become more square in shape; the superior borders of the laminae change from being sloped in the upper vertebrae to being more horizontal in the lower vertebrae; and the inferior articular facets come to adopt a more posterior position, closer to the site of the future spinous process.

The neural arches of T11 and T12 adopt a transitional morphology between that of the more typical thoracic arches above and the lumbar arches below. The transverse processes are reduced in size and may not be obvious in T12 and the laminae are more square in shape, with a more vertical posterior edge in the position of the synchondrosis. In T12, the direction and morphology of the superior articular facets is essentially thoracic in nature, while the inferior articular facets are fundamentally lumbar, indicating the transitional nature of this vertebra.

Once neurocentral fusion has occurred, then the identification of individual vertebrae essentially follows the guidelines given above for the adult.

Lumbar vertebrae

The lumbar centra can be separated from any others not only by their size and robusticity, but also because the height of the centrum is increased and the transverse diameter exceeds the anteroposterior diameter (Fig. 6.48). Only the L5 centrum can be identified with any certainty as it adopts adult morphology early in fetal life, being markedly wedge-shaped, with the anterior height exceeding the posterior height. As with the thoracic centra, we have been unable to establish any means of identifying the superior from the inferior surface.

The lumbar half neural arches can be separated from any others by the lack of transverse processes, the robusticity and virtually horizontal position of the pedicles, a reduction in size of the superior articular facets, which adopt a more posterior position, the location of the inferior articular facets on the posterior surface of the laminae close to the position of the future posterior synostosis, and the square, blade-like shape of the laminae (Fig. 6.49).

Sacral vertebrae

The upper sacral centra are readily identifiable by the presence of the paired billowed surfaces on their lateral borders for articulation with the neural arch posteriorly and the costal element anteriorly. The centra decrease in size from S1 to S5 and the superior surface has a greater area than the inferior surface (Fig. 6.41).

The neural arches of the upper sacral vertebrae are readily identifiable, due to the presence of two billowed articular surfaces, which gives the structure a club-like appearance. The anterior area is for articulation with the costal element, while the more medially located surface is for articulation with the centrum (Fig. 6.41). Once fusion of the various elements commences, identification essentially follows the guidelines given above for the adult.

It is unlikely that the **coccygeal** components of the developing column can be identified in isolation until much later in the skeletal development and so their identification is probably somewhat inconsequential.

Sideing/orientation of juvenile vertebra

Centra

Orientation of the anterior arch of the atlas is difficult, as it is essentially a square piece of bone. The anterior surface is somewhat convex, while the posterior surface is slightly concave and bears the midline atlanto-axial articulation. Identifying the superior from the inferior border is very difficult and relies heavily on being able to place the bone in its correct anatomical position to judge a 'best fit' scenario.

Orientation of the dens relies on being able to identify the slightly convex base that articulates with the centrum of C2 inferiorly and the forked appearance of the superior aspect. In addition, the intradental sulcus is most obvious on the posterior aspect. Correct orientation of the centrum of C2 is very difficult, as it is essentially a rectangular block. The superior and inferior articular surfaces are obvious, but distinguishing anterior from posterior is very difficult.

Orientation of the cervical centra relies on being able to identify the superior metaphyseal surface, which has a smaller horizontal area compared to the relatively larger inferior metaphyseal surface. In addition, the anterior aspect of the body slopes downwards, producing a wedge-shaped appearance.

We have been unable to identify any reliable means for distinguishing between the upper and lower metaphyseal surfaces of the thoracic and lumbar juvenile centra. However, the anterior and posterior aspects can always be separated, due to the convexity of the anterior margin, the concavity of the posterior margin and the more dorsally located neurocentral junctions (Fig. 6.50).

Unlike the cervical centra, the sacral centra display a relatively larger superior metaphyseal surface compared to the smaller inferior surface. In addition, the centra are always wider anteriorly and narrower posteriorly.

Neural arches

Sideing of the arches of the atlas rely on being able to identify the relatively larger superior articular facet, which is rounded from the smaller, more oval-shaped inferior facet. The posterior arch passes backwards from the articular facet.

In the axis, the laminae slope inferolaterally on their outer aspect, leaving a distinct concavity on the inner aspect at the junction between the neurocentral region and the laminae proper.

In the cervical half-neural arches, the laminae also slope inferolaterally and the superior facet faces posterolaterally, while the inferior facet slopes anteromedially. In the thoracic segment, the transverse process is always on the same aspect of the bone as the superior articular facet and it generally slopes downwards from the inferior border. The superior articular facet tends to be perched on the superior border, while the inferior facet is entirely located on the dorsal surface of the laminae. The sideing of half-lumbar arches is more difficult and relies on the fact that the superior border is more horizontal and the inferior border is somewhat hook-shaped.

For the sacral half arches, the superior articular facets are considerably larger than the inferior facets, which lie at the lateral extent of the inferior border of the lamina.

The costal elements of the sacral vertebrae are pyramidal in shape, with a concave anterior surface and a billowed posterior articular surface. The upper surface of the first is non-articular, while its lower surface is metaphyseal. Both surfaces of at least the second segment are metaphyseal in nature and so more difficult to orientate.

Bones of a similar morphology

The centra may be confused with developing sternebrae, but the latter are much thinner and at an early stage the morphology is not distinct, whereas the centra are always clearly defined. Half-neural arches can be confused with ribs because of their angulation but their size and the lack of a well-defined long shaft

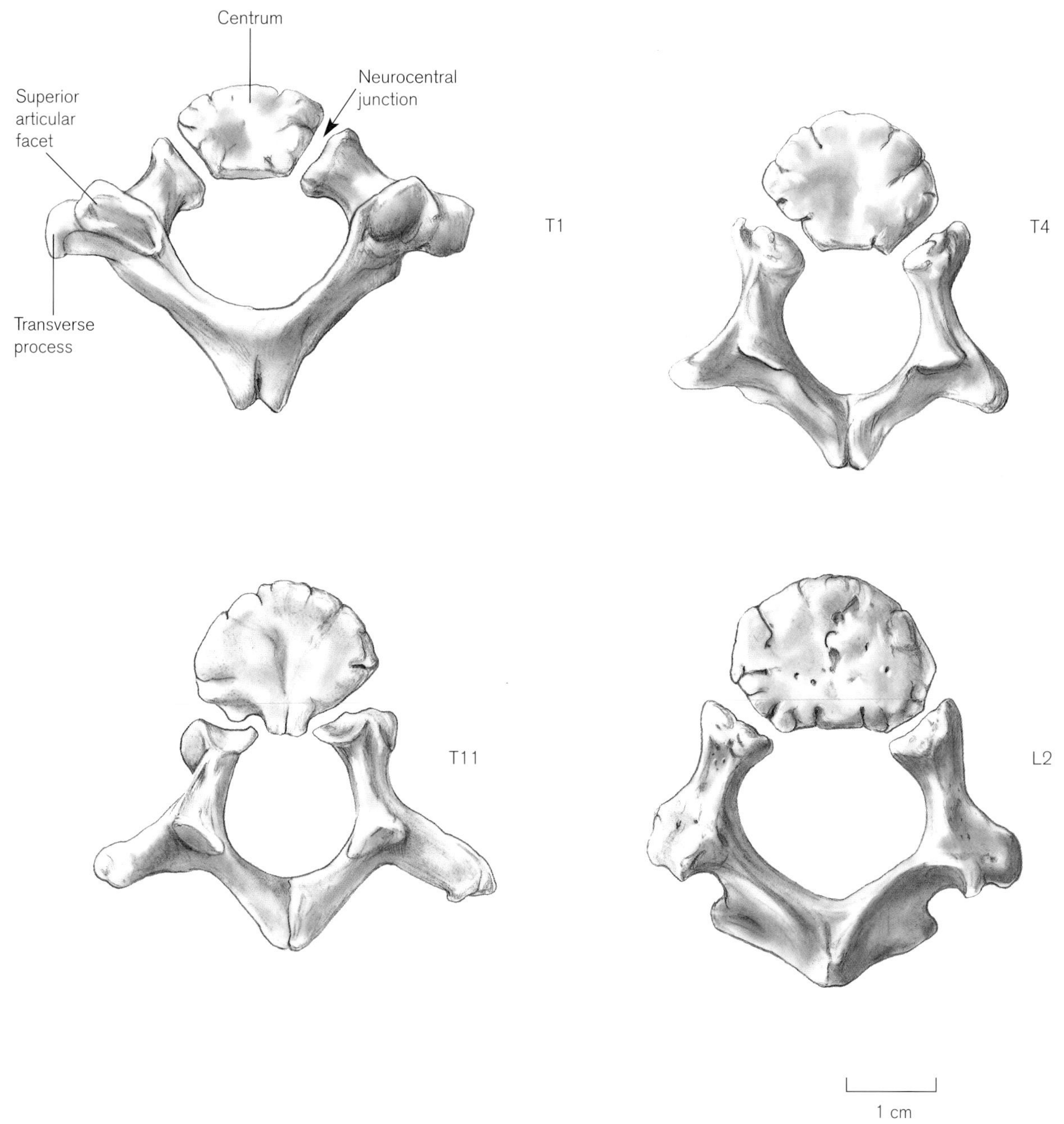

Figure 6.50 The thoracic and lumbar vertebrae in a child of between 2 and 3 years.

should remove the chances of confusion. The anterior arch of the atlas could be confused with the body of the hyoid bone (see Chapter 5), although the latter displays a more deeply scooped posterior surface.

Morphological summary

Fetal

Mth 2	Ossification centres appear for lateral masses of C1 and neural arches of C2–T2
Mth 3	Ossification centres appear for centra of C4–S2; neural arches of T3–L2; costal elements (ribs) in thoracic region
Mth 4	Ossification centres appear for centra of C2–3 and S3–4; neural arches of L3–3; paired centres for odontoid process. All primary ossification centres for the presacral vertebrae are present by this age
Mth 5	Ossification centres appear for centrum of S5 and neural arches of S4–5
Mth 6	Ossification centres appear for costal process of C7 and for lateral elements of S1–3
Mth 7	Intradental fusion
Mth 8	Ossification centres for Co1 and cornua appear

Birth All primary centres of ossification are present with the exception of the more distal coccygeal segments. Intradental fusion has occurred

1 yr Posterior fusion of the laminae commences in the thoracic and lumbar regions

2 yr Development of the anterior arch of the atlas. Ossification commences in ossiculum terminale. Fusion of posterior synchondrosis in C3–7 and complete in most thoracic and upper lumbar vertebrae. Transverse processes starting to develop in lumbar region. Annular rings may be present

3–4 yrs Foramen transversarium complete in all cervical vertebrae. Midline sulcus on posterior surface of dens filling in. Fusion of posterior synchondrosis of axis and dentoneural synchondrosis. Neurocentral fusion in C3–7, all thoracic and lumbar vertebrae. Neurocostal fusion in S1 and S2. Co2 appears

4–5 yrs Posterior fusion of the atlas. Dentocentral fusion commencing in the axis. Commencement of fusion of neurocostal elements of S1 and S2 to centra. Laminae unite in L5

5–6 yrs Neurocentral fusion in the axis. Axis complete, apart from fusion of ossiculum terminale. Costal fusion can commence in C7. Primary centres fused in all thoracic vertebrae. Primary centres fused in all lumbar vertebrae, apart from mamillary processes. Primary centres fused in all sacral segments, apart from region of posterior synchondrosis. Anterior arch of atlas fuses. Posterior fusion complete in lumbar segment. Development of unco-vertebral joints of Luschka in cervical region

6–8 yrs Mamillary processes develop in lumbar segment. Commencing fusion of posterior synchondrosis in sacrum

10 yrs Co3 appears. Continued fusion of posterior synchondrosis in sacral region. Costal fusion complete in C7

12 yrs Dens complete following fusion of ossiculum terminale. Costal elements start to fuse above and below in the sacrum

Puberty Co4 appears. All epiphyses appear. Posterior sacrum is completed

Early 20s Most epiphyses fused and column is virtually complete, except for fusion between bodies of S1 and S2

25+ yrs Column complete

Metrics

There are very few studies that have considered age-related change in the size of the components of the developing vertebral column. Most are clinical in nature and are therefore recorded from radiographs rather than dry bone (Hinck *et al.*, 1965, 1966; Locke *et al.*, 1966; Brandner, 1970). Fazekas and Kósa (1978) have examined age-related change in fetal dry bones but restricted their analysis to the maximum length of the vertebral arch of the atlas and the axis (Table 6.1).

Table 6.1 Maximum length of the fetal vertebral half arch of the atlas and the axis

	Maximum length of vertebral half arch (mm)	
Age (weeks)	Atlas	Axis
14	3.5	4.2
16	4.2	5.0
18	5.3	5.9
20	6.2	7.4
22	7.0	7.7
24	7.9	9.2
26	8.2	9.7
28	9.0	10.3
30	10.2	12.2
32	11.0	13.3
34	11.4	14.7
36	11.9	16.1
38	13.1	17.2
40	15.0	18.2

Adapted from Fazekas and Kósa (1978).

CHAPTER SEVEN

The Thorax

The thoracic skeleton is an osteo-cartilaginous framework that surrounds and protects the principal viscera of respiration and circulation. However, its primary function probably resides in its intimate involvement with the mechanism of respiration. First, the thorax offers a large surface area for muscle attachment and second its dynamics permit an active participation in altering thoracic dimensions and thus influencing internal thoracic pressure. Detailed information on the role of the thoracic cage in respiration can be found in various texts of functional anatomy (MacConaill and Basmajian, 1969: Basmajian, 1974: Williams *et al.*, 1995).

The thoracic cage comprises an anterior midline sternum, twelve thoracic vertebrae posteriorly and a lateral series of 12 pairs of ribs (Fig. 7.1). Ribs 1–10 articulate with the thoracic vertebral column behind and with the sternum in front via their costal cartilages, but the eleventh and twelfth ribs do not articulate anteriorly and are therefore termed floating ribs.

The thoracic inlet is reniform in shape and is the region where soft tissue structures pass from the neck into the thorax and vice versa. The boundaries of this inlet are the superior margin of the manubrium in front, the body of the first thoracic vertebra behind and the first ribs and their costal cartilages laterally. In life, this space is partly filled by the bilateral suprapleural membranes, which form the roof of the thoracic cavity.

The thoracic outlet is the region where soft tissue structures pass from the thorax into the abdomen and vice versa. The boundaries of the outlet are the xiphoid process anteriorly, the body of the twelfth thoracic vertebra behind and the costal (chondral) margin and lower ribs laterally. In life, this space is filled by the muscular thoracic diaphragm, which forms the floor of the thoracic cavity.

I. THE STERNUM

The adult sternum

The adult sternum is a composite structure displaying three distinct segments – a superior manubrium, a middle mesosternum (corpus or body) and an inferior xiphoid process (Figs. 7.1 and 7.2).[1] The manubrium articulates with the mesosternum via either a primary or a secondary cartilaginous joint (Smith, 1991b). These two bones do not lie in the same plane but form an angle so that their line of articulation is prominent and can be readily palpated in the living body. This junction is known as the sternal angle (angle of Louis) and marks the location of the second costal cartilages laterally. The mesosternum articulates with the xiphoid process via either a primary or a secondary cartilaginous joint which will usually synostose with advancing age. This is a relatively frail joint, which can readily fracture during excessive or sustained cardiopulmonary resuscitation.

The manubrium

The manubrium is the thickest and strongest portion of the sternum and is therefore the area that is most likely to survive inhumation. It is broad and thick along its superior margin and narrows towards its inferior articulation with the mesosternum (Jit *et al.*, 1980).

[1]The ancient anatomists likened the sternum to a sword, so that the upper portion (manubrium) reminded them of a handle and the term is derived from the Latin 'manus' meaning 'hand'. The mesosternum reminded them of the main blade of the sword and so its older name is the gladiolus which is a diminutive of the Latin 'gladius' meaning a sword, hence the origin of the term 'gladiator'. The name xiphoid is derived from the Greek 'xiphos', which also means sword-like. The combined term of 'sternum' is also derived from the Greek and refers to the breast of man but not to that of woman (Field and Harrison, 1957; Skinner, 1961; Simpson, 1969).

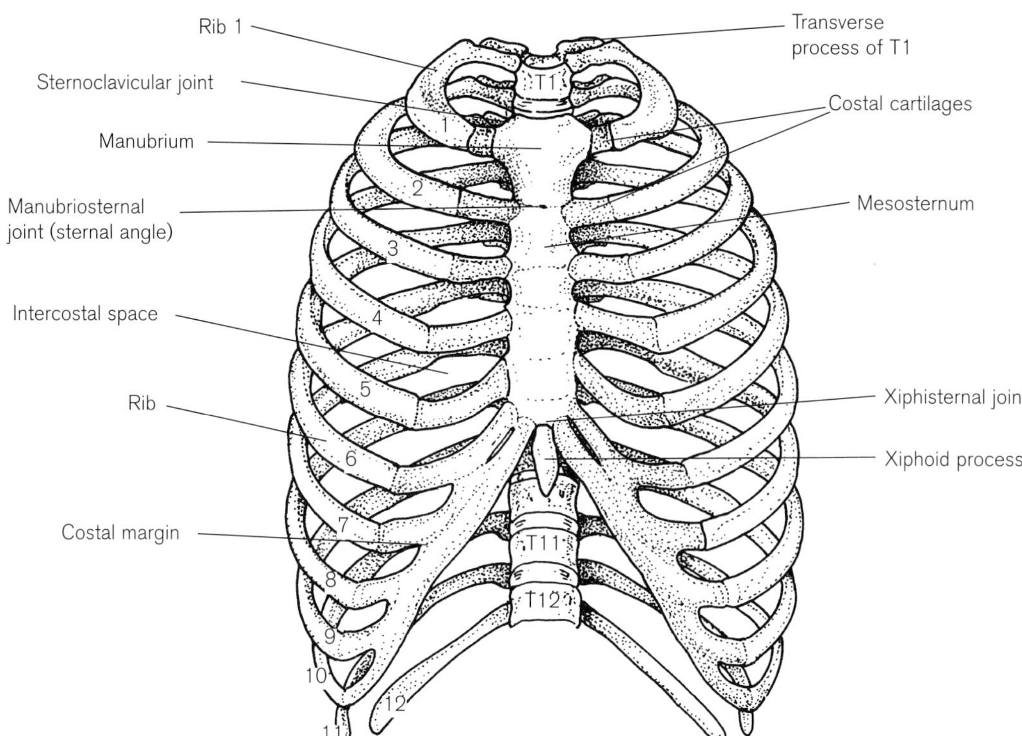

Figure 7.1 The adult thoracic skeleton.

The superior border has a central **suprasternal** (jugular) **notch** and lateral oval facets for the synovial articulation with the clavicle. Small facets may occasionally be seen on the superior border between the jugular and clavicular notches and these mark the site of articulation with the **suprasternal ossicles** (Fig. 7.3) (Carwardine, 1893; Cobb, 1937; Moore *et al.*, 1988). The presence of these ossicles is very variable and they are generally considered to be phylogenetic remnants of the epicoracoids of other mammals, although Gladstone and Wakeley (1932b) suggested that they may represent the sternal segments of cervical ribs.

The lateral borders of the manubrium are each marked by a depression for the articulation with the first costal cartilage above (a primary cartilaginous joint) and a small demi-facet for articulation with the upper half of the second costal cartilage below (a synovial joint). The anterior surface is relatively smooth, convex from side to side and somewhat concave from above to below. It displays two ill-defined lateral hollows below the clavicular level, from which the pectoralis major muscles arise. The vertical slightly raised area between these hollows forms a 'T'-shaped ridge with a transverse thickening that extends between the clavicular facets. Thus, the thickest part of the manubrium is that region extending between the clavicles that serves to withstand the transmission of forces from the upper appendicular to the axial skeleton. The sternocleidomastoid muscles arise from the front of the manubrium, superior to the attachment for the pectoral muscles. Both the sternohyoid and sternothyroid muscles take their attachment from the posterior surface, which is relatively featureless and concave both from side to side and from above to below.

In the living, the manubrium is to be found at the level of the third and fourth thoracic vertebrae and forms the anterior boundary of the superior mediastinum. The immediate relations of the upper part are therefore the thymus, left brachiocephalic vein and the brachiocephalic, left common carotid and left subclavian arteries, while its lower part is closely related to the arch of the aorta. Due to its close association with the major arteries, the manubrium can bear some evidence of arterial pathologies such as aneurysms (Kelley, 1979a; Ortner and Putschar, 1985). The lateral boundaries of the manubrium come into direct contact with the parietal pleurae (Fig. 7.2b). It is interesting to note that at birth, the superior margin of the manubrium lies opposite the body of the second thoracic vertebra and so it is one to one-and-a-half vertebral levels higher than its final adult position (Crelin, 1973).

Fractures of the manubrium are relatively rare (0.5% incidence) and most commonly arise following

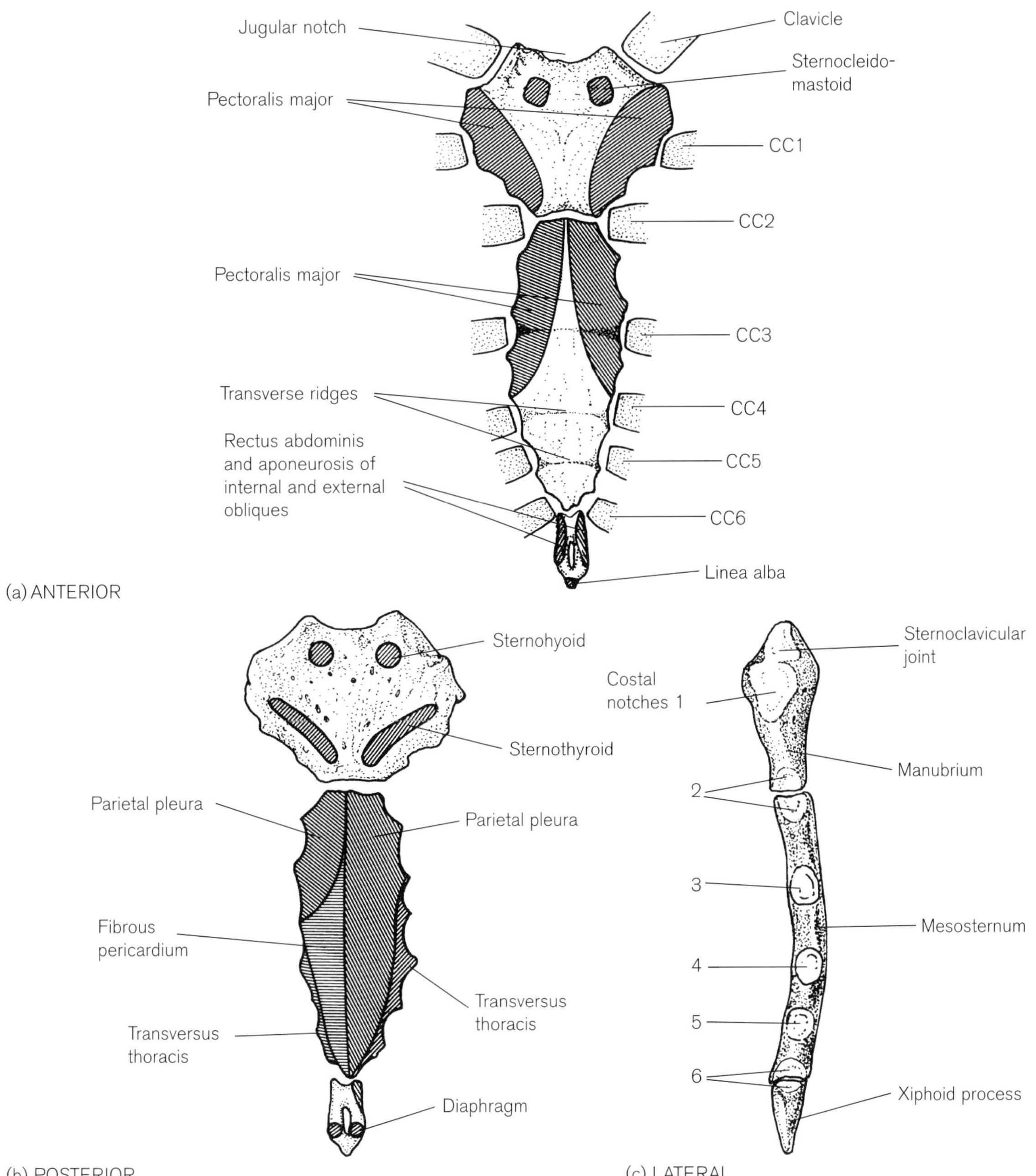

Figure 7.2 The adult sternum.

direct violence. There is no doubt that prior to the compulsory introduction of car seat belts in the UK, manubrial fractures following impact with the steering wheel were more common (Helal, 1964). In cases of indirect violence, e.g. falling onto the head or neck, the type and location of sternal injury is dependent upon the form of the manubriosternal joint (see below). As the manubrium is forced backwards with flexion of the vertebral column, there is a sudden rise in intra-thoracic pressure, which forces the lower sternum upwards and forwards. With the presence of a moveable manubriosternal joint, dislocation is the most common outcome; however, if the joint has synostosed, then fracture tends to occur in the lower regions of the body of the sternum (Stuck, 1933; Fowler, 1957).

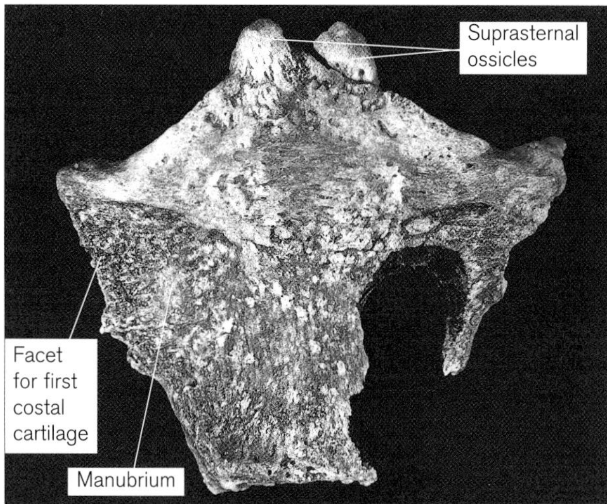

Figure 7.3 Suprasternal ossicles in a female of 65 years. Note that the right ossicle has fused with the manubrium although the left is only partly fused posteriorly but is open anteriorly.

The mesosternum

The mesosternum is longer, thinner and narrower than the manubrium. Its anterior surface is virtually flat but is frequently marked by three transverse ridges indicating the site of fusion of individual juvenile sternebrae (Fig. 7.2). The superior surface is oval for articulation with the manubrium, while the lower end is somewhat pointed and often continuous with the xiphoid process (Hatfield *et al.*, 1984). The lateral border has a small notch at its superior extremity for articulation with the lower half of the second costal cartilage. Below this, at least four costal notches mark the site of articulation between the body of the sternum and costal cartilages 3–6 (costal cartilages 7 and 8 occasionally articulate directly with the sternum) (Cunningham, 1890). Each of these joints is synovial in nature. The inferior extremity of the lateral border of the mesosternum bears a small demi-facet for articulation with the upper half of the costal margin. Ribs 6–8 are somewhat transitional in nature in that they may be classified as either vertebrosternal or vertebrochondral ribs, depending upon whether the costal cartilage of that rib articulates directly with the sternum or via the chondral margin. This pattern of articulation will dictate the number and position of costal notches on the lateral border of the mesosternum and considerable variation is often seen in the lower third of the mesosternum (Watts, 1990).

In the living, the body of the adult sternum lies opposite the fifth to ninth thoracic vertebrae and forms the anterior boundary of the inferior mediastinum. Its anterior surface gives rise to the pectoralis major muscles and its borders give attachment to the external intercostal membranes from the ridges between the costal notches. The posterior surface is in close contact with the parietal pleurae on either side and on the left with the fibrous pericardium surrounding the heart (Fig. 7.2). In addition, the transversus thoracis muscle arises from the lateral borders of the posterior surface.

The mesosternum is constructed from two plates of cortical bone, separated by a trabecular cavity that contains red marrow and is haemopoietic in nature. The subcutaneous nature of the mesosternum makes it an ideal site for biopsy and a sample of bone marrow can be readily aspirated via sternal puncture when a wide-bore needle is inserted through the cortex into the marrow cavity. It is perhaps not surprising, therefore, to find that the posterior surface of the mesosternum (and often the manubrium too) is a common site for haematogenous metastases (Walther, 1948; Steinbock, 1976).

The mesosternum does not readily fracture (except in old age) but when it does, it its usually as a result of impact trauma and presents as a comminuted fracture just distal to the manubriosternal joint. Atraumatic fractures have been reported in the elderly following calcification in the costal cartilages associated with a thoracic kyphosis (Sapherson and Mitchell, 1990).

The xiphoid process

This is morphologically the most variable component of the sternum and is frequently cartilaginous, even into advanced age. It is also known, but not so commonly, as the ensiform process, which is derived from the Latin meaning 'a little sword', metasternum, processus xiphoideus or xiphisternum. The xiphoid process may be broad, narrow, bifid, pointed, perforated, curved or deviated to one side and usually becomes continuous with the lower border of the mesosternum in advancing years. At the superior angle of the lateral border of the xiphoid process there is a small demi-facet for articulation with the lower half of the costal margin. The rectus abdominis muscles and the aponeuroses of the external and internal oblique muscles are attached to the anterior surface of the xiphoid process while its inferior extremity gives attachment to the linea alba and the aponeuroses of the internal oblique and transversus abdominis muscles. The posterior aspect gives origin to two anterior muscular slips of the thoracic diaphragm.[2]

[2]The xiphoid process lies in close approximation to the anterior surface of the liver and it is not uncommon for middle-aged patients to consult their general practitioners with a suspicious 'lump' that is always feared to be more sinister than simply ossification of the xiphoid process.

Maldevelopment in the sternal region results in two well-documented clinical conditions (Meschan, 1975; Ozonoff, 1979; Yochum and Rowe, 1987). Pectus excavatum or 'funnel chest' is a rare congenital condition where the lower part of the sternum is displaced posteriorly and the xiphoid process projects forwards. In some cases, the mesosternum may be displaced so far posteriorly that it almost makes contact with the vertebral column. This results in a gross displacement of the heart and impinges on the pleural cavities and, of course impairs respiratory performance. Therefore two of the symptoms to accompany this abnormality are shortness of breath (dyspnoea) and cyanosis. The second well-documented maldevelopment in this region arises usually as a result of rickets and is called pectus carinatum or 'pigeon chest'. In this case, the sternum projects forwards while the lateral regions of the chest are flattened, resulting in a keel-like condition. Pigeon chest can also arise from premature obliteration of the joints between the individual sternebrae in the child (see below).

Early development of the sternum

The sternum was originally considered to be an embryological derivative of the mesenchymal somite arrangement that gives rise to the vertebral column, ribs, intercostal and anterior abdominal musculature. However, it was clearly shown by Chen (1952a, 1952b, 1953) in mice and Seno (1961) in chicks, that the sternum is in fact developed from the same lateral somatopleuric mesenchyme that gives rise to the pectoral muscles and so is fundamentally of appendicular rather than axial derivation. The bilateral mesenchymal precursors of the sternum develop immediately ventral to the primordia for the clavicle and ribs but are in fact independent from them in their development (Gumpel-Pinot, 1984). The line of division between the somite-derived structures and the lateral plate mesodermal structures is the future chondro–sternal junction (Ogden *et al.*, 1979a).

At approximately 6 weeks of fetal life a pair of **lateral sternal plates** can be identified embedded in the anterior chest wall, which are independent of both each other and the developing ribs (Fig. 7.4). These mesenchymal plates first become associated with the upper six or seven ribs on each side and eventually fuse to their anterior extremities. Similar condensations then appear and connect the anterior ends of ribs 8–10, which eventually fuse with that of the seventh rib above. As the ribs increase in length, so the sternal plates migrate medially towards each other and it is then that chondrification commences. Around the ninth fetal week, the sternal plates begin to fuse with each other in the midline and do so in a cranio–caudal direction (Ogden, 1979: England, 1990). These plates should only fuse once the heart has descended into the thorax and a failure of fusion results in the clinical condition of ectopia cordis, where the heart is exposed to the exterior. A rare condition of cleft sternum is strongly associated with ectopia cordis (Chang and Davis, 1961; Moore, 1988) and, not surprisingly, there is a strong correlation between developmental abnormalities in this region and congenital heart defects in general (Fischer *et al.*, 1973; Lees and Caldicott, 1975).

Three mesenchymal masses appear at the superior extremity of the lateral plates around 6 weeks of fetal life. The **presternal mass** (median sternal anlage) lies inferior to the paired **suprasternal masses** and will

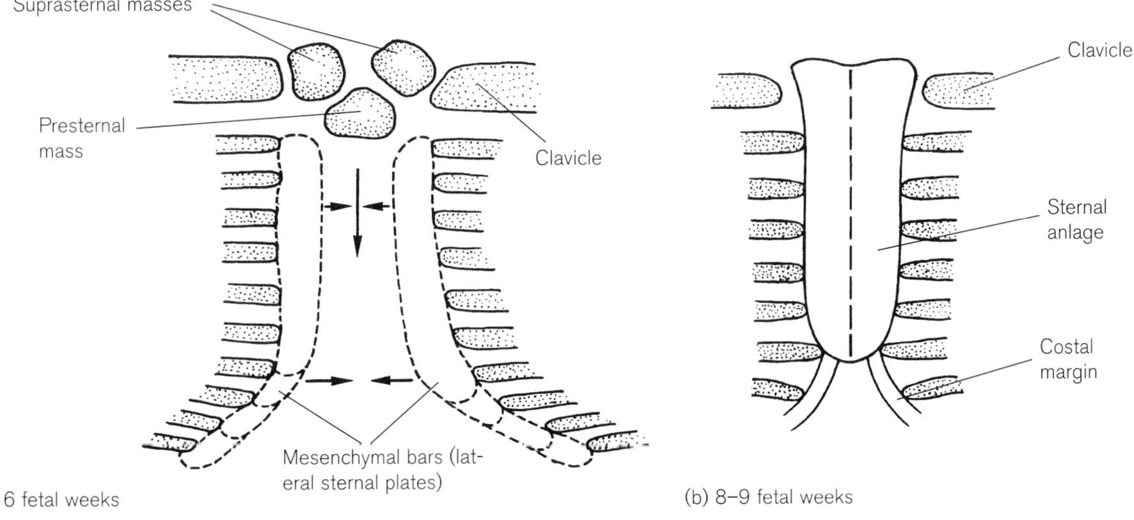

Figure 7.4 A diagrammatic representation of the embryological development of the sternum (redrawn after Larsen, 1993).

eventually fuse with all but the most lateral part of the suprasternal section to form the upper part of the manubrium, while the remainder of the two lateral masses take part in the formation of the sternoclavicular joint (Whitehead and Waddell, 1911; Jewett *et al.*, 1962; Klima, 1968; Eijgelaar and Bijtel, 1970). The pre sternal mass appears later than the lateral sternal plates and it is thought to be embryologically derived from the pectoral girdle (Currarino and Silverman, 1958).

Ossification

In the cartilaginous state, the sternum is a continuous non-segmented structure (Fig. 7.4b). However, once ossification commences, this ceases to be the case and the future development is a reflection of true metamerism. The ribs are segmental structures and their influence has been shown to be directly responsible for the relatively late ontogenetic segmentation of the sternum. Removal of the rib anlage in the experimental condition, results in the development of a non-segmental sternum (Chen, 1952b). It has been suggested that the tips of the ribs inhibit the spread of chondroblastic proliferation to the adjacent cartilage of the sternum and therefore the cartilage remains relatively immature in these locations and so is resistant to ossification (Currarino and Silverman, 1958). Premature synostosis is rare at these junctions but it can be detected as early as 6 months *postpartum* and results in a pigeon chest deformity.

The segmentation of the sternum may arise as a result of the high magnitude of compressive hydrostatic stress in the regions of the developing sternum adjacent to the costal facets. These stresses have been shown to slow the process of endochondral ossification so that the initial zones of bone formation occur away from these areas in the intercostal regions of the developing sternum (Wong and Carter, 1988).

It is generally agreed that ossification commences in the sternum once sternal bar fusion has begun. As union takes place in a craniocaudal direction, so the appearance of the centres of ossification also occurs in this direction. Should ossification commence before plate fusion has fully taken place, then two centres of ossification may result, one in each bar remnant.

Primary centres

The primary centre of ossification for the manubrium is generally the first to develop and this occurs within the fifth fetal month (Paterson, 1904; Flecker, 1932a; Noback and Robertson, 1951; Last, 1973; Fazekas and Kósa, 1978; Ogden, 1979; England, 1990). It is not uncommon for the manubrium to develop from more than one centre of ossification,

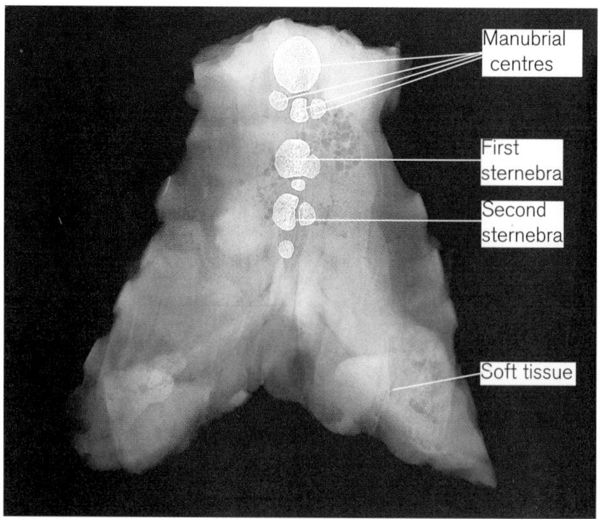

Figure 7.5 Radiograph of the sternal plate from a male aged 9 months (*postpartum*). Note the multiple centres for the developing manubrium and the irregular morphology of the centres in the mesosternum.

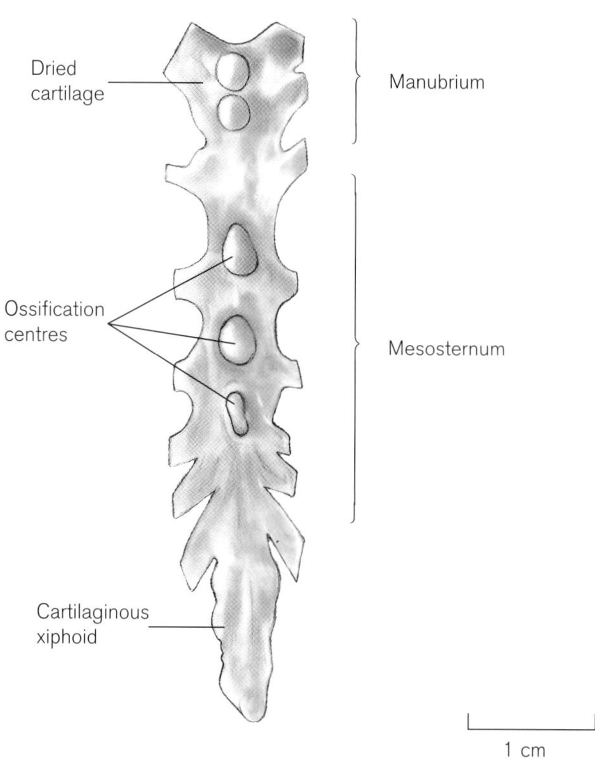

Figure 7.6 The ossification centres of the sternum at 8 fetal months.

although there is generally one major centre and a variable number of smaller centres (Ashley, 1956a; Smith, 1991b). These centres will, however, quickly coalesce to form one major centre (Fig. 7.5). Currarino and Swanson (1964) found that the manubrium developed from two centres, one above the other, in 90% of children suffering from Down's syndrome.

In the early stages of development, the manubrium is difficult to identify as it is represented by little more than small, undifferentiated bone nodules (Fig. 7.6). However, by approximately 6 months *postpartum* it starts to adopt a more recognizable appearance, with relatively flat anterior and posterior surfaces, straight sides for the first costal cartilage articulation and a small oval facet inferiorly for the manubriosternal joint (Fig. 7.7).

The mesosternum ossifies from a variable number of ossification centres. As a rule, either a single or multiple centres will arise in the area of the cartilaginous mesosternum, at regular intervals between the sites of costal cartilage attachment. Ashley (1956b) suggested that the variability in the pattern of fusion indicated that the mesosternum was 'held in a plastic stage of phylogenetic development', as similar variations are found throughout many primate groups. These sites of ossification develop into sternebrae, and so the first sternebra develops in the midline between the sites of articulation of the second and third costal cartilages. Similarly, the second sternebra develops between the sites of articulation of the third and fourth costal cartilages and so on. In total, there are four sternebrae that will eventually fuse to form the adult mesosternum (Fig 7.8). The first and often the second sternebra will develop from single centres of ossification, while the third and fourth may develop from paired centres. A higher frequency of bilateral centres is to be expected in the lower sternebrae, due to the relatively late fusion of the sternal plates in this region (Fig. 7.5).

It has been proposed that much of the morphological variation seen in the sternum may result from the pattern and number of ossification centres. Ashley's (1956a) type I sterna are narrow with parallel sides and they may result from each sternebra forming from a single centre. Type II sterna also have parallel sides but are much wider than type I and it has been proposed that they may arise from sternebrae that form from bilateral ossification centres. Type III sterna are

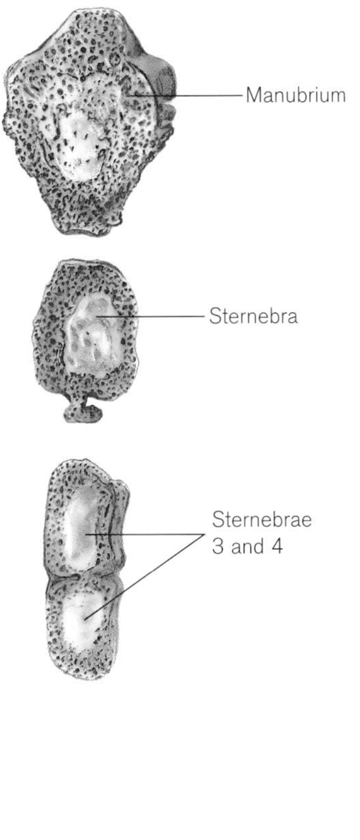

(a) Male aged 3 years 4 months

(b) Female aged 8 years 7 months

Figure 7.7 The developing ossification centres of the sternum.

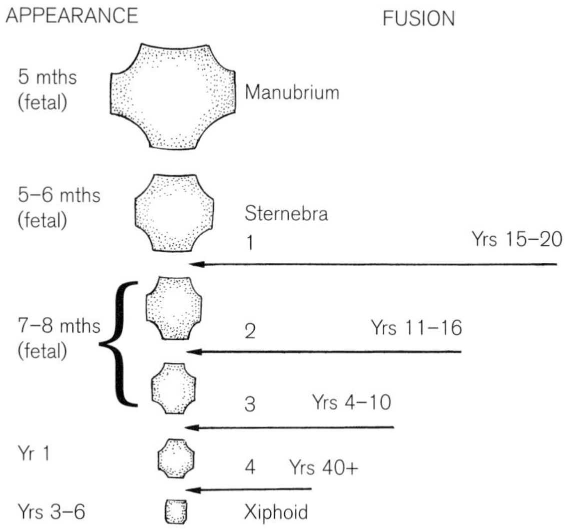

Figure 7.8 Times of appearance and fusion of the primary ossification centres of the sternum.

intermediate in form, being narrow in the upper part and wider in the lower part (piriform) and it is proposed that they may develop from upper sternebrae formed from single centres and lower sternebrae that form from bilateral centres (Wong and Carter, 1988).

A midline sternal foramen is a relatively common defect found in the region of sternebrae 3 and 4 (Jit and Bakshi, 1984) and it is not uncommon for it to be mistaken for a gun-shot wound in the forensic situation. It is thought to result from a defective or delayed fusion of the plates, resulting in bilateral ossification at that level, with concomitant non-fusion of the ossification centres (Cooper *et al.*, 1988). A sternal foramen has been identified in approximately 4% of European and some 13% of East African remains (Ashley, 1956a) and it has generally been found to be more common in males than in females. That a sternal foramen is a developmental defect is verified by the fact that it is not traversed by any anatomical structure (McCormick, 1981).

The ossification centre for the first sternebra generally appears in the fifth or sixth month of fetal life, with centres for the second and third appearing by the seventh or eighth month and that for the fourth sternebra possibly not appearing until the first year *postpartum*. Odita *et al.* (1985) summarized that any fetus with two ossified sternal segments (including the manubrium) is at least 30 weeks of age. The presence of three segments indicates an age of around 34 weeks and four segments an age of around 37 weeks.

Therefore, at birth, the sternum is generally represented by four centres of ossification as the xiphoid will not commence ossification until between the third and sixth year. However, the sternebrae will not become recognizable in isolation until after 6 months *postpartum*, when they start to take on their characteristic flattened appearance in the anteroposterior plane and are roughly oval or rectangular in outline (Fig. 7.7).

The fusion of the primary ossification centres occurs in a well-documented caudocranial direction (Fig 7.8). The line of fusion of adjacent sternebrae is found at the level of the chondrosternal junction. In fact, the superior half of each costal notch is formed from the sternebra above, while the inferior half is formed from the sternebra below. As a rule, sternebrae three and four are the first to fuse, although there is some confusion in the literature concerning when this actually happens. Paterson (1904) reported it to be between 11 and 15 years, Girdany and Golden (1952) said it was between 4 and 8 years, while Hodges (1933) and Jit and Kaur (1989) stated it to be between 6 and 10 years. There is clearly variation in the timing of this event and we have found fusion in a male child as young as 3 years and 4 months (Fig. 7.7a). This unit comprising the fused third and fourth sternebrae will then fuse to the second sternebra around the time of puberty (11–16 years) and this in turn, will finally fuse to the first sternebra towards the end of puberty (15–20 years). It is not uncommon for the manubrium and first sternebra to fuse so that the manubriosternal joint is displaced to occur effectively at the junction between the first and second sternebra at the level of the third costal cartilage (Watts, 1990).

Pattern of fusion

We have found that when two adjacent sternebrae fuse, the posterior surface fuses first, followed by the anterior surface and the lateral surface, bearing the costal notches, is the last to attain adult form. McKern and Stewart (1957) noted that in the sterna of males between the ages of 17 and 18 years, the delimitation of the individual sternebrae was clear and that only the lower two-thirds were fused. Complete fusion of the mesosternum does not arise until later in adulthood, often approaching 30 years, where remnants of fusion can be found in the middle of the costal notches. The remains of the site of sternebral fusion may persist as transverse lines seen on the anterior surface of the adult bone (Fig 7.2). Because of the considerable variation in both the time of appearance of the centres and their subsequent pattern of fusion, the sternum is probably of limited value in the accurate determination of age at death in the juvenile.

Secondary centres

In addition to these primary centres of ossification, a variable number of small secondary centres may occur.

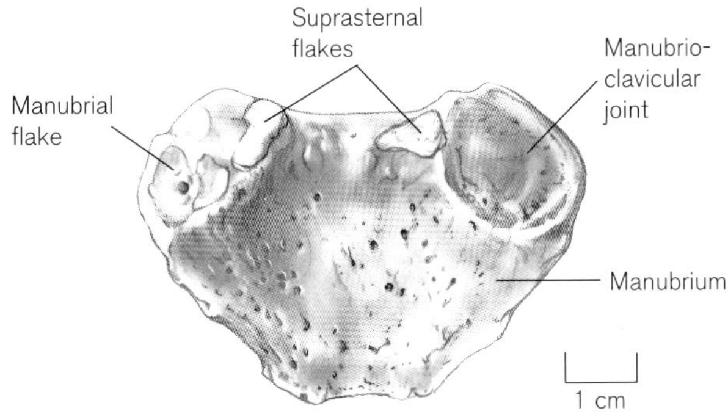

Figure 7.9 The manubrial secondary centres of ossification (approx. 12–14 years).

These are small, flake-like epiphyses that may not exist as separate entities, but rather fuse to the primary centres as they develop. The appearance and subsequent fusion of these centres are very variable and probably of limited value in age determination. They occur at sites of articulation, namely the sternoclavicular joints and the chondrosternal joints. These epiphyses are not well documented and in fact only Stewart (1954) and McKern and Stewart (1957) seem to have paid much attention to them. This is unfortunate as their sample did not contain individuals younger than 17 years of age and so little is documented concerning the earlier development of these centres.

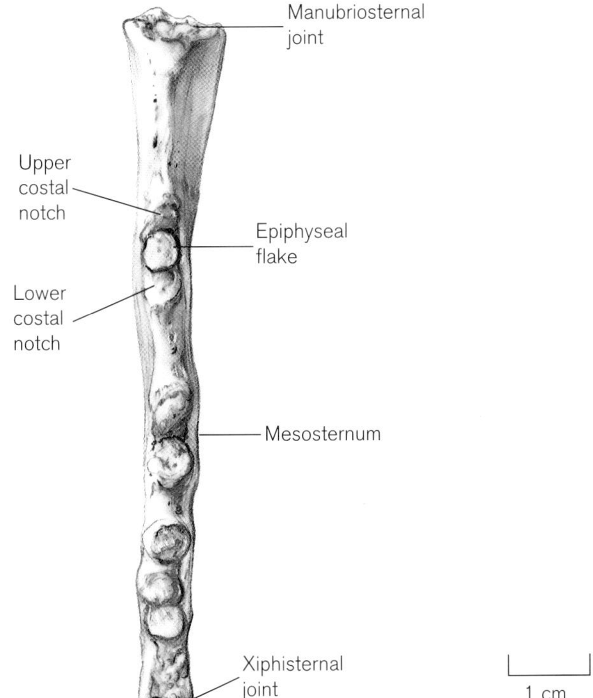

Figure 7.10 The epiphyseal flake of the mesosternal costal notch in a male of approximately 17 years.

Stewart (1954) and McKern and Stewart (1957), noted that a small, flake-like epiphysis was present on the clavicular surface of the manubrium. We have found that it is not uncommon for more than one epiphyseal flake to form and these fuse as patches in various areas of the articular surface (Fig 7.9). Two epiphyses consistently appear, however, at the anterior and superior margins of the manubrium (suprasternal flakes). It is likely that these are phylogenetic remnants of the epiphyses associated with the embryological presternal and suprasternal masses. McKern and Stewart (1957) noted that these epiphyses fused around 19 years of age, but we have found evidence of epiphyseal fusion in individuals as young as 12 years of age.

Epiphyseal activity was also recorded by McKern and Stewart (1957) in the region of the first costal articulation. They noted that in the immature bone there is a clear interarticular groove separating the articular surfaces of the clavicle above from the first costal cartilage below. With age, this groove gradually obliterates, or indeed a separate ossific nodule may appear, so that by the age of 22–23 years the groove disappears. While this is happening, a thin plaque of bone may be found in the pit of the first costal notch on the manubrium, and McKern and Stewart found this in individuals between the ages of 18 and 24 years.

Plaques of bone also appear in the remainder of the costal notches. The plaque forms in the pit of the notch, smoothing over the gap that quite often exists between the superior half of the notch formed from the sternebra above and the lower half of the notch being formed from the sternebra below (Fig 7.10).

The manubriosternal joint

The manubriosternal joint is generally described as either a primary or, more commonly, a secondary cartilaginous joint. The difference between these two classifications is the presence or absence of a fibrocartilaginous disc between two plates of hyaline cartilage. Unlike hyaline cartilage, fibrocartilage does not ossify and so secondary cartilaginous joints tend to remain patent even into late adult life. If the fibrocartilaginous disc is to develop, then a fibrous lamina will appear early in fetal life and the joint will progress to become secondary cartilaginous in form (Fig 7.11). If, however, for some reason, the lamina does not develop, then a primary cartilaginous joint ensues. In the absence of the fibrocartilaginous barrier, the ossification centres for the manubrium and first sternebra may become juxtaposed and union of the centres will occur (Fig 7.12). This leads to matrical synostosis of the manubriosternal joint, where there is incomplete demarcation between the manubrium and mesosternum either externally or internally as can be witnessed on X-rays (Fig 7.13). As the potential for this type of fusion arises in the fetus through non-development of a fibrous lamina, its presence should not be considered pathological in nature. It has been shown that the junction between the manubrium and sternum can slip to the level of the third costal cartilage. This arises when a fibrous lamina develops in this location and not at the level of the second costal cartilage, which represents the normal pattern (Paterson, 1900).

With age, the secondary cartilaginous form of the manubriosternal joint may show what is termed 'sclerotic synostosis' when the fibrocartilage pad breaks down and as the two areas of hyaline cartilage become opposed, fusion can then occur across

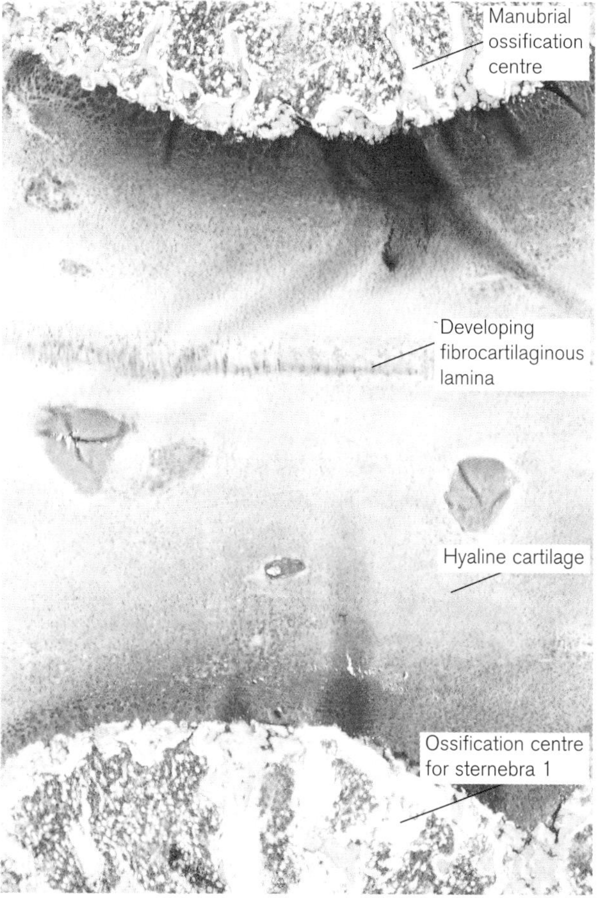

Figure 7.11 Histological (H&E) appearance of the manubriosternal joint in a male aged 9 months (*postpartum*). This shows normal development and a secondary cartilaginous joint will be present in the adult. This is the same specimen as is shown in the radiograph in Fig. 7.5.

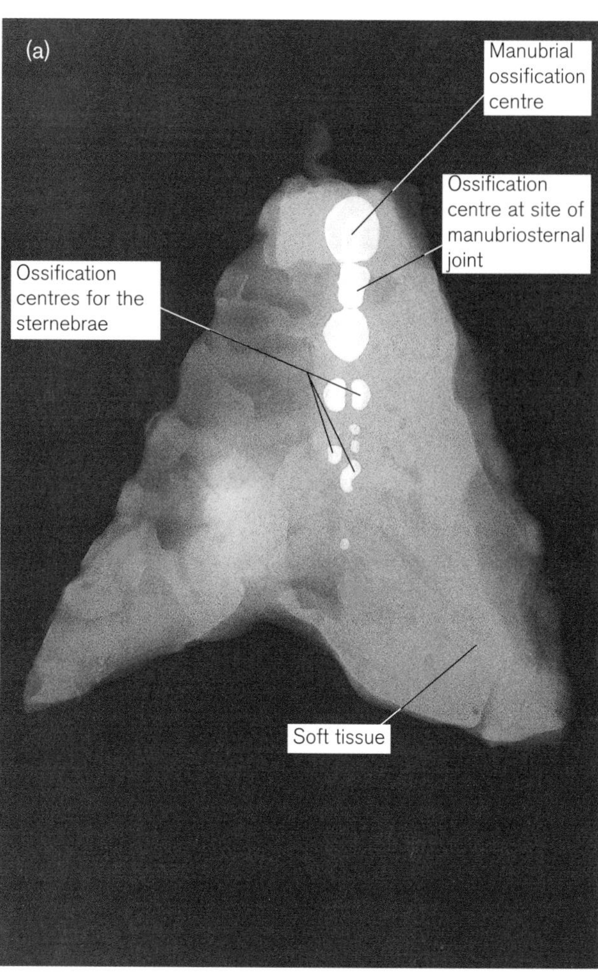

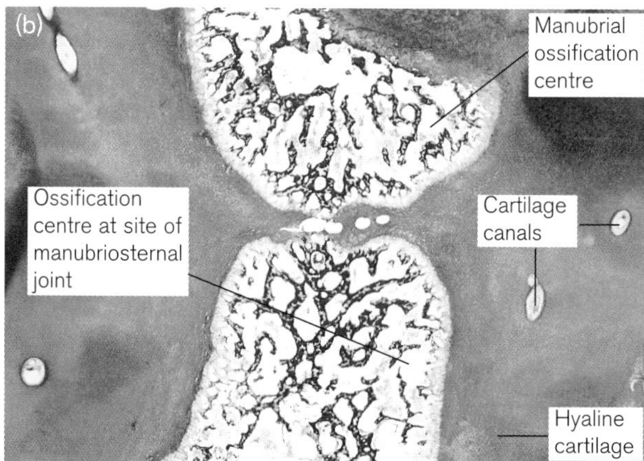

Figure 7.12 Matrical manubriosternal synostosis in a 40 week fetus (male). (a) PA radiograph; (b) histological section, Masson's stain x1 obj. Note that an ossification centre is present at the normal site of the manubriosternal joint, and in the histology there is no fibrous lamina present.

the joint (Fig 7.14). Interestingly, the sclerotic form of manubriosternal fusion is predominantly found in females of advancing years. Sclerotic fusion is degenerative in nature and cannot be confused with matrical synostosis, which is a developmental phenomenon (MacLaughlin and Watts, 1992). For further information, readers are directed to Trotter (1934a), Ashley (1954, 1956c) and Smith (1991b).

In summary, the configuration and final shape of the sternum is heavily dependent upon its embryological development. It is a highly variable structure and probably of limited value as an accurate indicator of chronological age for this very reason.

Practical notes

Orientation

Reliable orientation of the manubrium can only occur after approximately 6 months *postpartum* as before this time, it is represented by little more than bony nodules. The bone is flattened in an anteroposterior direction and the posterior surface will be smoother (Fig. 7.7). Paired, vertical lateral articular facets for the first costal cartilage can be clearly identified as extending for almost half the length of the bone and tend to be located more towards the superior pole. The upper aspect of the manubrium is always broader and more robust than the lower regions. The

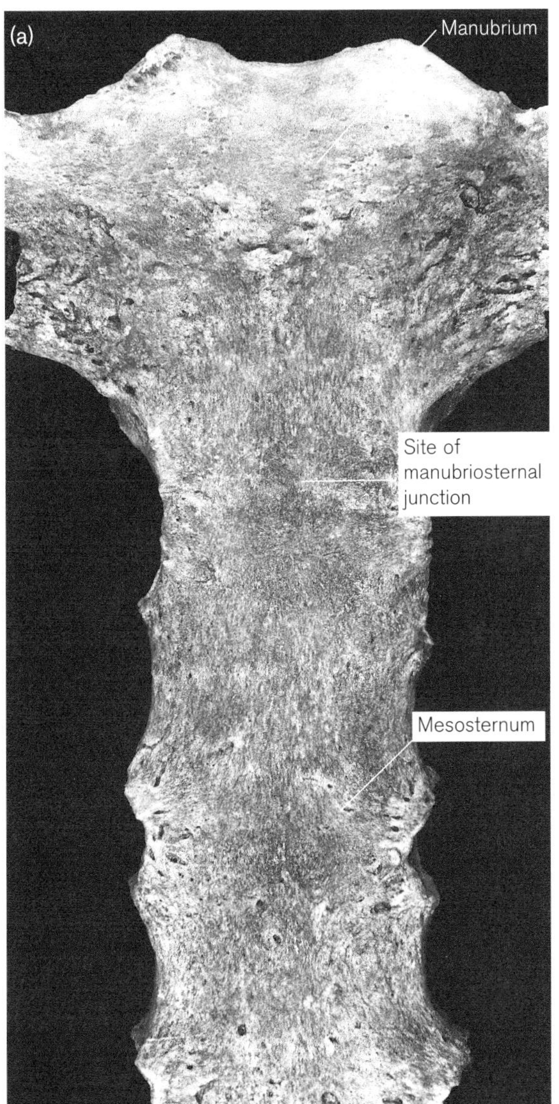

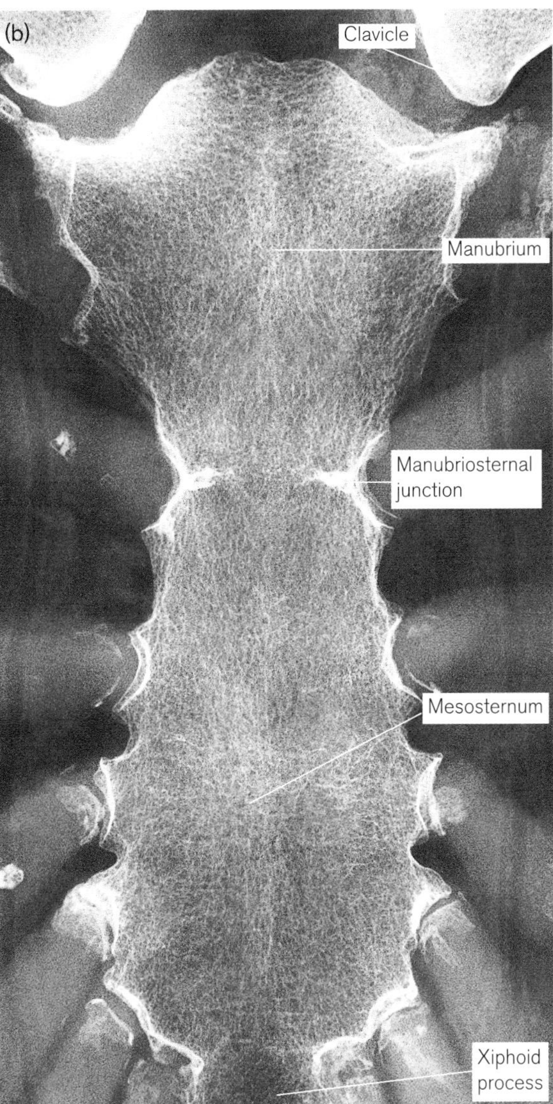

Figure 7.13 Matrical manubriosternal synostosis in a female aged 57 years. (a) External appearance of the bone; (b) PA radiograph. Note the continuity of internal architecture between the manubrium and the mesosternum on the radiograph.

superior border is rounded and smooth and may show the concavity of the jugular notch, while the inferior extremity is rougher in appearance and tends to be more clearly defined as an articular joint surface.

Reliable orientation of the sternebrae is difficult below 2–3 years and the positive identification of a particular segment is extremely difficult unless all the sternebrae are represented and then the attribution will be based on size, with the first tending to be the largest and the fourth the smallest. Each sternebra is flattened in the anteroposterior direction and takes on a roughly rectangular shape when unpaired, but becomes somewhat square in outline when fused with a centre from the opposite side (Fig. 7.7). The posterior surface is generally flatter than the anterior aspect and the height of the bone is generally in excess of its width.

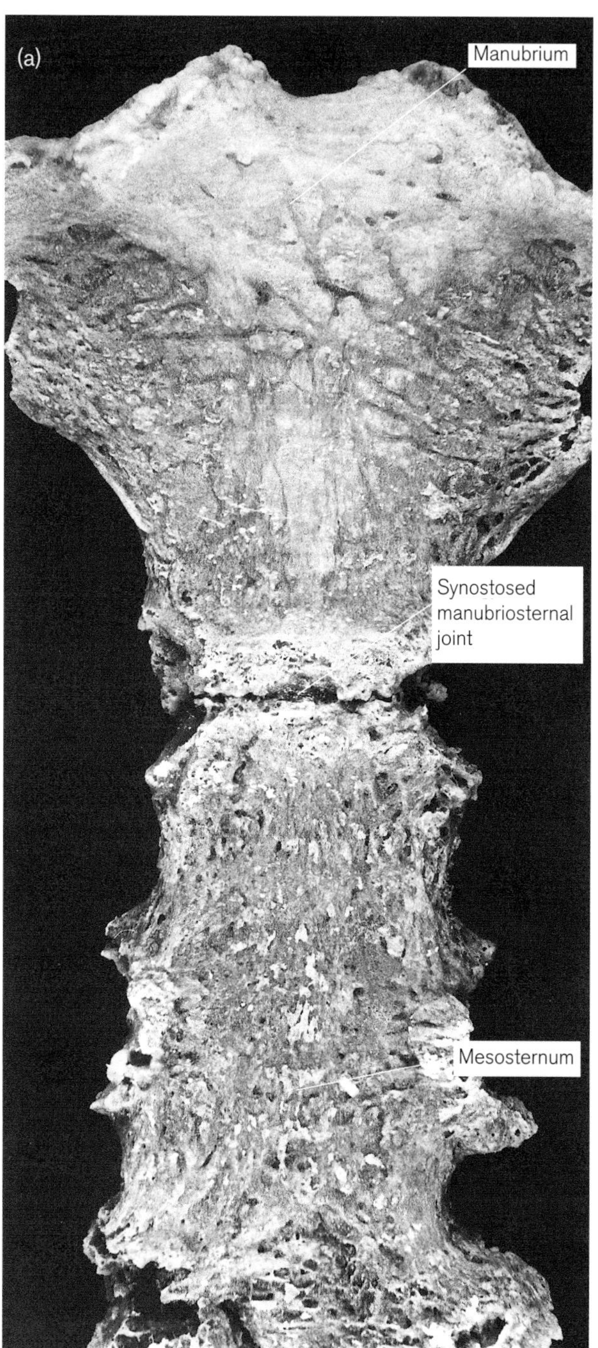

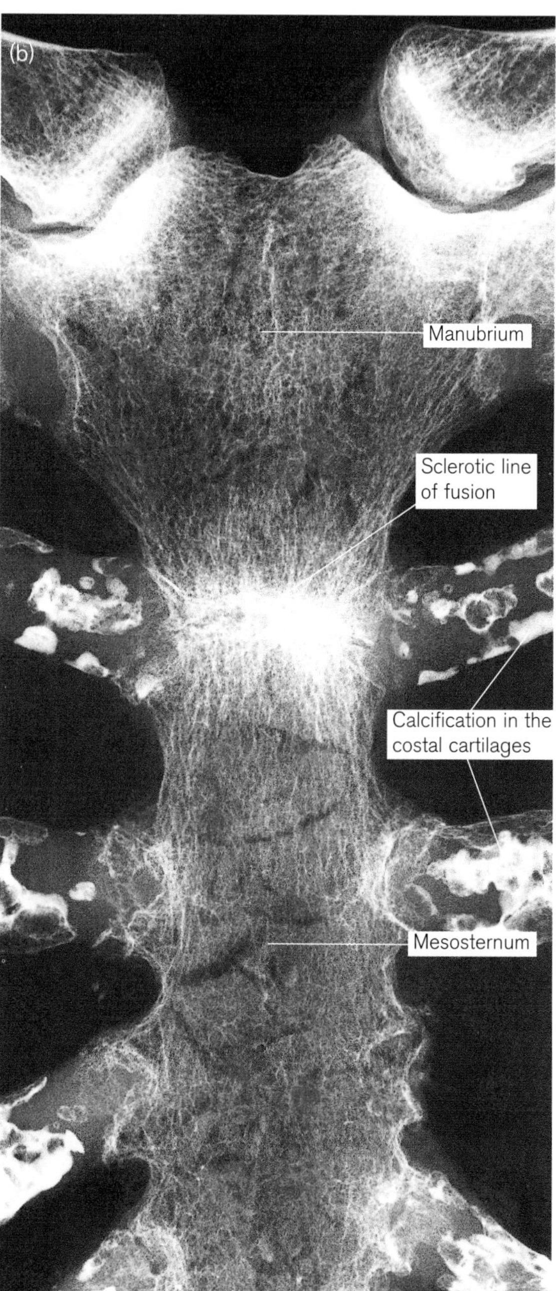

Figure 7.14 Sclerotic manubriosternal synostosis in a female aged 85 years.

Bones of a similar morphology

A neonatal basi-occiput may be confused with a more mature manubrium. However, the former will possesses a deep concavity for the anterior boundary of the foramen magnum, a mediolateral concavity of the intracranial surface, evidence of part of the occipital condyle and a thickened, D-shaped anterior extremity at the spheno-occipital synchondrosis (see Chapter 5). A basi-occiput and a manubrium from the same individual could never be confused, as the latter will always be smaller and thinner.

The early sternebrae are similar in their morphology to the vertebral centra, but close examination will show that the sternal structures are flatter, more irregular in shape and do not possess the well-developed vascular foramina and radiating grooves seen in the centra (see Chapter 6).

Morphological summary

Fetal

Mth 5	Primary centre develops for the manubrium
Mth 5–6	Primary centre develops for first sternebra
Mth 7–8	Primary centres develop for sternebrae 2 and 3
Birth	The sternum is represented by four centres of ossification
Yr 1	Primary centre develops for sternebra 4. The manubrium can be identified in isolation
3–6 yrs	Ossification can commence in the xiphoid. All sternebrae can probably be identified in isolation
4–10 yrs	Sternebrae 3 and 4 fuse
11–16 yrs	Sternebra 2 fuses to 3 and 4. Epiphyses appear and commence fusion
15–20 yrs	Sternebra 1 fuses to rest of mesosternum. Epiphyses continue to fuse
21 yrs +	Sternum essentially complete, although lines of fusion between sternebrae may persist until 25 years
40 yrs +	Xiphoid process fuses to mesosternum

Metrics

We have been unable to locate any metrics based on the developing sternum that have been derived from material of a documented age at death.

II. THE RIBS AND COSTAL CARTILAGES

The adult ribs and costal cartilages

As a general rule, the adult skeleton has 24 ribs (12 pairs), which articulate via synovial joints with the thoracic vertebrae behind and pass anteriorly around the chest wall to terminate in the ventral hyaline costal cartilages (Fig 7.15). There is evidence to suggest that the higher primates tend towards an overall reduction in the total number of ribs, with a concomitant reduction in the vertical dimension of the thoracic cavity (Tredgold, 1897). In man, the number of ribs are by no means constant and may be either increased by the presence of a cervical or lumbar pair, or reduced by the agenesis of the twelfth pair (Gladstone, 1897; Sycamore, 1944). A cranial shift in the sequence is more common than a caudal shift, so that cervical ribs are more common than lumbar ribs (Steiner, 1943). Lumbar ribs are generally asymptomatic but cervical ribs can produce an array of clinical symptoms. These range from paraesthesia along the medial border of the forearm and wasting of the muscles of the hypothenar eminence to vascular changes and even gangrene if the subclavian artery is severely impaired. Accessory ribs have been considered in Chapter 6 and more detailed information can be found in Gladstone and Wakeley (1932a). In addition, a rare condition of 'intra-thoracic' ribs can arise (Weinstein and Mueller, 1965) and it is thought that these develop as a result of incomplete fusion of the sclerotomes in the embryo (see below). Pelvic, iliac, sacral and coccygeal accessory ribs have also been encountered in the clinical literature. While these are generally asymptomatic congenital anomalies, it is possible that they may cause some interference with urinary and obstetrical functions (Halloran, 1960; Sullivan and Cornwell, 1974; Kaushal, 1977; Lame, 1977; Pais *et al.*, 1978; Greenspan and Norman, 1982; Dunaway *et al.*, 1983).

As with all anatomical structures that manifest in a segmental series, there is often reference to a 'typical' member, which generally occurs in the middle range of the series. The more peripheral members tend to adopt individual characteristic appearances and patterns of articulation and are therefore termed 'atypical'. The ribs follow this pattern, in that a 'typical' rib occurs somewhere in the middle of the series, e.g. ribs 4–8, while the 'atypical' ribs are at the extremities, e.g. ribs 1, 2, 11 and 12. Although the term 'typical' does apply, as there is indeed a basic morphology to these ribs, each has its own particular characteristics that allow individual identification, certainly in the adult situation (see below).

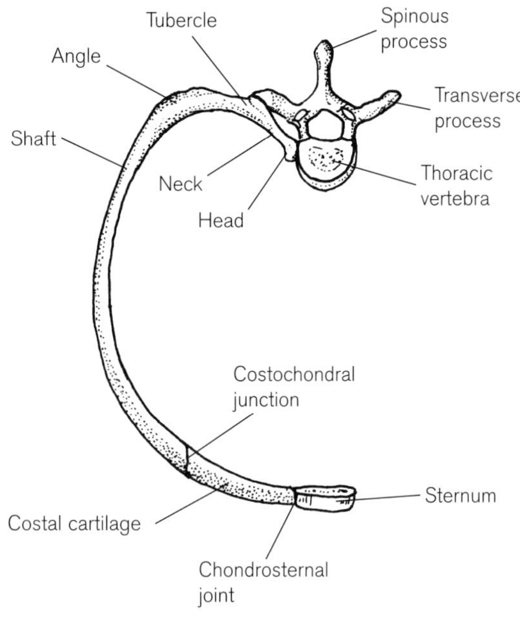

Figure 7.15 The articulations of a typical right adult rib.

Typical ribs

Figure 7.16 shows that the vertebral (posterior) end of a 'typical' adult rib has an expanded **head**, with two articular facets that correspond with the facets on the bodies of the two thoracic vertebrae with which it articulates. The facets are separated by an **interarticular crest**, which is attached to the intervertebral disc by a ligament. The head passes into a more slender **neck**, which has a rough ridge on its superior aspect (crest of the neck) for the attachment of the superior costotransverse ligament. The neck has a smooth inner pleural surface but may be ridged externally by the attachment of the inferior costotransverse ligament.

The remainder of the bone is the **shaft** or body and this joins the neck at the **tubercle**, which presents a posterior articular facet for the synovial joint with the vertebral transverse process. An anterior non-articular region of the tubercle is the site of attachment of the lateral costotransverse ligament. The articular and non-articular regions of the tubercle are closely related in the upper ribs, but the distance between them increases as the thoracic cage is descended.

The shaft passes outwards from the tubercle for a short distance, and then turns abruptly forwards, forming the **angle** of the rib, and beyond this the shaft continues in a forward and inferomedial direction. It has a superior rounded border that is sharper in front than behind and an inferior border that is less sharp in front than behind. These borders are the sites of attachment of the intercostal muscles. The inner smooth surface of the rib is covered by parietal pleura and the outer surface bears various markings for the attachments of muscles. The inferior border is characterized by a **subcostal groove**, which is more pronounced posteriorly and houses the intercostal neurovascular bundle.

The anterior extremity of the rib is somewhat cup-shaped for the reciprocal surface of the costal cartilage. A slight bend in the shaft may be noticed close to the anterior extremity and this is termed the anterior angle. For a more detailed description of 'typical' rib morphology, see Frazer (1948).

Atypical ribs

The atypical ribs are readily identifiable because of their individual characteristics. These include ribs 1, 2, 10, 11 and 12 (Fig 7.17).

The **first rib** articulates with the body and transverse process of the first thoracic vertebra posteriorly and passes anteriorly in a tight curve across the apex of the lung to terminate in its costal cartilage. This rib is the most readily identifiable because of its shape and size, being short, hook-shaped, flat, relatively broad and not possessing a subcostal groove. It has flat superior and inferior surfaces and outer and inner borders. The head is more rounded than a typical rib and has only one facet for articulation with the body of the first thoracic vertebra. The neck is more elongated, the tubercle more pronounced and there is no posterior angle.

The superior surface has a posterior groove for the passage of the subclavian artery and brachial plexus into the axilla and an anterior groove for the passage of the subclavian vein into the neck. The lowest trunk of the brachial plexus in fact causes the groove said to be formed by the subclavian artery (sulcus subclaviæ). Jones (1910) even went as far as to suggest that the name be changed to 'sulcus nervi brachialis' in deference to its neurological origin. It has been shown that if sufficient pressure is exerted on the developing bone by this trunk of the brachial plexus, then normal ossification can be impaired. In this situation, a rudimentary rib may develop, characterized by a fibrous band in the region of the nerve trunk (Jones, 1910). As occurs with the supraclavicular nerves and the clavicle (see Chapter 8), the first rib can be pierced by a foramen, which allows transmission of a branch of the first dorsal nerve (Thomson, 1885).

An intervening scalene tubercle (Lisfranc's) is present on the inner border, separating the two subclavian grooves and offers attachment to the scalenus anterior muscle. The more anterior, venous, groove is not constant in position and an anterior displacement can result in compression syndromes, causing difficulty in cannulation of the subclavian vein (Wayman *et al.*, 1993).

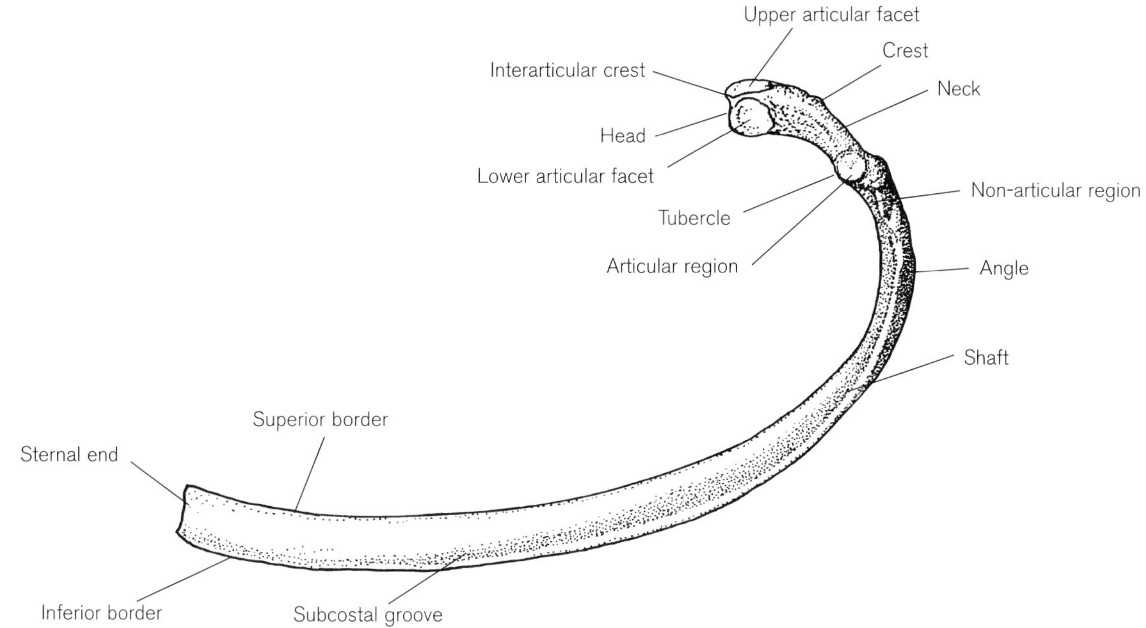

Figure 7.16 A typical right adult rib.

The inferior surface of the first rib is said to be unremarkable, displaying few characteristics. However, Cave (1929) noted that the course of the first intercostal nerve and its branches could be detected in some cases. The main trunk of the nerve can cause a wide depression midway along the shaft, passing in an oblique inferomedial direction (sulcus diagonalis). In addition to this, the collateral muscular branch of the nerve can cause a shallow groove that lies more posterior to the main trunk and traverses the width of the shaft (sulcus transversus).

Thoracic outlet (costoclavicular) syndrome is a blanket term for vascular and neurological complications in this region. These can be attributed to a variety of congenital anomalies such as a hypoplastic first rib, cervical rib or exostoses on the first rib (Roos, 1976).

The **second rib** articulates with the transverse process and upper demi-facet on the body of the second thoracic vertebra and with the lower demi-facet on the body of the first thoracic vertebra. It passes around the thoracic wall at a more oblique angle than the first rib and so is not as hooked in shape. The head has two articular facets, like a typical rib, but the upper is often very small. The angle is only a short distance from the tubercle. A prominent thickening of bone is found on the outer surface of the shaft about half way along, and this is the site of attachment for the serratus anterior muscle. A subcostal groove is present but is generally restricted to the posterior region of the shaft.

The **tenth rib** is not always readily identifiable. The head may possess one or two articular facets and an articular facet may or may not be present on the tubercle. This rib is therefore transitional between the typical ribs above and the truly atypical ribs below.

The **eleventh** and **twelfth** ribs do not articulate with the transverse processes of a thoracic vertebrae, so there are no articular facets on the tubercles. They possess a single facet on the head for articulation with the vertebra of the corresponding number. The eleventh rib is longer than the twelfth and may show a subcostal groove close to the region of the posterior angle. The twelfth rib possesses neither an angle nor a subcostal groove. Both ribs have a free pointed end with a short costal cartilage, which is embedded in the musculature of the abdominal wall.

In the living, ribs 1, 2, 11 and 12 are the least likely to fracture as the first two are partly protected by the clavicle and the latter two are more mobile and so offer little resistance to force. In general, the juvenile thorax is more elastic and pliable than that of the adult and so rib fractures are not common. However, direct injuries to the chest may drive the broken ends of the ribs inwards, causing a tear in the underlying pleura that will lead to a pneumothorax (collapsed lung). In indirect violence, e.g. compression, the ribs normally fracture just in front of their angles and the broken ends tend to slide outwards, thus sparing the pleura. In relation to fractures, it is also important to note that the lower ribs and their costal margin overlap the upper abdominal viscera,

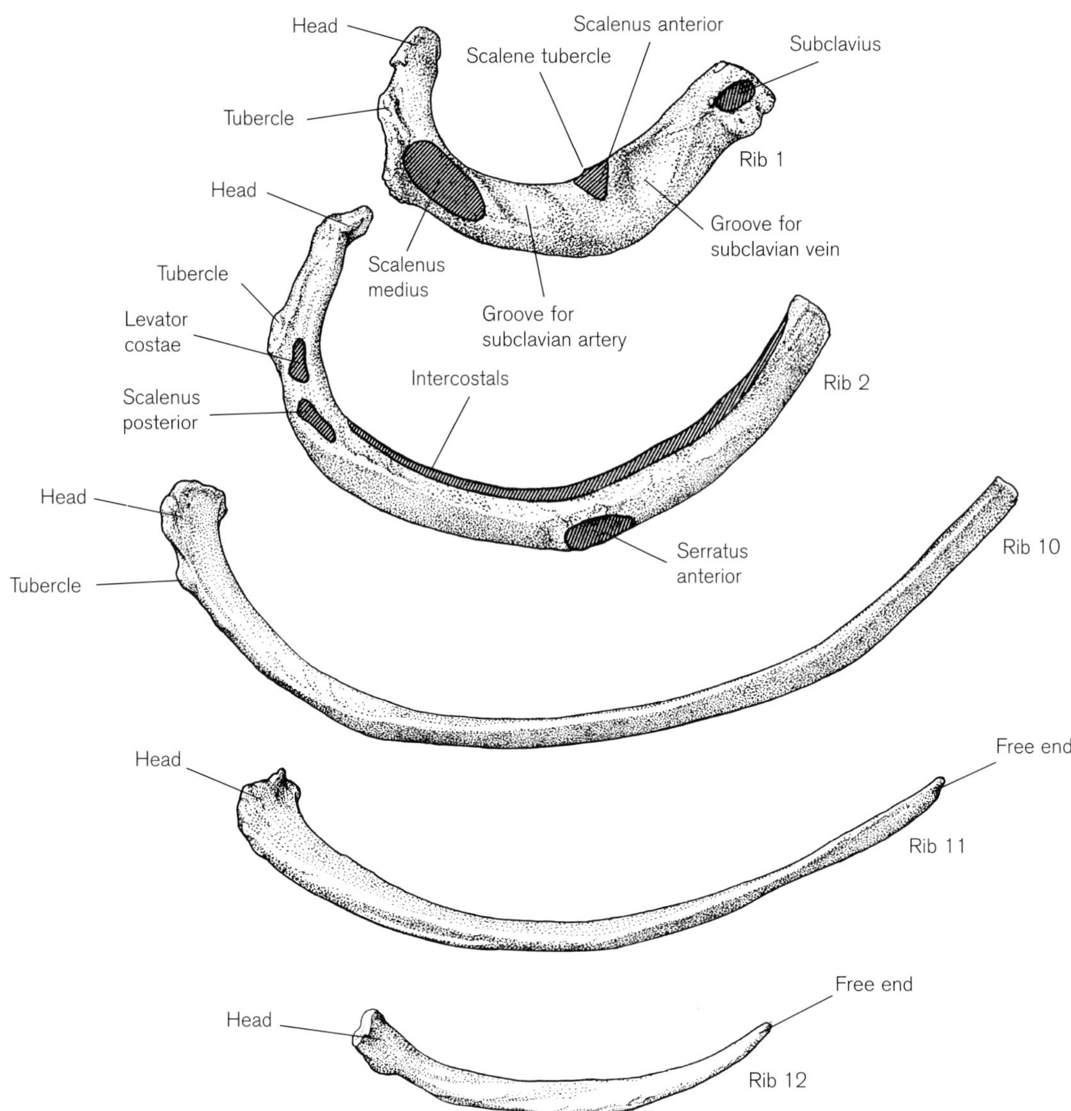

Figure 7.17 The atypical right adult ribs.

so that fracture can lead to lacerations of the liver, spleen, kidneys, etc.

Surprisingly, there is very little detailed information available on the **individual identification** of a rib within the costal sequence. Most anatomical and osteological text books describe the atypical ribs in some detail, but ribs 3–9 are considered together under the heading of 'typical ribs' with little or no attempt to identify individual differences. However, being able to identify the location of a specific rib within the sequence has considerable importance, e.g. establishing the number of individuals that are present or matching knife or gun-shot wounds with corresponding marks in clothing (Mann, 1993).

It is generally recognized that the length of adult ribs increase from 1 to 7 with either the seventh or the eighth rib being the longest in the series, before they decrease in length again until the twelfth rib is reached. Similarly, the rib width is reported to increase from 1 to 7 and then decrease again until rib 12 (Anderson, 1884). Although this allows some degree of placement of individual ribs within a series, it is of little value in identifying individual bones, especially when the series is incomplete.

Dudar (1993) devised a technique for the identification of rib number and tested the results on a series of ribs of known number. His technique involved the initial removal of the atypical ribs 1, 2, 10, 11 and 12, while the remainder (ribs 3–9) were then examined on the basis of three characteristics – change in the horizontal angle of the rib (i.e. more or less hooked), a change in the inferior angle in the vertical plane (i.e.

whether or not the rib points downwards) and a change in the twist of the superior external border (i.e. whether or not the border approaches the vertical plane). Although changes in these three factors formed the basis of the method, the practicality of identification was still achieved by stacking the ribs and checking which two showed the greatest similarities, i.e. by identifying rib 2, rib 3 could be found and then rib 4, and so on.

Mann (1993) also offered a method for sideing and sequencing human ribs using features such as maximum (relative) rib length, the size and shape of the articular facets, the distance between the articular facets and rib angle and the height of the rib heads relative to one another. However, both these methods rely on a comparison between adjacent ribs and therefore are of limited value in identifying isolated bones. To achieve a more reliable sequencing procedure, morphological factors that have a sound functional basis must also be taken into consideration, as indicators of only shape and size may not prove to be sufficiently definitive.

Although most osteologists will have their own preferred method of sequencing, it is always tempting to devise one's own definitive method, and it is certainly true in this situation that the intuition of experience is difficult to distil into written instructions.

The atypical ribs (1, 2, 11 and 12) are easy to identify and so do not require further consideration. However, ribs 3–10 are not easy to correctly identify in isolation. Although rib 10 is transitional and as such is not always easy to assign, when placed on a horizontal surface with its inferior border downwards the head is always in direct contact with the surface. In this way, rib 10 can be separated from all other lower ribs whose heads are raised above the horizontal surface as a result of the obliquity of the shafts. The horizontal shaft of this rib is an indication of its limited involvement in active respiration. It is also a relatively short rib, which may, or indeed may not, show an articular facet on the tubercle and may show either one or two articular facets on the head.

This then leaves ribs 3–9 to be identified. Rib 3 can always be removed from this series as its shape bears some similarity to rib 2, in that it is moderately hooked, whereas in ribs below number 3, the hook shape begins to open out. Thus, the upper three ribs clearly reflect the tight curve of the thoracic shape around the upper lobes of the lung and below this level, the lungs increase in diameter considerably and so the ribs must increase in size and alter in shape to accommodate these changes.

Ribs 4–9 can be considered on the basis of three functional considerations – ventral articulation with either the sternum directly or via the costal margin (vertebrosternal or vertebrochondral), functional involvement with respiration (i.e. bucket handle action during breathing) and increase in size and robusticity due to an increase in lateral body weight that requires to be transferred to the axial skeleton via the articulation at the head of the rib.

Ribs 4–6 articulate directly with the sternum via their costal cartilages, while ribs 7–9 articulate via the costal margin. When placed on a horizontal surface, ribs 4–6 show an obliquity in the region of the anterior angle, with the superior border directed inwards and the inferior border outwards. However, in ribs 7–9 the superior and inferior borders are in the same plane and the anterior aspect of the shaft is essentially vertical. In addition to this, those ribs that articulate with the sternum tend to have a broader and flatter ventral extremity, while those that articulate with the costal margin tend to be narrower and more rounded, or even pinched, in appearance. This is presumably related to the fact that the former ribs articulate via their own costal cartilage and so convey greater individual stresses, while the latter have a more communal insertion via the chondral margin, so that forces are more dissipated.

The upper ribs tend to be more horizontal in position, while the lower ribs take on an obliquity so that when examined in the living, the head of a lower rib is considerably higher in position than its anterior extremity. When these ribs are placed on a flat surface, this manifests by the heads of the ribs rising above the horizontal plane. The heads of ribs 4 and 5 remain close to the horizontal surface, while the remainder rise above it, with the maximum elevation being achieved in either rib 7 or 8. In rib 9, the obliquity is not so well developed and the head of this rib tends to be lower than either 7 or 8.

The upper ribs carry less lateral body weight than the lower ribs and so the head and neck of an upper rib tends to be more gracile than that of a lower rib. Ribs 4–6 show a gracile head compared to ribs 7–9 (most obvious in rib 4), with a slender neck and poorly developed crest region.

Following these basic guidelines, each rib may be placed into a functional category and by now stacking one on top of the other within that category, the best fit and thus the rib order can be achieved. This method of identification certainly holds true if the individual is in excess of 2 years of age, but individual rib identification is more difficult in younger individuals (see below).

Costal cartilages

The 12 pairs of costal cartilages are the persistent, unossified ventral extensions of the cartilaginous models that preceded the fully ossified ribs. These relatively flat bars of hyaline cartilage extend anteriorly from the ventral aspect of the ribs and contribute considerably to the mobility and elasticity of the thorax. The upper seven pairs articulate directly with the sternum via synovial joints, while the eighth to tenth articulate with the lower border of the cartilage above to form the costal (chondral) margin (Briscoe, 1925). The lowest two (11 and 12) have free, pointed ends that terminate in the musculature of the anterior abdominal wall.

The costochondral junction is not a joint *per se*, as the two elements of rib and cartilage merge together, with the convex tip of the cartilage being received into a reciprocal recess in the anterior end of the rib. The periosteum and perichondrium are continuous and there is no active movement across this joint. In diseases such as rickets, the lack of calcification leads to proliferative changes in the costal cartilages, which become especially marked at the costochondral junctions, leading to a condition known as 'rickety rosary' (Ozonoff, 1979).

The first chondrosternal joint between the first costal cartilage and the manubrium is a primary cartilaginous articulation, which therefore retains the potential to synostose with age (Resnick *et al.*, 1981; MacLaughlin, 1990b; Watts, 1990, 1991; MacLaughlin and Watts, 1992). It is interesting to note that if manubriocostal synostosis occurs with the first rib, then manubriosternal synostosis will not develop (Fig. 7.18). Reciprocally, when matrical manubriosternal fusion occurs, then manubriocostal fusion will not result. This reciprocal agreement is necessary to retain mobility and elasticity in the upper regions of the sternal complex, as fusion must by necessity impair free movement. The intimate relationship between the manubrium and the first and second costal cartilages is apparent following sternal fracture when the manubriocostal complex remains intact (Fowler, 1957).

The second costal cartilage articulates with both the manubrium above and the mesosternum below via a synovial joint. Although the articulation straddles the manubriosternal joint, it is more firmly attached to the manubrium above as it tends to remain with the manubrium–first rib complex following fracture (Fowler, 1957). The second costal cartilage is also the most frequently affected in Tietze's syndrome. It is believed that the characteristic anterior buckling of the cartilage is caused by contracture of the ligament directly behind the cartilage (Beck and Berkheiser, 1954).

The anterior ends of cartilages 3–7/8 articulate with the shallow costal notches on the lateral margins of the mesosternum by synovial joints. The interchondral joints between contiguous surfaces of the sixth to ninth costal cartilages are enclosed in a thin fibrous capsule that is lined by a synovial membrane. The articulation between the ninth and tenth is rarely synovial and a joint cavity may in fact be absent (Williams *et al.*, 1995).

Suppurative infection of the costal cartilages is not uncommon and becomes established after cartilage necrosis following trauma or ischaemia. Mild forms respond well to antibiotic treatment, whereas a more established form can lead to a retrosternal abscess and more widespread infection (Elson, 1965).

Early development of the ribs

To fully understand the early development of the ribs, it is advised that the relevant section in Chapter 6 is read, as only a brief summary will be considered here.

The rib primordia arise from the costal downgrowths of the neural arch portion of the vertebral anlage and are almost entirely derived from the caudal half of the sclerotome (Sensenig, 1949; Ogden, 1979; Verbout, 1985). This embryological origin explains why each typical rib essentially articulates with only one vertebra, namely that which also develops from the same caudal sclerotome portion and why there is only a minor articulation with the vertebra above. By the time the tenth rib is reached, there is no articulation with the vertebra above as the rib remains fully within the realms of its embryological cohort. It also explains why the rib has a more intimate relationship with the neural arch portion of the vertebra than with its centrum (Fig. 7.19).

The rib primordia penetrate into the body wall between two adjacent segmental myotomes and eventually become associated with the sternal mesenchymal plates, as described earlier (Fig. 7.4). The junction between the sclerotome derivatives (ribs) and the lateral plate mesoderm derivatives (sternum) persists as the chondrosternal articulations.

Chondrification commences in the posterior section of the rib primordium around day 36 of intra-uterine life. It progresses ventrally, and as growth also occurs in this direction, the sternal plates become approximated and eventually meet and fuse in the midline. By the time these plates have finally met, ossification has commenced in the ribs. Once ossification begins, the synovial costovertebral joints commence development and so the rib separates from the vertebral anlage (Tsou *et al.*, 1980). Failure of this joint formation will result in congenital costovertebral fusion and whilst this is generally asymptomatic when restricted to one segment, if several segments are involved then respiratory limitations may ensue.

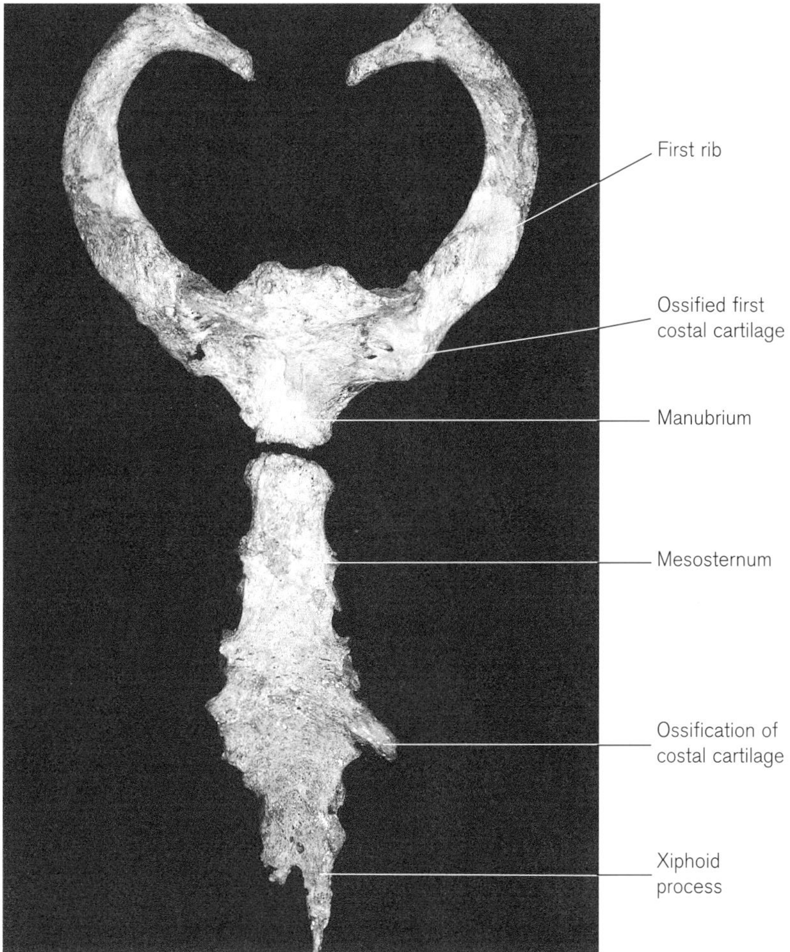

Figure 7.18 Bilateral manubriocostal fusion in a male aged 56 years. Note that the manubriosternal joint is patent.

The shape of the developing ribs is said to be greatly influenced by the structures that they grow around. Therefore, the upper ribs are modified by the shape of the underlying lung buds and developing heart, while the lower ribs grow to accommodate the shape of the abdominal viscera, such as the liver (Geddes, 1912).

Rib abnormalities, such as bifidity, flaring, fusion or bridging, generally arise from irregular segmentation either in association with the vertebral anlage or with abnormal segmentation in the sternum (Sycamore, 1944; White *et al.*, 1945; Martin, 1960; Barnes, 1994). These abnormalities are relatively common and generally asymptomatic. Congenital fusion of ribs should not, of course, be confused with post-traumatic fusion of fractures. The latter is a more common event and identification of an intercostal callus formation should prevent confusion (Steinbock, 1976; Mann and Murphy, 1990).

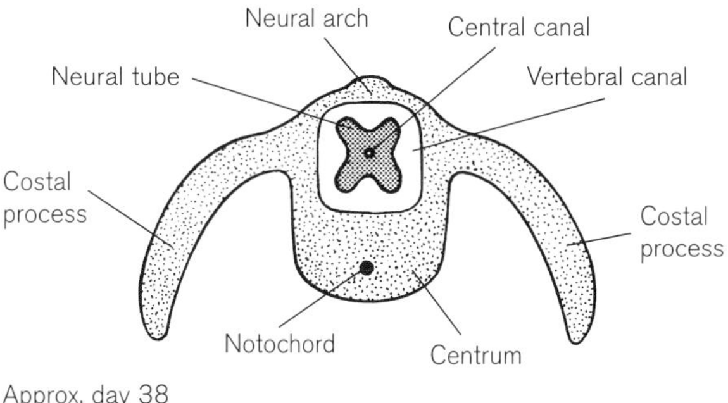

Figure 7.19 A diagrammatic representation of the embryological origins of a developing rib.

Ossification

Primary centres

Primary centres of ossification first appear in ribs 5–7 in the region of the posterior angle between the eighth and ninth weeks of fetal life (Geddes, 1912; Frazer, 1948; Noback and Robertson, 1951; Last, 1973; Fazekas and Kósa, 1978; Ogden, 1979). Ossification centres then appear in a bidirectional manner, with the primary centre for the first rib appearing before that of the twelfth (Frazer, 1948; Noback and Robertson, 1951). By the eleventh and twelfth weeks of intra-uterine life, each rib (often with the exception of the twelfth) possesses a single primary centre of ossification (Flecker, 1932a). The rib therefore commences ossification in advance of its corresponding vertebra, indicating that in terms of development it is divorced from the primitive mesenchymal vertebra, at a very early fetal age (Fazekas and Kósa, 1978; Ogden, 1979).

Ossification of the cartilage model then ensues, with more rapid development occurring in a ventral, rather than a dorsal, direction. The ventral progression of ossification slows down in the fourth fetal month, when the proportion of bone to costal cartilage seems to reach equilibrium, reflecting that of the future adult situation (Fazekas and Kósa, 1978).

Between this stage in the ossification process and the presence of secondary centres of ossification at puberty, the only obvious development in the ribs is a change in shape and size. This reflects the gradual development of the juvenile thorax as its ventral aspect descends while its posterior attachment to the vertebral column remains constant and so comes to adopt a more active role in the mechanism of respiration. It has long been recognized that the ribs of the neonate are more horizontal in position than those of the adult (Fig 7.20). Breathing is essentially a diaphragmatic and anterior abdominal wall process in the newborn, with the thorax *per se* offering little more than a relatively fixed container in which the diaphragm's descent induces the movement of air in and out of the respiratory organs (Crelin, 1973). An increase in the obliquity of the rib shaft, and thus a general descent of the thorax, results in a decrease in dependency on diaphragmatic breathing and an increase in direct thoracic involvement (England, 1990). In the neonate, the transverse diameter of the thorax is relatively smaller than in the adult, but this situation changes at approximately the time when the child begins to walk (Williams *et al.*, 1995). The effect of these mechanical factors can in fact be detected in the juvenile rib series, and may act as useful corroborative evidence in the determination of age at death (see below).

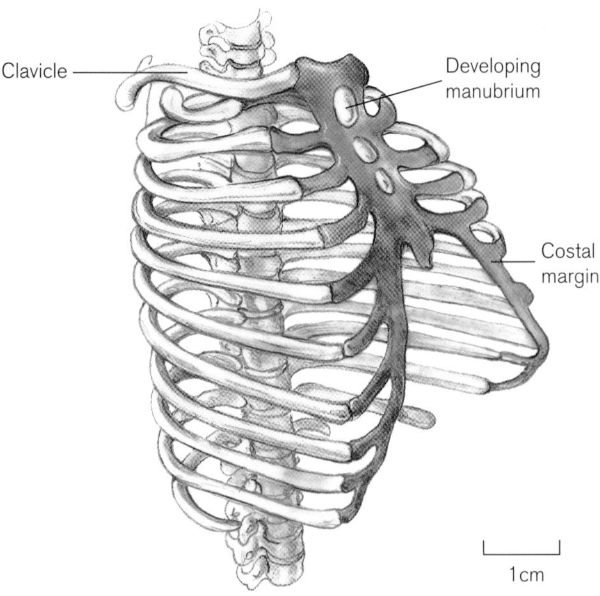

Figure 7.20 The articulated perinatal thoracic skeleton. Note the virtually horizontal ribs and therefore the relatively high position of the thorax.

Secondary centres

There is very little detailed information concerning the secondary centres of ossification, either in their time of appearance or their time and order of fusion. Stevenson (1924) went so far as to say that the ribs were of little value in age determination. Presumably this was because of the variability in timings and in the fact that these epiphyses are probably the smallest and least readily identifiable in the human body. It is also often very difficult to interpret their status of union as the appearance of many of the surfaces is much the same both before and after union. It is often only when the epiphysis is actually in the process of fusing that it is readily identifiable (McKern and Stewart, 1957).

Secondary centres of ossification will occur at the sites of articulation. In addition, a centre may be present for the non-articulating area of the tubercle and these are generally the first to appear at the early stages of puberty (12–14 yrs). It is unlikely that these epiphyses exist as separate structures, but rather that they fuse with the non-articulating area of the tubercle as they are being formed. Therefore, fusion will also occur at an early age. Ribs that do not possess a tubercle, as they do not articulate with a transverse process (ribs 11, 12 and often 10) will naturally not show epiphyses in this area. The non-articular epiphysis for rib 1 is slightly different in that once it has fused it continues posteriorly and expands to also become the epiphysis for the articulating region of the tubercle (Fig 7.21). This arises because of the close proximity of the two surfaces in this rib. In ribs where

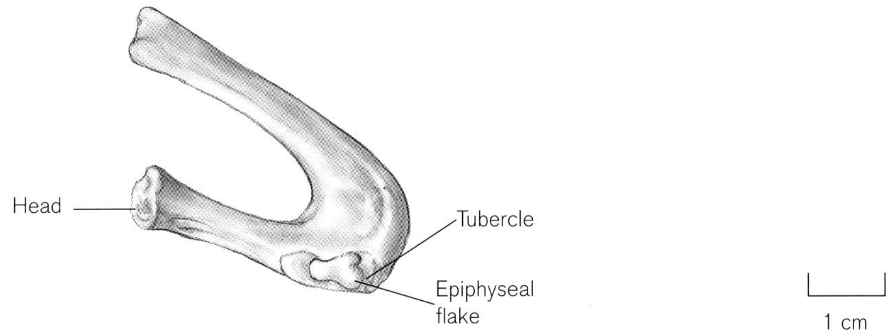

Figure 7.21 Epiphyseal fusion on the tubercle of rib 1 (right) in a male of approximately 17 years.

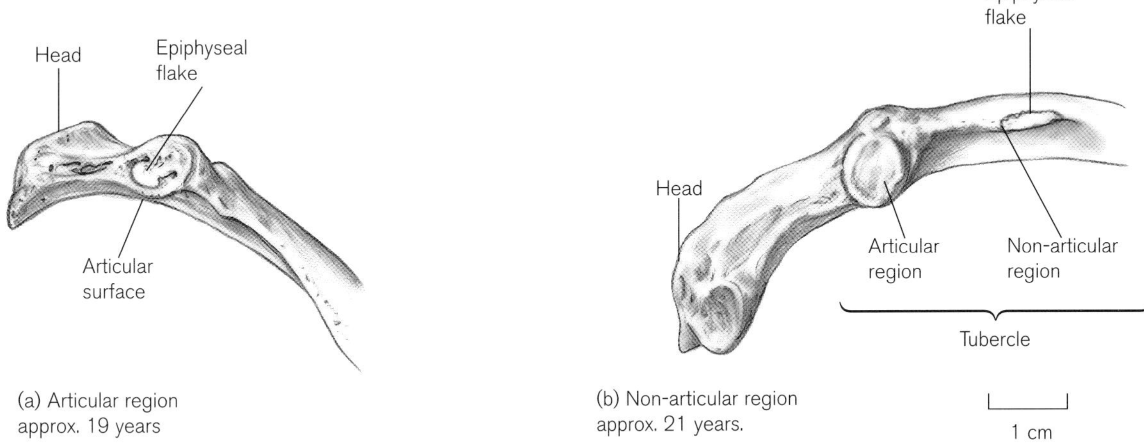

Figure 7.22 Epiphyseal fusion on the articular and non-articular regions of the right rib tubercle.

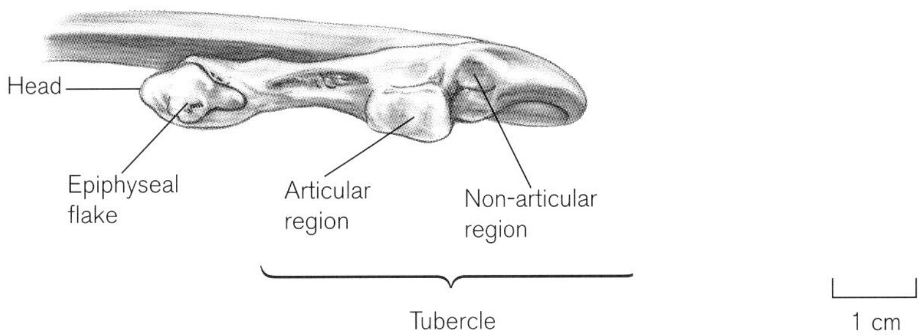

Figure 7.23 Epiphyseal fusion on the head of a right rib (approx. 22 years).

the two areas are further apart, then two separate centres of ossification will arise and fuse independently.

The epiphysis for the articulating region of the tubercle is next to develop, and in the same way it appears to fuse to the surface while it is actually forming, so it probably never achieves a separate existence (Fig. 7.22). The appearance and fusion of these epiphyses appears to follow no specific pattern in terms of the sequence of ribs. It is said that they appear and unite in the eighteenth year (Stevenson, 1924), but more detailed information is not available.

The epiphyses for the heads of the ribs are the last to form, with the first of these showing complete fusion around 17 years of age (McKern and Stewart, 1957). The epiphysis appears as a nodule of bone in the superior articular facet and then gradually spreads outwards into the crest and downwards into the inferior facet (Fig. 7.23). Epiphyses for the heads

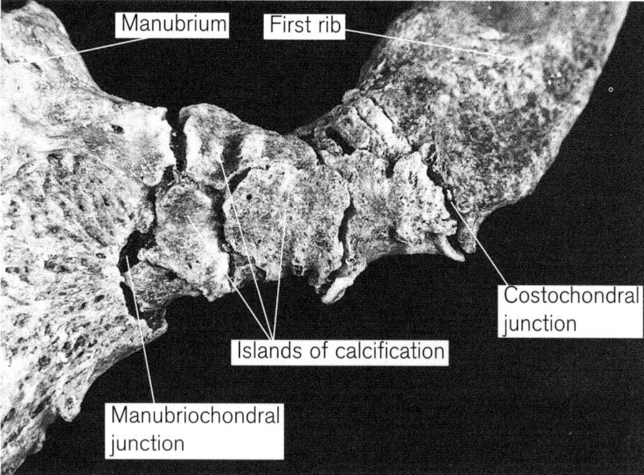

Figure 7.24 Islands of calcification in the first costal cartilage in a female aged 62 years.

of the ribs initially appear in the upper and lower members of the series so that the upper and lower ribs are generally more advanced in terms of maturity than the middle ribs. It is generally recognized that complete fusion of the epiphyses of the heads of the ribs is completed by years 22–25 (Fawcett, 1911b; Stevenson, 1924; Hodges, 1933; McKern and Stewart, 1957).

Age changes in rib ends and within the costal cartilages

The costochondral junction is the region where the bone of the rib merges into the hyaline cartilage of the costal cartilages. This junction represents a developmental anomaly in that the progressive juvenile ossification process falls short of its cartilaginous anlage. Therefore, with increasing age it is perhaps not surprising that continued ossification may proceed in a ventral direction. This process occurs in two ways – morphological alteration of the ventral rib end, and direct ossification of the costal cartilages.

Işcan (1985) and Işcan *et al.* (1984, 1985) developed a component phase analysis system to determine age and establish sex differences in the metamorphosis of the ventral extremity of the fourth rib. For a full description of this technique, it is advised that the original papers be consulted.

Hyaline cartilage has the ability to mineralize and retains this property even into old age. The value of costal cartilage calcification in the prediction of age at death and sex determination has been extensively examined and again it is advised that the original texts are consulted (McCormick, 1980, 1983; McCormick

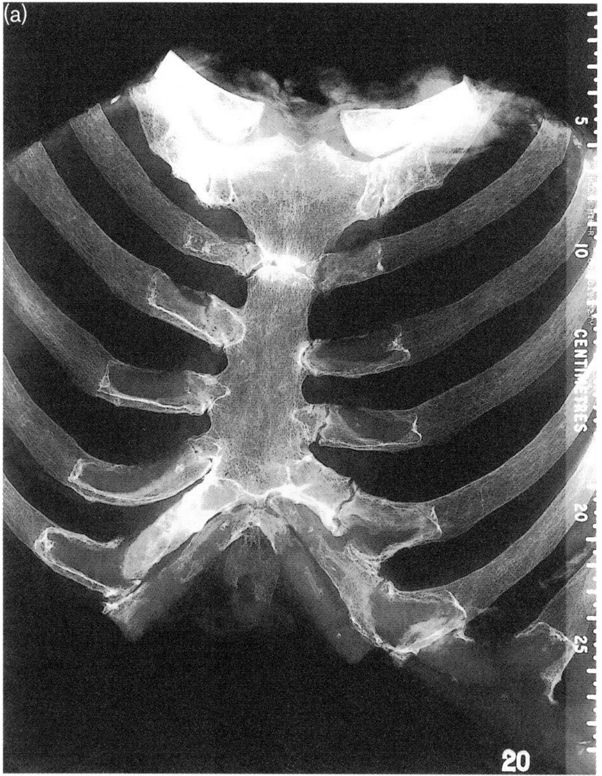

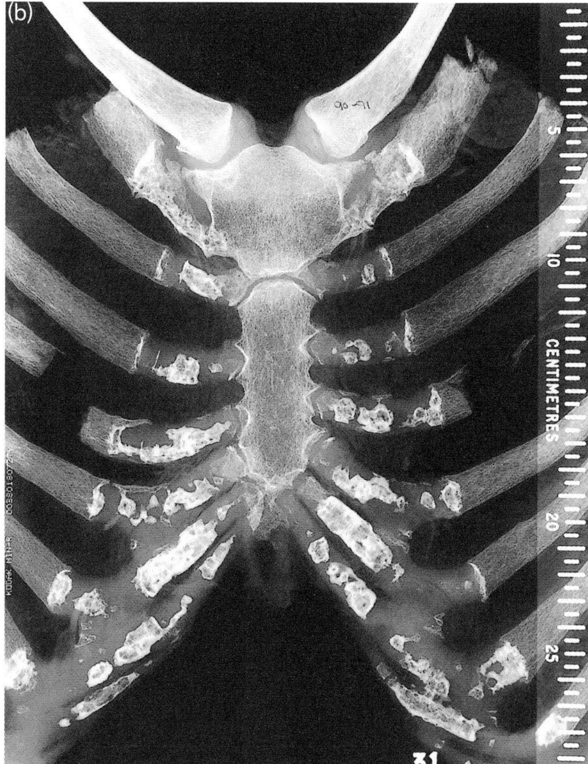

Figure 7.25 Male and female patterns of calcification in the costal cartilages. (a) Male – calcification is characterized by tongues of trabecular bone which form characteristic 'claw'-like extensions at the ventral extremity of the rib. (b) Female – calcification is characterized by discrete islands of dense sclerotic calcium deposits.

et al., 1985; McCormick and Stewart, 1988; Rao and Pai, 1988; Watts, 1990; Powell, 1991; Peace, 1992; Loth, 1995). Patterns of calcification differ between the first and all other costal cartilages. The appearance of the calcification in the first costal cartilage is identical in males and females and occurs as perichondral islands of bone that can span the full distance between the ventral end of the rib and the lateral margin of the manubrium (Fig. 7.24). All other costal cartilages ossify in a specific way depending upon the sex of the individual (Fig. 7.25). Female calcification tends to be characterized by dense sclerotic deposits of bone, while the male pattern is characterized by trabecular-type bone formation, which often extends ventrally from the rib end (King, 1939; Vastine and Vastine, 1946; Sanders, 1966; Navani *et al.*, 1970; Rao and Pai, 1988; Powell and MacLaughlin, 1992). It is believed that this highly specific sexual dimorphism (94% accuracy) occurs as a result of both hormonal influences and chemotactic factors, which influence subsequent vascular invasion (Peace, 1992). In addition, there is believed to be a genetic predisposition towards the pattern of calcium deposition in the costal cartilages (Vastine and Vastine, 1946).

Practical notes

Identification of individual juvenile ribs

To understand the functional basis for the identification and orientation of individual juvenile ribs, it is advised that the section on the identification of individual adult ribs is read. From the late fetal age, all ribs are readily identifiable, as they have already achieved close to the basic adult morphology. As a result, the identification of a rib is not at issue, only the identification of the specific bone within its series. It should, however, be borne in mind that the cortical shell of juvenile ribs is extremely thin and that both pre- and post-mortem deformation can be major contributory factors in the misidentification of single bones (Caro and Borden, 1988).

Fetal and perinatal

In the fetal and perinatal skeleton, rib 1 is readily identifiable, as it bears the characteristic shape that it will maintain through to adult life. Ribs 2–6 can be identified as their heads generally lie in contact with the horizontal plane when they are placed, inferior border downwards, on a flat surface. Ribs 2 and 3 are somewhat hook-shaped, although this is not as pronounced as in rib 1. The hook shape starts to straighten out in rib 4, as the shaft takes on a more gentle curve. In this way, ribs 2 and 3 can be separated from ribs 4–6. Ribs 7–9 are characterized by the fact that their heads have risen above the horizontal plane and so when the rib is placed on a flat surface, the head is elevated. Either rib 7 or 8 will attain the greatest elevation and this is again a phenomenon that is maintained through to adult life.

Ribs 10–12 in the fetal and perinatal skeleton are identifiable first by their smaller size and the general lack of definition in the region of the head. The head of rib 10 is in the horizontal plane and so lies in direct contact with a flat surface. This also occurs in ribs 11 and 12, but the latter two are markedly more rudimentary in terms of their development.

The fact that so many of the heads of fetal and perinatal ribs will lie in direct contact with a flat surface is readily explained by the common observation that fetal or neonatal ribs lie more horizontally, rather than obliquely in the thorax. It is for this reason that the neonate depends almost entirely on its diaphragm for respiration, as thoracic involvement cannot occur until the ribs adopt a more oblique angle and the thorax descends (Fig 7.20).

Young child

In the young child, up until approximately 2–3 years of age, the major change that occurs is a descent of the ventral aspect of the thorax by an increasing obliquity of the ribs. This becomes apparent in the morphology of the infant ribs by an increase in the torsion of the shaft and therefore an inclination of the heads to rise above the horizontal plane when the rib is placed, inferior border downwards, onto a flat surface. Within the first year, the heads of ribs 5 and 6 will start to rise, so that by the end of the second or third year of life, all ribs except 1, 2 and 10–12 will show significant shaft torsion that results in an inclination of the heads above the horizontal plane and this persists into the adult situation.

Sideing of juvenile ribs

Typical ribs

As with adult remains, fetal and juvenile ribs are most readily sided by identification of the basic rib morphology. The head of the rib will be posterior and the slightly concave, cup-shaped surface for the costochondral junction will be anterior. The inner surface is concave, the outer surface is convex and the inferior border carries the subcostal groove.

In the absence of the extremities of the rib and given only the shaft, then sideing becomes more difficult. Ribs 2–6 show a twist or torsion at the ventral extremity, so that the outer surface faces more obliquely upwards. This is presumably due to the fact that these ribs articulate directly with the sternum. In the lower ribs, the region of the subcostal groove may be of value in identifying the anterior from the posterior extremities when only the shaft is present. Ventral to the region of the posterior angle, the subcostal groove is deeper posteriorly and becomes more shallow anteriorly. Those ribs that lack a subcostal groove (ribs 1, 11 and 12) are naturally more difficult to side when fragmentary.

Atypical ribs

In the event of being unable to identify the characteristic morphology of the superior surface of the first rib, when the rib is placed on a horizontal surface, the tip of the head should be in contact with that surface. In this situation, the rib is in its correct position, in that the inferior surface faces downwards and the superior surface faces upwards. If the first rib is placed on a flat surface with the inferior surface facing upwards, then the head of the rib and the outer border will be elevated from the horizontal surface. This general rule holds true from the earliest prenatal stage to the adult situation.

Although the eleventh rib does not posses a readily identifiable subcostal groove, if the inner surface of the rib is examined, a change in shape may be identified, which may aid in side identification. It will be seen that passing from the tubercle in a ventral direction, the shaft increases in height in the region just beyond the posterior angle by an addition of a ledge of bone on the inferior margin. Again, this morphology holds true from the earliest prenatal material to the adult situation.

The twelfth rib is probably the most difficult to side, but it is possible if the rib is intact. If placed on a horizontal surface, the superior border faces more outwards, while the inferior border faces more inwards. In this way, when looking at the outer surface of the rib, the superior border will overhang the inferior border.

Bones of a similar morphology

Although it is unlikely that the ribs will be confused with any other bone in the body, even when fragmented, some confusion may occur with a fibular shaft fragment, which can be mistaken for the neck region of a rib. Similarly, it is possible for an isolated region of the neck of the acromion of the scapula to be mistaken as a first rib. However, the real difficulty lies in establishing the individual identity of the bone.

Morphological summary

Fetal	
Wks 8–9	Ossification centres appear for ribs 5–7
Wks 11–12	Ossification centres present in all ribs
Birth	All primary ossification centres present
12–14 yrs	Epiphyses appear in non-articular region of the tubercle
Around 18 yrs	Epiphyses appear for articular region of the tubercle
17–25 yrs	Epiphyses appear and fuse for head region
25 yrs +	Ribs are fully adult

Metrics

Using regression equations, Fazekas and Kósa (1978) calculated the body length (and thus the age at death) of a fetus from rib lengths (Tables 7.1 and 7.2). The cord length of the rib was defined as 'the distance between the articular part of the head and the sternal end of the rib'. They concluded that using this cord length, the body length and thus age of the fetus could best be established using ribs 1, 3 and 10.

> "We can easily determine the body length of fetuses in the following way:
>
> 1. by adding 3 to the double of the value of the length of the first rib measured in millimetres and expressing the value in centimetres, we obtain the body length in centimetres.
> 2. the cord distance in millimetres of the third rib corresponds to the body length in centimetres.
> 3. by adding 3 to the value of the tenth rib measured in millimetres and expressing it in centimetres, we obtain the approximate body length of the fetus in centimetres" (Fazekas and Kósa, 1978).

Table 7.1 Calculation of fetal body length from the cord length of the ribs

Body length = Rib 1 (length in cm)	× 20.53 + 2.68 cm
Body length = Rib 2 (length in cm)	× 12.70 + 0.64 cm
Body length = Rib 3 (length in cm)	× 11.84 − 2.13 cm
Body length = Rib 4 (length in cm)	× 8.52 + 1.27 cm
Body length = Rib 5 (length in cm)	× 8.18 − 0.33 cm
Body length = Rib 6 (length in cm)	× 7.97 + 0.00 cm
Body length = Rib 7 (length in cm)	× 7.67 + 1.43 cm
Body length = Rib 8 (length in cm)	× 8.15 + 1.93 cm
Body length = Rib 9 (length in cm)	× 8.87 + 2.65 cm
Body length = Rib 10 (length in cm)	× 10.07 + 3.44 cm
Body length = Rib 11 (length in cm)	× 12.08 + 5.14 cm
Body length = Rib 12 (length in cm)	× 21.13 + 7.09 cm

Adapted from Fazekas and Kósa (1978).

Table 7.2 Fetal rib length (in mm) from 12–40 weeks

	Ribs											
Age (weeks)	1	2	3	4	5	6	7	8	9	10	11	12
12	3.2	6.2	8.3	9.5	11.5	11.0	9.7	9.0	6.0	4.2	3.0	–
14	4.2	9.0	11.0	11.9	13.2	14.0	13.2	10.1	10.0	8.2	6.6	3.1
16	7.1	13.0	16.7	19.6	21.3	22.5	21.9	19.4	16.9	14.1	11.6	5.9
18	9.2	16.1	20.5	24.5	26.0	27.2	26.3	25.4	22.3	19.3	13.6	6.8
20	11.6	20.4	26.3	30.0	31.7	33.4	33.1	30.5	27.3	23.6	15.4	7.8
22	12.4	21.8	27.4	31.0	33.8	35.1	33.8	31.9	29.3	25.9	18.5	9.0
24	14.0	23.4	29.4	32.2	36.1	38.5	37.4	35.0	31.3	27.0	21.1	10.7
26	15.3	26.3	32.1	37.1	40.2	40.7	40.5	38.0	34.6	28.5	22.5	11.8
28	16.0	27.4	35.1	39.5	42.3	43.9	44.5	41.6	37.9	31.0	24.0	12.5
30	16.7	29.2	37.1	41.7	44.9	46.7	46.3	42.7	39.1	32.7	25.8	13.7
32	17.7	31.8	41.0	46.1	48.8	52.5	52.2	48.9	42.8	37.1	30.2	16.8
34	19.1	32.6	43.5	49.4	52.7	54.2	53.0	49.6	44.6	38.7	32.4	17.7
36	20.4	35.2	45.2	53.0	55.7	57.3	58.4	51.9	47.2	39.4	34.0	18.3
38	22.1	37.4	49.1	55.7	59.4	60.4	60.8	56.4	52.0	45.9	35.2	19.4
40	24.0	38.7	50.5	56.9	60.3	61.6	63.4	59.8	53.4	47.2	37.4	21.1

Adapted from Fazekas and Kósa (1978).

CHAPTER EIGHT

The Pectoral Girdle

The human pectoral (upper limb) girdle comprises a ventral **clavicle**, which articulates with the scapula laterally and the manubrium medially, and a **scapula**, which articulates laterally with the humerus at the shoulder joint. Therefore, the girdle only articulates with the axial skeleton anteriorly and under normal conditions has no posterior bony connection with the vertebral column (see below). As such, the clavicle serves as a strut to steady and brace the upper limb to the thorax, while the scapula achieves maximum mobility by being held in position by muscles and ligaments only. Therefore, the pectoral girdle serves to increase upper limb mobility and so release it for prehensile and manipulative activities.

This basic skeletal arrangement can be identified to a variable extent in most mammals in situations where the upper limb is not solely devoted to propulsive activities, but also incorporates some degree of limb abduction, e.g. swimming, climbing, flying and burrowing. However, in mammals where the main function of the forelimb is to absorb the stress of body weight on landing during forward locomotion (e.g. horse, cat and dog) the scapula requires to be free to act as a shock absorber and, as the forelimb displays no abductive capacity, the clavicle is essentially superfluous to requirements and may in fact be absent or rudimentary (Jenkins, 1974; Rojas and Montenegro, 1995). The human pectoral girdle is therefore a product of specific phylogenetic requirements and it is appropriate to look to other texts for details on the anatomy and evolution of this region for comparative purposes (Watson, 1917; Miller, 1932; Steindler, 1935; Oxnard, 1969; Wake, 1979; Romer and Parsons, 1986; Hildebrand, 1988; Aiello and Dean, 1990; Inuzuka, 1992).

I. THE CLAVICLE

The adult clavicle

Despite the lack of a medullary cavity, the clavicle is classified as a long bone and articulates with the manubrium medially and the acromion process of the scapula laterally. It passes horizontally across the root of the neck and is subcutaneous throughout most of its length. It possesses a double curve in the horizontal plane, which gives rise to the supposed derivation of its name – clavicula being the Latin diminutive of 'clavis' meaning a key (Field and Harrison, 1957).[1]

There are four principal functions attributed to the clavicle

- to provide a bony framework for muscle attachment
- to act as a strut, holding the glenohumeral joint in a parasagittal plane thereby increasing the range of potential movement of the shoulder joint
- to transmit the supportive stresses of the upper limb to the axial skeleton
- to protect the axillary neurovascular bundle as it passes from the neck into the upper limb (Inman *et al.*, 1944; Copland, 1946; Gurd, 1947; Abbot and Lucas, 1954; Howard, 1965; Moseley, 1968; Ljunggren, 1979).

Despite these, the clavicle is not considered to be essential, as total resection (claviculectomy) results in little impairment of function providing that the

[1]Other sources state that the Roman key was no different from that of modern day and that this is an unsatisfactory explanation for the derivation of the term. Other authors state that the name is derived from the Latin meaning 'to shut or close' (claudere) as the clavicle is said to close the thorax. Or, perhaps it is in deference to the morphological similarity of the bone to a curved catch that was used to fasten or shut a window (Skinner, 1961).

muscle ends are re-attached (Copland, 1946; Gurd, 1947; Abbot and Lucas, 1954; Wood, 1986). Jockeys display a disproportionate number of clavicular fractures and the long period of time required for the fracture to heal delays return to work and to riding in general. A complete surgical excision of the lateral fragment results in no functional loss and the jockey can return to work more quickly with no fear of repetition of such an injury (Middleton *et al.*, 1995).

Congenital absence of the clavicles is rare and tends to show a familial tendency. The patient suffers from no power loss in the upper limb and no restriction in movement. In fact, bilateral absence of the clavicle results in hypermobility in this region so that the shoulders can be approximated in the midline when the arms are brought forward and the scapular borders can be made to overlap when the arms are brought behind (Carpenter, 1899; Schorstein, 1899). In these circumstances, the muscles that would normally attach to the bony clavicle instead find anchorage in an oblique fibrous band.

The clavicle possesses anterior and posterior borders, superior and inferior surfaces and medial and lateral articular extremities (Fig. 8.1). The double curvature of the shaft separates the bone into a medial two-thirds and a lateral one-third. The medial two-thirds is somewhat quadrilateral in cross-section and is convex anteriorly, thereby clearing the position of the axillary

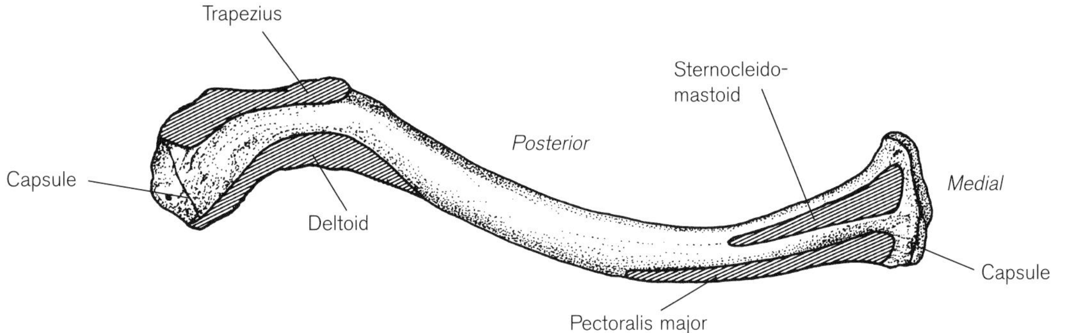

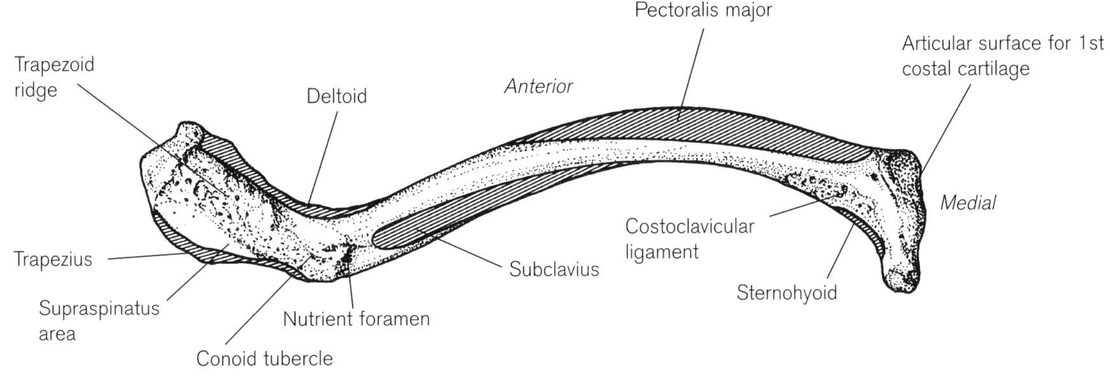

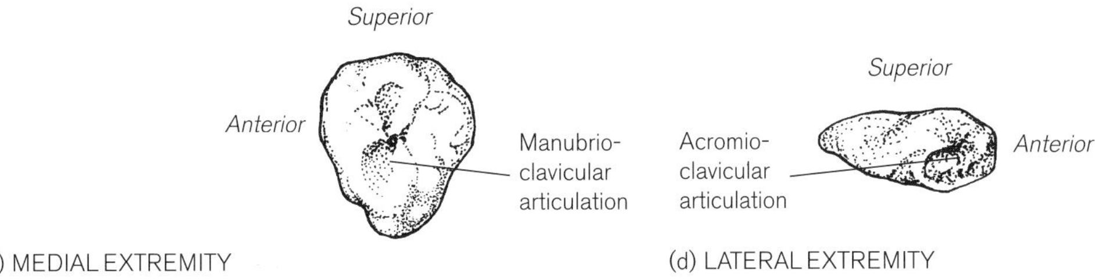

Figure 8.1 The right adult clavicle.

sheath, which lies directly behind the bone. The lateral one-third of the clavicle is somewhat flattened in shape and concave anteriorly as it passes slightly backwards to reach the scapula.

The **superior surface** is smoother than the inferior surface and is predominantly a site for muscle attachment (Fig. 8.1a). The muscles clearly separate into those that are attached to the medial aspect of the bone (sternocleidomastoid and pectoralis major) and those that are attached more laterally (trapezius and deltoid). The intervening area (middle third) that is devoid of muscle attachments has often been used by anaesthetists as a suitable anatomical site for administering a supraclavicular block to the brachial plexus. It is also the site chosen for the taking of blood when venous pressure is low, as the subclavian vein cannot collapse at this point as it is supported by the clavicle and its fascial coverings. The site is also critical to a clear understanding of the fracture pattern that is seen in this bone (see below). A groove may sometimes be found on this surface between the attachments of trapezius and deltoid. This is caused by a venous communication between the cephalic and external jugular veins and represents an embryological remnant of a previously large venous channel (Frazer, 1948).

The **inferior surface** of the clavicle shows well-developed sites of attachment for both muscles and ligaments (Fig. 8.1b). At the medial end, extending from the inferior surface onto the anterior border is the articular facet for the first costal cartilage. This is generally continuous with the sternal articular surface, but an entirely separate facet can arise and has only been reported in man, although its function is not yet fully understood (Redlund-Johnell, 1986). Posterolateral to this is a roughened area for the attachment of the very strong **costoclavicular** (rhomboid) **ligament**. This is a major stabilizer of the clavicle and binds its inferior surface tightly to the first rib and its costal cartilage. The clavicular attachment of the ligament can be so strong as to produce a deep depression (**rhomboid fossa**) that can be detected on radiographs and may be confused with soft tissue lesions such as a tumour (Pendergrass and Hodes, 1937; Shulman, 1941; Treble, 1988) or syphilitic gummata (Steinbock, 1976).

The small sternohyoid muscle may attach to the posterior border of the expanded sternal extremity, but it rarely leaves any mark on the bone. The pectoralis major muscle extends from the anterior border onto the inferior surface and posterior to it lies the subclavius muscle, which occupies a groove along the axis of the inferior surface. The function of this muscle is to stabilize the clavicle during movements of the shoulder (Cave and Brown, 1952). Subclavius cannot be palpated due to its deep location, which can serve in a protective role to prevent fragments of a comminuted fracture from piercing the subclavian vessels (Ellis and Feldman, 1993). In active young males in particular, both the tendons of the subclavius and scalenus anterior muscles can cause intermittent obstruction of the subclavian vein. Removal of the former muscle alleviates the situation, with little impairment to the functional integrity of the girdle (McCleery *et al.*, 1951).

The subclavius groove is bounded by anterior and posterior ridges that give attachment to the anterior and posterior layers of the clavipectoral fascia, respectively. The tendinous intersection of the omohyoid muscle is bound to the posterior ridge by a fascial sling that is derived from the deep lamina of the investing layer of deep cervical fascia. Last (1973) suggested that in the fetus, the omohyoid muscle originally belongs to the strap-like group of infrahyoid muscles but, by a process of migration, its attachment moves laterally along the clavicle to adopt its final position at the suprascapular notch. The truth of this statement is somewhat dubious and no other references can be found that relate to such an unusual and extensive form of muscle migration. It is interesting to note, however, that the muscles all share the same fascial confinements and the same nerve supply (ansa cervicalis).

The clavicular nutrient foramen is usually found on the posterior border in the medial two-thirds, lateral to the point of maximum posterior concavity. In the majority of cases it is a single foramen (64%), although it can be double, triple or quadruple (Parsons, 1916). The nutrient artery is derived from the suprascapular artery as it passes deep to the inferior belly of the omohyoid muscle. Other foramina may be present in the shaft of the clavicle, but these will be seen to pass directly through the bone (canaliculi claviculare). These are formed by the passage of the supraclavicular nerves that become entrapped during the early development of the bone (Turner, 1874). After exiting from the bone, the nerves continue on their course to supply the skin over the pectoralis major muscle.

The other supportive ligament of the clavicle is the **coracoclavicular ligament** at the lateral extremity of the bone (Cockshott, 1992; Haramati *et al.*, 1994). This ligament is separated into two parts – the conoid part (cone–shaped), which stretches from the coracoid process of the scapula to the conoid tubercle on the inferior surface of the clavicle, and the trapezoid part that passes as a more horizontal sheet from the trapezoid line on the coracoid process to the trapezoid ridge on the inferior surface of the clavicle. The **conoid tubercle** lies more posterior and medial to the **trapezoid ridge** and occasionally a groove marking the passage of the subclavian artery may be visible just medial to the tubercle (Ray, 1959). A joint can exist between the coracoid process and the clavicle, although it is not common (Lewis, 1959; Aiello and Dean, 1990; Nalla and Asvat, 1995). It is equally represented in males and females and in an extensive study, Kaur and Jit (1991) did not find it to be present before 13 years of age. Instead of a true joint, a bony or cartilaginous communication can occur and although this rarely causes symptoms, some limitation of shoulder motion may result from interference with free scapular rotation (Liebman and Freedman, 1938; Chung and Nissenbaum, 1975; Chen and Bohrer, 1990). Cho and Kang (1998) found that the joint was not present in individuals younger than 40 years of age and suggested that its presence was significantly correlated with increasing age. Interestingly, they did not find any significant correlation with the size of the scapulae and the presence of the joint.

The deltoid muscle attaches anterior to, and the trapezius muscle posterior to, the trapezoid ridge. There is a smooth area of bone located between the trapezoid ridge and the trapezius attachments and this marks the site where the supraspinatus muscle passes in close proximity to the clavicle as it extends from the supraspinous fossa of the scapula to the greater tubercle of the humerus. The subacromial bursa may occupy this position.

The **medial** (sternal) **extremity** of the clavicle is roughly oval in shape and may extend onto the inferior surface for articulation with the first costal cartilage (Fig. 8.1c). Only the lower part of the sternal face is in contact with the manubrium as the remainder of the surface projects upwards beyond the sternum into the jugular fossa. The joint is synovial with an intra-articular fibrocartilaginous disc, which is firmly bound by the joint capsule and a series of strong ligaments, thereby adding to the mobility of the joint. The anterior and posterior sternoclavicular ligaments support their respective aspects of the joint, while the interclavicular ligament joins the upper margins of the two clavicles. It is in this ligament that suprasternal ossicles may develop (Chapter 7). The costoclavicular ligament is the major support to this joint, tightly binding the inferior surface of the clavicle to the upper surface of the first rib and its costal cartilage (Kennedy, 1949; Cave, 1961). Due to the strength of this ligament in particular, the joint rarely dislocates, but if it does, then it tends to be displaced anteriorly (Salvatore, 1968). Following dislocation, it is common for the costoclavicular ligament to tear, although it is unlikely to result in any long-term functional impairment of the joint (Cyriax, 1919).

The **lateral extremity** of the clavicle may be either narrow or broad and spatulate-like in appearance and articulates with the acromion process of the scapula at the acromioclavicular joint (Fig. 8.1d) (Terry, 1934; Keats and Pope, 1988). The articular facet is oval in shape and small in comparison to the sternal face. The joint is synovial in nature and may also contain an intra-articular fibrocartilaginous disc. This joint is held in position by the strong coracoclavicular ligament inferiorly and the much weaker acromioclavicular ligament superiorly. An unknown mechanism, whereby atraumatic osteolysis of the most lateral aspect of the clavicle can arise following spinal cord injury, has been reported in the literature (Roach and Schweitzer, 1997). This bony condition (abbreviated to AODC – atraumatic osteolysis of the distal clavicle) has also been reported in association with hyperparathyroidism, progressive systemic sclerosis, rheumatoid arthritis and even as a result of repetitive stress-related activities, such as weight-lifting (Madsen, 1963; Halaby and DiSalvo, 1965; Cahill, 1992).

Movements of the clavicle are passive and brought about by movements of the scapula. A specific movement at the acromial end results in an opposite movement at the sternal end, as the clavicle acts like a seesaw being bound down by its coracoclavicular ligament laterally and the costoclavicular ligament medially (Inman *et al.*, 1944). These ligaments bind the ends of the clavicle so tightly that the most common injury is fracture that generally occurs at the weakest site, i.e. between the two ligaments, in the area not protected by muscle attachments and at the junction of the two shaft curvatures.

This is the most frequently broken bone in the skeleton and almost 80% of all clavicular fractures will occur at the junction between the medial and lateral segments, with only 15% of fractures arising at the lateral and 5% at the medial extremities (Neer, 1960; Allman, 1967; Rowe, 1968). Fracture generally arises following indirect violence such as a fall on the outstretched hand or a fall onto the shoulder. Following a fracture, the trapezius muscle is unable to support the weight of the limb and the lateral fragment is depressed and drawn medially by the teres major, latissimus dorsi and pectoralis major muscles. Despite the difficulty in immobilizing the bone, the fracture will generally reunite under any circumstances as the clavicle displays a remarkable healing capacity (Ghormley *et al.*, 1941). Healing of the fracture site is rapid, with infants showing union in around 2 weeks, children in 3 weeks, young adults in 4–6 weeks and mature adults by around 6 weeks (Rowe, 1968). Non-union after 4–6 weeks is rare (Ghormley *et al.*, 1941). Clavicular fractures are not however to be considered lightly, as various complications can arise, e.g. pneumothorax (3%), re-fracture (2%), death (2%) and haemothorax (1%). The presence of the subclavius muscle ensures that rupture of the major vessels is rare following fracture, although this is said to have been the cause of death of Sir Robert Peel when he was thrown from his horse in Hyde Park.

Fractures of the lateral extremity represent almost one-half of all the clavicular fractures that do not unite, although they only represent some 15% of clavicular fractures as a whole (Gurd, 1941; Neer, 1968). This non-union can result in a resorption of the lateral fragment of the clavicle (Yochum and Rowe, 1987) and is generally more common in the elderly (Robinson, 1998).

The close proximity of the clavicle to the important axillary neurovascular sheath can result in a number of clinical syndromes. Bateman (1968) likened the clavicle to the constriction found in an hourglass, where the structures are funnelled together before dispersing again on either side of the bone. He summarized that supraclavicular lesions tended to result in neurological disruptions, while a combination of neurological and vascular disorders were indicative of lesions either behind the clavicle or in the infraclavicular region.

Sternocostoclavicular hyperostosis is a clinical condition that has been found almost exclusively in the Japanese. Its aetiology is uncertain but may be bacterial in origin, as it is often found associated with pustulosis palmaris and plantaris (Beck and Berkheiser, 1954; Resnick *et al.*, 1981; Chigra and Shimizu, 1989). The patient generally presents with pain in the upper part of the chest and shoulder girdle. Radiological examination reveals a periosteal and endosteal hyperossification of the sternum, clavicles, upper ribs and surrounding soft tissues. In this condition, the clavicles are often described as being symmetrically enlarged and club-like.

The adult clavicle tends to survive inhumation successfully due to its thick shell of compact bone and so it is of some value in both forensic and anthropological investigations (Lin, 1991). It can be useful in sex determination (Thieme and Schull, 1957; Iordanidis, 1961; Jit and Singh, 1966; Steel, 1966; Singh and Gangrade, 1968), age at death estimation (Walker and Lovejoy, 1985; Kaur and Jit, 1990; Stout and Paine, 1992), stature estimation (Jit and Singh, 1956), racial evaluation (Terry, 1932), establishing handedness (Longia *et al.*, 1982; Steele and Mays, 1995) and personal identification (Sanders *et al.*, 1972).

The clavicle is unusual in one further aspect. It is generally recognized that the left bone is usually longer than the right within any one individual, although the right is generally the more robust. Many authors have attributed this to different factors including differential loading, ligamentous asymmetry or dominant vascularity. Most recently, Mays *et al.* (1999) concluded that such asymmetry was due to an inhibition of longitudinal growth due to a bias in mechanical loading, particularly via axial compression.

Early development of the clavicle

The girdle bones are almost entirely derived from the lateral plate mesoderm of the trilaminar embryonic disc. Consistent with the fact that the embryo develops in a cephalocaudal direction, the pectoral girdle develops in advance of the pelvic girdle and larger elements tend to chondrify before their smaller counterparts (Glenister, 1976). Mesenchymal cells migrate to the site where the future clavicle will develop and maintain a lateral continuity with the mesenchymal condensation that will form the scapula (Hamilton and Mossman, 1972). As the scapula develops from the midcervical region, the embryological and fetal clavicle does not adopt a horizontal position until the shoulders have fully descended (Noback, 1944; Corrigan, 1960a; McClure and Raney, 1975). Migration of the shoulder commences in the first year and continues until approximately 4 years of age (Terry, 1959) but until full descent is achieved, the clavicle remains elevated at its lateral extremity.

The blastemal stage of clavicular development arises in fetal week 5, with a fibrocellular proliferation that commences laterally and spreads medially (Gardner, 1968). These cells further condense into a mesenchymal rod that is certainly recognizable by the end of the fifth fetal week (Fawcett, 1913; Gardner and Gray, 1953; Andersen, 1963; Wall, 1970; O'Rahilly and Gardner, 1975). By around 10 fetal weeks, cavitation of the acromioclavicular joint is complete (Uhthoff, 1990c).

Ossification

Primary centre(s)

There is much controversy over the mode of development of the clavicle during the sixth and seventh fetal weeks. The most widely accepted view is that ossification commences directly within the membranous structure of the blastemal stage, or at least in a matrix that some authors describe as 'precartilaginous' (Fawcett, 1910c, 1913; Fitzwilliams, 1910; Hanson, 1920a; Golthamer, 1957; Gardner, 1968; Ogden *et al.*, 1979b; Ogata and Uhthoff, 1990a). This membranous (dermal) origin for the clavicle was previously taken as firm evidence that the clinical condition of craniocleidodysostosis (see later) arose from an early

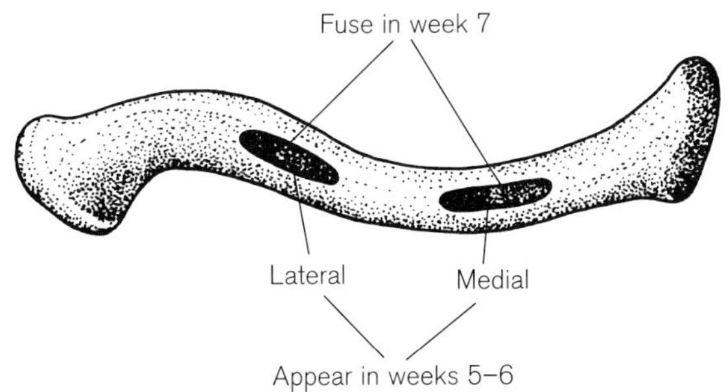

Figure 8.2 Location of the clavicular primary centres of ossification.

defect in bones formed via intramembranous ossification. This is now considered to be too simplistic a viewpoint, as the condition is more likely to be inherited as an autosomal dominant with a high degree of penetrance (Lasker, 1946; Marie and Sainton, 1968). Although no longer held to be true, some authors have reported that all ossification of the clavicle takes place in true hyaline cartilage (Koch, 1960; Alldred, 1963). It has been widely accepted that the lateral aspect of the clavicle may develop from a membranous tissue (as evidenced by its more flattened appearance), while the more medial aspect develops via true endochondral ossification (given its tubular appearance, the presence of an articular disc and a medial epiphysis). This dual origin has also been used to explain the presence of paired centres of ossification.

At around day 39, in the sixth week of intrauterine life, ossification commences in the precartilage anlage. Although some authors consider that there is only a single primary ossification centre (Koch, 1960; Gibson and Carroll, 1970), most agree that there are two primary centres (Fig 8.2), one medial and one lateral (Mall, 1906; Fawcett, 1913; Hanson, 1920a; Golthamer, 1957; Alldred, 1963; Andersen, 1963; Gardner, 1968; Wall, 1970; O' Rahilly and Gardner, 1972; Ogden *et al.*, 1979b; Ogata and Uhthoff, 1990a). Congenital absence of the lateral half of the clavicle seems to lend some support to a double origin of ossification (Terry, 1899), as does duplication of the lateral half (Rutherford, 1921). Some authors consider the lateral centre to be the larger (Andersen, 1963; Gardner, 1968) whilst others state that the medial centre is the larger (Mall, 1906; Ogata and Uhthoff, 1990a). A bony bridge forms shortly after ossification commences and the two centres have generally fused by fetal week 7, when vascular invasion of the ossified matrix commences (Fawcett, 1913; Andersen, 1963; Wall, 1970).

An inferior displacement of one of the primary centres of ossification can lead to the development of an accessory clavicle (os subclaviculare). This is generally an asymptomatic rudimentary structure (Golthamer, 1957; Twigg and Rosenbaum, 1981). Qureshi and Kuo (1999) suggested that the duplication of the lateral half might be indicative of a previous fracture or injury to the bone. They reported that following lateral physeal separation, full reconstitution of the lateral part could occur.

Once the osteoid matrix has been laid down in the precartilage model, then the medial and lateral extremities develop chondrogenous zones of hyaline cartilage so that bone length increases from this stage by true endochondral ossification via growth plates (Gardner, 1968; Gibson and Carroll, 1970). The sternal end grows more rapidly than the acromial end, so that some 80% of the total bone length is derived from growth at the medial end (Ogden *et al.*, 1979b; Rönning and Kantomaa, 1988; Rojas and Montenegro, 1995). This explains the disproportionate morphology of the bone in terms of the proportions of the double curvatures and the lateral position of the nutrient artery, which is directed away from the growing end (Ogden *et al.*, 1979b).

The shaft of the clavicle adopts a distinctive 'S' shape by about 8–9 fetal weeks (Andersen, 1963) and achieves adult morphology by 11 fetal weeks (Fig. 8.3) (Ogata and Uhthoff, 1990a). Increases in bone width then continue by subperiosteal apposition in the shaft and true endochondral ossification at the medial and lateral extremities gives rise to an increase in bone length. This unusually early attainment of adult morphology indicates that the clavicle is not greatly influenced by postnatal mechanical stresses and forces. It is therefore a bone of both considerable

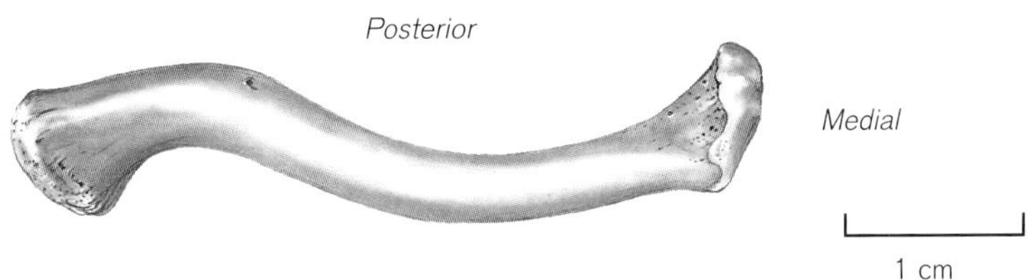

Figure 8.3 The right perinatal clavicle. Note the remarkable morphological similarity to the adult form at this very early stage.

phylogenetic and ontogenetic morphological stability (Corrigan, 1960a). An unusual radiological phenomenon of a unilateral 'wavy clavicle' has been reported in the absence of either trauma or congenital abnormality and it has been suggested that its aetiology may lie in the exaggerated effect of pulsations of the right subclavian artery as it passes deep to the bone (Levin, 1990; Freiberger, 1991).

Studies on the fetal growth of the clavicle both by direct examination of the bone (Fazekas and Kósa, 1978) and by ultrasound (Yarkoni *et al.*, 1985) have shown that the clavicle grows at a surprisingly linear rate of approximately 1 mm per week (Table 8.1). By term, the clavicle measures some 40–41 mm and then growth appears to slow down, although later growth spurts can be identified between 5–7 years of age and again at puberty (Black and Scheuer, 1996b).

There are two other congenital conditions that affect the clavicle and require some further consideration. The patient with craniocleido (cleidocranial) dysostosis presents with an exaggerated development of the transverse diameter of the cranium concomitant with a retarded ossification of the fontanelles. In addition, the clavicles are either hypoplastic, or indeed absent, leading to marked hypermobility of the shoulder joints (Barlow, 1883; Fitzwilliams, 1910; Heindon, 1951; Tachdjian, 1972; Yochum and Rowe, 1987). In some instances, only medial and lateral clavicular stumps may develop for the appropriate muscular attachments with an absence of the central section. This can lead to abnormal pressure on the brachial plexus and subclavian arteries, leading to neurological and vascular disturbances. This condition tends to have an autosomal dominant inheritance, although there are some rare cases where it appears to be recessive (Jarvis and Keats, 1974; Dore *et al.*, 1987).

Table 8.1 Fetal clavicular measurements

	Maximum clavicular length (mm)	
Age in weeks	Fazekas and Kósa*	Yarkoni *et al.*†
12	8.2	–
14	11.1	–
16	16.3	17.0
18	19.4	19.0
20	22.7	21.0
22	24.5	23.0
24	26.9	25.0
26	28.3	27.0
28	30.3	29.0
30	31.3	31.0
32	35.6	33.0
34	37.1	35.0
36	37.7	37.0
38	42.6	39.0
40	44.1	41.0

*Data derived from Fazekas and Kósa (1978) – dry bone.
†Data derived from Yarkoni *et al.* (1985) – ultrasound.

Fairbank (1949) found that the most common alteration to the clavicle was the absence of the lateral end, whilst Forland (1962) reported that most commonly the central segment would be absent but that medial and lateral stumps would prevail. This latter proposition would corroborate the fact that craniocleidodysostosis generally affects those bones that form early in fetal life and, as the medial and lateral extremities of the clavicle develop later, then perhaps they are less affected. Alternatively, it may simply be an indication that the only true functional requirement of the clavicle is to provide a site for muscle attachment.

Although congenital pseudo-arthrosis of the clavicle is rare, it has received a considerable amount of attention in the clinical literature (Rossignol, 1948; Sakellarides, 1961; Jinkins, 1969; Owen, 1970; Herman, 1973; Shalom *et al.*, 1994). This condition is generally detected shortly after birth and certainly by 6 years of age, presenting as a painless lump over the clavicle. It does not represent a birth injury, as there is no reactive bone at the site and no callus formation and some authors have taken its presence as being representative of non-union between the two primary centres of ossification. There is no evidence of a genetic link, it is not sex specific and predominantly affects the right-hand side. In fact, Behringer and Wilson (1972) found that 94% of all cases occurred unilaterally on the right. This pseudo-arthrosis generally occurs just lateral to the midline of the bone (Alldred, 1963), so that the sternal fragment is larger (Wall, 1970). The ends of the bone may be covered by cartilage and may even possess a synovial lining (Quinlan *et al.*, 1980). The aetiology of this condition is unknown, although Lloyd-Roberts *et al.* (1975) suggested that it might be concerned with the relatively higher position of the fetal right subclavian artery. This would result in the right clavicle being subjected to exaggerated arterial pulsation in the region of the midshaft and this may affect the development of a bony bridge between the ossification centres and so alter the normal ossification process. Although painless, except in advancing age, when the condition may cause some aching, surgery is often recommended solely on the grounds of aesthetics (Tachdjian, 1972; Ozonoff, 1979).

Secondary centres

Following the pattern displayed by all other major long bones of the limbs, the adult clavicle is derived from a shaft (primary centre(s) of ossification) and medial (sternal) and lateral articular extremities that develop from secondary ossification centres (Todd and D' Errico, 1928). The medial epiphysis is flake-like in appearance and fairly rudimentary in nature, while the lateral epiphysis rarely exists as a separate structure, if indeed it is ever present.

The **medial** metaphyseal surface of the developing shaft of the clavicle bears the characteristic ridge-and-furrow appearance indicative of vascular activity. Arteries gain access to this region from the periosteal vascular network and penetrate into the zone of hyaline cartilage at the articular extremity (Haines *et al.*, 1967). Ossification commences in the epiphyseal cartilage mass around puberty (13–14 years – Ogden *et al.*, 1979b) and has been reported as early as 11 years in females and 12 years in males (Flecker, 1932b).

Despite formation at an age which is in accordance with the appearance of other secondary centres in the skeleton (Dawson, 1925), the medial end of the clavicle is, for some unknown reason, a slow-maturing epiphysis and fusion to the diaphysis will not occur until at least 10 years after its initial formation (McKern and Stewart, 1957). In fact, it is usually attributed to being the final epiphysis to fuse.

The medial epiphysis generally appears as a small nodule in the centre of the sternal cartilage mass of the clavicle (Fig. 8.4). The nodule then begins to flatten out and spread over the articular face, first in a posterior and superior direction. At this stage, the epiphysis may be a separate structure or it may have commenced fusion in the centre of the flake with the metaphyseal surface. The epiphysis rarely covers the entire articular surface and often falls short of the anterior diaphyseal rim (Black and Scheuer, 1996b). Fusion between the diaphysis and the epiphysis is said to begin around 16–21 years (although it has been reported as early as 11 years) and completion may not take place until close to 30 years of age (Stevenson, 1924; McKern and Stewart, 1957; Jit and Kulkarni, 1976; Szilvassy, 1980; Webb and Suchey, 1985; MacLaughlin, 1990a; Black and Scheuer, 1996b). In summary, a medial end of a clavicle with no evidence of a fused/fusing epiphysis is likely to have come from an individual less than 18 years of age. The presence of a well-defined fusing flake will occur in individuals between the ages of 16 and 21 years and an epiphysis that covers most of the articular surface will probably occur in an individual between 24 and 29 years. Complete epiphyseal fusion is unlikely to be seen before 22 years and is always complete by 30 years.

The age at which epiphyseal ossification commences, initiation of fusion begins and total fusion occurs, shows a considerable degree of variation. It is likely that much of this variation can be explained in terms of individual maturation timings that are influenced by predisposing hereditary and environmental factors (Galstaun, 1930). Therefore, timings should always be taken as an indication of the estimated chronological age of the individual, but never considered to be evidence of the true age.

Trauma at the medial end of the juvenile clavicle, e.g. dislocation, can result in a separation of the medial epiphysis so that it forms as a separate bone (Denham and Dingley, 1967). Alternatively, the medial end may be resorbed and in this situation the sternal end of the diaphysis will glaze over so that a smooth articular surface is still formed.

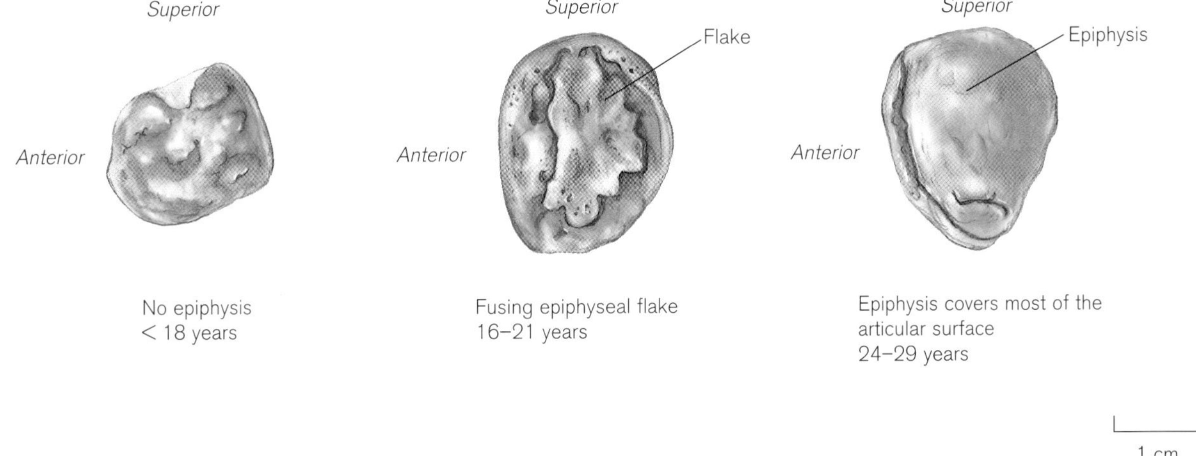

Figure 8.4 Epiphyseal union at the medial end of the right clavicle.

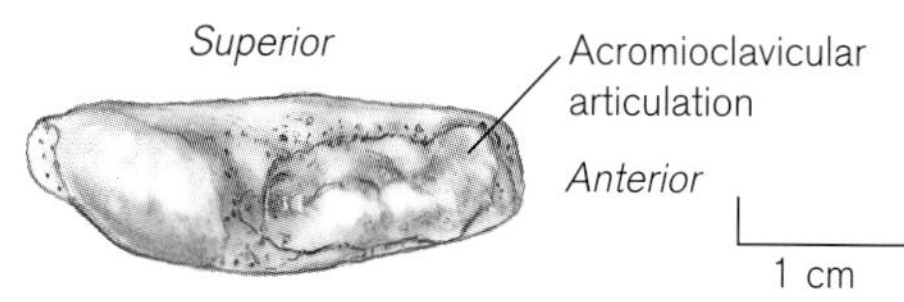

Figure 8.5 The lateral epiphyseal surface of the right clavicle.

Although there are a number of texts that state that no epiphysis forms at the **lateral** (acromial) end of the clavicle, there are a sufficient number of reports that claim the opposite to be true. When, and if, a lateral epiphysis develops, it tends to be a transitory structure forming around 19 or 20 years of age and fusing within months of its formation (McKern and Stewart, 1957; Gardner, 1968). Alternatively, the vascular ridge-and-furrow articular surface of the juvenile diaphysis (Fig. 8.5) may simply glaze over as bone is laid down to smooth the articular surface and so a separate entity may never exist (Todd and D'Errico, 1928).

Practical notes

Sideing

The early attainment of the adult-like form ensures that it is relatively easy, not only to identify a juvenile clavicle, but also to be sure of its side. Correct orientation relies on being able to identify the superior and inferior surfaces, the anterior and posterior borders and the medial and lateral extremities.

Bones of a similar morphology

A small cross-sectional fragment of a clavicle may be confused with a shaft of one of the long bones in the early stages of development, but the configuration of the medullary cavity should prevent a misidentification. Fragments of the lateral end of the clavicle can also be confused with rib fragments.

Morphological summary

Fetal

Wks 5–6	Primary ossification centres appear
Wk 7	Two centres fuse to form a single mass
Wks 8–9	Clavicle becomes 'S' shaped
Wk 11	Clavicle adopts adult morphology
Birth	Clavicle is represented by shaft only and is essentially adult in its morphology
12–14 yrs	Medial epiphyseal flake forms
16–21 yrs	Fusion of flake commences at medial extremity
19–20 yrs	Lateral epiphysis may form and fuse
29+ yrs	Fusion of medial epiphysis will be complete in all individuals

Metrics

Fazekas and Kósa (1978) measured fetal clavicular length on dry bone specimens, and although their sample was not strictly documented, the results agreed closely with that of Yarkoni *et al.* (1985), who measured the living bone by ultrasound (Table 8.1). Only Black and Scheuer (1996b) appear to have examined a substantial number of postnatal clavicular lengths from documented juvenile material (Table 8.2).

Table 8.2 Clavicular measurements from documented juveniles

	Maximum clavicular length (mm)		
Documented age	*n*	Mean	Range
Birth–6 months	11	44.4	38.8–54.5
7 months–1 year	9	54.1	48.0–60.9
1 year–1.5 years	11	59.5	54.3–66.0
1.5 years–2 years	4	63.0	61.4–64.6
2–3 years	13	66.5	58.5–72.6
3–4 years	7	73.4	69.1–77.0
4–5 years	8	74.4	65.3–82.0
5–6 years	2	75.9	74.7–77.0
6–7 years	4	86.5	85.4–88.8
7–8 years	1	89.5	–
8–9 years	3	89.0	78.5–98.7
9–10 years	0	–	–
10–11 years	2	103.7	103.0–104.0
11–12 years	2	105.0	104.5–105.0
12–13 years	3	106.4	102.5–111.3
13–14 years	2	118.6	117.0–120.1
14–15 years	2	118.5	113.5–123.5
15–16 years	3	137.7	127.0–154.0

Adapted from Black and Scheuer (1996b).

II. THE SCAPULA

The adult scapula

The scapula is thought to derive its name from the Greek, 'skapto' meaning 'I dig', with reference to its spade-like appearance (Field and Harrison, 1957).[2] It is classified as a flat bone and is located on the posterolateral aspect of the thoracic wall. It articulates with the humerus at the shoulder (glenohumeral) joint, with the clavicle at the acromioclavicular joint and is

[2]Nowhere in classical writing does the singular term 'scapula' arise except in reference to a surname of the Cornelian family (Simpson, 1969). In the works of Galen and Aristole, the scapula was referred to as the 'omoplate' a word derive from the Greek 'omos' meaning shoulder and in some languages the scapula may still be referred to in this way (Vallois, 1928, 1946; Iordanidis, 1961).

suspended from the vertebral column, ribs and skull by muscles. The scapula is not a common site for fractures, as much of the bone is deeply buried in muscle, which effectively cushions it from direct impact (Rowe, 1968; Wilber and Evans, 1977; Heyse-Moore and Stoker, 1982; Hollinshead, 1982). When fractures do occur, it is usually in association with other traumatic injuries (Imatani, 1975; McGahan *et al.*, 1980; Thompson *et al.* 1985; Ada and Miller, 1991; Gupta *et al.*, 1998).

The morphology of the bone is largely dictated by its functions, which are first, to provide an articular surface for the upper limb and second, to provide a large surface area for the muscles, which facilitate mobility at that joint (Anetzberger and Putz, 1996). The thinness of the bone in conjunction with its relatively large surface area means that it does not tend to survive inhumation successfully, which is unfortunate given its potential value for anthropological and forensic investigations. The adult scapula displays sexual dimorphism (Bainbridge and Tarazaga, 1956; Olivier and Pineau, 1957; Hanihara, 1959; Iordanidis, 1961) and exhibits age-related change (Graves, 1922; McKern and Stewart, 1957). Indeed, it can also be used (albeit with limited success) to predict handedness (Schulter-Ellis, 1980), race (Flower, 1879; Hrdlička, 1942a; Wolffson, 1950) and stature (Shulin and Fangwu, 1983).

Although the scapula is essentially a triangular bone, there is some considerable variation in its basic morphology (Graves, 1921; Gray, 1942; Hrdlička, 1942a, b; Khoo and Kuo, 1948; Wolffson, 1950). It possesses three borders (medial, lateral and superior), three angles (superior, inferior and lateral), two surfaces (ventral and dorsal) and three bony projections (spine, acromion and coracoid) (Fig. 8.6). Detailed descriptions of the scapular muscles and their actions can be found in all major anatomical texts (Frazer, 1948; Last, 1973; Williams *et al.*, 1995).

In the adult, the **medial** (vertebral) **border** (Fig. 8.6a) lies adjacent to thoracic vertebrae 2–7 and dorsal to the outer surfaces of the corresponding ribs. This border is usually convex (Gray, 1942) and runs from the superior angle at the level of T2 to the inferior angle at T7. The upper one-third lies opposite the supraspinous fossa and is the site of attachment for the levator scapulae muscle. There is a small flattened area opposite the root of the spinous process, where the rhomboid minor muscle attaches. The rhomboid major muscle is attached to the lower two-thirds of the medial border at the level of the infraspinous fossa. These three muscles act together to elevate and retract the scapula and, with trapezius, suspend the scapula from the vertebral column.

In Sprengel's deformity (a maldescent of the fetal scapula), an omovertebral bone may persist, which connects the medial border to the spinous processes, transverse processes or laminae of the mid-cervical vertebrae (see below).

The **lateral** (axillary) **border** (Fig. 8.6a) is a sharp and somewhat concave ridge that runs from the glenoid mass above and passes onto the dorsal surface as it descends towards the inferior angle. At the upper limit of the border, below the neck of the scapula, is a roughened area for the attachment of the long head of the triceps muscle. The attachment of the teres minor muscle may be interrupted by the passage of the circumflex scapular vessels, which lie in a distinct groove on the lateral border and are covered by a fibrous arch from which muscle fibres arise. These vessels form part of the extensive scapular anastomosis, which is of considerable clinical importance in ligation or indeed stenosis of the axillary or subclavian arteries. The teres major muscle arises from the lower part of the lateral border as it passes down towards the inferior angle.

The **superior border** (Fig. 8.6b) is sharp and the shortest of the three margins of the scapula. It slopes downwards from the superior angle at the junction with the medial border to the root of the coracoid process laterally. The suprascapular notch lies on this border, medial to the coracoid process and it is converted into a foramen in the living by the transverse scapular ligament (Van Dongen, 1963). Some fibres of the omohyoid muscle take origin from the ligament, which acts like a bridge enabling the suprascapular nerve to pass under it and the suprascapular vessels to pass over it, thereby gaining access to the supraspinous fossa. Occasionally, the ligament may become ossified so that a true bony suprascapular foramen is formed (Edelson, 1995a). The presence of a bony canal has been shown to cause weakness at the shoulder joint, due to entrapment of the suprascapular nerve (Gray, 1942; McClure and Raney, 1974; Rengachary *et al.*, 1979; Ganzhorn *et al.*, 1981; Garcia and McQueen, 1981; Pate *et al.*, 1985). This manifests as a weakness in abduction (supraspinatus muscle) and lateral rotation of the arm (infraspinatus muscle). The mechanism of the trauma to the suprascapular nerve tends to arise more from a kinking of the nerve against the upper bony boundary (called the sling effect) rather than from compression, due to the restrictions of the small bony canal (Rengachary *et al.*, 1979).

The **superior angle** (upper medial angle) lies at the junction between the superior and medial borders at the level of the second thoracic vertebra (Fig. 8.6a, b). It is not generally palpable in the living as it is covered by the upper fibres of the trapezius muscle. A

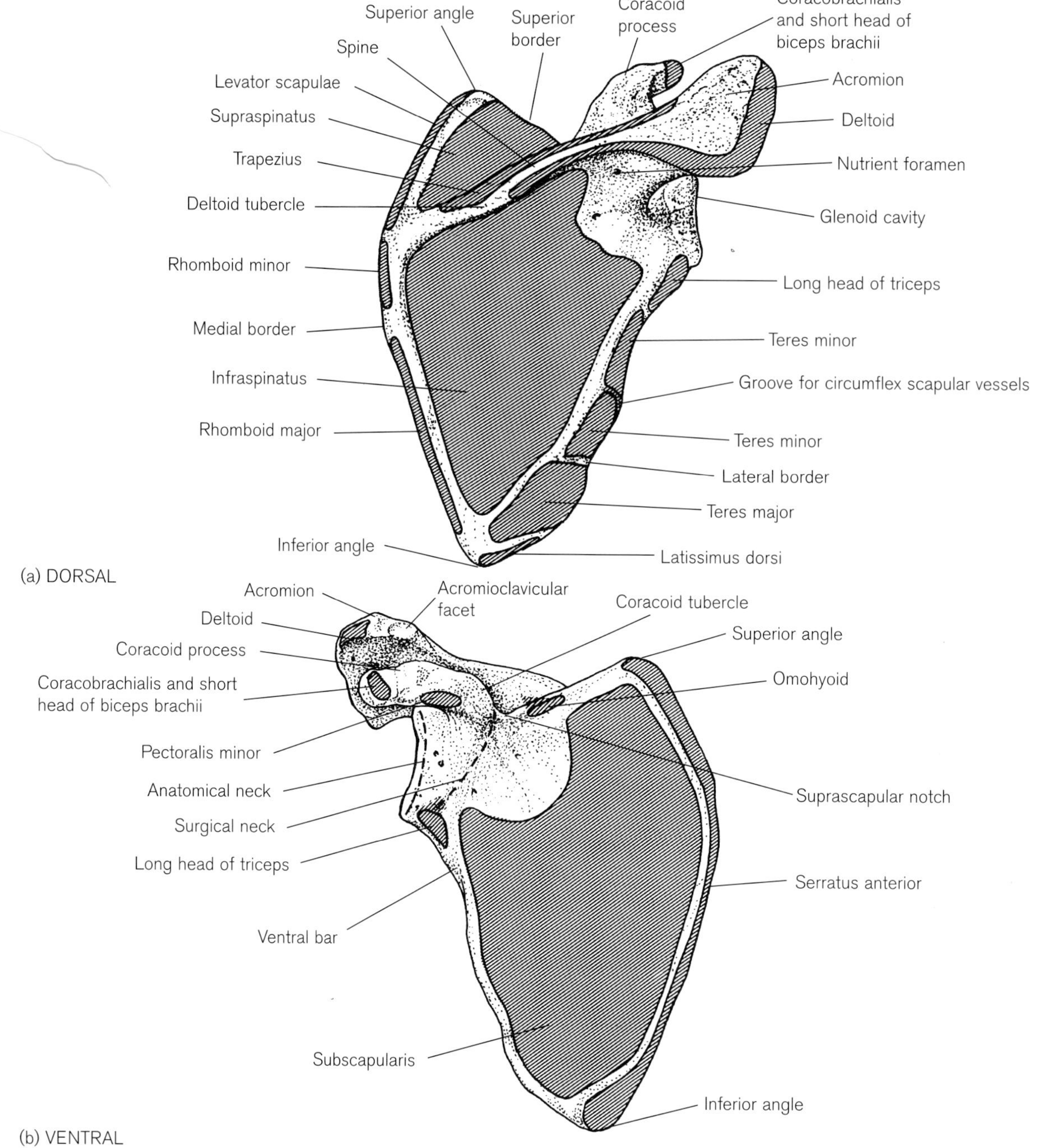

Figure 8.6 The right adult scapula.

costal facet is sometimes found associated with the ventral surface of the scapula at this site (Gray, 1942; Bainbridge and Tarazaga, 1956). These facets appear to be more common in the male and normally articulate with the dorsal surface of the second rib although, depending upon the shape of the scapula and the position of the superior angle, an articulation can occur with the third rib (Gray, 1942). This exostosis, sometimes known as the tubercle of Luschka, can give rise to a loud snapping sound on movement of the shoulder joint (Parsons, 1973).

The **inferior angle** (Fig. 8.6a, b) is formed at the junction of the medial and lateral borders and lies dorsal to the seventh rib. Although it is covered by the upper border of latissimus dorsi, this angle is still palpable in the living. It is usually more robust than the

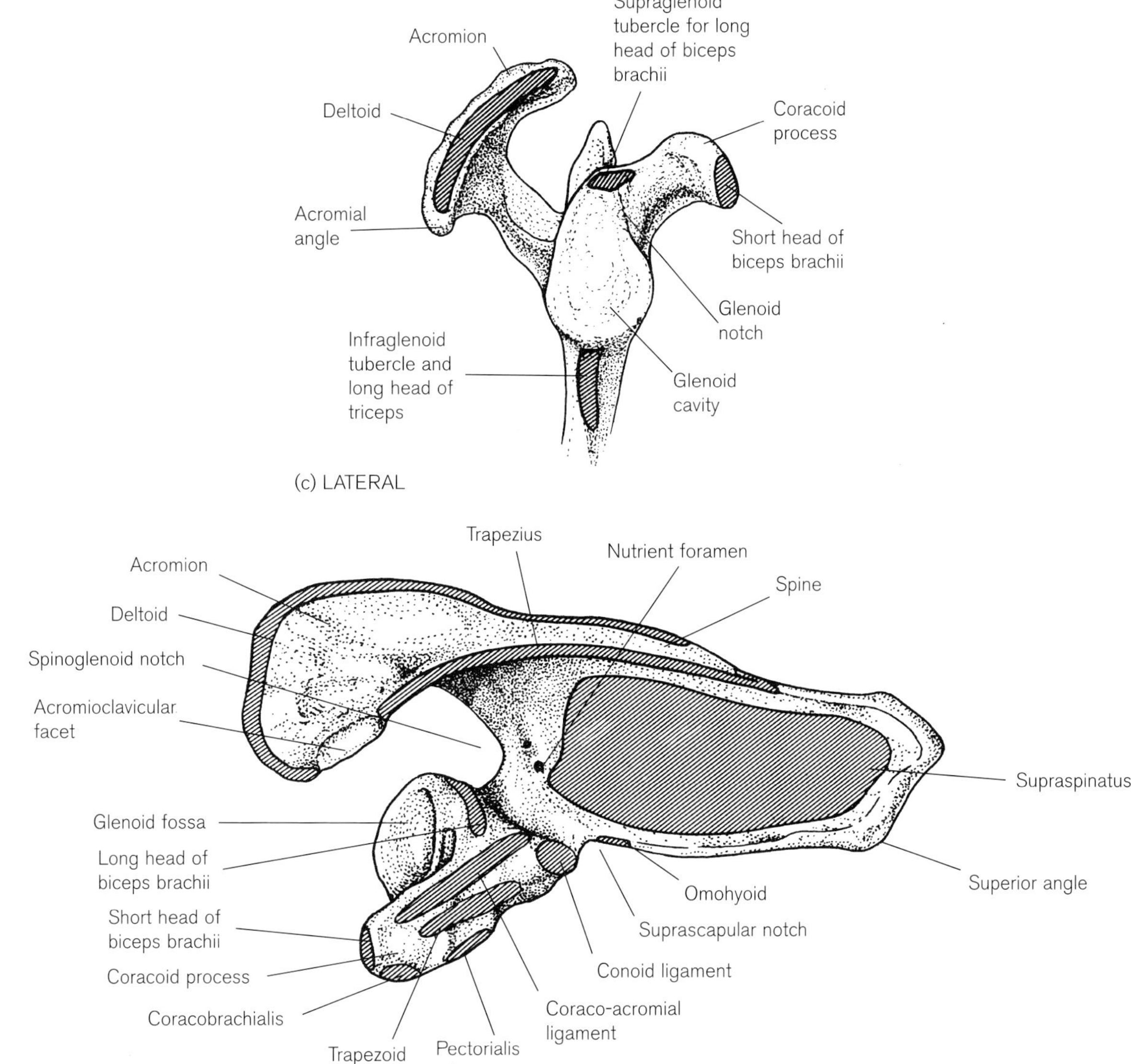

Figure 8.6 *(Continued).*

superior angle due to the larger mass of muscle fibres that insert on both its ventral and dorsal surfaces. Costal facets have also been identified on the ventral surface at the inferior angle but their incidence is less frequent than is seen at the superior angle (Gray, 1942; Bainbridge and Tarazaga, 1956). A separate infrascapular bone has also been reported (McClure and Raney, 1974), although it is said to fuse with the main body of the scapula by 20 years (Keats, 1992) as it is epiphyseal in nature (see below). Sickle shaped scapulae with a hook-like process arising from the region of the inferior angle have been identified in Pierre Robin syndrome (Bezirdjian and Szucs, 1989).

The **lateral** (upper lateral) **angle** comprises the head (glenoid mass) and neck of the scapula (Fig. 8.6b). The anatomical neck lies around the glenoidal rim and the surgical neck is represented by a line drawn from below the glenoid mass to the lateral boundary of the suprascapular notch. The **glenoid cavity** (fossa[3]) is the site of the synovial articulation with the head of the humerus, thus forming the shoulder joint. The head of

[3]The term 'glenoid' is said to be derived from the Greek meaning 'a shallow socket' but Homer used the term to mean 'a mirror'. It is thought that perhaps the glistening cartilaginous surface of the glenoid suggested a reflective surface (Skinner, 1961).

the scapula is usually pear-shaped (Gray, 1942) being broader in its inferior diameter and tapering towards its superior pole, where it lists slightly anteriorly (Fig. 8.6c). Superior to the glenoid cavity and at the root of the coracoid process is the supraglenoid tubercle for the attachment of the tendon of the long head of the biceps brachii muscle. The majority of anatomical texts state that the origin of the long head of the biceps is simply the supraglenoid tubercle. It is clear, however, that whilst around 50% of the fibres of the tendon do arise from this bony region, the remainder of the tendon arises directly from the glenoidal labrum (Vangsness *et al.*, 1994).

The articular surface of the glenoid cavity is shallow and covered with hyaline cartilage, which is thinnest in the centre and thickest around the periphery. The surface is deepened by the presence of a fibrocartilaginous collar (glenoidal labrum), which is triangular in cross-section with a sharp, free inner margin and a thick base that is attached around the edge of the glenoid cavity. The loose fibrous joint capsule attaches outside the labrum and has at least three openings, which form bursae under the tendons of supraspinatus, infraspinatus and the long head of biceps brachii. The relatively weak capsule is supported by partial fusion of the tendons of muscles that form the rotator cuff – supraspinatus, infraspinatus, subscapularis and teres minor. The supraspinatus tendon is most frequently torn in rotator cuff injuries, which is relatively common in active bowling sports activities, e.g. baseball pitchers and cricket bowlers (Carola *et al.*, 1992). Rotator cuff injuries are also common in instances of bipartite acromion processes (see below), where the patient may present with shoulder pain, particularly in abduction, a decreased range of motion, muscle weakness and clicking in the joint (Warner *et al.*, 1998). Acromial fractures resulting from a direct downward force on the apex of the shoulder may also give rise to rotator cuff injury (Dennis *et al.*, 1986). Surgical intervention may include removal of the loose part of the acromion (Mudge *et al.*, 1984).

The laxity of the joint capsule is a reflection of the general instability of the joint, which is perhaps one of the most readily dislocated in the entire body. The shoulder joint has sacrificed much of its stability to maximize its mobility and in so doing has had to incorporate various surrounding structures to lend it some support. The rotator cuff muscles and surrounding ligaments shore up the anterior, posterior and superior aspects of the joint so that the inferior aspect becomes the weakest region. Dislocation generally happens when the arm is in full abduction and the head of the humerus can ride over the virtually unsupported inferior margin of the joint (Kanagasuntheram *et al.*, 1987). Inferior dislocation may damage the axillary nerve, resulting in sensory loss and paralysis of the deltoid muscle.

The glenoid cavity is almost always concave in shape to receive the convex head of the humerus, although in exceptionally rare circumstances the cavity can be convex and in this situation the head of the humerus is reciprocally concave (Brailsford, 1953). The glenoidal rim is normally notched in the superior ventral region and this corresponds closely with the junction between the 'coracoid' and 'true scapular' origins of the developing articular surface (see below). This glenoid notch (incisura acetabuli) is said to arise as a result of pressure caused by the tendon of the subscapularis muscle (Martin, 1933). It is interesting to note that when the notch is present then the glenoidal labrum is not attached along the rim of the bone, but in fact bridges it, presumably to allow passage of the tendon (Prescher and Klümpen, 1997). These authors suggested that such an anatomical arrangement represented a 'locus minoris resistentiae' and predisposes the joint to Bankart lesions (recurrent dislocations of the shoulder joint–Bankart, 1938). They did not detect any side or sex preference for the presence of a glenoidal notch (Prescher and Klümpen, 1995). Bainbridge and Tarazaga (1956) reported the presence of a small tubercle in the centre of the glenoid cavity, which was surrounded by a crescentic depression, but the aetiology of this is unknown.

The **ventral** (costal) surface is concave both from above to below and from medial to lateral (Fig. 8.6b). Much of the appearance of a concavity arises from both a bending forwards of the upper third at a site that corresponds to the spinous process on the dorsal surface, and a built-up longitudinal pillar of bone along the lateral border. This thick bar does not correspond with the lateral border, but is a mechanical buttress which supports an otherwise weak bone and prevents buckling, due to the antagonistic action of many strong muscles (deltoid and serratus anterior in particular) (Anetzberger and Putz, 1996).

Along the medial border is the attachment for the serratus anterior muscle and this area is clearly delimited by a ridge, which is the site of attachment for the strong fascia on the surface of the subscapularis muscle. The serratus anterior attachment site widens at the level of the superior angle to receive the upper two muscular digitations and again at the inferior angle to receive the bulk of the muscle. The remainder of serratus anterior attaches along the thin strip of the medial border between the two angles. Damage to the long thoracic nerve, which lies on the medial wall of the axilla, results in paralysis of the serratus anterior muscle and subsequent 'winging' of the scapula (Moore, 1992). Often the affected arm cannot be abducted further than the horizontal position, because the serratus anterior is unable to rotate the inferior angle of the scapula. Serratus anterior is also called the Fencer's muscle, due to its involvement in the lunge movement.

The majority of the costal surface is given over to the attachment of the subscapularis muscle. This attaches along the lateral border (lateral to the buttress) and may pass onto the dorsal surface between the teres minor and major muscles. It does not attach to the inferior angle or as far as the medial border. To increase the available surface area for attachment, intramuscular tendons arise, which may leave ridges on the surface of the bone. These ridges always run superolaterally in the direction of the subscapular muscle fibres (Gray, 1942).

The area around the glenoid mass is bare of muscular attachment and is separated from the overlying muscle by the subscapular bursa. A nutrient foramen is usually found in this position and it is directed laterally towards the glenoid mass. Numerous other nutrient foramina can occur, but their position and number are variable (Gray, 1942).

The **dorsal surface** of the scapula is divided by the spinous process into a smaller supraspinous fossa and a larger infraspinous fossa (Fig. 8.6a). These two areas are continuous via the spinoglenoid notch (Fig. 8.6d), which passes between the lateral border of the spinous process medially and the glenoid mass laterally. Due to differences in development (see below), the two fossae lie in different planes and meet at an angle of approximately 130° (Frazer, 1948). It is this difference in muscle planes that gives rise, in part, to the apparent concavity seen in the subscapular fossa.

The supraspinatus muscle arises from the whole of the upper region of the spine and all of the **supraspinous fossa** with the exception of the region adjacent to the glenoid mass (Fig. 8.6d). The tendon of the muscle then passes under the acromion process, over the shoulder joint and inserts into the superior facet on the greater tubercle of the humerus. The tendon of supraspinatus is separated from the coraco-acromial ligament, acromion process and deltoid muscle by the subacromial bursa. Injury to the supraspinatus tendon can result in degeneration and calcified deposits, as the blood supply to the tendon is precarious. Calcification and subsequent infiltration of calcium deposits into the subacromial bursa causes severe pain, particularly in abduction of the arm at the shoulder joint due to the related subacromial bursitis (Kanagasuntheram *et al.*, 1987).

A large nutrient foramen can usually be found in the supraspinous fossa at the thickest part of the lateral boundary of the spinous process. It is for the passage of a branch of the suprascapular artery which pierces the base of the spine at its medial third before dividing into medial and lateral vascular cones, which supply the spinous process (Brookes and Revell, 1998). The foramen is usually non-directional and is considered to be the site of the initial nucleus of ossification (see below). The position and number of other accessory nutrient foramina can vary (Gray, 1942).

The suprascapular vessels enter the supraspinous fossa by passing over the transverse scapular ligament and then, in the company of the suprascapular nerve, they gain access to the infraspinous fossa under the spinoglenoid ligament (fused fascial sheaths of the supra- and infraspinatus muscles). This fibro-osseous tunnel is a potential site for nerve entrapment (Cummins *et al.*, 1998).

The **infraspinous fossa** is somewhat concave under the spinous process, but the majority of the surface is convex from side to side (Fig. 8.6a). A deep hollow passes down the length of the lateral aspect parallel to the axillary border. The infraspinatus muscle arises from the whole of the fossa, with the exception of the region around the glenoid mass, the medial and lateral borders and the inferior angle. The teres minor muscle passes from the lateral border onto the dorsal surface, as does the teres major, which occupies a larger oval area near the inferior angle. The circumflex scapular groove on the lateral border is often continued onto the dorsal surface. The subscapularis muscle may also pass onto this surface for a short distance between the attachments of the two teres muscles. Some authors consider that the nutrient supply to the scapula arises from a branch of the subscapular artery, which pierces the lateral pillar of bone in the infraspinous fossa (Crock, 1996).

The **spine** of the scapula is located on the dorsal surface in the upper one-third and forms a demarcation between the supra- and infraspinous fossae (Fig. 8.6a). It passes from its root at the medial border, across the width of the scapula to end in a thick, free lateral border, which forms the medial boundary of the spinoglenoid notch. The root of the spine lies at the level of the spinous process of the third thoracic vertebra and the crest of the spine is subcutaneous throughout almost its entire length. The upper margin of the spine turns superiorly at its medial extremity and continues as a ridge parallel to the medial border of the supraspinous fossa. As it passes laterally, the upper margin is concave in shape and becomes the medial border of the acromion process where the articular facet for the acromioclavicular joint is located (Fig. 8.6d). The lower margin of the spine turns inferiorly at its medial extremity and forms a ridge that is parallel to the medial border of the infraspinous fossa for a short distance. The triangular area of the medial border that is delimited by the divergence of the upper and lower margins of the spinous process is the site of attachment for the rhomboid minor muscle. As the lower margin of the spine passes laterally, it forms a small, downward projection, the deltoid tubercle, before becoming continuous with the posterior border of the acromion process laterally.

The **acromion process** forms the lateral free extension of the spinous process (Fig. 8.6d). It lies both above and behind the articulated head of the humerus, and with the coracoid process, helps to form an incomplete bony cup to prevent upward or backward dislocation of the shoulder joint. The acromion is usually quadrilateral in shape, although it can also be triangular or falciform in appearance (Macalister, 1893b; Gray, 1942; Bainbridge and Tarazaga, 1956). Its posterior border is continuous with the lower margin of the spine and its medial border is continuous with the upper margin of the spine. The lateral border is longer than the medial border and forms the acromial angle at its junction with the posterior border. This bony prominence can be felt under the skin and is commonly called the 'tip' of the shoulder. It is from this position that clinicians measure the length of the upper limb (Lumley, 1990). The derivation of acromion arises from the Greek '*acros*' meaning uppermost or top, therefore 'acromion' literally means the top of the shoulder.

The **acromioclavicular joint** is located on the medial border of the acromion. This small, oval facet faces upwards and medially and both surfaces of the joint are covered with fibrocartilage. The capsule surrounds the joint and a fibrocartilaginous intra-articular disc may sometimes occur (de Palma, 1957). The superior surface of the joint is strengthened by the parallel fibres of the acromioclavicular ligament. This is a planar joint and movement is therefore restricted, although axial rotation of approximately 30° has been reported (Kapandji, 1974). Although Gray (1942), Finnegan (1978) and Williams *et al.* (1995) mention the occasional presence of an accessory articular facet on the inferior surface of the acromion, they do not offer either an aetiological or a functional explanation for its presence. It is likely that this represents a pathological impingement facet caused by the superior displacement of the humeral head, which ruptures the supraspinatus tendon (Wilson and Duff, 1943; Weiner and MacNab, 1970; Ozaki *et al.*, 1988; Uhthoff *et al.*, 1988; Ogata and Uhthoff, 1990b; Patte, 1990; Miles, 1996, 1999). Although generally associated with osteo-arthritic change, this phenomenon can also be found in younger individuals who are involved in strenuous physical activity, such as athletes (Penny and Welsh, 1981).

The inferior surface of the acromion is smooth due to the presence of a subacromial bursa, but is roughened along the medial margin and towards the tip for the attachment of the **coraco-acromial ligament**. The ligament may also attach to the undersurface of the acromion, often to its lateral margin (Wood Jones, 1953; Miles, 1998). An extremely rare muscle, termed the 'sternoscapularis', has been reported as having an attachment to the medial aspect of the acromion (Huntington, 1905). With age, the acromion can adopt a hooked appearance, which is generally thought to result from calcification of the acromial attachment of the coraco-acromial ligament (Edelson, 1995b). The upper surface of the acromion is roughened by the presence of the 'acromial rete' (Frazer, 1948) and displays at least four distinct ridges that pass towards the lateral border. These are for the attachment of the septa in the multipennate central mass of the deltoid muscle. Occasionally, a congenital fibrotic band can replace some of the anterolateral deltoid fibres, which causes an abduction contracture (Chung and Nissenbaum, 1975).[4]

The deltoid muscle arises from the anterior surface of the lateral end of the clavicle and the fibres then pass onto the anterior then lateral and finally posterior borders of the acromion (Fig 8.7). The deltoid attachment then continues along the lower border of the spine of the scapula and becomes aponeurotic by the time it reaches the deltoid tubercle. The anterior fibres of deltoid arise from its clavicular and anterior acromial attachment, the middle fibres from the lateral acromial attachment and the posterior fibres from the posterior acromial and spinous attachments. The anterior fibres are responsible for flexion and medial rotation of the arm at the shoulder joint, the middle fibres for abduction and the posterior fibres for extension and lateral rotation at that joint. The trapezius insertion also has both clavicular and scapular sites of attachment. The upper fibres of trapezius insert onto the posterior border of the lateral end of the clavicle, the middle fibres attach to the medial border of the acromion and the upper margin of the spinous process, while the lower fibres pass upwards and attach onto a hook-shaped region around the deltoid tubercle on the spinous process. Thus, the deltoid tubercle is misnamed as this represents the point of convergence of the lower

[4]The deltoid muscle takes its name from its triangular shape that is reminiscent of the fourth letter of the Greek alphabet. The term is said to have originally described the mouth of the River Nile (the delta of the Nile) and so was first a geographical, rather than an anatomical, term (Skinner, 1961).

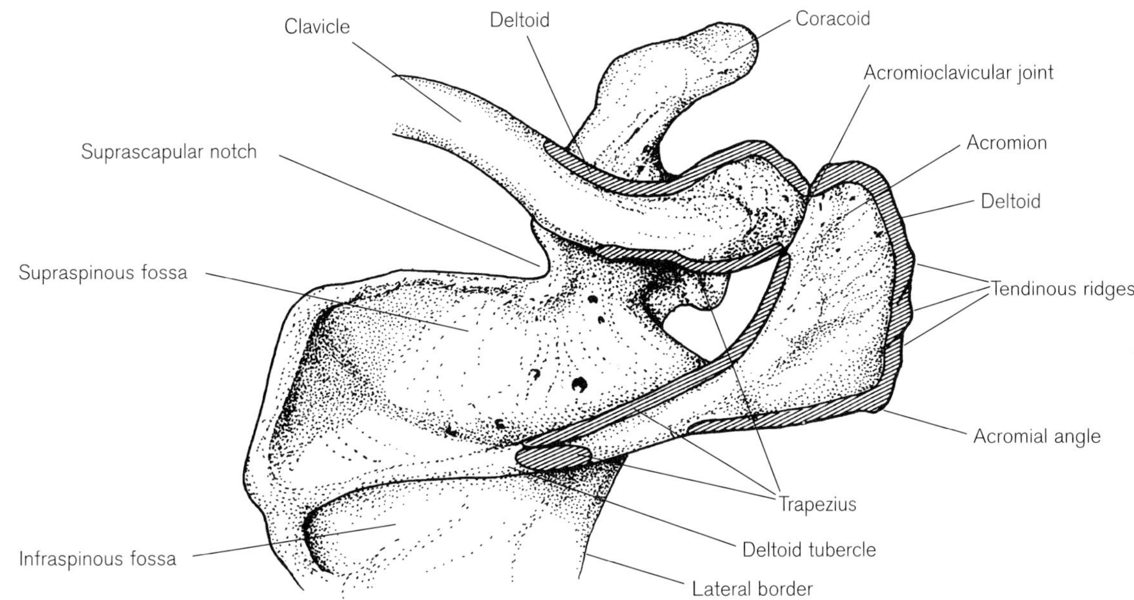

Figure 8.7 The scapular attachments of the trapezius and deltoid muscles.

and middle fibres of trapezius and the hook-like site of attachment ensures that the fibres are free to fan out and not overlap each other, thus avoiding impairment of function (Last, 1973).

There are few reports in the clinical literature concerning anomalies of the spine of the scapula but there are several for the acromion process. Perhaps the most common is a bipartite acromion (os acromiale), which is the result of failure of one of the outer portions of the acromion to unite with the more medial part (McClure and Raney, 1975; Uri *et al.*, 1997). The acromial epiphyseal line generally runs from in front of the acromial angle to the posterior aspect of the acromioclavicular facet and it is generally non-union of this epiphysis that results in the condition (see below). Patients with an os acromiale tend to display rotator cuff disturbances and may also suffer from nerve impingement problems (Edelson *et al.*, 1993). Persistent pain, resulting from soft tissue damage, can be alleviated by a total acromionectomy (Bosley 1991). A double acromion process has been reported (McClure and Raney, 1974) but this situation appears to be unique in the literature. An elongation of the acromion process has also been reported by the same authors, where the acromion extends down to the level of the surgical neck of the humerus rather like a hood. In this relatively rare situation, the only symptom appears to be a considerable limitation in the range of abduction.

The **coracoid process** projects anteriorly and slightly laterally from the superior border of the scapula and can be palpated in the lateral part of the infraclavicular fossa (Fig. 8.6d).[5] The phylogenetic origins of the coracoid process and its homologous structure in the pelvic girdle have been considered at some length in the literature and further discussion is outwith the remit of this text (Watson, 1917; Hanson, 1920b; Romer, 1959; Cauna, 1963; Maderson, 1967; Ciochon and Corruccini, 1977; Wake, 1979; Hildebrand, 1988).

The root of the coracoid is marked by the supraglenoid tubercle laterally and the lateral border of the suprascapular notch medially. From here, the process passes almost vertically upwards and then bends sharply at its tubercle to pass almost horizontally to the tip, which is drawn slightly downwards due to muscular sites of attachment (Fig. 8.6c).

The inferior surface of the coracoid process is smooth due to the passage of the supraspinatus tendon and the intervening subcoracoid bursa, while the superior surface is roughened for both ligamentous and muscular attachments. The ligaments associated with the coracoid process are indispensable to the structural integrity and stability of the pectoral girdle.

[5]Its shape has been likened to a 'bent little finger' but its name is thought to be derived from the Greek '*korax*' and '*oides*' meaning, 'shaped like a crow'. It is likely that the early anatomists thought the process resembled a crow perched on the shoulder with its body and head curving forwards (Field and Harrison, 1957). Or perhaps it was that it bore some similarity to the shape of the beak of the crow. This Greek word was also used to describe anything that was hooked or pointed and it is likely that Galen adopted this term for the bony scapular process from its resemblance to a door handle, rather than to a raven's beak (Skinner, 1961).

The coracoclavicular ligament has been considered in some detail on the section on the clavicle, but briefly it consists of both conoid and trapezoid parts. The conoid part attaches to the tubercle at the angle of the coracoid process and the trapezoid part attaches to a smooth narrow line that passes away from the tubercle towards the tip (Fig. 8.6d). In some instances, these ligaments can be replaced by either an articulation or by a bar of bone, which unites the coracoid to the clavicle (Lane, 1888; Anderson, 1891; Gowland, 1915; Gradoyevitch, 1939; Nutter, 1941; Wertheimer, 1948; Hall, 1950a; McClure and Raney, 1975). In the case of a diarthrodial articulation, a triangular bony outgrowth arises from the inferior surface of the clavicle, which meets a similar-shaped outgrowth from the upper surface of the coracoid (Vallois, 1926; Bainbridge and Tarazaga, 1956). This condition can cause some pain and limitation of movement in the shoulder joint, as well as numbness or tingling in the upper limb due to neurovascular involvement (Chung and Nissenbaum, 1975).

The entire length of the lateral border of the coracoid process gives attachment to the coraco-acromial ligament, which serves to form a tough superior protection for the shoulder joint and has an active involvement in preventing upwards dislocation of the humeral head. The coracohumeral ligament attaches to the coracoid process below the coraco-acromial ligament and it blends with the supraspinatus tendon to offer support to the superior aspect of the shoulder joint.

The remainder of the superior surface and the medial border of the coracoid receives the insertion of the pectoralis minor muscle, whose tendon may leave a groove as it passes across the process (Steele and Bramblett, 1988). The tip of the coracoid receives the insertion of the coracobrachialis muscle medially and gives rise to the origin of the short head of the biceps brachii muscle laterally.

Fractures of the coracoid process are not common (Rowe, 1968; Hollinshead, 1982) but they can arise following repeated direct trauma via the coracobrachialis, biceps brachii and pectoralis minor muscles (Boyer, 1975). The majority of fractures tend to occur posterior to the attachment of the coracoclavicular ligament (Ogawa *et al.*, 1997). McClure and Raney (1974, 1975) reported a case of a double coracoid process, but this does not appear to have been commented upon by any other author and its aetiology is unknown. One other anomaly associated with the coracoid process is the presence of a connection with the sternum. This has been reported in marsupials (Broom, 1897), but only Finder (1936) has identified the condition in man. In this single case, a bony projection (*os coracosternale vestigiale*) was seen arising from the base of the coracoid process medial to the glenoid cavity and it passed upwards and medially towards the sternum. It is important to note that the patient in question also presented with Sprengel's deformity and spina bifida of the lower four cervical vertebrae. Although no other author seems to have come across this condition in man, Lane (1886) reported an incidence of an unusual 'coracoclavicular sternal' muscle.

Early development of the scapula

There is a paucity of detailed information concerning the embryological development of the scapula. The upper limb bud arises as a localized differentiation of the lateral plate mesoderm opposite somites 8–10, which corresponds with future cervical vertebrae 5–7 (Streeter, 1942; O'Rahilly *et al.*, 1956; O'Rahilly and Gardner, 1975; Ogden, 1979; Ozonoff, 1979). The mesenchymal forerunner of the scapula begins to condense around day 33 and is clearly recognizable by day 37 (Lewis, 1901). The scapular anlage (attached to the clavicle via a blastemal connection) then migrates caudally so that by day 44 it lies opposite the first rib, by day 48 it has reached the fifth rib and by day 52 the lower angle has reached the fifth intercostal space (Lewis, 1901; O'Rahilly and Gardner, 1972; Gardner, 1973).

Failure of normal scapular descent results in a congenital elevation of the scapula known as 'Sprengel's deformity'. The aetiology of this maldescent is uncertain (Engel, 1943), although there may be some predisposing genetic factor (Tachdjian, 1972). It has even been described as an atavistic representation of a normal condition that was present in man's simian ancestors (Terry, 1959) but this would necessitate it being a bilateral phenomenon and it is usually unilateral. The author who originally described the clinical manifestations of the condition (Sprengel, 1891) suggested that it arose following malpositioning of the fetus *in utero*.

Sprengel's deformity is usually diagnosed in early childhood when the patient presents with an asymmetry at the base of the neck and elevation of the affected shoulder. It is likely that a radiological investigation will reveal that the scapula is not only elevated but also hypoplastic, retaining its fetal form (Livingstone, 1937; Chung and Nissenbaum, 1975; Ogden *et al.*, 1979c). The affected scapula is elevated, reduced in length, occupies a position that is closer to the midline than in the normal situation and the inferior angle is somewhat tilted posteriorly and medially so that the glenoid cavity faces inferiorly. In this position, the mobility of the shoulder joint is affected and the clavicle may not develop its normal characteristic 'S' shape as it is elevated laterally and not in its normal position, which necessitates morphological compensation for the proximity of the neurovascular structures of the upper limb (Chung and Nissenbaum, 1975).

The deformity can be either uni- or bilateral (McClure and Raney, 1975) but the incidence tends to be greater on the left. Although some authors state that there is no sex specific predilection (Tachdjian, 1972), Ozonoff (1979) considered it to be three times more common in the female. Sprengel's deformity is rare, although it is the most common of all congenital malformations in the shoulder region. In approximately 25% of cases, there is a physical connection between the medial border of the scapula and the cervical part of the vertebral column. This may occur by either a fibrous band or a cartilaginous strip, which may ossify to form an 'omovertebral' bone (Smith, 1941; Jeannopoulos, 1952). Some authors consider this bone to be homologous with the suprascapular bone of lower vertebrates and therefore essentially epiphyseal in nature (Willett and Walsham, 1883; Smith, 1941). The omovertebral connection is generally wedge-shaped, being broader medially and attaches to either the spinous processes, transverse processes or laminae of cervical vertebrae 4–7 (Tachdjian, 1972; McClure and Raney, 1975; Calder and Chessell, 1988). The omovertebral bone may fuse with the vertebral column or it may form a diarthrodial joint (Jeannopoulos, 1952). Corrective surgery is possible, but a significant complication is the subsequent traction that is placed on the brachial plexus by a 'guillotine-like' action of the straightened clavicle (Woodward, 1961; Robinson *et al.*, 1967; Cavendish, 1972; Ross and Cruess, 1977; Conforty, 1979). Maldescent of the juvenile scapula can also arise as a deformity following obstetrical brachial plexus paralysis (Pollock and Reed, 1989).

While this condition is normally attributed to failure of descent of the scapula from the neck to the thorax, other authors have attributed it to direct maldevelopments of the vertebrae. For example, Fairbank (1914) remarked that 'the only explanation which seems to account for the deformities is . . . faulty segmentation of the mesoblast'. Von Bazan (1979) on the other hand, recognized that this was a relatively common embryological maldevelopment and suggested that it arose from a disturbance of the development of the notochord with abnormal inductive influence on the formation of the upper limb buds. The justification for these propositions is that Sprengel's deformity is normally associated with some form of vertebral maldevelopment (Müller and O'Rahilly, 1986).

The evidence for the cervical origin of the scapula has recently been confirmed through genetic research in mice (Aubin *et al.*, 1998). They showed that if the *Hoxa* 5 gene is incorrectly expressed, abnormal development of the vertebral column in the region of C3–T2 could occur. In addition, they found that the normal development of the acromion process of the scapula could also be affected.

The early embryological scapula is said to be somewhat convex on its ventral surface due to the virtual absence of a supraspinous fossa (Frazer, 1948). In the early stages, the supraspinatus muscle is rudimentary and only attaches along the upper limits of the base of the spinous process. However, as the muscle mass increases, so the supraspinous fossa develops in response to the muscle activity. As a result, the two developing plates (supra- and infraspinous) meet at an angle, resulting in an apparent subscapular concavity.

Chondrification of the mesenchymal scapular plate commences in week 6 (Last, 1973) and ossification may begin around day 57 in the eighth week (Andersen, 1963; O'Rahilly and Gardner, 1972). Cavitation of the glenohumeral joint commences in the seventh fetal week and is generally completed by the tenth week (Uhthoff, 1990c).

Ossification

Primary centres

The principal primary centre of ossification for the scapula is said to arise in the vicinity of the surgical neck towards the end of the second month of fetal life, around 7–8 weeks (Mall, 1906; Hess, 1917; Noback, 1944; Frazer, 1948; Noback and Robertson, 1951; Andersen, 1963; Last, 1973; Meschan, 1975; Birkner, 1978; Basmajian and Slonecker, 1989). Only Fazekas and Kósa (1978) seem to be in any disagreement with this, stating that ossification commences somewhat later, around the twelfth week.

The primary ossification centre is said to arise in the perichondrium on the ventral aspect of the scapula (Frazer, 1948). However, perichondral ossification is normally initiated via muscle related activity, but as this region of the scapula is devoid of muscle attachments, then this mode of ossification is unlikely. However, Laurenson (1964a) has reported that perichondral ossification can commence in advance of normal endochondral ossification when acting in a protective capacity, to prevent damage to well-established nerve pathways. In the fetal scapula, the supraspinous fossa is not well developed and the centre of ossification would correspond closely to the site of the suprascapular nerve as it passes over the superior border. We have consistently found that the largest nutrient foramen is situated in the lateral aspect of the supraspinous fossa at the junction with the spinous process and corresponds closely with the proposed site for the appearance of the primary nucleus of ossification (Fig. 8.6d). It is therefore possible that ossification in the scapula is initially perichondral before becoming truly endochondral in nature. The suprascapular artery is the principal arterial source for the entire scapular region and the aforementioned foramen lies directly in its path, where it passes inferiorly towards the spinoglenoid notch. Therefore, it is likely that a branch directly from the suprascapular artery in the supraspinous fossa is the principal nutrient artery that initiates endochondral ossification. Although other nutrient foramina are present in the lateral aspect of both the infraspinous and subscapular fossae, they tend to be both smaller and more variable in position and so are unlikely to be the source of primary ossification.

Ossification expands bidirectionally and reaches the level of the base of the spine by week 9 and the glenoid mass by week 12 (Corrigan, 1960b; Andersen, 1963; Ogden and Phillips, 1983). This pattern of ossification leads to proximal (vertebral) and distal (glenoidal) epiphyseal formation at the end of radiating cones of endochondral ossification (Fig. 8.8). Growth rates are accelerated in the vertebral cone, which results in a greater expansion of the medial border compared to that for the lateral mass (Noback, 1944; Ogden and Phillips, 1983). The spaces between the two endochondral cones are then filled by membranous ossification so that much of the 'blade' of the scapula is said

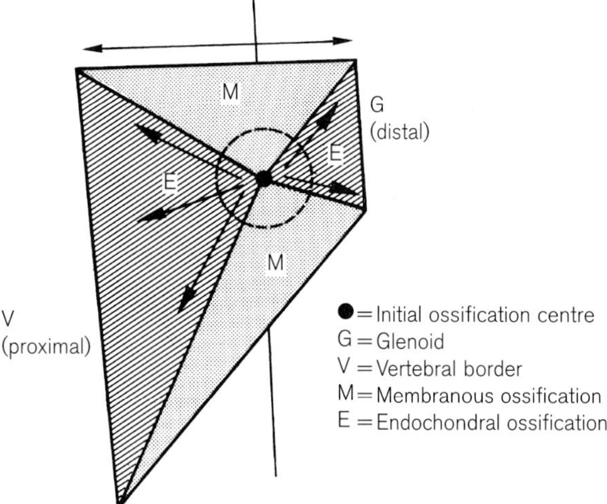

Figure 8.8 Pattern of ossification in the early scapula (redrawn after Ogden and Phillips, 1983).

to form via intramembranous ossification, thereby explaining its relatively flat morphology. The scapula achieves close to adult morphology by 12–14 fetal weeks and alters little until birth (Corrigan, 1960b; Fazekas and Kósa, 1978; Ogden and Phillips, 1983).

Corrigan (1960b) reported that the concept of 'parturitional proportions' should be considered in relation to growth of the scapula and clavicle, as these dimensions are important in the safe passage of the shoulder region at birth. He found these dimensions to be among the least variable of all measurements of the neonatal clavicle and scapula. Obstetric shoulder arises following trauma to the shoulder region as the fetus passes through the pelvic cavity and this can lead to fractures (most commonly of the clavicle), displacement of the glenohumeral joint or paralysis of upper limb muscles following damage to the brachial plexus. If the trauma passes undetected, then the deformity will persist throughout life and often leads to altered growth at the proximal end of the humerus and to abnormal development of the glenoid cavity (Brailsford, 1953).

At birth, the acromion process, coracoid process, medial border, inferior angle and glenoid articular surface remain cartilaginous (Fig. 8.9) (Frazer, 1948; Corrigan, 1960b; Last, 1973). The superior margin is often scalloped, the medial margin is convex and the lateral margin is concave. The subscapular fossa is gently concave and the supra- and infraspinous fossae are relatively flat. The infraspinous surface of the spinous process is sharply inclined, while the supraspinous surface is more horizontal. The spinous process ends in a bulbous lateral extension, which bears an epiphyseal surface on its more dorsal aspect. The glenoidal surface is almost oval in shape and slightly convex, with the articular surface extending onto the superior and ventral aspects for articulation with the coracoid process. A notch on the ventral surface clearly demarcates the coracoid from the true scapular regions of the glenoid surface. The glenoidal notch is said to arise due to the pressure of the tendon of subscapularis as it passes in front of the joint on its way to attachment at the lesser tubercle of the humerus (Martin, 1933). The vascular foramina are prominent and the principal foramen is located in the supraspinous fossa at the junction with the spinous process laterally. There is a discernible thickening of the lateral border extending from the glenoid surface above to the inferior angle below.

The primary centre for the coracoid usually appears in the centre of the process within the first year of life (Cohn, 1921a; Smith, 1925; Camp and Cilley, 1931; Hodges, 1933; Elgenmark, 1946; Girdany and Golden, 1952; Harding, 1952a; Smith, 1954; Andersen,

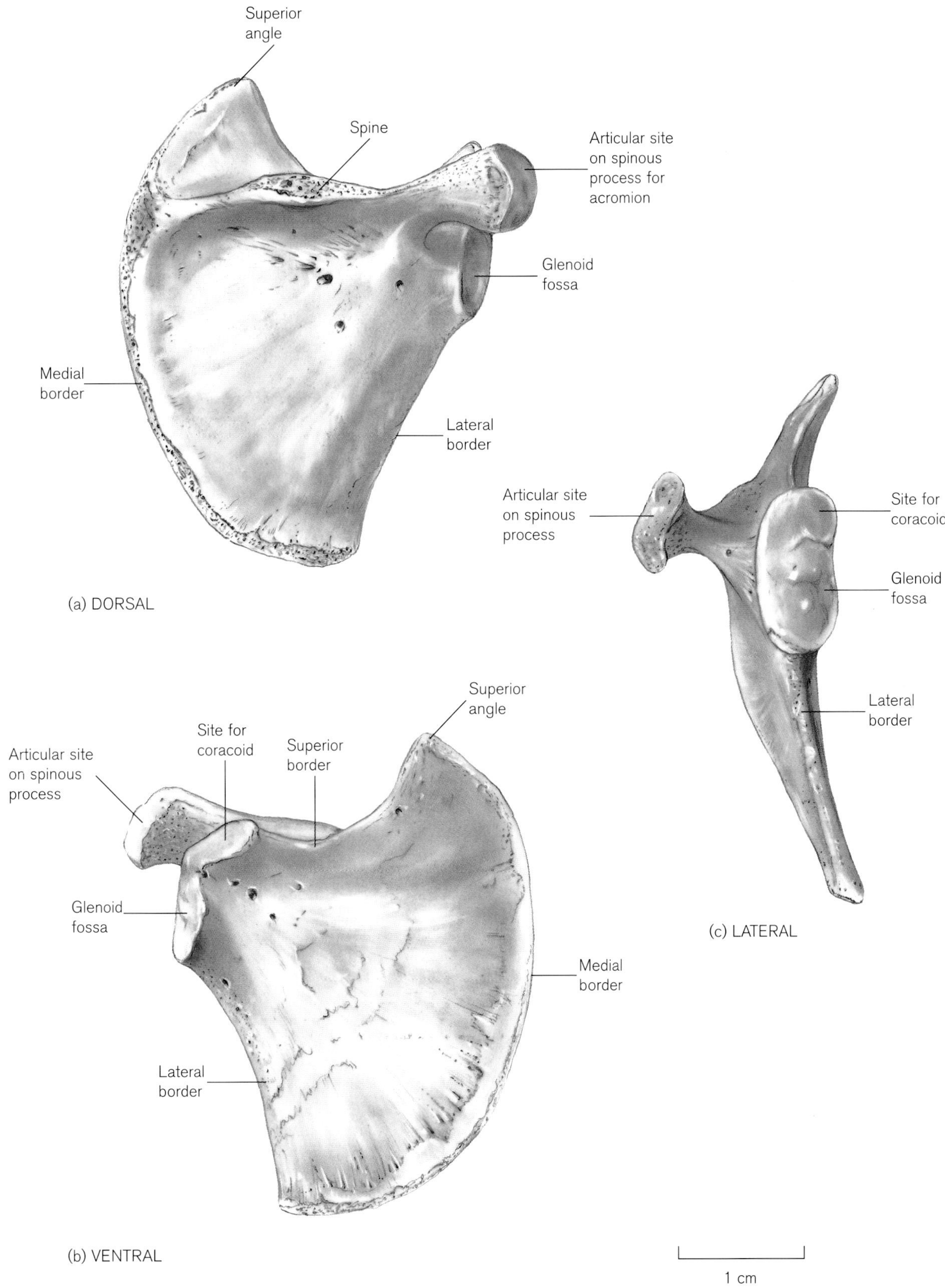

Figure 8.9 The right perinatal scapula.

1962; Garn *et al.*, 1967b; Birkner, 1978; Ogden and Phillips, 1983) although it can be present before birth (Fawcett, 1910c; Hess, 1917; Menees and Holly, 1932; Smith, 1954). The centre is always present by the second year and is certainly recognizable by the third year (Cohn, 1921a) if not before. Depending upon its time of ossification, the coracoid process can usually be identified as a separate structure within the first year, but becomes easier to recognize as it increases in size and the growing surfaces approach the main body of the scapula. The coracoid is hook-shaped, with a broad base and a pointed apex (Fig. 8.10). The base has a large billowed surface for articulation with the body of the scapula and a smaller articular surface on the posterolateral aspect for the subcoracoid centre. The infero-anterior surface is concave and smooth due to the passage of the supraspinatus tendon and the position of the subcoracoid bursa, while the superior surface is ridged for muscular and ligamentous attachments. The posterior surface bears the trapezoid ridge for the attachment of the trapezoid element of the coracoclavicular ligament.

The coracoid centre enlarges progressively and as it nears the scapula (generally in the second year) it develops a bipolar physis (growth plate) permitting growth at both the scapular and coracoid surfaces. Ogden and Phillips (1983) considered this to be a reflection of 'the independence of scapula and coracoid, from an evolutionary standpoint, in most vertebrates'.

Fusion of the coracoid to the scapula generally occurs at around 14–15 years (Andersen, 1963) and commences in the region of the coracoid angle (Fig. 8.11). It is completed along the dorsal border in advance of the ventral border and the final area of the coracoid to show union is on the ventral surface of the scapula adjacent to the glenoid mass. This area finally fuses following invasion by a tongue of bone from the subcoracoid centre (Fig. 8.11c). Fusion with the sub- or infracoracoid process requires further consideration (see below). An extremely rare instance of non-fusion of the coracoid has been reported by Gunsel (1951).

Secondary centres

The scapula is said to have at least seven secondary centres of ossification – three associated with the coracoid process, one for the inferior aspect of the glenoid, one at the inferior angle, one (or, more realistically, several small islands) associated with the vertebral border and at least one for the acromion process.

The **subcoracoid** (infracoracoid) centre appears between 8 and 10 years of age (Frazer, 1948; Birkner, 1978; Basmajian and Slonecker, 1989) and is the first of the scapular secondary centres to commence

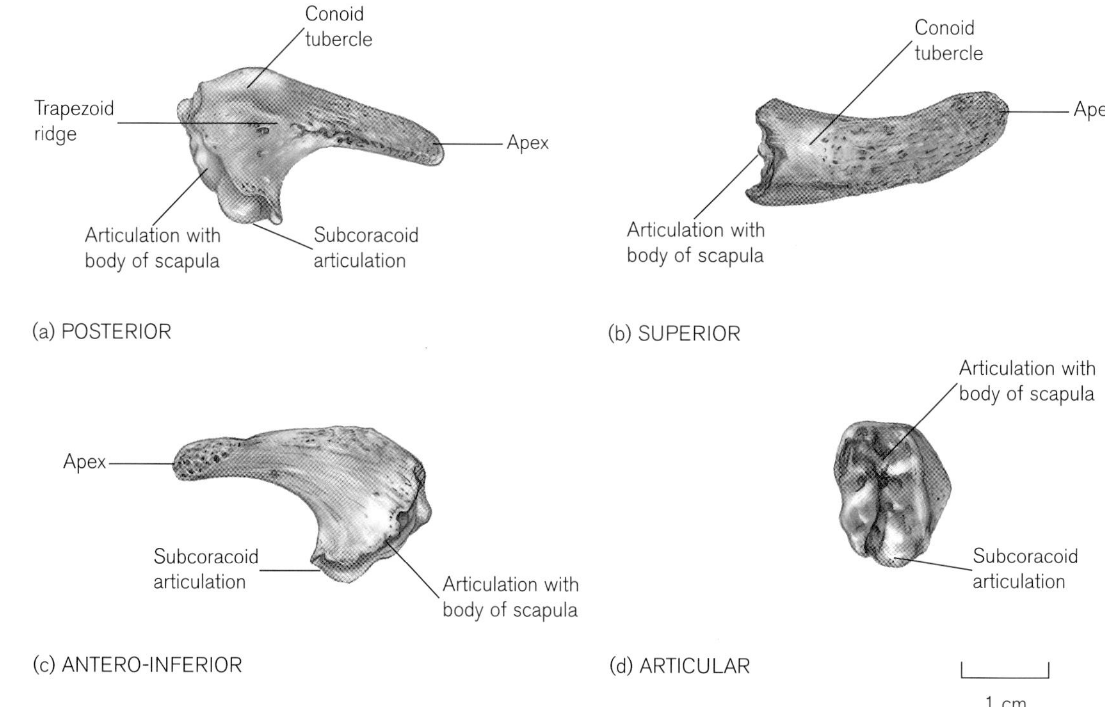

Figure 8.10 Right unfused coracoid process in a female aged 12 years.

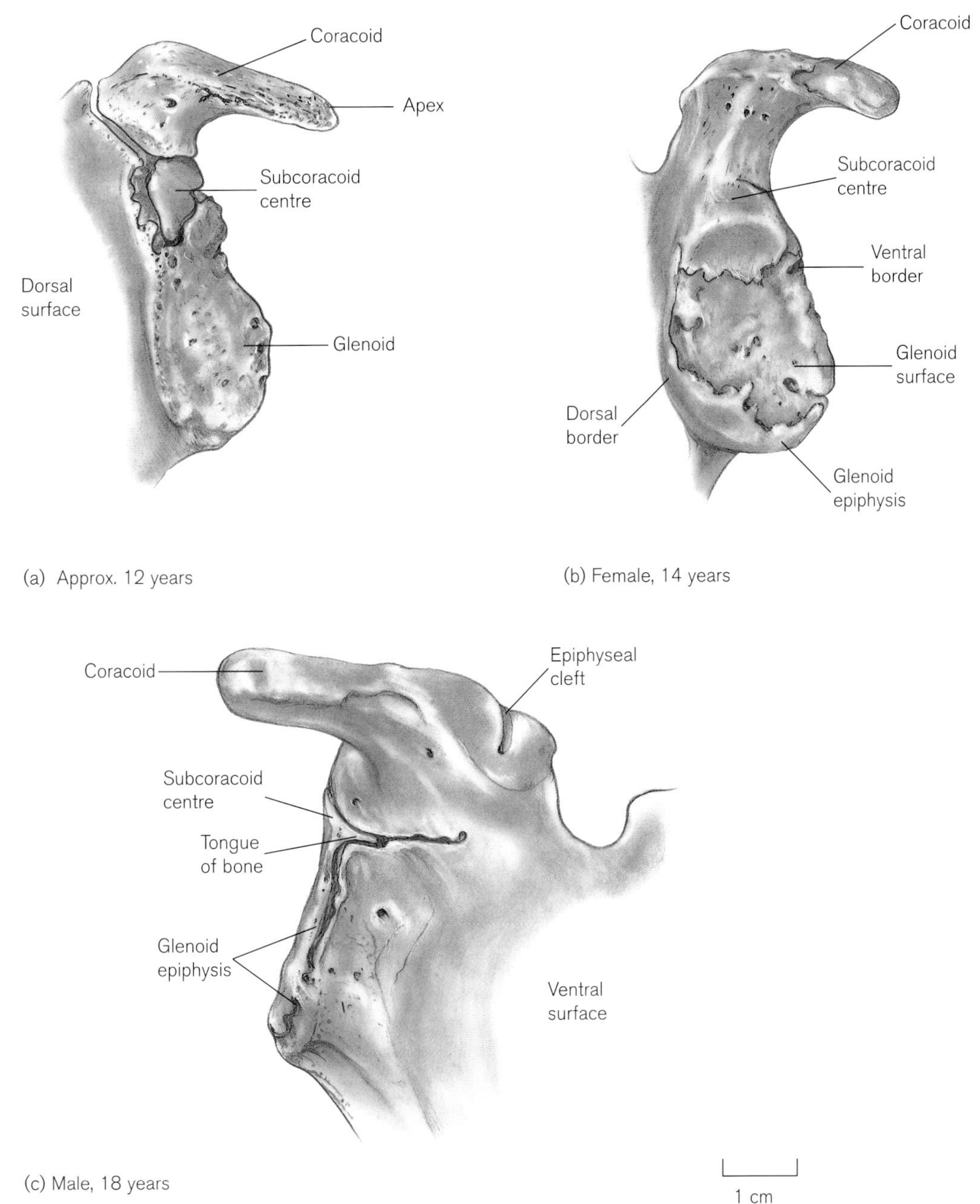

Figure 8.11 Development of the right subcoracoid centre.

ossification (Fig. 8.11). It is located in the superior third of the glenoid surface and is dorsal to the base of the coracoid process. It has a double epiphyseal surface for articulation with both the coracoid process anteriorly and the remainder of the scapula inferiorly. Both of these epiphyseal surfaces commence fusion simultaneously around 14 to 15 years (Hodges, 1933; Williams *et al.*, 1995). Complete fusion between the coracoid and the subcoracoid occurs before complete fusion of the subcoracoid to the remainder of the scapula, as the inferior part of the epiphysis gradually spreads downwards across the upper region of the glenoidal face. The subcoracoid centre is said to be responsible for the formation of the upper third of the glenoidal articular surface. Complete fusion is generally achieved by 16–17 years in both sexes and an indentation remains in the ventral rim of the adult glenoid, which represents the junction between the subcoracoid, coracoid and scapular ossification centres. It is likely that the early commencement of ossification in the subcoracoid centre occurs as a result of the action of the long head of the biceps brachii muscle, which partly attaches to the supraglenoid tubercle on the subcoracoid mass. It is unlikely that this centre is ever recognizable as a separate centre of ossification.

The secondary centre for the remainder of the **glenoid** surface appears around 14–15 years of age, as small islands of ossification around the periphery of the lower aspect of the glenoid rim (Hodges, 1933; Johnston, 1961; Birkner, 1978). These islands eventually coalesce to form a horseshoe-shaped epiphysis, which attaches around the rim of the lower two-thirds of the glenoidal surface and ultimately fuses with the down growths from the subcoracoid centre (Fig. 8.12). The epiphysis then spreads from the periphery towards the centre of the glenoidal articular surface and complete fusion probably occurs between 17 and 18 years of age. The absence or maldevelopment of this centre gives rise to glenoid dysplasia and an increased incidence of congenital posterior dislocation of the shoulder joint. This hypoplasia or aplasia of the articular surface generally presents as a dentate-shaped glenoidal rim (Sutro, 1967; Chung and Nissenbaum, 1975). Given the size and fragile nature of this secondary epiphysis, it is again unlikely to exist as a recognizable structure in isolation from the glenoid mass.

The epiphysis for the **angle of the coracoid process** is said to appear around 14–15 years of age and fuse by about 20 years (Flecker, 1932b; Hodges, 1933; Francis, 1940; Garn *et al.*, 1967b; Haines *et al.*, 1967; Birkner, 1978). However, it is again unlikely that this epiphysis is ever a separate structure, as it appears to form as an outgrowth from the medial part of the coracoid process, which is in fact 'scapular' in origin (Fig. 8.13). Following fusion of the coracoid process to the scapula, the thin, scale-like epiphysis passes forwards and laterally across the angle and superior surface of the coracoid process, where it eventually meets and fuses with the **epiphysis of the apex** (Fig. 8.13). This latter epiphysis is also flake-like in appearance and is said to appear between 13 and 16 years and to fuse by 20 years of age (Hodges, 1933; Flecker, 1942; Birkner, 1978). Frazer (1948) reported accessory epiphyseal islands associated with the trapezoid ridge on the superior surface of the coracoid, but did not give any ages for either their appearance or fusion.

There is a considerable amount of variation, not only in the times of appearance and fusion of the **acromial epiphyses**, but also in their number and pattern of coalescence (Figs. 8.14 and 8.15). Some authors state that there are two secondary centres of ossification, some say four and some say that it is a site of multifocal ossification, but all agree that they appear between 14 and 16 years of age (Macalister, 1893b; Struthers, 1896; Stevenson, 1924; Camp and Cilley, 1931; Francis, 1940; Flecker, 1942; Frazer, 1948; Girdany and Golden, 1952; McKern and Stewart, 1957; Last, 1973; Williams *et al.*, 1995). What is clear is that there is a polarization in the literature depending upon whether the topic under discussion is the normal development of the acromion process or the aetiology of a bipartite

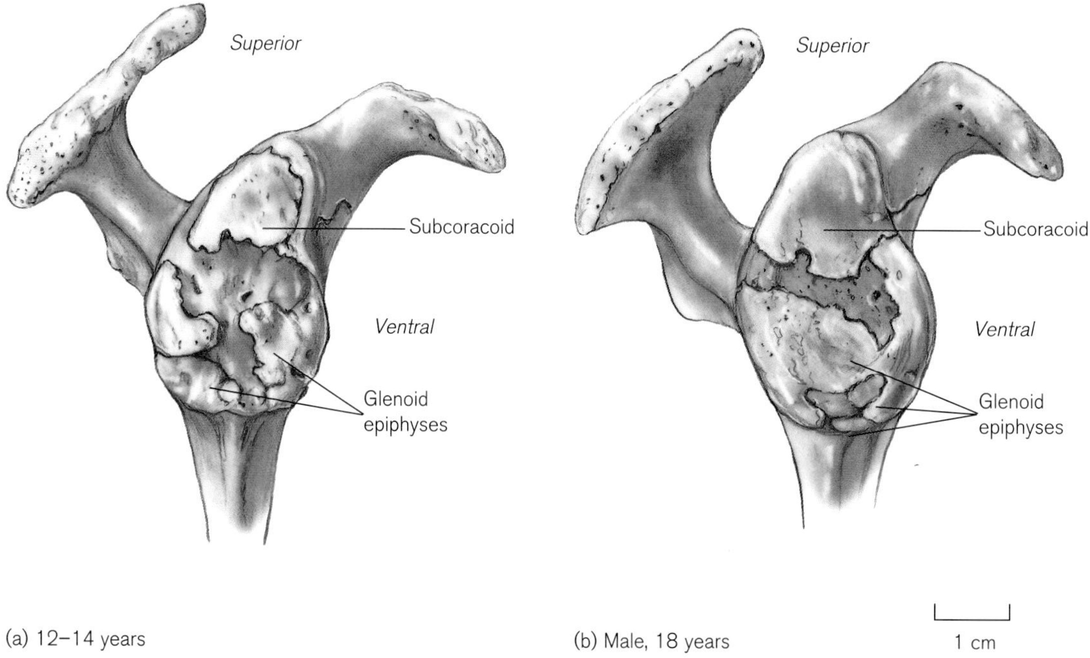

Figure 8.12 Right glenoid epiphyses.

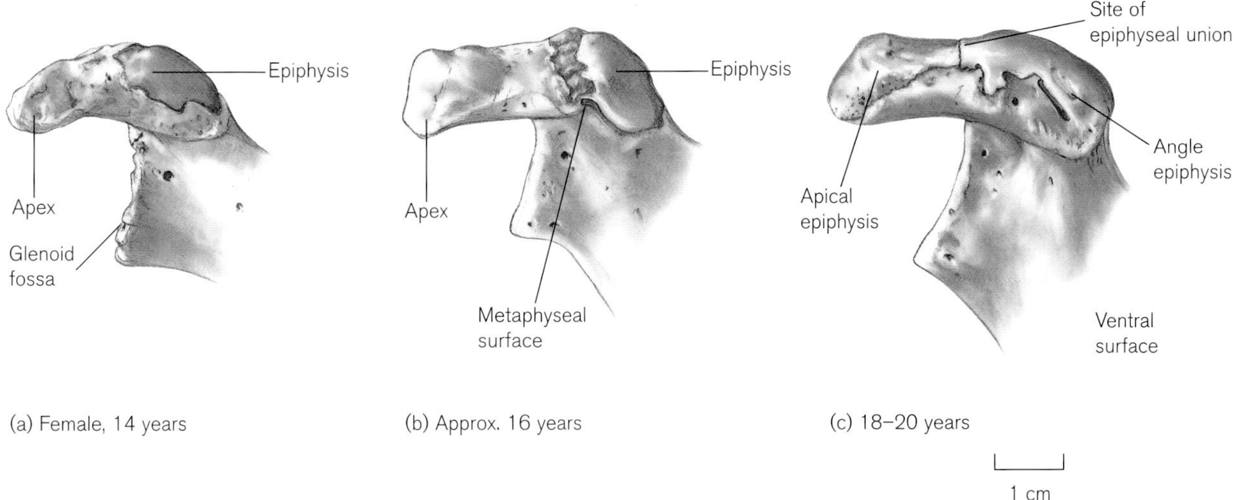

Figure 8.13 The epiphyses of the apex and angle of the right coracoid process.

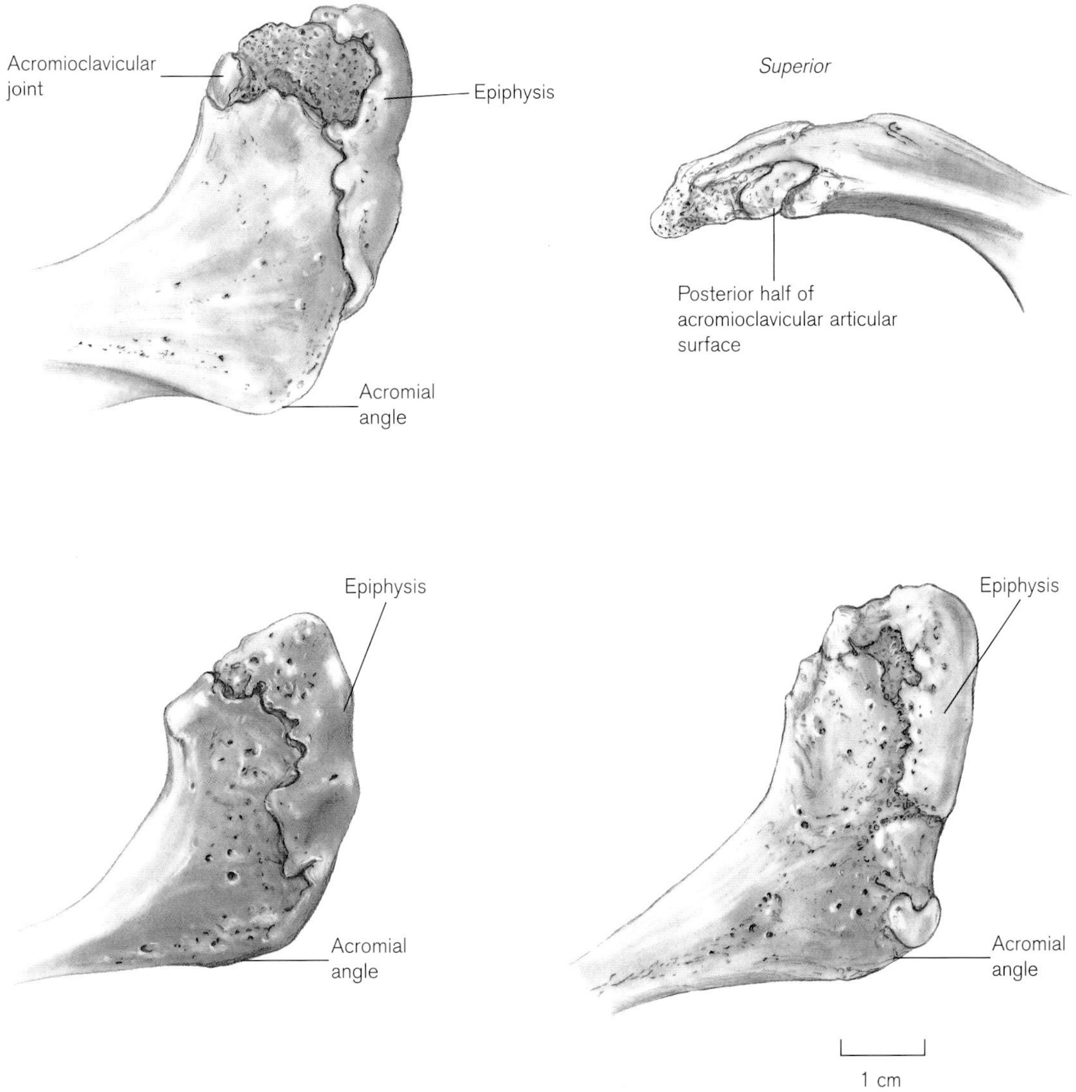

Acromioclavicular joint

Epiphysis

Acromial angle

Superior

Posterior half of acromioclavicular articular surface

Epiphysis

Acromial angle

Epiphysis

Acromial angle

1 cm

Figure 8.14 Variations in the appearance of the right acromial epiphyses.

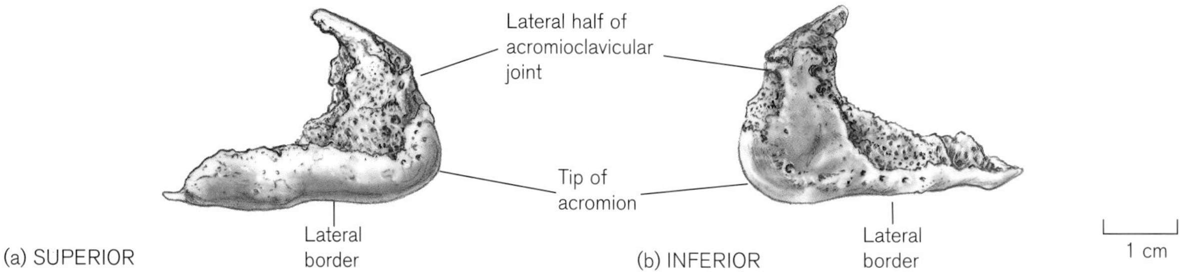

Figure 8.15 Right unfused acromial epiphysis.

acromion process (os acromiale). Papers and texts that deal with the latter state that there are usually four centres, while those of the former state that there are either two or three secondary centres (Frazer, 1948; Last, 1973; Basmajian and Slonecker, 1989; Williams *et al.*, 1995) and this corresponds with the situation that we have encountered in our investigation of juvenile remains (Fig. 8.14). The base of the acromion process develops from the lateral extension of the spinous process and generally extends from just medial to the acromial angle across to incorporate the most dorsal third of the acromioclavicular articular facet. An epiphysis (or, more likely, several foci of secondary ossification) develops along the lateral border of the acromion forming a cap that usually extends as far as the apex of the acromion. A second centre forms to fill the gap along the remainder of the anterior and medial borders and indeed a separate centre may form for the acromioclavicular facet. Although this basic pattern was present in all the scapulae we have examined, there is still a considerable amount of variation (Fig. 8.14). **Fusion** of the epiphysis will generally occur by 18–20 years of age.

The acromial epiphysis is distinct in appearance and can probably be identified as a separate structure by around mid- to late puberty (Fig. 8.15). It generally presents as a comma-shaped cap of bone with a rounded and thicker lateral border that forms a prominence at its lateral extremity (tip of the acromion). The anterior border bears the lateral half of the articular surface for the acromioclavicular joint. The lateral border has a shell of compact bone and this extends for a short distance onto the superior surface and for a greater distance on the inferior surface, thereby forming a distinct plateau.

A bipartite acromion results from a mal-union of the epiphyseal centres to the basal part of the acromion that developed from the spinous process (Miles, 1994). The condition is often bilateral (Symington, 1900; Liberson, 1937) and results in a usually quadrangular separate piece of bone that articulates with the acromial base. The junction between the two pieces generally arises close to the acromial angle and passes across the middle of the process, often bisecting the acromioclavicular joint (Miles, 1994). This condition is often asymptomatic (Chung and Nissenbaum, 1975), although it has been associated with an elevated incidence of rotator cuff injury (Mudge *et al.*, 1984; Warner *et al.*, 1998). Some authors have stated that rather than being a developmental defect or in fact the result of traumatic injury, a bipartite acromion can result from repeated occupation-related trauma (Stirland, 1984), which prevents bony union. Many of the original texts on the bipartite acromion state that the acromion arises from four distinct regions – a pre-acromion, meso-acromion, meta-acromion and a basi-acromion (Liberson, 1937) or some similar combination (Macalister, 1893b; Folliason, 1933). It is generally held that when non-union arises, it is usually between the meso and meta-acromial portions (Liberson, 1937). What is in general agreement is that the secondary centres for the acromion arise between 14 and 16 years of age and complete fusion does not tend to occur before 20 years of age, with the most concentrated period of activity being between 18 and 20 years (Garn *et al.*, 1967b; Ogden and Phillips, 1983). The last site of fusion is to be found on the inferior surface of the acromion, close to the lateral border.

The last scapular epiphyses to commence union are those associated with both the medial border and the inferior angle. Rather than a single centre, it is more likely that the **medial border epiphysis** arises from several small islands, which eventually coalesce to form a fragile narrow strip that commences union in the region of the inferior tip. The islands are said to appear around 15–17 years of age and fusion is generally completed by 23 years of age (Stevenson, 1924; Hodges, 1933; Girdany and Golden, 1952; McKern and Stewart, 1957; Birkner, 1978; Basmajian and Slonecker, 1989). Fissures can often be found along the medial border in the adult bone and these may represent the sites of incomplete fusion of the epiphyses. It is unlikely that a separate epiphyseal strip can be recovered, as it probably fuses to the medial border as it is forming.

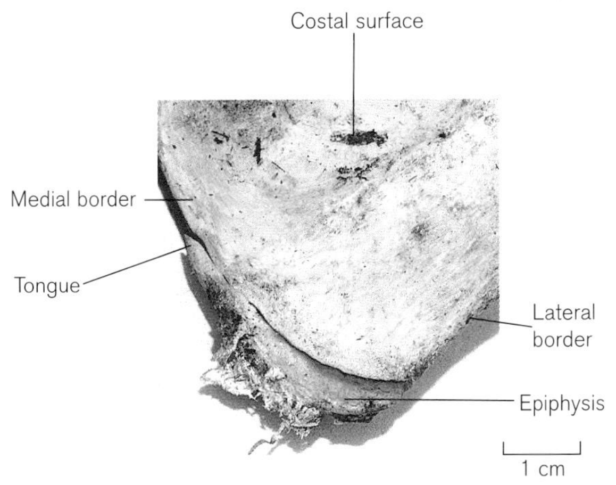

Figure 8.16 Epiphysis at the inferior angle of the left scapula in a male aged 17–19 years.

The **inferior angle** of the scapula develops from a secondary centre of ossification, which also appears around 15–17 years of age and generally fuses by 23 years (Stevenson, 1924; Camp and Cilley, 1931; Flecker, 1932b; Hodges, 1933; McKern and Stewart, 1957; Birkner, 1978; Basmajian and Slonecker, 1989). It is a small, crescentic epiphysis that fuses directly at the angle of the scapula and then sends a small tongue for a variable distance along the medial border (Fig. 8.16). A separate infrascapular bone has been reported (McClure and Raney, 1974), where non-union of the epiphysis has occurred. Further, the inferior angle of the scapula may completely fail to develop and this will result in a notched and somewhat foreshortened inferior extremity (Khoo and Kuo, 1948).

While there is much variation in the time of onset, the duration and the final time of closure of the epiphyses of the scapula, there does appear to be a fairly regular order within the individual (Fig 8.17). At the same time as the coracoid commences fusion with the scapula, the subcoracoid also begins to fuse with both the coracoid and the scapula simultaneously. Before the subcoracoid centre has completed fusion, the ossification centre for the lower two-thirds of the glenoid will commence fusion. Upon completion of the entire glenoid surface, a flake will appear at both the angle and the tip of the coracoid process. Whilst the flake at the coracoid angle is in the process of fusing, the acromion process will commence fusion with the lateral aspect of the spinous process. The epiphyses for the inferior angle and the vertebral border lag behind and do not commence fusion until all other scapular epiphyses have ceased fusion (Stewart, 1934a).

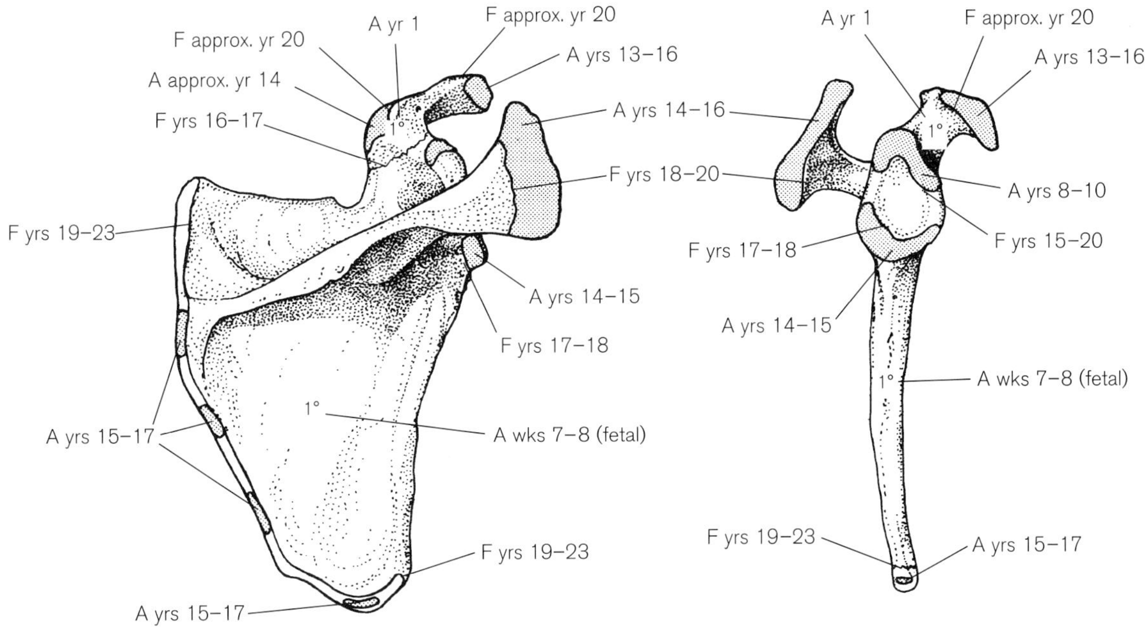

Figure 8.17 Times of appearance (A) and fusion (F) of the scapular centres of ossification.

Practical notes

Sideing

The main body of the juvenile scapula achieves close to adult morphology by 12–14 weeks of intra-uterine life (Fazekas and Kósa, 1978; Ogden and Phillips, 1983) and so is readily identifiable by birth. Therefore, the same criteria are used to identify side in both juvenile and adult scapulae. The sideing of juvenile coracoids is not easy and primarily relies on being able to identify the articular surface for the subcoracoid and separate the superior from the inferior surfaces. Sideing of the acromial epiphysis relies on the recognition of the differences between the superior and inferior surfaces, identification of the tip at the junction between the lateral and anterior borders and the position of the acromioclavicular facet. Sideing of the inferior angle epiphysis relies on being able to distinguish between the costal and dorsal surfaces, which is extremely difficult. The medial aspect of the epiphysis is characterized by a tongue of variable length that courses along the medial border. It is unlikely that any of the other scapular epiphyses can be identified in isolation, either because of their flake-like appearance or because they fuse shortly after formation.

Bones of a similar morphology

Fragmented areas of a juvenile scapula may be confused with various bones of the skull or pelvis due to their flat morphology. The orientation of the bone formation along the extended medial cone should prevent misidentification and due to the nature of the spine, this tends to persist to some degree even in badly fragmented remains. If an area of spine is present, then the bone cannot be confused with any other in the skeleton. However, the similarity of the perinatal scapula to the isolated lateral occipital is quite remarkable, although on close examination the differences probably outweigh the similarities (see Chapter 5).

Morphological summary

Fetal

Wks 7–8	Primary ossification centre appears
Wks 12–14	Main body of the scapula has adopted close to adult morphology
Birth	Majority of main body of scapula ossified but acromion, coracoid, medial border, inferior angle and glenoidal mass are still cartilaginous
Yr 1	Coracoid commences ossification
Yr 3	The coracoid is recognizable as a separate ossification centre
8–10 yrs	Subcoracoid centre appears
13–16 yrs	Coracoid, subcoracoid and body of scapula start to fuse Epiphyses appear for glenoid rim Epiphyses for angle and apex of coracoid appear Acromial epiphysis appears
15–17 yrs	Fusion complete between coracoid, subcoracoid and body of scapula Epiphyseal islands appear along medial border Epiphysis for inferior angle appears
17–18 yrs	Fusion of glenoid epiphyses complete
By 20 yrs	Fusion of acromial and all coracoid epiphyses complete
By 23 yrs	Fusion complete at both inferior angle and along medial border; therefore, all scapular epiphyses fused and full adult form achieved

Metrics

There are several reports on measurements of fetal and juvenile scapulae but it is important to note that most ages are unavoidably derived either from fetal crown-rump lengths or from assessment of dental development. Table 8.3 shows fetal data from 12 weeks to term (Fazekas and Kósa, 1978) and Table 8.4 shows less detailed information from Hrdlička (1942c) spanning the age range of 16 weeks to birth.

Table 8.3 Fetal scapular dimensions (cm)

Age (weeks)	Scapular length	Scapular width	Length of spine
12	0.45	0.30	0.35
14	0.71	0.51	0.58
16	1.16	0.90	1.02
18	1.50	1.15	1.24
20	1.72	1.39	1.54
22	1.88	1.54	1.70
24	2.09	1.75	1.84
26	2.23	1.85	1.95
28	2.31	1.94	2.12
30	2.45	2.06	2.22
32	2.66	2.23	2.38
34	2.81	2.33	2.53
36	2.93	2.44	2.60
38	3.31	2.68	2.91
40	3.55	2.95	3.16

Scapular length: maximum distance between superior (upper medial) and inferior angles.
Scapular width: distance between the margin of the glenoid fossa and the medial end of the spine.
Length of spine: maximum distance between the medial end of the spine and the tip of the acromion process.
Adapted from Fazekas and Kósa (1978).

Table 8.5 (Vallois, 1946) shows both fetal and juvenile results, while Table 8.6 (Saunders *et al.*, 1993a) covers the age span from birth to 12 years of age.

Table 8.4 Scapular dimensions (cm) in fetal and neonatal remains

Approximate age	Total height	Infrascapular height	Breadth
16 weeks	1.0	0.9	0.83
18 weeks	1.39	1.14	1.10
22 weeks	1.83	1.57	1.46
28 weeks	2.32	1.95	1.85
32 weeks	2.48	1.99	1.96
Term	2.99	2.48	2.37
Birth	3.48	2.86	2.86

Total height: maximum distance between the superior and inferior angles.
Infrascapular height: diameter from a point at which the axis of the spine intersects the vertebral border to the lowest point of the inferior angle.
Breadth: diameter from the centre of the posterior margin of the glenoid fossa to the point at which the axis of the spine intersects the vertebral border.
Adapted from Hrdlička (1942c).

Table 8.5 Fetal and juvenile scapular dimensions (cm)

Age	Scapular height	Scapular breadth
Fetal		
2 months	0.5	0.4
3 months	0.8	0.6
5 months	2.3	1.85
6–7 months	3.6	2.7
8–9 months	3.7	2.9
Birth	4.65	3.4
2 years	6.1	4.6
2–4 years	6.65	4.5
4–6 years	8.0	5.4
6–8 years	9.1	6.1

Scapular height: distance between superior (upper medial) and inferior angles.
Scapular breadth: maximum distance between glenoid margin and medial border.
Adapted from Vallois (1946).

Table 8.6 Juvenile scapular dimensions (cm)

Age	*n*	Scapular length	*n*	Scapular width
Birth–6 months	1	3.93	7	3.11
6 months–1 year	15	4.92	16	3.70
1–2 years	19	6.04	19	4.33
2–3 years	10	6.78	8	5.98
3–4 years	5	6.39	5	5.60
4–5 years	3	8.10	3	5.68
5–6 years	3	9.17	3	6.18
6–7 years	6	9.73	7	6.61
7–8 years	1	9.40	2	6.33
8–9 years	1	11.70	1	8.25
9–10 years	2	12.00	2	7.73
10–11 years	1	12.10	2	8.73
11–12 years	1	12.10	1	8.20

Scapular length: distance between superior (upper medial) and inferior angles.
Scapular width: distance between margin of glenoid fossa and medial end of spine.
Adapted from Saunders *et al.* (1993a).

CHAPTER NINE

The Upper Limb

The human upper limb comprises the arm, forearm and hand and is connected with the axial skeleton by the two elements of the pectoral girdle. The humerus articulates directly with the scapula at the shoulder joint and is indirectly joined to the thorax by scapular muscles and the clavicle.

One intriguing, but unlikely, view of the limbs suggested that they developed from specialized placodal ectoderm similar to that of the tactile sense organs of the body wall of earlier forms, with the limb being a modified tentacle adapted to carry the organ for exploratory movements (Cauna, 1963). However, Jarvik (1965, 1980) and Maderson (1967) argued that evidence from palaeontology and embryology supported the classical 'fin-fold' theory of the primary locomotor function of appendages.

In tetrapods, the primary function of the forelimbs is to support the anterior part of the body. However, in some orders of mammals they have become secondarily modified to assume a wide variety of forms to undertake such activities as climbing, burrowing, swimming and flying. In the early primates, the forelimbs were also primarily used for support, but in more advanced forms they became increasingly adapted for climbing, clinging and feeding. These movements were aided by modifications of the shoulder girdle, rotation of the forearm bones to allow pronation and supination, and opposition of the thumb to the fingers. Only in humans, with the adoption of upright posture and bipedal locomotion, were the upper limbs completely released from their supportive role. This allowed the hand to be freed and to develop manipulative dexterity.

Early development of the limbs

Given the basic underlying pattern of the pentadactyl limb, it is not surprising that the development of the upper and lower limbs initially follow a very similar course. For this reason, the early development of both limbs is considered together. Accounts of the histogenesis of human embryonic and early fetal limb development can be found in Bardeen and Lewis (1901), Lewis (1901), Bardeen (1905) and Streeter (1942, 1949). Correlation of Carnegie stages, crown-rump length and age in post-ovulatory days during the embryonic period are reported by O'Rahilly and Gardner (1975) and Uhthoff (1990b).

The upper limb buds are first recognizable at stage 12 (about 26 days of intra-uterine life) as slight elevations and then as definite ridges opposite the seventh to twelfth somites in the region of the caudal cervical segments C3/4–T1 (O'Rahilly and Gardner, 1975; Müller and O'Rahilly, 1986) (Fig. 9.1). At stage 14 (about 32 days) the upper limb buds are rounded projections curving ventrally and medially and tapering towards the tip. By stage 15 the hand plate is recognizable and by stage 16, internal mesenchymal condensations for the humerus, radius and ulna have formed (O'Rahilly *et al.*, 1956).

The lower limb buds are recognizable at stage 13 (about 28 days) opposite somites 25–29 at the L4–S2 level (Fig. 9.1). In the early stages, the development of the upper limb is in advance of the lower limb by about 2 days. The footplate is recognizable at stage 16 (about 37 days) and mesenchymal condensations for the femur, tibia and fibula have formed by stage 17 (about 41 days).

Up to stage 19 (about 7 weeks), the longitudinal axes of the limbs are parallel, with the pre-axial borders facing cranially and the post-axial borders facing caudally (Fig. 9.2). There are several discrepancies in the accounts of embryological limb rotation, but most describe the upper and lower limbs rotating in opposite directions. However, O'Rahilly and Gardner (1975) stated that the changes in position are complex and ill-understood and involve growth changes in all components of the limbs, including their

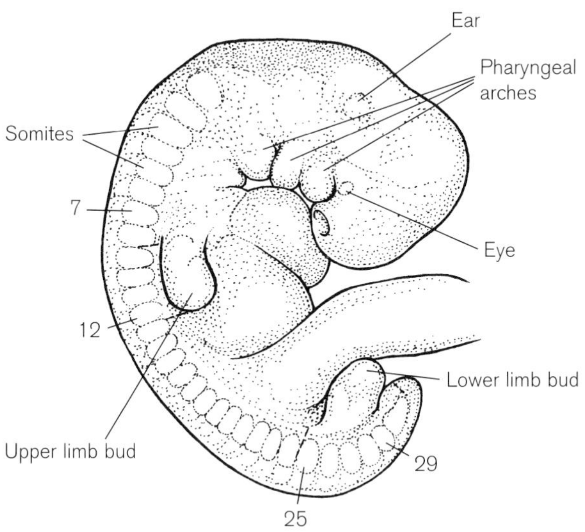

Figure 9.1 Stage 12–13 embryo (about 26–28 days) showing somites and limb buds (redrawn after O'Rahilly and Gardner, 1975).

girdles. The changes in position of the palms of the hands and soles of the feet from stages 17 to 23 (6–8 weeks) are shown in Fig. 9.3.

Much of the present knowledge of early limb development comes from experimental work on amphibian, reptilian and avian models (Amprino, 1984) and it has been assumed that similar mechanisms occur in the human embryo. At the site of the limb bud, the ectoderm forms an **apical ectodermal ridge** (AER) covering a core of mesenchymal cells derived from somatopleuric mesenchyme. These

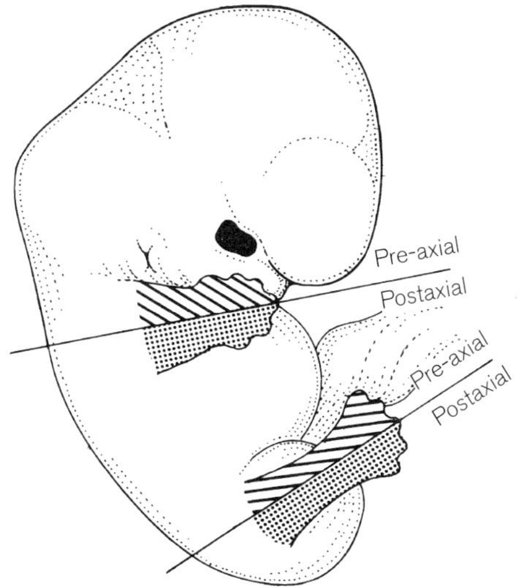

Figure 9.2 Stage 19 embryo showing pre- and postaxial borders of the developing limbs (redrawn after O'Rahilly and Gardner, 1975).

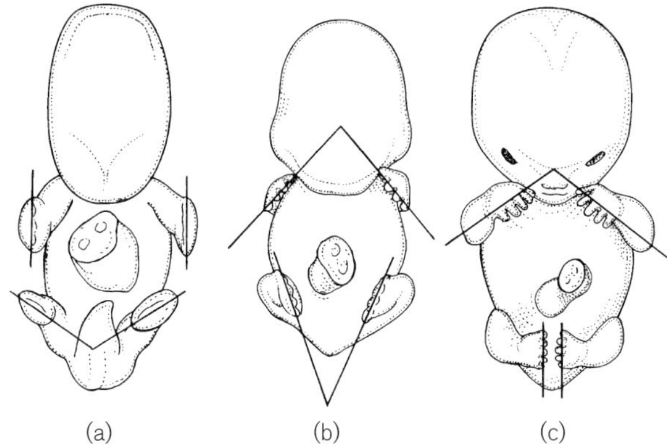

Figure 9.3 (a) Stage 17; (b) stage 19; (c) stage 23 embryos to show rotation of the developing limbs (redrawn after O'Rahilly and Gardner, 1975).

tissues form the **progress zone**, which remains at the distal tip until the digits are formed. It is thought that the epithelium controls the developmental stage of the limb, while the mesenchyme controls the type of limb that will ultimately form. Within the progress zone, mesenchymal cell populations receive specific assignments, which in turn affect the overlying ectoderm. Three axes have been identified during early development. A line from the base of the bud to the centre of the AER constitutes the **proximodistal** axis of the limb. The border rostral to this is known as the pre-axial border and that caudal to it, the postaxial border. The **craniocaudal** axis is controlled by a small cell population on the postaxial border called the **zone of polarizing activity** and the **dorsoventral** axis is thought to be controlled by the ectoderm.

Limb muscle precursor cells have been identified in the lateral halves of the somites and they migrate into the limb anlagen, colonizing the limb bud in a proximodistal direction. The patterning of the musculature is controlled by the somatopleuric mesenchyme. Movements of the embryo are essential for the correct migration and orientation of both myoblasts in the limb and the orientation of the trabeculae in the developing bones. Study of overlapping *Hox* gene domains are gradually providing explanations of the mechanism of control of limb development (Gumpel-Pinot, 1984; Dollé *et al.*, 1989; Izpisua-Belmonte *et al.*, 1991; Tabin, 1992).

Differentiation of the human limb buds occurs between about weeks 5 and 8 and so has a short duration of only 1 fetal month. It is clear, therefore, that the critical period of sensitivity for limb growth and development is a relatively narrow window in fetal life. For this reason, the introduction of any teratogenic agent such as thalidomide, or indeed any interruption to normal developmental processes within this period can lead to congenital limb malformations.

Limb deformities have been classified into three broad categories: (1) reduction defects, where all or part of a limb is absent, (2) duplication defects where supernumerary elements are present and (3) dysplastic defects, which represent all other malformations (Lewin, 1917; Kanavel, 1932; O'Rahilly, 1946; Smitham, 1948; O'Rahilly, 1951, 1959; Frantz and O'Rahilly, 1961; Glessner, 1963; Poznanski *et al.*, 1971a; Field and Krag, 1973; Larsen, 1993).

A different classification incorporating a possible functional explanation of some congenital limb reduction deformities has been suggested by McCredie (1976, 1977). This is the concept of 'sclerotome subtraction' and is based on much earlier work by Inman and Saunders (1944) who studied the segmental distribution of the sensory nerve supply to skeletal structures in the limbs. In a combined clinical and experimental study using observations of location of referred pain radiating from a variety of lesions affecting skeletal and ligamentous structures, they built up so-called 'sclerotome' maps, unfortunately adopting a term that is used for a quite different embryological structure. They defined their 'sclerotome' as a longitudinal band of skeletal elements, which began proximally at the neuraxis and extended distally towards the periphery and which was supplied by one spinal segmental sensory nerve. Although the 'sclerotomes' were definitely segmental in distribution, they did not appear to coincide with either the myotomes or dermatomes. Nor, in fact, were they related to either a major peripheral nerve or to the vascular tree. Because of its longitudinal orientation, a sclerotome can cross joints and subdivide the bones of both the limbs and their girdles. McCredie demonstrated that whole, partial or multiple sclerotomes could be subtracted from the maps and matched with the radiograph of a limb deformity. For example, subtraction of the C6 sclerotome would remove the thumb and most of the radius. It was further suggested that these skeletal structures are linked anatomically through segmental levels of innervation and embryologically related to tissues derived from the neural crest. Recently, McCredie and Willert (1999) studied the radiographs of 203 children with thalidomide embryopathy and observed that in over 73% of the sample there was a concordance between the longitudinal reduction deformities (dysmelia) and the sclerotome maps published by Inman and Saunders (1944). This concept radically challenges the traditional teaching of skeletal anatomy.

The mechanism by which teratogens such as thalidomide could affect the limb has been the subject of much discussion. The idea that the neural crest was the target organ for the action of thalidomide at the embryological stage of development has been criticized by O'Rahilly and Gardner (1975), Gardner and O'Rahilly (1976), Poswillo (1976) and Wolpert (1976), mainly on the grounds that it does not conform to accepted principles of morphogenesis whereby the mesenchymal condensations for the skeletal components precede the ingrowth of peripheral nerve fibres into the limbs. Cameron and McCredie (1982) demonstrated axons and immature Schwann cells earlier than previously observed in the equivalent stage in the rabbit limb. They suggested that this might provide an anatomical framework by which neurotropic influences could act upon the limb at the mesenchymal stage of development.

More recently, Tabin (1998) has proposed an alternative model for thalidomide defects, which conforms to current concepts of limb development. According to the progress zone model, the proximodistal location of structures within a limb is controlled by **fibroblast growth factor** (FGF) produced by the AER. Initially, the limb is thought to carry only a proximal identity but under the influence of FGF on the progress zone, mesenchyme is directed towards a more distal fate. If thalidomide were to block mesenchymal proliferation in the limb bud, then a greater proportion of cells would remain under the influence of the FGF and the whole limb would become specified to form distal segments. Tabin suggested that in this way the mesenchyme cells forget their original proximal fate and the entire limb becomes progressively distalized.

Whilst the pharmacological mechanisms are still not fully understood, events such as the thalidomide tragedy have stimulated further research into the more mainstream theories of limb development. Fortunately, it is rare to be able to study such specific teratogenic effects on human development.

I. THE HUMERUS

The adult humerus

The humerus forms the skeleton of the arm and articulates proximally at the shoulder joint with the scapula (Chapter 8) and distally at the elbow joint with the radius and ulna. It is a long bone consisting of a proximal rounded head, a shaft and an irregular distal end.

The **head** (Fig. 9.4, 9.5a), which faces medially and slightly posteriorly, forms almost a third of a sphere and is separated from the rest of the bone by the **anatomical neck**, to which the greater part of the capsule of the shoulder joint is attached. The **lesser tubercle** is a rounded eminence which lies below and

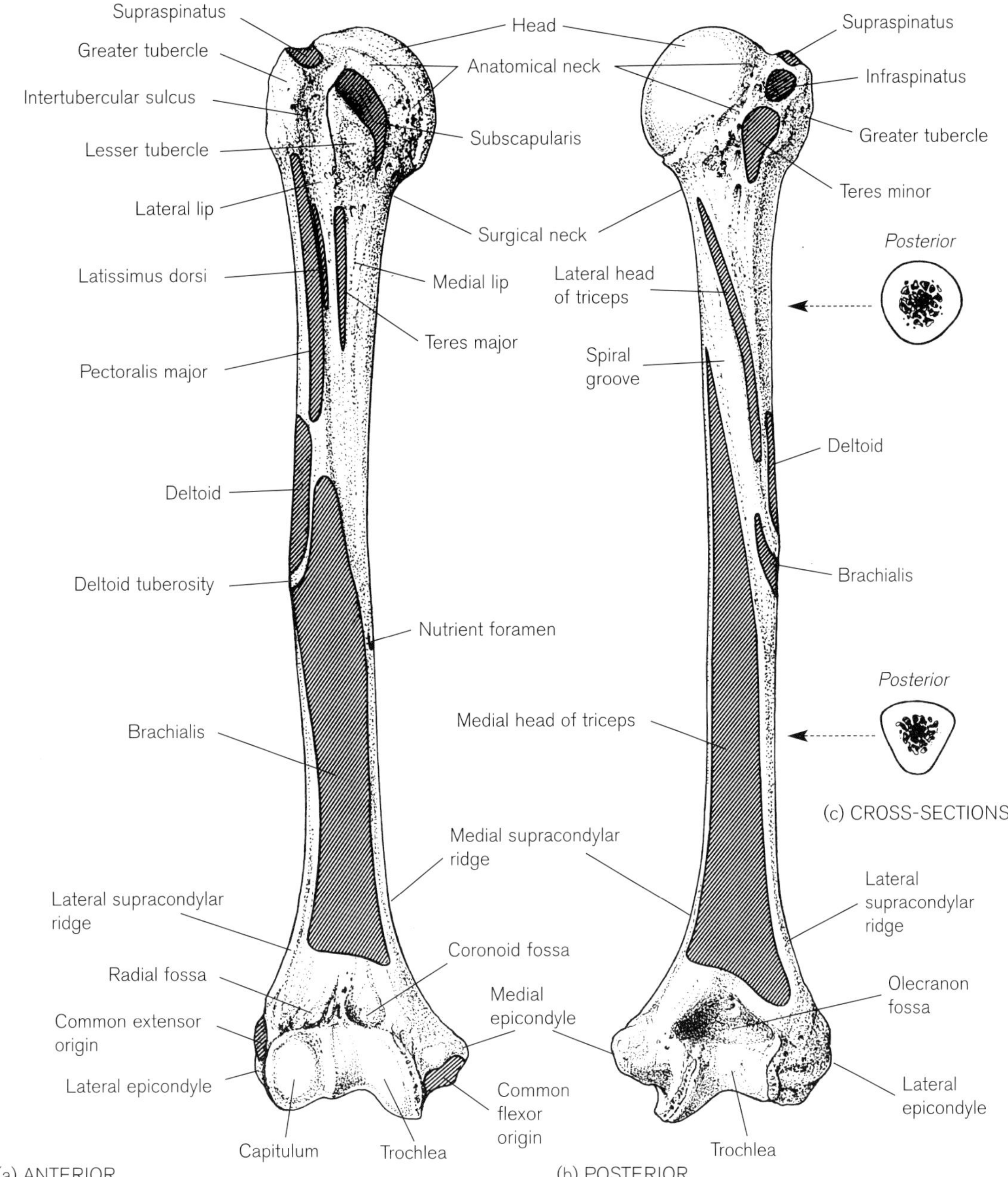

Figure 9.4 Right adult humerus.

anterior to the head and provides attachment for the subscapularis muscle. Meyer (1928) described a supratubercular ridge extending obliquely distally and anteriorly from the articular cartilage of the head, which was present in 17% of humeri. The **greater tubercle** faces laterally and bears three facets on its upper surface for the supraspinatus, infraspinatus and teres minor muscles. These three muscles, together with subscapularis, form the 'rotator-cuff' muscles, which stabilize the shoulder joint during movement. As both the capsule and the ligaments of the joint are of limited mechanical value, these muscles are the main factor responsible for maintaining the head of the bone against the glenoid surface of the scapula and preserving the stability and integrity of the joint (see also Chapter 8). The blood supply of the upper end of the humerus is derived from arteries that originate at the base of the neck of the bone (Crock, 1996) and give off vessels which enter through the numerous accessory nutrient foramina (Laing, 1956). Dislocation of the shoulder joint, which is nearly always anterior and subglenoid, can result in damage both to the axillary nerve, which innervates the deltoid and pectoralis minor muscles and skin of the upper arm, and to the

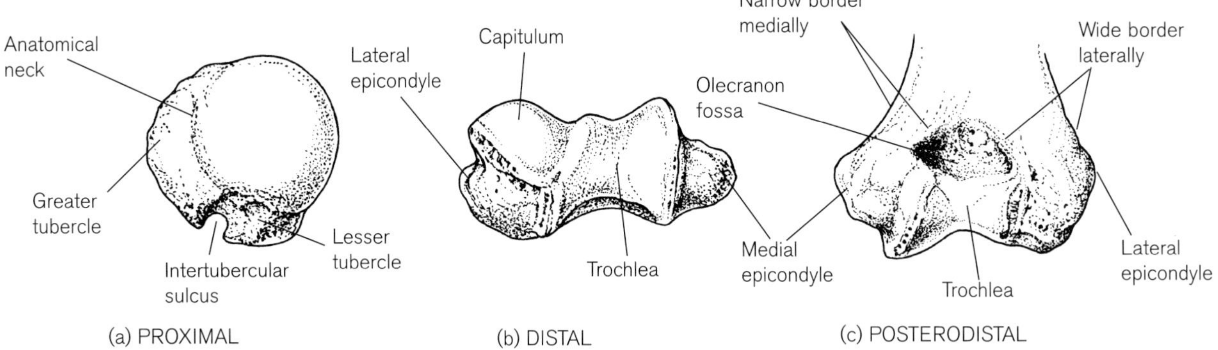

Figure 9.5 Right adult humerus.

anterior and posterior circumflex humeral vessels. Recurrent anterior dislocation can result in a humeral head defect, an area of depression or flattening on the posterolateral surface of the head, which can vary from a groove to the loss of one-third of the total articular surface. Its pathology and aetiology are discussed by Hill and Sachs (1940) and Adams (1948, 1950). Recurrent dislocation can also result in muscle paralysis particularly of the deltoid, which can ultimately alter the shape of the **deltoid tuberosity** (see below) resulting in an enthesopathy. Pathology of the humeral head and both tubercles in an archaeological population has been described by Miles (1996), who ascribed the lesions to the clinically recognized condition of acromial impingement disorder. Musculoskeletal markers manifesting on the humerus have been investigated in skeletal assemblages from a variety of geographical and temporal situations (Churchill and Morris, 1998; Peterson, 1998; Steen and Lane, 1998; Wilczak, 1998). In older studies, the variations in entheses have been attributed to age, sex, hormonal levels, genetics and life styles. More recent studies have concentrated on markers of occupational stress, but methodological problems, especially the determination of accepted standards, make them difficult to evaluate (Robb, 1998; Stirland, 1998).

Between the two tubercles lies the **intertubercular sulcus**, which is continued distally as the **bicipital groove** that occupies the upper quarter of the shaft. In most texts the two terms tend to be used synonymously, although Meyer (1928) and Vettivel *et al.* (1992) distinguish between them. The attachment of the latissimus dorsi muscle occupies the floor of the sulcus over which runs the tendon of the long head of the biceps brachii in its synovial sheath. The **medial lip** of the sulcus is continuous with the lesser tubercle and is the site of attachment of the teres major muscle. The **lateral lip** of the groove is continuous with the greater tubercle and serves as an attachment for pectoralis major. Vettivel *et al.* (1992, 1995) and Selvaraj *et al.* (1998) have used measurements of the sulcus both as an indicator of handedness and as a correlate of the length of the humerus. The **surgical neck** is the junction of the proximal end of the bone and the top of the shaft and is a frequent site of fracture, which is most commonly seen in elderly women following rarefaction of the bone (Adams and Hamblen, 1992).

Dokládal (1977, 1978) has described variability in the shape of the shaft of the humerus, but in general the cross-section of the upper half is cylindrical, while the lower half is triangular (Fig. 9.4c). The anterior surface bears a rounded ridge that is continuous proximally with the lateral lip of the intertubercular sulcus. About half way down the shaft on the lateral side is a roughened area, the **deltoid tuberosity**, for the attachment of the deltoid muscle. Fracture by muscle action is more common in the shaft of the humerus than in any other bone and usually occurs just below the attachment of deltoid. Posteriorly, from just below the head to the deltoid tuberosity, and running distally and laterally, is a roughened line to which the lateral head of the triceps muscle is attached. Below this line is the **radial** (spiral) **groove**, which houses the radial nerve and the profunda brachii vessels. Fractures of the shaft in this area can damage these structures and occur most commonly in persons over 50 years of age (Klenerman, 1966). Injury to the nerve results in a loss of extension at the wrist, metacarpophalangeal and interphalangeal joints. The lower third of the shaft is smooth on both sides and provides attachment for the brachialis muscle anteriorly and the medial head of the triceps muscle posteriorly. The dominant **nutrient foramen** is usually found on the medial aspect of the middle third of the shaft (Lütken, 1950; Carroll, 1963; Mysorekar, 1967) and the entrance is directed distally.

The shaft of the humerus is twisted about its long axis so that a line through the axis of the head and greater tuberosity between the attachments of the supraspinatus and infraspinatus muscles makes an angle with a line through the plane of the elbow joint (centre of the capitulum and the trochlea – see below). Mean torsion is about 73° and always in a medial (internal) direction (Martin, 1933; Krahl and Evans, 1945). Evidence from comparative anatomy suggests that the primary hereditary torsion has imposed upon it a secondary torsion caused by opposing muscle actions that act during ontogeny, possibly at the proximal epiphyseal level (Evans and Krahl, 1945; Krahl, 1948; Krahl, 1976). Two different methods of expressing the angle of torsion have been used. Some authors include in their measurements the 90° rotation that the entire upper limb undergoes during ontogeny. Even without this, humeral torsion appears to be measured, not as the direct angle between the two axes, but as 90° minus this angle and is thus expressed differently from the measurement of torsion in the femur or tibia (see Chapter 11). Larson (1988), in a study of the mechanics of the shoulder in primates, suggested that the high degree of torsion present in humans translated the lateral facing glenohumeral joint to a more medial facing elbow joint. This has made it possible to manipulate the hands in front of the body by pronation and supination of the forearm without changing the position of the shoulder.

The **distal end** (Figs. 9.4, 9.5b, c) is irregular in shape and has bony projections at either side, the lateral and medial epicondyles, from which the lateral and medial supracondylar ridges extend upwards onto the shaft. The medial ridge is longer and leads from the more protuberant condyle, whereas the lateral ridge has more prominent muscle markings. The extensor muscles of the forearm originate from the **lateral epicondyle** and extend upwards onto the supracondylar ridge. The **medial epicondyle** is the site of attachment for the superficial flexor muscles of the forearm and the long flexors of the digits. The ulnar nerve passes directly posterior to the medial epicondyle and can be damaged as a result of a blow to the medial side of the elbow.

The supracondylar process (spur) is an anomalous hook-like extension of varying size that extends distally from the medial ridge and is usually connected to the medial epicondyle by a fibrous band (the ligament of Struthers).[1] It has been identified in the embryo (Adams, 1934), is not uncommon in neonatal bones and is considered by some anthropologists to be a non-metric trait (Finnegan, 1978; Saunders, 1989), where it is said to occur in 1% of populations of European descent (Terry, 1921, 1923, 1930; Hrdlička, 1923; Keats, 1992). The ligament may become ossified and thus form a foramen through which passes the brachial artery, or its branches, and the median nerve to reach the forearm. A large spur may exert pressure on the neurovascular bundle, especially with the forearm in the extended and supinated position and this can cause pain, paraesthesia or even obliterate the radial pulse (Barnard and McCoy, 1946; Kessel and Rang, 1966; Symeonides, 1972). Occasionally, it may fracture and this can also produce neurovascular complications (Doane, 1936; Kolb and Moore, 1967; Newman, 1969).

Between the epicondyles lie the medial **trochlea** and the lateral **capitulum**[2] which face anteriorly from the line of the shaft and which articulate with the ulna and the radius respectively to form the elbow joint. The pulley-shaped trochlea, which articulates with the trochlear notch of the ulna, extends from the anterior surface, round the distal end onto the posterior surface. The capitulum, a rounded eminence, is limited to the anterior and distal surfaces, and articulates with the head of the radius. Above them anteriorly lie the **coronoid fossa** and the shallower **radial fossa**, which accommodate the coronoid process of the ulna and the head of the radius during full flexion of the elbow joint. Posteriorly, there is a deep **olecranon fossa** (Greek, meaning 'elbow and head') into which the olecranon of the ulna fits during extension at the elbow joint.

The septal aperture (foramen olecrani), a foramen of variable size between the olecranon and the coronoid fossae, has been viewed as a nonmetric trait by anthropologists (Hrdlička, 1932; Finnegan, 1978; Saunders, 1989) and some studies have shown it to be population-specific (Hrdlička, 1932; Akabori, 1934; Trotter, 1934b; Ming-Tzu, 1935; Glanville, 1967). It may merely be a reflection of incomplete ossification, as Ming-Tzu (1935) and Godycki (1957) found it present more frequently in the gracile humeri of females and Benfer and McKern (1966) also found it to be negatively correlated with the robusticity of the bone. Glanville (1967) favoured a more mechanical explanation as, although it had a higher frequency in an African than a European population, this was associated with a wider range of flexion and extension at the elbow joint. Benfer and Tappen (1968) have studied

[1]Frequently, eponymous terms were not originally described by the individual whose name is associated with the structure. The spur was described by Robert Knox in 1841 and 1842–3. His lectures on the anomaly, which he found both in human cadavers and in a performing jaguar that died in Edinburgh (together with libellous remarks about physiologists), make fascinating reading. The spur was illustrated in *Quain's Anatomy* in 1848. Sir John Struthers described it and his name has been associated with it ever since.

[2]*Capitulum* meaning 'little head' in Latin, is still referred to as the capitellum in the clinical literature. The nomina term is now capitulum.

the occurrence of the perforation in non-human primates and believe that the explanation is more complex. Although genetic and developmental factors may be primarily responsible for the presence of the perforation, the robusticity of the humerus has an inhibitory effect on the expression of this trait.

The adult humerus displays some sexual dimorphism, especially in head dimensions (Dwight, 1905; Thieme and Schull, 1957; Steel, 1962; Singh and Singh, 1972a; France, 1983, 1988; Dittrick and Suchey, 1986; MacLaughlin, 1987; Holman and Bennett, 1991; Işcan *et al.*, 1998). It has long been suggested that the so-called 'carrying angle' (valgus angle) between the axis of the humerus and the forearm during supination is also a sexually dimorphic feature and it has been measured in many studies (Potter, 1895; Mall, 1905; Atkinson and Elftman, 1945; Steel and Tomlinson, 1958; Smith, 1960; Beals, 1976). As with the angle of torsion, different bony points are used to measure the carrying angle and it is expressed in two different ways, either as the medial (acute) angle between the long axis of the humerus and forearm, or as the lateral (obtuse) angle. Although some authors have reported a difference between males and females, the differences do not appear to be statistically significant and the wide range and extensive overlapping preclude its usefulness as an indication of sex.

Age-related change, mostly using radiographic methods, has been investigated by Schranz (1959), Acsádi and Nemeskéri (1970), Bergot and Bocquet-Apel (1976) and MacLaughlin (1987). Estimation of stature from humeral length can be made using the figures of Breitinger (1937) for north European males only, Telkkä (1950) and Trotter and Gleser (1952, 1958, 1977) for Blacks and Whites, Genovés (1967) for Mesoamericans and for other populations in Krogman and Işcan (1986), but results are obviously not as accurate as those achieved using the lower limb bones. Data on extrapolation of maximum bone length from fragments of the humerus can be found in Steele and McKern (1969) and Rao *et al.* (1989). Calculation of living stature can then be attempted, but the accuracy of reconstruction will be compromised if the data is from different populations. Some attempt has been made, using long bone lengths and calculation of the brachial index (radial length × 100/humeral length) to establish racial affinity and metrics may be found in Krogman and Işcan (1986).

It has long been accepted that there is asymmetry in the dimensions of the long bones (Schultz, 1937; Schell *et al.*, 1985) and some studies suggest that this appears to be congenital but decreases with age (Pande and Singh, 1971; Ruff and Jones, 1981; Stirland, 1993). It is tempting to assume that asymmetry is directly related to handedness (Schulter-Ellis, 1980) but doubts have been expressed about the causes of asymmetry (Glassman and Bass, 1986) and it is difficult to prove without independent documentary verification, which is rarely available. However, strong circumstantial evidence is provided by the work of Vettivel *et al.*, (1992, 1995) and Selvaraj *et al.* (1998). They reported that significant differences in measurements of the intertubercular sulcus and the presence or absence of a supratubercular ridge of Meyer in right and left non-matched humeri closely parallels the handedness of the population from which the bones were drawn. Similarly, Steele and Mays (1995) found a distribution of lateral asymmetries in length in the humerus and humerus-plus-radius in an archaeological population that closely parallels handedness in modern populations. Asymmetry in the measurement of the greater tubercle and its relation to activity-related change is discussed by Stirland (1993).

Early development of the humerus

Details of the early development of the humerus may be found in Bardeen and Lewis (1901), Lewis (1901), Gray and Gardner (1951), Gardner and Gray (1953) and O'Rahilly and Gardner (1975). The mesenchymal humerus is visible at stage 16 (about 8–11 mm CRL/37 days (O'Rahilly *et al.*, 1956; O'Rahilly and Gardner, 1975). The cartilaginous humerus begins to form during stages 16 and 17 (about 8–14 mm CRL/37–41 days) and is complete before the end of the eighth week of embryonic life. Chondrification has reached the head of the humerus by 44 days and the epicondyles by 48 days. By 51 days, the neck and both tubercles are discernible (Gardner and Gray, 1953), as are the condyles (Gray and Gardner, 1951). The humerus reaches 2.2 mm and 3.3 mm at 51 and 54 days, respectively, and at the end of the fetal period it is about 4.8 mm in length (Streeter, 1949; O'Rahilly and Gardner, 1975).

Ossification

Primary centre

The definitive study on the later development of the prenatal humerus from the end of the embryonic period is by Gray and Gardner (1969). A bony collar appears in the midshaft at stage 21 (week 8 – Gray and Gardner, 1969; O'Rahilly and Gardner, 1975) and by week 7 the primary ossification centre can be seen histologically, although it is not visible radiologically until about 2 weeks later. The main nutrient foramen becomes apparent near the middle of the bone on the anterior surface at about the ninth to tenth week. Skawina and Wyczólkowski (1987) found that 88% of fetuses had a single artery, usually situated in the mid-shaft region. There may also be accessory foramina, some of them posteriorly. At first, periosteal bone occupies more of the length of the diaphysis but, by the beginning of the fifth month, periosteal and endochondral bone formation are co-extensive. By the sixth month, ossification extends proximally to the region of the anatomical neck and distally into the olecranon fossa and the epicondyles. From this period, the morphology of the humeral diaphysis is sufficiently distinct to permit identification and, for the remainder of the fetal period, growth of the bone by apposition and resorption takes place as it enlarges in length and width. Remodelling, indicated by the presence of osteoclasts external to the compacta, begins in the second trimester on the anterolateral part of the proximal metaphysis with bone deposition on the lips, and removal from the floor of the intertubercular groove. At the distal end, remodelling starts a little later along the supracondylar lines. At term, 79% of the length of the bone is occupied by ossified shaft and 21% by the cartilaginous extremities (Gray and Gardner, 1969).

The perinatal humerus (Fig. 9.6) is rounded in the proximal half, waisted in the middle and triangular in the distal half. At the proximal end, the shaft slopes slightly towards the medial side. When viewed from the proximal end, the metaphyseal surface is raised medially and the superior end of the intertubercular sulcus is visible anteromedially. A ridge on the anterior border continues proximally as the prominent lateral lip of the intertubercular sulcus, the medial lip of which is less obvious and often eroded. There is usually a nutrient foramen on the anteromedial surface just below the middle of the bone, and often one or more posteriorly at the proximal end below the metaphyseal surface. The entrances of all the foramina slope distally. The distal end is widely flared and on the anterior surface the coronoid fossa forms a slight dip medially. Posteriorly, the lateral border of the olecranon fossa is wider than the medial border. The distal metaphyseal surface is dumb-bell-shaped with circular lateral and oval medial surfaces connected by a bridge of bone anterior to the olecranon fossa.

During the third year, the proximal metaphyseal surface changes from a smooth, rounded surface to an angulated one as it begins to reflect the shape of the proximal composite epiphysis. By puberty, there is a sharp peak on the posterolateral edge of the metaphysis, which fits into the posterior notch of the epiphysis (see below). At the distal end, the radial fossa develops before the end of the first year, and between the ages of 4 and 6 the region of the deltoid tuberosity usually becomes apparent as a roughened patch of bone. Krahl (1948) reported that, with increasing age, the bicipital groove twists from lateral to medial. Posteriorly, the groove for the radial nerve is rarely visible before puberty.

In children, fracture of the humeral shaft can occur at either end, but proximal damage is not so frequent as in adults. At the distal end, supracondylar fractures are the second most common type of injury after that to the forearm bones and most occur between the ages of 5 and 10 years (Wilkins, 1984).

Secondary centres

The **proximal epiphysis** of the humerus is described in most anatomical texts as being ossified from three centres, one each for the head, the greater and the lesser tubercles, although much doubt has been expressed about the independent formation of the lesser tubercle. The separate centres coalesce early in childhood to form a compound epiphysis, which fuses with the shaft at cessation of growth in length. The growth plate is characteristically cone-shaped, the medial part being intra-articular and lying within the capsule of the shoulder joint. Most of the information concerning times of appearance comes from radiological studies (Puyhaubert, 1913; Davies and Parsons, 1927; Flecker, 1932b, 1942; Hasselwander, 1938; Elgenmark, 1946; Kelly and Reynolds, 1947; Christie, 1949; Hansman, 1962; Garn *et al.*, 1967b). However, Gray and Gardner (1969) demonstrated histologically that epiphyseal vascularization is present in the fetal period long before the onset of ossification. Early studies showed that the ossification centre for the **head** can be present at birth but usually appears by 6 months *post-partum* (Spencer, 1891; Davies and Parsons, 1927; Menees and Holly, 1932). Christie (1949) found that the early appearance of the head was positively correlated with weight at birth, and was present more commonly in black females. Lemperg and Liliequist (1972) reported that in Swedish children the humeral head was ossified in over 50% of newborns and a definite correlation existed between time of appearance and weight at birth. Kuhns *et al.* (1973a) and Kuhns and Finnstrom (1976) related the appearance of the humeral head to maternal history, birth weight, size as detailed by head circumference and body length, as well as maturity judged by neurological examination. The earliest sign of ossification was at 36 weeks *in utero* but there was wide variability in the onset of ossification and this was only slightly affected by the sex of the neonate. The centre for the humeral head therefore remains unossified in a significant percentage of infants at term and is too variable a feature to be used

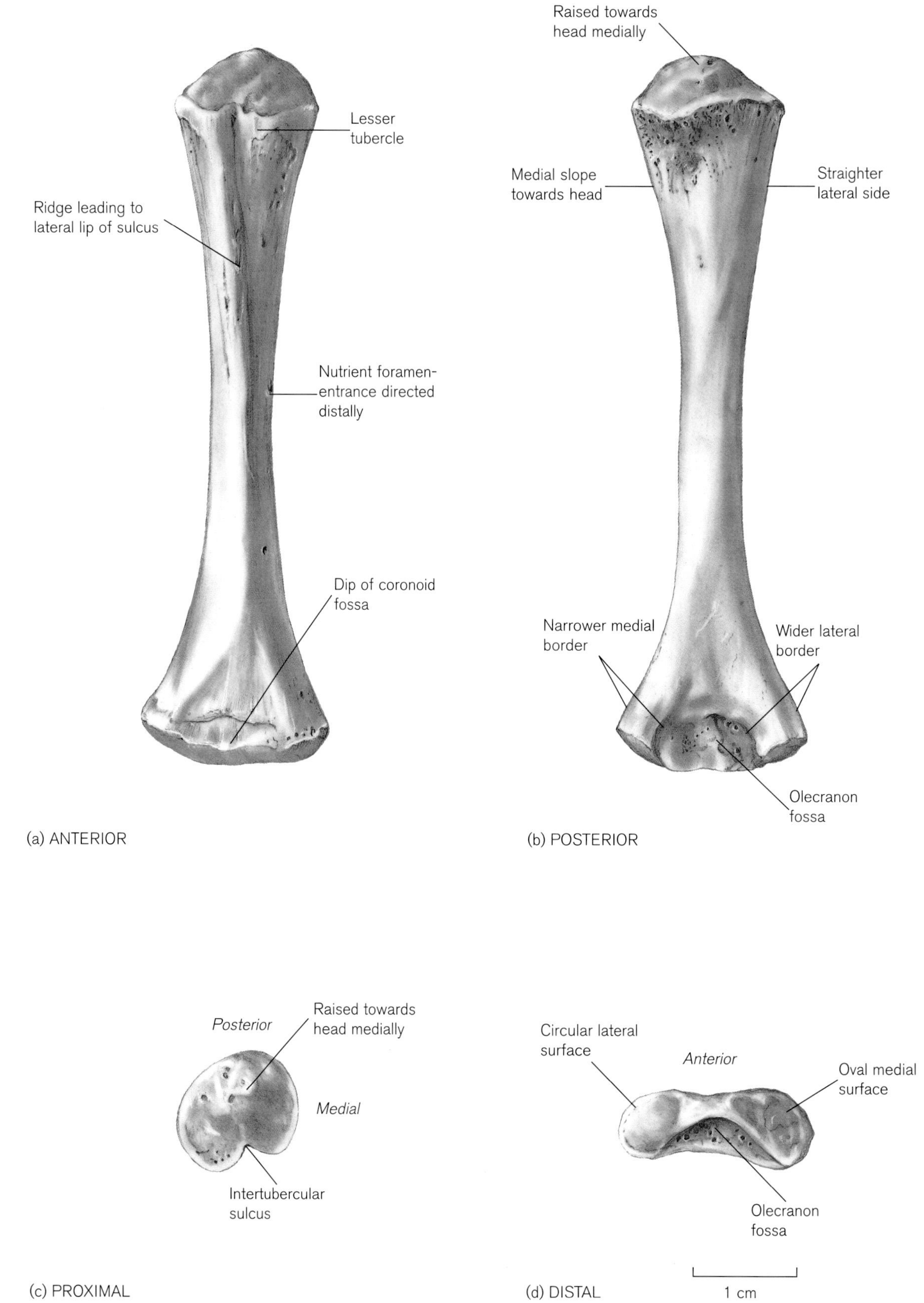

Lesser tubercle
Ridge leading to lateral lip of sulcus
Nutrient foramen-entrance directed distally
Dip of coronoid fossa
(a) ANTERIOR
Raised towards head medially
Medial slope towards head
Straighter lateral side
Narrower medial border
Wider lateral border
Olecranon fossa
(b) POSTERIOR
Posterior
Raised towards head medially
Medial
Intertubercular sulcus
(c) PROXIMAL
Circular lateral surface
Anterior
Oval medial surface
Olecranon fossa
(d) DISTAL
1 cm

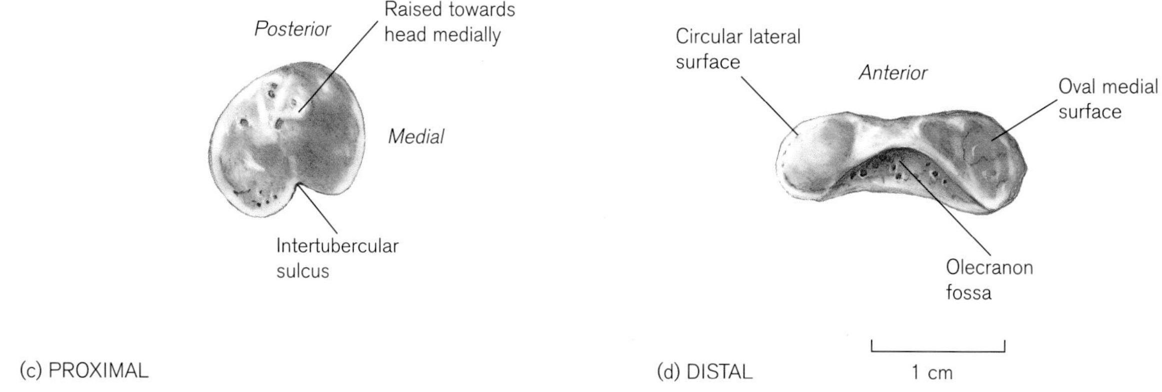

Figure 9.6 Right perinatal humerus.

as a reliable indicator of maturity at birth. From about the end of the first year, the epiphysis for the head is an almost spherical nodule with a smoothly curving, pitted articular surface. It may have the beginning of a bridge of bone to the greater tubercle, which appears as a small downward-pointing beak, or it may remain unjoined to the tubercle for the first few years (Fig. 9.7a).

Reported appearance times for the centre for the **greater tubercle** are very variable and range from 3 months *postpartum* to 3 years. Most accounts agree that it is present earlier in girls than in boys (Elgenmark, 1946; Hansman, 1962; Garn *et al.*, 1967b). The centre appears laterally and at an angle to that of the head, so that the characteristically conical shape of the proximal epiphysis is present from an early stage. A separate centre for the **lesser tubercle** is described in most anatomy texts but the original source for this information is not well documented. Most radiological accounts (Ogden *et al.*, 1978; Caffey, 1993) only illustrate two centres for the proximal end. Cohn (1924) and Paterson (1929) doubted its separate existence, assuming it to be a downgrowth from the secondary centre for the head. However, Cocchi (1950), described a distinct third centre appearing between the ages of 4 and 5 years. This was not visible radiographically on a normal AP view as its demonstration required a special axillary projection with the upper limb outwardly rotated. If indeed this third centre has a separate existence in all individuals, it is probably of fairly short duration.

The coalescence of the secondary centres to form a single **compound proximal epiphysis** is described in numerous radiological accounts as occurring between 5 and 7 years and this is the age reported in most anatomy texts. However, Ogden *et al.* (1978) stress that 'studies of postnatal development are virtually non existent' and that the 'appearance of ossification centres in the proximal humerus is not settled'. In their histological study, they describe bone bridging as early as 2 years, long before it can be demonstrated radiologically, which could account for the wide range of reported times of appearance in the literature. We have several compound proximal humeral epiphyses of documented ages younger than 3 years. The morphology of the recently formed compound epiphysis is consistent with either the lesser tubercle appearing as a separate centre, or as a downgrowth from the capital epiphysis. It is an irregularly shaped bone, with the head joined to the greater tubercle at a constricted waist leaving definite anterior and posterior notches (Fig 9.7b). The lesser tubercle is attached to the anterior border of the head. At about 7–8 years, the three parts of the epiphysis become more completely fused together and form an irregularly shaped cap (Fig. 9.7c). The area between the greater and lesser tubercles consolidates to form the floor of the intertubercular sulcus anteriorly, although the junction between the head and greater tubercle persists as an obvious posterior notch. The whole articular surface is formed from porous-looking bone and the metaphyseal surface is deeply divided by a Y-shaped groove into its three constituent parts. By puberty, the three parts consolidate further. The surface of the head is smooth and delimited from the tubercles by an obvious anatomical neck, but there is still a pronounced posterior notch (Fig. 9.7d). From this stage until fusion, the epiphysis takes on the appearance of the adult bone.

Incidence of damage to the proximal humerus is uncommon in children compared to that seen in adults, and subluxation of the glenohumeral joint is rare. Displacement of the entire epiphysis may occur during delivery (Michail *et al.*, 1958; Broker and Burbach, 1990) and is not often seen after the age of 5 years. After this age, fractures may include a posteromedial fragment of the metaphysis (Dameron and Rockwood, 1984) or rarely, avulsion of the lesser tuberosity in adolescents (Paschal *et al.*, 1995). Hook-like projections called epiphyseal spurs are sometimes seen at the lateral edge of the epiphysis during childhood and adolescence. They can be mistaken for avulsion fractures but are normal transient phenomena that disappear during late puberty (Keats and Harrison, 1980).

Fusion of the proximal epiphysis coincides with cessation of growth in length. This is the growing end of the bone and it is responsible for 80% of growth in length of the shaft (Ozonoff, 1979; Ogden, 1984d; Pritchett, 1991). Information on ages of closure from radiographic data are given by Davies and Parsons (1927), Paterson (1929), Flecker, (1932b, 1942), Hasselwander (1938) and Hansman (1962). These range from 12 to 19 years in females and 15.75 to 20 years in males. The only figures available from observations on skeletal material are those of Stevenson (1924), who does not distinguish between the sexes, and McKern and Stewart's (1957) report on the Korean War dead, which considers only the upper end of the range for males, from 17 to 24 years. They give 24 years for complete union and it thus appears that, from this incomplete set of data, there is, a discrepancy (for males, at least) between the appearance of fusion radiographically and those observations made directly on bone, which give an age of about 2 years later.

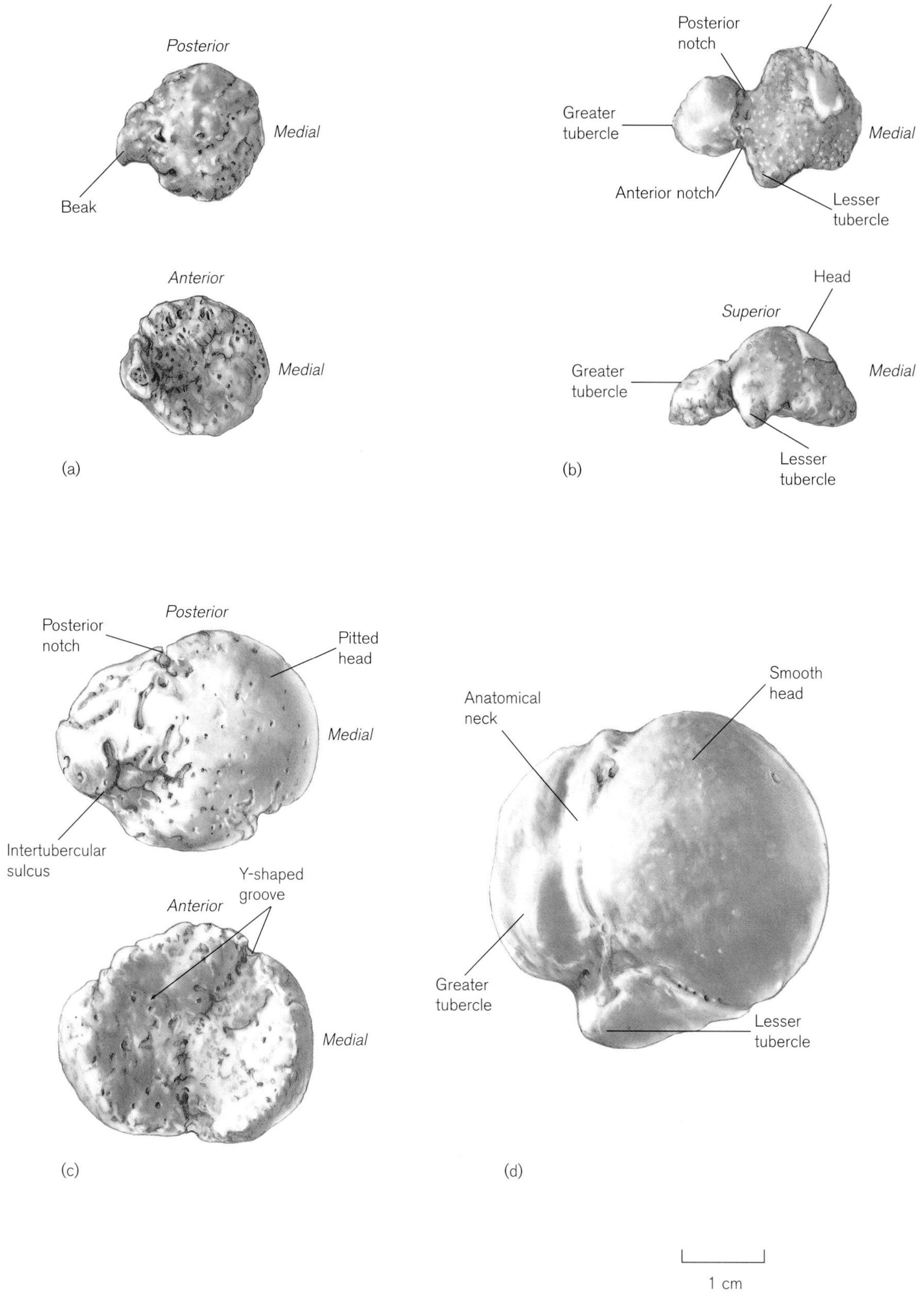

Figure 9.7 Development of the right proximal humeral epiphysis. (a) Head only ossified – 3 years; (b) early compound epiphysis – also 3 years; (c) later compound epiphysis – 8 years; (d) mature epiphysis – adolescent.

The stages of closure first described by Stevenson, have been used by many authors but the only information on the pattern of closure is from McKern and Stewart (1957), who state that, 'the last site of union for the proximal end appears as a slight groove, posterolaterally'. Ogden *et al.* (1978) suggest that the pattern of closure is variable and may begin in the central region of the epiphysis. In a series of juvenile skeletons, we have found a regular pattern of fusion around the periphery. It usually commences in the region of the posterior notch between the head and the greater tubercle by small bridges of bone that eventually coalesce and this was also reported in a specimen by Haines *et al.* (1967). The next area to fuse is anteriorly at the junction of the anatomical and surgical necks. Fusion then progresses medially, thus attaching the head to the shaft, leaving the area under both tubercles open. Bridges of bone at the lateral lip of the sulcus consolidate and fusion spreads to the floor of the sulcus. The last areas remaining open are laterally and posteriorly around the greater tubercle. It thus appears that the pattern of fusion reflects the separate existence of the different parts of the proximal epiphysis.

The **distal epiphysis** of the humerus develops from four separate ossification centres, which appear in the following order: capitulum, medial epicondyle, trochlea and lateral epicondyle. Ranges for the appearance of these centres can be found in Davies and Parsons (1927), Flecker (1932b, 1942), Hasselwander (1938), Francis *et al.* (1939), Francis, (1940), Elgenmark (1946), Haraldsson (1959) and Hansman (1962). The most useful developmental account is a radiological atlas of the paediatric elbow (Brodeur *et al.*, 1981), which illustrates stages of maturation at 6-monthly intervals, distinguishing between early and late developers. There is also a radiological and histological study by McCarthy and Ogden (1982a).

The capitulum may appear as early as 6 months *postpartum* and is nearly always present by 2 years. It begins as a spherical nodule of bone and by about 3 years its radiological appearance is hemispherical, with a straight superior margin. It appears to be tilted downwards anterior to the lower end of the diaphysis, as the growth plate is always wider posteriorly (Silberstein *et al.*, 1979). A recovered capitular fragment is a substantial wedge-shaped nodule of bone, which is thickest at its lateral base and thinner towards the medial apex. The articular surface is convex anteroposteriorly and the metaphyseal surface is flat. The anterior border is straight and the posterior border is pitted and pointed (Fig. 9.8a).

The medial epicondylar epiphysis can normally be seen on a radiograph by 4 years of age, but is slow to develop. Silberstein *et al.* (1981a) described its appearance as spherical, ovoid, or occasionally multicentric, but it would be difficult to recognize as an isolated epiphysis. The trochlear epiphysis develops initially as multiple foci in the eighth year and soon becomes joined at its lateral edge to the capitulum, from which it is separated by a groove (Fig. 9.8b). The lateral epicondyle is visible on a radiograph at the level of the capitular ossification at the outermost edge of the cartilaginous epiphysis at about 10 years of age (Silberstein *et al.*, 1982). It is occasionally double, but more normally appears as a semilunar sliver, which matures fairly rapidly into a triangular shape with the apex directed medially. The distal part fuses to the lateral edge of the capitulum and often has a nodular articular surface (Fig. 9.8c).

There is a complex pattern of **fusion** but, unlike the proximal end, once the separate centres coalesce, the composite epiphysis does not remain separate from the shaft for very long. The combined capitulum, trochlea and lateral epicondyle is usually united by 10 years in girls and 12 years in boys (Haraldsson, 1959). Brodeur *et al.* (1981) illustrate this fusion as beginning at about 11.5 years in girls and about a year later in boys. Fusion with the shaft begins posteriorly, leaving a line open above the capitulum, lateral trochlea and proximal lateral epicondyle and is usually complete by about 15 years. The centre for the medial epicondyle remains separate from the rest of the compound epiphysis, being isolated from it by a non-articular part of the shaft (Fig. 9.8d). The medial epicondyle is the last of the elbow epiphyses to unite with the shaft, but reported ages of fusion cover a wide time range (Paterson, 1929; Flecker, 1932b, 1942; Hansman, 1962) so that it is not a useful indicator of age. Hansman gives a range of 11–16 years in females and 14–19 years for males, but the Brodeur *et al.* (1981) atlas shows that fusion usually occurs by about 15 years of age. It fuses from below upwards, the superior and anterior surfaces being the last to unite, leaving a temporary notch anterosuperiorly (Fig. 9.8e).

After supracondylar fracture, avulsion of the lateral epicondyle is the most common injury at the distal end of the humerus in children (Rutherford, 1985; De Jager and Hoffman, 1991; Nicholson and Driscoll, 1993). If fracture separation of the whole distal epiphysis including the medial epicondyle occurs, it is usually in the young child, when the epiphysis is composed predominantly of cartilage. In the older child the medial epicondyle often remains with the shaft (Wilkins, 1984). The late and separate fusion of the medial epicondyle, with its characteristic notch, can lead to a mistaken diagnosis of fracture in

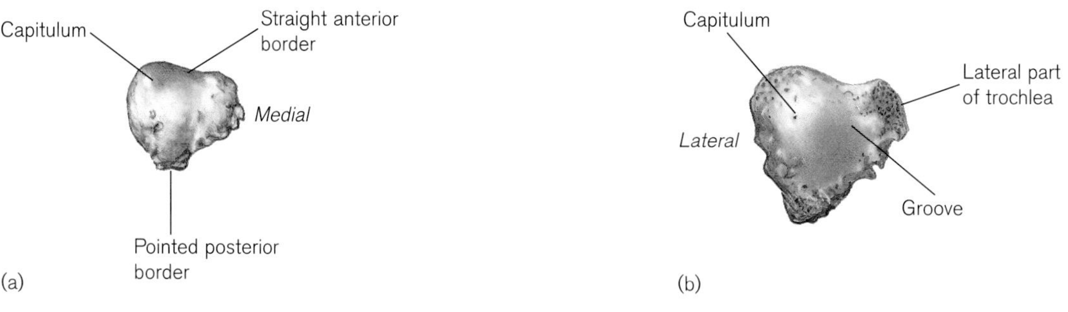

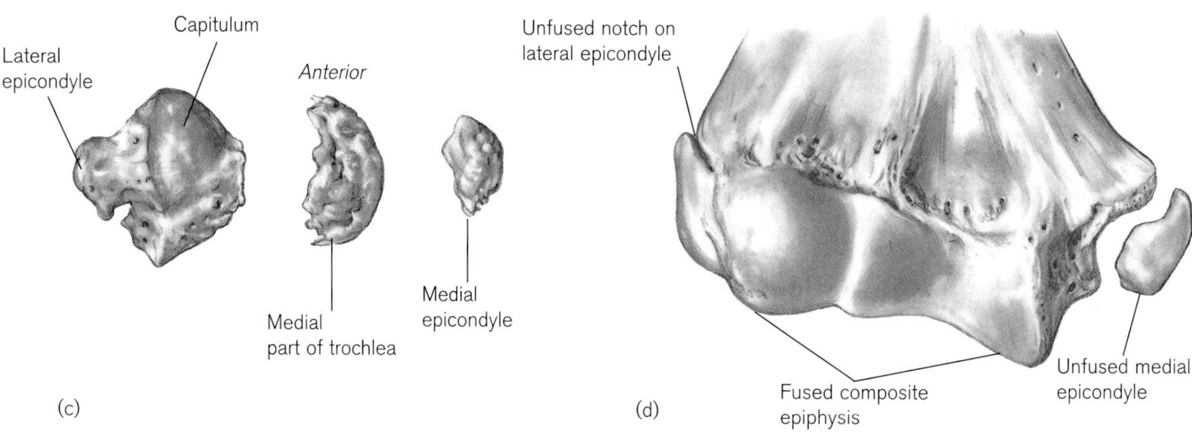

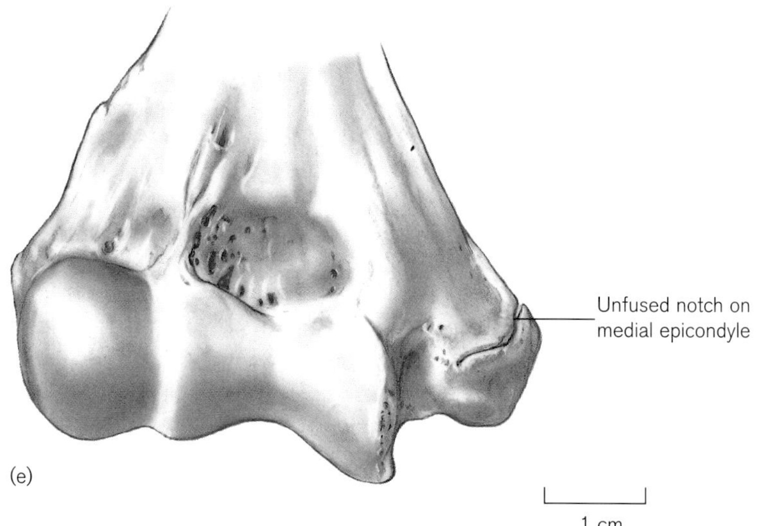

Figure 9.8 Development of the right distal humeral epiphysis. (a) Early capitulum – 7 years; (b) later capitulum – 8 years; (c) three separate parts of epiphysis – late childhood; (d) main part of compound epiphysis fused – adolescent; (e) almost mature distal end – late adolescent.

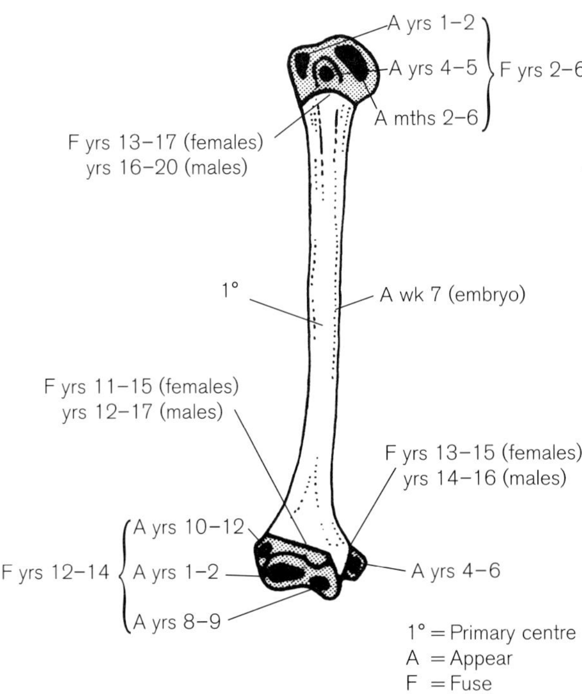

Figure 9.9 Appearance and fusion times of the humeral ossification centres.

adolescence, but avulsion by muscular action is possible and in the USA is sometimes known as 'Little Leaguer's elbow' (Larson and McMahan, 1966).

The appearance and fusion of the humeral ossification centres are summarized in Fig. 9.9.

Practical notes

Sideing

Diaphysis – the neonatal or infant humerus can be sided using the following features. Proximally, the anterior ridge in the middle of the shaft leads up to the lateral lip of the intertubercular sulcus. The medial border slopes slightly towards the head, whereas the lateral border is straighter. The nutrient foramen is usually on the anteromedial side, with its entrance directed distally. Distally, the lateral border of the olecranon fossa is wider than the medial side (Fig. 9.6b).

Proximal epiphysis – the lesser tubercle is attached to the head anteriorly and the greater tubercle extends laterally from this, separated by anterior and posterior notches (Fig. 9.7).

Distal epiphysis – in a young skeleton, the capitulum is usually the only recognizable separate part of the distal epiphysis that is recovered. It is a wedge-shaped nodule of bone, wider at the lateral end. The anterior border is straight and the posterior border is pointed and pitted with nutrient foramina (Fig. 9.8). Once the other parts of the epiphysis have fused to the capitulum, it can be sided in the same manner as the distal end of the adult bone.

Bones of a similar morphology

Perinatal diaphyses – the six major long bones of the limbs can be divided into two groups: the femur, humerus and tibia are larger and look more robust than the radius, ulna and fibula. Taking the bones of a single individual, in the first group, the femur is considerably longer than the humerus and tibia, which are about equal in length (Table 9.1). The humerus can be distinguished from the tibia as it is flattened distally and bears the obvious olecranon fossa posteriorly whereas the tibial shaft is triangular and has flared proximal and distal ends (Figs. 9.6 and 11.17). From birth onwards, the rate of growth in the lower limb starts to accelerate and the tibia increases in length faster than the humerus.

Proximal humeral fragment – this may be confused with a proximal femoral fragment or a proximal or distal tibial fragment (Fig. 9.10). The metaphyseal surface of the humerus is roughly circular, with the notch of the intertubercular sulcus visible anteriorly, whereas the metaphyseal surface of the proximal femur is larger and continuous posteriorly onto the lesser trochanteric surface of the shaft. After the neonatal period, the humerus assumes its characteristic peaked proximal end and the femur begins to develop a neck. The proximal tibia is distinguished from the proximal humerus by its more oval metaphyseal surface, the presence of the tuberosity and, if enough of the shaft is present, the very large nutrient foramen posteriorly. The distal tibial metaphyseal surface is similar in size to that of the humerus but is flatter and has a 'D'-shaped outline with a straight lateral border. The metaphyseal surface of the humerus is raised medially towards the head.

Table 9.1 Means and ranges for maximum lengths of diaphyses of major long bones at 10 lunar months

	Mean (mm)	Range (mm)
Humerus	64.9	61.6–70.0
Radius	51.8	47.5–58.0
Ulna	59.3	55.0–65.5
Femur	74.3	69.0–78.7
Tibia	65.1	60.0–71.5
Fibula	62.3	58.0–68.5

Adapted from Fazekas and Kósa (1978).

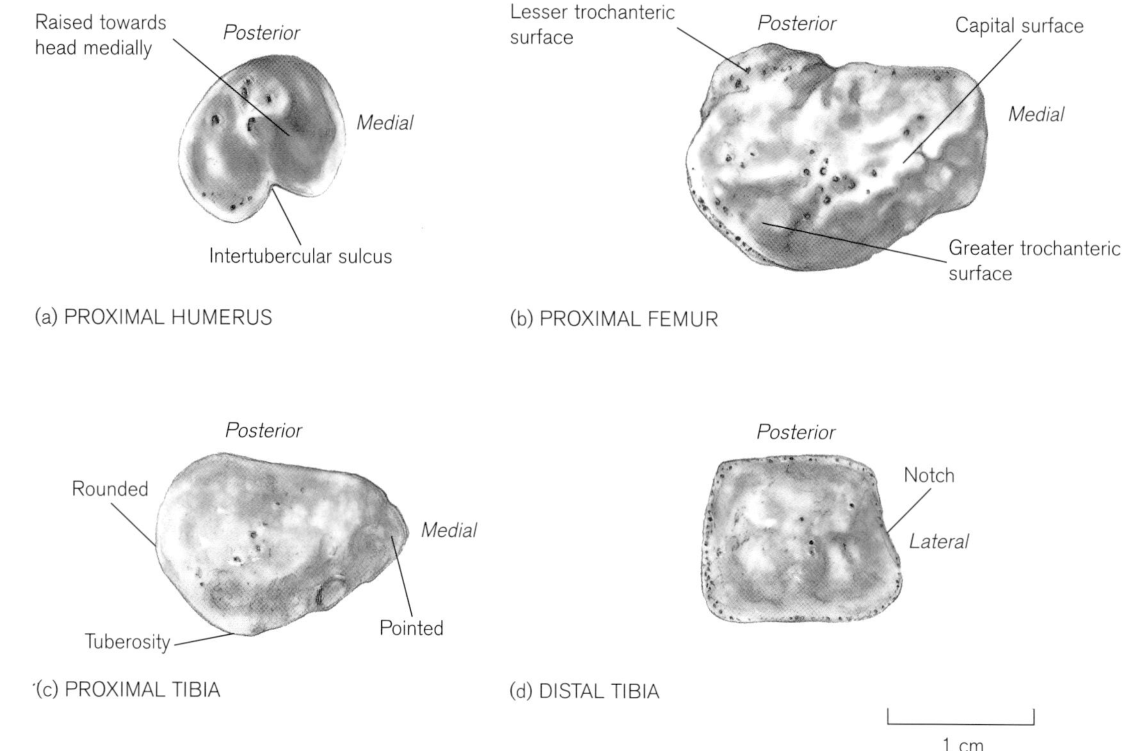

Figure 9.10 Metaphyseal surfaces of right perinatal humeral, femoral and tibial diaphyses.

Distal humeral fragment – this can be recognized by the characteristic olecranon fossa posteriorly.

Proximal humeral and femoral head epiphyses – superficially these may look similar but, for a single individual at an early stage, the capital femoral epiphysis is about 1.5 times larger than that of the humerus (Fig. 9.11a and b) and the latter often has either a small laterally pointed beak, which is the beginning of the bridge to the greater tubercle, or has already assumed its tripartite appearance (Figs. 9.7a, b). Later, the composite epiphysis and the femoral head are of similar size, but the humeral epiphysis has assumed its characteristic cap shape with a tripartite groove on its metaphyseal surface. The femoral head epiphysis is more circular, with a flattened lateral border. The fovea is visible on the articular surface and the beak-shaped projection can be seen on the relatively flat metaphyseal surface (Fig. 9.11c–f).

Morphological summary (Fig. 9.9)

Fetal

Wk 7	Primary ossification centre appears
Wks 36–40	Secondary ossification centre for the head may be visible
Birth	Usually represented by shaft only
2–6 mths	Secondary centre for head appears
1–2 yrs	Secondary centre for greater tubercle appears; secondary centre for capitulum appears
4+ yrs	Secondary centre for medial epicondyle appears and possibly that for lesser tubercle
2–6 yrs	Centres for head, greater and lesser tubercles fuse to form composite epiphysis
By yr 8	Secondary centre for trochlea appears
Yr 10	Secondary centre for lateral epicondyle appears
11–15 yrs	Distal composite epiphysis joins shaft in females
12–17 yrs	Distal composite epiphysis joins shaft in males
13–15 yrs	Medial epicondyle fuses to shaft in females
14–16 yrs	Medial epicondyle fuses to shaft in males
13–17 yrs	Proximal epiphysis fuses in females
16–20 yrs	Proximal epiphysis fuses in males

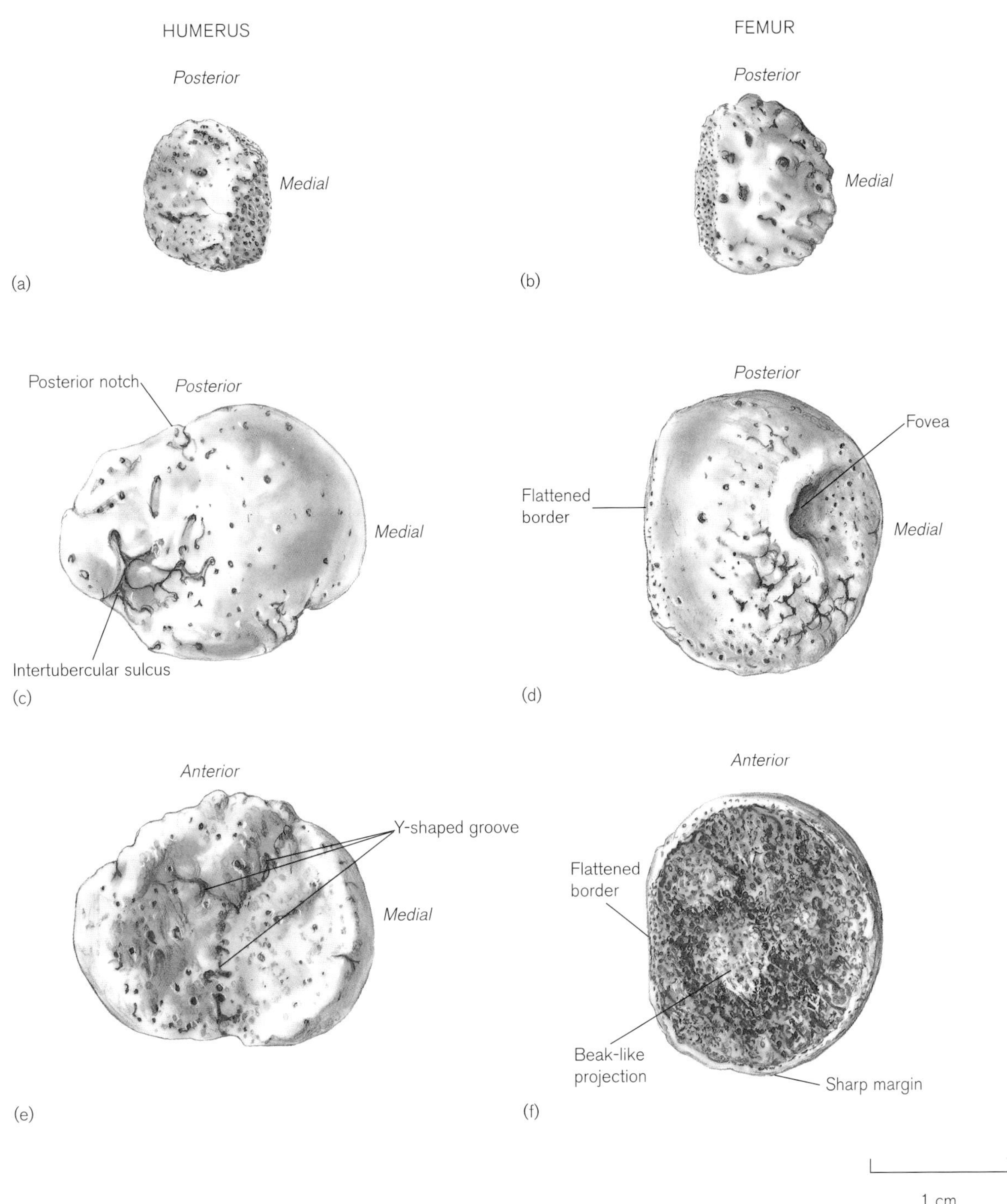

Figure 9.11 Right humeral and femoral proximal epiphyses. Articular surfaces of (a) humeral head epiphysis and (b) femoral head epiphysis – 3 years, male. Articular surfaces of (c) humeral proximal epiphysis and (d) femoral head epiphysis – 8 years, female; (e) and (f) metaphyseal surfaces of (c) and (d), respectively.

Metrics

Fazekas and Kósa (1978) measured the length and the distal width of the humeral diaphysis throughout fetal life (Table 9.2) and the length of the humerus as measured on ultrasound is taken from Jeanty (1983, Table 9.3). Mehta and Singh (1972) measured the length of the ossified shaft of the humerus prepared from fetuses of crown–rump lengths between 65–290 mm (about 12–36 weeks). Trotter and Peterson (1969) recorded the length and weight of the perinatal humeral diaphysis (Table 9.4).

Scheuer *et al.* (1980) gave linear and logarithmic regression equations for age on humeral diaphyseal length, as measured on radiographs from 24 fetal weeks to 6 weeks postnatal (Table 9.5). Data showing the length of the humerus at 6-monthly intervals (2-monthly for the first half-year) from birth to the cessation of growth are shown in Table 9.6. These data from Maresh (1970) from the University of Colorado longitudinal growth study have become the most commonly used modern population with which archaeological studies are compared, and they are particularly useful during the adolescent period. From ages 10–12 years double sets of figures give the lengths of the diaphysis with and without epiphyses, so that comparisons can be made depending on the state of fusion of the specimen. Pritchett (1988), using the Colorado data from age 7 years, to maturity, charted growth and predictions of growth from the upper limb bones. The length of the humerus is 18% of standing height in girls at age 7 years, increasing to 19% at age 15 years and the humerus grows at about 1.2 cm per year during this period. The equivalent figures for boys are 18%, 20% (at age 20 years) and 1.3 cm.

Diaphyseal length data for some archaeological populations from Africa, Europe and North America are given in Appendix 3. Most of the age at death estimates are based on dental development.

Table 9.2 Length and width of the fetal humeral diaphysis

Age (weeks)	Length (mm)	Distal width (mm)
12	8.8	1.9
14	12.4	2.2
16	19.5	4.7
18	25.8	6.1
20	31.8	7.8
22	34.5	8.3
24	37.6	9.3
26	39.9	9.9
28	44.2	10.9
30	45.8	11.9
32	50.4	12.5
34	53.1	13.6
36	55.5	14.4
38	61.3	15.7
40	64.9	16.8

Length: maximum length.
Width: maximum mediolateral width at distal end.
Adapted from Fazekas and Kósa (1978).

Table 9.3 Length of the fetal humerus as measured by ultrasound

	Length (mm) Percentile		
Age (weeks)	5th	50th	95th
12	3	9	10
14	5	16	20
16	12	21	25
18	18	27	30
20	23	32	36
22	28	36	40
24	31	41	46
26	36	45	49
28	41	48	52
30	44	52	56
32	47	55	59
34	50	57	62
36	53	60	63
38	55	61	66
40	56	63	69

Adapted from Jeanty (1983).

Table 9.4 Length and weight of the perinatal humerus

	Length (mm)	Weight (g)
White male	65.2	2.47
White female	61.2	1.90
Black male	62.2	1.91
Black female	65.4	2.01
Mean	63.5	2.10

Adapted from Trotter and Peterson (1969).

Table 9.5 Regression equations of age on maximum humeral length (mm)

Linear	Age (weeks) = (0.4585 × humerus) + 8.6563 ± 2.33
Logarithmic	Age (weeks) = (25.069 $\log_e$ × humerus) − 66.4655 ± 2.26

Adapted from Scheuer *et al.* (1980).

Table 9.6 Humeral length (mm) – 2 months–18 years

	Male			Female		
Age (years)	*n*	Mean	SD	*n*	Mean	SD
Diaphyseal length						
0.125	59	72.4	4.5	69	71.8	3.6
0.25	59	80.6	4.8	65	80.2	3.8
0.50	67	88.4	5.0	78	86.8	4.6
1.00	72	105.5	5.2	81	103.6	4.8
1.5	68	118.8	5.4	84	117.0	5.1
2.0	68	130.0	5.5	84	127.7	5.8
2.5	72	139.0	5.9	82	136.9	6.1
3.0	71	147.5	6.7	79	145.3	6.7
3.5	73	155.0	7.8	78	153.4	7.1
4.0	72	162.7	6.9	80	160.9	7.7
4.5	71	169.8	7.4	78	169.1	8.3
5.0	77	177.4	8.2	80	176.3	8.7
5.5	73	184.6	8.1	74	182.6	9.0
6.0	71	190.9	7.6	75	190.0	9.6
6.5	72	197.3	8.1	81	196.7	9.7
7.0	71	203.6	8.7	86	202.6	10.0
7.5	76	210.4	8.9	83	209.3	10.5
8.0	70	217.3	9.8	85	216.3	10.4
8.5	72	222.5	9.2	82	221.3	11.2
9.0	76	228.7	9.6	83	228.0	11.8
9.5	78	235.1	10.7	83	234.2	12.9
10.0	77	241.0	10.3	84	239.8	13.2
10.5	76	245.8	11.0	75	245.9	14.6
11.0	75	251.7	10.7	76	251.9	14.7
11.5	76	257.4	11.9	75	259.1	15.3
12.0	73	263.0	12.8	71	265.6	15.6
Total length including epiphyses						
10.0	76	258.3	11.2	83	256.1	14.6
10.5	76	263.7	11.6	75	262.9	16.1
11.0	75	270.0	11.5	76	269.6	16.4
11.5	77	276.3	12.7	75	278.5	17.3
12.0	76	282.0	13.8	75	287.5	18.2
12.5	67	289.2	13.1	65	294.0	17.7
13.0	69	296.6	15.3	69	301.0	17.5
13.5	69	305.0	16.6	62	305.7	17.4
14.0	69	313.3	16.8	64	311.7	16.1
14.5	64	321.4	17.6	42	314.9	17.1
15.0	60	329.0	16.7	57	315.6	17.0
15.5	52	336.5	16.5	12	323.2	19.6
16.0	60	341.0	14.5	40	316.5	18.5
16.5	38	343.4	15.3	3	–	–
17.0	50	347.1	14.6	18	315.4	17.3
18.0	28	350.6	15.6	4	–	–

Adapted from Maresh (1970).

II. THE RADIUS

The adult radius

The radius forms the skeleton of the lateral part of the forearm. It articulates proximally with the capitulum of the humerus at the elbow joint, distally with the scaphoid and lunate bones of the carpus at the wrist joint and medially with the ulna, at both the proximal and distal radio-ulnar joints. It is a long bone consisting of a proximal head, a shaft and an expanded distal end.

The **head** is disc-shaped with an **articular fovea** for the capitulum of the humerus, is tilted slightly laterally from the line of the shaft and connected to the head by a constricted **neck** (Fig. 9.12). The head is encircled by the annular ligament, a strong band that is attached to the anterior and posterior margins of the radial notch of the ulna. The peripheral **articular circumference** of the head is deeper on the anteromedial aspect. The detailed morphology of the combined lateral ligament of the elbow joint and the annular ligament have been described by Martin (1958). Ring (coronary) arteries from the radial recurrent and interosseous arteries surround the base of the neck of the bone, from which regular radiate arteries spread out to supply the head (Crock, 1996). Below the neck on the medial side is the **radial** (bicipital) **tuberosity**, which is roughened on its posterior aspect for the attachment of the tendon of the biceps brachii muscle.

Fracture of the head of the radius, usually caused by a fall on the outstretched hand, is one of the most common fractures of young adults. Forward dislocation of the head is rare (Adams and Hamblen, 1992).

The **shaft** curves gently laterally and anteriorly, and widens considerably towards the distal end. In cross-section, it is circular in its proximal quarter, becoming triangular in the distal half and roughly quadrangular at the distal end (Fig. 9.12c). It is described as having three borders, but it is not always easy to identify them throughout their length as they do not fit well with the usual description. The **anterior border** begins at the lower edge of the radial tuberosity and is a well-marked oblique line running laterally and bearing part of the origin of the flexor digitorum superficialis muscle. The middle and lower sections of the border, rounded and sharp respectively, are actually on the lateral edge of the bone. The **posterior border** also begins at the lower edge of the tuberosity and is a rounded ridge running distally in a mediolateral direction. Its middle section is the sharpish posterior oblique line, but its lower third is not well defined. The **interosseous border** runs straight down the medial side of the bone.

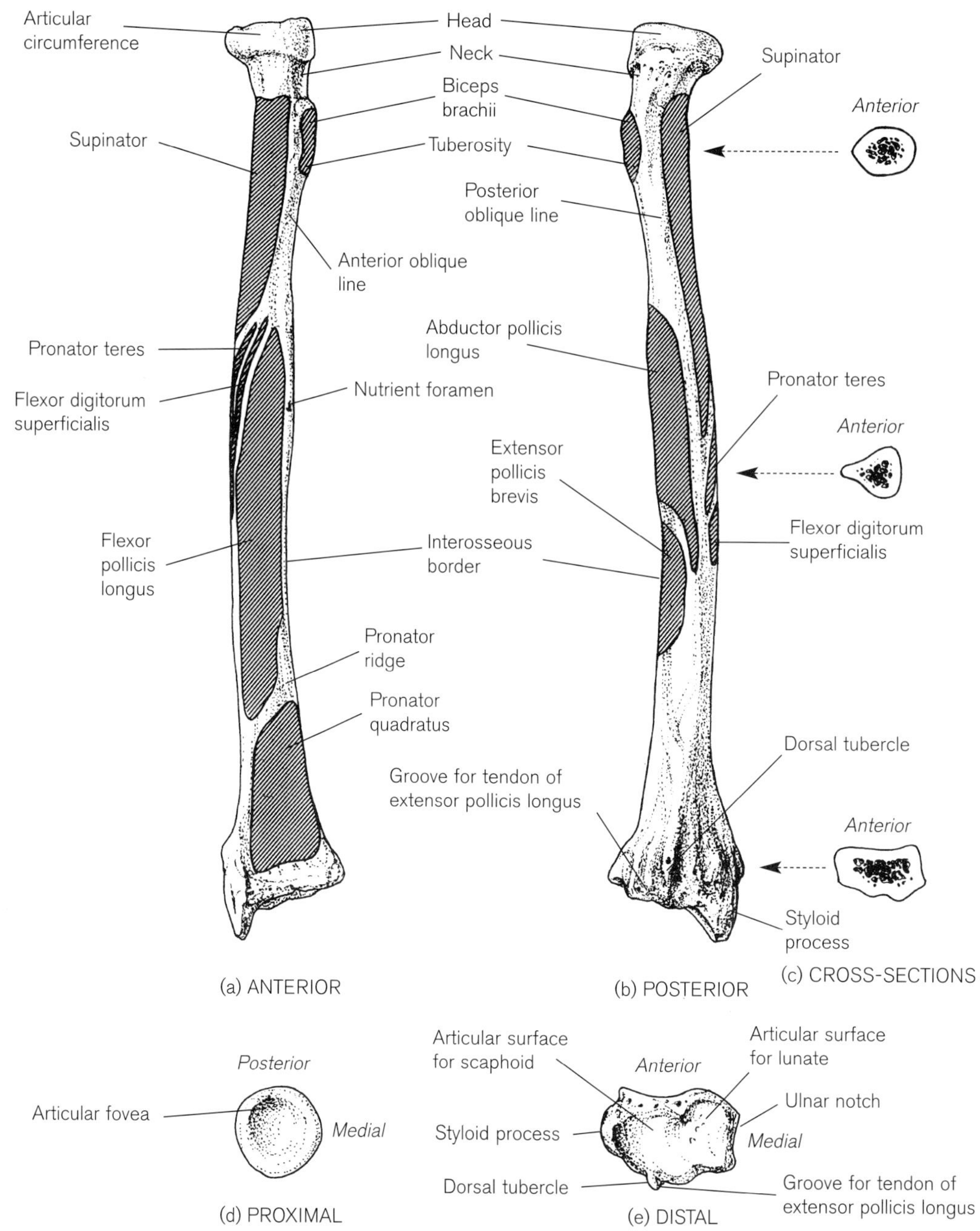

Figure 9.12 Right adult radius.

It is rounded in its upper section and then becomes a sharp edge to which is attached the interosseous membrane connecting it to the ulna. The upper quarter of the shaft, both anteriorly and posteriorly, above the oblique lines, provides attachment for the supinator muscle. The **anterior surface** lying between the anterior and interosseous borders, is slightly hollowed in the middle two quarters, for the attachment of flexor pollicis longus. The lower quarter curves forward distally, may show a faint pronator ridge and has the pronator quadratus muscle attached to it. The **lateral surface** lies between the anterior and posterior borders and at the point of maximum curvature, about the middle of the bone, is a roughened area for the pronator teres muscle. The **posterior surface**, actually facing posteromedially, is hollowed in the middle third and has the abductor pollicis longus muscle attached above and the extensor pollicis brevis muscle below. There is nearly always a single dominant nutrient foramen on the proximal half of the shaft and, in over 75% of cases, it is on the anterior surface (Shulman, 1959; Mysorekar, 1967). The entrance slopes proximally.

Fractures of the midshaft are most common in young adults, whilst fractures at the distal end are most often seen in older adults. The majority of the latter are Colles'[3] fractures, usually occurring in osteoporotic female patients over the age of 50. The distal fragment, about 2.5 cm above the wrist joint, is displaced posteriorly, causing a 'dinner-fork' deformity. Much less commonly, the fragment is anteriorly displaced and is known as a 'reverse Colles' or Smith's fracture (Adams and Hamblen, 1992). The middle and lower end of the radius are common sites to measure bone mineral density because of ease of access and relatively high levels of cancellous bone (Kanis, 1994).

The interosseous border divides distally to enclose a triangular area forming the **ulnar** notch, for articulation with the head of the ulna during pronation and supination. The anterior surface has a thickened ridge at its lower end. The lateral surface extends distally as the **styloid process**. The posterior surface bears a prominent **dorsal** (Lister's) **tubercle** with a marked groove on its medial aspect for the passage of the tendon of the extensor pollicis longus muscle. The tubercle divides the dorsal surface into a lateral part for the long tendons of the wrist and thumb and a medial part for the extensors of the fingers. The **inferior carpal articular surface** (Fig. 9.12e) is divided by a faint ridge into a medial quadrangular and a lateral triangular area with which the lunate and scaphoid carpal bones, respectively, articulate. Blood supply of the lower end of the bone comes from arteries that penetrate the surface and are distributed in a radiate fashion (Crock, 1996).

There are no common anomalies of the radius *per se*. Congenital partial or complete absence of the radius can occur and is usually associated with abnormalities of the hand (Wakeley, 1931; Evans *et al.*, 1950). Complete absence of the bone is more common than partial absence and occurs more frequently in males than females. A radio-ulnar synostosis may occur and can present with either, the proximal radius assimilated with the ulna leaving no recognizable radial head or, with the two bones connected by a bony bar, proximal to which a rudimentary radial head may be seen (Hughes and Sweetnam, 1980). This anomaly prevents pronation or supination and therefore severely restricts the functional range of the limb. Both these abnormalities probably occur at the embryological 5–6 week stage when the normal separation of the anlagen of the two bones fails to occur during development of the proximal radio-ulnar joint.

[3]Abraham Colles was a Dublin surgeon who first described the fracture in 1914 – see Jones, A.R. (1950) *J Bone Joint Surg* **32B**: 126–130.

Sexual dimorphism of the radius has been investigated by Steel (1962), Singh *et al.* (1974a), Allen *et al.* (1987), Berrizbeitia (1989) and Holman and Bennett (1991). Estimation of stature, in the absence of lower limb bones, can be made using the figures of Breitinger (1937), Telkkä (1950), Trotter and Gleser (1952, 1958, 1977), Genovés (1967) and those in Krogman and Işcan (1986). Rao *et al.* (1989) reported data for northern Indian populations to calculate the length of the radius from fragments and so estimate living stature. Attempts have been made, using long bone lengths and the brachial index, to establish racial affinity and metrics may be found in Krogman and Işcan, 1986.

Early development of the radius

The mesenchymal radius is identifiable at stage 16 (about 37 days of intra-uterine life (O'Rahilly *et al.*, 1957). The cartilage anlage starts to form by stage 17 (about 41 days) and by the end of the embryonic period, the head, neck and styloid process are all clearly defined (Gray and Gardner, 1951; O'Rahilly *et al.*, 1957; O'Rahilly and Gardner, 1975). By stage 21 there is evidence of early bone collar formation and enlargement of cartilage cells in the centre of the shaft.

Ossification

Primary centre

Ossification in the diaphysis is evident during week 7 (O'Rahilly and Gardner, 1972). By 3 lunar months, ossification has reached as far as the radial tuberosity and by 5 months it has extended into the neck proximal to the tuberosity, although the tuberosity itself is still only partially ossified and consists largely of cartilage (Gray and Gardner, 1951). There is a single nutrient foramen in 95% of cases, which is normally situated in the middle of the proximal half of the shaft (Skawina and Wyczółkowski, 1987). From an early fetal period, the morphology of the radial diaphysis is sufficiently distinct to permit identification.

The perinatal radius (Fig. 9.13) is rounded in its proximal half and triangular in the distal half and has a very slight lateral curvature. At the proximal end, the neck is directed laterally and the metaphyseal surface is circular and almost flat. Posteriorly, the oblique line is usually visible as a rounded ridge in the middle two quarters and the interosseous border forms a sharp edge. The roughened tuberosity is obvious on the medial side. The shaft flares towards the distal end and its anterior surface is flattened, smooth and slightly concave. The nutrient foramen usually occurs just

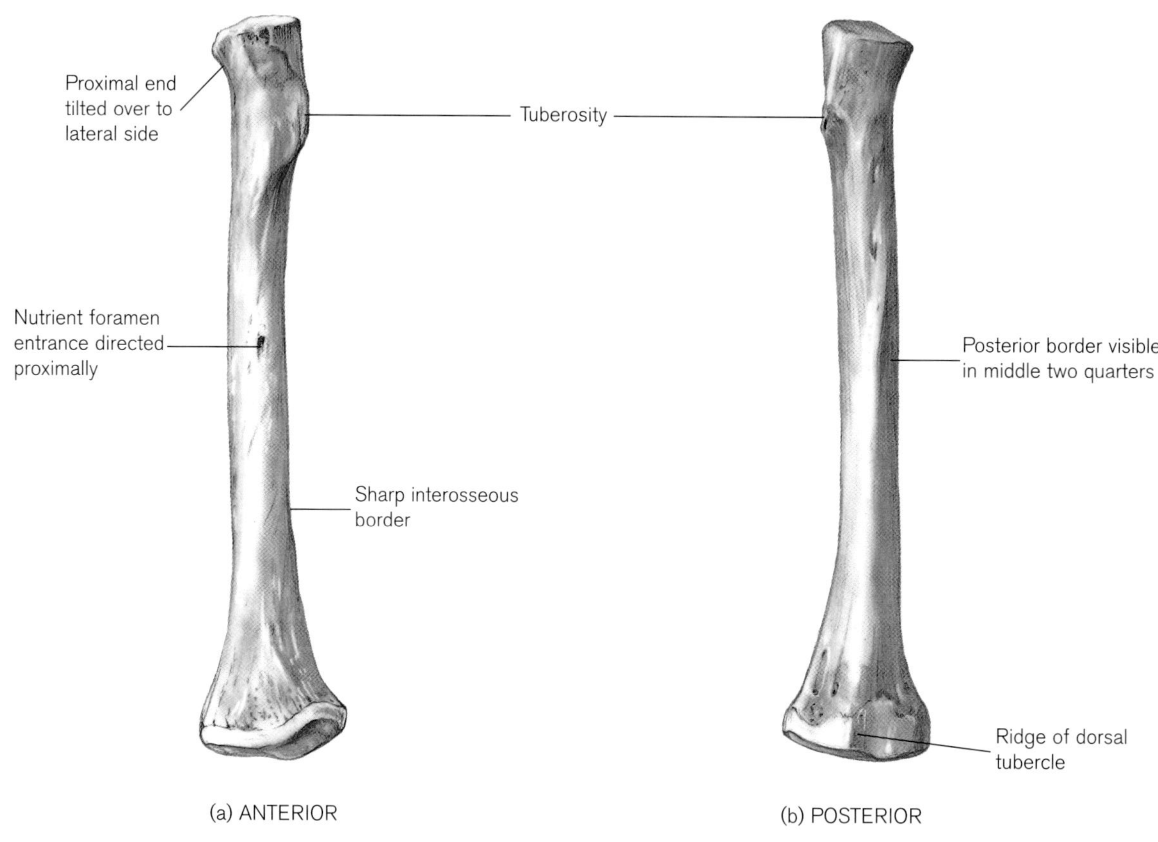

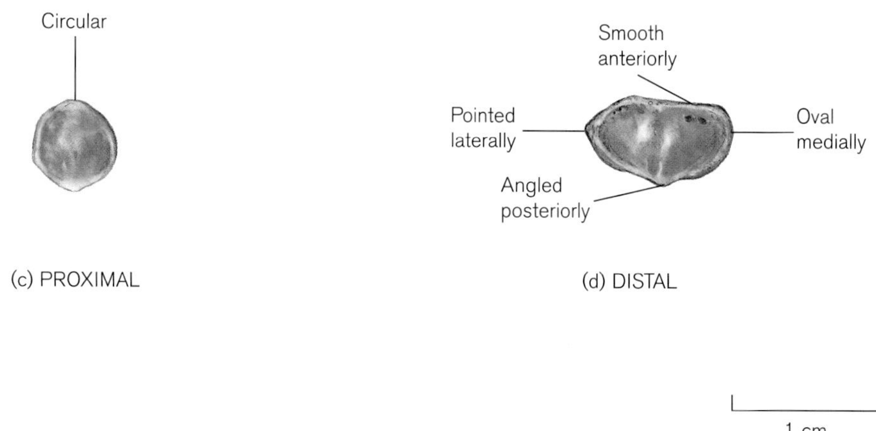

Figure 9.13 Right perinatal radius.

above the centre of the anterior surface, towards the medial side, and the entrance slopes proximally. The distal metaphyseal surface is oval or triangular with pointed lateral and rounded medial ends. The anterior border is smooth and the posterior border is angled (Fig. 9.13d).

During the first year, a more pronounced lateral curvature develops. The distal metaphyseal surface becomes more angulated posteriorly and flattened medially at the base of the triangle for the ulnar notch. By about 4 years, the anterior oblique line (the attachment for pronator teres) can be identified. The dorsal tubercle and the groove for the tendon of extensor pollicis longus become apparent with the development of the distal epiphysis and both features extend onto the shaft at about the time of puberty.

The radius is the most commonly fractured bone in children and the injury usually occurs following a fall on the outstretched hand. In a series of 2094 children's long bone fractures, 45% involved the radius and of these, 75–82% of fractures occurred in the distal third (O'Brien, 1984).

Secondary centres

The **distal epiphysis** of the radius normally develops from a single centre, which usually appears during the first year and is always present by the middle of the third year. Age ranges for appearance are given by Davies and Parsons (1927), Flecker (1942), Elgenmark (1946), Hansman (1962) and Garn *et al.* (1967b). Detailed radiological standards for girls and boys can be found in the Greulich and Pyle (1959) atlas and a more recent radiological developmental study, including injury patterns, has been described by Ogden *et al.* (1981). Epiphyseal displacements of the distal radius and ulna are amongst the most common injuries of the growth mechanism in childhood.

The distal ossification centre appears first as a rounded bony nodule, which only gradually takes on the recognizable shape of the distal epiphysis. It begins to flatten out towards the ulnar side during the second year and soon the lateral part becomes thicker so that the epiphysis assumes a triangulated wedge-shaped appearance (Fig. 9.14a). By about 7–8 years the anterior border is straight and the posterior border is angulated in the region of the dorsal tubercle. The medial border is flattened and the thick lateral end is beginning to ossify into the styloid process (Fig. 9.14b). The latter may develop from a separate centre and even remain unfused throughout life (Keats, 1992). By puberty, the ossified area occupies most of the epiphysis and the metaphyseal surface begins to 'cap' the end of the shaft. The dorsal tubercle becomes obvious and bears a groove on its medial side and the medial border forms a definite ulnar notch (Fig. 9.14c). From this stage until fusion, the epiphysis takes on the appearance of the end of the adult bone. Small hook-like projections called epiphyseal spurs, which may simulate avulsion fractures, sometimes develop at the lateral edge of the epiphysis. They are normal variants, probably caused by isolated islands of ossification and disappear by the time of fusion (Harrison and Keats, 1980).

The distal radius is the growing end of the bone and is responsible for 75–80% of the growth in length of the shaft (Ozonoff, 1979; Ogden, 1984d; Pritchett, 1991) and the epiphysis is one of the last of the major long bones to fuse. Figures for ages of **fusion** from radiographic observations are given by Paterson (1929), Hasselwander (1938), Flecker (1942) and Hansman (1962). The Greulich and Pyle (1959) radiological wrist atlas gives a series of maturity indicators for the distal end of the radius. They show that fusion begins in the middle of the epiphysis and is usually complete by 15–16 years in females and 17–18 years in males. However, McKern and Stewart (1957) report that 100% fusion was not found in males until the age of 23 years so that, as with the humerus, there is a discrepancy between radiographic and osteological observations.

The **proximal epiphysis** of the radius normally appears at 5 years of age. It is one of the few epiphyses that is not spherical on first appearance and forms as a flat disc, although it may occasionally develop from two centres lying side by side (Brodeur *et al.*, 1981). Early authors, Puyhaubert (1913), Davies and Parsons (1927) and Flecker (1932b) give ages for appearance of the centre but do not distinguish between the sexes. Francis *et al.* (1939), Elgenmark (1946), Hansman (1962) and Garn *et al.* (1967b) all give separate figures for males and females, which demonstrate that appearance is usually earlier in females and the paediatric elbow atlas (Brodeur *et al.*, 1981) has staged radiographs for boys and girls. A detailed radiological account of early development correlated with possible injury patterns can be found in McCarthy and Ogden (1982b). The epiphysis of the radial head (Fig. 9.15a) first appears as a flat sclerotic nucleus slightly posteriorly placed and elliptical in shape when first formed, being wider laterally than in the anteroposterior plane. It has a smooth articular surface and a roughened metaphyseal surface. Ossification gradually expands, first in an elliptical fashion, towards the edge of the epiphysis until its margins and those of the shaft attain the same width, although the joint space is wedge-shaped, being wider on the lateral side. This is related to the fact that, prior to ossification, the metaphyseal surface is not parallel to the

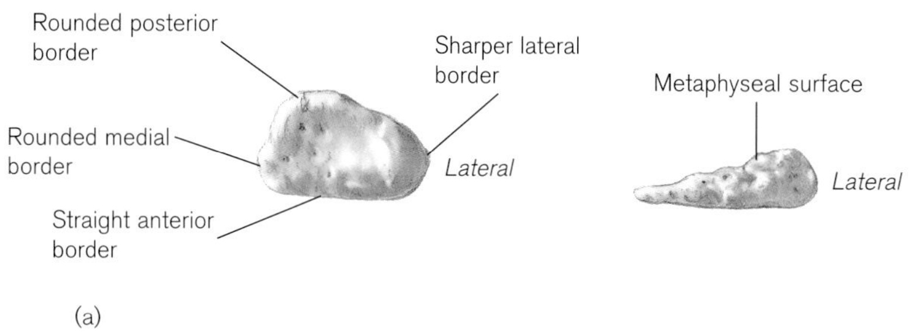

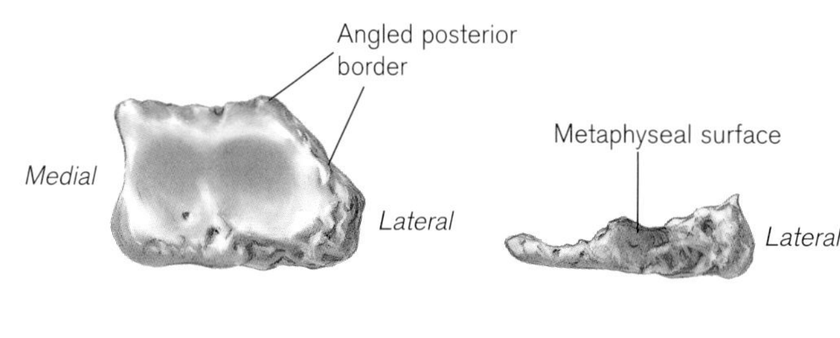

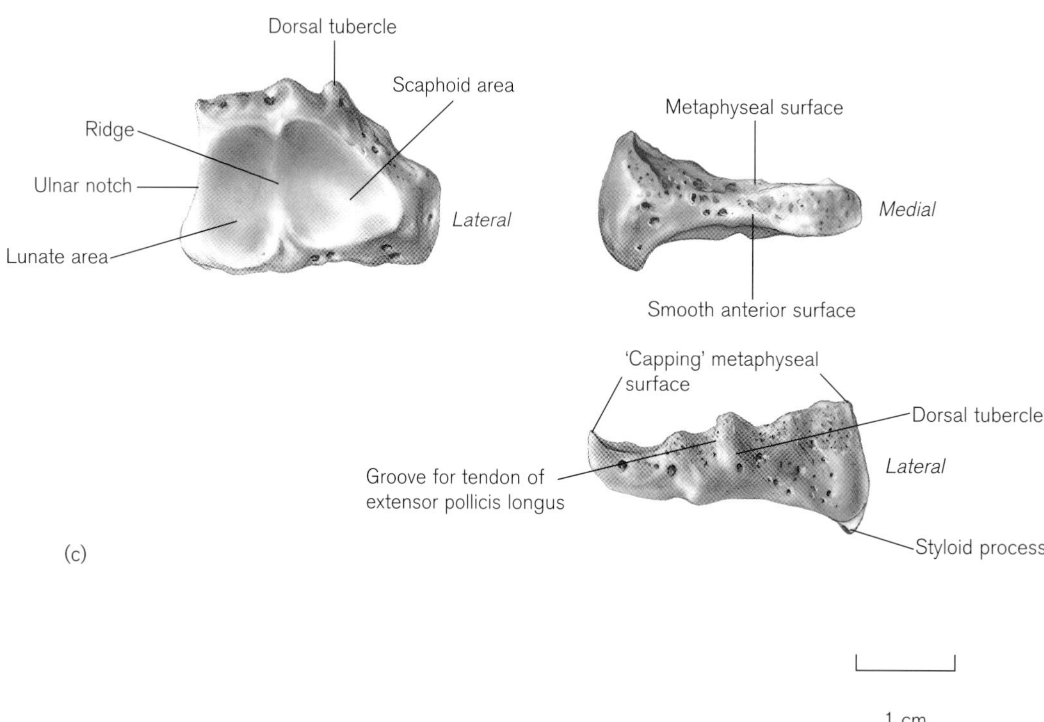

Figure 9.14 Development of the right distal radial epiphysis. (a) Early stage – 7 years; (b) later stage –10 years; (c) mature epiphysis – adolescent. Left row articular surface. Right row (a) and (b) posterior surfaces; (c) anterior and posterior surfaces.

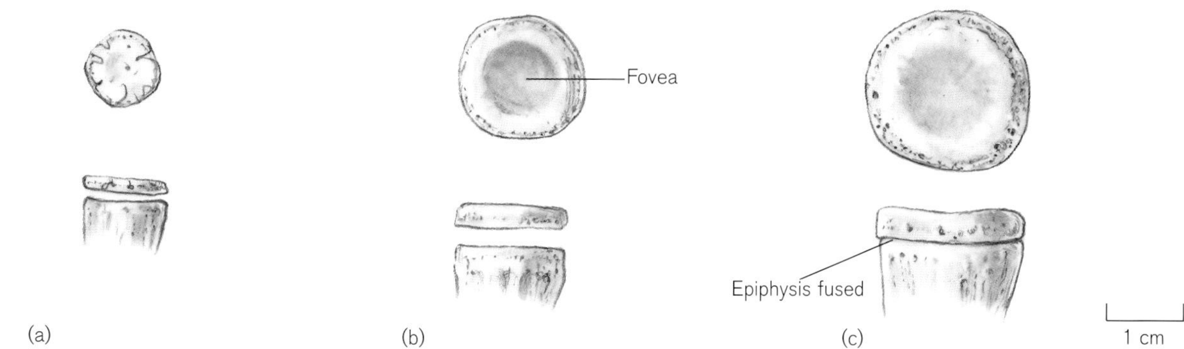

Figure 9.15 Development of the right proximal radial epiphysis. (a) Early stage – 7 years; (b) later stage – 10 years; (c) fused epiphysis – late adolescent. Top row – proximal surface. Bottom row – anterior surface.

articular surface of the capitulum and therefore a line drawn through the long axis of the radial neck projects lateral to the capitulum (Brodeur *et al.*, 1981). The indentation of the fovea is not usually obvious until 10–11 years of age (McCarthy and Ogden, 1982b) and this deepens as the epiphysis matures towards fusion at adolescence (Figs. 9.15b, c).

The so-called 'pulled elbow' occurs when the radial head is subluxated out of the annular ligament. It usually occurs in early childhood when a child is suddenly swung by the arm or steps down from a curb while being held by the hand.[4]

Ages for fusion of the proximal epiphysis are variable, especially in females, as this is affected by menarche, but all accounts agree that fusion occurs earlier in girls than in boys. Brodeur *et al.* (1981) show a range from radiographs of 11.5–14 years in females and from 13.5–16 years in males. Direct observations on dry bone are incomplete as McKern and Stewart (1957) were able to report ages of fusion during the last part of the range for males only. Even though the proximal radius falls into their Group I of early union, they only found 100% fusion at 19 years. A photograph shows an almost fused epiphysis, with the epiphyseal line still open medially over the tuberosity, and in a series of juvenile skeletons, we have confirmed that this is usually the last part of the head to fuse.

The tuberosity of the radius often has the appearance of new bone formation but both Davies and Parsons (1927) and Flecker (1932b) noted that there is no evidence for a separate epiphysis at this site, as described by Frazer (1948). However, it is possible that it is a flake epiphysis similar to those for the tubercles of the ribs whose epiphyses look very similar before and after union (see Chapter 7). They have a short independent life, fusing soon after their formation and are therefore only identifiable during the process of fusion. The appearance and fusion times of the radial ossification centres are summarized in Fig. 9.16.

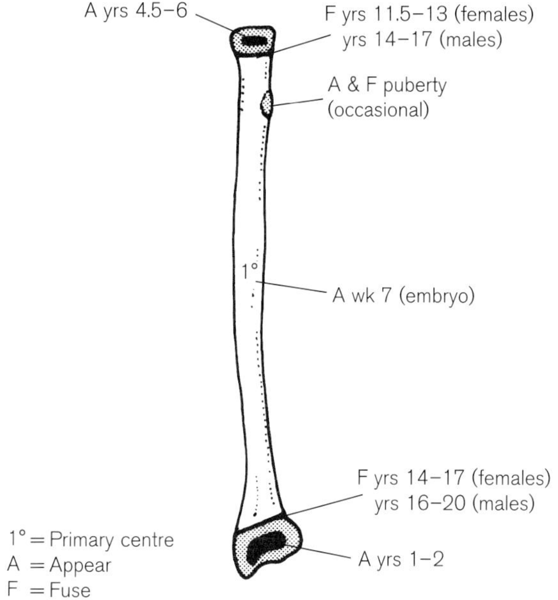

Figure 9.16 Appearance and fusion times of the radial ossification centres.

Practical notes

Sideing

Diaphysis – the perinatal or infant radius (Fig. 9.13) can be sided using the following features. Proximally, the bone tilts laterally and the radial tuberosity is on the medial side. In the shaft, the sharp interosseous border is on the medial side. At the distal end, the anterior surface is smooth and slightly concave, whereas the posterior surface is angulated at the dorsal tubercle. The nutrient foramen is usually on the anterior surface of the proximal half of the bone with its entrance directed proximally.

[4]The Dutch call this 'zondags armpje' – literally 'Sunday arm' – due to the obligatory walk with impatient parents.

Distal epiphysis – (Fig. 9.14) is wedge-shaped with the thicker end lateral, the anterior border straight and the posterior border rounded or angled. At a later stage, the styloid process can be seen laterally and the dorsal tubercle and groove are on the posterior surface.

Proximal epiphysis – we have not been able to distinguish a right from a left proximal radial epiphysis prior to fusion with the shaft.

Bones of a similar morphology

Perinatal diaphyses – of the diaphyses of the six major long bones, the radius, ulna and fibula are smaller and look less robust than the femur, humerus and tibia (Table 9.1). The radius always remains the shortest of all the long bones. Its tuberosity and flared distal end are characteristic.

Proximal radial fragment – this is distinctive (Fig. 9.13), with the constricted neck and circular metaphyseal surface tilted to the lateral side. The tuberosity is obvious just below this. The distal ulna and both ends of the fibula have surfaces of much the same size, but they are all at right angles to the shaft.

Distal radial fragment – this is similar to the distal ulnar, proximal fibular or distal fibular fragments. The radial metaphyseal surface is bigger than either the ulna or fibula and has an oval outline, which is usually angled posteriorly. The shaft is flared and has a curved anterior surface (Fig. 9.17).

Morphological summary (Fig. 9.16)

Fetal	
Wk 7	Primary ossification centre appears in shaft
Birth	Represented by shaft only
1–2 yrs	Secondary centre for distal epiphysis appears
Yr 5	Secondary centre for head appears
By yr 8	Styloid process forms on distal epiphysis
10–11 yrs	Proximal epiphysis shows foveal indentation
11.5–13 yrs	Proximal end fuses in females
14–17 yrs	Proximal end fuses in males
Puberty	Flake for tuberosity may form as separate centre
14–17 yrs	Distal end fuses in females
16–20 yrs	Distal end fuses in males

Metrics

Fazekas and Kósa (1978) measured the length of the radial diaphysis throughout fetal life (Table 9.7) and the length of the fetal radius as measured by ultrasound is taken from Jeanty (1983 – Table 9.8). Trotter and Peterson (1969) recorded the length and weight of the perinatal radial diaphysis (Table 9.9).

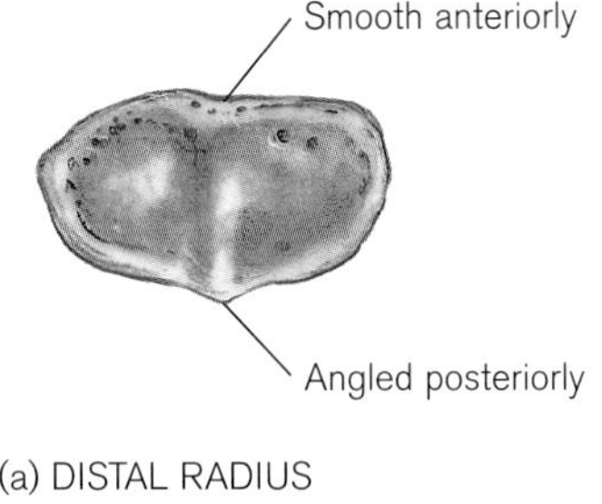

(a) DISTAL RADIUS

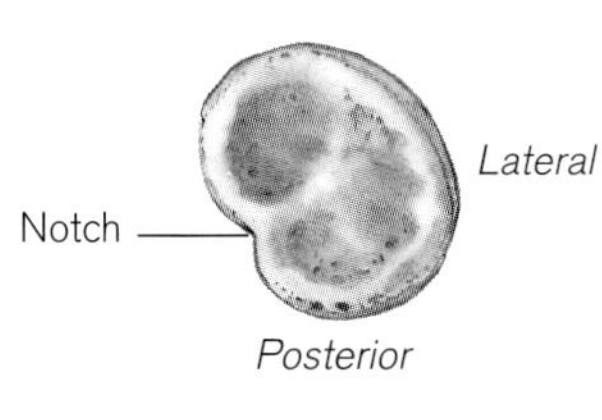

(b) DISTAL ULNA

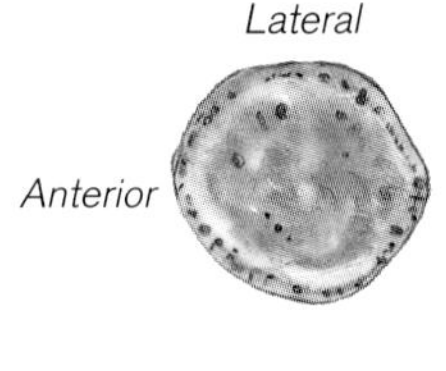

(c) PROXIMAL FIBULA

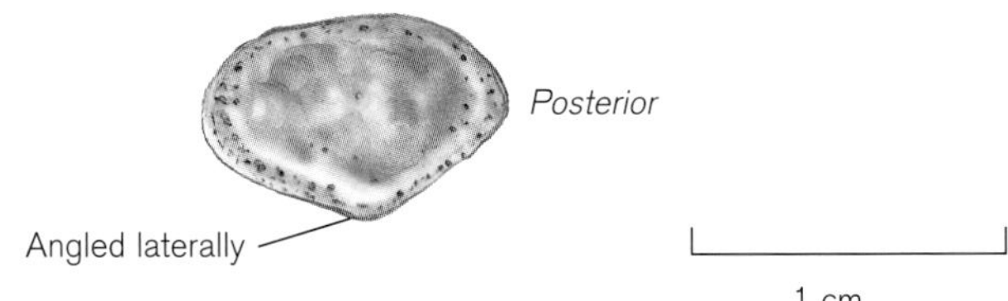

(d) DISTAL FIBULA

Figure 9.17 Metaphyseal surfaces of right perinatal radial, ulnar and fibular diaphyses.

Table 9.7 Length of the fetal radial diaphysis

Age (weeks)	Length (mm)
12	6.7
14	10.1
16	17.2
18	21.5
20	26.2
22	28.9
24	31.6
26	33.4
28	35.6
30	38.1
32	40.8
34	43.3
36	45.7
38	48.8
40	51.8

Length: maximum length.
Adapted from Fazekas and Kósa (1978).

Table 9.8 Length of the fetal radius as measured by ultrasound

	Length (mm) Percentile		
Age (weeks)	5th	50th	95th
12	–	7	–
14	8	13	12
16	9	18	21
18	14	22	26
20	21	27	28
22	24	31	34
24	27	34	38
26	30	37	41
28	33	40	45
30	34	43	49
32	37	45	51
34	39	47	53
36	41	48	54
38	45	49	53
40	46	50	54

Adapted from Jeanty (1983).

Scheuer *et al.* (1980) gave linear and logarithmic regression equations for age on radial diaphyseal length, as measured from radiographs from 24 fetal weeks to 6 weeks postnatal (Table 9.10). There are data from three postnatal longitudinal studies. Ghantus (1951), using the Brush Foundation material at Western Reserve, measured the diaphyseal lengths at 3-monthly intervals for the first year and 6-monthly intervals for the second year (Table 9.11). Gindhart (1973), using the Fels Research Institute series, gave the length of the radial diaphysis at 3-monthly intervals for the first year, 6-monthly intervals from 1–12 years and yearly intervals from 12–18 years (Table 9.12). Data for the length of the radius at 6-monthly intervals (2-monthly for the first half year) from birth to the cessation of growth are from the University of Colorado (Maresh, 1970). They have become the most commonly used modern population with which archaeological studies are compared and are particularly useful during the adolescent period. From ages 10–12 years double sets of figures give the lengths of the diaphysis with and without epiphyses, so that comparisons can be made depending on the state of fusion of the specimen (Table 9.13). Pritchett (1988), using the Colorado data from age 7 years, to maturity, charted growth and predictions of growth from the upper limb bones. The length of the radius is 13% of standing height in girls at age 7 years, increasing to 14% at maturity and the radius grows at about 0.9 cm per year during this period. The equivalent figures for boys are 14%, 15% and 1.0 cm.

Diaphyseal length data from some archaeological populations from Africa, Europe, and North America are given in Appendix 3. Most of the age at death estimates are based on dental development.

Table 9.9 Length and weight of the perinatal radius

	Length (mm)	Weight (g)
White male	53.4	0.81
White female	48.9	0.62
Black male	50.8	0.67
Black female	52.8	0.70
Mean	51.5	0.70

Adapted from Trotter and Peterson (1969).

Table 9.10 Regression equations of age on maximum radial length (mm)

Linear	Age (weeks) = (0.5850 × radius) + 7.7100 ± 2.29
Logarithmic	Age (weeks) = (25.695 $\log_e$ × radius) − 63.6541 ± 2.24

Adapted from Scheuer *et al.* (1980).

Table 9.11 Radial diaphyseal length (mm) – 3 months–2 years

	Male			Female		
Age (months)	*n*	Mean	Range	*n*	Mean	Range
3	100	65.90	58–73	100	62.85	54–70
6	100	73.10	66–81	100	69.73	60–78
9	100	80.01	73–90	100	76.18	66.5–84
12	100	85.72	75.5–95	100	81.73	71–91
18	100	94.84	84–107	100	91.70	82–103
24	100	102.37	95–115.5	100	99.44	88–112

Adapted from Ghantus (1951).

Table 9.12 Radial diaphyseal length (mm) – 1 month–18 years

	Male			Female		
Age	*n*	Mean	SD	*n*	Mean	SD
1 month	138	55.84	2.89	123	54.00	2.72
3 month	117	62.42	3.02	102	59.85	3.31
6 month	200	69.72	3.42	176	66.93	3.74
9 month	115	75.84	4.13	105	73.50	4.55
1.0 years	198	82.29	4.64	169	79.52	4.51
1.5 years	117	92.52	6.89	106	89.44	4.87
2.0 years	183	100.20	5.10	162	97.46	5.00
2.5 years	110	107.52	5.33	104	104.28	5.67
3.0 years	179	114.44	5.92	166	110.80	5.94
3.5 years	101	119.97	5.67	111	117.13	6.51
4.0 years	184	125.97	6.55	175	122.88	6.76
4.5 years	99	131.42	6.53	92	128.83	7.61
5.0 years	182	137.54	7.18	165	134.32	7.56
5.5 years	86	142.30	7.67	79	140.66	8.00
6.0 years	184	148.85	8.11	165	145.30	8.32
6.5 years	107	153.14	8.51	89	150.45	9.07
7.0 years	172	159.10	8.73	157	155.28	9.10
7.5 years	100	163.81	8.81	89	160.36	9.63
8.0 years	163	168.93	8.89	153	165.38	9.81
8.5 years	99	173.57	9.35	94	169.58	10.77
9.0 years	164	179.45	9.43	145	175.06	10.54
9.5 years	85	183.47	9.63	90	180.31	11.46
10.0 years	148	188.52	10.29	139	185.39	11.75
10.5 years	17	192.34	7.62	17	186.03	13.14
11.0 years	140	198.63	10.74	127	196.20	12.90
11.5 years	14	202.27	7.54	14	199.25	16.18
12.0 years	130	208.59	12.36	116	208.81	13.50
13.0 years	119	220.17	14.25	106	217.72	12.26
14.0 years	118	234.45	15.56	101	223.30	11.15
15.0 years	98	245.23	14.56	91	226.75	11.36
16.0 years	87	253.42	11.97	76	228.34	10.31
17.0 years	73	255.90	12.40	60	227.98	11.33
18.0 years	64	255.70	12.27	45	230.89	11.71

Adapted from Gindhart (1973).

III. THE ULNA

The adult ulna

The ulna forms the skeleton of the medial part of the forearm. It articulates proximally with the trochlea of the humerus at the elbow joint and laterally, both proximally and distally, with the radius at the superior and inferior radio-ulnar joints. It is a long bone, consisting of an expanded proximal end, a shaft and a head at the distal end.

The bulky proximal end (Fig. 9.18, 9.19a, b) consists of a pronounced, anteriorly facing **trochlear** (sigmoid/semilunar) **notch**, composed superiorly of the **olecranon** and inferiorly by the **coronoid process**. The upper part of the trochlear notch, formed from the anterior surface of the olecranon, and the lower part, formed from the upper surface of the coronoid process, are separated from each other by a constriction. In 75% of ulnae this has a non-articular strip of bone, the **fossa nudata**, filled by fibrous connective tissue and its development is discussed by Haines (1976). An indistinct vertical ridge also separates the notch into two parts, whose medial portion is wider than the lateral. The upper section of the lateral part is smaller than the lower, so that all these surfaces reciprocally fit the trochlea of the humerus during flexion and extension at the elbow.

The olecranon extends directly from the shaft and terminates in an anteriorly projecting beak, which occupies the olecranon fossa of the humerus when the elbow is in full extension. Behind this is a quadrangular surface area, which forms the point of the elbow and provides attachment for the triceps brachii muscle. The posterior surface is subcutaneous. If the olecranon is fractured and becomes displaced, extension of the elbow is compromised and it is necessary to re-attach the triceps muscle. The coronoid process projects anteriorly and bears a tubercle on its medial side, to which is attached part of the medial collateral ligament

Table 9.13 Radial length (mm) – 2 months–18 years

	Male			Female		
Age (years)	*n*	Mean	SD	*n*	Mean	SD
Diaphyseal length						
0.125	59	59.7	3.3	69	57.8	2.8
0.25	59	66.0	3.3	65	63.4	2.8
0.50	67	70.8	3.5	78	67.6	3.4
1.00	72	82.6	4.0	81	78.9	3.4
1.5	68	91.4	4.4	83	87.5	4.0
2.0	68	98.6	4.7	84	95.0	4.5
2.5	71	105.2	4.8	82	101.4	5.0
3.0	71	111.6	5.3	79	107.7	5.2
3.5	73	116.9	6.2	78	113.8	5.5
4.0	72	123.1	5.6	80	119.2	5.7
4.5	71	128.2	5.6	78	125.2	6.6
5.0	77	133.8	6.1	80	130.2	6.9
5.5	73	138.9	6.4	74	134.6	7.2
6.0	71	143.8	5.9	75	140.0	7.4
6.5	72	148.3	6.4	81	144.7	7.8
7.0	71	153.0	6.7	86	149.3	8.0
7.5	76	157.9	6.9	83	154.3	8.4
8.0	70	162.9	7.1	85	158.9	8.7
8.5	72	166.8	6.6	82	162.8	8.8
9.0	76	171.3	7.4	83	167.6	9.3
9.5	78	176.1	7.7	83	172.2	10.2
10.0	77	180.5	7.9	84	176.8	10.4
10.5	76	184.4	8.4	75	181.8	11.8
11.0	75	188.7	8.5	76	186.0	11.7
11.5	76	193.0	9.2	75	192.0	12.1
12.0	74	197.4	9.6	71	196.9	12.7
Total length including epiphyses						
10.0	76	193.0	8.1	83	189.3	11.4
10.5	76	197.7	8.9	75	195.0	13.0
11.0	75	202.6	8.9	76	200.0	13.0
11.5	77	207.3	9.7	75	206.7	13.5
12.0	77	212.3	10.3	75	213.5	14.2
12.5	71	218.0	10.2	67	218.8	14.2
13.0	73	223.7	11.8	70	223.6	13.1
13.5	73	230.2	12.9	63	227.8	12.7
14.0	75	236.9	13.5	64	231.4	11.8
14.5	69	242.8	14.1	42	233.5	11.7
15.0	61	248.7	13.4	57	234.5	11.7
15.5	52	255.0	12.8	12	237.4	15.2
16.0	61	257.7	11.7	40	235.0	11.8
16.5	38	259.8	11.3	3	–	–
17.0	50	261.8	11.2	18	233.8	11.8
18.0	28	263.2	12.8	4	–	–

Adapted from Maresh (1970).

of the elbow joint. Just distal to this are the ulnar heads of the flexor digitorum superficialis and pronator teres muscles and an occasional head of flexor pollicis longus. The lower part of the coronoid process, the **tuberosity of the ulna**, is a roughened triangular area for the brachialis muscle. Just below the lateral side of the trochlear notch is the oval **radial notch**, for articulation with the circumference of the head of the radius. Inferior to the notch the bone is hollowed out, which allows space for the tuberosity of the radius during the movements of pronation and supination. The posterior border of this area forms a sharp, raised ridge, the **supinator crest** and from here, and the hollow anterior to it, is attached the supinator muscle.

The upper three-quarters of the **shaft** is triangular in cross-section and the lower quarter is rounded (Fig. 9.18c). Three borders and three surfaces may be distinguished throughout most of the shaft. The **interosseous** (lateral) **border** begins proximally at the junction of two lines that extend from the supinator crest and the anterolateral margin of the coronoid process. It continues in its middle two-quarters as the sharp attachment for the interosseous membrane connecting it to the radius, but distally it becomes indistinct.

The rounded **anterior border** begins proximally, medial to the ulnar tuberosity and curves medially to end at the base of the styloid process. The subcutaneous **posterior border** is also rounded and runs from the apex of the olecranon, curving sinuously, to reach the styloid process. An aponeurosis for the flexor and extensor carpi ulnaris muscles is attached to it. The grooved **anterior surface** lies between the interosseous and anterior borders, is covered by the flexor digitorum profundus muscle in its proximal three-quarters and has the pronator quadratus muscle attached to it distally. The main nutrient foramen is always found on the proximal two-thirds of the shaft. Between 73% and 80% are on the anterior surface and the rest are on the anterior or interosseous borders (Shulman, 1959; Mysorekar, 1967). The entrance of the foramen slopes proximally. The **medial surface** lies between the anterior and posterior surfaces, is rounded and smooth and gives attachment to the flexor digitorum profundus muscle proximally; distally, there is a roughened area for the pronator quadratus muscle. The **posterior surface** has the anconeus muscle attached in the proximal third as far down as a posterior oblique line and below this a vertical line divides it into a wider medial and a narrow lateral strip. The former is covered by extensor carpi ulnaris and the latter provides attachment from proximal to distal for the abductor pollicis longus, extensor pollicis longus and extensor indicis muscles.

The **distal end** (Fig. 9.19c) is composed of a rounded **head** separated by a roughened area from a prominent, posteromedially directed **styloid process**. There is a groove on the lateral side of the styloid

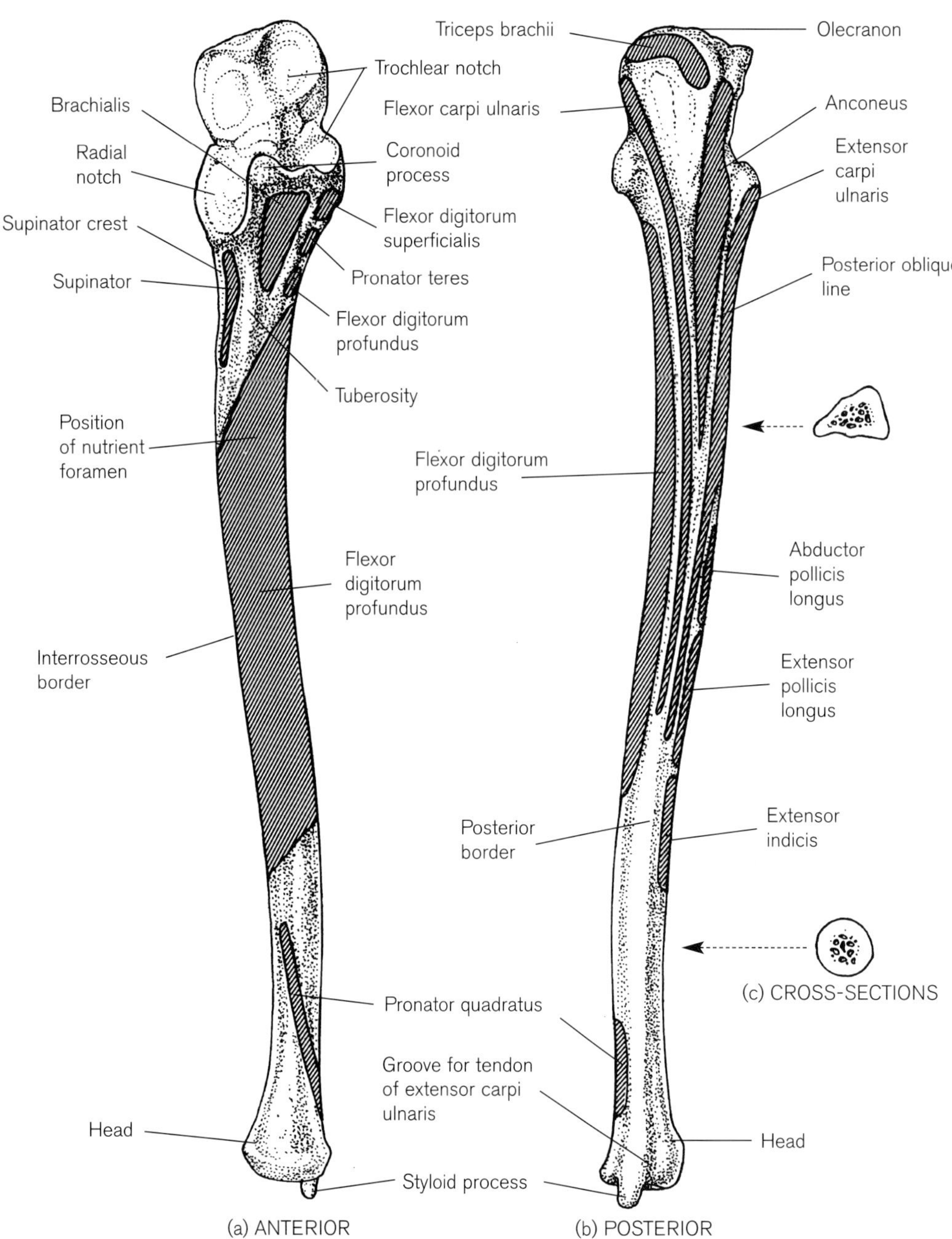

Figure 9.18 Right adult ulna.

process, which accommodates the tendon of extensor carpi ulnaris. The head bears a convex **articular surface** on its lateral side, which articulates with the ulnar notch of the radius at the inferior radio-ulnar joint. An intra-articular disc attached to the roughened area separates the smooth surface of the head from the lunate and triquetral bones of the carpus. The ulna is therefore not part of the wrist joint and, in contrast to the radius, is sometimes spared damage, when there is a fall on the outstretched hand. The Monteggia injury (Bruce *et al.*, 1963) involves a fracture of the shaft of the ulna, accompanied by anterior dislocation of the head of the radius.

As with the humerus and radius, the ulna may be congenitally absent (see above). An unusual case, observed in a prehistoric archaeological specimen, has been reported by Mann *et al.* (1998).

Occasional skeletal anomalies in the elbow region include accessory bones in a variety of positions. Anteriorly, small nodules of bone can be associated with either the coronoid process or lie in a paratrochlear position. They have been named ‘os cubiti anterior’

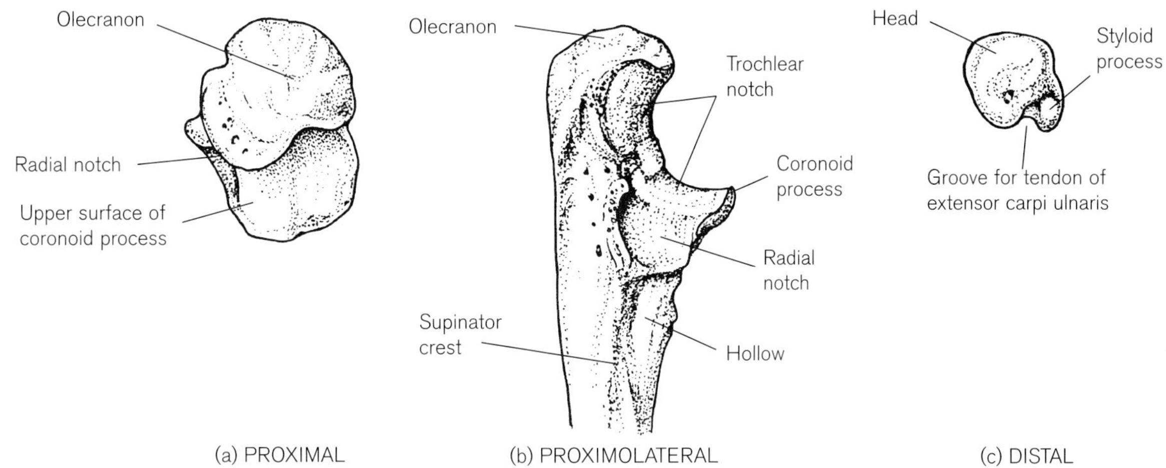

Figure 9.19 Right adult ulna.

(Simril and Trotter, 1949) or 'fabella cubiti' (Schwarz, 1957). Posteriorly placed nodules of bone, termed 'patella cubiti', have been described by Gunn (1928), Levine (1950) and Kohler *et al.* (1968) and could be regarded as sesamoid bones in the tendon of the triceps brachii muscle. Zeitlin (1935) argued that they are the result of traumatic early separation of epiphyseal ossification centres in childhood. Other authorities (Kohler *et al.*, 1968) regard them as true accessory bones, to be distinguished from persistent, non-united epiphyses (see below).

Sexual dimorphism of the ulna was investigated by Godycki (1957), using the dividing groove of the trochlear notch, and by Singh *et al.* (1974b) and Holman and Bennett (1991), using measurements that reflected the robusticity of the bone. Estimation of stature from the ulna can be attempted using tables from Telkkä (1950), Trotter and Gleser (1952, 1958, 1977), Allbrook (1961), Genovés (1967) and from data in Krogman and Işcan (1986). The ulna should only be used in the absence of other long bones, as it has the largest standard error of estimate. Rao *et al.* (1989) give data for northern Indian populations to calculate the length of the ulna from fragments and so estimate living stature.

Early development of the ulna

The mesenchymal ulna is identifiable at stage 16 (about 37 days of intra-uterine life) and the cartilage anlage starts to form at stages 17–18 (between 41 and 44 days; O'Rahilly and Gardner, 1975). Chondrification in the olecranon is usually obvious at 48 days and in the styloid process by 51 days. By stage 21 there is evidence of early bone collar formation in the shaft (Gray and Gardner, 1951; O'Rahilly and Gardner, 1975).

Ossification

Primary centre

Ossification in the centre of the diaphysis is first seen during week 7 (O'Rahilly and Gardner, 1972). By 3 lunar months, it has reached the level of the radial tuberosity proximally and by 5 months has extended almost to the coronoid process and radial notch. There is a single nutrient foramen that is located on the proximal half of the shaft in over 90% of fetuses (Skawina and Wyczólkowski, 1987). The morphology of the ulna is sufficiently distinct to permit identification from early fetal life. At term, ossification extends over half the distance between the coronoid and superior limit of the olecranon process (Gray and Gardner, 1951).

The perinatal ulna (Fig. 9.20) looks relatively more robust than in childhood or the adult. The shallow trochlear notch with a truncated olecranon is recognizable at the bulky proximal end and the radial notch is obvious on the lateral side. The shaft is flattened mediolaterally in its proximal half and becomes more triangular distally. In the middle two-quarters of the bone, the posterior border is prominent and the interosseous border forms a sharp edge, but the anterior border is not very obvious. The nutrient foramen, whose entrance slopes proximally, is usually on the anterior surface at the junction of the proximal and middle thirds of the bone. At the distal end, the shaft flares slightly towards the oval metaphyseal surface. A faint notch on its posteromedial surface marks the position where the tendon of extensor carpi ulnaris runs towards the styloid process. The supinator crest may be visible on the perinatal bone or become obvious during the first year of life.

During early childhood, the ulna takes on a more elongated sigmoid curvature and becomes more

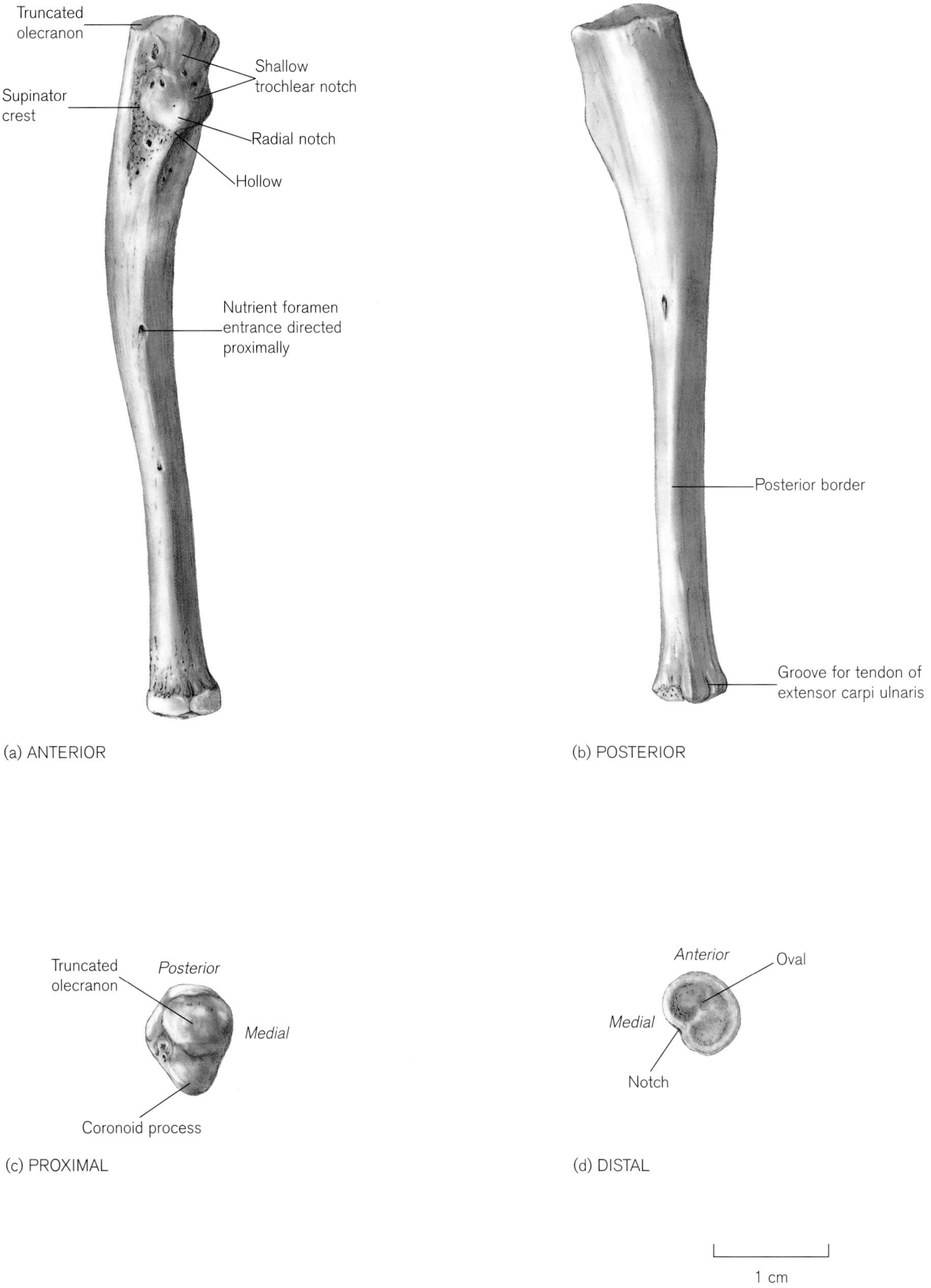

Truncated olecranon
Shallow trochlear notch
Supinator crest
Radial notch
Hollow
Nutrient foramen entrance directed proximally
(a) ANTERIOR
Posterior border
Groove for tendon of extensor carpi ulnaris
(b) POSTERIOR
Truncated olecranon
Posterior
Medial
Coronoid process
(c) PROXIMAL
Anterior
Oval
Medial
Notch
(d) DISTAL
1 cm

Figure 9.20 Right perinatal ulna.

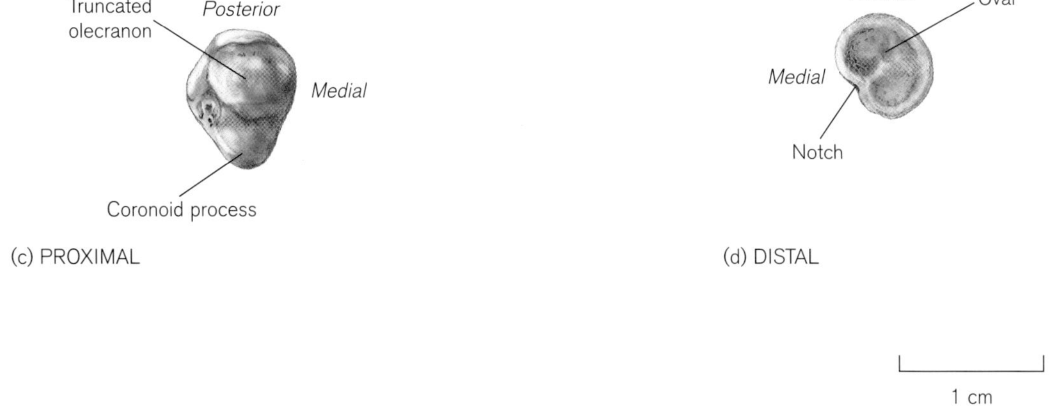

gracile with increasing age. As a result, the slenderness of the lower half of the shaft makes the ulna one of the least likely long bones to survive inhumation without damage.

The trochlear notch appears very wide until about 8 or 9 years of age, as its margins are much less well developed during childhood. Superiorly, it appears truncated over the olecranon as the epiphysis is unossified and inferiorly the coronoid process is not very prominent. The tuberosity is represented by a ridge and hollow and, as a result, the characteristics of the tuberosity in young children are less clearly defined than in the adult (Evans, 1951).

Secondary centres

The **distal epiphysis** of the ulna appears between 5 and 7 years, which is considerably later than that of the distal radius (1–2 years). Age ranges for appearance are given by Davies and Parsons (1927), Flecker (1932b), Hasselwander (1938), Elgenmark (1946), Hansman (1962) and Garn *et al.* (1967b). Detailed radiographic standards for girls and boys can be found in the Greulich and Pyle (1959) atlas and a more recent radiological developmental study has been described by Ogden *et al.* (1981). Appearance is normally 1 year to 18 months earlier in girls than in boys.

The ossification centre appears radiologically as an oval bony nodule with smooth margins. The metaphyseal surface soon begins to accommodate itself to the shaft of the bone and becomes flattened and circular in outline with the medial side being thicker than the lateral side (Fig. 9.21a). About 3 years after its first appearance (8–10 years), ossification spreads into the styloid process and the metaphyseal surfaces of the diaphysis and epiphysis show reciprocal undulations as the growth plate narrows. Occasionally, there is a separate centre for the styloid process (Davies and Parsons, 1927), which may remain separate throughout life (Keats, 1992). Defects (epiphyseal clefts) have been reported in the distal ulna (Harrison and Keats, 1980). They appear just before puberty but disappear during

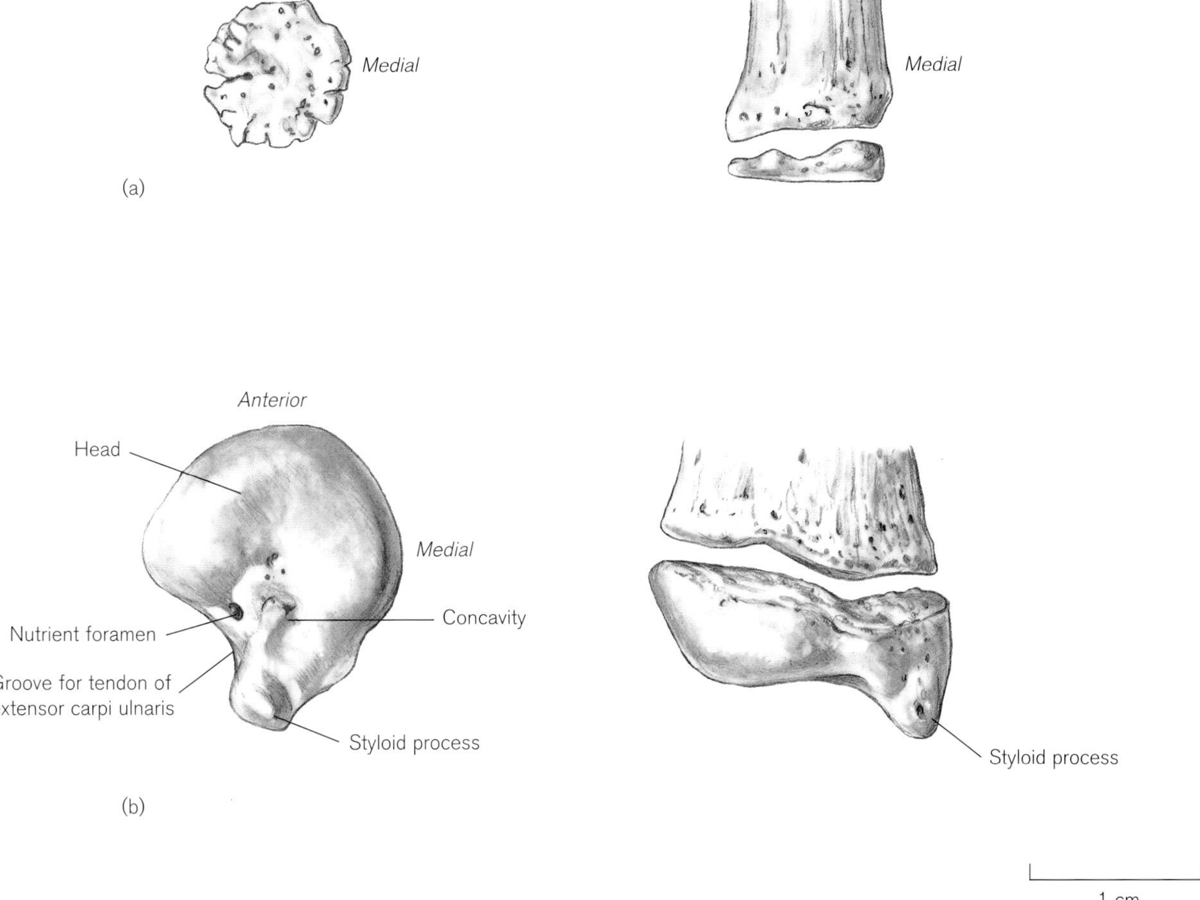

Figure 9.21 Development of the right distal ulnar epiphysis. (a) Early stage – 7 years; (b) later stage – adolescent.

fusion and are viewed as normal variants. By puberty, the epiphysis takes on the appearance of the adult bone (Fig. 9.21b). The articular head is well formed and separated from the styloid process by a shallow concavity pitted with nutrient foramina. The posterolateral end of the concavity bears a groove for the tendon of extensor carpi ulnaris and often has a large nutrient foramen. The articular edge of the epiphysis is now deeper on the anterolateral side.

Fusion of the distal ulnar epiphysis precedes that of the distal radius, beginning in the centre of the epiphyseal plate at 14–15 years in females and 17–20 years in males. This is the growing end of the bone, responsible for 75–85% of growth in length of the shaft (Ozonoff, 1979; Ogden, 1984d; Pritchett, 1991). Ranges of fusion times are given by Paterson (1929), Flecker (1932b) and Hansman (1962). The Greulich and Pyle (1959) radiographic standards show complete fusion, with epiphyseal line obliteration soon afterwards, at 16–17 years in females and 17–18 years in males. Thus, the distal ulnar epiphysis has a shorter independent life than its fellow radial epiphysis, appearing about 4 years later and fusing a year earlier. As with the distal radial epiphysis, McKern and Stewart's (1957) observations on male skeletal material show complete union to be later than that described in radiological accounts. They give 23 years for 100% fusion of their specimens, the last traces of peripheral fusion being proximal to the styloid process.

The **proximal epiphysis** of the ulna also appears several years after that for the proximal radius and is usually present by 8 years in females and 10 years in males. The coronoid process and most of the olecranon are formed by extension of ossification from the primary centre in the diaphysis. The olecranon epiphysis forms the superior lip of the articular surface of the trochlear notch and most of the area of bone to which the triceps muscle is attached. Ranges for ages of appearance can be found in Davies and Parsons (1927), Paterson (1929), Flecker (1932b), Hansman (1962) and Garn *et al.* (1967b). A detailed radiological description can be found in Cohn (1921b) and Brodeur *et al.* (1981). The account by McCarthy and Ogden (1982b) is based on specialized radiographic techniques and includes possible injury patterns.

The early epiphysis is often composed of a complex collection of ossific nodules and early accounts usually recognize at least two (Fawcett, 1904; Davies and Parsons, 1927; Paterson, 1929). Fawcett described an anterior, or 'beak' centre, which formed part of the articular surface of the trochlear notch, and a second centre which formed the apex of the olecranon process. This description equates with the 'articular' and 'traction' epiphyses of Porteous' (1960) account. Birkner (1978) illustrated the various forms that the olecranon may take in 8–10 year-old children and Brodeur *et al.* (1981) note that the epiphysis is often composed of two, three or more centres, with the upper nucleus, adjacent to the tip, being smaller than the lower. They state that the olecranon has the most predictable age of appearance and final fusion of all the elbow epiphyses and its development is therefore a relatively reliable indicator of age.

The pattern of **fusion** at the proximal extremity is very variable. Small bony foci may join together before fusing with the shaft, or the smaller proximal articular epiphysis may fuse first, leaving the larger traction part to fuse later. A whole epiphysis (Fig. 9.22a) is a rough, flattened oval piece of bone with a beak pointing to the lateral side. Most of the underside is formed by the irregular metaphyseal surface, but has adjoining it a smooth semilunar part that is the superior rim of the articular surface of the trochlear notch. The upper surface has a rounded, 'bun-like' appearance posteriorly, marking the site of attachment of the tendon of triceps brachii. Fusion starts first on the articular surface at the lateral side and then proceeds posteriorly and medially. The postero-inferior surface is always the last part to remain open (Fig. 9.22b). Silberstein *et al.* (1981b) called the line of fusion the 'wandering physeal line of the olecranon', from its appearance on a lateral radiograph. The epiphyseal plate is first seen proximal to the elbow joint and as the epiphysis increases in size, so the line migrates distally, frequently ending up at the level of the middle of the joint, leaving a wedge-shaped line open inferiorly. Their elbow atlas shows the epiphyseal plate to be half closed by 13 years in females and 14 years in males. It can be complete by 12–14 years in females and 13–16 years in males. Again, McKern and Stewart (1957) find that 100% fusion is later in their skeletal material than is stated in the radiological accounts. Their observations show that the olecranon epiphysis fuses at 19 years in males and is the latest in the range of their Group I early union.

There are reports in the literature of persistent, unfused olecranon epiphyses in the adult (O'Donoghue and Sell, 1942; Retrum *et al.*, 1986; Skak, 1993). They are usually asymptomatic unless injured after trauma to the elbow, when they can be diagnosed from a lateral radiograph. Kohler *et al.* (1968) distinguish this appearance from 'patella cubiti' (see adult).

The appearance and fusion times of the ulnar ossification centres are summarized in Fig. 9.23.

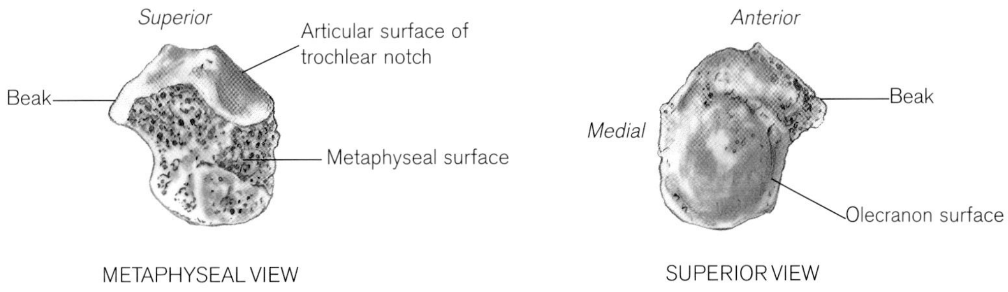

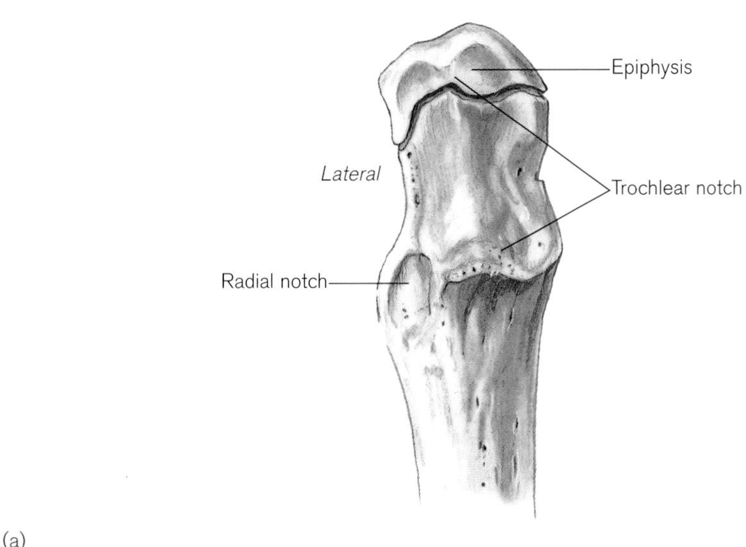

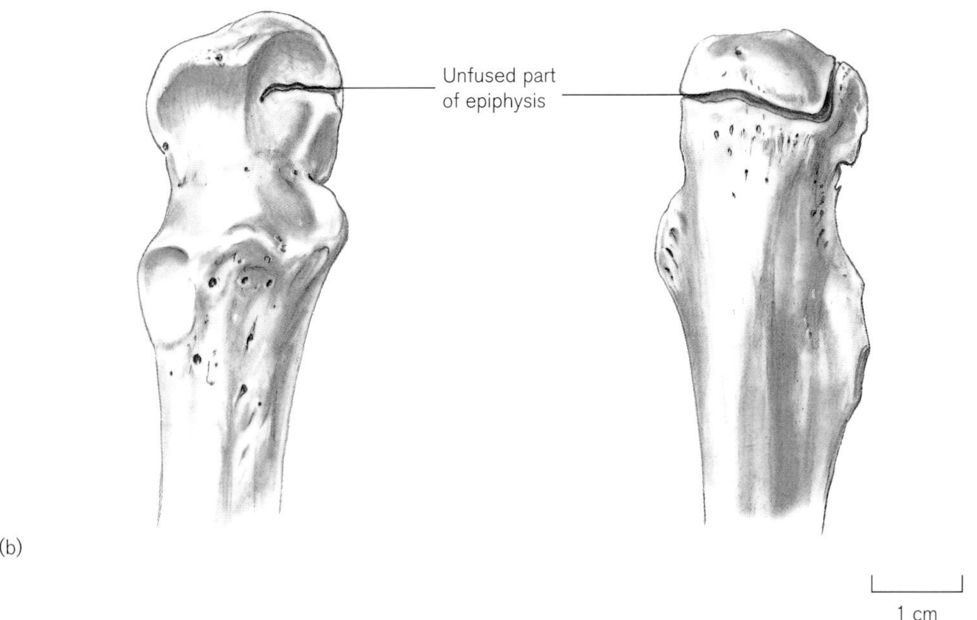

Figure 9.22 Development of the right proximal ulnar epiphysis. (a) Early adolescent; (b) late adolescent.

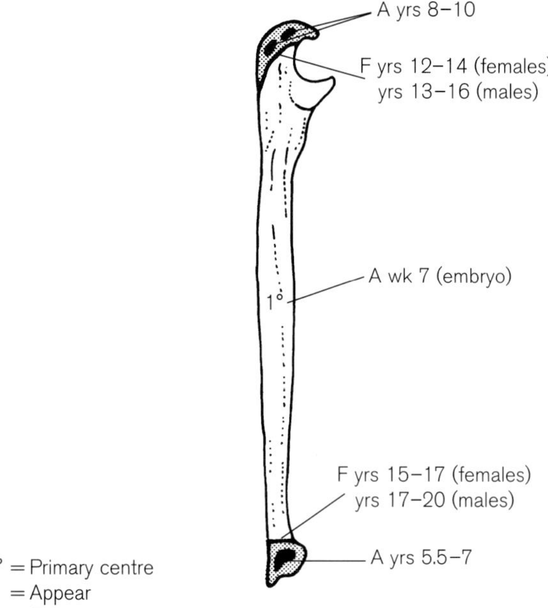

Figure 9.23 Appearance and fusion times of the ulnar ossification centres.

Practical notes

Sideing

Diaphysis – the perinatal or infant ulna can be sided using the following features. Proximally, the trochlear notch bears the articulation for the radius on its lateral side. In the shaft, the sharp interosseous border is lateral and the nutrient foramen is usually in the centre of the anterior upper half with its entrance directed proximally. Distally, the medial surface is slightly concave and the metaphyseal surface is oval with a notch on the lateral side for the tendon of extensor carpi ulnaris (Fig. 9.20).

Distal epiphysis – it is difficult to side a distal epiphysis until the styloid process has developed. Looking at the articular surface, the right epiphysis is comma-shaped, with the rounded head towards the top and the groove for the tendon on the left (Fig. 9.21b).

Proximal epiphysis – looking at the metaphyseal proximal epiphysis with the trochlear articular surface superiorly, the beak points to the opposite side from which the bone comes (Fig. 9.22a).

Bones of a similar morphology

Perinatal diaphyses – of the diaphyses of the six major long bones, the radius, ulna and fibula are smaller and look less robust than the femur, humerus and tibia. Up to the age of about 2 months the ulna and fibula are of similar length but the radius is considerably shorter (See Table 9.1). The ulna is distinguishable from the fibula as it is more robust and has the characteristic trochlear notch at the proximal end, whereas the fibula is a slim bone of even width throughout its length (Figs. 9.20 and 11.25). After the neonatal period, the fibula is considerably longer than the ulna, as the lower limb increases in length more rapidly than the upper limb.

Proximal fragment – this is distinctive as it bears both trochlear and radial notches (Fig. 9.20a and c).

Distal fragment – is similar to a proximal fibula, distal fibula or possibly a distal radius. The proximal fibula has a slight neck and the metaphyseal surface is circular, whereas the distal ulna is more oval and may show a notch posteromedially. The distal fibula is flattened mediolaterally and is considerably more gracile than the ulna. The shaft of the radius flares and curves anteriorly towards its end and the metaphyseal surface is angled and larger than that of the ulna (Fig. 9.17).

Morphological summary (Fig. 9.23)

Fetal	
Wk 7	Primary ossification centre appears
Birth	Represented by shaft only
5–7 yrs	Secondary centre for distal end appears
About 8–10 yrs	Styloid process forms on distal epiphysis
	Secondary centre(s) for olecranon appear(s)
12–14 yrs	Proximal epiphysis fuses in females
13–16 yrs	Proximal epiphysis fuses in males
15–17 yrs	Distal epiphysis fuses in females
17–20 yrs	Distal epiphysis fuses in males

Metrics

Lengths of fetal bones were recorded by Fazekas and Kósa (1978) throughout fetal life (Table 9.14) and the length of the fetal ulna as measured on ultrasound is taken from Jeanty (1983–Table 9.15).

From radiographs, Scheuer *et al.* (1980) gave linear and logarithmic regression equations for age on ulnar diaphyseal length from 24 fetal weeks to 6 weeks postnatal (Table 9.16). Ghantus (1951), using the Brush Foundation longitudinal growth study at Western Reserve, Cleveland, measured the diaphyseal lengths at 3-monthly intervals for the first year, and 6-monthly intervals for the second year (Table 9.17). Data showing the length of the ulna at 6-monthly intervals (and 2-monthly for the first half-year) from birth to the cessation of growth (Table 9.18) are taken from Maresh (1970). These data, from the University of Colorado longitudinal growth study, have become the most commonly used modern population with which archaeological studies are compared. They are particularly useful during the adolescent period as from

Table 9.14 Length of the fetal ulnar diaphysis

Age (weeks)	Length (mm)
12	7.2
14	11.2
16	19.0
18	23.9
20	29.4
22	31.6
24	35.1
26	37.1
28	40.2
30	42.8
32	46.7
34	49.1
36	51.0
38	55.9
40	59.3

Length: maximum length.
Adapted from Fazekas and Kósa (1978).

Table 9.15 Length of the fetal ulna as measured by ultrasound

	Length (mm) Percentile		
Age (weeks)	5th	50th	95th
12	–	8	–
14	4	13	17
16	8	19	24
18	13	24	30
20	21	29	32
22	24	33	37
24	29	37	41
26	34	41	44
28	37	44	48
30	38	47	54
32	40	50	58
34	44	53	59
36	47	55	61
38	48	57	63
40	50	58	65

Adapted from Jeanty (1983).

Table 9.16 Regression equations of age on maximum ulnar length (mm)

Linear	Age (weeks) $= (0.5072 \times \text{ulna}) + 7.8208 \pm 2.20$
Logarithmic	Age (weeks) $= (26.078 \log_e \times \text{ulna}) - 68.7222 \pm 2.10$

Adapted from Scheuer *et al.* (1980).

Table 9.17 Ulnar diaphyseal length (mm) – 3 months–2 years

	Male			Female		
Age	*n*	Mean	Range	*n*	Mean	Range
Mths						
3	100	73.55	65–82.5	100	70.58	61–80
6	100	81.03	73–90.5	100	77.67	69–87
9	100	88.20	80–98	100	84.70	75–93
12	100	94.84	85–104.5	100	90.73	80–102
18	100	104.99	93–115	100	101.62	90–115
24	100	112.64	102–125	100	109.79	79–124

Adapted from Ghantus (1951).

the ages 10–12 years double sets of figures give the lengths of the diaphysis with and without the epiphyses. Comparisons can therefore be made depending on the state of fusion of the specimen.

Table 9.18 Ulnar length (mm) – 2 months–18 years

	Male			Female		
Age (years)	*n*	Mean	SD	*n*	Mean	SD
Diaphyseal length						
0.125	59	67.0	3.5	69	65.3	3.1
0.25	59	73.8	3.4	65	71.2	3.1
0.50	67	79.1	3.7	78	75.7	3.8
1.00	71	92.6	4.4	81	89.0	4.0
1.5	68	102.3	4.6	83	98.9	4.4
2.0	68	109.7	4.9	84	107.1	4.8
2.5	71	116.6	5.2	82	113.8	5.2
3.0	71	123.4	5.6	79	120.6	5.4
3.5	73	129.1	6.4	78	127.2	5.7
4.0	72	135.6	5.6	80	133.1	5.8
4.5	71	141.0	5.6	78	139.3	6.6
5.0	77	147.0	6.1	80	144.6	7.1
5.5	73	152.6	6.7	74	149.1	7.2
6.0	71	157.5	6.2	75	154.9	7.4
6.5	72	162.2	6.8	81	159.9	7.9
7.0	71	167.3	7.0	86	164.8	8.3
7.5	76	172.2	7.4	83	170.1	8.5
8.0	70	177.3	7.4	85	174.9	8.7
8.5	72	181.6	7.1	82	179.1	8.8
9.0	76	186.4	7.9	83	184.3	9.5
9.5	78	191.7	8.3	83	189.7	10.4
10.0	77	196.2	8.5	84	194.4	10.6
10.5	76	200.4	8.8	75	200.0	12.4
11.0	75	205.1	9.2	76	204.7	12.0
11.5	76	209.8	9.9	75	211.3	13.1
12.0	74	214.5	10.2	70	216.4	13.3
Total length including epiphyses						
10.0	76	202.2	9.0	83	203.8	12.3
10.5	76	208.0	9.7	75	210.2	13.8
11.0	75	213.3	10.2	76	215.5	13.3
11.5	77	219.5	11.3	75	222.6	13.8
12.0	77	224.9	11.7	75	229.7	14.7
12.5	71	231.5	11.8	67	235.4	14.4
13.0	73	237.9	13.2	70	240.0	13.3
13.5	73	245.1	13.9	63	244.4	13.1
14.0	75	252.3	14.6	65	248.1	12.1
14.5	69	259.0	14.7	42	250.2	11.8
15.0	61	265.1	14.0	57	251.0	12.2
15.5	52	271.9	13.1	12	255.0	15.1
16.0	61	274.8	12.2	40	252.3	12.0
16.5	38	277.3	12.1	3	–	–
17.0	50	279.4	11.7	17	250.2	12.3
18.0	28	281.6	13.5	4	–	–

Adapted from Maresh (1970).

Diaphyseal length data from some archaeological populations from Africa, Europe and North America are given in Appendix 3. Most of the age at death estimates are based on dental development.

IV. THE HAND

Given not only the functional, but also the evolutionary and the clinical importance of the hand, it is not surprising that there is almost an unsurpassed volume of literature relating to this region of the skeleton. Much of the information lies outwith the scope of this book and readers are directed to more specialized and specific texts. Understandably, the functional anatomy of the hand assumes considerable importance in the literature (Wood Jones, 1941; Phillips, 1986; Jenkins, 1990; Meals and Seeger, 1991), particularly in the light of both comparative and evolutionary research (Martin and Saller, 1959; Tuttle, 1967; Marzke, 1971; Lewis, 1974, 1977; Susman, 1979; Wake, 1979; Napier, 1980; Aiello and Dean, 1990), but it is perhaps in the clinical fields of injury, repair and rehabilitation that the literature is most actively updated (Kaplan, 1965; Rank *et al.*, 1973; Conolly and Kilgore, 1975; Pulvertaft, 1977; Sandzen, 1980; Birch and Brooks, 1984; Burke, 1989; Lister, 1993). In the post-1957 thalidomide years, congenital deformities of the upper extremity were studied extensively (Lenz and Knapp, 1962; Kajii *et al.*, 1973; Kelikian, 1974; Blauth and Schneider-Sickert, 1981; Lenz, 1988). Further, the importance of the hand in relation to manual dominance is not only well recognized in the anthropological, but also in the psychological literature (Wilson, 1891; Revesz, 1958; Hicks and Kinsbourne, 1976; Coren and Porac, 1977; Plato *et al.*, 1980; Plato and Norris, 1981; Annett, 1985). However, in the anthropological literature, it is probably the area of maturation of the hand that has assumed the greatest importance. Therefore, readers are directed to the literature written by some of the principal contributors in this field for the discussion of factors such as communality indices, genetic linkage, environmental influences, bilateral symmetry and population variation (Acheson, 1954; Baer and Durkatz, 1957; Koski *et al.*, 1961; Garn and Rohmann, 1962a; Roche, 1962; Garn *et al.*, 1963; Massé and Hunt, 1963; Roche, 1970; Andersen, 1971; Falkner, 1971; Haas *et al.*, 1971; Blanco *et al.*, 1972; Himes and Malina, 1977; Takai, 1977).

The adult hand

The adult hand articulates at the wrist (radiocarpal) joint with the radius and comprises at least 27 bones – eight carpals, five metacarpals and 14 phalanges (Figs. 9.24 and 9.25).

Carpals

These small, irregularly shaped bones are arranged in two transverse rows with four bones in each and they form a broad base for the firm support of the hand. Two bones of the proximal row (scaphoid and lunate) articulate with the radius to form the radiocarpal (wrist) joint, there being no direct articulation with the ulna. The distal row articulates with the metacarpals that form the substance of the palm of the hand. The proximal and distal rows articulate with each other at the transverse midcarpal joints. The carpal bones are wedged together and tightly bound by interosseous ligaments to form a deeply concave palmar arch and a more gently convex morphology to the dorsum of the hand. This palmar/dorsal-shaped incongruity is partly brought about by the considerably smaller palmar surface area of each carpal compared to its relatively larger dorsal surface area. The shape and position of the scaphoid and trapezium bones in particular, further deepen the lateral (radial) side of the palmar concavity as they are turned forwards and as a result carry the thumb in front of the plane of the rest of the digits. The medial (ulnar) side is deepened by the presence of the hook of the hamate and the elevated position of the pisiform bone.

The pillars of the palmar carpal arch are bound together by the **flexor retinaculum** (a thickening of the deep fascia), which attaches to the aforementioned prominent medial and lateral bony projections. Specifically, these are the tubercles of the scaphoid

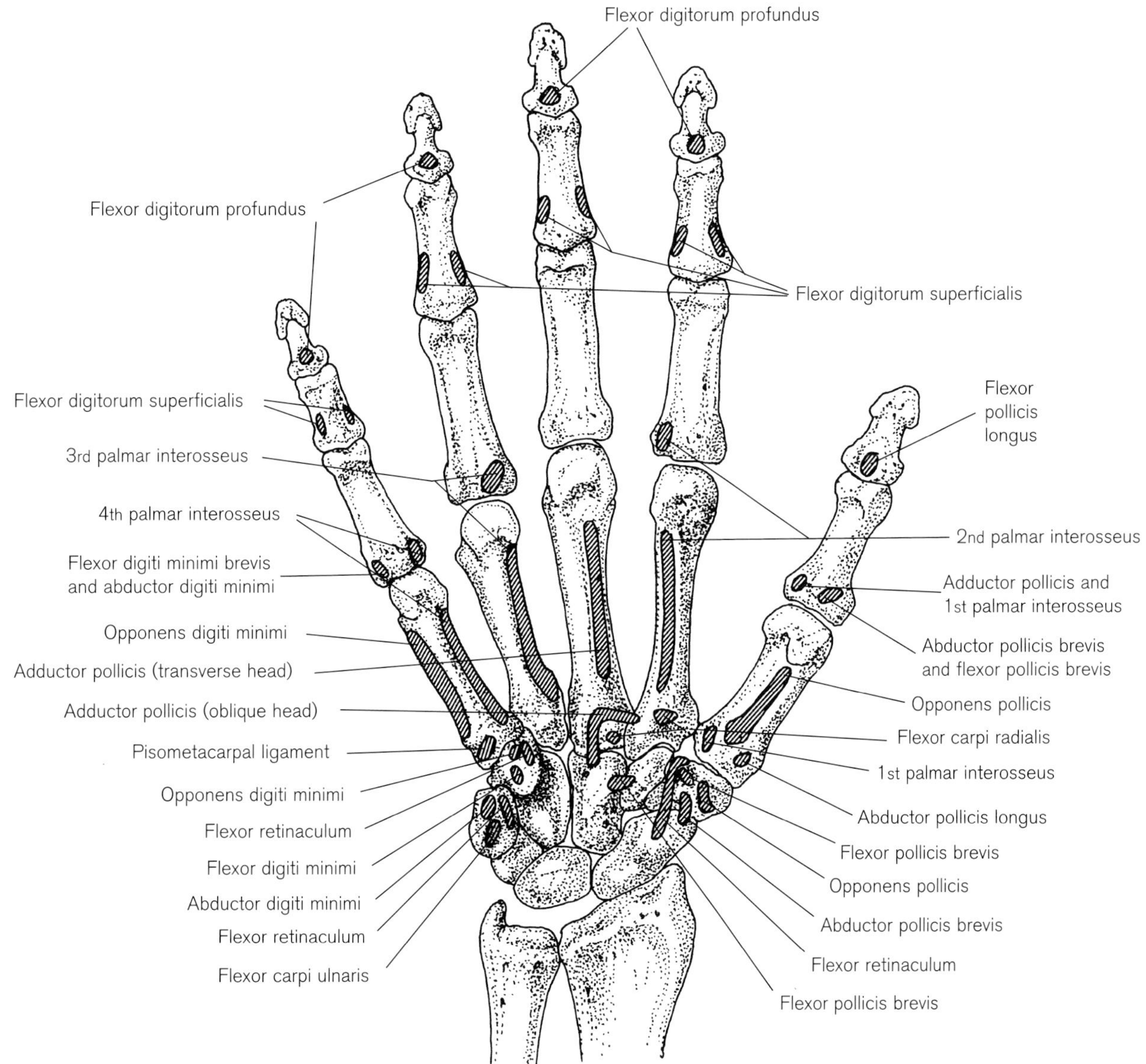

Figure 9.24 The palmar surface of the right adult hand showing sites of muscle attachment.

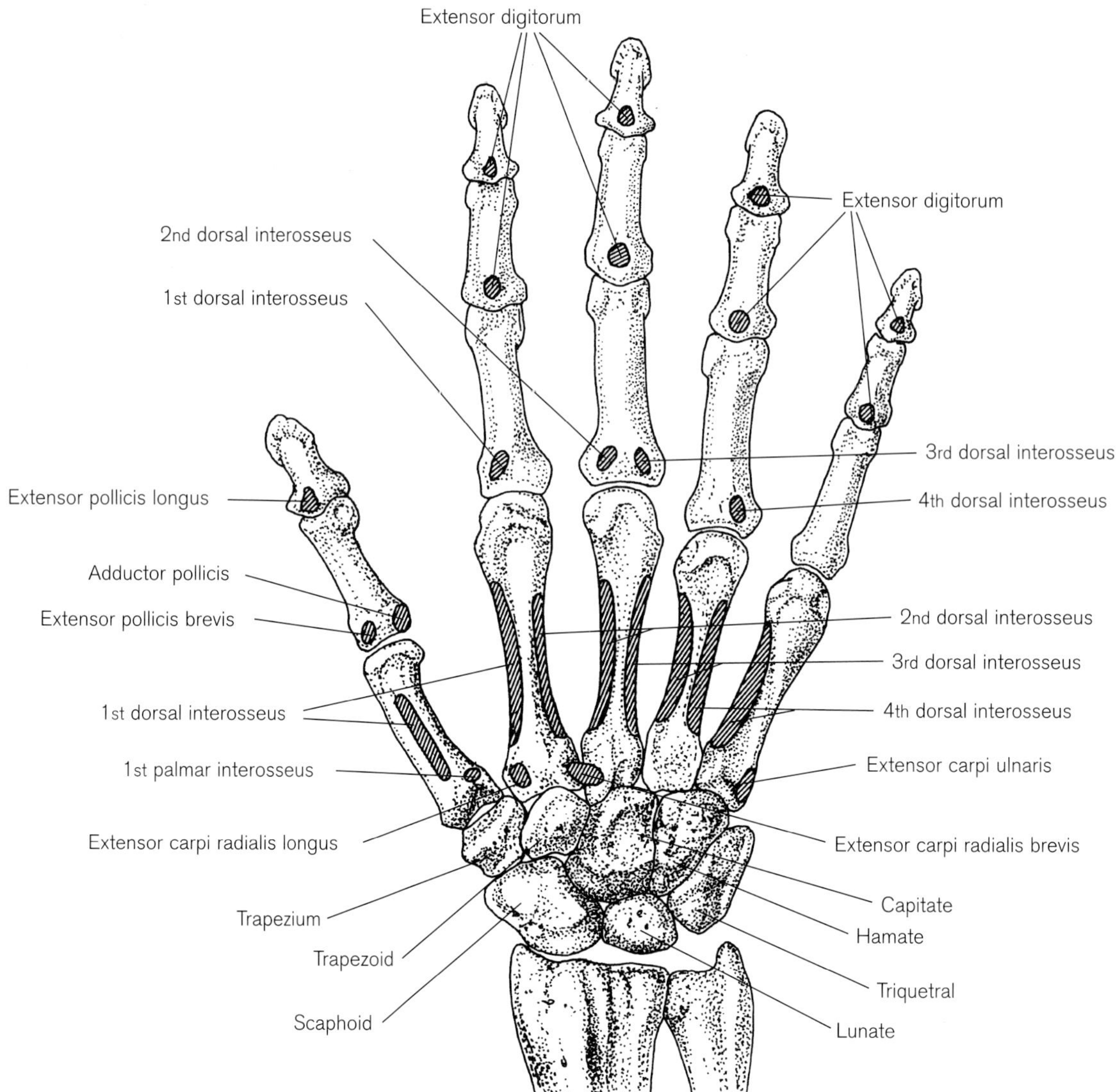

Figure 9.25 The dorsal surface of the right adult hand showing sites of muscle attachment.

and trapezium laterally and the pisiform, hook of the hamate and pisohamate ligament medially. The areas of the scaphoid and trapezium that lie lateral to the flexor retinaculum, and the area of the hamate that lies medial to it, are occupied by the sites of attachment of the muscles of the thenar and hypothenar eminences, respectively (Frazer, 1908; Eyler and Markee, 1954). The flexor retinaculum acts as a roof, converting the carpal arch into a carpal tunnel through which pass the median nerve, the eight tendons of the long flexor muscles of the fingers and those of the flexor carpi radialis and flexor pollicis longus muscles. Any lesion that significantly reduces the size of the carpal tunnel may result in compression of the median nerve and lead to carpal tunnel syndrome. Most commonly, this can arise from tenosynovitis of the tendon sheaths, dislocation of the lunate bone or arthritic change and it is most prevalent in females between the ages of 40 and 60 years. Symptoms are often more common at night and may present as a tingling (paraesthesia), absence of tactile sensation (anaesthesia) or diminished sensation (hypoaesthesia) in the lateral 3.5 fingers. There is often a progressive loss of co-ordination and strength in the thumb, which can result in difficulty performing fine movements. In severe cases of compression, there may be wasting or atrophy of the thenar muscles and a procedure called carpal tunnel release may be necessary, which involves either partial or complete division of the flexor retinaculum (Ellis, 1992).

The first reported naming of the carpal bones was by Lyser in 1653 (McMurrich, 1914), but subsequent renaming has introduced some confusion and, as a result, the literature is not always consistent. From lateral to medial, the proximal row of carpal bones is comprised of the **scaphoid** (os scaphoideum or navicular), **lunate** (os lunatum or semilunar), **triquetral** (os triquetrum or cuneiform) and **pisiform** (os pisiforme), while the distal row is comprised of the **trapezium** (os trapezium or multangulum major), **trapezoid** (os trapezoideum or multangulum minor), **capitate** (os capitatum or os magnum) and **hamate** (os hamatum or unciform) (Holden, 1882; Turner, 1934). It has been remarked upon (Wood-Jones, 1941) that the human carpals are remarkably primitive (constant) in form and comparative anatomy reveals more profound changes in function than in structure (Napier, 1980; Kanagasuntheram *et al.*, 1987; Aiello and Dean, 1990). It is worth bearing in mind that the carpal bones can vary significantly in their appearance so that they may prove to be of some value in the forensic evaluation of personal identity (Greulich, 1960).

The **radiocarpal joint** (wrist) is commonly described as being ellipsoidal in shape, with the concavity being formed by the distal articular surface of the radius and the convexity by the scaphoid and lunate distally (Frazer, 1948; Lewis *et al.*, 1970; Last, 1973; Williams *et al.*, 1995). Collateral, radiocarpal and ulnocarpal ligaments (Mayfield *et al.*, 1976) strengthen the articular capsule of the joint. It is difficult to isolate the movements that are possible at this joint from those that occur at the midcarpal and intercarpal sites of articulation. The active movements that can occur at the radiocarpal complex are flexion (approx. 85°), extension (approx. 85°), adduction or ulnar deviation (approx. 45°), abduction or radial deviation (approx. 15°) and circumduction (MacConaill, 1941; MacConaill and Basmajian, 1977; Williams *et al.*, 1995).

The **midcarpal** (transverse carpal) **joint** is a compound sinuous articulation between the proximal and distal carpal rows. Both the radiocarpal and midcarpal joints are directly involved in flexion, with the greatest degree of movement occurring in the latter joint. Conversely, in extension at the wrist, a greater proportion of movement occurs at the radiocarpal joint and this is witnessed by the fact that the articular surfaces extend further onto the dorsal surface of the proximal carpal row than they do onto the palmar surface. The greater degree of movement in adduction compared to abduction is explained by the relative shortness of the styloid process of the ulna, which does not tend to impair movement as much as that of the radial styloid. Adduction occurs at the radiocarpal joint, whereas abduction takes place almost entirely at the midcarpal joint. The **intercarpal articulations** occur between adjacent carpal bones within each carpal row and are generally described as planar joints, which are tightly bound by an extensive network of intercarpal ligaments (Kauer, 1974; Voorhees *et al.*, 1985).

Each carpal bone can be considered to have six surfaces, at least two of which (palmar and dorsal) will be non-articular. The **scaphoid** is the largest of the carpal bones in the proximal row and it articulates with five bones - the radius proximally, the lunate medially and the trapezium, trapezoid and capitate distally.[5] The distal part of its palmar surface bears a rounded tubercle, which is directed somewhat anterolaterally and is the site of attachment for the lateral aspect of the flexor retinaculum and some fibres of the abductor pollicis brevis muscle. At this point, it is crossed by the tendon of the flexor carpi radialis muscle, which can leave a poorly defined groove on the bone, lateral to the site of attachment of the retinaculum. The tubercle is palpable in the living and can be detected in the 'anatomical snuffbox', which is that area on the lateral aspect of the wrist that is defined within the boundaries of the tendons of extensor pollicis longus medially and extensor pollicis brevis and abductor pollicis longus laterally. The styloid process of the radius, the scaphoid, trapezium and base of the first metacarpal all lie in the floor of the snuff box, which is crossed by the radial artery. At this point, the artery gives rise to the dorsal carpal branch, which supplies the posterior aspect of the carpal bones. The narrow dorsal surface of the scaphoid is rough, grooved and pierced by numerous vascular foramina.

The articular facet for the radius encroaches upon the dorsal surface and so it is narrowed to little more than a strip, to which are attached the dorsal ligaments of the wrist. The radial collateral ligament attaches to the slightly roughened lateral surface. The radial articular surface is convex and directed somewhat proximally and laterally and extends for some distance onto the dorsal aspect of the bone. The articular facet for the lunate is relatively flat, semilunar in shape, narrow and directed medially. A well-defined ridge separates it from the deeply concave facet that faces medially and distally for articulation with the capitate. A small roughened area is present between the radial and lunate facets and this is the site of attachment for the strong interosseous ligament that binds the scaphoid to the lunate. The articular surface for the trapezium and trapezoid bones tend to be continuous, convex and directed distally, although a poorly defined ridge can

[5]The term 'scaphoid' is said to be derived from its resemblance to a boat, which is also the origin of its older name 'navicular' and hence the origin of the word 'navy' pertaining to boats. However, it may even be derived from the Latin word 'scaphium' meaning a bowl of drinking vessel, perhaps in deference to the deeply concave distal articular surface (Simpson, 1969).

sometimes be found separating the two areas of articulation. The interosseous ligament that binds the scaphoid to the capitate attaches to the area of bone between the trapezoid and capitate articular surfaces.

The scaphoid is one of the most common sites of carpal fracture and it tends to occur following a fall onto the outstretched hand (Barr *et al.*, 1953). Non-union of the fracture is common and avascular necrosis is a frequent complication following an interrupted blood supply to the proximal pole of the bone as the vascular supply tends to enter from the distal extremity (Obletz and Halbstein, 1938; Gasser, 1965; Gelberman and Menon, 1980; Crock *et al.*, 1981; Panagis *et al.*, 1983; Crock, 1996). Fracture of the scaphoid can be confused with a congenital bipartite bone. In this situation, there is no evidence of a fracture line, as the contiguous surfaces are smooth and the division will normally follow an oblique line across the waist of the bone (Waugh and Sullivan, 1950). A full appreciation of the normal anatomical variants of the scaphoid is therefore critical to a successful clinical diagnosis of injury or anomaly (Waterman, 1998).

The **lunate** derives its name from its broadly crescentic outline. It lies in the middle of the proximal row and is somewhat obliquely placed. Its position can readily be identified, particularly in thin individuals, as in hyperflexion of the wrist joint, the lunate rises above the level of the other carpals. It articulates with five bones – the radius proximally, the scaphoid laterally, the triquetral medially and the capitate and hamate distally. It has a relatively broad, triangular, non-articular palmar surface and a much diminished non-articular dorsal surface, due to the dorsal prolongation of the radial articular facet. The lateral surface is narrow and bears a flat semilunar facet for articulation with the scaphoid. Immediately proximal to this facet is a roughened groove for the attachment of the interosseous ligament that binds the two bones together. The proximal surface is convex for articulation with the radius laterally and with the articular disc of the inferior radio-ulnar joint medially. Rarely, a ridge is present on the proximal surface of the lunate, delimiting the two sites of articulation. The medial surface presents a roughly square four-sided facet for articulation with the triquetral and this is separated from the deeply concave distal facet for articulation with the capitate, by a curved semi-lunar ridge, which represents the site of articulation with the hamate. Although both non-articular surfaces possess vascular foramina, they are particularly abundant on the dorsal surface (Gelberman *et al.*, 1980). An extremely unusual case of bilateral absence of the lunate bone has been reported by Kobayashi *et al.* (1991). The total absence of a bone is normally associated with an anomaly of the ulnar or radial ray but in this case all other skeletal elements were normal.

The **triquetral** (meaning three-sided) or carpal cuneiform (meaning wedge-shaped) is a somewhat pyramidal-shaped bone with a base that articulates with the lunate, an apex that points distally and medially, a lateral surface that articulates with the hamate, a medial surface that is essentially non-articular and a palmar surface that bears a single oval facet for articulation with the pisiform. The articular facet for the lunate is almost square in shape and is directed proximally and laterally. The concavo-convex articular surface for the hamate is directed somewhat laterally and distally and is broader proximally and narrower distally. The dorsal and medial surfaces are virtually confluent and roughened dorsally for the attachment of the ulnar collateral ligament of the wrist and smoother proximally for the site of articulation with the disc of the inferior radio-ulnar joint.

The **pisiform** derives its name from its 'pea-like' nodular shape and it is generally considered to possess all the attributes of a sesamoid bone as it forms within the tendon of the flexor carpi ulnaris muscle. It carries one articular facet on its dorsal surface for the triquetral bone and its long axis runs distally and laterally in the direction of the hook of the hamate (Robbins, 1917). The flexor carpi ulnaris tendon attaches to its palmar surface and it continues distally as the pisometacarpal and pisohamate ligaments. Indeed, the attachment of the latter ligament may be so well developed that it forms a distinct tubercle and an ossific bridge in this location results in pisohamate fusion (Cockshott, 1963). The flexor retinaculum is attached to the palmar aspect of the lateral surface and the abductor digiti minimi tendon and the extensor retinaculum are attached to the medial and distal aspects, respectively, of this bone. The ulnar artery may leave a faint depression on the medial surface. The pisiform is readily palpable in the living at the base of the hypothenar eminence and, as such, it is vulnerable to fracture following a fall onto the outstretched hand (Fleege *et al.*, 1991). The ulnar nerve, if it comes into contact at all with the pisiform, is confined to the distal portion, where it lies palmar to the ridge for the attachment of the flexor retinaculum (Robbins, 1917).

The **trapezium** is the most lateral of the distal row of carpal bones and articulates with four bones – the first and second metacarpals distally, the scaphoid proximally and the trapezoid medially.[6] The palmar surface

[6]The term 'trapezium' is derived from the Greek 'trapezion' meaning 'small table'. Thus, the the four-sided bone became known as the trapezium as two of the four sides (proximal and distal) are almost parallel. It is also known as the multangulum major in older texts, due to its irregular outline that produces many angles.

of the trapezium is characterized by a well-defined tubercle laterally and a deep groove in the middle of the surface that runs in a somewhat mediodistal direction. The tubercle gives attachment to the superficial layer of the flexor retinaculum, while the deeper layer attaches to the medial lip of the groove that houses the tendon of the flexor carpi radialis muscle. Thus, it can be said that the tendon essentially passes through the retinaculum as it splits to accommodate its passage. The tubercle can be detected on deep palpation in the living, but it is generally masked by muscles of the thenar eminence. The superficial head of the flexor pollicis brevis muscle arises from the distal region of the lateral aspect of the tubercle, the abductor pollicis brevis from the proximal region and the opponens pollicis arises between these two. The dorsal surface is somewhat roughened and elongated in shape and is closely related to the passage of the radial artery. The tubercle on the dorsal surface marks the site of attachment for the first carpometacarpal ligament. The lateral surface of the trapezium is non-articular and roughened for the attachment of the radial collateral ligament and capsular ligament of the first carpometacarpal joint. The proximal surface bears a shallow, hollowed out articular site for the scaphoid and a distinct interarticular ridge separates this from the relatively shallow, concave facet for the trapezoid on the medial surface.

The most distal extremity of the trapezium extends between the bases of the first and second metacarpals and presents a small quadrilateral facet that is directed somewhat distally and medially for articulation with the lateral aspect of the base of the second metacarpal. The distal surface that articulates with the first metacarpal at the sellar (saddle-shaped) first carpometacarpal joint has received much attention. It is the unique form and function of the thumb, in terms of its mobility and dexterity, that has resulted in the considerable degree of interest expressed in this joint. The two articular surfaces are not congruent and this facilitates a large degree of joint movement (MacConaill and Basmajian, 1977). Flexion and extension are said to occur in a plane that is parallel to the plane of the hand, while abduction and adduction occur in a plane that is at right angles to that of flexion and extension. Flexion of the thumb brings about a concomitant medial rotation which, when combined with abduction, brings the pad of the thumb into contact with the pads of the other fingers (Bunnell, 1938; Terry, 1943; Haines, 1944; Napier, 1955; Jacobs and Thompson, 1960; Forrest and Basmajian, 1965; Kuczynski, 1974). This action of opposition is unique to the primates and has naturally been widely researched in the evolutionary and comparative literature (Montagu, 1931; Musgrave, 1971; Vlček, 1975; Susman and Creel, 1979; Napier, 1980; Trinkaus, 1983, 1989).

The action of opposition is of paramount importance with regards to the functional integrity of the thumb in the precision grip (Napier, 1956). Osteoarthritic change at the joint or paralysis of the thenar muscles, which can arise following suicide attempts by slashing of the wrists, tend to leave the mobility of the thumb severely impaired and the hand is rendered virtually useless as a precision instrument (Jacobs and Thompson, 1960; Forrest and Basmajian, 1965; Leach and Bolton, 1968). Most clinicians operate under the principle that all attempts should be made to ensure the integrity of the thumb in, for example, industrial accidents involving the hand. Often however, it cannot be saved and unless some attempt at restitution of a thumb is attempted, the hand will become a tool of limited dextrous value. Pollicization of the index finger is a successful operation, which involves the reorientation of the index finger and fashioning it into a makeshift pollex (Jeffery, 1957; Clark *et al.*, 1998).[7]

The **trapezoid** also derives its name from the Greek meaning 'small table', but it is further defined by the fact that none of the sides are actually parallel. It is also known in older texts as the multangulum minor because of its irregular outline. It is a small bone, characterized by a dorsal non-articular surface, roughly four times the size of its palmar surface, around which is a virtually continuous cylinder of articular surfaces. The palmar surface continues onto the lateral surface for a short distance, where the slightly convex facet for articulation with the trapezium can be found. This surface is continuous with the proximal slightly convex facet for articulation with the scaphoid, which is in turn continuous only towards the upper surface with the small square facet for articulation with the distal aspect of the lateral surface of the capitate. This surface is then continuous with the distal aspect, which bears the largest facet for articulation with the grooved head of the second metacarpal. The facet is somewhat triangular in outline, convex from medial to lateral and concave from palmar to dorsal. The palmar surface of the trapezoid gives attachment to the

[7]The importance of the thumb in terms of man's dexterity has been recognized throughout history. It is reported that during the Gallic wars, Caesar ordered the thumbs to be removed from his captured prisoners because he said that he would no longer fear them as warriors. Similarly, the same fate was carried out by the Athenians during the Peloponesian wars on the oarsmen of hostile galleys before the prisoners were returned to their homes. Thus, they maintained their power grips and could row but were of no value as fighting soldiers as they could not hold their weapons efficiently (Terry, 1943).

deep head of the flexor pollicis brevis muscle, which arises as a large fasciculus from the adductor pollicis muscle (Day and Napier, 1961).

The **capitate** is the largest of the carpal bones and its name is probably derived from the proximal 'head-like' articular region. Being the largest of the carpal bones it is not surprising that it articulates with the largest number of other bones, seven in total – the second, third and fourth metacarpals distally, the scaphoid and lunate proximally, the trapezoid laterally and the hamate medially. The dorsal surface is roughly triangular in shape and comes to a point that is directed both distally and medially between the bases of the third and fourth metacarpals. Its distal border is obliquely aligned in response to both the styloid process of the third metacarpal and the larger medial projection of the distal articular surface of the second metacarpal. The distal articular surface is roughly triangular in shape, being broader towards the dorsal and narrower towards the palmar surfaces. The slightly concave facet for the second metacarpal is directed somewhat laterally and the very small facet for articulation with the fourth metacarpal is restricted to a small area on the dorsal rim. The lateral surface displays a concave strip distally for articulation with the trapezoid and a somewhat spherical surface proximally for articulation with the scaphoid. These two areas can be continuous but more often than not, they are separated by a deep depression that houses a strong interosseous ligament. A large articular strip is present on the posterior aspect of the medial surface for articulation with the hamate, which is deeper proximally and narrows towards its distal limit. The area directly anterior to this is roughened for the exceptionally strong interosseous ligament that binds the capitate to the hamate. The medial aspect of the head of the capitate articulates with the deeply concave distal facet of the lunate. The palmar surface of the capitate is small and roughened for ligamentous attachment, although it also gives rise to some of the fibres of the oblique head of the adductor pollicis muscle.

Both the term **hamate** and unciform refer to the hook-like appendage of this bone. It is the most medial of the carpals in the distal row and articulates with five bones – the fourth and fifth metacarpals distally, the lunate and triquetral proximally and medially, and the capitate laterally. The hamulus (hook) projects from the distal part of the palmar surface and is deeply concave on its lateral aspect. This arises due to its immediate relation to the synovial coverings of the flexor tendons that pass to the little finger. The base of the hamulus can often be traversed by a groove brought about by the presence of the deep terminal branch of the ulnar nerve. The medial aspect of the flexor retinaculum attaches to the tip of the hamulus and lateral to this, the opponens digiti minimi attaches distally and the flexor digiti minimi proximally. The upper border also gives attachment to the pisohamate ligament, which is considered to be a continuation of the flexor carpi ulnaris tendon. The hamulus can be detected in the living following deep palpation lateral and slightly distal to the position of the pisiform.

The distal surface of the hamate presents as a roughly square facet that is separated by a dorsopalmar ridge into a larger medial facet for articulation with the base of the fifth metacarpal and a smaller lateral facet for articulation with the base of the fourth metacarpal. The true proximal extent of the hamate is thin and wedge-shaped and only comes into direct contact with the lunate when the hand is adducted. The articular facet covers the lateral surface for the capitate in all but the palmar and distal angle, which is the site of attachment for the strong capitohamate interosseous ligament. The proximomedial surface is represented by a broad articular strip, which is convex proximally and concave distally for articulation with the triquetral. As with all the other carpal bones, the dorsal surface is roughened for ligamentous attachment and displays numerous vascular foramina.

The prominent position of the hook of the hamate makes it susceptible to injury and although fracture can arise following a fall on the outstretched hand, it more commonly results from traumatic impact during sports activities, particularly those that involve the swinging of a bat or a club (Bray *et al.*, 1985; Foucher *et al.*, 1985; Norman *et al.*, 1985; Stark *et al.*, 1989; Failla, 1993; Wakely and Young, 1995). An untreated hook fracture generally results in weakness of the hand, particularly in the tendons associated with the medial two fingers and this will dramatically affect the strength of the power grip. A fracture of the hook can also lead to numbness of these fingers along with paralysis of the hypothenar muscles.

Metacarpals

The five metacarpals extend in a somewhat radiating manner (Figs. 9.24 and 9.25) from their proximal articulation with the distal carpal row (carpometacarpal joints) to their distal articulation with the base of the proximal row of phalanges (metacarpophalangeal joints). They are numbered in sequence from the lateral side, although there is considerable debate over the true phylogenetic and ontogenetic derivation of the first metacarpal (see below). The metacarpals are defined as long bones as they posses a tubular shaft with proximal (base) and distal (head) synovial articular extremities. Presumably, it is as a result of this morphology that, like the other long bones of the skeleton, the metacarpals have been utilized in the estimation of living stature (Himes *et al.*, 1976; Kimura, 1976; Himes *et al.*, 1977; Musgrave and Harneja, 1978; Kobyliansky *et al.*, 1985).

The common length formula for the metacarpals is that the second is the longest followed in a decreasing sequence by the third, fourth and fifth, with the first metacarpal being the shortest (Martin and Saller, 1959; Garn *et al.*, 1975a; Susman, 1979; Arias-Cazorla and Rodriguez-Larralde, 1987). Deviations from this normal pattern have been used as an indication of skeletal malformations (Poznanski *et al.*, 1972).

The cross-sectional morphology of the **shaft** of the thumb differs markedly from that seen in metacarpals 2–5. The former is more robust and triangular, while those of the remaining metacarpals range from more of a egg-shape in the second metacarpal to oval in the fifth (Lazar and Schulter-Ellis, 1980). The volar (palmar) surface of the shafts of metacarpals 2–5, are concave longitudinally, which corresponds with the natural concavity of the palm, while the dorsal surface is either straight or slightly convex in nature.

The metacarpal **bases** articulate via complex carpometacarpal joints with the distal carpal row. The saddle-shaped nature of the first of these joints is characteristic and the anatomy of its structure is well-documented (Williams *et al.*, 1995). The remaining carpometacarpal joints are often described as planar in terms of functional morphology, but in reality they are more complex than that. There is a limited degree of movement present at these joints and it is often restricted to a gliding motion, which is best developed at the articulation between the fifth metacarpal and the hamate. In addition, there are small, planar intermetacarpal joints between contiguous surfaces of the metacarpals, which permit slight gliding of the articular surfaces, particularly when the hand is cupped. As with most long bones, it is interesting to note that the most sexually dimorphic region of a metacarpal is reported to be in its proximal articulation, i.e. a measurement of the base (MacLaughlin, 1987). Scheuer and Elkington (1993) found that by measuring only the base of a metacarpal, sex could be correctly assigned to 76% of their sample (Elkington, 1989).

The metacarpal **heads** are generally classified as ellipsoidal in nature and articulate with the shallow concavities at the base of the proximal phalanges. The surfaces are not regularly convex and can be almost bicondylar in some cases, when a well-defined dividing trough is present on the palmar aspect. The heads are distinctly asymmetrical, being smaller in their transverse than their anteroposterior dimensions, with the articular surface extending further proximally on the palmar than the dorsal surface. The prominence of the knuckles, which is best seen in full flexion of the digits at the metacarpophalangeal joints, is formed by the dorsal aspect of the heads of the metacarpals. These joints are strengthened by palmar, deep transverse metacarpal and collateral ligaments which, whilst providing support to the joint, also permit a considerable degree of mobility. Flexion is possible to almost 90°, while extension from the standard anatomical plane is limited to only a few degrees, as are abduction and adduction. The first metacarpophalangeal joint is the most mobile (and the most likely to develop osteo-arthritis), followed in a sequence of decreasing mobility by the second, fifth, fourth and then the third (Parsons, 1895; Harris and Joseph, 1949; Joseph, 1951a; Long, 1968).

The **first metacarpal** articulates with the trapezium proximally and the first proximal phalanx distally. Due to its volar rotation, it is removed from the immediate vicinity of the second metacarpal and so does not possess an intermetacarpal articulation at its base. As a rule, this bone is shorter and more robust than the other metacarpals, with a shaft that is somewhat flattened dorsally and is convex towards the palmar surface in the transverse plane. In the longitudinal plane, the shaft is relatively straight dorsally and gently concave on the volar surface. The palmar surface of the shaft is unequally marked by a rounded ridge into a larger lateral and a smaller medial area. The opponens pollicis muscle attaches to the whole length of the larger lateral aspect of the palmar surface of the shaft, while the lateral head of the first dorsal interosseous (sometimes referred to as the abductor indicis muscle) arises from the smaller medial aspect of this surface. The nutrient foramen is generally located on the distal aspect of the anteromedial surface of the shaft and is directed distally, although additional foramina can occur on both the anterolateral and the dorsal surfaces (Singh, 1959a; Patake and Mysorekar, 1977). A small flattened tubercle is present on the lateral side of the proximal end of the shaft for the attachment of the abductor pollicis longus muscle. A poorly defined site of attachment for the origin of the first palmar interosseous muscle is found on the medial aspect of the proximal end of the shaft, anterior to the site of attachment for the first dorsal interosseous muscle.

The first carpometacarpal joint, between the thumb and the trapezium, is probably one of the most important joints in the hand as the majority of the movements of the first digit occur here (Coonrad and Goldner, 1968). The joint *per se* has been discussed above but the articular surface of the base of the first metacarpal merits some description. The articular surface is concavo-convex in appearance and is separated into two quite distinct areas. The larger lateral aspect articulates with the ventrodorsal convexity of the trapezium, while the smaller medial area articulates with the distally projecting medial side of the saddle-shaped joint. Therefore, the articular surface on the medial aspect of the first metacarpal extends further distally towards the shaft. The junction between the two basal articular surfaces is marked by a poorly defined ridge, which corresponds with a well-developed styloid process on its palmar surface, which is displaced somewhat medially. This process deepens the antero-posterior concavity of the base of the metacarpal so that it forms a better fitting joint with the saddle shape of the trapezium.

The head of the first metacarpal is less convex than those of the other metacarpals but is considerably broader. On the palmar surface, the medial and lateral angles are enlarged to form two articular eminences for the sesamoid bones that form in the tendons of adductor pollicis and the first palmar interosseous muscles medially and flexor pollicis brevis laterally (Fawcett, 1897; Patterson, 1937; Sinberg, 1940; Hubay, 1949; Garn and Rohmann, 1962b; Lewis, 1965; Onat and Numan-Cebeci, 1976).

Using regression equations, Scheuer and Elkington (1993) were able to assign the correct sex to 94% of their sample using only measurements of the first metacarpal. They found this to be the most dimorphic of the metacarpals, which was attributed to its involvement in grip and the associated muscle requirements for that function.

The **second metacarpal** is of vital importance in the maintenance of the integrity of the hand, both in terms of the power and the precision grip. Next to the thumb it is the most powerful of the digits (Plato and Norris, 1980) and its clear and unobstructed view on radiographs has resulted in it playing an important part in the monitoring of bone mass with age, particularly in relation to postmenopausal women and the development of osteoporosis (Smithgall *et al.*, 1966; Virtama and Helela, 1969; MacLennan and Caird, 1973; Evans *et al.*, 1978; Horsman *et al.*, 1981; Moermann, 1981; Plato and Purifoy, 1982; Plato *et al.*, 1982, 1984; Kusec *et al.*, 1988; Edmonds, 1990).

The second is the longest of the metacarpals and it articulates at its base with, from lateral to medial, the trapezium, trapezoid and capitate bones, while its medial side articulates with the lateral aspect of the base of the third metacarpal at the intermetacarpal joint. The shaft is gently convex dorsally and concave ventrally in its long axis and is said to be somewhat prismoidal in cross-section, with medial and lateral surfaces that are separated by a palmar ridge, each of which are in turn separated from the dorsal surface by medial and lateral interosseous ridges. The dorsal surface is broad distally, narrows proximally and is covered by the extensor tendons of the index finger. The lateral surface gives rise to the medial head of the first dorsal interosseous muscle and the medial surface gives attachment to the second palmar interosseous ventrally and the second dorsal interosseous more dorsally (Stack, 1962). The nutrient foramen varies in position, being found in roughly equal proportions on both the anteromedial and anterolateral surfaces (Singh, 1959a; Patake and Mysorekar, 1977), although it is always directed proximally.

The base is characteristically grooved to correspond in shape with the ventrodorsal inclination of the trapezoid. The medial edge of the deep groove is more prolonged than the lateral edge and it articulates with the capitate, while the lateral side of the base has a small quadrilateral facet for articulation with the trapezium. Immediately behind this facet, on the dorsal surface, is a small tubercle for the insertion of the extensor carpi radialis longus tendon. A corresponding tubercle on the medial aspect of the dorsal surface gives attachment to some of the fibres of the extensor carpi radialis brevis muscle. The flexor carpi radialis tendon attaches to a small tubercle on the more lateral inclination of the palmar aspect of the base, while the oblique head of the adductor pollicis attaches to the medial aspect. The medial side of the base articulates with the base of the third metacarpal by a strip-like facet that is somewhat constricted in the middle, due to the presence of the interosseous ligament.

The head of the second metacarpal is characteristically asymmetrical. Most of this asymmetry arises from the large site of attachment of the second metacarpophalangeal ligament on the dorsolateral aspect of the head. This large attachment site appears to pare away part of the rounded articular surface so that on profile the lateral aspect of the head has a steeper slope than the medial aspect (Landsmeer, 1955). The medial and lateral ligamentous impressions are in close proximity to tubercles on the dorsal aspect of the metacarpal and because of the larger volume of the lateral ligament in the second digit, the lateral dorsal tubercle is located further away from the metacarpophalangeal joint than is the medial tubercle, resulting in a well-defined proximolateral sloping of the dorsal non-articular surface (Landsmeer, 1955).

Adding further to the asymmetry of the head is the larger palmar prolongation of the articular surface on the lateral aspect. This is commonly (incidence of approximately 40%) a site of articulation for a sesamoid bone in the head of the first dorsal interosseous muscle (Hubay, 1949). Following sports-related hyperextension injuries, it has been known for this sesamoid to become entrapped within the metacarpophalangeal joint (Sweterlitsch *et al.*, 1969).

The **third metacarpal** forms the so-called axis of the hand and as such is considered to be the most stable element of the hand (Marzke and Marzke, 1987). The shaft gives attachment to the medial head of the second dorsal interosseous muscle laterally and to the lateral head of the third dorsal interosseous medially. In its distal two-thirds, the palmar ridge that separates these two attachments provides a site of origin for the transverse head of the adductor pollicis muscle. The extensor tendon of the middle finger covers the dorsal surface of the shaft. The nutrient foramen tends to occur more frequently on the lateral aspect and is again directed proximally, away from the growing end of the bone (Patake and Mysorekar, 1977).

The base of this metacarpal is easily recognized by the presence of a styloid process that projects from the lateral aspect of the dorsal surface. The embryological origin of this styloid process is said to be homologous with a group of cells, which fuse with the capitate in Old-World monkeys, but instead fuses with the third metacarpal in man. It is said to stabilize the hand against forces directed towards the palmar aspect of the metacarpal head and so prevent hyperextension of the bone and palmar subluxation of its base (Marzke and Marzke, 1987). A relatively common supernumerary carpal bone, sometimes referred to as the ninth carpal bone, the styloid bone or the hunchback carpal bone is found in the angle between the base of the third metacarpal, the capitate and the trapezoid bones (Bassoe and Bassoe, 1955). The origin of this bony mass is uncertain but it may well be related to the development of the styloid process of the third metacarpal, although some authors believe it to be acquired rather than congenital (Dorosin and Davis, 1956). When present it can cause limitations in digit extension, caused by slipping of the extensor tendons over the prominence (Kootstra *et al.*, 1974). Symptoms also include an occasional ache and easy fatigue in the muscles at the wrist, although it is frequently asymptomatic (Carter, 1941; Curtiss, 1961).

The base of the third metacarpal has a single articulation site with the capitate, which is convex in its palmar aspect and concave in its dorsal portion, where it becomes continuous with the styloid process. The lateral aspect articulates with the second metacarpal via a strip like articulation, which is constricted in the midline for the attachment of the interosseous ligament. The medial aspect articulates with the lateral surface of the base of the fourth metacarpal, usually via two discrete oval sites, but the palmar one may be absent or, less frequently, a narrow bridge may join the two facets. The tendons of the flexor carpi radialis and oblique head of the adductor pollicis attach to the palmar aspect of the base, while the extensor carpi radialis brevis tendon attaches to a tubercle on the lateral extent of the dorsal aspect directly distal to the styloid process. Infrequently, the brachioradialis tendon may attach to the dorsal aspect of the base of this metacarpal, deep to the insertion of extensor carpi radialis brevis (Sañudo *et al.*, 1996). A smaller tubercle is present on the medial border of the dorsal surface for the attachment of the interosseous ligament that connects the third and fourth metacarpals.

The head of the third metacarpal is roughly symmetrical and rarely if ever articulates with any sesamoid bones (Hubay, 1949). There is, however, still a tendency for the lateral metacarpophalangeal ligament to be stronger than its medial counterpart, so the head of the metacarpal does tend to be more pared away on the lateral aspect, but it is not so well defined as in the second metacarpal (Landsmeer, 1955). On the dorsal surface, the lateral tubercle does tend to be slightly further removed from the metacarpophalangeal joint than the medial tubercle, so that there is still a tendency for a proximolateral sloping of the non-articular surface, but again this is not as pronounced as is found for the second metacarpal.

Although not the shortest, the **fourth metacarpal** is generally the most slender of the five bones. The lateral surface of its shaft gives attachment to the third palmar interosseous and the medial head of the third dorsal interosseous, while its medial surface gives origin to the lateral head of the fourth dorsal interosseous. The nutrient foramen is generally located on the lateral aspect and is directed proximally (Patake and Mysorekar, 1977).

The base articulates with the third metacarpal laterally via two discrete oval facets (see above). The more dorsal of these is usually the larger and not infrequently, the more ventral may be absent due to the presence of the well-developed interosseous ligament that binds the two metacarpals to the capitate and the hamate. The base articulates medially with the lateral aspect of the base of the fifth metacarpal via a single elongated and slightly concave facet, which is continuous with that on the proximal surface for the hamate, quadrangular in shape and convex towards the palmar surface, but concave towards the dorsal aspect.

The head of this metacarpal is roughly symmetrical, although the dorsal surface does show a somewhat lateral inclination. The impressions for the metacarpophalangeal ligaments are roughly equal on both sides and as a result the dorsal tubercles are effectively equidistant from the joint cavity, although there is a slight tendency for the lateral tubercle to be located more distally (Landsmeer, 1955). Sesamoid bones are rarely associated with this metacarpal (Hubay, 1949).

The **fifth metacarpal** is generally more robust than the fourth. Its shaft gives attachment to the opponens digiti minimi medially, while the lateral surface is separated by a longitudinal ridge into a palmar aspect for the attachment of the fourth palmar interosseous and a dorsal aspect for the attachment of the medial head of the fourth dorsal interosseous. The nutrient foramen is generally located on the lateral aspect and is directed proximally (Patake and Mysorekar, 1977).

The base is readily recognized as there is no medial articular site, only a well-defined tubercle for the attachment of the extensor carpi ulnaris tendon. The lateral side of the base articulates via a strip-like facet with the medial surface of the fourth metacarpal and this facet is continuous proximally with that between the fifth metacarpal and the hamate. This latter facet is somewhat concave from side to side and convex from palmar to dorsal and extends quite high onto the dorsal surface. On the lateral palmar aspect of the base, a small tubercle is sometimes present, representing the site of attachment of the pisometacarpal ligament. As this is in reality the continuation of the flexor carpi ulnaris tendon, it is inappropriately named.

The head of this metacarpal is asymmetrical on its palmar aspect, due to the frequent occurrence of a sesamoid bone in the abductor digiti minimi tendon, which articulates with the medial palmar aspect of the head and so frequently ensures that the medial surface is larger than the lateral (Hubay, 1949). Relatively small impressions are present on both medial and lateral sides for the metacarpophalangeal ligaments and although the dorsal tubercles are roughly equidistant from the joint surface, there is a tendency for the lateral to be more distal in location.

Phalanges

The **phalanges** form the skeleton of the fingers and tend to be named rather than numbered (probably to prevent clinical confusion). From lateral to medial they are: the thumb, index, middle, ring and little fingers. The thumb is also known as the pollex from the Latin 'polleo' which means 'to be strong', in deference to the fact that it is the strongest digit. In older texts, the fingers may be referred to as index, medius, annularis and minimus (Holcomb *et al.*, 1958). It is generally recognized that of the fingers, the middle is the longest and the little finger is the smallest, with the ring being longer than the index in males, while the opposite tends to occur in females (Blincoe, 1962).[8]

There are only two phalanges associated with the thumb (proximal and distal) but under normal conditions there are three for every other digit (proximal, middle and distal) (Drinkwater, 1916). The controversy over the phylogenetic origin of the bones of the thumb is well documented, with some authors stating that the first metacarpal is indeed a phalanx because of its atypical epiphyseal formation, and while this theory may carry some plausibility, it is no longer the most accepted explanation. Phalangeal reduction has been studied in many animal groups, and while this offers an attractive phylogenetic scenario it does not fully explain the presence of only two phalanges in the Palaeozoic Stegocephali (Windle, 1892), nor the not so uncommon occurrence of a triphalangeal thumb (trimerous digit) in man (Windle, 1892; Jones, 1941; Lapidus *et al.*, 1943; Wilkinson, 1951; Abramowitz, 1959). In the case of a triphalangeal thumb, the terminal phalanx is usually shortened and an accessory element (middle phalanx) is present between this and the basal phalanx. This has led some authors to suggest that the normal terminal polliceal phalanx may represent two fused phalanges. Other authors have suggested that either the triphalangeal thumb is in fact a duplicated digit with an absent thumb, or that the middle phalanx is not a true phalanx but in fact the remnant of a base of one of the phalanges of a bifid thumb (Lapidus *et al.*, 1943). Triphalangeal thumbs can occur as a sporadic disorder but are more often seen as a dominant familial trait (Le Minor, 1995). In researching the genes that regulate the differentiation of the developing forelimb, a gene has been identified that seems to be responsible for triphalangeal thumbs (Zguricas *et al.*, 1994).

While correct identification of a proximal, middle or distal phalanx causes little or no problems in the adult, both the identification of side and correct assignation to a specific digital ray are extremely difficult and correct identification relies very heavily on subtle changes in bone morphology. This, of course, does not apply to the phalanges of the thumb, as they are sufficiently distinct to permit ready identification. However, there are very few texts which even attempt to illustrate or describe individual phalanges other than in the terms of proximal, middle or distal. Although some authors have been bold enough to identify individual phalanges, they tend not to disclose their secret formula to the rest of the academic community. Given an intact hand, most investigators

[8]The term 'phalanx' takes its origin from the Greek, meaning 'an array of soldiers in close formation' (Field and Harrison, 1957; Simpson, 1969). Aristotle was the first to apply this term to the bones of the digit, as they are arranged one behind the other, reminding him of the ranks of the Macedonian phalanx.

could probably assign individual bones with some degree of reliability, but when they are isolated finds, it is often only those who have extensive experience in hand bone identification that will be in any way successful. As it is so difficult to achieve positive identification even in the adult, so it is understandably even more complicated, if indeed not impossible, to attempt to do so in the juvenile. For the purposes of identification, we have been unable to locate any text that describes individual morphological differences in developing phalanges. For this reason alone, we have limited our detailed descriptions of the development of the phalanges and their ultimate adult morphology to the identification of proximal, middle and distal only (Figs. 9.24 and 9.25). Although we have access to a considerable number of documented fetal and juvenile remains, many are not represented by known finger rays and so any attempt at description could be misleading at best. This is certainly one area of osteological identification that would benefit from further investigation. It should be borne in mind, of course, that next to the ribs, the phalanges are probably the most common bones to be confused with animal remains and so sometimes even assigning them as 'human' can be difficult in certain circumstances (Stewart, 1959; Angel, 1974; Brothwell, 1981).

Each phalanx can be described as having a base, shaft and head, a convex dorsal surface and a concave palmar surface. The **proximal phalanx** of the thumb is usually the shortest, followed in increasing size by the fifth, second and fourth, with the third generally being the longest. Although the second and fourth proximal phalanges may be of similar length, it is generally found that the second is longer.

The **base** of a proximal phalanx articulates proximally with the head of a metacarpal at the metacarpophalangeal (MCP) joint. This is usually described as an ellipsoidal joint but is in reality almost bicondylar, particularly on the palmar aspect. The base displays a characteristic single concave oval facet, which is longer in its transverse than in its palmodorsal aspect. The joint is strengthened by a palmar ligament, which is firmly attached to the base of the proximal phalanx and strong collateral ligaments, which attach to the posterior tubercle and an adjacent depression on the heads of the metacarpal (Landsmeer, 1955, 1976). They pass obliquely distally and forwards to attach to the side of the ventral aspect of the base of the proximal phalanx. Extension is limited to a few degrees but flexion can occur up to 90° and although abduction and adduction are limited to only a few degrees in most of the joints, as much as 30° can occur in the index finger, which is considered to be the most mobile at this joint. Adduction arises through the action of the palmar interosseous muscles and abduction is via the dorsal interosseous muscles. The first palmar interosseous inserts onto the medial aspect of the base of the first proximal phalanx via a sesamoid bone, while the second and third mainly insert into the dorsal digital expansion. However, some fibres of the second may insert onto the medial aspect of the base of the second proximal phalanx and some fibres of the third may pass to the lateral aspect of the base of the fourth proximal phalanx. The fourth palmar interosseous inserts onto the lateral aspect of the base of the fifth proximal phalanx. The first dorsal interosseous muscle inserts onto the lateral aspect of the base of the second proximal phalanx, the second dorsal interosseous inserts onto the lateral aspect of the third proximal phalanx and the third muscle may not reach as far as the medial aspect of the base of the third proximal phalanx but may insert into the dorsal digital expansion. The fourth dorsal interosseous most commonly inserts into the dorsal digital expansion, but occasionally some fibres may insert into the medial aspect of the base of the fourth proximal phalanx.

The base of the first proximal phalanx is the site of attachment for a number of muscles involved in the movement of the thumb. The extensor pollicis brevis tendon inserts onto its dorsal aspect, the abductor pollicis brevis, flexor pollicis brevis and adductor pollicis insert onto its lateral aspect and the remainder of the adductor pollicis inserts onto its medial aspect. Similarly, the medial aspect of the base of the fifth proximal phalanx is the site of attachment for muscles that move the little finger, namely the flexor digiti minimi brevis and the abductor digiti minimi.

The **shaft** of a proximal phalanx generally tapers towards its distal end. The dorsal surface is usually described as being somewhat convex, both along its long axis and from side to side (Schulter-Ellis and Lazar, 1984). This surface is virtually covered by the dorsal digital expansion, which attaches to the base of the middle phalanx and the dorsal aspect of the base of the distal phalanx (Haines, 1951). However, Stack (1962) showed that there is some attachment to the proximal phalanx by collateral wing tendons, which pass to both the medial and lateral aspects of the dorsal surface. The palmar surface of the shaft is said to be flat from side to side but gently concave along the long axis of the bone. The shafts are bounded by sharp margins on either side which form the site of attachment for the fibrous flexor sheaths. This strong attachment helps to form a bed for the flexor tendons and keeps them firmly in position. The flexor sheath is not so strongly developed in the first digit and so the sides of the first proximal phalanx are not so well defined.

The **heads** of the proximal phalanges are shaped like grooved pulleys, which extend further onto the palmar than the dorsal surface. This forms the site of articulation with the distal phalanx in digit 1 and the middle phalanges at the proximal interphalangeal (PIP) joint in the remainder of the digits. These are uni-axial hinge joints that restrict movement to only flexion and extension. The latter tends to be limited to only a few degrees of movement, explaining the reduced encroachment of the articular surface on the dorsal aspect, while flexion is much more extensive (Kuczynski, 1968). The bicondylar area is unevenly separated by an intercondylar concavity into a larger medial area in phalanges 2 and 3 and a larger lateral surface in phalanges 1, 4 and 5 (Kuczynski, 1968). A pit and a more flattened area are present on both the medial and the lateral aspects of the head and this is the site of attachment for the collateral ligaments of the PIP joint.

Where the capsule of an interphalangeal joint supports a flexor tendon (flexors digitorum superficialis and profundus for the PIP joint and only the latter for the DIP joint), it may become thickened into a single sesamoid body, which nestles in the palmar surface of the intercondylar area (Bradley, 1906). This serves to raise the tendon above the line of the joint and so increase the leverage and therefore the power of the muscle (Frazer, 1948).

The **middle phalanges** articulate with the proximal phalanges at the PIP joint and with the distal phalanges at the distal interphalangeal (DIP) joint. It is generally found that the middle phalanx of the third finger is both the longest and the most robust. This is followed in order of decreasing length by that of the fourth, second and finally fifth middle phalanges (there being, of course, no middle phalanx for the first digit). The middle phalanx of the fifth digit is generally the most gracile.

The **base** of a middle phalanx has two small concave articular facets separated by a smooth intercondylar ridge that allow the joint to articulate closely with the pulley-shaped head of the proximal phalanx. A relatively large tubercle that produces an elevation on the dorsal surface of the joint represents the site of attachment of the tendons of the extensor digitorum muscle via the dorsal digital expansion. The palmar surface of the base displays two small concavities on either side of a midline elevation and these are the sites of attachment of the split tendon of the flexor digitorum superficialis tendon.

The **shaft** of a middle phalanx also tapers towards its distal end and, like the proximal phalanx, it is somewhat tunnel-shaped in cross-section, with a rounded dorsal surface and a flat palmar surface. The sides of a middle phalanx are also raised, due to the attachment of the flexor tendon sheath, which binds down the tendon of the flexor digitorum profundus tendon.

The **head** of the middle phalanx is pulley-shaped and therefore similar in its morphology to the head of the proximal phalanx, although it is obviously much smaller. The anatomy of the DIP joint is very similar to that of the PIP joint as it is also a uni-axial hinge joint that is capable of significant degrees of movement in only one plane. During flexion at the MCP joint, extension at the interphalangeal joints is brought about by the lumbrical muscles[9] which arise from the tendons of the flexor digitorum profundus muscle and insert into the dorsal digital expansion (Long and Brown, 1964; Goldberg, 1970).

The **distal phalanges** (sometimes referred to as the 'ungual phalanges' from the Latin meaning 'claw or nail') are distinctive because of their non-articular free distal extremity and are often said to be somewhat triangular in shape, being widest proximally and then tapering towards the distal pole. In fact, it is quite appropriately described as being 'harpoon'-shaped, given the two barb-like extensions that pass proximally from either side of the distal extremity. The polliceal distal phalanx is not only the longest but also significantly more robust than any of the other distal phalanges.

Abnormal shortness of the first distal phalanx is known as brachymegalodactylism and is recognized as an autosomal dominant with 40% penetration (Straus, 1942; Goodman *et al.*, 1965; Poznanski *et al.*, 1971a).[10] In approximately 74% of cases, a sesamoid bone is present at the polliceal interphalangeal joint, but it occurs within the capsule of the joint and not in the tendon of the flexor pollicis longus muscle (Joseph, 1951b).

It is interesting to note that in the remaining four digits there is very little difference in the length of the distal phalanx but they do differ significantly in robusticity, with the third being the most robust, followed in decreasing order by the second, fourth and finally the fifth, which is the most gracile. The distal phalanx articulates proximally at the DIP joint with the head of the middle phalanx and its base bears two sometimes quite indistinct concave articular facets. The dorsal surface is smooth and its base is the site of attachment for the extensor pollicis longus tendon in the thumb and the extensor digitorum tendons in the other digits. The distal pole of the phalanx is smooth

[9]These muscles derive their name from their 'worm-like' appearance in deference to the genus *Lumbricus*, e.g. Lumbricus terrestris (earthworm).

[10]Interestingly, palm readers and mystics call this the 'murderer's thumb', as it was considered to be a clear indicator of homicidal inclinations!

and sits deep to the fingernail. The palmar surface is rougher and the base is flattened to take the insertion of the flexor digitorum profundus tendon in the medial four digits and the flexor pollicis longus tendon in the thumb (Wilkinson, 1953). In the thumb, the principal central tendon insertion and the two lateral fasciculi may insert onto separate well-defined tuberosities. In the terminal phalanges of the fingers, the roughening for the flexor tendon attachment is limited proximally by a transverse bony ridge, while distally the tendon attaches more than halfway from the articular margin to the base of the palmar tuberosity (Wilkinson, 1951). The palmar tuberosity (tuberositas unguicularis) at the distal pole of the phalanx is the site of attachment of the digital fibro-fatty pad, which secures the pulp of the fingertip.

Early development of the hand

Around day 33 of intra-uterine life, the hand plate becomes recognizable as a flattened area of mesenchyme that lies parallel to the median plane (O'Rahilly and Gardner, 1975; Larsen, 1993). By day 37, it clearly shows areas of mesenchymal condensations that will form the region of the carpus, which is surrounded by a **crescentic flange** that will go on to form the **digital plate** (Streeter, 1948). By day 38, the **digital rays** are visible as thickenings in the digital plate and the tips of the future fingers project beyond the crescentic flange, giving it a somewhat crenulated appearance (Fig. 9.26). By day 41, the finger rays are well established and the radial, median and ulnar nerves have penetrated into the hand plate (Blechschmidt, 1969; Uhthoff, 1990b). Between days 38 and 44 the interdigital notches have formed as a result of specific pre-programmed location cell necrosis (apoptosis) as the apical ectodermal ridge thins in this region (Kelley, 1970, 1973; Hurle and Colvee, 1982). It has been experimentally shown in chick embryos that if Janus green is injected at a critical time, then necrosis is inhibited and this results in soft tissue syndactyly (Menkes and Deleanu, 1964; Christ *et al.*, 1986). It has also been shown in mice that following amniotic sac puncture, a transient period of bradycardia is induced, which may produce temporary hypoxia in the distal extremities. When this was performed at a critical gestational age that corresponded with the normal time for chorionic villus sampling in the human, mitotic activity and not apoptosis was observed in the interdigital spaces. It has been postulated that this might explain the phenomenon of syndactyly, which can occur following amniotic sac puncture (Chang *et al.*, 1998).

By day 47 the hand has become tilted so that the pre-axial border is more medial than the postaxial border, i.e. the palm faces caudally and medially and the limb has undergone horizontal flexion so that it lies in a parasagittal, rather than a coronal plane (O'Rahilly and Gardner, 1975; Larsen, 1993). By day 48, certain areas of the mesenchymal mass of the future carpal area begin to chondrify. Chondrification progresses in a well defined proximodistal direction in the hand so that the carpals are formed first and followed in succession by the metacarpals, proximal phalanges, middle and finally distal phalanges, which commence chondrification around day 50 (Senior, 1929; Saunders, 1948; O'Rahilly *et al.*, 1957). Of the carpal bones, the capitate and hamate are the first to commence chondrification around day 41, while the lunate at day 47 and the pisiform at day 50 are the last to commence cartilage anlagen formation (O'Rahilly *et al.*, 1959). By day 52 the digits develop **palmar swellings** (tactile pads) and the embryological hands now meet in the midline anterior to the cardiac eminence (Larsen, 1993).

From around 48–56 days, **interzones** appear between the chondrifying bone primordia (Fig. 9.27). This presumptive joint area then develops a distinct three-layered appearance, with future articular cartilage at both ends and a central zone that will differentiate into synovial tissues. Cavitation of this central

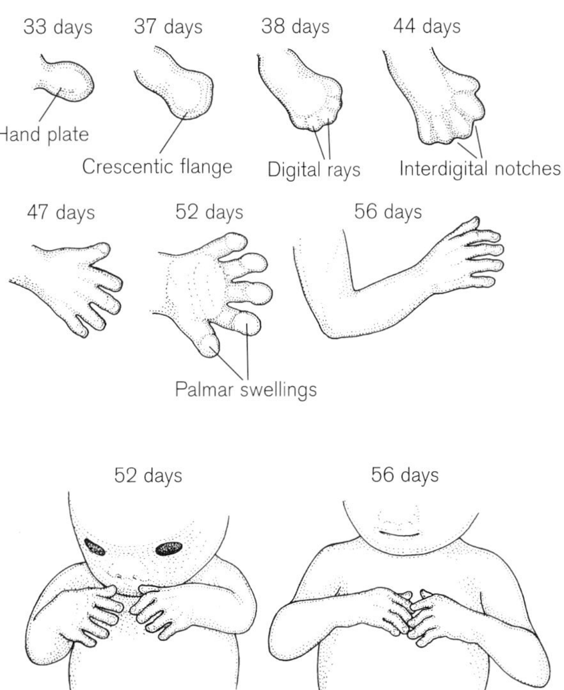

Figure 9.26 The development of the upper limb between 5 and 8 embryonic weeks (redrawn after Larsen, 1993).

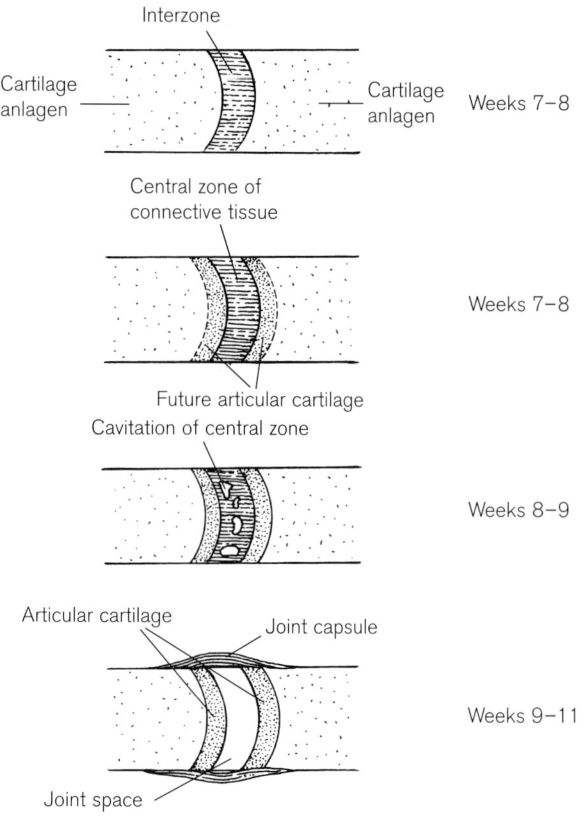

Figure 9.27 Diagrammatic representation of the embryonic development of a synovial joint (redrawn after Larsen, 1993).

zone into a true joint space occurs between weeks 9 and 11 (Whillis, 1940; O'Rahilly, 1949; Gray *et al.*, 1957; O'Rahilly *et al.*, 1957; O'Rahilly and Gardner, 1975). It is at this stage that not only are all of the joints in the hand formed, but also the fate of the future carpal pattern is set. So-called 'carpal fusions' are not uncommon but in reality they are really a non-separation of chondrifying zones so that no intercarpal joint space is formed. McCredie (1975) described congenital carpal fusion as arising from 'a disorder of organization of mesenchyme in week 5' and proposed that the structure responsible for organizing the fate of the mesenchyme was the penetrating nerve.

It is generally accepted that in isolated developmental situations, carpal coalitions occur within the same carpal row, whereas if the condition is syndrome-related, then the coalitions may cross between the proximal and distal rows (Oner and de Vries, 1994). The coalition of carpal bones and the presence of supernumerary elements that most likely develop from aberrant ossification of small cartilage tags, have been the subject of much debate. Some authors have attempted to explain their presence in terms of phylogenetic evolution, reflecting a primitive atavistic phenomenon, whereas they are in reality more likely to be ontogenetic variants, although there is some evidence for a racial and therefore a genetic predisposition (Pfitzner, 1893; Dwight, 1904, 1907b, 1909; Johnston, 1906; Bizzaro, 1921; Cave, 1926; Hardman and Wigoder, 1928; Schultz, 1936; White, 1944; Rushforth, 1949; O'Rahilly, 1953a, 1956/57; Hughes and Tanner, 1966; Kohler *et al.*, 1968; Levine, 1972a; McCredie, 1975; Garn *et al.*, 1976a; Carlson, 1981). The nomenclature for these coalitions and supernumerary elements is confusing. O'Rahilly, (1953a) describes 28, while Kohler *et al.* (1968) describe 27 separate accessory ossicles and to prevent confusion they are probably best described in terms of their anatomical location, e.g. the os lunatotriquetrum, which is by far the most common carpal coalition (McConnell, 1906/07; Smith, 1908b; Saunders, 1942; Curr, 1946/47; Minnaar, 1952; O'Rahilly, 1953b; Wetherington, 1961; Szaboky *et al.*, 1969; Garn *et al.*, 1971). It has a reported incidence of 2–6% in Negroes and 0.1–0.5% in Caucasians (Silverman, 1955; Hughes and Tanner, 1966) and although generally asymptomatic, it can permit more extensive ulnar and radial deviation (Dean and Jones, 1959). The lack of a joint space may result in a loss of plasticity of the region and so the bone may be more susceptible to fracture (McGoey, 1943). Cavitation of the joint space between the lunate and triquetral bones occurs around 46–48 days and so from around the sixth week of embryonic life, the template has been set for the possibility of lunatotriquetral fusion (Gray *et al.*, 1957).

At approximately day 47, an independent area of chondrification appears at the distal end of the scaphoideum (forerunner of the scaphoid) between the trapezium, trapezoid and capitate. This is known as the 'centrale' and is visible in all embryos up to day 56 (Cihák, 1972; Caughell *et al.*, 1990). Around day 50, an interzone appears between the scaphoideum and the centrale, which eventually narrows until no visible dividing line can be detected around 3–4 fetal months (Fazekas and Kósa, 1978). If however, the interzone persists and a joint space does form, then the result will be a separate os centrale (O'Rahilly, 1954; Gerscovich and Greenspan, 1990). Some authors have considered this to be the phylogenetic remnant of a primitive central carpal row (Poznanski and Holt, 1971). The presence of an os centrale is often associated with developmental abnormalities such as Holt Oram syndrome and hand-foot-uterus syndrome (Poznanski *et al.*, 1970). However, in the majority of circumstances the cartilaginous centrale fuses with the scaphoideum and forms the part of the future scaphoid that articulates with the trapezium and the trapezoid. It habitually fuses on its palmar surface first and the dorsal surface eventually fuses some time later (Gray *et al.*, 1957). A tripartite scaphoid can develop when the scaphoideum arises in two parts (naviculare radiale and naviculare ulnare) and remains separate from the centrale (Pfitzner, 1895, 1900).

By day 56, the sesamoids of both the first metacarpophalangeal joint and the interphalangeal joints of the thumb are present either as blastemal condensations or have commenced chondrification (Gray *et al.*, 1957). Even at this early stage of development, the adult shape of the MCP sesamoids is established, with the lateral being more ovoid in shape and the medial more spherical (Gray *et al.*, 1957).

Interzones should be present in all joints by around day 56 (Gray *et al.*, 1957). Failure of joint formation in the digits results in the congenital fusion of one phalanx to another within a digit and this is known as symphalangism. It is an autosomal dominant condition, which manifests most frequently in the proximal interphalangeal joints and in particular that of the fifth digit (Freud and Slobody, 1943; Schwarz and Rivellini, 1963; Elkington and Huntsman, 1967; Harle and Stevenson, 1967). It is not surprising that the incidence of this condition is strongly linked to congenital carpal fusions and in particular to both triquetrohamate and capitohamate fusion (Ozonoff, 1979). The absence of the joint space does not result in digital fusion in the fetus, but is delayed until around 6–7 years of age, when epiphyseal activity would be accelerated resulting in premature and abnormal fusion.

It is interesting to note that up until the time of ossification it is reported that the male hand is in advance of the female hand in terms of maturation and development (Garn *et al.*, 1974). However, it is clear that once ossification commences, the female hand is in advance of the male hand by a matter of weeks initially, but by the end of adolescence this margin has increased to at least 2 years (Pryor, 1923; Garn *et al.*, 1975b). Garn (1962) and Garn *et al.* (1969) suggested that this sex-related delay in development could be explained by partial X-chromosome involvement, although other authors cited the retarding influence of the Y-chromosome as being responsible for the differences (Tanner *et al.*, 1959).

Ossification

We have been unable to discover a single text that describes in any detail, the morphology of the individual developing hand bones. The majority of descriptions refer to the radiological appearance of the bones and this often has little or no bearing on the true appearance of the dry bone. For this reason, our descriptions of the developing bones have had to rely on a relatively small sample size of juvenile hands of documented age at death, while the remainder is based on radiographic appearances.

There are a total of 48 separate centres of ossification in the hand (Fig. 9.28). Of these, 27 (29 if the sesamoids of the thumb are included) are primary centres and 19 are secondary. However, the pattern of ossification is quite unlike any other region of the skeleton (except that of the foot), as some primary centres arise in the early fetal period and the remainder do not occur until after birth, while the appearance of the secondary centres of ossification are interspersed between the sequential appearance of the primary centres. Therefore, for the sake of both clarity and conformity with the other chapters, the centres will still be considered under the headings of 'primary' and 'secondary', but the reader should be aware that there is no direct time continuity between these two sections. It should also be appreciated that there has been a considerable amount of research dedicated to the radiographic identification of appearance and fusion times in the hand and this has resulted in many slightly conflicting reports of the time of a specific event (see Chapter 2). It is certain that much of this interest has resulted not only from the ready availability of the hand for radiography but also the large number of centres of ossification provides a considerable amount of information regarding growth and maturity over an extended period of time. There is certainly a considerable amount of individual variability in the timing of events in the hand and when this is coupled with racial variation and environmental factors, it is clear that it is impossible to arrive at a universal date for the appearance of a specific centre or its ultimate fusion. Therefore, we have attempted to summarize much of the information available so that a relatively broad time spectrum of events is presented (Fig. 9.28). These timings should not, of course, be considered definitive.

Primary centres

Ossification first appears in the distal phalanges, followed closely by the metacarpals, proximal phalanges and finally the middle phalanges (Noback and Robertson, 1951). There is reported to be a tendency for the central digits to ossify in advance of the more marginal fingers (Gray *et al.*, 1957).

It is somewhat surprising that the first centres of ossification to appear in the hand occur in the **distal phalanges** as early as fetal weeks 7–9 (Hill, 1939; Flecker, 1942; Brailsford, 1943; Gray *et al.*, 1957; Jit, 1957; O'Rahilly *et al.*, 1959; Kjar, 1974; O'Rahilly and Gardner, 1975; Fazekas and Kósa, 1978; MacLaughlin-

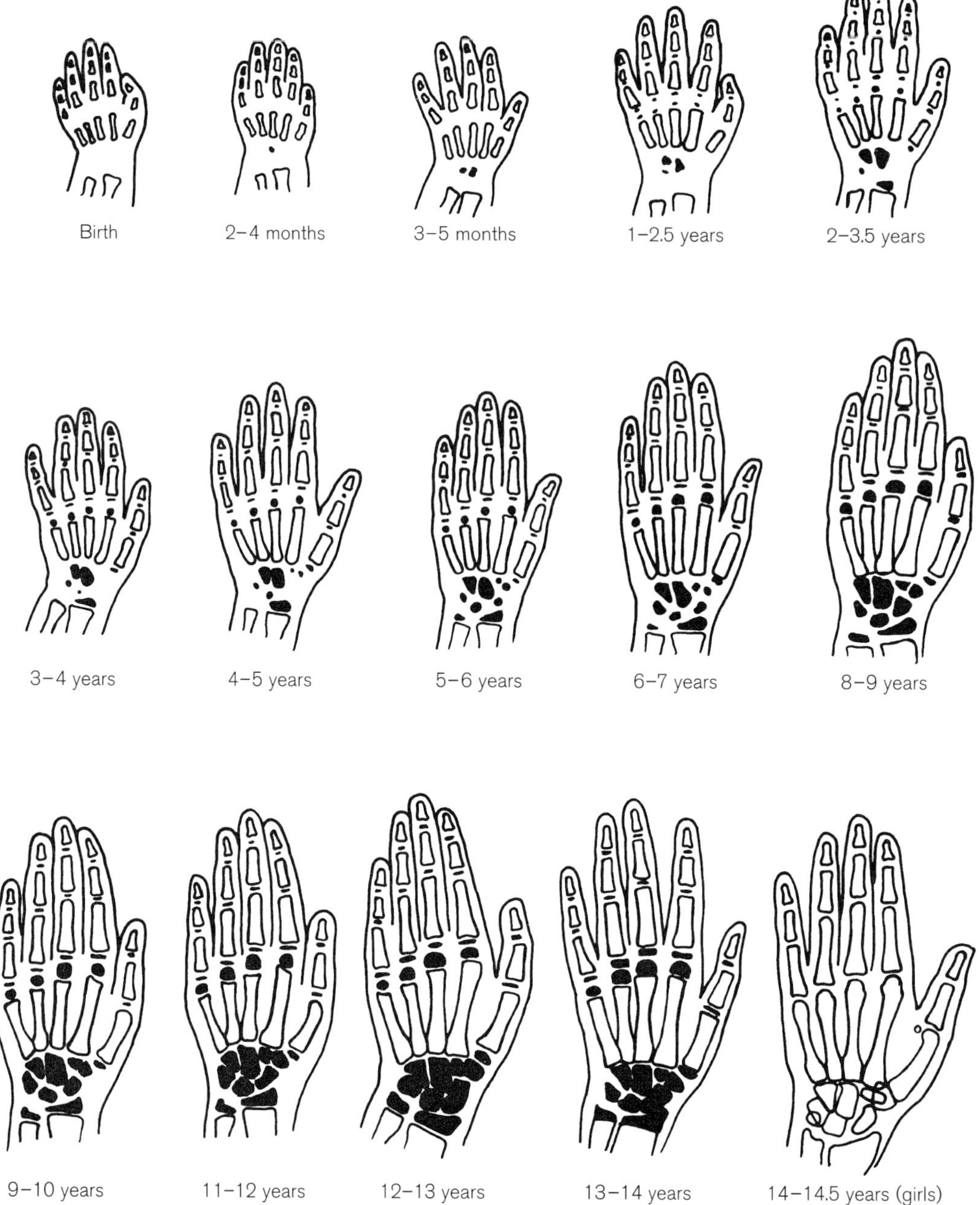

Figure 9.28 Various stages of osseous development in the hand from birth to the end of adolescence (redrawn after Birkner, 1978).

Black and Gunstone, 1995; Williams *et al.*, 1995). The ossification of a distal phalanx starts at the tip and progresses proximally. A shell of subperiosteal bone is deposited rather like a thimble over the cartilaginous phalanx while the ungual tuberosity forms by intramembranous ossification on the exterior of the subperiosteal cap (Dixey, 1881; Schuscik, 1918; Frazer, 1948; Gray *et al.*, 1957; Last, 1973). In all other phalanges, ossification commences with the development of a bony subperiosteal collar in the region of the midshaft. This precedes vascular invasion and the commencement of true endochondral ossification (O'Rahilly *et al.*, 1959).

Ossification in the **metacarpals** occurs shortly after that of the terminal phalanges, between fetal weeks 8 and 10 (Gray *et al.*, 1957; O'Rahilly *et al.*, 1959; O'Rahilly and Gardner, 1975) and commences in metacarpals 2 and 3 first, followed by 4 and 5 and finally by the first metacarpal. In all aspects of ossification and fusion the first metacarpal behaves more like a proximal phalanx than a metacarpal (Jit, 1957; Kjar, 1974; MacLaughlin-Black and Gunstone, 1995).

The primary centres of ossification for the **proximal phalanges** appear very shortly after that for the first metacarpal, in fetal weeks 9–11 (Flecker, 1942; Brailsford, 1943; Gray *et al.*, 1957; O'Rahilly *et al.*, 1959). The proximal phalanges of digits 2, 3 and 4 are the first to appear, followed by that for the thumb and finally that for digit 5 (Jit, 1957; Kjar, 1974; MacLaughlin-Black and Gunstone, 1995).

The **middle phalanges** are the last of the long bones of the hand to commence ossification. The phalanx for digits 2–4, appear in fetal weeks 10–12, while that for the fifth digit may not appear until close to term (Gray *et al.*, 1957). This relatively late appearance for this primary centre, in conjunction with premature epiphyseal fusion, may partly explain its susceptibility to growth disorders and its unique involvement in conditions such as brachymesophalangia (Hertzog, 1967). In this possibly autosomal recessive inherited disorder, it is typically the middle phalanx of digit 5 that is affected and it appears both wider and shorter than in the normal situation (Blanco *et al.*, 1973; Garn *et al.*, 1976b; Buschang and Malina, 1980; Cybulski, 1988). Not only has a higher incidence of brachymesophalangia-5 has been reported in Asiatic groups (Sutow and West, 1955; Pryde and Kitabatake, 1959; Garn *et al.*, 1967c; Hertzog, 1967), but it also tends to be prevalent in disorders such as Down's syndrome (Roche, 1961; Garn *et al.*, 1972a; Greulich, 1973).

In summary, the primary centres of ossification for the metacarpals and phalanges are all present (with the possible exception of the middle phalanx of digit 5) by the beginning of the fourth fetal month and they are individually recognizable, certainly in a radiograph, by the fifth month (Gunstone, 1992). From this stage until birth no further primary ossification centres develop.

From the earliest fetal age, the first metacarpal is stunted in length compared to the other metacarpals, and it is much more robust (Fig. 9.29). It is certainly identifiable from an early fetal age as it bears a somewhat rounded distal end with a flattened proximal end that is almost circular in outline and clearly metaphyseal. The remainder of the developing metacarpals are true to the standard morphology of a long bone, bearing a diaphysis which is virtually cylindrical in outline, slightly waisted in the middle but expanded at both ends. Unlike other long bones, however, they only bear a metaphyseal surface at their distal extremity, thus in the early stages of development the distal extremities are flat and the proximal are rounded until they develop their characteristic basal form.

From early fetal life, the second metacarpal is usually the longest of the five and it can be readily identified by birth, as its distal end is displaced somewhat laterally, while its proximal end shows a medial displacement, thereby giving the bone a slightly sinuous outline (Fig. 9.29). The bone retains this morphology until approximately 3.5–4.5 years of age when the lateral aspect of the base begins to develop and expand proximally. The second metacarpal adopts its characteristic condylar-shaped proximal extremity around 4–5 years of age, concomitant with the appearance of the ossification centre for the trapezoid.

At birth, the third metacarpal is slightly shorter than the second, with a flat distal extremity that is somewhat rectangular in outline with a gently rounded distal extremity (Fig. 9.29). There is no sinuous shape to the diaphysis. Due to its lack of any specific morphology, this metacarpal is not easily distinguished until the intermetacarpal articular sites start to develop. From approximately 5–6 years of age, the proximal surface adopts a roughly triangular outline, although the reciprocal concave lateral border for the second metacarpal may be present slightly earlier at 4 years of age. The styloid process is the most characteristic trait of this metacarpal but it does not develop until around 11–12 years of age and then appears as a slowly developing proximal elongation of the dorsolateral surface (Fig. 9.30).

The fourth metacarpal is considerably shorter than either the second or third and only marginally longer than the fifth (Fig. 9.29). The morphology of the fourth metacarpal is not distinct until the intermetacarpal articulations develop around 4–5 years of age. The fifth metacarpal can be identified at an early age by a number of factors – it is the shortest (true from early fetal life); the proximal end is slightly bulbous and deviates laterally (true from approximately the first year); there is no articular region on the medial side (identifiable around 4–5 years). These intermetacarpal articulations probably develop at different ages for different joints, but they are certainly apparent in some specimens by 4 years of age.

At birth, the proximal phalanges look too robust and too wide to be associated with the heads of the appropriate metacarpals (Fig. 9.29). The first proximal phalanx is shorter than the others and has three virtually straight sides with a curved distal surface. The remainder of the proximal phalanges are somewhat dumb-bell-shaped with expanded proximal and distal extremities and a constriction in the midshaft. The distal surface is rounded and notched, while the

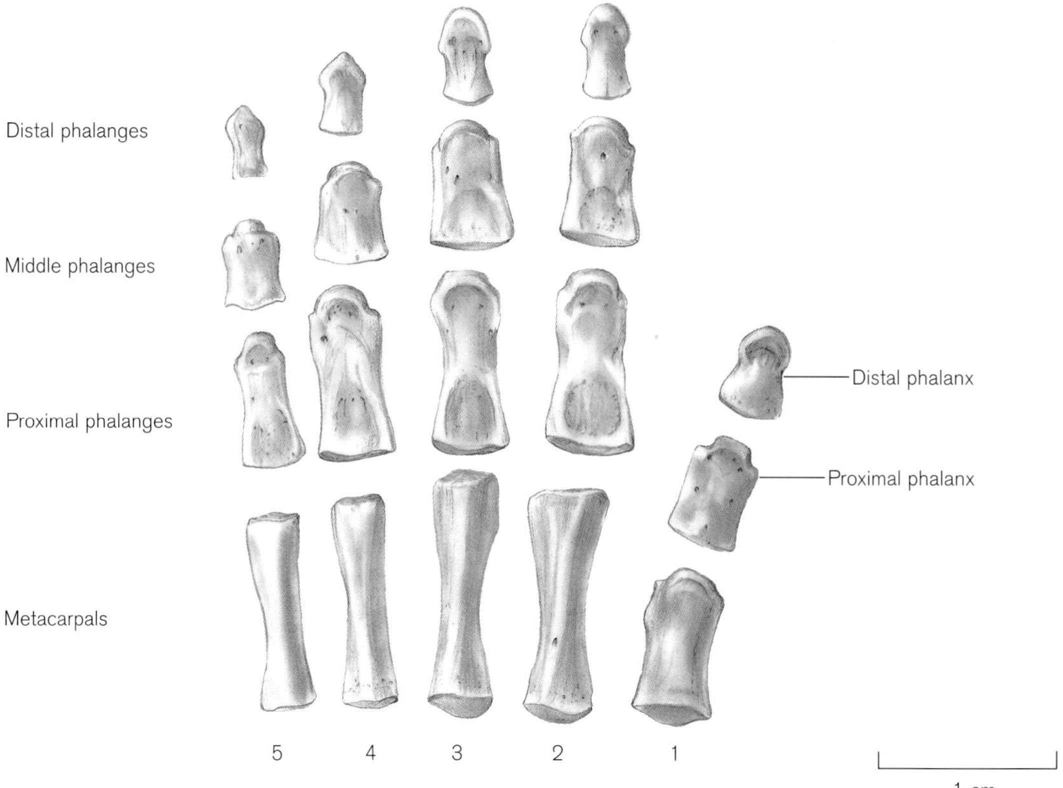

Figure 9.29 The right perinatal hand.

proximal surface is flat with a transversely oval outline that shows a slight concavity on the palmar surface.

The middle phalanges are smaller than their proximal counterparts and they lack the distinctive constriction in the midshaft region (Fig. 9.29). This makes them somewhat dome-shaped, with a rounded but notched distal extremity and medial and lateral borders that flare proximally to terminate at the transversely oval proximal surface, which does not display the concavity seen in the proximal phalanges.

From even the fetal stage of development, the distal phalanges are harpoon-shaped with rounded or pointed distal margins that are flattened on the volar (palmar) surface and display the characteristic barb-like structures that abut onto the shaft (Fig. 9.29). The first distal phalanx is more robust than the others and although it is not necessarily longer, it is obviously wider.

The second group of primary centres of ossification in the hand form the carpal bones and these are almost exclusively postnatal in terms of their time of appearance, although Menees and Holly (1932) have reported that the capitate was present at birth in approximately 4% of their male sample and 8% of their female sample, while the hamate was also present in almost identical percentages (Hess and Weinstock, 1925; O'Rahilly *et al.*, 1959). The order of appearance of ossification in the carpal region is well documented, although dysharmonic patterns do arise in situations of congenital malformations or environmental adversities (Dreizen *et al.*, 1958; Johnston and Jahina, 1965; Poznanski *et al.*, 1971b). Maturation in the hand, and particularly in the carpal region, has assumed considerable clinical significance as a reflection of the state of skeletal maturation in the rest of the body. For this reason, several atlases of skeletal development in the hand are available (Poland, 1898; Todd, 1937; Vogt and Vickers, 1938; Speijer, 1950; Sutow and Ohwada, 1953; Greulich and Pyle, 1959; Tanner and Whitehouse, 1959; Schmid and Moll, 1960; Acheson, 1966; Pyle *et al.*, 1971; Meschan, 1975; de Roo and Schröder, 1976; Tanner *et al.*, 1983; Himes, 1984).

The normal sequence of appearance for the carpal bones is that the capitate appears first, followed closely by the hamate and later by the triquetral and then the lunate. The trapezium, trapezoid and scaphoid all appear at approximately the same time and so their order can be interchangeable, dependent upon the sample under investigation. It is interesting

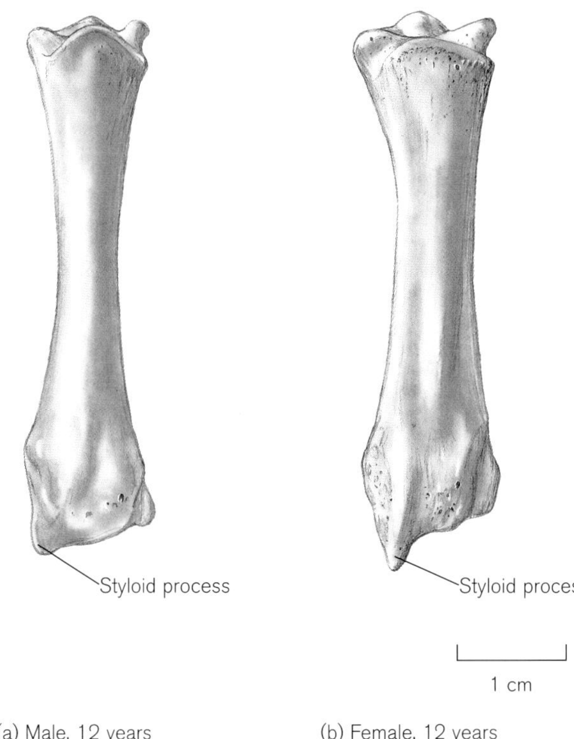

Figure 9.30 The development of the styloid process of the right third metacarpal.

to note that the pattern of appearance of the carpal centres follows an almost circular route. It starts with ossification in the capitate, moves laterally into the hamate and triquetral, before moving proximally into the lunate and finally completing the circuit with the virtually simultaneous appearance of the scaphoid, trapezium and trapezoid. It is not known whether or not any functional significance can be attributed to this pattern. Last (1973) reported that the carpals ossify in order according to their ultimate adult size, with the largest usually forming first and the smallest last, but this is not strictly true, given that both the lunate and the triquetral are smaller than the scaphoid but they ossify in advance of it by almost 2 years. The sesamoids of the thumb and the pisiform bone are the last primary centres to appear (Beresowski and Lundie, 1952).

When disarticulated, the carpal bones are really only identifiable once they take on their adult form. While it is possible to positively identify each bone from radiographs because of its anatomical position, this information is clearly lost when the specimen is only represented by dry bone (Fig. 9.28). Until virtually adult morphology is achieved, carpal bones are represented by small, undifferentiated nodules of bone.

The **capitate** is the first carpal to undergo ossification and although a bony centre can be present at birth it most frequently appears between the second and third postnatal month in girls and the third and fourth months in boys (Holden, 1882; Hess and Weinstock, 1925; Pryor, 1925; Davies and Parsons, 1927; Paterson, 1929; Francis *et al.*, 1939; Hill, 1939; Pyle and Sontag, 1943; Elgenmark, 1946; Harding, 1952a; MacKay, 1952; O'Rahilly *et al.*, 1959; Hansman, 1962; Stuart *et al.*, 1962; Acheson, 1966; Garn *et al.*, 1967b; Birkner, 1978). It commences as a small, rounded nodule of bone that soon develops a vertically aligned long axis with that of the third metacarpal. Its articular surface with the hamate starts to flatten around 10 months in girls and 12 months in boys and by 1 year in girls and 1.5 years in boys it is said to resemble a reversed 'D' (Pyle *et al.*, 1971). By 1.5 years in girls and 2 years in boys, the articular surface with the hamate begins to show a distinct concavity, but in real terms the bone is fairly indistinct before 2 years of age (Todd, 1937). At around 2.5 years in girls and 3 years in boys the lateral surface of the capitate shows a distinct indent, which marks the site of attachment of the large interosseous ligament between the trapezoid and scaphoid articular surfaces (Todd, 1937). The capitate can usually be identified in isolation by 3–4 years of age. At 3 years in girls and 4 years in boys the facet for the second metacarpal has formed an obtuse angle with the articular facet for the trapezoid. The articular surface for the second metacarpal has flattened by 4 years in girls and 5 years in boys and the bone continues to expand, particularly in a vertical direction. At approximately 8.5 years in girls and 9.5 years in boys, there is a sharp angle of demarcation between the articular facets for the second and third metacarpals. The bone has virtually reached its full adult proportions by 11.5 years in girls and 14 years in boys and is essentially adult by 13 years in girls and 15 years in boys (Pyle *et al.*, 1971).

The ossification centre for the **hamate** appears very shortly after that for the capitate at around 3–4 months in girls and 4–5 months in boys (Holden, 1882; Hess and Weinstock, 1925; Pryor, 1925; Davies and Parsons, 1927; Paterson, 1929; Francis *et al.*, 1939; Hill, 1939; Pyle and Sontag, 1943; Elgenmark, 1946; Harding, 1952a; MacKay, 1952; O'Rahilly *et al.*, 1959; Hansman, 1962; Stuart *et al.*, 1962; Acheson, 1966; Garn *et al.*, 1967b; Birkner, 1978). It appears as a small, roughened nodule, slightly distal to the capitate and aligned with the space between the fourth and fifth metacarpal bones (Pyle *et al.*, 1971). Some authors have suggested that it can develop from two separate foci of ossification, which reflects its functional position of supporting two metacarpal bases (Frazer, 1948). This somewhat rounded ossific nodule develops a long oblique axis by 6 postnatal months in females and 7 months in males. The capitate surface becomes somewhat flattened around 7 months in girls and 9 months in boys, while flattening of the triquetral surface begins around 10 months and 12 months respectively. The developing hamate assumes the shape of an inverted triangle with a convex capitate margin at approximately 1 year in girls and 1.5 years in boys, but the bone is essentially featureless, like the capitate, until around 2 years of age. The articular surface adjacent to the metacarpals flattens around 3 years in girls and 4 years in boys and the triquetral facet becomes well-defined by 4 years and 5 years respectively. It is at this stage that the hamate can be identified in isolation. By 6 years in females and 7 years in males, the triquetral surface shows an indentation and the metacarpal sites are flat. It is not until 7 years in females and 8 years in males that the bone is clearly wedge-shaped with a squared corner at the capitate-metacarpal junction. By 9 years in girls and 11 years in boys the saddle shape of the articular surface for the fifth metacarpal is well defined. The concavity of the triquetral surface is clear by 10 years in girls and 12 years in boys and the saddle-shaped surface for metacarpal 4 is clearly defined. At this stage, the hamulus is visible radiographically but it is not distinct until 11 years and 14 years, respectively. The hamate reaches adult morphology and proportions by 12 years in girls and 15 years in boys (Pyle *et al.*, 1971).

There is a gap of at least a year until the third carpal centre appears. This is for the **triquetral** and is said to form in the first year by some authors (Davies and Parsons, 1927; Francis *et al.*, 1939) in the second year by others (Robinow, 1942; Pyle and Sontag, 1943; Elgenmark, 1946; Harding, 1952a; O'Rahilly *et al.*, 1959; Acheson, 1966; Garn *et al.*, 1967b; Pyle *et al.*, 1971; Fazekas and Kósa, 1978) and even in the third year by others (Holden, 1882; Pryor, 1925; Paterson, 1929; Frazer, 1948; Hansman, 1962; Stuart *et al.*, 1962; Birkner, 1978; Williams *et al.*, 1995). Not surprisingly, Johnston *et al.* (1968) reported that the variability of time of onset of ossification of the triquetral rendered it of little value in estimating the skeletal age of an individual. It is probably as a result of the considerable degree of variation in timings of events in the hand, that many authors have abandoned estimating skeletal age on the basis of appearance and relied more heavily on the number of centres present at any one time, rather than on which specific bone is present (Sontag *et al.*, 1939; Garn and Rohmann, 1960; Lee *et al.*, 1966; Kjar, 1974; MacLaughlin-Black and Gunstone, 1995). Greulich and Pyle (1959) found that the triquetral became recognizably triangular by around 3.5 years in girls and 4.5 years in boys and by 6 months later the hamate and lunate surfaces had begun to flatten, while the non-articular margin remained convex. A distinct corner was present at the hamate–lunate junction by 6 years in girls and 7 years in boys and by a year later the bone was distinctly wedge-shaped. The concavity of the hamate surface was visible by 8.5 years in girls and 10 years in boys and it is at this stage that the triquetral can be identified in isolation. They reported that there was little change in either the size or shape of the bone after 12 years in girls and 15 years in boys.

The **lunate** is the fourth carpal to commence ossification and it does so around 3 years in girls and 4 years in boys (Pryor, 1925; Davies and Parsons, 1927; Paterson, 1929; Robinow, 1942; Harding, 1952a; MacKay, 1952; Hansman, 1962; Stuart *et al.*, 1962; Acheson, 1966; Pyle *et al.*, 1971) and often from more than one focus of ossification (O'Rahilly *et al.*, 1959). The lunate develops a long transverse axis with a bevelled lateral border, a pointed scaphoid region and a rounded triquetral half by 4 years in girls and 5 years in boys. The lunate can be identified in isolation at around 9–10 years of age. Little change in size and shape occurs after 12.5 years in girls and 15 years in boys.

The centres of ossification for the trapezium and trapezoid appear at approximately the same time and there is some conflict in the literature as to which appears first, although the majority seems to agree that it is the **trapezium**. This is said to appear around 4 years in girls and 5 years in boys (Acheson, 1966) and it soon develops a long axis, which is directed towards the second metacarpal joint. The margin adjacent to the first metacarpal flattens within the next year and by 6 years in girls and 7 years in boys the bone has developed a squared outline. The concavity of the saddle joint is visible radiologically by 9 years in girls and 10 years in boys and, at this stage, the bone can be positively identified in isolation. The projection of the distal surface between the two metacarpals is well defined by 11.5 years in girls and 14 years in boys. The bone reaches its full adult shape and size by 12.5 years in girls and 15 years in boys (Pyle *et al.*, 1971).

The **trapezoid** commences ossification at approximately the same age as the trapezium and its angular outline is well defined radiologically by 5 years in girls and 6 years in boys. The convexity of the second metacarpal surface is visible by 7 years in girls and 8 years in boys and the proximal margin is concave by 8.5 and 10 years, respectively. It is at this stage of development that the dry bone can be positively identified in isolation. The bone reaches adult proportions by 12.5 and 15 years, respectively.

The **scaphoid** commences ossification around 5 years in girls and 6 years in boys and a long axis is visible very shortly afterwards (Paterson, 1929; Sawtell, 1929; Lurie *et al.*, 1943; Frazer, 1948; Harding, 1952a; MacKay, 1952; Hansman, 1962; Acheson, 1966; Garn *et al.*, 1967b; Pyle *et al.*, 1971). By approximately a year later, the area next to the radial styloid process has flattened and the long axis is clearly aligned with the centre of the radiocarpal joint (Pyle *et al.*, 1971). Within the next year (7 for girls and 8 for boys) the scaphoid becomes distinctly 'teardrop'-shaped, with the pointed end lying nearest to the styloid process of the radius and the distal surface has become rounded. The capitate surface is concave and the trapezium and trapezoid surfaces are flattened with a distinct demarcation angle between them by 8.5 years in girls and 10 years in boys. An indent is clearly visible between the radial and trapezial surfaces by 9.5 years in girls and 11 years in boys and it is at this stage that the dry bone can be identified in isolation. The scaphoid tubercle does not become radiologically distinct until 11 years in girls and 14 years in boys. The bone reaches its adult shape and size by approximately 12.5 years in girls and 15 years in boys.

A non-traumatic divided scaphoid (os scaphoideum bipartitum) is well documented and probably arises from dual centres of ossification which fail to unite. The division between the two centres occurs across the waist of the bone and it has often been associated with a free os centrale (Dwight, 1907b; Boyd, 1933; O'Rahilly, 1953a).

The **sesamoids** are the last bones in the hand to commence ossification. The **pisiform** appears radiologically by 8 years in females and by 10 years in males (Francis, 1940; Michelson, 1945; Frazer, 1948; Harding, 1952a; O'Rahilly *et al.*, 1959; Hansman, 1962; Pyle *et al.*, 1971). The bone enlarges to adult size by 12.5 years in females and 15 years in males (Pyle *et al.*, 1971). The sesamoids associated with both the thumb and the fifth digit appear between 11 and 15 years of age in girls and 13 and 18 years in boys (Paterson, 1929; Francis, 1940; Lurie *et al.*, 1943; Kelley and Reynolds, 1947; Joseph, 1951b; Harding, 1952a; MacKay, 1952; Garn and Rohmann, 1962b; Hansman, 1962; Stuart *et al.*, 1962; Garn *et al.*, 1967b; Onat and Numan-Cebeci, 1976; Birkner, 1978).

Secondary centres

Appearance

There are four morphologically distinct groups of epiphyses in the long bones of the hand – the heads of the metacarpals and the bases of the proximal, middle and distal phalanges. Unlike the situation found in the other long bones of the skeleton, where epiphyses arise at both the proximal and distal poles, in the hand, they tend to be restricted to one end of the bone, although in rare circumstances true supernumerary epiphyses have been documented. It is a general rule that with the exception of the first metacarpal, the heads of all other metacarpals ossify from a separate secondary centre of ossification. The first metacarpal behaves like a proximal phalanx, as all phalanges ossify from a single centre that forms the shaft and the distal articular surface, while the base of the bone at its proximal extremity forms from a separate secondary centre of ossification.

There are several reports in the literature that state the **order of appearance** of the secondary centres and, of course, few of these actually agree. Therefore, we have summarized the views of the following papers and presented the most frequently reported pattern for secondary centre ossification (Francis *et al.*, 1939; Pyle and Sontag, 1943; Harding, 1952a; Greulich and Pyle, 1959; Garn and Rohmann, 1960; Stuart *et al.*, 1962; Acheson, 1966; Garn *et al.*, 1967b; Birkner, 1978). The general rule is, that the secondary centres in the bases of the proximal phalanges are the first to appear, followed closely by those for the metacarpal heads, then the middle phalangeal bases and finally by the distal phalangeal bases (Fig. 9.31). There is, however, a considerable degree of individual and population-related variation within this general pattern (Garn and Rohmann, 1960; Garn and McCreery, 1970; Pyle *et al.*, 1971).

After birth, it is clear that the capitate and hamate centres of the wrist are consistently the first evidence of continued ossification but that the base of the third proximal phalanx follows them very shortly at around 10 months in girls and 14 months in boys (Pyle and Sontag, 1943; Elgenmark, 1946; Hansman, 1962; Stuart *et al.*, 1962; Garn *et al.*, 1967b). The ossification for the base of the second proximal phalanx appears at approximately 14 months in girls and 19 months in boys, while that for the fourth proximal phalanx appears at approximately the same time but marginally later. The head of the second metacarpal appears around 16 months in girls and 22 months in boys, followed by that for the base of the distal phalanx of the first digit at approximately 17 months in girls and 22 months in boys. The head of the third metacarpal appears around 17 months in girls and 24 months in boys, while the fifth proximal phalangeal base appears shortly afterwards at 17 months in girls and 2 years 1 month in boys. The head for the fourth metacarpal appears around 18 months in girls and 2 years 1 month in boys, while that for the base of the middle phalanx of the third digit appears around 19 months and 2 years 4 months, respectively. Ossification of the base of the fourth middle phalanx, the head of the fifth metacarpal and the base of the second middle phalanx all appear around the same time of 19 months in girls and 2 years 5 months in boys. Although the appearance of the triquetral is somewhat variable, it is approximately at this stage of development when the capitate, hamate, heads of metacarpals 2–5, bases of proximal phalanges 2–5, bases of middle phalanges 2–4 and the base of the first distal phalanx have been formed (i.e. 2 years in girls and 2.5 years in boys). The bases of the distal phalanges of the third and fourth digits appear next at approximately 2 years in girls and 2 years 8 months in boys and the centres for the base of the first metacarpal and the base of the first proximal phalanx coincide at approximately 2 years 1 month in girls and 3 years 2 months in boys. It has been reported that it is not uncommon for the epiphysis at the base of the first proximal phalanx to be formed from more than one focus of ossification (Roche and Sunderland, 1959). It is around this time that the ossification centre appears for the distal end of the radius. The distal phalanx of digit 2 appears around 2 years 4 months in girls and 3 years 7 months in boys, while the centres for the bases of the distal and middle phalanges of digit 5 are the last to appear, at approximately 2 years 5 months in girls and 3 years 7 months in boys. Therefore, by 2.5 years in girls and approximately 3.5 years in boys the secondary ossification centres for the long bones of the hand are all present and it is only the centres for the lunate, trapezium, trapezoid, scaphoid and pisiform bones that are still not present.

The **metacarpal heads** appear as small undifferentiated rounded nodules of bone until approximately 5 or 6 years of age. After this time, they become recognisable as metacarpal heads with rounded articular distal surfaces, flattened proximal metaphyseal surfaces and roughly square-shaped outlines. From this age onwards, they continue to approach the adult morphology. Identification of individual metacarpal heads is difficult and confidence will be greatest when only one individual is present (Fig. 9.32). Due to their larger size, the second and third heads can be readily separated from those of the fourth and fifth metacarpals. When the distal articular surfaces are viewed from above, the head of the second metacarpal is almost stellate in appearance, displaying prolongations from each corner. The ventrolateral corner is well developed because of the presence of a sesamoid bone and although the dorsomedial aspect also looks well developed it is mainly due to the fact that its contemporary dorsolateral prolongation is foreshortened, due to the

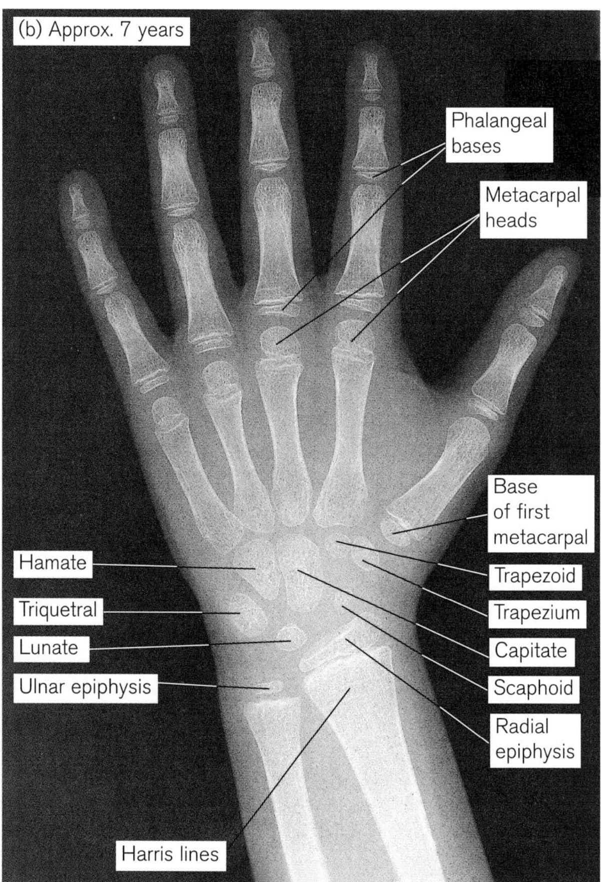

Figure 9.31 Radiographs of the developing hand and wrist.

intrusion of the large second metacarpophalangeal ligament that attaches to this surface. The head of the third metacarpal appears more square in outline, principally due to the lesser development of the ventrolateral corner. However, the dorsomedial prolongation is still well developed, again due to the foreshortening of the dorsolateral corner by the attachment of the relatively strong third metacarpophalangeal ligament. The heads of the third and fourth metacarpals are more difficult to identify, although they are noticeably smaller than those of the more lateral metacarpals. They are both almost square in outline but that of the fifth metacarpal displays a slight paring away of the dorsomedial angle of the synovial articular surface. The ventromedial corner can show evidence of prolongation due to the presence of the sesamoid in the abductor tendon. Despite this, the only way to ensure correct identification of a metacarpal head is to be able to fit it securely to a specific metacarpal shaft and this can be achieved only from approximately 9–10 years of age.

The proximal metaphyseal surfaces of the metacarpal heads are quite distinctive (Fig. 9.32). Those of the second and third metacarpals are floral-shaped with rounded corners and distinct waistings that form petal-like shapes. As a result, four deep crevasses are clearly defined on this surface. The proximal surfaces of metacarpals four and five are flatter and although they do still display the characteristic roundings and constrictions, they are less well developed.

Brailsford (1953) described the epiphyses of the **proximal phalanges** as ‘flattened discs having a slightly convex distal surface and a slightly concave proximal surface’. This is certainly true, but there are several details that have not been included and it is somewhat ironic that it is easier to side juvenile proximal phalangeal epiphyses than the equivalent fused adult bone. The epiphysis of the first proximal phalanx is noticeably wider in its transverse than in its ventrodorsal plane (Fig. 9.33). It is almost oval in outline, although the palmar surface is gently concave and the dorsal border is clearly convex. When viewed from the front, this epiphysis displays a slightly sinuous outline with a distally orientated prolongation laterally that will fuse with the shaft and a proximally oriented prolongation medially. As for all these epiphyses, and in agreement with Brailsford (1953), the proximal surface is markedly concave, while the distal metaphyseal surface is very gently convex.

Despite a concavity along the ventral border, the epiphysis of the second proximal phalanx is virtually square in outline (Fig. 9.33). When viewed from the front, it is clearly wedge-shaped, being thicker on its

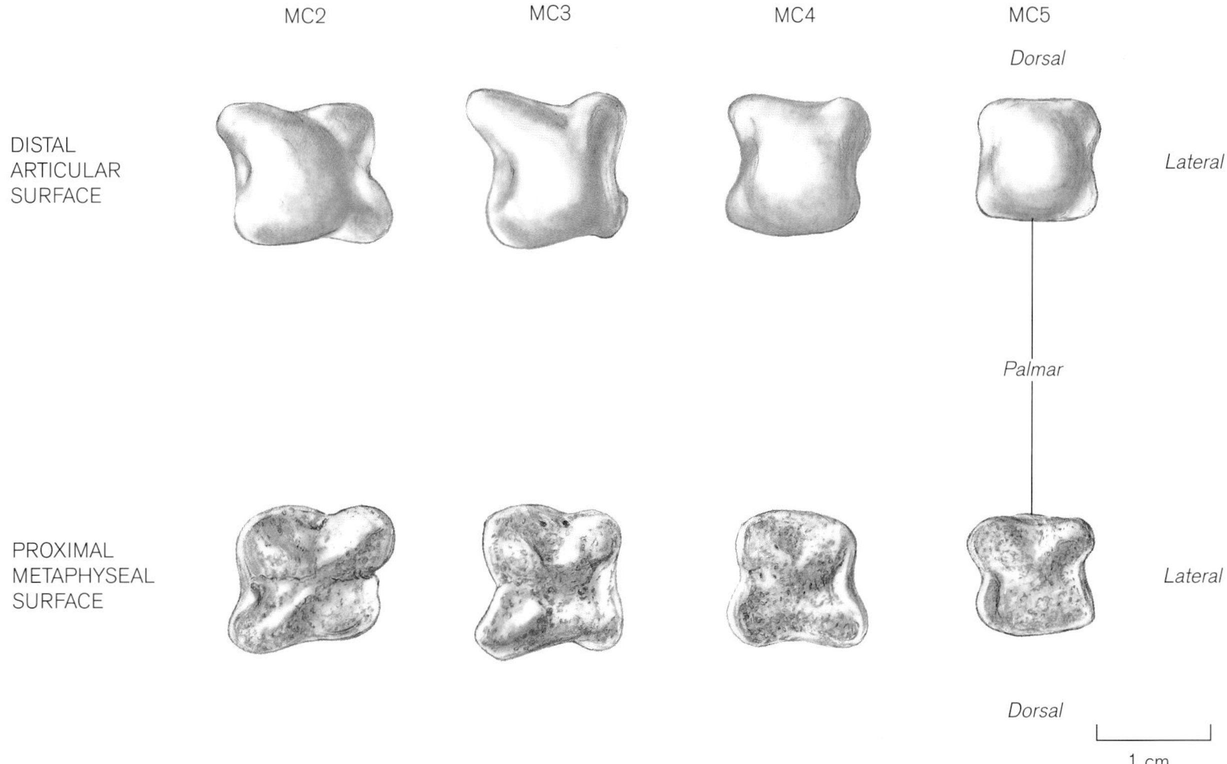

Figure 9.32 The distal and proximal surfaces of right metacarpal heads 2–5.

lateral than its medial aspect. The base of the third proximal phalanx also displays this wedge shape and the concavity along the ventral border, but it is clearly wider in its transverse than in its ventrodorsal plane. In addition, the lateral border is more blunt and the medial border tends to end anteriorly in a sharper projection. The epiphysis of the fourth proximal phalanx displays a semicircular outline with a concave ventral border, which has a more prominent projection on the medial aspect. The epiphysis of the fifth proximal phalanx is the smallest and adopts a more oval outline, with only a gentle hint of a concave ventral border. The lateral aspect of this border is more blunt, while the medial aspect is more pointed.

Brailsford (1953) described the epiphyses of the **middle phalanges** as 'plano-convex shaped discs – the convex surface being opposed to the slightly concave distal extremity of the proximal phalanx'. This description is not quite true, as the discs are essentially biconvex proximally, with a separating ridge that runs from a promontory on the ventral to a similar promontory on the dorsal border (Fig. 9.34). The epiphysis is essentially oval in outline, being longer in the transverse plane, although the ventral border is more gently convex, while the dorsal border is more obviously rounded. The distal metaphyseal surface is convex from ventral to dorsal, with the latter showing a steeper slope down to the dorsal border. From medial to lateral, the distal surface shows a roughly central hollow (corresponding to the ridge on the proximal surface), flanked by a medial and a lateral elevation that correspond with the concavities of the proximal surface. We have found that attempting to side these epiphyses or indeed assign them to a specific ray, is extremely difficult and in our opinion it cannot be done with any degree of confidence.

Brailsford (1953) described the epiphyses of the **distal phalanges** simply as 'biconcave discs about the same width as the base of the diaphyses of the terminal phalanges'. This description is somewhat misleading, as the epiphyses of the middle phalanges are more obviously biconcave and further, the epiphyses tend to be wider than diaphyses (Fig. 9.35). The proximal articular surfaces of the epiphyses of the distal phalanges are concave from ventral to dorsal and slightly convex from medial to lateral. Although essentially biconcave, a delimiting ridge is not so clearly defined

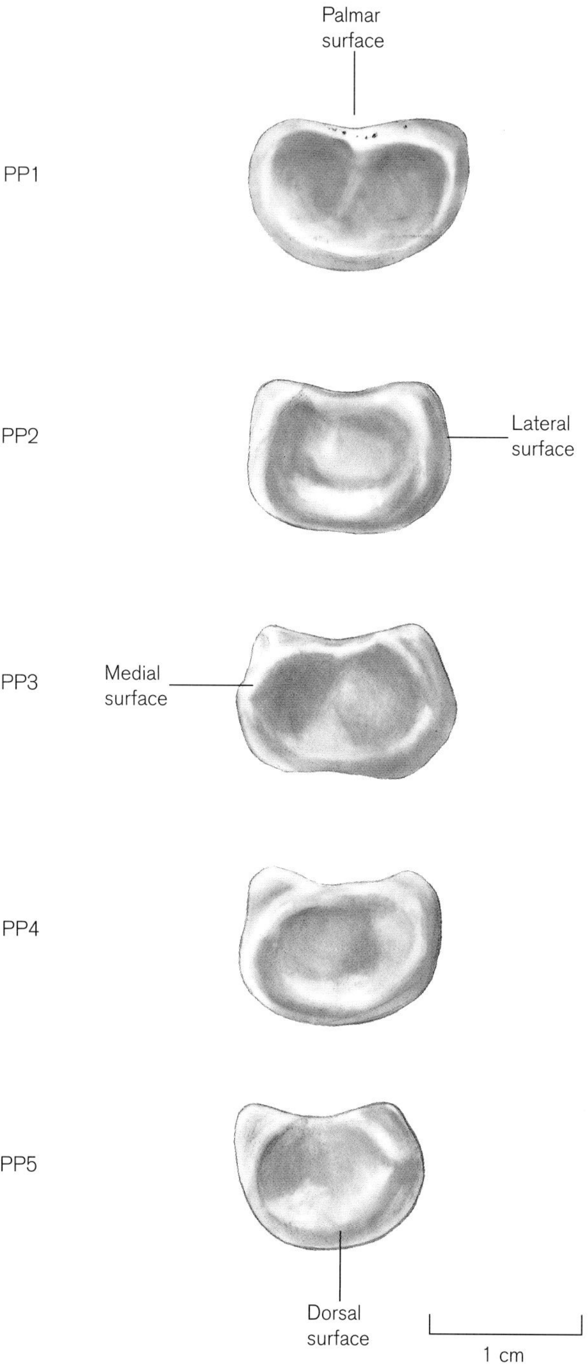

Figure 9.33 The epiphyses of the right proximal phalanges.

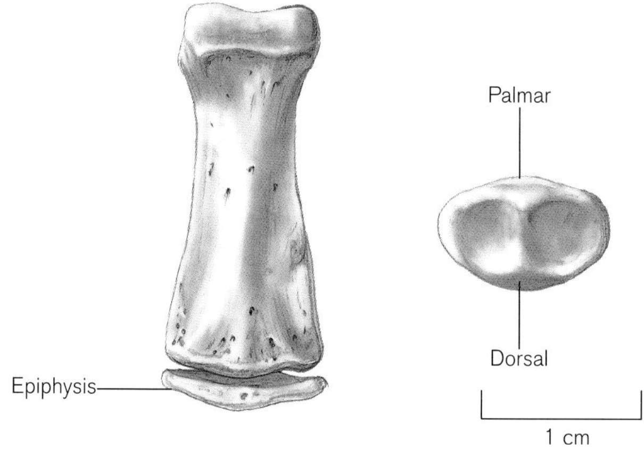

Figure 9.34 The right middle phalangeal epiphysis.

as seen in the articular surface of the middle phalanges. At around 10–11 years of age, the ventral border develops a medial and a lateral tongue of bone that pass upwards towards the diaphysis of the phalanx and so form a stable cup-shape in which the diaphysis sits. These tongues presumably form in response to the attachments of the profundus flexor tendon. The dorsal surface does not respond in a similar manner and in fact it dips somewhat proximally, thereby forming a sloping distal metaphyseal surface, which is clearly convex from ventral to dorsal and concave from medial to lateral. We have been unable to correctly assign epiphyses to specific distal phalanges with any degree of reliability, with the exception, of course, of that for the thumb (Fig. 9.35). This is a much larger epiphysis than for any of the other terminal phalanges, is distinctly oval in outline and clearly biconcave. Yet, in all other ways it is identical to the other epiphyses for terminal phalanges.

The epiphysis for the **base of the first metacarpal** is sufficiently different from all the other hand epiphyses to merit a separate description (Fig. 9.36). It is well developed by 7–8 years of age, but can probably not be accurately identified until around 9–10 years. The distal metaphyseal surface is virtually circular in outline and almost planar, although there is a slight slope down towards the dorsal border. The lateral border of the epiphysis develops an upward-projecting tongue of bone that fits into a corresponding recess on the lateral aspect of the diaphysis. The proximal aspect of the ventral border ends in the well-developed styloid process, which is connected to a corresponding process on the dorsal surface and thereby demarcates the bicondylar articular surface.

Fusion

Not surprisingly, the order of **fusion** of the secondary to the primary centres does not mirror their order of

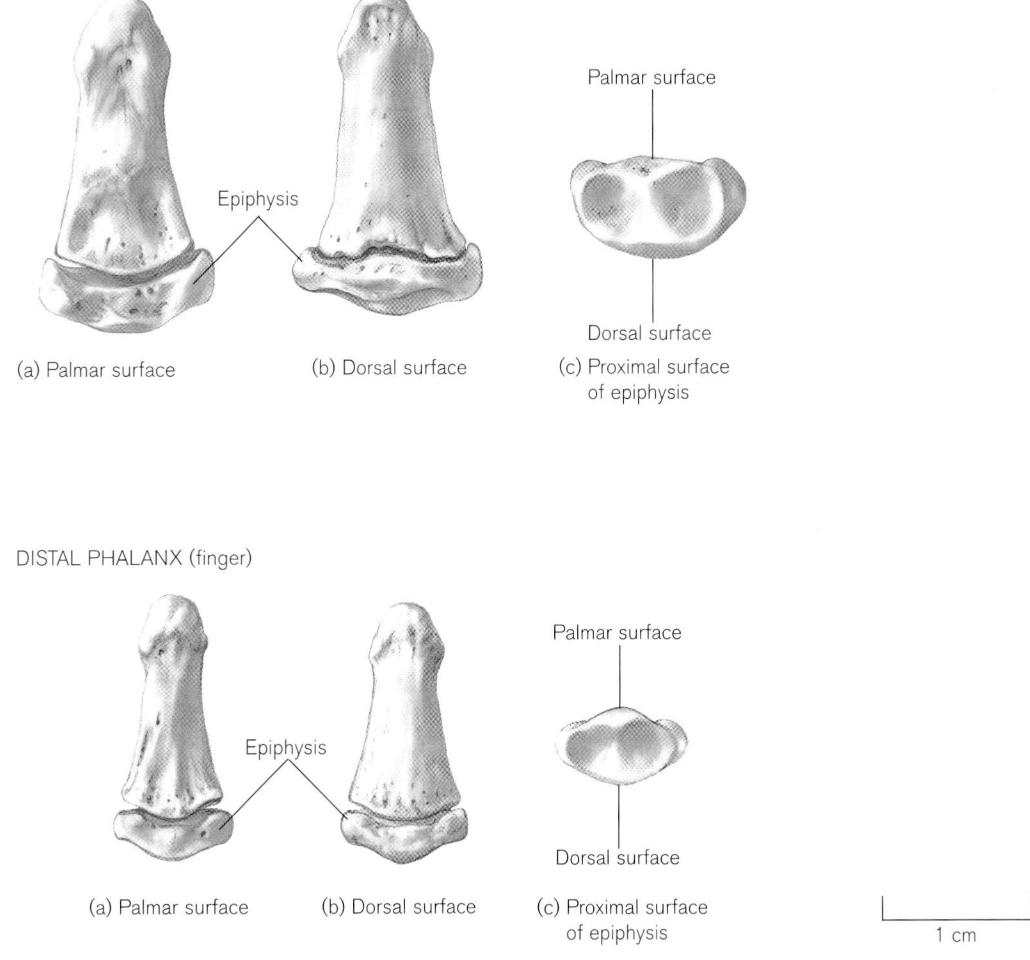

Figure 9.35 The right distal phalangeal epiphyses.

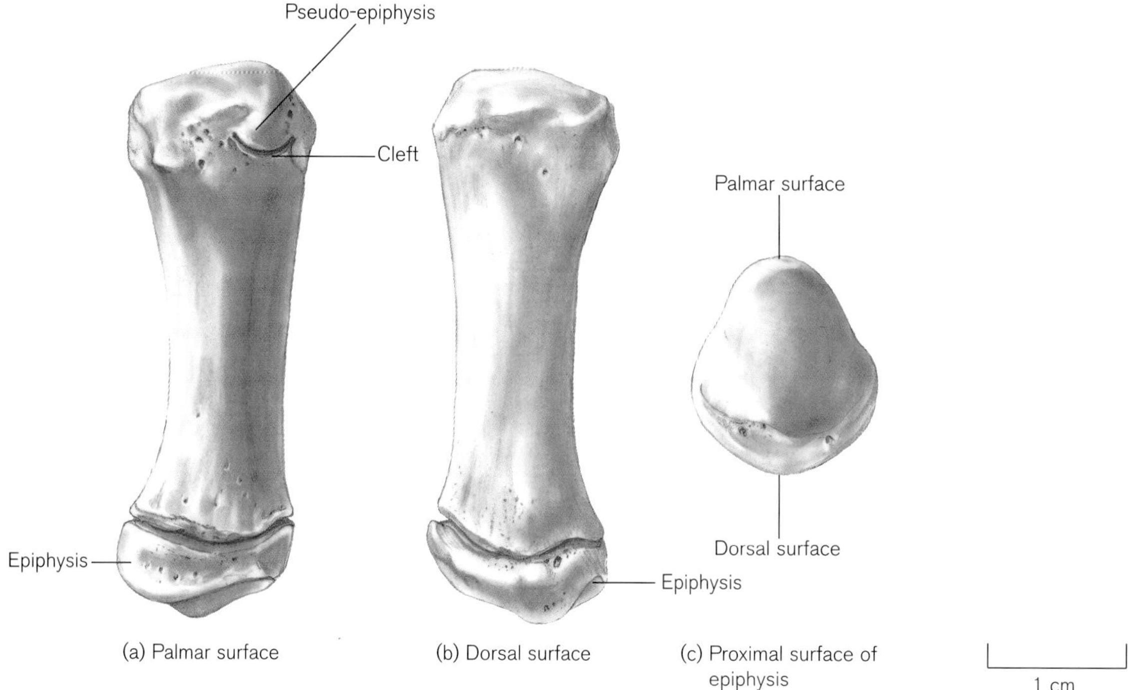

Figure 9.36 The right first metacarpal epiphysis.

appearance and there is much disagreement in the literature. Moss and Noback (1958) state that fusion first occurs in the distal phalanges, with no clear preference for a specific digit or phalanx. Garn *et al.* (1961b) and Hansman (1962) both state that the distal epiphyses commence fusion first, followed by the proximal phalanges and the base of the first metacarpal, followed then by the middle phalanges and finally by the remainder of the metacarpals. Joseph (1951b) reported that the first digit commenced fusion in advance of all others and the subsequent pattern was for the distal phalanx to fuse first, followed by the metacarpal base and finally by the proximal phalangeal base, while in all the other digits the pattern was for the distal phalanx to fuse first, followed by the middle phalanges, then the proximal phalanges and finally by the remaining metacarpals.

In many ways, it is a purely academic concern as to which epiphysis fuses first as it takes only a matter of 2–4 months for an epiphysis to complete the process of fusion and so many studies may well have missed this critically small window of time (Moss and Noback, 1958). Further, it takes only some 13 months for the entire hand to complete epiphyseal fusion from start to finish (Moss and Noback, 1958).

To summarize digital fusion, it can be stated that the distal phalanges are probably the first to commence union at approximately 13 years and 7 months in girls and 16 years in boys and that the first digit seems to fuse about a month in advance of the other distal phalangeal bases (Hellman, 1928; Sidhom and Derry, 1931; Noback, 1954; Moss and Noback, 1958; Noback *et al.*, 1960; Garn *et al.*, 1961b). The base of the first metacarpal behaves like the bases of the proximal phalanges in many ways and so it is perhaps not surprising that they tend to commence fusion around the same time (Thomson, 1869; Broom, 1906). The base of the first metacarpal completes fusion with the diaphysis by approximately 14 years 1 month in girls and 16 years 4 months in boys, while fusion at the bases of the proximal phalanges occurs between 14 years 2 months and 14 years 5 months in girls and between 16 years 2 months and 16 years 6 months in boys. Fusion of the bases of the middle phalanges range from 14 years 3 months to 14 years 6 months in girls and 16 years 4 months to 16 years 6 months in boys. The heads of metacarpals 2–5 are reported to fuse between 14 years 5 months and 15 years in girls and around 16 years 6 months in boys, with a tendency for metacarpal 5 to be the last bone in the hand to complete epiphyseal fusion.

The epiphyses of the hand have been a contentious issue for hundreds of years, particularly in relation to the so-called 'pseudo-epiphyses' which tend to present as notches or clefts at the non-epiphyseal end of a hand (or foot) long bone and in the position that corresponds with the position of an epiphyseal plate were it to be present (Fig. 9.37). The head of the first metacarpal, the lateral aspect of the base of the second metacarpal and the medial aspect of the base of the fifth metacarpal are reported to be the most common sites for this phenomenon (Colwell, 1927; Lachman, 1953; Dreizen *et al.*, 1965; Lee and Garn, 1967; Levine, 1972b). Albinus was probably the first to note this in 1737.

Pseudo-epiphyses were first described in the mid-1700s (Nesbitt, 1736; Albinus, 1737) and many papers, particularly radiological, have been concerned with their relevance to specific clinical conditions such as Down's syndrome, hypothyroidism, achondroplasia, etc. (Lee and Garn, 1967). Clinicians are also interested in identifying these anatomical variants as they can mimic pathological conditions (Keats and Harrison, 1980). However, some anatomists and anthropologists have been obsessed with the importance of these pseudo-epiphyses in relation to phylogenetic development, seeing the retention of bipolar epiphyses as atavistic evidence for man's evolution from lower life forms (Thomson, 1869; Broom, 1906; Wakeley, 1924).

It is, however, clear that these structures represent normal stages in the physeal invasion of the primary centre into the head of the metacarpal and depending upon their stage of development at a specific time they will appear in a number of guises. In fact, this phenomenon is actually present in most samples within a particular age range and can actually lend some weight to the observation that it is a normal stage in the development of the bone. For example, ossification into the head of the first metacarpal commences in advance of the appearance of the secondary centre at the proximal pole and its ossification progresses at a much faster rate, indicating that it is different from secondary ossification processes (Ogden *et al.*, 1994). If there is a central invasion into the distal cartilaginous pole, then a mushroom-shaped advancing column of bone can be seen, which is connected by a stalk to the principal ossification centre (Haines, 1974; Ogden *et al.*, 1994). Proximal to this mushroomed head is a circular notch, which is the constriction where it joins to the shaft and this gives the structure the appearance of an epiphysis. However, the ossification front may be displaced to one side (usually medial), which results in a notch on the lateral side of the bone and as this develops it leaves a deep crescentic cleft on the lateral side, which is referred to as the epiphyseal notch or cleft (Lee and Garn, 1967). These notches can be identified in the first year but do not become well defined until years 2–3 and so they can remain potentially identifiable until the completion of fusion (Fig. 9.38). Complete fusion occurs with the remainder of the structures of the hand at approximately 12 years in females and 14 years in males (Lee and Garn, 1967). These pseudo-epiphyses are therefore transient structures that ultimately align with the remainder of the bone and form a completely normal adult morphology so that retrospective confirmation of their presence

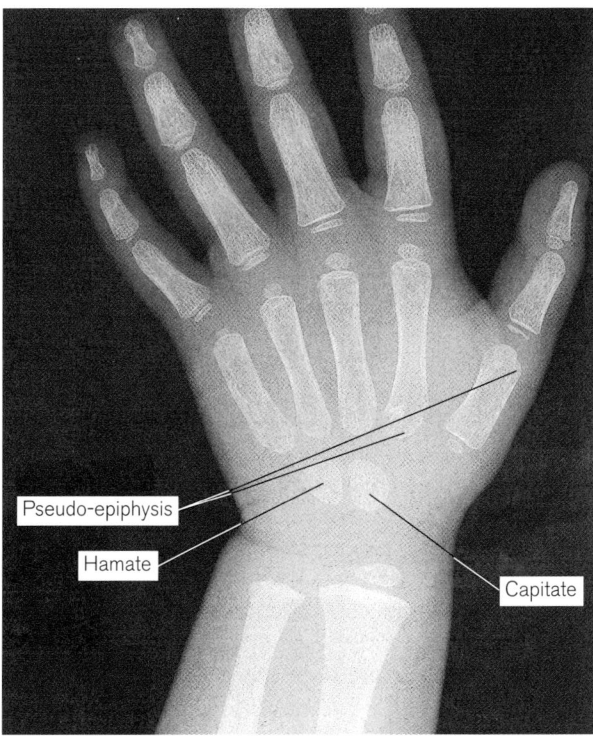

Figure 9.37 Radiograph from a girl of 3 years showing pseudo-epiphyses at the head of the first metacarpal and the base of the second metacarpal.

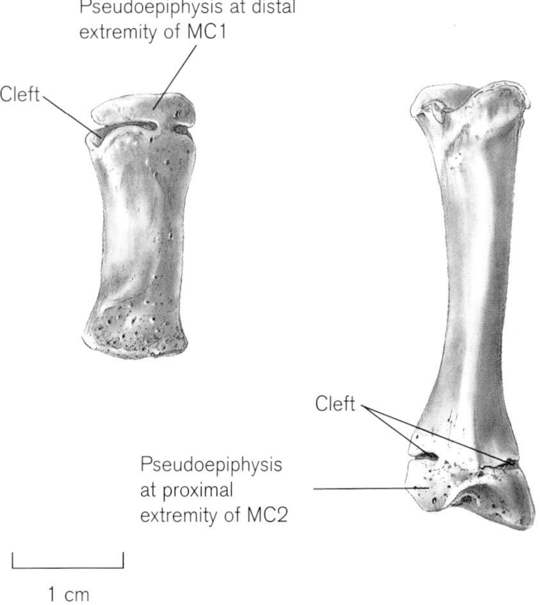

Figure 9.38 Pseudo-epiphyses as seen on the dorsal surface of the first and second metacarpals in a girl aged 8 years and 7 months.

is not possible (Snodgrasse *et al.*, 1955). It is clear from the histological investigations of Haines (1974) and Ogden *et al.* (1994) that the region of the pseudo-epiphysis is associated with an area of cartilage that displays discontinuity of cell columns and so the normal linear progression of ossification is impeded in this region, resulting in so-called 'tide lines', which temporarily halt ossification (Ogden *et al.*, 1994).

These pseudo-epiphyses are therefore not truly epiphyses at all but normal progressions of the ossification process. However, true supernumerary epiphyses do exist, although they are rare, but they do present in the normal form of an epiphysis as an entirely separate node of ossification in an island of hyaline cartilage (Posener *et al.*, 1939).

There are a number of anomalies that appear in the skeletal development of the hand, which relate in particular to the development of the epiphyses. For example, cone-shaped epiphyses have been well documented in the clinical literature and although their aetiology is unknown, it has been linked to conditions such as brachymesophalangia (Arkless and Graham, 1967; Hertzog *et al.*, 1968; Garn *et al.*, 1972b). The epiphysis is best described as possessing a conical projection of the distal border so that it points towards the proximal border of the diaphysis and it has been somewhat artistically likened to 'the indentation in the bottom of a wine bottle' (Giedion, 1965; Wetherington, 1982, 1983). Interestingly, it shows an incidence that is four times greater in the female than in the male (de Iturriza and Tanner, 1969).

Ivory or sclerotic epiphyses are described as epiphyses that appear dense on radiography, making the internal architecture difficult to discern. It is a transitory phase as the epiphysis generally continues to grow and fuse as a normal adult bone. It is thought that the growing epiphyses are particularly sensitive to metabolic alterations and this condition may be radiographic evidence of growth disturbances (Kuhns *et al.*, 1973b; Shaw and Bohrer, 1979).

Abnormalities of epiphyseal growth and/or fusion can result in a number of clinical conditions that seem to affect the fifth digit in particular. Brachymesophalangia has been discussed earlier, but conditions such as clinodactyly, where the fifth finger is tilted or crooked, occurs as a growth deformity at the level of the distal interphalangeal joint (Ozonoff, 1979). Angular deformities can also arise as a result of a condition known as delta phalanx, which is a manifestation of polydactylism. In this condition, a tubular bone of the extremity with a proximal epiphysis becomes the site of origin of an extra skeletal ray. The tethering of the proximal epiphysis by the supernumerary ray creates a peculiar D-shaped phalanx (Jones, 1964; Watson and Boyes, 1967).

Practical notes

Sideing

It is a general rule that sideing of the bones of the hand can only be achieved with any degree of confidence as the bone approaches adult morphology around the time of puberty. Before this period, the bones are sufficiently lacking in strong identifiable features for sideing to be extremely difficult, if not impossible. Certainly, we have found it very difficult to side adult phalanges, so the prospect of correctly assigning side to juvenile hand remains seems to be almost akin to the search for the Holy Grail. Metacarpals and carpals become more recognizable as puberty approaches and so it is possible, in some cases, that the recognition of developing features that would permit identification of side in the adult, might be observed in the juvenile.

Sideing the juvenile first metacarpal relies on being able to identify:

- the nutrient foramen, which is generally located on the distal aspect of the anteromedial surface of the shaft and is directed distally
- demarcation of the volar surface into a larger lateral and a smaller medial area
- identification of the tubercle on the lateral aspect of the proximal extremity for the attachment of the abductor pollicis longus muscle. Once the basal epiphysis is present, then side is easy to establish, as it follows the adult morphology.

Correct identification of side for the second metacarpal relies almost entirely on the development of the base of the bone. However, the head does show marked asymmetry in relation to the attachments of the second metacarpophalangeal ligament, which tends to pare away the dorsolateral aspect. The nutrient foramen is of no value in side identification as it is found with approximately equal frequency on both the anteromedial and anterolateral surfaces.

Identification of side for the third metacarpal is heavily dependent upon identification of the styloid process on the dorsolateral aspect. The nutrient foramen is usually found on the lateral aspect, although variation in its position does not make it a very reliable indicator.

The fourth metacarpal is probably the most difficult to side in the juvenile as correct assignation depends on the morphology of the base. Some additional information may be gleaned from the nutrient foramen, which is generally located on the lateral aspect.

Sideing of the fifth metacarpal also relies heavily on the identification of the non-articular medial surface of the base. The head of the metacarpal tends to be asymmetrical on the palmar aspect, due to the presence of a sesamoid bone on the medial articular surface, which therefore tends to be larger than that of the lateral aspect. The nutrient foramen is generally located on the lateral aspect.

The capitate cannot be identified with any degree of certainty until approximately 3–4 years of age and it is probably not until around 12 years that side can be attributed with any degree of reliability. By an early stage, the bone adopts the shape of a reversed 'D', with a flattened medial surface for articulation with the hamate and a slightly wider distal transverse diameter.

The hamate can probably be identified in isolation from approximately 4–5 years of age, but side cannot be established with confidence until after 9 years of age, when the bone has adopted its characteristic wedge-shaped appearance. In the early years of puberty the hamulus begins to develop and this is located on the palmar surface in a somewhat mediodistal location.

It is unlikely that any of the remainder of the carpals can be attributed correctly to a side until puberty has commenced and the adult morphology is well established (around 12 years in girls and 14–15 years in boys).

Bones of a similar morphology

It is obvious that the appearance of the bones of the hand and the foot are morphologically close and therefore most likely to cause some confusion. It is highly unlikely that any carpal could ever be confused with a tarsal bone, as the latter are considerably larger and much more robust. The metatarsals are generally longer than the metacarpals and the shafts and heads are more slender and slightly compressed in the mediolateral plane. With the exception of the phalanges of the big toe (which are actually larger than those of the thumb), the remaining pedal phalanges are considerably shorter, less well defined and more irregular than their manual counterparts. The pedal phalanges tend to be more rounded in cross-section of the shaft, while the phalanges of the hand show a roughly semicircular outline, due to the volar flattening caused by the close proximity of the long flexor tendons.

Morphological summary

Fetal	
7–9 wks	Primary ossification centres appear for distal phalanges
8–10 wks	Primary ossification centres appear for metacarpals
9–11 wks	Primary ossification centres appear for proximal phalanges
10–12 wks	Primary ossification centres appear for middle phalanges
Birth	All 19 primary centres for the long bones of the hand are present (ossification centres for capitate and hamate can be present)
2–3 mths (female) 3–4 mths (male)	Ossification centre appears for capitate
3–4 mths (female) 4–5 mths (male)	Ossification centre appears for hamate
1–2 yrs	Ossification centre appears for triquetral
10–17 mths (female) 14 mths–2 yrs (male)	Epiphyses for bases of proximal phalanges 2–5 appear
17 mths (female) 22 mths (male)	Epiphysis for base of distal phalanx 1 appears
16–19 mths (female) 22 mths–2.5 yrs (male)	Epiphyses for heads of metacarpals 2–5 appear
19 mths (female) 2.5 yrs (male)	Epiphyses for bases of middle phalanges 2–4 appear
2 yrs (female) 2–3 yrs (male)	Epiphyses for bases of distal phalanges 3–4 appear Epiphyses for base of metacarpal 1 and proximal phalanx 1 appear
2.5 yrs (female) 3.5 yrs (male)	Epiphyses for bases of distal and middle phalanges of 5 appear
3 yrs (female) 4 yrs (male)	Ossification centre appears for lunate; the capitate can now be recognized if in a dry bone state
4 yrs (female) 5 yrs (male)	Ossification centre appears for trapezium; the hamate can now be recognized if in a dry bone state
5 yrs (female) 6 yrs (male)	Ossification centres appear for trapezoid and scaphoid
8 yrs (female) 10 yrs (male)	Ossification centre appears for pisiform; triquetral can now be recognized if in a dry bone state
9–10 yrs	Trapezium, trapezoid and lunate can now be recognized if in a dry bone state
9.5–11 yrs	Scaphoid can now be recognized if in a dry bone state
10–12 yrs	Hook of hamate appears and fuses to body
12 yrs	Pisiform can now be recognized if in a dry bone state

11–15 yrs (female) 13–18 yrs (male)	Sesamoid bones commence ossification
13.5 yrs (female) 16 yrs (male)	Distal phalangeal epiphyses fuse
14–14.5 yrs (female) 16.5 yrs (male)	Base of metacarpal 1 fuses proximal and middle phalangeal epiphyses fuse
14.5–15 yrs (female) 16.5 yrs (male)	Heads of metacarpals 2–5 fuse

Metrics

All of the available information on size changes in the bones of the developing hand comes from radiographs. Fazekas and Kósa (1978) gave measurements on the fetal first metacarpal from 16 fetal weeks to term and this is summarized in Table 9.19. Table 9.20 shows the dimensions of all the long bones of the developing hand, as taken from a sample of fetuses with crown–rump lengths that ranged from 15–104 mm (Garn *et al.*, 1975a). Table 9.21 shows the change in length and minimum shaft width in the fourth middle phalanx and third proximal phalanx of 40 Australian children aged between 3 and 13 years (Roche and Hermann, 1970). Table 9.22 shows the values for the length and width of the second metacarpal in a sample of 923 Japanese children aged between 6 months and 18 years (Kimura, 1976). Table 9.23 shows the maximum length and the midshaft width of the second metacarpal in a sample of 326 Guamanian children aged between 5 and 17 years of age (Plato *et al.*, 1984). Table 9.24 shows variations in the lengths of the second metacarpal in a sample of 2056 Japanese children between 6 and 19 years of age (Kimura, 1992). Finally, Table 9.25 shows the values for the lengths of all the developing metacarpals and phalanges in a sample of 1290 Nigerian children aged between 3 and 16 years of age (Odita *et al.*, 1991).

Table 9.19 Diaphyseal length of metacarpal (from 16–40 weeks)

Age (weeks)	Diaphyseal length (mm)
16	1.8
18	2.3
20	3.1
22	3.7
24	4.3
26	4.6
28	5.1
30	5.9
32	6.3
34	7.2
36	8.1
38	8.9
40	9.3

Length = maximum length of the diaphysis.
Adapted from Fazekas and Kósa (1978).

Table 9.20 Maximum metacarpal and phalangeal lengths (mm) in fetuses with a crown–rump length (CRL) of 15–104 mm

CRL	MC1	MC2	MC3	MC4	MC5
15–29 mm	0.44	0.76	0.77	0.71	0.67
30–44 mm	0.86	1.31	1.29	1.17	1.12
45–59 mm	1.34	2.11	1.99	1.64	1.58
60–74 mm	2.06	3.31	3.04	2.70	2.56
75–89 mm	2.21	3.36	3.15	2.89	2.63
90–104 mm	3.34	5.50	5.18	4.75	4.23
	PP1	PP2	PP3	PP4	PP5
15–29 mm	0.35	0.41	0.45	0.43	0.36
30–44 mm	0.64	0.76	0.82	0.77	0.69
45–59 mm	0.97	1.04	1.08	1.05	0.95
60–74 mm	1.32	1.66	1.77	1.65	1.41
75–89 mm	1.46	1.88	2.04	1.80	1.54
90–104 mm	2.18	3.37	3.19	3.22	2.30
		MP2	MP3	MP4	MP5
15–29 mm		0.30	0.31	0.29	0.24
30–44 mm		0.53	0.59	0.57	0.49
45–59 mm		0.67	0.81	0.69	0.59
60–74 mm		0.93	1.11	1.02	0.90
75–89 mm		1.06	1.23	1.23	1.02
90–104 mm		1.87	1.93	1.84	1.29
	DP1	DP2	DP3	DP4	DP5
15–29 mm	0.30	0.18	0.22	0.21	0.15
30–44 mm	0.74	0.52	0.61	0.60	0.51
45–59 mm	1.03	0.69	0.66	0.66	0.51
60–74 mm	1.36	1.01	1.05	1.02	0.85
75–89 mm	1.39	0.98	1.09	1.07	0.95
90–104 mm	2.01	1.35	1.55	1.46	1.34

Adapted from Garn *et al.* (1975a).

Table 9.21 Maximum length and minimum shaft width (in mm) for the developing fourth middle and third proximal phalanges

		Male		Female	
Age (years)	Bone	Length	Width	Length	Width
3	MP4	13.6	5.4	13.2	5.3
4	MP4	14.5	5.5	14.2	5.5
5	MP4	15.3	5.9	14.9	5.7
6	MP4	16.1	6.0	15.5	5.8
7	MP4	16.8	6.2	16.4	5.9
8	MP4	17.4	6.4	17.3	6.1
9	MP4	18.2	6.5	17.8	6.3
10	MP4	18.7	6.8	18.5	6.4
11	MP4	19.3	6.9	19.4	6.6
12	MP4	20.2	7.0	20.3	6.8
13	MP4	21.1	7.3	20.9	6.9
3	PP3			22.2	6.2
4	PP3			23.5	6.6
5	PP3			25.0	6.9
6	PP3			26.3	7.0
7	PP3			27.7	7.3
8	PP3			29.1	7.5
9	PP3			30.3	7.6
10	PP3			31.9	7.9
11	PP3			33.5	8.0
12	PP3			35.4	8.2
13	PP3			36.9	8.4

Adapted from Roche and Hermann (1970).

Table 9.22 Variation in maximum length and midshaft width (in mm) of the second metacarpal between 6 months and 18 years 6 months of age

	Bone length		Bone width	
Age (years:months)	Male	Female	Male	Female
0.7–1.6	21.9	22.9	4.3	4.0
1.7–2.6	29.2	30.0	5.0	4.7
2.7–3.6	32.6	33.3	5.2	5.0
3.7–4.6	35.8	35.6	5.4	5.2
4.7–5.6	37.4	38.5	5.5	5.4
5.7–6.6	39.8	40.9	5.8	5.4
6.7–7.6	43.9	45.2	5.9	5.7
7.7–8.6	48.1	46.9	6.1	5.8
8.7–9.6	49.3	49.6	6.3	6.2
9.7–10.6	51.3	50.8	6.5	6.3
10.7–11.6	53.3	54.4	6.8	6.8
11.7–12.6	55.2	57.0	7.2	7.1
12.7–13.6	57.4	57.9	7.8	7.2
13.7–14.6	59.9	58.4	8.1	7.4
14.7–15.6	62.2	58.9	8.5	7.3
157–16.6	63.7	59.4	8.7	7.4
16.7–17.6	64.6	59.5	8.8	7.6
17.7–18.6	65.0	59.4	8.9	7.6

Adapted from Kimura (1976).

Table 9.23 Maximum length and midshaft widths (in mm) of the developing second metacarpal

	Male		Female	
Age (years)	Length	Width	Length	Width
5	38.37	4.63	39.80	5.30
6	40.30	5.14	41.30	5.20
7	42.85	5.37	44.00	5.59
8	46.67	5.57	46.43	5.70
9	45.60	5.80	47.18	5.72
10	51.65	5.90	50.45	5.96
11	52.03	6.39	52.93	6.14
12	53.37	6.35	55.05	6.65
13	55.29	6.73	59.02	6.71
14	57.25	7.15	63.36	7.04
15	60.42	7.67	63.08	7.03
16	63.40	6.90	61.38	6.72
17			64.55	7.35

Adapted from Plato *et al.* (1984).

Table 9.24 Variations in the maximum length of the second metacarpal (in mm) in children from three regions of Japan

Region	Age (years)	Male	Female
Takamatsu	6	40.8	42.8
	7	43.2	43.6
	8	45.2	45.3
	9	46.7	48.8
	10	48.7	49.6
	11	52.6	53.4
	12	55.1	55.2
Kagoshima	7	42.0	43.2
	8	44.7	46.4
	9	45.9	47.3
	10	48.0	49.2
	11	48.8	53.7
	12	53.1	55.8
	13	56.9	55.8
	14	56.9	58.4
	15	61.2	58.6
	16	64.5	59.9
	17	62.4	60.4
	18	64.8	58.3
	19	65.6	61.4
Okinawa	7	42.4	42.4
	8	44.9	45.1
	9	48.2	48.1
	10	49.4	50.6
	11	52.2	53.6
	12	54.6	56.1
	13	59.1	57.8
	14	60.6	59.5
	15	62.0	60.5
	16	62.6	60.2

Adapted from Kimura (1992).

Table 9.25 Mean values for maximum metacarpophalangeal lengths (in mm) in Nigerian children

	MALE AGE (years)													
Bone	3	4	5	6	7	8	9	10	11	12	13	14	15	16
MC1	23.7	25.0	27.6	30.5	31.2	32.9	35.2	36.9	38.8	40.7	44.0	46.4	48.1	48.9
MC2	38.0	40.3	43.5	47.7	48.4	51.3	54.2	57.1	60.0	62.2	67.1	70.9	72.0	75.2
MC3	36.6	38.7	42.4	46.1	46.9	49.8	52.3	55.0	57.4	59.2	63.0	66.9	69.1	70.8
MC4	32.4	34.2	37.4	40.4	41.6	43.9	45.9	47.9	50.3	51.9	55.9	58.6	60.9	62.6
MC5	28.8	30.7	33.5	36.8	37.6	39.6	42.1	43.7	46.2	47.9	51.3	54.2	56.2	47.5
PP1	17.3	18.0	19.5	20.7	21.3	23.1	23.8	25.9	26.5	28.5	29.3	32.1	32.4	33.2
PP2	23.6	24.6	26.6	28.0	29.0	30.1	31.4	33.0	34.3	35.9	38.0	40.8	42.1	43.6
PP3	27.1	28.0	30.2	37.1	32.6	34.3	35.9	37.4	39.1	40.8	43.3	46.4	47.9	49.0
PP4	25.4	26.7	28.3	30.1	30.7	32.3	33.6	35.1	36.6	38.1	41.2	43.5	44.8	45.7
PP5	19.7	20.1	21.6	22.8	23.4	24.5	25.4	27.0	28.2	29.4	31.6	33.8	35.2	35.9
MP2	12.7	13.2	14.6	15.4	16.2	16.7	17.8	18.7	19.3	19.9	21.5	22.6	23.4	24.3
MP3	16.1	16.7	18.5	19.3	20.2	21.0	22.2	23.6	23.8	25.2	26.8	28.2	29.2	29.9
MP4	15.8	16.4	17.8	18.6	19.4	20.1	21.2	22.1	22.8	23.9	25.7	27.1	27.7	28.2
MP5	11.0	11.3	12.6	13.1	13.6	14.2	15.1	16.1	16.0	16.9	18.9	19.4	20.1	19.8
DP1	13.2	13.7	14.7	15.8	16.4	17.3	18.2	19.6	19.9	20.8	22.0	23.0	23.8	24.3
DP2	8.9	9.2	10.4	10.8	12.1	12.1	12.6	13.5	13.8	14.5	15.9	16.3	16.8	17.0
DP3	9.9	10.6	11.3	11.9	12.7	13.4	14.0	15.0	14.9	15.7	17.3	17.7	18.3	18.6
DP4	10.2	10.8	11.6	12.3	13.1	13.8	14.3	15.4	15.4	16.5	17.6	18.1	18.6	19.0
DP5	8.7	9.2	10.0	10.6	11.1	11.7	12.2	13.0	13.1	14.4	15.2	15.7	16.2	16.1
	FEMALE AGE (years)													
Bone	3	4	5	6	7	8	9	10	11	12	13	14	15	16
MC1	24.8	26.3	28.6	30.4	32.1	34.3	36.5	39.2	40.3	42.2	43.6	44.3	43.6	44.1
MC2	38.7	40.4	44.2	47.1	50.0	53.2	56.3	60.3	62.2	64.3	66.9	68.7	66.1	67.4
MC3	37.9	39.2	43.1	45.8	48.5	51.1	54.2	57.8	59.4	61.8	63.5	64.9	62.9	65.1
MC4	33.0	34.5	37.7	40.2	42.6	45.0	47.7	50.4	52.5	54.6	55.4	57.3	55.9	57.3
MC5	29.6	31.2	33.8	36.2	38.5	41.2	43.3	46.5	48.0	50.0	50.9	52.4	51.3	53.3
PP1	17.4	18.3	19.4	20.6	21.8	23.6	25.0	27.4	28.0	29.4	30.7	30.8	30.7	32.1
PP2	23.7	24.8	26.4	27.8	29.2	31.0	32.8	35.3	36.4	38.5	39.4	40.4	40.1	41.3
PP3	27.3	28.2	30.1	32.0	33.3	35.2	37.3	39.9	41.6	43.8	44.7	45.4	45.2	46.7
PP4	25.4	26.4	28.2	29.8	31.2	32.7	34.5	37.3	38.7	40.7	41.6	42.8	41.8	43.5
PP5	19.5	20.2	21.3	22.4	23.5	24.9	26.5	28.9	29.9	31.1	32.7	33.4	33.3	34.4
MP2	13.1	13.6	14.7	15.3	16.2	17.0	18.3	19.4	19.9	21.1	21.8	22.4	22.3	22.6
MP3	16.7	17.2	18.4	19.3	20.4	21.2	22.8	24.7	25.2	26.2	26.9	27.5	28.0	26.1
MP4	15.9	16.5	17.6	18.5	19.5	20.5	21.8	23.5	24.1	25.4	26.0	26.1	26.6	26.3
MP5	10.9	11.4	12.2	12.8	13.6	14.0	15.1	16.7	17.0	17.9	18.3	18.8	19.2	19.6
DP1	13.1	13.7	14.6	15.9	16.4	17.6	18.9	20.4	20.1	21.0	21.8	21.7	21.8	23.0
DP2	8.8	9.9	10.3	11.0	11.5	12.3	13.0	14.2	14.3	14.6	15.3	15.4	15.4	15.8
DP3	9.8	10.6	11.3	11.8	12.6	13.5	14.3	15.6	15.5	16.0	16.9	16.7	17.2	17.7
DP4	10.1	10.9	11.5	12.2	12.8	13.9	14.5	15.8	15.9	16.6	17.2	17.1	17.5	18.0
DP5	8.6	9.4	9.8	10.3	10.8	11.7	12.1	13.4	13.3	13.7	14.5	14.6	14.5	15.6

Adapted from Odita *et al.* (1991).

CHAPTER TEN

The Pelvic Girdle

The pelvic girdle is formed by the articulation of the two innominate bones with the midline sacrum and coccyx, thereby forming the junction between the trunk and the lower limbs (Fig. 10.1). It is divided into a greater (false) pelvis above and a lesser (true) pelvis below by an oblique plane (pelvic inlet). The **false pelvis** houses abdominal viscera and is bounded anteriorly by the abdominal wall, laterally by the iliac fossae and posteriorly by the fifth lumbar vertebra. The **pelvic inlet** (brim) is formed by the promontory and alae of the sacrum posteriorly, the iliopectineal lines laterally and the pubic crest and symphysis anteriorly (Fig. 10.2). The **true pelvis** houses the urinary bladder, the rectum and the internal genitalia. Its longer posterior wall is formed by the sacrum and coccyx, its shorter anterior wall by the pubic symphysis and body of the pubis and its lateral walls by the inner aspect of the innominates and the obturator fascia and muscles that cover the obturator foramen. The **pelvic outlet** is roughly diamond-shaped and is bounded by the coccyx posteriorly, the ischial tuberosities and sacrotuberous ligaments laterally and the pubic symphysis anteriorly (Fig. 10.3). An artificial line drawn between the two ischial tuberosities, roughly delimits the urogenital triangle anteriorly from the anal triangle posteriorly. The urogenital region contains the external genitalia and terminal parts of the urogenital passages and the anal region contains the anal canal, bounded on each side by an ischiorectal fossa. The true pelvis above is separated from the structures of the perineum and anal region below by the pelvic diaphragm, which is principally formed by the levatores ani muscles.

The shape of the adult female pelvis reflects a functional compromise between the biomechanical refinements imposed by bipedalism and the biological requirements to ensure safe parturition. As the adoption of erect posture preceded encephalization, so the primary determinant of human pelvic shape probably lies in the modifications required for the optimal transfer of body weight in an erect position to permit efficient bipedal locomotion (Reynolds, 1931; Davies, 1955; Krukierek, 1955; Snell and Donhuysen, 1968; Schultz, 1969; Leutenegger, 1972; Abitbol, 1987; Lovejoy, 1988). Body weight is initially concentrated on the first sacral segment before being transmitted via the sacro-iliac joints to the acetabulum and thence to the femoral heads. This weight tends to depress the anterior part of the sacrum and this is counteracted to a considerable degree by the action of the sacrotuberous ligament. There are three trajectory systems of pressure lamellae within the substance of the innominate that reflect the characteristically human pathway of body weight transfer (Fig. 10.1). The first passes from the lower part of the auricular surface of the sacro-iliac joint to the superior border of the acetabulum (inferior auriculo-acetabular trajectory pathway) and this is said to be the main pathway for transmitting compressive force (Kapandji, 1987). The second passes from the upper part of the auricular surface to the inferior border of the acetabulum (superior auriculo-acetabular trajectory pathway) and this is said to counteract shearing stress. The third set passes from the auricular region to the ischial tuberosities (sacro-ischial trajectory pathway) and is said to be the main pathway involved in transmitting body weight in the sitting position. The tie-rods of these transmission arches are the superior pubic and ischiopubic rami, which resist inward collapse of the bones. However, due to the curvatures of the vertebral column, body weight tends to fall somewhat anterior to the sacro-iliac joints, which imposes a rotatory force on the sacrum encouraging it to tilt backwards and the sacral promontory to fall forwards. These actions are resisted primarily by the strength of the sacrotuberous and sacrospinous ligaments.

The shape and size of the pelvic cavity have, of course, received a great deal of attention in obstetrical (Willson *et al.*, 1971; Pritchard and MacDonald,

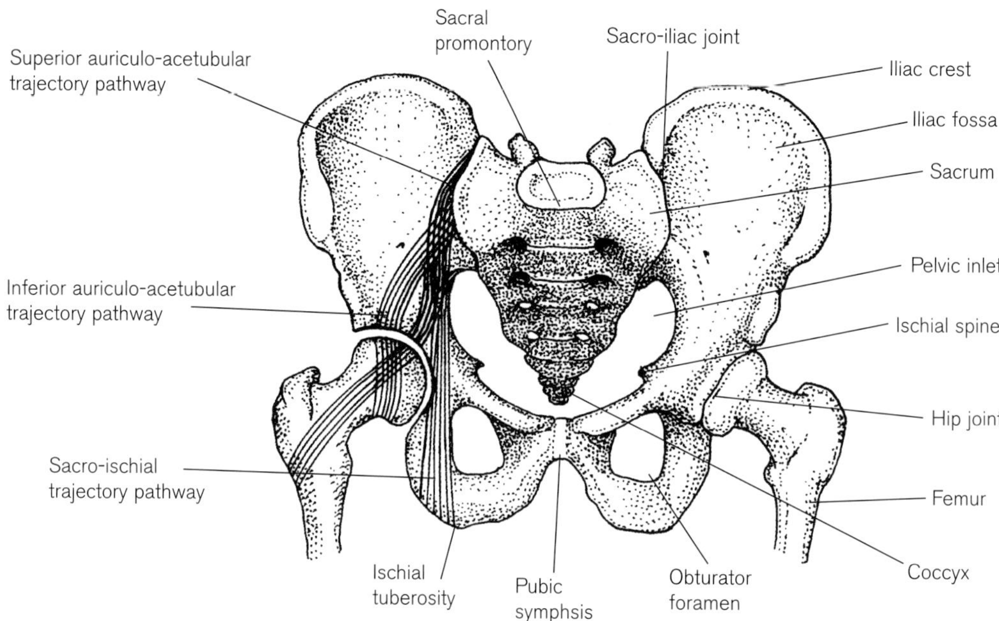

Figure 10.1 The adult pelvic girdle showing the internal trajectory pathways for body weight transfer on the right hand side.

1980), anthropological (Gebbie, 1981) and palaeontological literature (Mednick, 1955; Stewart, 1984; Rosenberg, 1992; Ridley, 1995). It was fashionable in the 1930s and 40s to classify female pelvic shape and size in an attempt to predict the success of parturition (Garson, 1881; Caldwell and Moloy, 1933; Greulich and Thoms, 1938; Caldwell *et al.*, 1940; Ince and Young, 1940; Thoms, 1940; Kenny, 1944; Torpin, 1951). Given the relatively high fetomaternal mortality rates prior to the 1950s it was important to preempt, prior to the onset of labour, any potential complications that might arise. Conditions such as rickets, scoliosis and tuberculosis could all influence maternal pelvic shape and thus increase the likelihood of cephalopelvic disproportion (Naegele, 1839; Reinberger, 1933; De Carle, 1957; Wells, 1975; Micozzi and de la Paz, 1977; Phelan *et al.*, 1978; Siegler and Zorab, 1981; Micozzi, 1982; Visscher *et al.*, 1988).

The pelvis is the area of the human skeleton said to display the greatest levels of sexual dimorphism and in fact the innominate is to be preferred over any other single bone for the accurate prediction of sex in the adult (Krogman, 1973; WEA, 1980; MacLaughlin, 1987; Knussmann, 1988). Despite a wealth of literature concerning sex differences in the fetal and juvenile pelvis, it is still generally held that while dimorphism may exist from an early age, it does not reach a sufficiently high level to permit reliable dis-

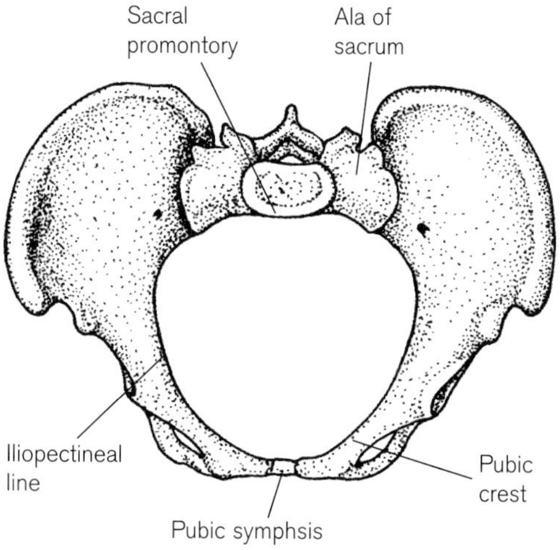

Figure 10.2 The adult pelvic inlet.

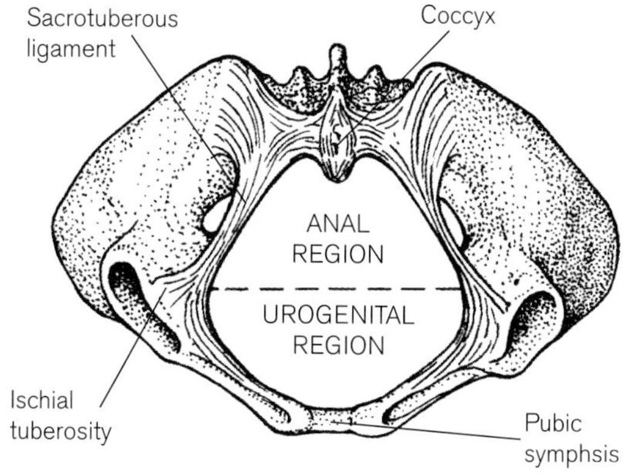

Figure 10.3 The adult pelvic outlet.

crimination of sex until after the extensive skeletal modifications of puberty have arisen (Thomson, 1899; Yamamura, 1939; Morton and Hayden, 1941; Morton, 1942a; Reynolds, 1945, 1947; Boucher, 1955, 1957; Imrie and Wyburn, 1958; Souri, 1959; Coleman, 1969; Choi and Trotter, 1970; Crelin, 1973; Sundick, 1977, 1978; Weaver, 1980; Bruzek and Soustal, 1981; Hunt, 1990; Mittler and Sheridan, 1992; Garmus, 1993; Schutkowski, 1993; Holcomb and Konigsberg, 1995; LaVelle, 1995). Interestingly, it has been shown that even in fetal innominates, the sex differences that do arise, tend to parallel those found in the adult, namely sciatic notch proportions, iliac proportions and pelvic inlet and outlet dimensions. Hromada (1939) identified two growth phases in the fetal pelvis where, between the second and the seventh fetal months, there were virtually no discernible sex differences in fetal pelvic dimensions, whereas the dimorphism became increasingly more apparent between 7 months and birth.

Differentiation in female pelvic growth at puberty is said to be restricted to those regions that are directly involved in the development of the birth canal (Wood and Chamberlain, 1986) and pubertal alterations occur rapidly under hormone induction over as short a period as 18 months (Greulich and Thoms, 1944). Therefore, from around mid-puberty, the secondary sexual differentiation of the pelvis is probably sufficiently advanced in the female to permit reliable evaluation of that sex. However, given the considerable volume of literature that is devoted to the subject of sex differences in the adult pelvis, it is advised that more specific literature is consulted (Straus, 1927a; Pons, 1955; Genovés, 1956; Gaillard, 1961; Acsádi and Nemeskéri, 1970; Stewart, 1970; Day and Pitcher-Wilmott, 1975; Singh and Potturi, 1978; Ubelaker, 1978; Kelley, 1979b; Stewart, 1979; Segebarth-Orban, 1980; Seidler, 1980; WEA, 1980; Brothwell, 1981; Novotony, 1983; Schulter-Ellis *et al.*, 1983; Rathbun and Buikstra, 1984; Krogman and Işcan, 1986; Novotny, 1986; Bass, 1987; MacLaughlin 1987; Suri and Tandon, 1987; MacLaughlin and Bruce, 1990a).

The adult innominate

As the sacrum has been described in Chapter 6, only the innominate will be considered here. Many of the older anatomical texts refer to the paired bones of the pelvis as the 'os coxae' (hip bones), but it is somewhat paradoxical to consider that the 'name' by which these bones are most commonly known (certainly in the English language) is derived from the Latin 'in nomen' meaning 'unnamed'.

The adult innominate is a large irregularly shaped bone, which has been likened to an aeroplane propeller by some authors (Woodburne and Burkel, 1988), as it bears two 'expanded and oppositely bent blades' (Figs. 10.4–10.6). It articulates with its counterpart from the opposite side anteriorly, via a secondary cartilaginous joint at the pubic symphysis and with the sacrum posteriorly via synovial sacro-iliac joints. Each innominate also articulates laterally at the acetabulum with the head of the femur at the synovial hip joint.

The adult innominate is formed from the fusion of three separate bones–the ilium above, ischium below and behind and the pubis below and in front. The three parts meet in the acetabulum and fuse during puberty to form the single adult bone.

The **ilium**[1] (Latin meaning 'flank') has an upper extremity, (crest), a lower extremity, which forms somewhat less than two-fifths of the articular surface of the acetabulum (Woodburne and Burkel, 1988), anterior and posterior borders and gluteal, iliac and sacropelvic surfaces (Figs. 10.4–10.6). The **iliac crest** is convex superiorly (Camacho *et al.*, 1993) and runs in a sinuous course from the anterior superior iliac spine (ASIS) in front to the posterior superior iliac spine (PSIS) behind. When viewed from above, it displays an inner pelvic concavity in the first two-thirds (iliac fossa) with a corresponding convexity on the outer or gluteal surface that predominantly arises due to the dorsal projection of the iliac tubercle. The course of the crest changes direction at the **spina limitans** (vertical ridge that separates the smooth region of the iliac fossa from the more roughened region of the sacropelvic surface), so that the posterior third of the crest is concave towards the gluteal surface at the gluteus medius site of attachment and convex in the non-articular sacro-iliac region. The iliac crest provides an expanded site for extensive muscle insertion and those that attach to the inner pelvic lip of the crest are (from anterior to posterior) the transversus abdominis, which attaches above the iliac fossa, quadratus lumborum, which attaches superior to the position of the spina limitans, and erector spinae, which attaches above the iliac tubercle of the sacro-iliac region. The muscles that attach to the outer gluteal lip of the crest are (from anterior to posterior) the tensor fascia latae and the iliotibial tract anterior to the iliac tubercle, external and internal oblique abdominal muscles, and latissimus dorsi, which has a very small site of attachment posterior to the internal oblique muscle (Figs. 10.5 and

[1] Ilium was also the alternative name given to the Asia Minor city of Troy after its founder, Ilus. Hence, Homer's *Iliad* refers to the particular events that occurred in the Greek wars pertaining to that city.

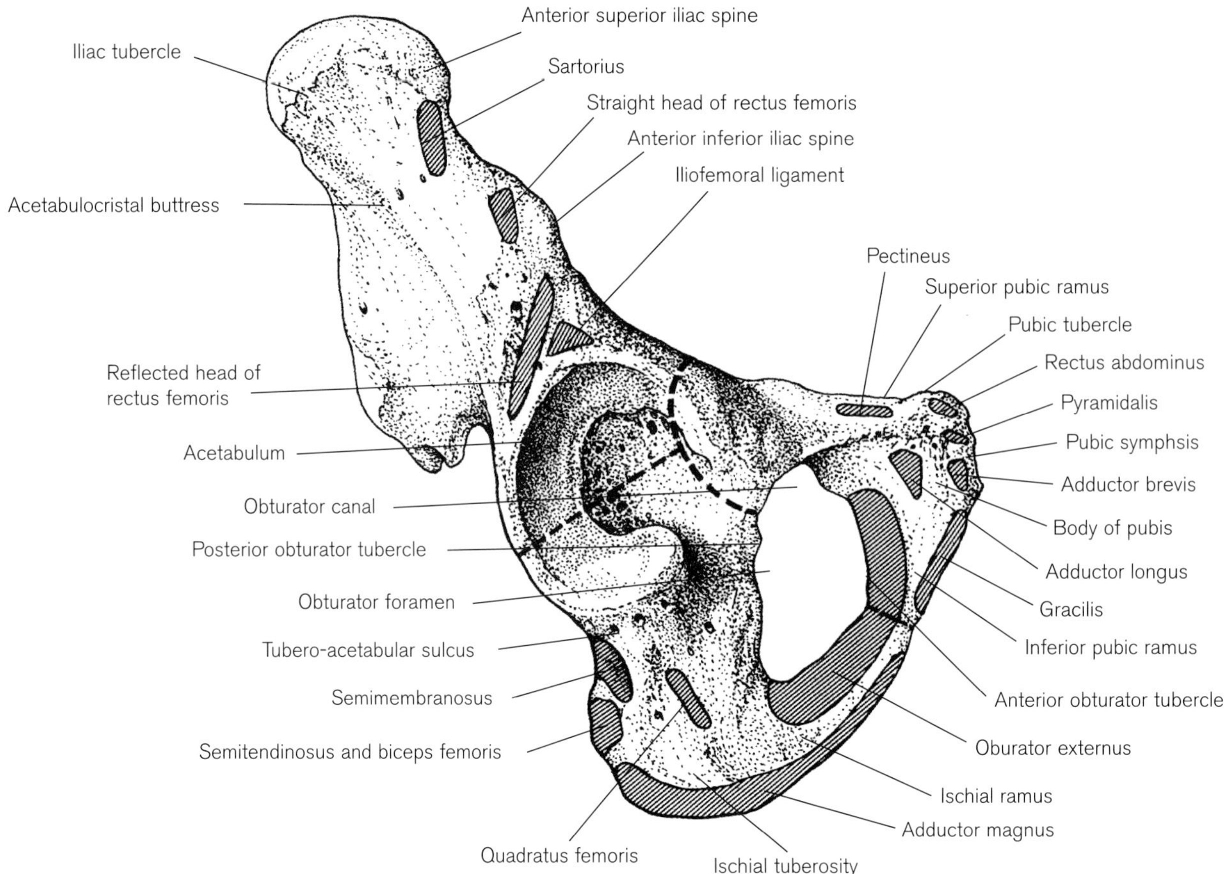

Figure 10.4 Lateral view of the right adult innominate.

10.6). The highest point of the iliac crest lies at approximately the level of the intervertebral disc between the fourth and fifth lumbar vertebrae and this is an important clinical landmark when performing a lumbar puncture. The high proportion of cancellous bone in the region of the iliac crest renders it an important site for aspiration of bone marrow and for removing pieces of bone for grafts, e.g. treating tibial fractures and inter-body spinal fusion (Dommisse, 1959; Whitehouse, 1977; Gross *et al.*, 1989; Behrman, 1992). In the autosomal dominant condition of onycho-osteodysplasia (nail-patella syndrome), horns of bone project dorsally from the iliac crest at the junction between the middle and posterior thirds (Beals and Eckhardt, 1969). These correspond with the site of attachment of the gluteus medius muscle, rarely cause any direct clinical symptoms and may give rise to a skin dimple (Fong, 1946; Zimmerman, 1961). The aetiology of the horns is unclear, but their presence has been recorded from birth.

The **anterior border** of the ilium descends from the anterior superior iliac spine to the anterior inferior iliac spine (AIIS), which lies directly above the acetabulum. The **ASIS** is readily palpated in the living and is the site of attachment for both the inguinal ligament and the sartorius muscle. Avulsion fractures of the ASIS tend to occur in adolescence as a result of strenuous athletic activity (Khoury *et al.*, 1985). The **AIIS** is divided into two areas, with the upper part being the site of attachment for the straight head of the rectus femoris muscle, while the lower part has a triangular depression for the attachment of the iliofemoral ligament and the reflected head of the rectus femoris muscle, which extends posteriorly from this position along a groove above the acetabulum (Fig. 10.4). The anterior inferior iliac spine is also a common site for avulsion fractures in athletes following abnormal contraction of the rectus femoris muscle (Yochum and Rowe, 1987). A rare congenital anomaly of 'pelvic digit' has been associated with the AIIS and other areas of the pelvis in the clinical literature. It presents as a bone formation, which resembles a finger and can even appear to have one or more joints (Greenspan and Norman, 1982; Granieri and Bacarini, 1996). Also known as 'iliac' or

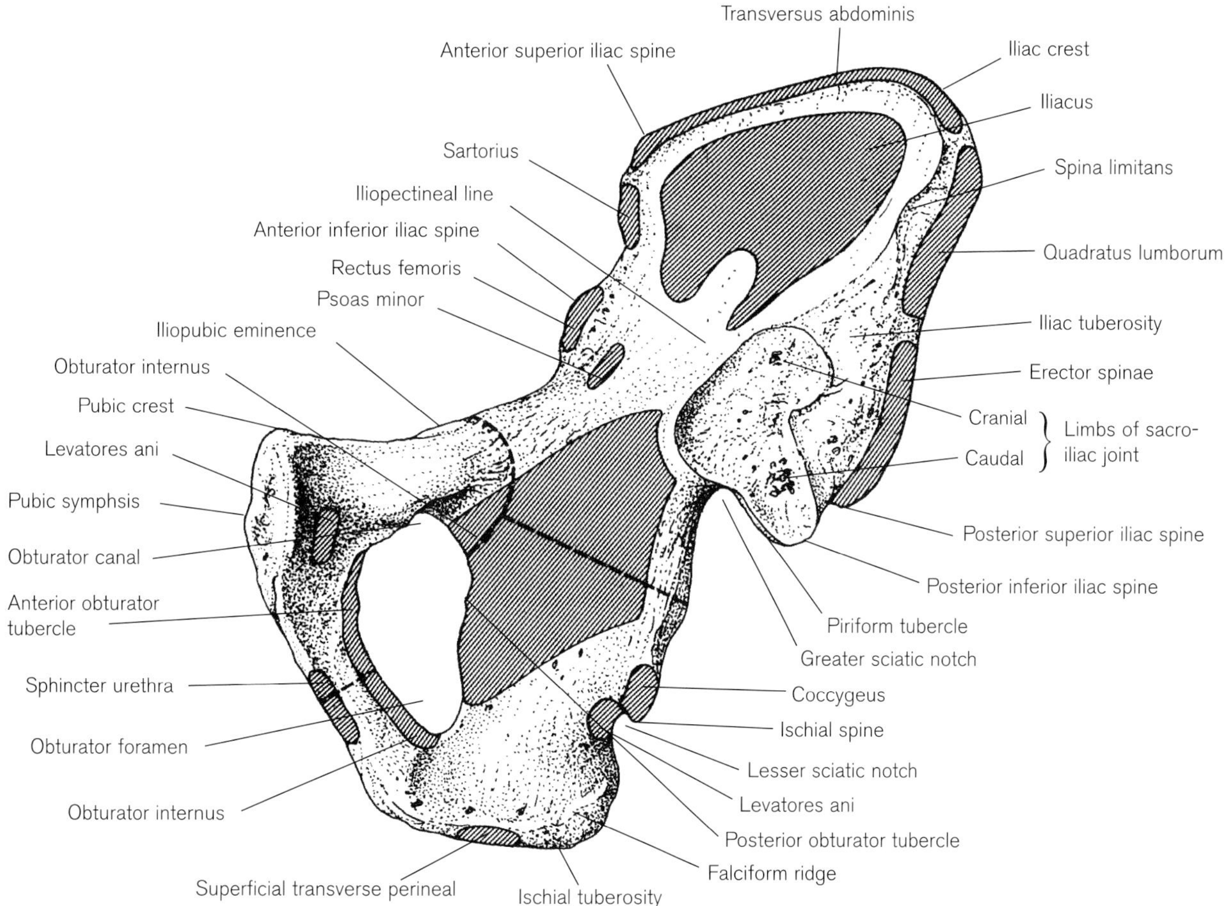

Figure 10.5 Internal (pelvic/medial) view of the right adult innominate.

'pelvic rib', it is generally asymptomatic and often discovered purely by chance (Sullivan and Cornwell, 1974; Lame, 1977; Dunaway *et al.*, 1983). The histological structure of the bone is identical to rib tissue and it has been hypothesized that this may represent an embryological remnant of either a sacral or a coccygeal rib (Reiter, 1944; Halloran, 1960; Kaushal, 1977; Pais *et al.*, 1978).

The **posterior border** of the ilium is considerably shorter than the anterior border and commences at the posterior superior iliac spine (PSIS) and descends a short distance to the posterior inferior iliac spine (PIIS). In females in particular, the posterior extension of the caudal limb of the sacro-iliac joint may project beyond the **PIIS** (St Hoyme, 1984), making the spine somewhat difficult to identify. In most individuals, the **PSIS** is firmly bound to the overlying skin and fascia so that it is readily located in the living as a skin dimple about 4 cm lateral to the median plane at the level of the second sacral vertebra. This provides a useful landmark for bone biopsy site identification, as the needle can be inserted 1 cm inferolateral to the dimple to be assured of an appropriate site for marrow aspiration (Gross *et al.*, 1989). The remainder of the posterior iliac border then bends sharply forwards and runs almost horizontally until it finally turns downwards and forwards to become continuous with the posterior border of the ischium. This recurve forms the greater sciatic notch, which is converted into a foramen in the living by the presence of the strong sacrospinous ligament. This foramen forms the main conduit for structures passing between the pelvis and the gluteal region, e.g. sciatic nerve, superior and inferior gluteal vessels, nerves and piriformis. Some small slips of the piriformis muscle can arise from the superior border of the greater sciatic notch and, with age, may leave a well-defined tubercle in this location (MacLaughlin and Bruce, 1986).

The **gluteal surface** faces backwards and laterally in its posterior part but laterally and slightly downwards in its anterior part. This change in direction is brought about by the presence of the **acetabulocristal buttress**, which extends between the iliac tubercle superiorly and the upper border of the acetabulum

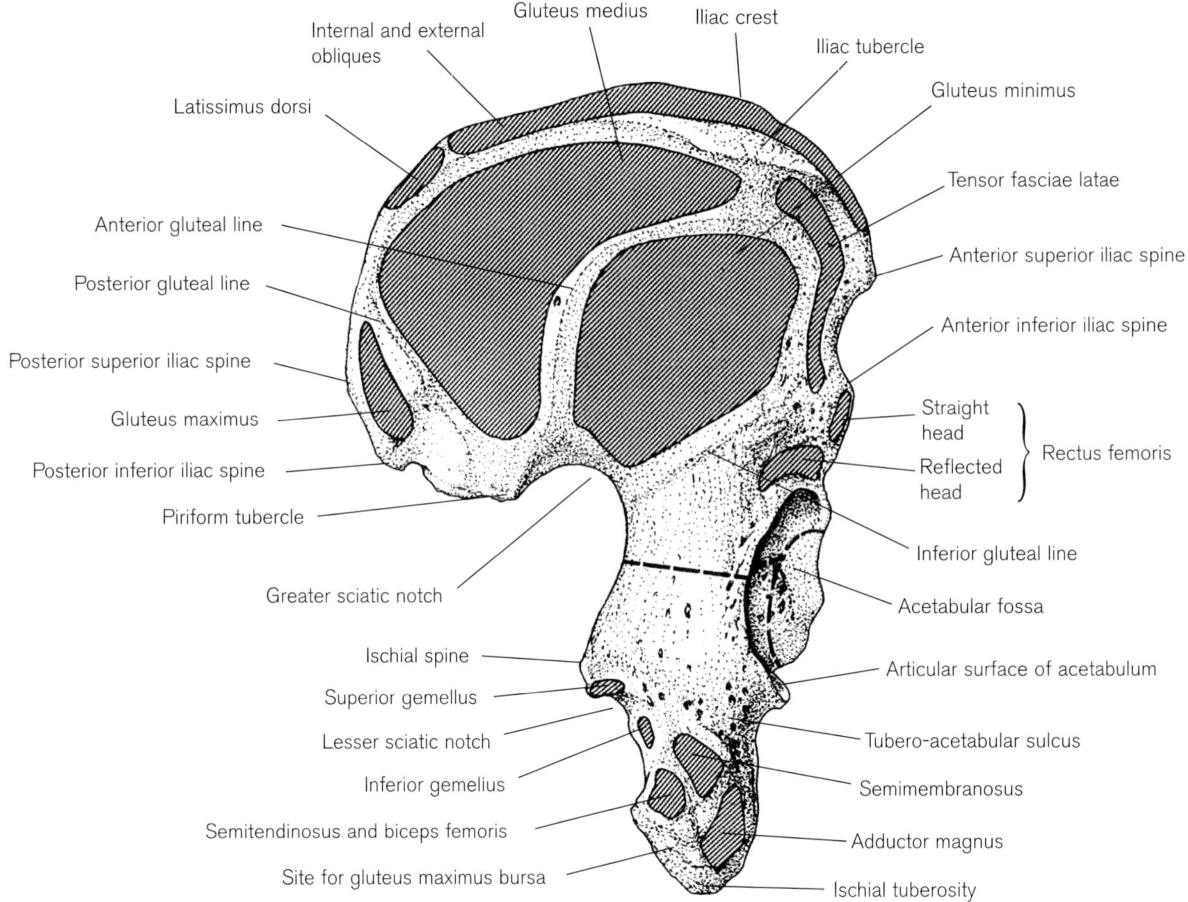

Figure 10.6 Posterior (gluteal) view of the right adult innominate.

inferiorly (Fig. 10.4). This strong bar develops in response to the stresses imposed on the bone by the muscles involved in erect posture and bipedal locomotion by counteracting the forces that would induce buckling of the bone (Wakeley, 1929; Aiello and Dean, 1990). The gluteal surface is bounded in front and behind by its anterior and posterior borders respectively, above by the iliac crest and below by the acetabulum anteriorly and its site of fusion with the ischium posteriorly. The attachments of the three gluteal muscles are delimited by posterior, anterior and inferior gluteal lines, which are not always well developed (Fig. 10.6) but are formed by the presence of tendinous fibres on the surfaces of these muscles. The posterior line is the shortest and commences anterior to the PIIS and ascends to reach the posterior aspect of the iliac crest. It is usually well defined in its upper limits, but becomes less distinct inferiorly. Gluteus maximus, the iliac head of piriformis and the sacrotuberous ligament, all arise from behind this line. The anterior line is the longest of the three and commences near the deepest part of the greater sciatic notch and ends near the iliac crest, just in front of the iliac tubercle. Gluteus medius arises between this and the posterior line. The inferior gluteal line is the most variable in its extent (Roberts, 1987) but generally passes from the apex of the upper border of the greater sciatic notch towards the upper part of the AIIS. Gluteus minimus arises between the anterior and inferior gluteal lines.

Although there are numerous small nutrient foramina around the periphery of the acetabulum, the principal nutrient foramen for this surface generally occurs in the mid-region of the anterior gluteal line, in the cleft between the attachments for the gluteus medius and minimus muscles. It is directed inferiorly and can often lead into a much larger vascular channel within the substance of the bone (Sirang, 1973). The lowest part of the gluteal surface becomes continuous with the posterior surface of the ischium behind the posterior border of the acetabulum. This marks the site of union of these bones during puberty and in the adult a distinct thickening of bone still remains in this area.

The hollowed-out anterior aspect of the ilium forms the **iliac surface** (fossa), which is the site of attachment for the iliacus muscle (Straus, 1929). This surface forms the posterolateral wall of the false pelvis and, in the living, it is closely related to the caecum, appendix and terminal part of the ileum on the right and the terminal part of the descending colon on the left. It is limited above by the iliac crest, anteriorly by the anterior border and behind by the medial border (spina limitans) that separates it from the sacropelvic surface (Fig. 10.5). The iliac surface is continuous with a shallow groove that runs between the AIIS and the iliopubic eminence, which is occupied by the converging fibres of the iliacus muscle laterally and the psoas major muscle medially (Frazer, 1948). A large laterally directed nutrient foramen is generally present in the postero-inferior aspect of this fossa and this houses a branch of the iliolumbar artery (Williams *et al.*, 1995). Interestingly, the radiographic image of this nutrient foramen has proved to be of some value in the identification of remains from mass disasters (Moser and Wagner, 1990) and can, somewhat misleadingly, simulate disease when viewed by computed tomography (Richardson and Montana, 1985).

The **sacropelvic surface** is bounded above by the iliac crest, in front by the spina limitans (medial border) and behind by the posterior border. It is separated into three areas – a dorsal and superior postauricular region for ligamentous attachment, a middle auricular region, which is the site of the synovial sacro-iliac joint, and a ventral and inferior pelvic region that lies between the auricular margin, the upper border of the greater sciatic notch and the iliopectineal line. The **postauricular region** is marked by a well-defined iliac tuberosity for the attachment of the strong sacro-iliac interosseous ligament and the more poorly defined dorsal sacro-iliac ligament (Weisl, 1954a). It is not uncommon to find accessory sacro-iliac articulations between the lateral sacral crest and the posterior inferior iliac spine and/or the iliac tuberosity (Derry, 1910; Trotter, 1937; Stewart, 1938; Hadley, 1952; Bowen and Cassidy, 1981). The **auricular** surface is roughly 'l'-shaped, with a shorter cranial limb that is directed dorsocranially and a longer caudal limb that is directed dorsocaudally (Weisl, 1954b). The cranial limb articulates with the lateral articular surface of the first sacral vertebra and the caudal limb with the smaller lateral articular surfaces of the second and occasionally third sacral vertebrae (Brooke, 1924; Schunke, 1938; Ali, 1989). Despite being a synovial joint, the sacro-iliac articulation displays limited movement in normal circumstances (often said to be 'locked'), due to the strength of the supporting ligaments, which hold the irregular articular surfaces in close apposition (Sashin, 1930; Cleaves, 1937; Dory and Francois, 1978; Beal, 1982; Bellamy *et al.*, 1983). However, increased joint movement has been reported during parturition probably as a result of alteration in hormone levels (Weisl, 1955). With increasing age, fibrous adhesions and gradual obliteration of the joint space can result in bony ankylosis (Sashin, 1930). This does not tend to happen before 50 years of age and is reported to be four times more common in the male (Brooke, 1924; Sashin, 1930; Weisl, 1954b; Oldale, 1990; Waldron and Rogers, 1990). Chronological changes in the morphological appearance of the auricular surface of the sacro-iliac joint have been used to predict age at death with some degree of accuracy (Lovejoy *et al.*, 1985b).

There is limited direct body weight transfer through the articular surfaces of the sacro-iliac joint as it is almost vertical in position in the living (Last, 1973) and so most of the stresses are borne by the supporting ligaments. As the skeletal effects of body weight transfer can manifest as sex differences, this passive role of the articular surfaces of the sacro-iliac joint is confirmed by the virtual lack of sexual dimorphism in the dimensions of the articular surfaces (Ali and MacLaughlin, 1991). The stresses placed on the supporting ligaments, particularly in the female, where pelvic dimensions change dramatically over a relatively short period of time at puberty, may partly explain the phenomenon of pre-auricular sulci as being growth, rather than parturition, related (Dee, 1981; St. Hoyme, 1984; MacLaughlin, 1987; Andersen, 1988; Tague, 1988; MacLaughlin and Cox, 1989; Spring *et al.*, 1989; Cox and Scott, 1992). It is now clearly established that, while a sulcus in this location is more common in females, it is not indicative of parity status, as was widely accepted in the past (Derry, 1908, 1911; Lang and Haslhofer, 1932; Jit and Gandhi, 1966; Houghton, 1974; Ullrich, 1975; Finnegan, 1978; Kelley, 1979c; Dunlap, 1982; Schemner *et al.*, 1995).

A strong bony buttress (iliopectineal line) runs obliquely downwards (55° to the horizontal plane – Moore, 1992) and forwards from the auricular region to the pubis and forms the lateral part of the pelvic brim that separates the lesser pelvis above from the true pelvis below (Fig. 10.2). The remainder of the pelvic surface of the ilium gives origin to the upper limits of the obturator internus muscle. It is not uncommon to find a well-developed nutrient foramen in the region of the deepest concavity of the greater sciatic notch, probably formed by a branch from the superior gluteal artery as it passes through the notch anterior to the piriformis attachment and onto the gluteal surface.

The **ischium** forms the lower posterior region of the innominate and comprises a body and a ramus. The body has an upper extremity, which fuses with the ilium (forming somewhat more than two-fifths of the acetabular surface), a lower extremity that gives rise to the ramus, and it can be described in terms of possessing femoral, dorsal and pelvic surfaces. The **femoral surface** of the body faces down, forwards and laterally and is bounded in front by the posterior margin of the obturator foramen (Fig. 10.4). The quadratus femoris muscle and part of the obturator externus attach to this surface in the region that is bounded by the acetabulum above and the ischial tuberosity behind. The tendons of both muscles then pass in the deep groove between the acetabulum above and the tuberosity below (tubero-acetabular sulcus, Stern and Susman, 1983) to attach to the posterior aspect of the femur. The **dorsal surface** of the ischial body faces backwards, laterally and superiorly and fuses with the lower extremity of the ilium above (Fig.10.6). The posterior border of this surface forms two notches, the lower region of the greater sciatic notch superiorly and the lesser sciatic notch inferiorly, which are separated by the ischial spine. The **ischial spine** projects downwards and slightly medially and is the site of attachment for the sacrospinous ligament, the coccygeus, levator ani and gemellus superior muscles. Its dorsal surface is crossed by the pudendal nerve and internal pudendal vessels as they pass from the gluteal region into the pudendal canal.[2] As these structures lie almost directly on the bone surface, fractures of the posterior wall of the pelvis can give rise to pudendal nerve damage, which can result in both incontinence and impotence (Dunn and Morris, 1968; Meschan, 1975). In obstetric practice the pudendal nerve can be blocked with local anaesthetic prior to forceps delivery by inserting a long needle through the vaginal wall, which is then guided by a finger to the ischial spine, which can be palpated *per vaginam* (Ellis, 1992). One of the main functions of the ischial spine is to provide a site of attachment for the muscles and ligaments that support the pelvic floor (Waterman, 1929; Elftman, 1932; Lawson, 1974; Oelrich, 1978; Tanagho, 1978). However, the ischial spines tend to protrude into the midline of the pelvic cavity, which can give rise to obstetric complications as it is in the region of the mid-pelvis that the progress of parturition is most frequently arrested (Oxorn, 1986; Abitbol, 1988a).

[2]The term 'pudendal' comes from the Latin 'pudere' meaning, literally translated, 'that of which one ought to be ashamed'. It is probably worth bearing in mind that pudenda normally only refers to the female external genitalia.

The tendon of obturator internus passes through the lesser sciatic notch and is separated from the bony surface by a bursa. The gemellus inferior muscle arises from the margin of this notch directly below the groove for the obturator internus tendon.

The **ischial tuberosity** marks the lowest limit of the dorsal surface of the ischium and is readily palpated in the living during flexion of the hip joint, although in extension it is fully covered by the gluteus maximus muscle. The tuberosity is clearly divided into upper and lower regions by the presence of a transverse ridge. The upper region gives rise to the semimembranosus muscle laterally and the long head of biceps femoris and semitendinosus medially. The lower region of the tuberosity tapers inferiorly and turns anteriorly to form the ischial ramus. The hamstring portion of the adductor magnus muscle attaches to the lateral aspect of this lower region of the tuberosity, while the medial aspect is covered by a fibro-adipose tissue that contains the gluteus maximus bursa. It is this lower medial area of the ischial tuberosity that supports the body in the upright sitting position (Williams *et al.*, 1995).

The **pelvic surface** of the ischium is smooth and relatively featureless, with the lower part of this wall forming the lateral wall of the ischiorectal fossa (Fig. 10.5). The obturator internus muscle is attached to the upper region and as the fibres converge on the lesser sciatic notch, they tend to cover most of this surface of the ischium, although they are separated from the bone by a bursa. A nutrient foramen is usually present on this surface around the level of the ischial spine and it transmits a branch of the obturator artery. The falciform ridge on the pelvic surface of the tuberosity is the site of attachment of the falciform process of the sacrotuberous ligament (Frazer, 1948).

The **ischial ramus** is the anterior prolongation of the lower extremity of the ischial body and it fuses with the inferior pubic ramus ventrally to form the ischiopubic ramus. The outer surface of the ischial ramus faces forwards and down towards the thigh, giving origin to the obturator externus muscle above, the anterior fibres of adductor magnus below and gracilis near the inferior border (Fig. 10.4). The inner/pelvic surface of the ischial ramus is smooth and partly subdivided into a pelvic and a perineal area (Fig. 10.5). The pelvic area is directed up and back and gives rise to part of the obturator internus muscle. The perineal area is directed more medially, with its upper part being related to the crus of the penis or clitoris and gives rise to the sphincter urethrae muscle, while its lower part is the site of attachment for the ischiocavernosus and superficial transverse perineal muscles.

The upper border of the ischial ramus completes the lower margin of the obturator foramen, while its free lower border provides attachment for the fascia lata of the thigh and the membranous layer of the superficial fascia of the perineum.

The **pubis** forms the ventral lower part of the innominate and articulates with its counterpart from the opposite side in the median plane. The **pubic symphysis** does not fuse in man and many of the great apes but it is a common occurrence in most other mammal groups (Todd, 1921a–e, 1923). It is thought that fusion is inhibited in man (perhaps hormonally) so that the pelvic girdle maintains the potential for some movement, which may be necessary to permit safe parturition. This would not, of course, explain the absence of fusion in the male.

The pubic bone is comprised of a body which lies anteriorly, a superior ramus which passes up and backwards to fuse with the ilium at the iliopubic eminence and an inferior ramus, which passes back, down and laterally to fuse with ramus of the ischium along the lower border of the obturator foramen. The anterior (outer) surface of the **pubic body** is the site of attachment for the adductor muscles of the thigh (Fig. 10.4). A roughened strip marks the medial extent of this surface and gives attachment to the ventral pubic ligament (Phenice, 1969; MacLaughlin and Bruce, 1987, 1990b; Budinoff and Tague, 1990). Adductor longus arises in the angle between this medial strip and the pubic crest, whereas gracilis arises at a somewhat lower level from a linear origin close to the medial border of the body and extends down onto the inferior ramus. Adductor brevis arises lateral to gracilis and the obturator externus muscle attaches to this surface around the limits of the obturator foramen. The smooth posterior surface of the pubic body forms the anterior wall of the true pelvis and lies in close approximation to the urinary bladder being separated from it by a retropubic pad of fat. The middle of this surface provides a site of attachment for the anterior fibres of the levatores ani muscles with obturator internus arising laterally (Fig. 10.5).

While the paired pubic bones are connected by superior and arcuate pubic ligaments, they are also separated by an intra-articular disc of fibrocartilage. A limited degree of movement occurs at the pubic symphysis, although repeated traumatic incidents can lead to lesions and weakness in the joint (Hunter, 1761a, b; Harris, 1974; Harris and Murray, 1974). The repeated trauma of childbirth was considered to be responsible for the appearance of pits on the posterior surface of the pubic body, but it is more likely that these depressions are related to osteoclast activity under the influence of oestrogen or may even result from ligamentous hyperplasia as a result of strain on the supporting ligaments of the joint (Lang and Haslhofer, 1932; Hall, 1950b; Morton and Gordon, 1952; Ullrich, 1975; Ashworth *et al.*, 1976; Putschar, 1976; Holt, 1978; Kelley, 1979c; Suchey *et al.*, 1979; Bergfelder and Herrmann, 1980; Tague, 1988; Cox and Scott, 1992).

The pubic bone is probably the most dimorphic region of the adult skeleton and it also displays considerable age-related change, which will be discussed below. Therefore, in both forensic and archaeological investigations, this is the region of the skeleton that is most likely to offer a reliable indication of both sex and age at death. It is therefore unfortunate that due to the thin covering shell of compact bone, this is one of the regions of the skeleton that frequently does not survive inhumation intact. In addition to this, the pubis is often the highest projecting bone in a burial and is therefore frequently damaged, either as a result of the collapse of the coffin, or the means of discovery (the bucket of an excavator is the common offender) or during the process of excavation.

The **pubic crest** is the rounded free upper border of the body between the symphysis medially and the **pubic tubercle** laterally (Fig. 10.4). The tubercle is the lower site of attachment for the inguinal ligament and the anterior loops of the cremaster muscle. Bergfelder and Herrmann (1980) and Cox and Scott (1992) both reported a positive correlation between the degree of development of the pubic tubercle and the parity status of the individual. The lateral head of the rectus abdominis muscle and the pyramidalis muscle arise from the lateral part of the pubic crest and so perhaps the positive correlation may lie with strain on the abdominal muscles during the advanced stages of pregnancy.

The **superior pubic ramus** arises from the lateral part of the pubic body, forming the upper boundary of the obturator foramen before it fuses with the ilium at the iliopubic eminence, where it forms approximately one-fifth of the articular surface of the acetabulum. The pectineal surface is triangular in cross-section and extends from the pubic tubercle anteriorly to the iliopubic eminence posteriorly. It is bounded in front by the rounded obturator crest and behind by the sharp pecten pubis, which gives rise to the pectineus muscle. The pelvic surface is smooth and featureless (Fig. 10.5). The obturator surface is crossed from behind forwards and downwards by the obturator groove, which is converted into a canal by the attachments of the obturator fascia and transmits the obturator nerve and vessels from the pelvic cavity to the medial aspect of the thigh.

The **inferior pubic ramus** arises from the lower lateral part of the pubic body and unites with the ischial ramus to complete the lower limit of the obturator foramen. The anterior surface is continuous with that of the pubic bone and it gives attachment to the gracilis, adductor brevis, obturator externus and adductor magnus muscles (Fig. 10.4). The internal surface of the ramus is directed medially towards the perineum and is the site of attachment for the crura of the penis or clitoris. The upper region of this surface gives rise to some fibres of the obturator internus muscle.

The **obturator foramen** lies in front of the acetabulum and is formed from only the pubis and ischium, with no iliac involvement. The name is derived from the Latin 'obturare' meaning 'to plug or stop up' and refers to the outlet to the adductor compartment. In the living, the foramen is covered by the obturator membrane, which is attached to its margins, except in the region of the obturator canal. The free superior end of the membrane stretches between the anterior and posterior obturator tubercles, with the former being located on the obturator aspect of the posterior margin of the pubic body and the latter at the anterior border of the ischium in front of the acetabular notch (Figs. 10.4 and 10.5). The canal is traversed by the obturator nerve and vessels. The obturator externus and internus muscles attach to the appropriate surfaces of the foramen.

The **acetabulum** (Latin meaning 'vinegar cup') is directed laterally, downwards and forwards and is the site of synovial articulation, with the head of the femur forming the hip joint. The acetabulum is separated into a horseshoe-shaped smooth articular surface surrounding a smaller, central non-articular roughened area. This area can occasionally be perforated and in such circumstances it is closed by a membrane (Frazer, 1948). The acetabular margin is deficient inferiorly at the acetabular notch and in the living this gap is bridged by the transverse acetabular ligament (Fig. 10.4). Vessels and nerves pass through the notch and under the ligament to gain access to the ligament of the head of the femur.

The non-articular floor (acetabular fossa) contains fibro-fatty tissue in the living condition and opens below at the acetabular notch, while the articular surface is covered by hyaline cartilage. The acetabulum is formed by the union of the three bones of the innominate with the pubis forming the upper and anterior one-fifth, the ischium forming the floor of the acetabular fossa and the lower and posterior two-fifths, while the ilium forms the remaining upper two-fifths of the articular surface. The depth of the acetabulum is considerably increased by the presence of a fibrocartilaginous labrum, which attaches around its margins and bridges the acetabular notch as the transverse ligament. The fibrous capsule attaches to the acetabulum outside the limits of the labrum and passes downward to surround the neck of the femur beyond the edge of the articular surface. This fact has a considerable importance in the diagnosis of many palaeopathological conditions (Steinbock, 1976; Ortner and Putschar, 1985; Roberts and Manchester, 1995). A roughly linear defect in the smooth outline of the articular surface, called an acetabular crease, has been reported in the literature, but its aetiology is uncertain (Finnegan, 1978).

Early development of the innominate

The lower limb buds appear around day 28 in the region of the lumbar and upper sacral cord segments (Fig. 10.7) (Bardeen and Lewis, 1901; O'Rahilly and Gardner, 1975) in response to inductive signals from adjacent somites 24–29 (Larsen, 1993, 1994). At this stage, the limb bud is comprised of a small proliferating mass of mesenchymal cells lying within a border of ectoderm (O'Rahilly *et al.*, 1956; Laurenson, 1964b; Yasuda, 1973; Langman, 1975).

Around days 34–36, a core of mesoblast cells starts to condense within an area that is defined by the positions of the obturator, femoral and sciatic nerves, which have already extended deep into the developing limb bud (Laurenson, 1963). It is interesting to note that the position of these major nerves is well-established *before* the condensation of the pelvic mesenchyme commences, so that the future cartilaginous anlage is forced to form around the already well established nerve pathways. In situations where a cartilaginous

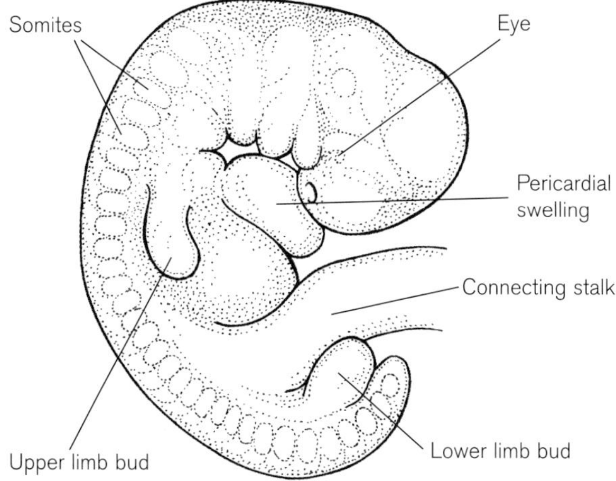

Figure 10.7 The human embryo in week 5 (CR length 8–14 mm).

model precedes nervous invasion, then it is the nerve that is forced to adopt a more circuitous route to reach its target. This somewhat precocious development of the three principal nerves of the lower limb may well explain their strikingly linear course from their origin to their target site in the adult (Laurenson, 1963).

The mesenchymal primordium extends in the form of three processes, an upper iliac, a lower posterior ischial (sciatic) and a lower anterior pubic (Fazekas and Kósa, 1978). The ischial and pubic mesenchymal masses meet and fuse inferiorly around the position of the obturator nerve, thereby forming the obturator foramen. Around days 36–38, the iliac process extends towards the vertebral mesenchymal primordium and fuses with the costal processes of the upper sacral vertebrae (Bardeen, 1905; Frazer, 1948; Fazekas and Kósa, 1978). Eventually, the pubic primordia meet in the midline anteriorly and fuse at the site of the future pubic symphysis.

Chondrification commences in this blastemal structure around weeks 6–7 of intra-uterine development (Bardeen, 1905; O'Rahilly and Gardner, 1975) and appears first in the iliac mass in the region of the acetabulum, cephalad to the greater sciatic notch (Fig. 10.8) (Laurenson, 1964b). Chondrification centres for the pubis and the ischium are well developed by 7–8 weeks and are separated by the course of the obturator nerve (Gardner and O'Rahilly, 1972). Towards the end of the second month, the three chondrification centres meet and fuse to form a shallow acetabulum, with the ischium and ilium fusing in advance of a union with the pubic mass (Adair, 1918). By the end of the second month, the two cartilaginous pubic masses meet and fuse in the midline in the region of the future symphysis (Adair, 1918; Frazer, 1948; Lloyd-Roberts *et al.*, 1959). In the eighth week, the anterior superior iliac spine, the ischial spine and the ischial tuberosity are well defined (Bardeen, 1905; Andersen, 1962). Therefore, the cartilaginous pelvis is approaching completion by the beginning of the third intra-uterine month (Adair, 1918).

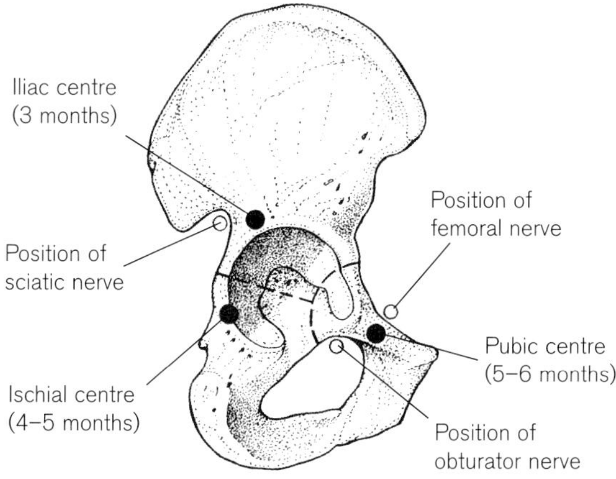

Figure 10.8 The position of the primary centres of ossification (and indeed chondrification) and the principal nerves of the lower limb in relation to the right innominate.

The embryological development and subsequent growth of the acetabulum has been of considerable interest, particularly in relation to congenital dislocation of the hip (Mezaros and Kery, 1980; Gepstein *et al.*, 1984; Portinaro *et al.*, 1994). This condition manifests as a deformity of the acetabulum and dislocation of the hip joint caused mainly by inversion of the fibrocartilaginous labrum and capsular contraction (Yochum and Rowe, 1987). Ponseti (1978a) noted that following unilateral congenital hip dysplasia, a cartilaginous ridge could be identified within the acetabulum (neolimbus of Ortolani). This was formed by a bulge of the acetabular cartilage that separated the cavity into two sections, with the more lateral of these forming the abnormal shallow site of articulation for the femoral head (Ortolani, 1948). The acetabulum may become shallow or even triangular in shape, with its base directed towards the obturator foramen and its apex looking up and back (Fairbank, 1930). Both Harrison (1957) and Ponseti (1979) have shown that the development of a cup-shaped acetabulum is directly influenced by the presence of the femoral head. If the head is displaced, then an abnormal shape of acetabulum will ensue. Chronic slippage of the femoral head can lead to a permanent dislocation and the development of a rudimentary secondary articulation site, usually located superior to the primary joint site on the dorsal surface of the wing of the ilium (Leffmann, 1959; Steinbock, 1976; Ortner and Putschar, 1985; Wakely, 1993). This condition is rare in fetuses younger than 20 weeks and has not been conclusively confirmed prior to the third trimester (Walker, 1983; Lee *et al.*, 1992). It has been suggested that complications at an early embryological stage, perhaps even at the time of limb rotation (6–8 weeks), may interfere with the ordered sequence of development and thereby initiate a train of events that ultimately manifest in an abnormal acetabular design (Badgley, 1949; Gardner and Gray, 1950; Ráliš and McKibbin, 1973). In theory, the fetal hip can dislocate as early as 11 weeks (Watanabe, 1974), as the joint cavity has formed and the hip flexors are active. It is at this time, however, that the acetabulum is at its deepest relative to the femoral head, so this is probably the most stable period in acetabular development (Ippolito *et al.*, 1984). Subsequent normal growth of the acetabulum relies heavily on growth at the triradiate cartilage and so any abnormality in this location will severely affect the appearance and function of the joint (Plaster *et al.*, 1991). Relative to the shape of the femoral head, the acetabulum is at its most shallow around the time of birth and so perhaps it is not surprising that the traumas associated with birth can easily give rise to congenital hip dislocation (Ráliš and McKibbin, 1973). After birth, the trend is reversed and the acetabulum deepens and adapts to the more globular femoral head so that the joint becomes more stable.

Frazer (1948) gives an account of an interesting feature of development of the acetabulum that does not appear to have been confirmed by any other text that we can find. He reports that in the embryo, only the ischium and ilium are involved in the articulation with the head of the femur and that the capsule is attached around their ventral margin, while the pubic cartilage remains extracapsular. Later, the pubis is reported to 'break through' the capsule and so becomes intracapsular, with the synovial cavity extending over it from the ilium. In this way, the original attachment of the capsule is only left on the ischium and this then forms the fibrous basis for the ligament of the head of the femur.

The embryological development of the sacro-iliac joint is particularly interesting. Cavitation of the joint begins in week 6 of intra-uterine life but from the seventh week it develops in a different way from other joints. There is a simultaneous presence of a synovial joint at the caudal part and a synarthrosis at the middle and cranial parts (McAuley and Uhthoff, 1990). A clear developmental difference is obvious between the caudal, cranial and middle segments at 14 fetal weeks. Cavitation at the caudal extremity leads to the formation of a joint space, whereas in the cranial region there is a rich vascular invasion of the tissues separating the sacral and iliac anlagen. In addition, it is interesting to note that at all times during embryological development, the iliac side of the joint is in advance of the sacral side (McAuley and Uhthoff, 1990). Further, it is clear that the iliac surface of the joint is covered by fibrocartilage, whereas the sacral side is covered by hyaline cartilage (Bowen and Cassidy, 1981; Uhthoff, 1990b).

The hip joint commences cavitation in week 7, this is complete by week 8 and the entire joint is fully formed by 18 weeks of intra-uterine life (Uhthoff, 1990b).

Ossification

Primary centres

Ossification centres virtually coincide in position with the earlier sites of chondrification and in the same order (Fig. 10.8) (Laurenson, 1964a). The centre for the ilium is the first to appear around the end of the second and the beginning of the third intra-uterine month (Bardeen, 1905; Mall, 1906; Hess, 1917; Adair, 1918; Flecker, 1932a, 1942; Hill, 1939; Noback, 1944; Francis, 1951; Noback and Robertson, 1951; Girdany and Golden, 1952; O'Rahilly and Meyer, 1956; Laurenson, 1964a; O'Rahilly and Gardner, 1972; Birkner, 1978). The centre of ossification appears in the perichondrium of the roof of the acetabulum (Fig. 10.8) in the vicinity of the future greater sciatic notch (Laurenson, 1964a). By around 9 weeks, the ossification has spread in a cranial direction, covering the internal and external surfaces of the iliac wing without invading the underlying cartilage. Ossification progresses in a radiating fan-like manner laying down bone on both an internal and an external shell (Laurenson, 1965; Birkner, 1978; Delaere *et al.*, 1992). There is evidence to suggest that, while the internal shell develops in advance of the external shell, the external shell tends to be thicker, probably by virtue of the action of the gluteal muscles (Delaere *et al.*, 1992). By 10–11 weeks, pores develop in the ossified shell and so invading osteoblasts and vascular elements gain access to the internal disintegrating cartilage and so form a primary marrow cavity. Laurenson (1964a) suggested that this unusual form of initial perichondral ossification, followed later by normal endochondral ossification (Burton *et al.*, 1989), is indicative of a protective reaction as it tends to occur in regions of the skeleton where the newly developed bone comes into direct contact with a well-established nerve trunk, e.g. the clavicle and ribs. In the ilium, the site of the initial ossification centre coincides with the location of the sciatic nerve. It is said that the ilium can be recognized by 4–5 fetal months by the presence of the upper border of the greater sciatic notch and the characteristic radiating appearance of the iliac shells (Francis, 1951; Laurenson, 1963).

Ossification of the ischium progresses by normal endochondral means (Laurenson, 1963) and the initial site appears in the body of the bone below and behind the position of the acetabulum around 4–5 intra-uterine months (Francis, 1951). The ischium is certainly identifiable in the third trimester of pregnancy when it appears as a comma or apple seed-shaped structure, which is broader superiorly and tapers inferiorly to the ramal surface, which points anteriorly. The superior, posterior and inferior borders are convex, while the anterior border is concave. The inner pelvic surface is smooth, while the outer surface bears a depression superiorly for the acetabular surface.

The pubic centre is the last to appear between 5 and 6 intra-uterine months (Fig. 10.8), and it commences in the region of the superior pubic ramus, anterior to the acetabulum and in close proximity to the passage of both the femoral and obturator nerves (Frazer, 1948). Although in the majority of cases, the pubis develops from a single centre of ossification, there are some reports that state that it can develop from two or more centres (Hess, 1917; Caffey and Madell, 1956). Even if multiple centres do develop, they are still restricted to the superior ramal region of the pelvis and they unite within the first few months of birth. However, during the process of fusion, they may adopt a sclerotic appearance on radiographs and so be incorrectly diagnosed as fracture sites (Caffey and Madell, 1956).

The pubis is rarely recovered from fetal remains as it is the last to commence ossification and so is both the smallest and most delicate of the pelvic elements. In the early stages it is reported to be dumb-bell-shaped or even in the form of a Turkish slipper (Fazekas and Kósa, 1978). The lateral (iliac) extremity is more rounded and club-like in appearance and is directed in an infero-oblique direction, while the

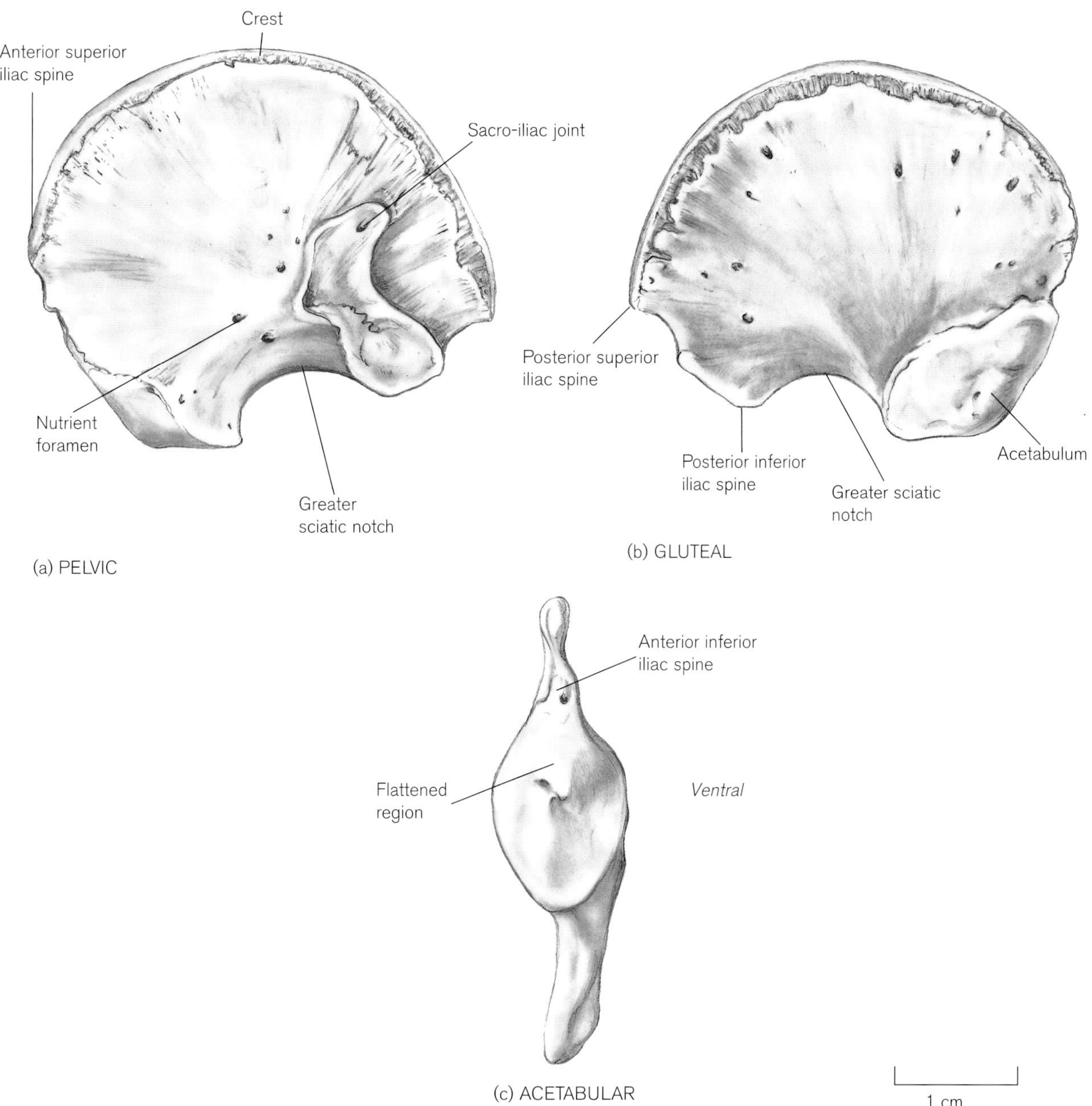

Figure 10.9 The right perinatal ilium.

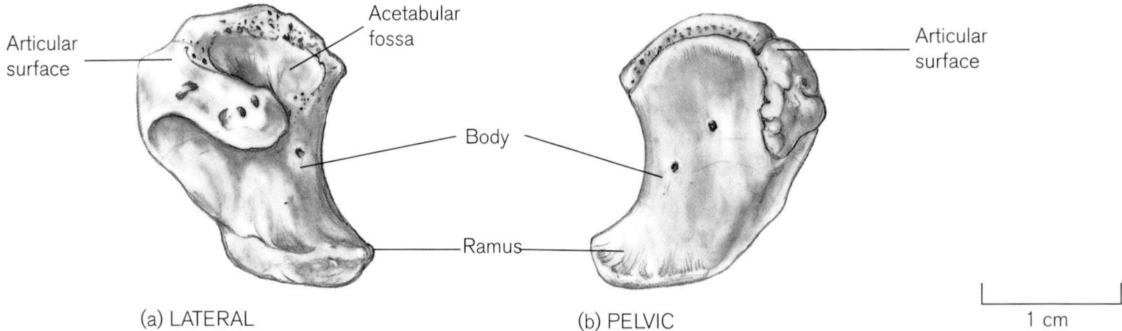

Figure 10.10 The right perinatal ischium.

medial (symphyseal) end is flatter and projects vertically downwards, forming the body of the pubis. The inner (pelvic) aspect is relatively featureless, while the outer region clearly shows the line of the pecten pubis passing superomedially across the upper region of the surface and the inferomedially orientated ventral arc of demarcation between the symphyseal surface medially and the lateral surface of the pubic body.

At birth, all three primary centres of ossification are well developed and readily identifiable and each has extended to such a point that it already forms part of the bony acetabular wall (Figs. 10.9–10.11). Although the morphology of the primary elements change little within the first few years after birth, each is reported to exhibit rapid growth in the first 3 months (Reynolds, 1945), which slows somewhat until 2–3 years of age (Miles and Bulman, 1995), then slows even further until the time of puberty, when the secondary sexually related growth changes occur concomitant with the normal adolescent growth spurt (Tanner, 1962). It is said that the pelvic organs descend fully into the pelvic cavity by 6 years of age and presumably this reflects the time at which the complex has grown sufficiently in all diameters to allow complete descent (Meschan, 1975).

Certainly by birth, the ilium has adopted most of the characteristic features of the adult bone (Fig. 10.9). Both the anterior and posterior superior iliac spines are well developed at this stage, although the region of the anterior inferior iliac spine is more poorly defined. Contrary to Wakeley (1929), we have found that both the acetabulocristal buttress and the thickened bar of bone that passes from the auricular surface to the acetabulum are present at birth. Although the crest is distinctly S-shaped, the characteristic concavities and convexities of the iliac and gluteal surfaces do not fully develop until the anterior border bends forward around 2 years of age. This alteration in blade morphology probably results from remodelling associated with body weight transfer in relation to upright posture and locomotion. This is also the time at which England (1990) reports that the sacrum descends between the ilia.

After birth, the appearance of the three centres alters very little, but recognizable changes do occur at the acetabular surface. At birth, the acetabular surface of the ilium is represented by a slight depression in the centre of the somewhat bulbous inferior extremity. By 6 months *postpartum*, the iliopectineal line can be distinguished as a distinct promontory on its ventral rim (Fig. 10.12) and by 4–5 years of age a well-defined plaque of bone is present on the ventral aspect of the depression, which represents the future non-articular region of the iliac acetabular fossa. Certainly by 6 years of age, although it can be earlier if ischiopubic fusion is imminent, there is a well-

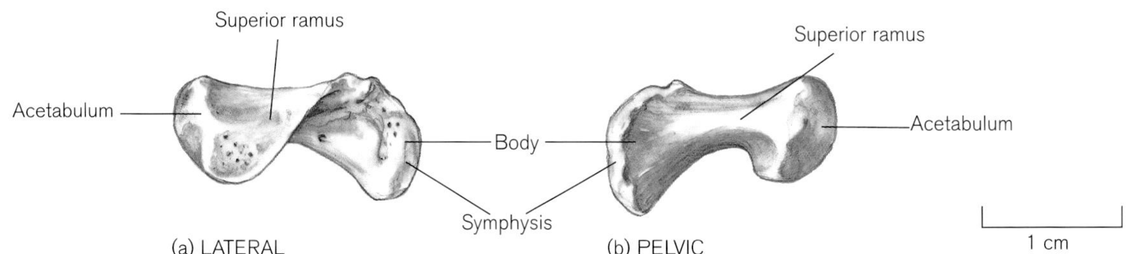

Figure 10.11 The right perinatal pubis.

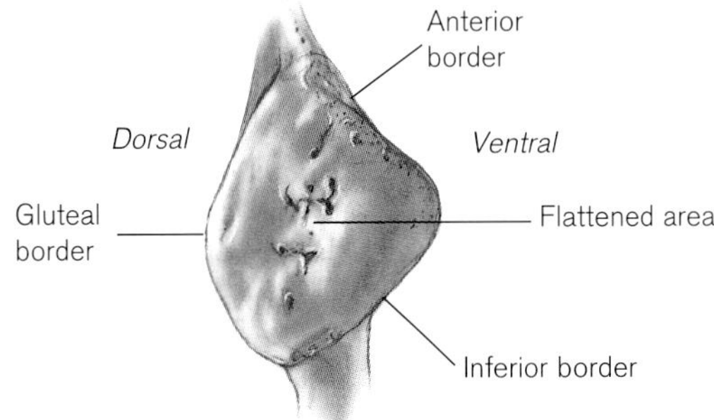

(a) 6 months

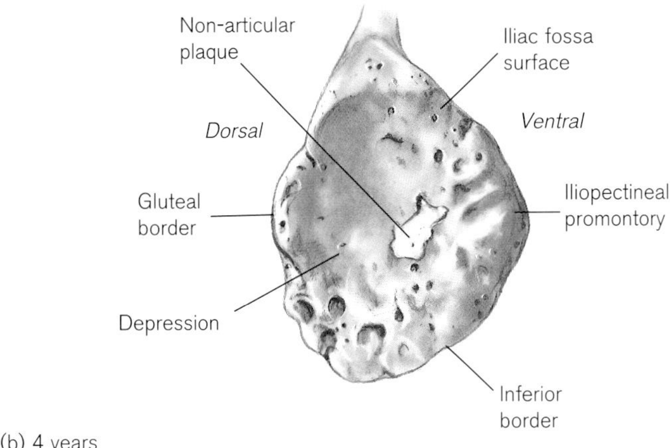

(b) 4 years

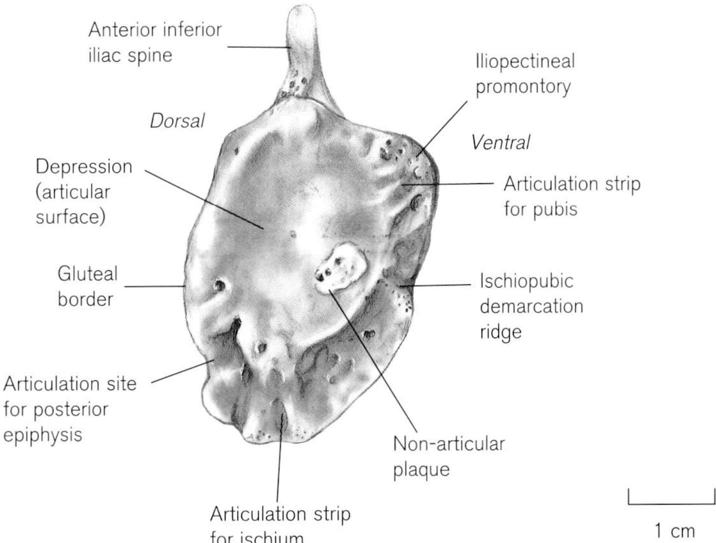

(c) 6 years

Figure 10.12 The development of the right iliac acetabular surface.

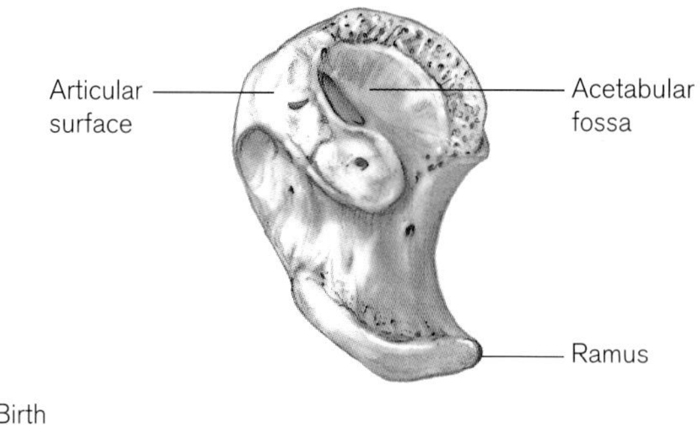

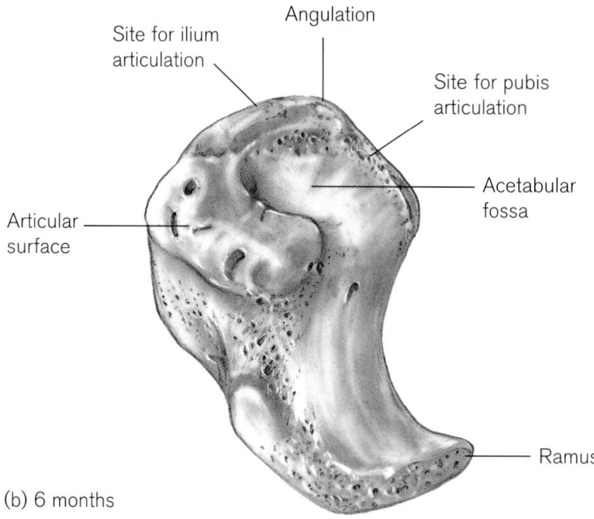

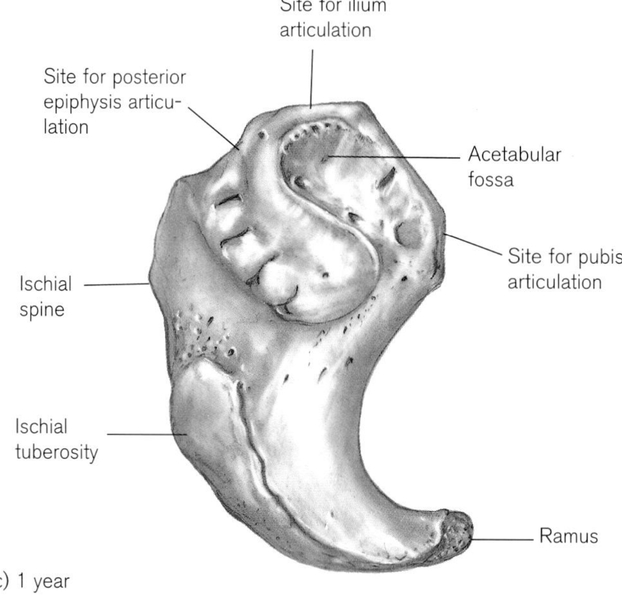

Figure 10.13 The development of the right ischium (with particular reference to the acetabular surface).

defined line of demarcation between the articulation sites for the pubis and the ischium. Thus, the immature ilial acetabular extremity is basically triangular in shape, bearing a somewhat dorsally located depression for the articular surface, which is bounded anteriorly and inferiorly by thick strips of metaphyseal bone for articulation with the pubis and ischium respectively (Fig. 10.12). The promontory for the iliopectineal line lies on the anterior border, superior to the line of demarcation between the pubic and ischial articulation sites. The plaque of non-articular bone lies on the anterior aspect of the acetabular depression, lateral to the ischiopubic demarcation line and inferior to the iliopectineal promontory. A highly convoluted area of bone is present at the inferodorsal margin at the point of contact with the descending margin of the greater sciatic notch, and this will be the future site of articulation for the posterior acetabular epiphysis. The gluteal margin of the acetabular extremity is scalloped in appearance and often becomes continuous superiorly with the anterior border of the ilium passing up towards the anterior inferior iliac spine.

In the ischium at birth (Fig. 10.10), the superior pole of the outer lateral surface bears the articular acetabular region, which is restricted to the posterior aspect as a strip of non-articular bone (acetabular fossa) occupies the anterior area. By around 6 months of age, the superior convex border of the ischium develops an angulation so that the site of articulation for the pubis lies anteriorly and that for the ilium lies superiorly (Fig. 10.13). By 1 year of age, the superior border is no longer convex but is straight, so that the articulation site for the ilium lies superiorly and almost horizontally and the site for the pubis lies anteriorly and almost vertically. The most posterior projection of the superior border is thickened and almost triangular in shape and this is the site of articulation for the future posterior acetabular epiphysis (Fig. 10.13). The ischial spine is also well developed by 1 year of age and initially presents as a rounded projection on the posterior margin.

The acetabular surface of the immature pubis is roughly oval in outline lying in a somewhat oblique plane. At 6 months of age it is somewhat raised from the remainder of the surface and occupies an anterior location (Fig. 10.14). This elevation is bordered on two sides by metaphyseal surfaces, with the superomedial aspect representing the site for articulation with the ilium and the inferomedial region being the site of articulation with the ischium. The demarcation between these two sites of articulation becomes detectable by around 3–4 years of age and becomes more clearly defined as the time for ischiopubic fusion approaches. By this age, the acetabular region is no longer elevated, but presents as a relatively flat surface that may even be concave in appearance. By 5–6 years of age, a non-articular plaque of bone becomes evident in the acetabular depression on the posterior margin adjacent to the region of articulation with the ischium (Fig. 10.14).

The primary centres of the ischium and the pubis are first to fuse in the region of the rami (Fig. 10.15) and although the timing is extremely variable, as it can arise as early as 3 years of age, it generally occurs between 5 and 8 years (Frazer, 1948; Birkner, 1978; Fazekas and Kósa, 1978; Caffey, 1993). As the time for fusion approaches, the ends of the synchondrosis become enlarged (Caffey and Ross, 1956; Birkner, 1978) but this 'heaped' appearance has normally diminished by 10 years of age (Davies and Parsons, 1927). Although of unknown function and aetiology, an accessory ossicle has been reported in the hyaline cartilage of the joint (Caffey, 1993). It is not clear which surface of the synostosis fuses first as we have found cases where the inner surface is fused but the outer is still open, and indeed cases where the opposite is true. At this early stage, fusion between the ischium and the pubis is restricted to the ramal region, as the vertical flange of the triradiate cartilage is still present between the two bones in the acetabular region and fusion here will not occur until puberty (see below).

Secondary centres

To understand the complex nature of secondary ossification centres in the pelvis, it is useful to consider each of the three constituent parts in terms of normal long bone development where proximal and distal epiphyses develop and fuse to a diaphysis. The secondary centres for the ilium appear at the crest (proximal) and the acetabulum (distal), the pubic secondary centres appear at the acetabulum (proximal) and at the body, crest and ramus (distal) and the ischial epiphyses occur at the acetabulum (proximal) and the ramus and tuberosity (distal). Accessory centres are also reported but they tend to be more variable, e.g. ischial spine and anterior inferior iliac spine.

Clearly, a factor common to all three pelvic elements will be the ossification of the secondary centres in the region of the acetabulum. Acetabular maturation is complex and this has been further complicated by misunderstandings and inconsistent use of nomenclature. An appreciation of the basic histological composition of the developing joint is essential before the pattern of ossification can be fully understood (Harrison, 1957; Walker, 1981). As with the end of any developing typical long bone, three types of cartilage are represented in the maturing acetabulum: growth,

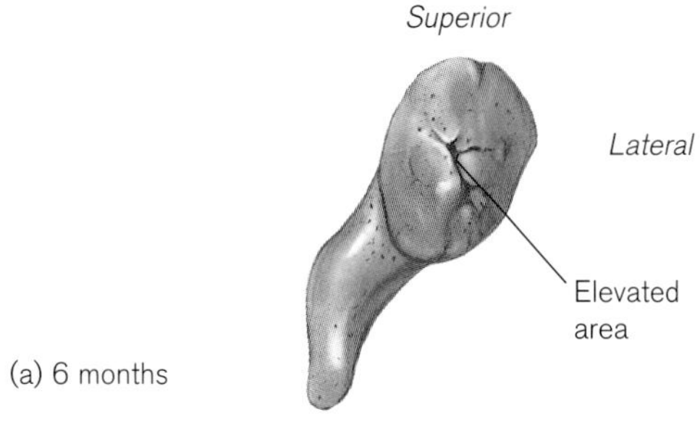

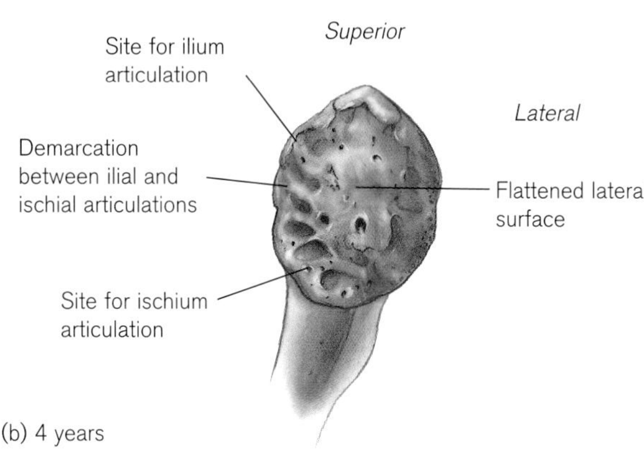

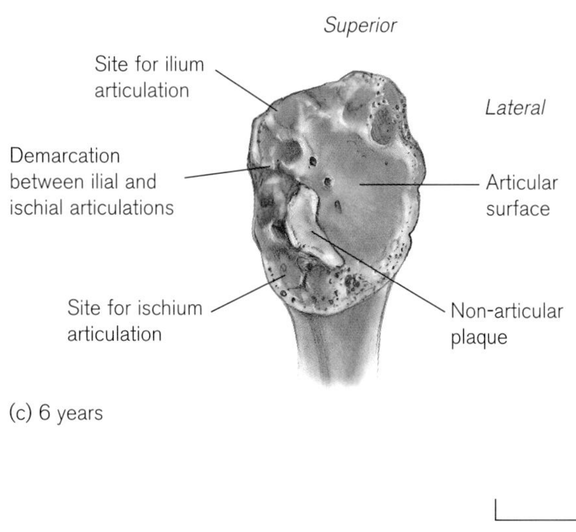

Figure 10.14 The development of the right pubic acetabular surface.

epiphyseal and articular cartilage. The cartilaginous acetabular anlage is composed of a cup-shaped articular area laterally (deficient inferiorly), which is connected to a medial triradiate unit that is interposed between the ilium, ischium and pubis (Harrison, 1957; Ponseti, 1978b, 1979). The articular cartilage lines the inner surface of the cup-shaped region of the anlage and will of course form the site of articulation for the head of the femur at the hip joint. The triradiate unit displays areas of growth cartilage adjacent to the surfaces of the three bony elements and each is separated from its counterpart on the opposite side by a strip of epiphyseal cartilage (Fig. 10.16). In this way, interstitial growth within the triradiate zone causes the acetabulum to expand during childhood and so accommodate the enlarging femoral head (Harrison, 1961).

The triradiate cartilage is comprised of three flanges (Fig. 10.17):

- the anterior flange is located between the ilium and pubis and is slanted superiorly
- the posterior flange is positioned between the ilium and the ischium and is more horizontally placed
- the vertical flange is located between the ischium and the pubis (Ponseti, 1978b).

To understand secondary ossification in the acetabulum it is important to visualize the spatial three-dimensional relationship between the laterally placed cup-shaped acetabular cartilage and the more medially located triradiate complex. Harrison (1957) emphasized the importance of establishing that the cup-shaped acetabular cartilage is not ossified by direct extensions from the triradiate unit but by separate ossicles that form within the cartilaginous zone around the acetabular rim. While Harrison's research was based on the development of the rat pelvis, there is a considerable amount of comparative research that shows a similar pattern throughout most mammals (Payton, 1935; Schultz, 1941b; Shapiro *et al.*, 1977).

There are generally three main epiphyses that form within the cup-shaped cartilage of the acetabulum and these will eventually expand to form both the outer rim of the acetabulum and much of the articular surface. As these centres enlarge they will ultimately meet with the ossifying triradiate epiphyses and fusion will occur. The first of the acetabular epiphyses to ossify is the **os acetabuli** (anterior acetabular epiphysis), which appears around 9–10 years of age as a triangular-shaped bone on the ventral acetabular rim, wedged between the pubis and the ilium (Zander, 1943; Ponseti, 1978b). It appears in the thick cartilage of the acetabulum adjacent to the pubis and as it matures it extends into the anterior flange of the

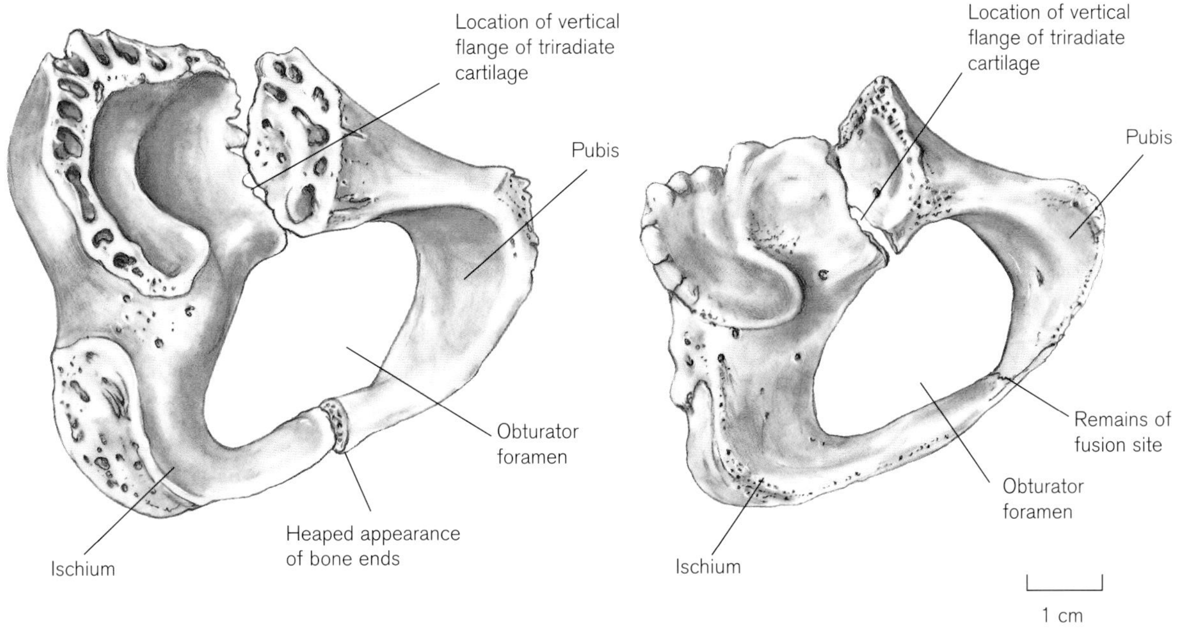

Figure 10.15 Right ischiopubic fusion.

triradiate zone between the pubis and the ilium (Fig. 10.18). This epiphysis forms the anterior aspect of the acetabular rim and extends downward to form both the acetabular articular surface of the pubic element and the upper anterior aspect of the ilium. In time, it will eventually expand upward to fuse with the superior epiphysis of the acetabulum and also with the anterior flange of the triradiate bone (Fig. 10.19).

When well developed and therefore close to the time of union, it is possible that the anterior epiphysis (os acetabuli) of the acetabulum may be identified in isolation (Fig. 10.18). It presents a flattened superior surface for articulation with the ilium, an inferior concave surface for articulation with the pubis, an expanding lateral surface that forms the articular acetabular surface and a triangular-shaped surface that forms at the iliopubic eminence.

A second acetabular epiphysis arises in the posterior acetabular rim at the junction between the ilium and the ischium. Although many radiological texts have also referred to this as the os acetabuli, it is clearly a different structure (Freedman, 1934). Some texts therefore suggest the use of the terms 'anatomical os acetabuli' for the anterior ossific nucleus and 'radiological os acetabuli, for that on the posterior acetabular rim (Zander, 1943). This is clearly not an ideal situation and so the term 'os acetabuli' tends now to be restricted to the anterior nodule, while the posterior structure has been referred to as the 'os marginalis

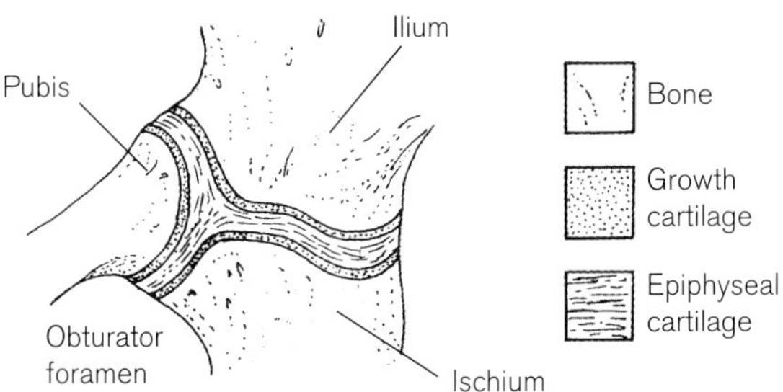

Figure 10.16 A diagrammatic representation of a sagittal section through the immature triradiate zone to show the arrangement of cartilage types.

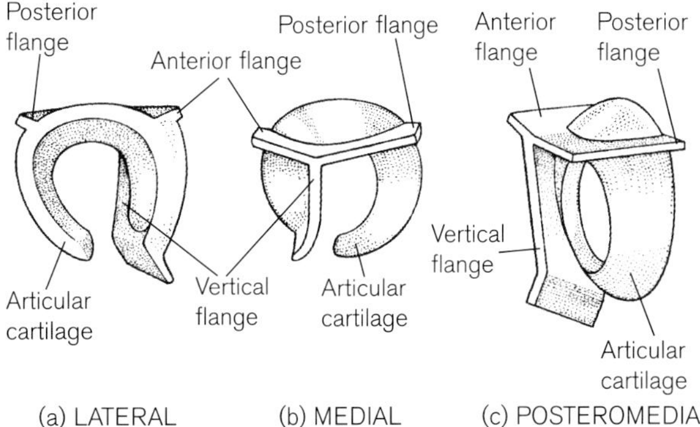

Figure 10.17 The right acetabular cartilaginous anlage (redrawn after Harrison, 1958).

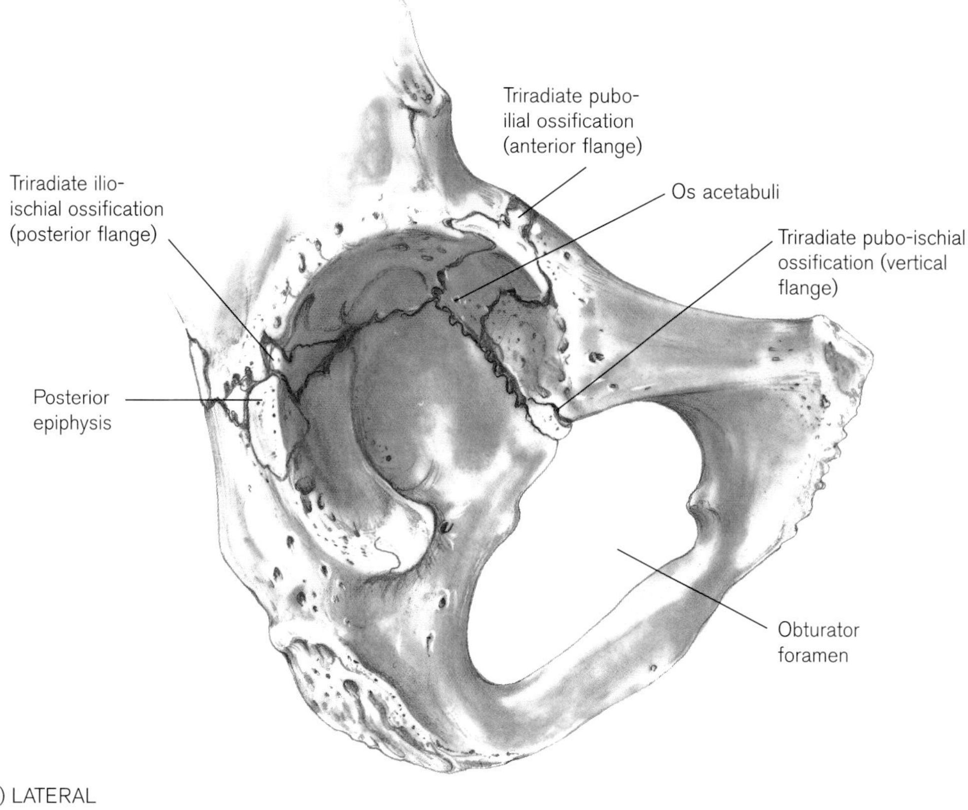

(a) LATERAL

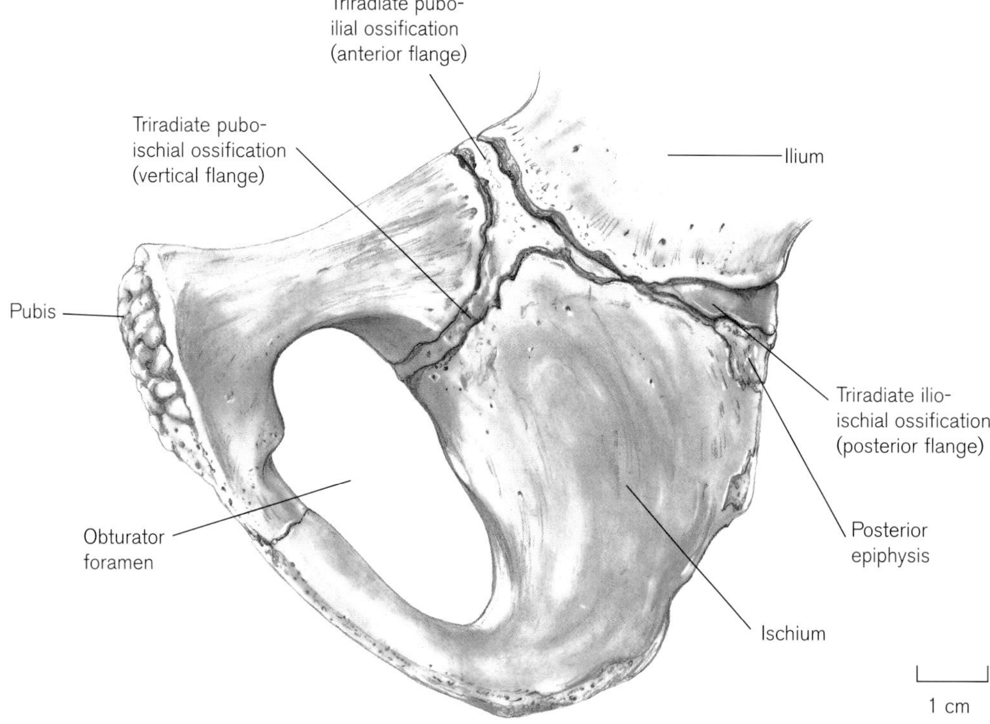

(b) PELVIC

Figure 10.18 Ossification of the right triradiate and acetabular epiphyses (approx. 15 years).

superior acetabuli,' or indeed the 'nucleus osseous superior marginalis acetabuli' (Zander, 1943). This **posterior epiphysis** tends to be larger than its anterior counterpart and frequently forms from the fusion of several smaller ossicles (Fig. 10.18). It appears around the age of 10–11 years in the posterior aspect of the acetabular cartilage and spreads superiorly and inferiorly to form not only the posterior rim of the acetabulum but also much of the acetabular articular surface of the ischium and a small part of the articular surface of the ilium, as well as fusing with the ossicles in the posterior limb of the triradiate cartilage.

A third, **superior epiphysis** appears in the upper rim of the acetabulum and this has been confusingly referred to as the 'acetabular epiphysis' (Figs. 10.19–21). This forms the upper rim of the acetabulum and much of the roof of the acetabular articular surface (Ponseti, 1978b; Johnstone *et al.*, 1982). This epiphysis does not extend into the triradiate zone but it does frequently pass upward as a tongue of bone to form the lower region of the anterior inferior iliac spine (Fig. 10.21). The epiphysis appears around 12–14 years of age but complete fusion involving the anterior inferior iliac spine may not, in our experience, be completed until 16 or 17 years of age.

From around 9 years of age, a variable number of small ossific islands appear within the true triradiate cartilage and it is likely that these represent the true central epiphyses of the ilium, ischium and pubis (Fig. 10.18). As these centres enlarge, they meet both the expanding acetabular epiphyses and the advancing borders of the three bones of the pelvis and ultimately fuse. There is a tendency for the pelvic aspect of the triradiate zone to fuse in advance of its acetabular aspect, although consolidation is generally complete by mid-puberty (Frazer, 1948). It is reported that acetabular fusion commences around 11 years in females and 14 years in males and is completed by 15

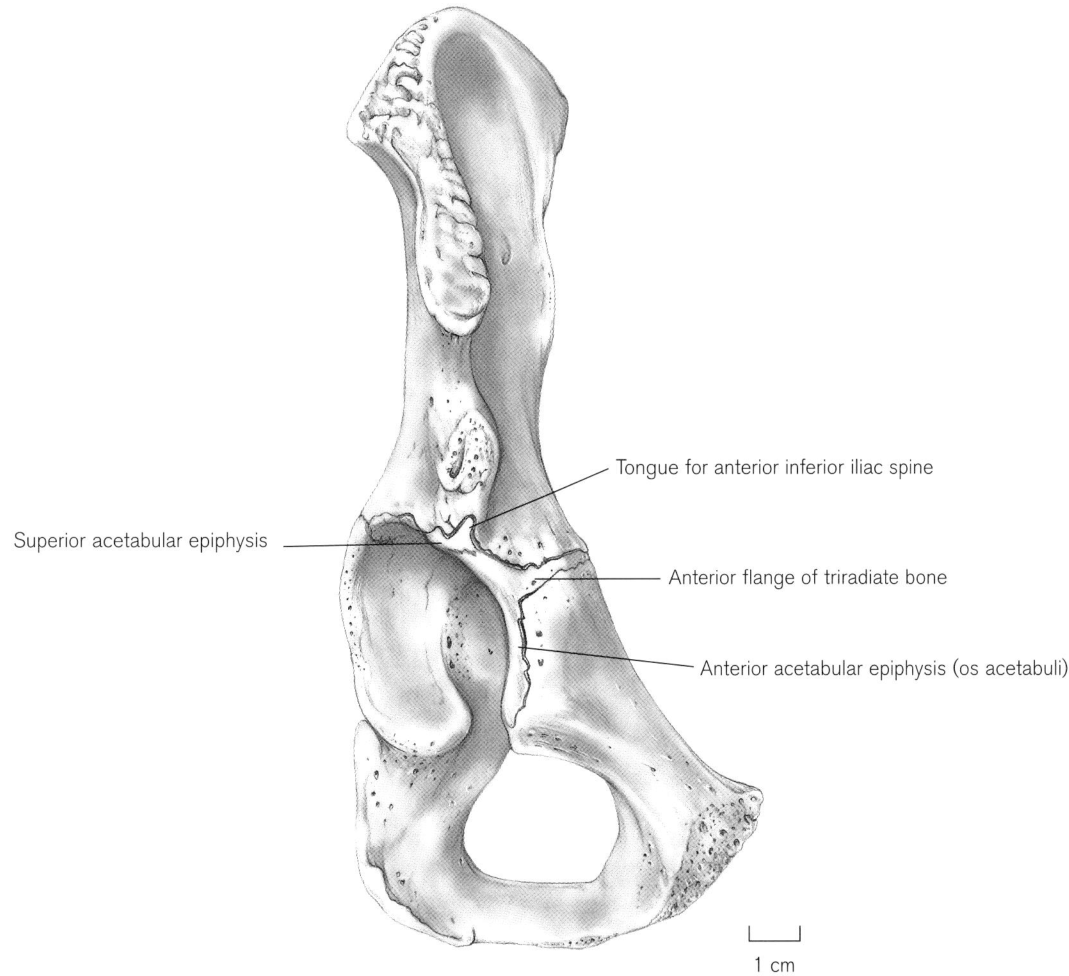

Figure 10.19 The development of the right anterior acetabular epiphysis (approx. 15 years).

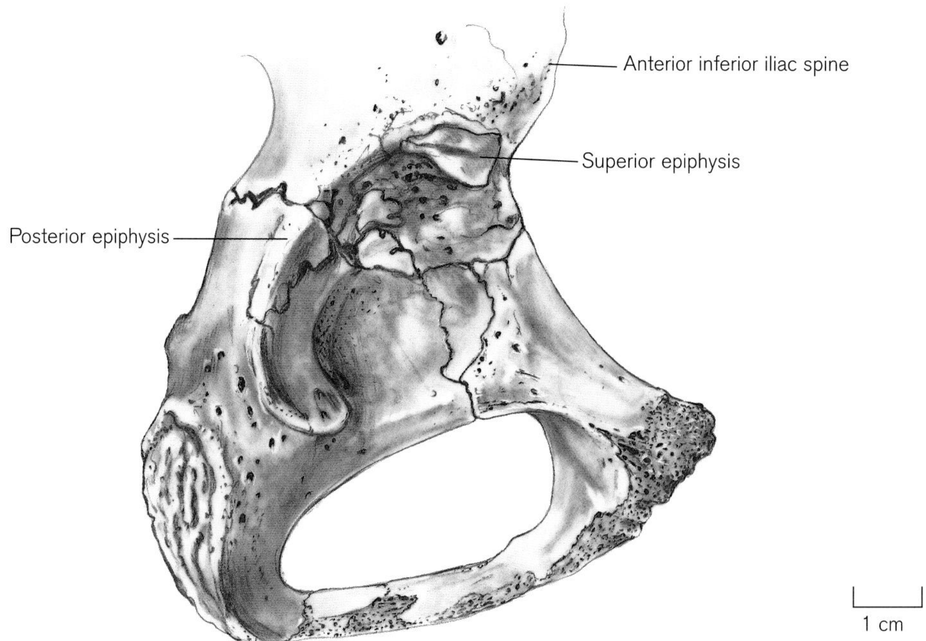

Figure 10.20 The right posterior and superior acetabular epiphyses (female aged 12 years).

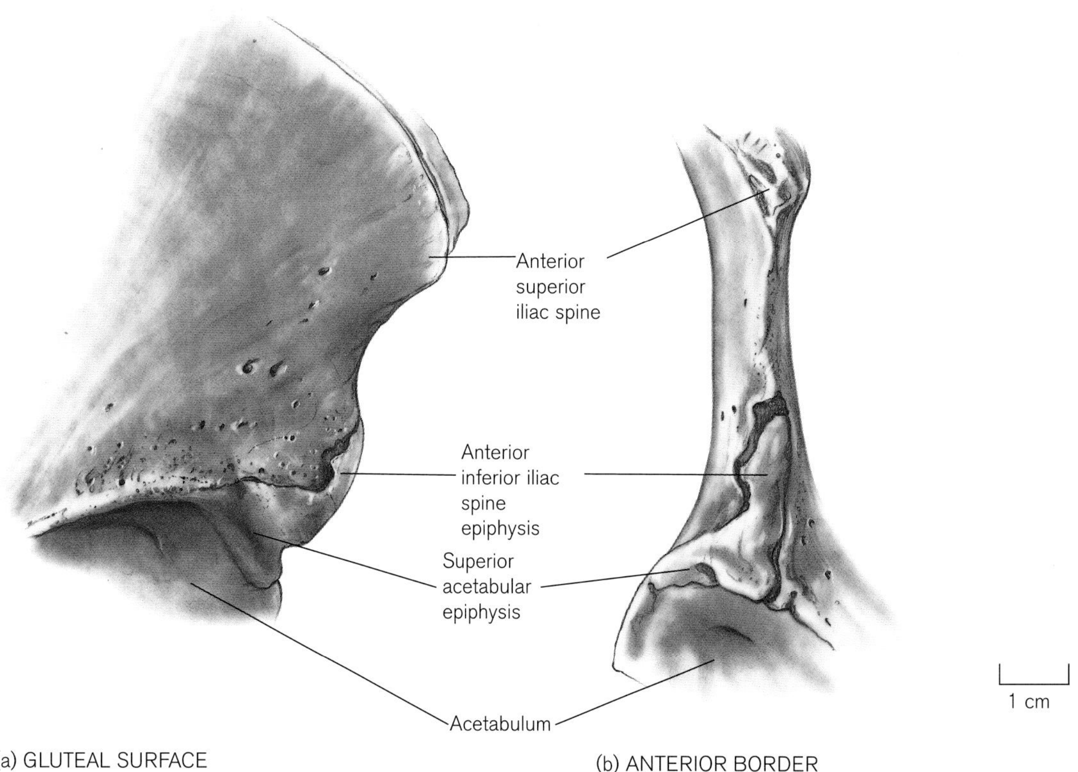

Figure 10.21 The prolongation of the right superior acetabular epiphysis to form the epiphysis for the anterior inferior iliac spine (female aged 14 years).

years in females and 17 years in males (Stevenson, 1924; Flecker, 1932b; Freedman, 1934; Johnston, 1961; Garn *et al.*, 1967b). In extremely rare circumstances, the epiphyses that form the rim of the acetabulum may persist as isolated nodules of bone (Zander, 1943). Other accessory shell-like ossicles may also develop in the cartilaginous walls of the acetabulum and in rare circumstances they too can persist as permanent separate structures (Denyer, 1904).

The formation of a strong supporting structure for the head of the femur is unquestionably of vital importance for the structural integrity of the hip joint in terms of efficient weight transfer and normal locomotion. It is thought that early maturation of the acetabulum may be desirable to enable the joint to withstand the considerable forces that pass through it as body mass and weight increase during puberty. Indeed, Greulich and Thoms (1944) reported that the radiographic appearance of prepubertal pelves was characterized by an 'acetabular constriction' caused by an inward projection of the pelvic wall in the region of the acetabuli. They suggested that this was a manifestation of the medially directed pressure transmitting through the femoral heads to a yielding cartilaginous junction. This radiographic appearance is known as 'juvenile beaking' and is a non-pathological condition resulting from plastic deformity of the triradiate region in relation to normal shear and rotational stress. However, if there is an abnormal progression of triradiate development the clinical condition of 'primary protrusio acetabuli' will arise and this can have many serious implications, not least being obstruction in the midpelvis which can lead to cephalopelvic disproportion during parturition (Alexander, 1965; Gusis *et al.*, 1990).

Trauma to the triradiate cartilage is relatively uncommon and is often difficult to diagnose immediately (Heeg, 1988). It generally arises following either a blow to the pubis or ischial ramus resulting in a sheering injury or by crushing/fracture or impaction-related trauma (Rodrigues, 1973; Blair and Hanson, 1979; Bucholz *et al.*, 1982). The younger the patient is at the time of injury (particularly under 10 years of age), the more likely it is that disruption or arrest of normal growth will occur (Rodrigues, 1973). Trauma to the cartilage initiates a bridge or graft across the physis, which can result in premature fusion leading to a shallow acetabulum and subluxation of the hip (Hallel and Salvati, 1977). It is only if this graft is broken or resorbed that normal growth can continue (Campbell *et al.*, 1959). It has also been shown in piglets that if the triradiate cartilage is crossed by an osteotome, for example during Pemberton osteotomy, this will also give rise to a bony bar that traverses the site of injury (Leet *et al.*, 1999). The triradiate cartilage can also be affected by conditions such as suppurative arthritis or even osteochondromas, which will also affect the normal growth of the cartilage (Wientroub *et al.*, 1981; Ortner and Putschar, 1985; Matsumo *et al.*, 1987).

The comparatively early union of the acetabulum restricts continued growth in the pelvis (St Hoyme, 1984) so that the majority of later pubertal alterations in pelvic shape and size tend to be restricted to the other epiphyseal sites away from the acetabulum. Although much of the initial research on pelvic growth was carried out on the rat pelvis (Harrison, 1965, 1968), it is generally recognized that growth at the caudal end of the ischium and at the pubic symphysis is four times faster than the rate of growth exhibited at the acetabulum. Perhaps it is not surprising then, that the joints in these locations continue to show a more prolonged period of growth-related activity and so have become useful as indicators of age at death (Todd, 1920; McKern and Stewart, 1957; Acsádi and Nemeskéri, 1970; Gilbert and McKern, 1973; WEA, 1980; Lovejoy *et al.*, 1985b; Meindl *et al.*, 1985; Katz and Suchey, 1986; Brooks and Suchey, 1990). This may also go some way towards explaining why the majority of the sexually dimorphic traits in the pelvis are restricted either to the posterior element, e.g. greater sciatic notch, or indeed to the anterior portion, e.g. pubis shape. Increased growth in these two regions in particular may well place undue strain on the ligaments that hold these joints in position and may therefore explain the frequency of pitting and grooving found in these regions in the female in particular where secondary sexual growth alterations are most prevalent (see above).

Following fusion of the acetabular centres, the order of the other secondary epiphyses of the pelvis is somewhat variable, but it is generally reported to be – from first to last – anterior inferior iliac spine, iliac crest, ischial tuberosity and pubic symphysis. The order of completion of fusion also tends to follow this pattern (Stevenson, 1924; Stewart, 1934a; Johnston, 1961).

The epiphysis for the **anterior inferior iliac spine** is reported to commence ossification around 10–13 years of age and fuse by around 20 years (Francis, 1940). However, there seems to be little information on the variation that can arise in the origin of this epiphysis, its pattern of fusion and its clinical relevance. Williams *et al.* (1995) only comment that 'The anterior inferior iliac spine may be ossified as an extension from this centre (os acetabuli) or from a separate centre.' We have found that in the majority of cases the inferior aspect of the anterior inferior iliac spine and the lower aspect of the anterior border of the ilium directly below it, form from an extension of the superior acetabular epiphysis (Fig. 10.21). The position of this epiphysis closely matches the site of attachment of the upper band of the iliofemoral ligament and, as this too passes up towards the AIIS, then perhaps it is not surprising that the lower aspect of the anterior border of the ilium forms in this way. The tongue-like expansion can be found in individuals from around 12 years of age, but it will have fused by around 16–18 years. The upper aspect of the AIIS can develop as a separate flake-like epiphysis that corresponds with the site of attachment for the straight head of the rectus femoris muscle and is therefore a true traction epiphysis (Fig. 10.22). This is a common site of avulsion fracture following violent muscular contraction in athletes (Jergensen, 1975; Fernbach and Wilkinson, 1981; Yochum and Rowe, 1987). This is also true for the ischial epiphysis as it too forms at the site of strong muscular attachment (biceps femoris, semimembranosus, semitendinosus and adductor magnus).

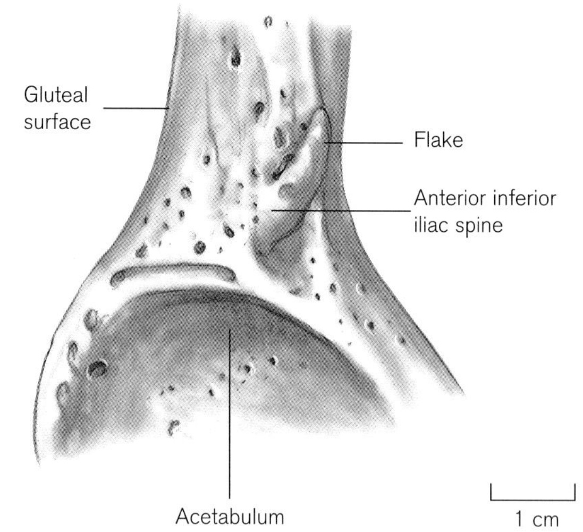

Figure 10.22 Epiphyseal flake on the superior aspect of the right anterior inferior iliac spine (approx. 19 years).

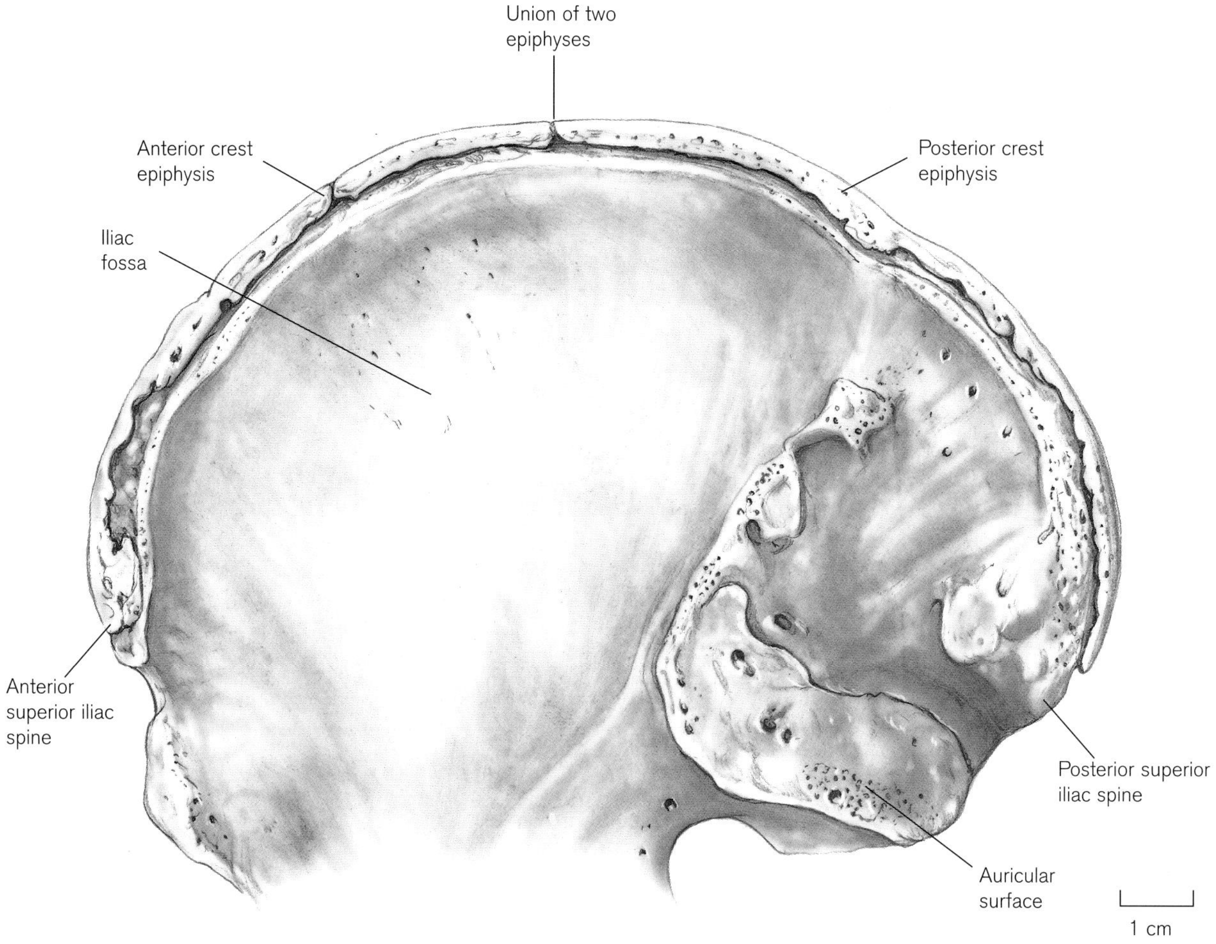

Figure 10.23 The right iliac crest epiphyses (approx. 16 years).

Despite Francis' (1940) report that the **iliac crest epiphysis** begins to ossify in the middle of the crest and extends outwards in each direction, it is generally recognized that it does indeed form from two separate ossification centres. The anterior epiphysis forms the anterior superior iliac spine and the anterior half of the crest of the ilium, while the posterior epiphysis forms the posterior superior iliac spine and the posterior half of the iliac crest (Stevenson, 1924; Frazer, 1948). The two epiphyses meet in the middle of the crest just posterior to the highest point (Fig. 10.23). The epiphysis obviously assumes the shape of the crest and so adopts a somewhat spiral growth pattern (Birkner, 1978). Unlike the other epiphyses of the innominate, that for the iliac crest is well formed before it commences fusion and so it tends to be somewhat delayed in terms of its maturation.

The iliac crest epiphyses are thin, flat, long, spiral and in the early stages, somewhat honeycombed in appearance (Fig. 10.24). The anterior epiphysis is roughly 's' shaped being concave medially at its ventral extent and concave laterally in its dorsal part. The anterior extremity is somewhat expanded and ends in a cap which passes inferiorly to cover the anterior superior iliac spine (Fig. 10.24). The posterior epiphysis is also somewhat s-shaped, being concave laterally in its anterior part and concave medially in its posterior region. It is broader in its posterior aspect, where it expands to cover the thickened area of bone over the non-articular region of the sacro-iliac articulation.

Ossification in the crest is said to commence around 12–13 years of age in girls and 14–15 years in boys (Flecker, 1932b; Galstaun, 1937; Francis, 1940; Buehl and Pyle, 1942; Lurie *et al.*, 1943; Garn *et al.*, 1967b; Jit and Singh, 1971), with the anterior epiphysis generally forming in advance of the posterior epiphysis (Zaoussis and James, 1958). Interestingly, Buehl and Pyle (1942) found that the onset of ossification in the crest consistently occurred within 6 months of the menarcheal date (on average 12.5–13 years), whereas Scoles *et al.* (1988) found that it occurred within 8 months of the onset of menses. The timing of epiphyseal fusion is extremely variable for the crest and this is perhaps not surprising as the epiphysis is almost completely formed before union commences (Kobayashi, 1967). The anterior and posterior epiphyses fuse to form a single cap for the crest, which tends to commence union initially on the pelvic aspect of the anterior superior iliac spine around 17–20 years of age in males (McKern and Stewart, 1957). The pelvic aspect of the anterior epiphysis fuses progressively from anterior to posterior until it reaches the junction with the posterior epiphysis (Fig. 10.25). However, the gluteal aspect of the anterior epiphysis is slower to close as it has a greater surface area to cover as it spreads over the thicker region of the iliac tubercle. The posterior epiphysis seems to commence union in the region of the posterior superior iliac spine and it is the gluteal aspect that fuses in advance of the pelvic aspect. The area of the crest directly superior to the sacro-iliac joint is often one of the last parts to fuse as again it has to spread over a wider surface area to cover the thickened bar of the crest in this region that marks the attachment of the erector spinae muscle. Partial fusion of the iliac crest is said to range from 15–22 years, with complete fusion occurring in 100% of individuals by 23 years of age (Galstaun, 1937; Lurie *et al.*, 1943; McKern and Stewart, 1957; Jit and Singh, 1971; Birkner, 1978; Webb and Suchey, 1985).

The maturation of the iliac crest epiphysis has proved to be of considerable clinical value in assessing an individual's remaining growth potential (Wagner *et al.*, 1995). This is particularly important when evaluating the necessity for, or indeed against, operative intervention in the management of conditions such as adolescent idiopathic scoliosis (Zaoussis and James, 1958; Urbaniak *et al.*, 1976; Scoles *et al.*, 1988). Risser (1948, 1958) has shown that the completion of fusion of the iliac crest epiphysis occurs simultaneously with the completion of vertebral growth, which is then concomitant with a static vertebral curvature.

Avulsion of the iliac crest epiphysis has been reported in athletes who undertake sudden contraction of the abdominal muscles (Goodshall and Hansen, 1973).

The **ischial epiphysis** appears as a small flake on the superior aspect of the ischial tuberosity between 13 and 16 years of age (Galstaun, 1937; Francis, 1940; Garn *et al.*, 1967b; Jit and Singh, 1971) and commences union (early in the development of the epiphysis) at the superior rim of the epiphyseal surface and often slightly directed towards the pelvic border that carries the ischial spine (Fig. 10.26). It is unlikely that this epiphysis is ever separate from the primary ischial centre apart from in its very earliest stages of development.

We have noted that in a small number of individuals there is a distinct bony gutter of communication (Fig. 10.27) between the upper medial border of the ischial tuberosity and the ischial spine and it is in these individuals that a billowed surface is seen on the lower aspect of the ischial spine. The presence of an epiphysis for the ischial spine has been reported as being somewhat variable (Frazer, 1948) and it is possible that an epiphysis may form only if a line of communication is retained between it and the ischial

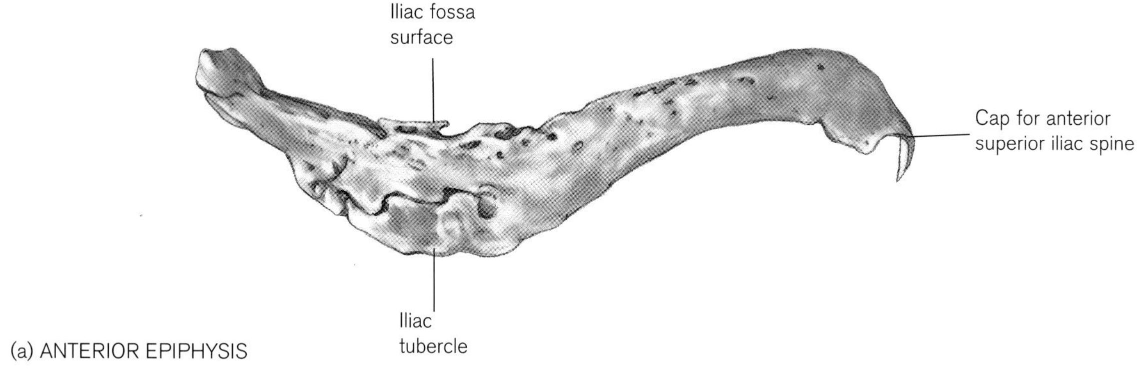

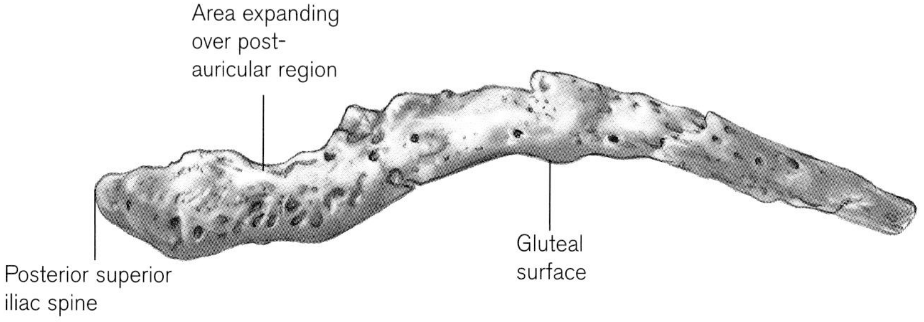

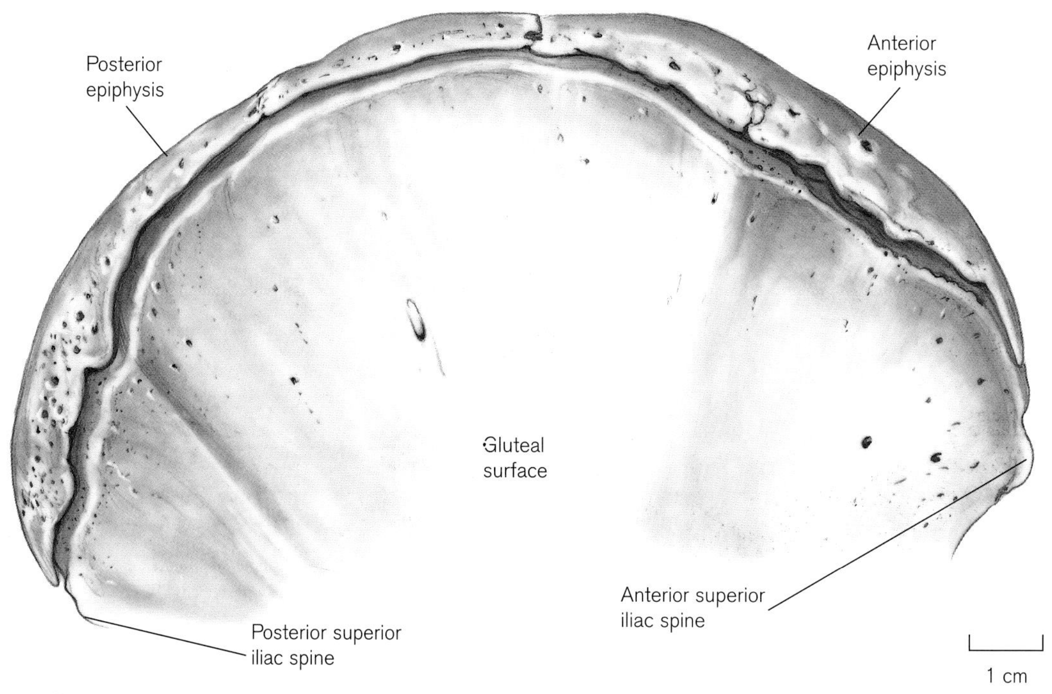

Figure 10.24 Isolated right iliac crest epiphyses and their position on the iliac crest (approx. 17 years).

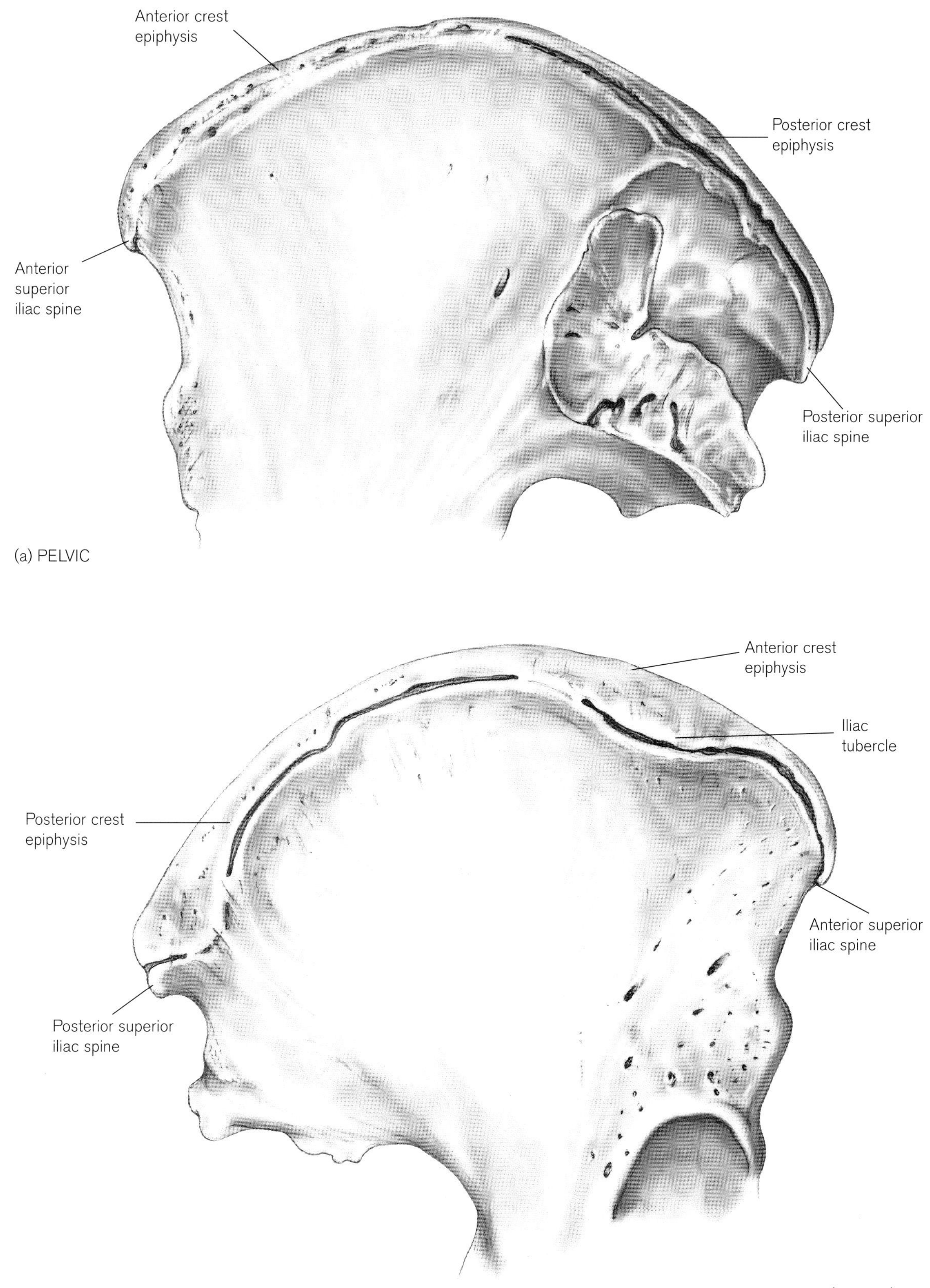

Figure 10.25 The right iliac crest epiphyses showing the commencement of fusion (approx. 19 years).

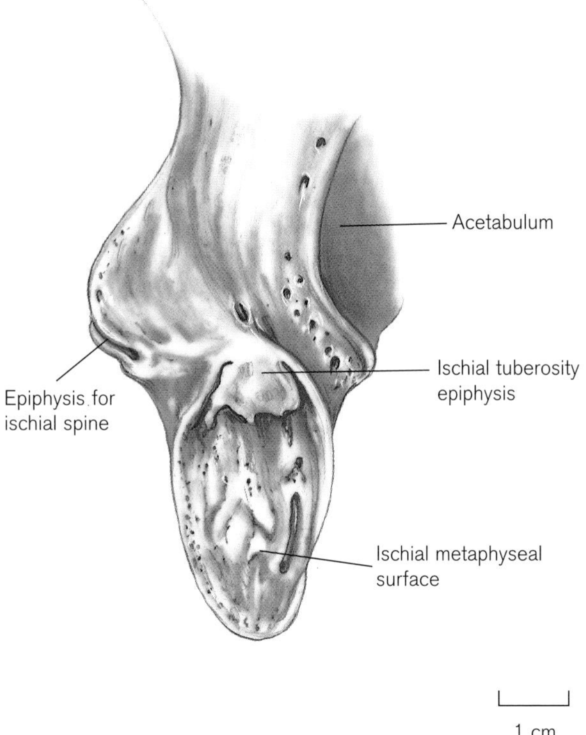

Figure 10.26 The right ischial epiphyses (female aged 14 years).

tuberosity (Fig. 10.26). As the superior border of the ischial tuberosity is the initial site of fusion for the flake-like epiphysis, it can be assumed that if an ischial spine epiphysis is to form, then it will occur in conjunction with that for the tuberosity.

The ischial epiphysis then spreads across the face of the tuberosity and extends down to its inferior pole, where it continues along the ischial ramus as the thin, tongue-like **ramal epiphysis**. The pelvic surface of the tuberal epiphysis commences union in advance of the lateral aspect so that generally by the time the ramal epiphysis has commenced development (Fig. 10.28) the pelvic border of the ischial tuberosity is well advanced in terms of fusion and this is said to occur between 16 and 18 years of age (Parsons, 1903; Stevenson, 1924; Stewart, 1954; Johnston, 1961; Jit and Singh, 1971). The ramal epiphysis continues forwards along the lower border of the ischial ramus and has generally reached half way along by around 19–20 years of age (Fig. 10.29). By this stage, the epiphysis for the ischial tuberosity has generally completed fusion on all borders and so is fully adult in appearance. The ramal epiphysis will continue edging slowly forwards along the ischiopubic ramus until it approaches the lower lateral aspect of the pubic body. The epiphyseal lines may remain visible for a number of years after fusion is completed and is said to occur by 20–21 years of age, although fusion in 100% of individuals may not occur until 21–23 years (Flecker, 1932b; Stewart, 1954; McKern and Stewart, 1957; Jit and Singh, 1971).

Avulsion of the ischial epiphysis is well documented as an athletic injury. It most commonly occurs in track athletes between the ages of puberty and 25 years of age and generally occurs as a result of uncoordinated extension at the hip joint, which puts excessive strain on the hamstring muscles (MacCleod and Lewin, 1929; Schlonsky and Olix, 1972).

Morphological changes at the **pubic symphyseal face** have been the subject of considerable attention in both the anthropological and forensic literature. This is mainly as a result of the prolonged period of age-related change displayed in this region, thereby making it a useful site for the determination of age at death from skeletal remains (Aeby, 1885; Cleland, 1889; Todd, 1920, 1921a–e, 1923, 1930b; Stevenson, 1924; Flecker, 1936a; Hanihara, 1952; Brooks, 1955; McKern and Stewart, 1957; Stewart, 1957; Acsádi and Nemeskéri, 1970; Gilbert, 1973; Gilbert and McKern, 1973; Hanihara and Suzuki, 1978; Suchey, 1979; WEA, 1980; Zongyao, 1982; Snow, 1983; Meindl *et al.*, 1985; Suchey, 1986; Katz and Suchey, 1986; Suchey *et al.*, 1986; Knussmann, 1988).

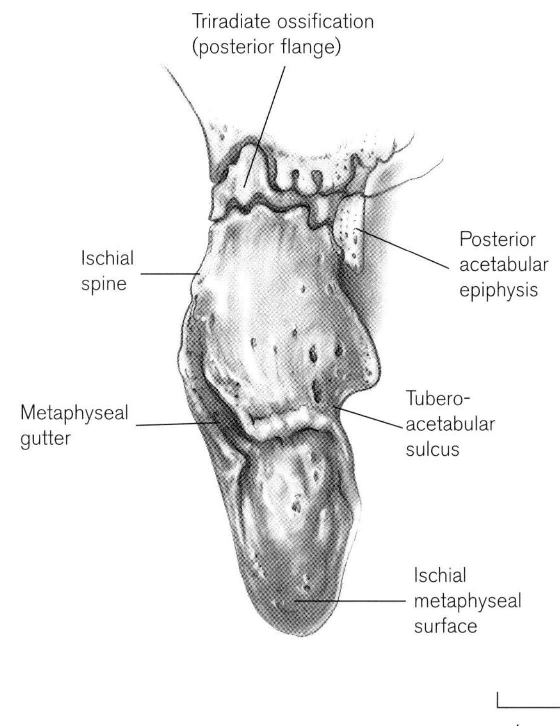

Figure 10.27 Communicating gutter between the right metaphyseal surface of the ischial tuberosity and the ischial spine (approx. 15 years).

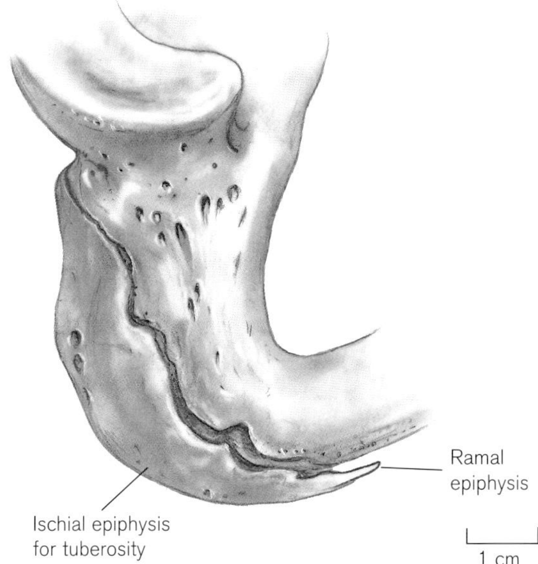

Figure 10.28 The right ischial tuberosity and ramal epiphyses (male aged 17 years).

It is reported that the epiphyseal structures associated with the human pubic bone represent remnants of the epipubis and hypo-ischium that occur in many animal groups (Parsons, 1903; Todd, 1921d). In fact, all mammalian pubic symphyses, with the exception of man and certain of the higher primates, fuse in the midline via a median bar of bone, which in most cases becomes continuous with the ischial epiphysis (Todd, 1921d; Dokládal, 1970). In the light of this comparative evidence, Todd (1920) proposed that the human symphysis pubis is retrogressive in nature, as the epiphyseal structures involved in the metamorphosis of the joint face represent bilateral vestiges of this median bar. Many authors have explained this strangely retrogressive phenomenon in terms of a functional requirement to resist fusion and maintain elasticity in this region for the purposes of expansion at parturition (Hunter, 1761a, b; Heyman and Lundqvist, 1932; Lang and Haslhofer, 1932; Crelin, 1954, 1969; Crelin *et al.*, 1957; Pinnell and Crelin, 1963; Putschar, 1976; Meindl *et al.*, 1985). This therefore suggests that the joint is a potential site of weakness in the biomechanics of the bony pelvic ring and so its structure probably reflects a compromise between the rigidity that is essential to maintain normal weight-related stress in conjunction with a certain degree of elasticity, which is essential for the safe passage of a relatively large fetal head.

In the juvenile, there is reported to be a continuous ischiopubic cap of cartilage that begins over the region of the pubic tubercle, lines the crest and ventral aspect of the face of the symphysis and then passes along the conjoint rami to the ischial tuberosity (Parsons, 1903; MacLaughlin, 1987). Ossification then commences in both ends of the cartilaginous strip with that of the ischium arising in advance of that at the pubic end.

McKern and Stewart (1957) noticed that the symphyseal face behaves as two distinct areas and named them the ventral and dorsal demifaces, which may be delimited by a longitudinal groove or ridge. They proposed that only the ventral aspects of the symphysis showed epiphyseal progression, whereas the dorsal aspect only reflects changes in the diaphyseal

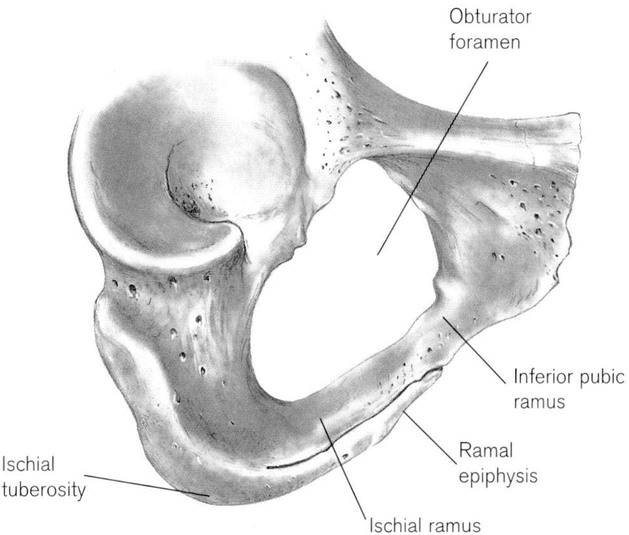

Figure 10.29 The right ischial ramal epiphysis (female aged 19 years).

structure. This morphological delimitation is based on an anatomical premise, where only the ventral aspect of the joint is separated by the interpubic disc of fibrocartilage as it is deficient over the posterior surface of the pubic face (Nemeskéri *et al.*, 1960; MacLaughlin, 1987; Williams *et al.*, 1995). Therefore it is not surprising that the majority of the methods that have employed symphyseal metamorphosis for the evaluation of age at death have relied strongly on the ventral structures of the joint which Todd (1921a–e; 1923) considered to be the vestiges of the phylogenetically older median bar.

What is termed the pre-epiphyseal stage by Meindl *et al.* (1985) is characterized by a well-marked ridge-and-furrow appearance of the joint surface (Fig. 10.30a). There is no build-up of bone along the ventral margin and the upper and lower limits of the joint surface are poorly defined. There is generally no epiphysis present for the pubic tubercle, which displays a classic juvenile appearance (Nemeskéri *et al.*, 1960). This morphological appearance is generally found in individuals up to approximately 20 years of age, but this will of course vary, depending upon the sex and genetic pool from which the individual originated. The first change to occur to this pre-epiphyseal joint is that by a process of gradual accretion, bone is laid directly onto the dorsal face initially, resulting in a smoothing over of the ridge-and-furrow appearance (Fig. 10.30b) and this tends to occur between 15 and 23 years of age (Suchey, 1986). The delimitation of the lower extremity of the joint tends to occur first (around 25 years of age) and this generally arises by the simple accretion of bone in that region. The upper extremity of the face commences delimitation around 23–27 years of age and can arise either by the fusion of a distinct superior ossific nodule in this region (Fig. 10.30c) or by gradual bone accretion (Todd, 1920). Todd (1921d) considered this superior ossific nodule to be homologous with the epipubis of other mammals. Not only does this nodule form the upper limit of the joint surface, but it also extends inferiorly to form the upper aspect of the ventral rampart, a bevelled area of built-up bone that develops along the ventral aspect of the joint separating the articular face medially from the outer surface of the pubic body laterally. The remainder of the rampart is formed either from an upgrowth from an inferior ossific nodule or by simple accretion of bone (Fig. 10.31). Todd (1921d) considered the ventral rampart formation to be homologous with changes that occur in the median bar of other Eutherian mammals and the inferior ossific nodule to be homologous with the hypo-ischium. The variable occurrence of an inferior ossific nodule was taken to be evidence of the removal of the ischium from the anterior midline articulation, which is typical for man and the higher primates.

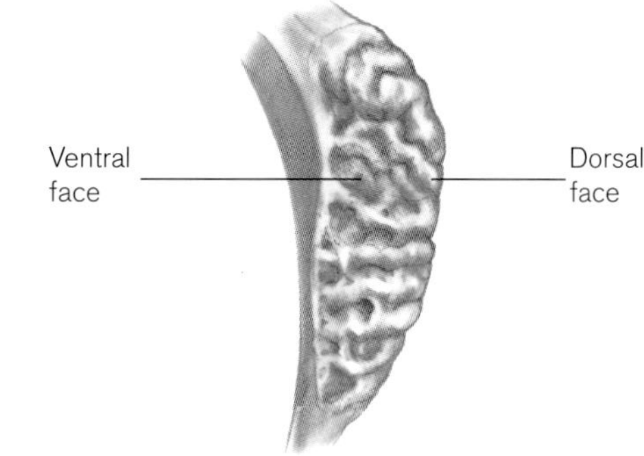

(a) The pre-epiphyseal stage (13 years)

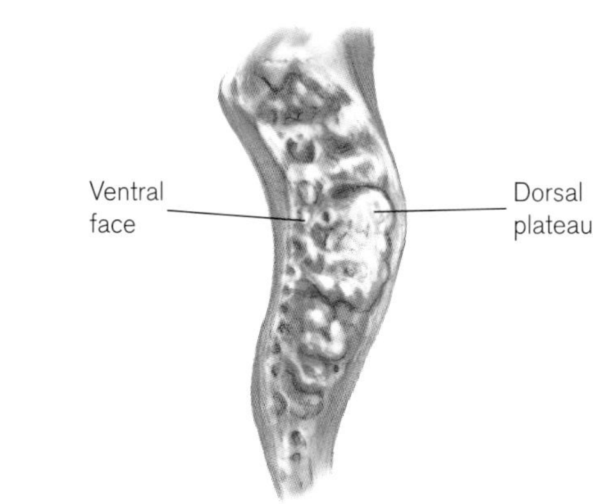

(b) Gradual infilling of the dorsal demiface (16 years)

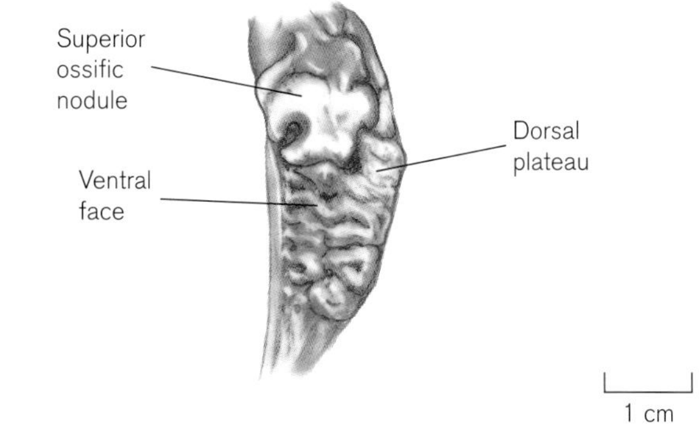

(c) The superior ossific nodule (23 years)

Figure 10.30 Age-related change in the right pubic symphysis.

Frequently, the upper and lower progressions of the rampart fail to meet and so leave a hiatus in the upper

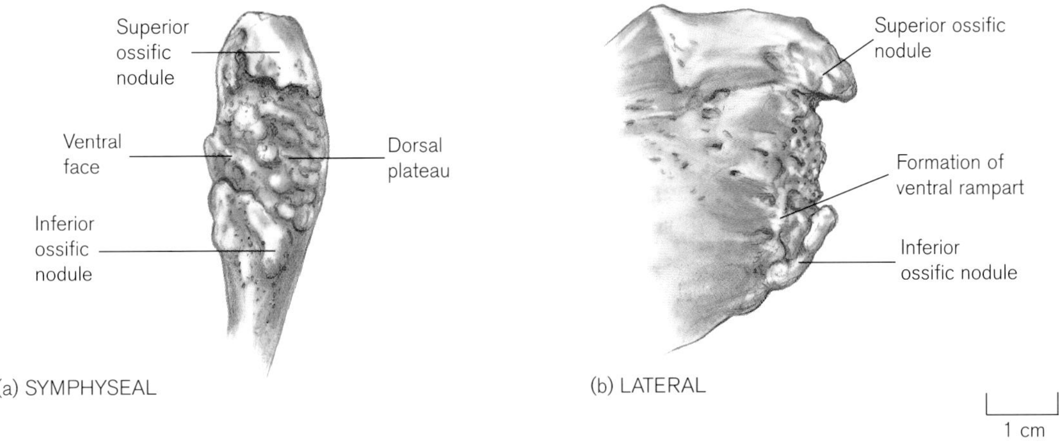

Figure 10.31 Symphyseal and lateral views of the right pubis to show development of the ventral rampart (26 years).

ventral rim (Fig. 10.32a – Todd, 1920; MacLaughlin, 1987; Brooks and Suchey, 1990). Active rampart formation generally occurs between 24 and 30 years of age, although it is often not completed until 35 years of age (Meindl *et al.*, 1985). The epiphysis for the pubic tubercle can appear as a separate flake between 23–25 years of age (Kobayashi, 1967) or indeed it may form from a backward prolongation of the superior ossific nodule (Parsons, 1903).

With increasing age, the dorsal plateau tends to show less dramatic maturation. A slight dorsal margin is said to develop in the middle of the border around 18 years of age and will continue to expand superiorly and inferiorly until the entire border is defined by a rim. This will tend to have occurred by 19–20 years of age (McKern and Stewart, 1957; Gilbert and McKern, 1973). The grooves and ridges of the dorsal face then start to fill in to form the characteristic plateau and vestiges of the billowed surface may remain evident until at least 22 to 25 years. By around 30 years of age, the dorsal plateau becomes flattened and slightly granular in appearance.

Thus, changes at the symphyseal face show a prolonged period of developmental activity and may not reach a fully matured appearance until 35–40 years of age (Fig. 10.32b). Beyond this age, the changes tend to be degenerative in nature, with breakdown of the symphyseal outline and general degeneration of the texture of the face.

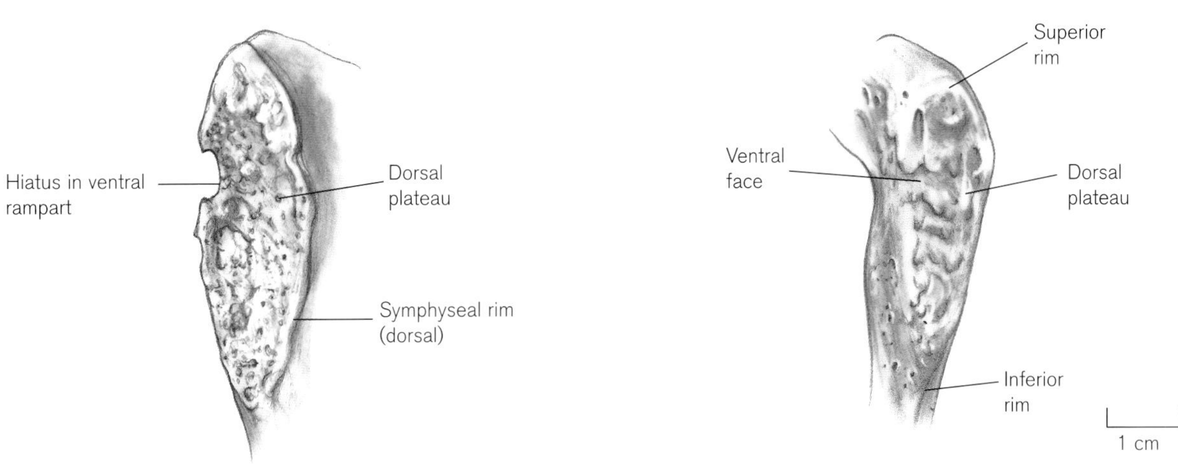

(a) The hiatus in the ventral rampart (25 years)

(b) The mature pubic symphyseal face (34 years)

Figure 10.32 Age-related change in the right pubic symphysis.

Practical notes

Sideing

As the three primary centres adopt close to adult morphology early in fetal development, it is not difficult to identify and side each of the elements. Sideing of the ilium (Fig. 10.9) relies on being able to identify the crest (superiorly), the acetabulum and greater sciatic notch (inferiorly) and the auricular regions (posteriorly) on the iliac surface. If the ilium is held with the iliac fossa facing and the greater sciatic notch inferiorly then the auricular surface will be on the side from which the bone originates, i.e. from the right side if the auricular surface is on the right of the specimen.

Sideing of the ischium (Fig. 10.10) relies on being able to identify the smooth pelvic surface (internally), the acetabular surface on the lateral surface (superiorly and posteriorly), the non-articular region (superiorly and anteriorly) and the thin arm of the ischial ramus inferiorly, which points anteriorly. If the specimen is held with the outer (acetabular) surface facing and with the ramal surface inferiorly, then the ramus will point to the side from which the specimen belongs.

Sideing of the pubis (Fig 10.11) is probably the most difficult and relies on being able to identify the pelvic from the lateral surfaces and the acetabular from the symphyseal surface. The symphyseal surface is longer and thinner than the acetabular extremity, which tends to be thicker and more club-shaped. The pelvic surface is relatively featureless, whereas the lateral surface shows a clear demarcation between the body ventrally and the superior ramus posteriorly. The upper border tends to be more linear than the inferior border, which is hooked by the passage of the obturator nerve and vessels. Therefore, if the specimen is examined with the lateral surface facing and the hooked border inferiorly, then the symphyseal face will point to the side from which the specimen originates.

Bones of a similar morphology

The immature ilium may be confused with any of the other flat bones of the skeleton if it is in a particularly fragmented state. However, the presence of two distinct compact shells surrounding coarse trabeculae should be sufficiently indicative of ilial origin. It is unlikely that either the ischium or the pubis would be confused with another bone, even from a very early stage.

Morphological summary

Fetal

Mths 2–3	Ilium commences ossification
Mths 4–5	Ischium commences ossification and ilium is recognizable
Mths 5–6	Pubis commences ossification
Mths 6–8	Ischium is recognizable in isolation
Birth	All three primary bony components are represented
By 6 mths	The ilium shows a prominence on its acetabular extremity formed by the development of the iliopectineal line and the angulation of the superior border of the ischium has occurred
By yr 1	The superior border of the ischium is square and the ischial spine, pubic tubercle and crest have developed
By yr 2	The anterior border of the ilium has bent forwards in the vertical plane
By yr 3–4	The demarcation of the iliac and ischial articulation sites are clearly defined on the pubis
By yr 4–5	The non-articular acetabular area is well defined on the ilium
By yr 5–6	The non-articular acetabular area is well defined on the pubis
5–8 yrs	Fusion of the ischiopubic rami occurs
9–10 yrs	The anterior acetabular epiphysis or 'os acetabuli' appears and ossific islands appear in triradiate cartilage
10–11 yrs	The posterior acetabular epiphysis commences ossification
10–13 yrs	Centre appears for the anterior inferior iliac spine
11–15 yrs	The acetabulum commences and completes fusion in females
12–14 yrs	The superior acetabular epiphysis appears and the iliac crest commences ossification in the female
13–16 yrs	The ischial epiphysis commences ossification
14–17 yrs	The acetabulum commences and completes fusion in males and the iliac crest commences ossification in the male
15–23 yrs	The dorsal plateau of the pubic symphysis may show gradual obliteration of the ridge-and-furrow appearance
16–18 yrs	The ischial tuberosity is complete
17–20 yrs	The iliac crest epiphyses commence fusion
19–20 yrs	The ischial epiphysis extends half way along the ramus
By 20 yrs	The anterior inferior iliac spine has fused
20–23 yrs	Both the ischial epiphysis and the iliac crest complete union
	The dorsal margin forms along the dorsal border of the pubic symphyseal surface

23–27 yrs	The epiphysis appears for the pubic tubercle and delimitation of the upper and lower borders of the symphyseal face commence
24–30 yrs	Active ventral rampart formation and obliteration of the ridge-and-furrow appearance of the ventral and dorsal aspects of the pubic symphyseal face
By 35 yrs	Ventral rampart is complete and the symphyseal rim is mature

Metrics

Although metrics are available from a number of sources, the majority of studies have involved undocumented material (Merchant and Ubelaker, 1977; Sundick, 1978; Hoppa, 1992; Miles and Bulman, 1995). However, some information is available from fetal remains from Fazekas and Kósa (1978) and Apuzzio et al (1992) from ultrasound studies (Tables 10.1 and 10.2). Table 10.3 shows some radiographic data from Abitbol (1988a).

Table 10.1 Dimensions of fetal ilium, ischium and pubis (in mm)

Age	Ilium		Ischium		Pubis
(weeks)	Length	Width	Length	Width	Length
12	4.8	3.2			
14	5.7	3.8			
16	9.7	7.8	3.1	2.2	
18	12.0	9.8	3.8	2.9	
20	15.6	12.6	5.5	3.5	3.6
22	16.5	14.2	6.4	4.3	4.5
24	18.3	15.6	7.5	5.6	5.5
26	19.6	17.1	8.7	6.0	6.0
28	21.3	19.1	9.7	6.6	6.6
30	22.1	20.1	10.3	7.6	8.0
32	25.1	22.2	12.1	8.1	9.9
34	26.8	24.6	13.2	9.3	12.4
36	28.7	26.0	16.2	10.4	14.1
38	32.1	28.5	17.2	11.6	15.0
40	34.5	30.4	18.5	12.4	16.6

Ilium length: max distance between the anterior to the posterior superior iliac spines.
Ilium width: max distance between the middle point of the iliac crest and the convexity of the acetabular extremity.
Ischium length: max distance between the convexity of the acetabular extremity and the tip of the ischial ramus.
Ischium width: max distance across the broad superior extremity.
Pubis length: max distance between the symphysis and the iliac articulation.
Adapted from Fazekas and Kósa (1978).

Table 10.2 Fetal iliac bone length as measured by ultrasound

Gestational age (weeks)	Iliac length (mm)	SD
13	6.25	0.96
14	7.77	1.21
15	8.46	1.74
16	9.57	1.46
17	10.30	1.50
18	12.10	2.56
19	11.70	1.48
20	14.18	1.33
21	15.20	1.50
22	15.80	2.50
23	17.18	2.36
24	19.36	2.54
25	18.50	3.03
26	19.86	2.97
27	20.17	3.43
28	21.74	1.91
29	23.51	3.45
30	24.18	1.54
31	23.55	2.81
32	25.30	3.15
33	26.30	3.86
34	25.88	2.45
35	26.80	2.39
36	26.36	3.26
37	29.83	2.86
38	28.36	2.31
39	29.63	2.33
40	31.50	3.78

Adapted from Apuzzio *et al.* (1992).

Table 10.3 Dimensions of the mid-pelvis from radiographs

Age	PSMP/ASMP × 100	Ischial prominence (cm)
Newborn	21	0
4 months	23	0
7 months	27	0
1 year	21	0
2 years	27–30	0
4 years	23–38	0
6 years	46–55	0
8 years	76–82	0
10 years	76	0.5
12 years	86	0.7
12 years	97	1.1
13 years	83	1.8
14 years	93	1.7

PSMP: posterior sagittal of mid-pelvis.
ASMP: anterior sagittal of mid-pelvis.
Adapted from Abitbol (1988a).

CHAPTER ELEVEN

The Lower Limb

The lower limb comprises the thigh, leg and foot and is connected to the axial skeleton via the pelvic girdle. The lower limbs support the weight of the entire upper body and are the principal organs of locomotion. To fulfil both of these functions satisfactorily, the morphology of the lower limb has been restrained by the necessity of maintaining strength and stability. In contrast, the upper limb has effectively relinquished these restrictions to free the limb and thereby maximize its mobility and prehensile capabilities. As a result, the bones of the lower limb tend to be more robust than their upper limb counterparts and the corresponding joints tend to be stronger and more stable (Williams *et al.*, 1995).

Man is the only habitual mammalian biped and while this activity is occasionally adopted in many of the other primate groups, it can also occur sporadically in other animal orders.[1] It is therefore not surprising that the lower limb has been studied extensively with regards to both its functional and comparative anatomy, its pivotal role in locomotion and, as such, its evolutionary significance regarding bipedalism. These topics are fundamentally outwith the scope of this text and readers are directed to some of the more important research and reference texts that cover these areas (Ellis, 1889; Morton, 1922; Straus, 1926; Keith, 1929; Elftman and Manter, 1935; Morton, 1942b; Lake, 1943; Eberhart *et al.*, 1954; Hicks, 1955; Bowden, 1967; Sigmon, 1971; Jenkins, 1972; Stott and Stokes, 1973; Zihlman and Brunker, 1979; Lewis, 1983; Sarrafian, 1983; Susman, 1983; Suzuki, 1985; Reynolds, 1987; Aiello and Dean, 1990; Day, 1991; Tardieu and Trinkaus, 1994; Tardieu, 1998).

Bipedality is a learned process and does not reach its full maturation until approximately 3 years of age. The transition from early walking to efficient bipedalism in the young child involves a change in the axis of the shaft of both the femur and the tibia and a change in the position of the foot (Walmsley, 1933; Elftman, 1945; Crelin, 1973). To understand the morphology of the lower limb, one needs to consider its involvement both in the act of standing and walking. The act of standing upright on two feet is a basically unstable occupation that man appears to achieve surprisingly well and with a comparatively small amount of energy expenditure (Abitbol, 1988b). The rectangular area of support through which the centre of gravity must fall is very small and so overbalancing is a constant potential problem (Zihlman and Brunker, 1979). For example, one needs only to observe the effects of alcohol on the control of equilibrium to understand how potentially unstable is this occupation. In the adult human, the centre of gravity passes roughly in the midline – through the dens of the axis, the anterior aspect of the body of T2, the middle of the body of T12, the posterior aspect of the body of L5, anterior to the second sacral vertebra, slightly posterior to the hip joint, anterior to the knee joint and anterior to the tibiotalar joint through the navicular (MacConaill and Basmajian, 1969; Sinclair, 1978). The centre of gravity then falls almost midway between the insteps of the feet and although there is some swaying action, it is normally contained within a circle of approximately 25 mm in diameter (Debrunner, 1985).

The primary unit of analysis in bipedal locomotion is the stride and this is separated into a stance and a swing phase. The stance phase, when the foot is in contact with the ground, accounts for some 60% of the stride, whereas the swing phase, when the foot is not in contact with the ground, accounts for the remaining 40%. When running, the stance phase can vary from 40% of the stride in jogging to only 27% in sprinting, so that in such circumstances there is also an aerial phase, when neither foot is in contact with

[1] It was Dr Johnson who was attributed with saying 'Sir, a woman's preaching is like a dog walking on his hinder legs; it is not well done, but you are surprised to find it done at all'.

the ground (Högberg, 1952). At the start of the walking cycle, the hip is flexed, the knee extended and the leg laterally rotated to bring the heel down in contact with the ground (heel strike). At heel strike, most of the body weight passes along the lateral aspect of the heel (the wear pattern on an old pair of shoes will bear witness to this – Barnett *et al.*, 1956), and as the remainder of the foot comes into contact with the ground (via plantar flexion) it is transferred along the fifth metatarsal (Barnett, 1956; Hooton, 1960). Following this stage, the foot rolls from lateral to medial across the ball of the foot (heads of the metatarsals) to what is called the 'mid-stance' phase. At mid-stance, the classic footprint pattern is achieved, where the pad of each toe, the ball of the foot, the lateral pedal margin and the heel are all in contact with the ground. At 'heel off', the heel is lifted away from the ground by plantar flexion and concomitant flexion occurs at the knee and hip joints. The metatarsals then leave the ground so that only the ball and the pad of the big toe remain in contact with the surface. The last aspect of the stance phase is the 'toe off', where the force of the muscles involved in plantar flexion of the big toe is used to propel the foot forward. In the swing phase, the foot is not in contact with the ground but is lifted upwards and extended forwards to the next 'heel strike'.

The **early development** of the lower limbs closely follows the basic pattern as seen in the upper limbs. Therefore, the development of both limbs has been considered together in the introduction to Chapter 9.

I. THE FEMUR

The adult femur

The femur forms the skeleton of the thigh and articulates proximally with the acetabulum of the innominate at the hip joint (Chapter 10) and distally with both the tibia and the patella at the knee joint. It is the largest and the most studied of the long bones (Humphry, 1889; Parsons, 1914; Pearson and Bell, 1919; Ingalls, 1924; Hrdlička, 1934a, b, 1938; Backman, 1957; Davivongs, 1963; Trotter *et al.*, 1968; Van Gerven, 1972; Lavelle, 1974). Many of the early reports are tabulations of measurements, indices and anomalies.

Proximally, the femur consists of a head, neck and two trochanters (Fig. 11.1). The **head** forms about two-thirds of a sphere and is directed anterosuperiorly and medially into the acetabulum. A pit (**fovea capitis**), situated below the centre of the head and containing nutrient foramina, provides attachment for the ligament of the head. The fovea is usually roughly circular with a smooth margin, but Schofield (1959) described an oval shape with an everted margin that is particularly characteristic of the Maori femur. The angle between the **neck** and the shaft varies throughout life (Humphry, 1889) from an average of 140° in early childhood (see below), to 125° during most of adult life and 120° in the elderly (Isaac *et al.*, 1997). Prasad *et al.* (1996a) reported the adult range to be 110° to 140° and Isaac *et al.* (1997) found that neck/shaft angle varied both with neck length and with total femoral length. These figures appear to concur with the well-known observation that the angle is usually smaller in women than in men, in order to accommodate a wider pelvis and shorter bones in the female. However, a survey of neck-shaft angles across a representative sample of recent and modern population samples recorded a wide degree of variability (Anderson and Trinkaus, 1998). There were no consistent patterns of sexual, side or geographic differences but the mean neck-shaft angles decreased significantly during ontogeny in populations whose lifestyle involved a large amount of physical activity.

The neck of the femur can be envisaged as a curved prolongation of the shaft that is masked by the presence of the **greater trochanter**, which projects superolaterally at the junction of the neck and shaft. The trochanter is a large, roughened knob of bone to which are attached the gluteus medius, gluteus minimus, piriformis and obturator internus muscles. On the posteromedial aspect of the trochanter is a deep pit, the **intertrochanteric fossa**, into which the tendon of the obturator externus muscle is attached. The posterior aspect of the neck often bears a groove produced by this tendon as it approaches the fossa. Finnegan (1978) viewed the rare occurrence of an exostosis in the fossa as a non-metric epigenetic trait.

The **lesser trochanter**, lying below the head and greater trochanter, is variable in position depending on the torsion of the shaft (see below) and is a smooth tubercle of bone to which is attached the tendon of the iliopsoas muscle. This is principally a trunk/thigh flexor but its role as a rotator of the hip has been much debated. Anteriorly, passing across the base of the neck, is the roughened **intertrochanteric line**, to which are attached the two distal ends of the Y-shaped iliofemoral ligament. Posteriorly, the trochanters are joined by the rough **intertrochanteric crest**, bearing in the centre a raised tubercle for the attachment of the quadratus femoris muscle, which is a lateral rotator of the hip. Formicola *et al.* (1990) described a rare skeleton from the Palaeolithic of Italy where bilateral absence of the lesser trochanter was replaced by a sagittally orientated ridge blending superiorly into the intertrochanteric crest.

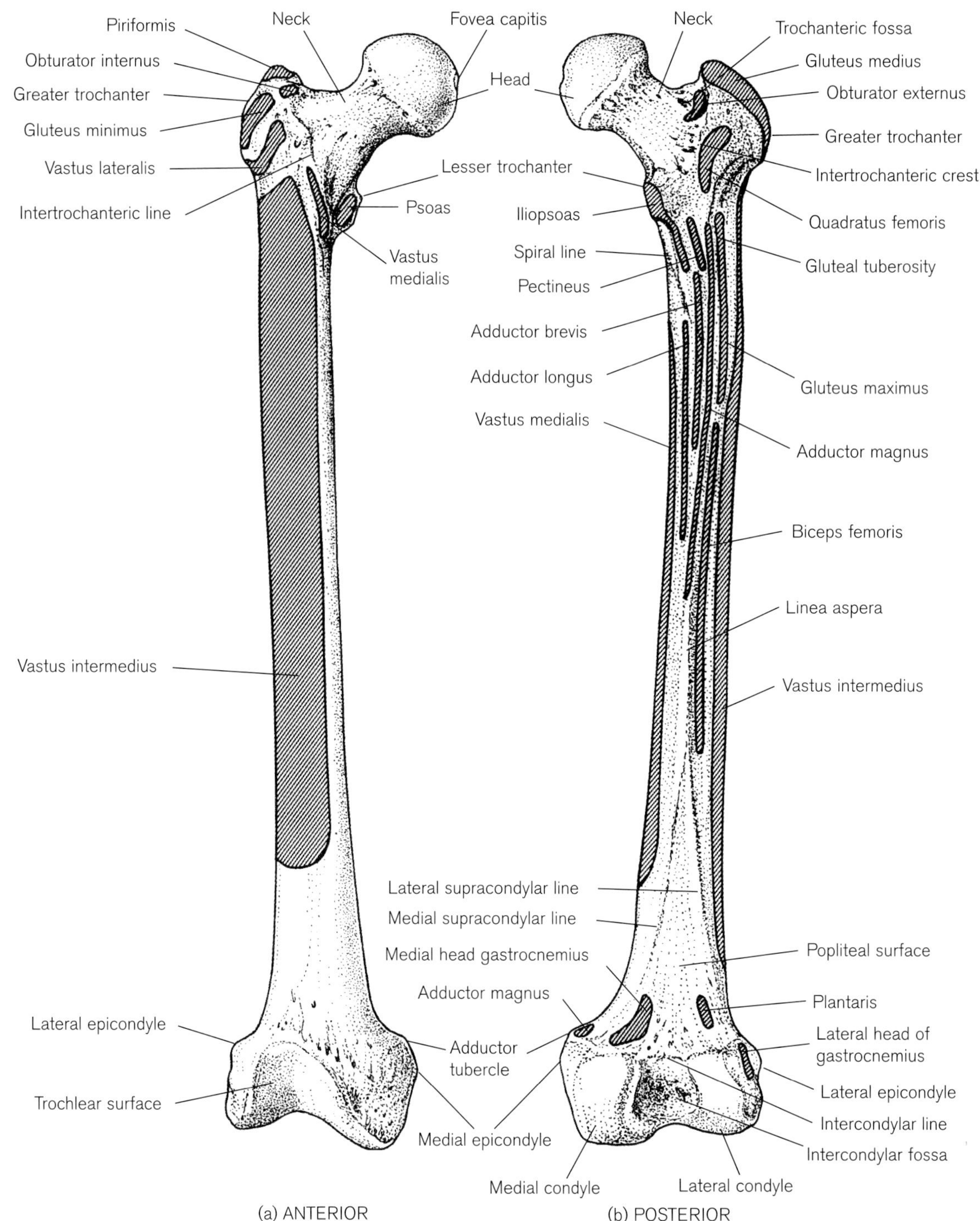

Figure 11.1 Right adult femur.

The capsule of the hip joint extends to the intertrochanteric line anteriorly but only reaches about half way down the neck posteriorly and this alignment has important consequences for the blood supply of the femoral head and neck. Early injection studies of the blood supply to the head (Trueta and Harrison, 1953; Trueta, 1957) have been revised and re-interpreted by Crock (1965, 1967, 1996). An arterial ring lies at the base of the neck from which ascending branches penetrate the capsule and give rise to both metaphyseal and epiphyseal arteries of the upper end of the bone. The blood supply is often compromised in various childhood conditions (see below), in fracture of the neck of the femur and dislocations of the hip joint

(Harty, 1957). A diagnosis of disturbance of blood supply causing abnormalities is common in the palaeopathological literature (Steinbock, 1976; Ortner and Putschar, 1985; Roberts and Manchester, 1995).

Both the proportions and the internal architecture of the head and neck of the femur are of great importance to its stability and weight-bearing properties and its failure in this regard leads to fractures of the neck. The cortical bone on the inferior surface of the neck is about twice as thick as that superiorly (Lovejoy, 1988). It was proposed that the stresses that occur due to weight bearing are compensated for superiorly by the abductors of the hip, which run parallel with the neck, but that inferiorly the cortex has to be thickened. This arrangement in humans, in contrast to the great apes, which have a cortex of more uniform thickness, is similar to that found in some fossil hominids, which are therefore thought to have been bipedal.

Internally, five groups of compressive and tensile trabeculae are commonly identified (Singh *et al.*, 1970), which, in the young adult, almost fill the neck except for a sparse area known as Ward's triangle. The changing radiographic patterns made by the trabeculae at different periods of life have been used, both by clinicians to investigate osteoporosis (Hall, 1961; Singh *et al.*, 1970), and by anthropologists as a means of establishing age at death (Acsádi and Nemeskéri, 1970; Lovejoy *et al.*, 1985a; Walker and Lovejoy, 1985). As well as the differential width of the cortex in the femoral neck, the inferomedial side is strengthened by the calcar femorale, a spur of bone projecting out from the cortex into the central cancellous tissue (Thompson, 1907; Dixon, 1910; Tobin, 1955; Harty, 1957; Garden, 1961). In normal circumstances it is thought to be important in weight transmission but, if a fracture should occur, it may act like a chisel and split the greater trochanter vertically (Thompson, 1907; Harty, 1957). The detailed trabecular anatomy of the proximal femoral neck, including the area of the calcar, has been studied by Whitehouse and Dyson (1974) using scanning electron micrographs. An appreciation of the clinical anatomy of the calcar femorale is important in the understanding of the biomechanics following total hip replacement. The literature on the calcar has been reviewed by Newell (1997), who revealed that its function appeared to be interpreted differently by anatomists and orthopaedic surgeons. Most early descriptions, perpetuated by radiographic images, were of a two-dimensional structure, but the current interpretation is based on neglected early work that described it as a three-dimensional, helical arrangement.

In some modern populations there appears to have been a change in recent times in femoral shaft/neck geometry and this is thought to be a factor in the present epidemic of femoral neck fractures. Duthie *et al.* (1998) found a significant increase in both femoral length and in the length and width of the femoral neck since 1900 and suggested that this could increase the risk of neck fracture. Ferris *et al.* (1989) and Walters and Price (1998) found differences both in bone mineral density and fracture sites to be related to femoral neck geometry.

There are several anomalies described around the head and neck of the femur. The anterior cervical (pubic) imprint (cervical fossa of Allen/empreinte of Bertaux) occurs on the anterior and inferior aspects of the medial side of the neck adjacent to the head, as a cancellous or ulcer-like impression in the bone (Walmsley, 1915a; Meyer,[2] 1924a, 1934; Odgers, 1931; Schofield, 1959; Kate, 1963; Kostick, 1963; Angel, 1964; Finnegan, 1978). Its presence has been variously ascribed to the mark of the anterior rim of the acetabular labrum, the attachment of the vertical limb of the iliofemoral ligament, the circular fibres of the zona orbicularis of the hip joint capsule and the tendon of the rectus femoris. None of these explanations appear to be very convincing and its aetiology remains uncertain. Poirier's facet is an extension of the articular surface of the head onto the anterior upper surface of the neck and is sometimes accompanied by a ridge of the upper surface of the neck known as the cervical eminence (Meyer, 1924a; Odgers, 1931; Schofield, 1959; Kostick, 1963). A posterior cervical imprint has also been described (Walmsley, 1915a; Kostick, 1963). Postural factors such as squatting had been suggested to account for these marks, but there now appears to be general agreement that this is an unlikely explanation as they occur with equal frequency in squatting and non-squatting peoples (Kate, 1963; Kostick, 1963; Trinkaus, 1975).

The **shaft** is twisted about its long axis so that a line passing through the centre of the neck makes an angle with that through the posterior surface of the condyles, and this is known as the angle of **femoral torsion**. Kate (1976) distinguished between torsion inherent in the neck and that due to torsion in the shaft itself. The angle measured normally includes both of these and usually varies between 9° and 15° (Elftman, 1945). Measurements can vary from −25° to +42°, but very large variations are probably due to difficulties of measurement and differences in methodology (Stirland, 1994), although smaller differences may be found between populations. Eckhoff *et al.* (1994a) found the range

[2]A.W. Meyer, of Stanford University, even investigated the positions in which his medical students slept to try and explain the existence of the cervical fossa.

of torsion to be greater in African femora than that previously reported in Caucasians and Orientals. Antetorsion (anteversion) – when the femoral head inclines upwards when the bone is laid down with the condyles on a flat surface – is much more common than its opposite, which is known as retroversion (retrotorsion). Increased positive torsion means that the position of the lesser trochanter appears more medially on the femoral shaft and is visible when the bone is viewed anteriorly. The mean anteversion angle for adult Whites is about 12°. Recent studies have compared different clinical methods using radiographs, CT scans and direct measurement in living patients (Ruwe *et al.*, 1992) and direct measurements on dry bone (Yoshioka *et al.*, 1987; Eckhoff, *et al.*, 1994a). Upadhyay *et al.*, (1987) developed an ultrasound method and Kirby *et al.* (1993), also using ultrasound on dry bone, have used four different methods of measuring anteversion, which they have compared to previous osteometric studies. Prasad *et al.* (1996b) investigated the angle of torsion and the degree of development of various markers on the femur in dry bones. Like the neck-shaft angle, torsion also changes with age during development (see below) and differences from the normal range are important in many pathological states, such as congenital dislocation of the hip, slipped capital epiphysis, Perthes' disease and other childhood disorders.

The shaft can be roughly divided into three parts (Fig. 11.1b). Posteriorly in the proximal third, the spiral line is continuous with the lower end of the intertrochanteric line and forms the upper limit for the attachment of the vasti medialis et lateralis muscles that cover the shaft. On the lateral side, the **gluteal tuberosity** (ridge) forms either a roughened ridge, or hollow, extending to the base of the greater trochanter to which the deep fibres of gluteus maximus and the horizontal part of adductor magnus are attached. The pectineus and adductor brevis muscles are attached between the spiral line and the tuberosity. Both a difference of terminology in this area, and a tendency to view anatomical variants as distinct non-metric traits, have caused confusion in descriptions of the upper end of the femur. Anatomists term the attachment for the gluteus maximus the gluteal tuberosity, but in most physical anthropology literature it is given the alternate name of the **third trochanter**. This is an oblong, rounded or conical bony projection lying along, or separated from, the superior end of the gluteal tuberosity (Hrdlička, 1938; Finnegan, 1978; Lozanoff *et al.*, 1985). It is often, but not always, accompanied by a so-called sub (hypo) trochanteric fossa (crural trough; Appleton, 1922; Schofield, 1959; Finnegan, 1978), which is a longitudinal hollow between the gluteal tuberosity and the lateral margin of the shaft. Lozanoff *et al.*, (1985) found that the incidence of a third trochanter was positively correlated with short femora, which had robust proximal diaphyses. Stirland (1996) found a significant difference in the incidence of both the third trochanter and the hypotrochanteric fossa between young and mature adult males. She suggested that these variations could be related to age and environmental factors, such as activity rather than to a genetic influence. While it is easy to see that both these structures would be associated with increased muscle bulk, the fact that they can develop to a considerable size in juvenile femora indicates that their occurrence may also have some genetic component. Opinion appears to be divided as to whether they have any positive correlation with age or sex. Hrdlička (1937), reporting on a large number of femora, found the incidence to be common in Native Americans and in females in particular. The presence of a third trochanter is often accompanied by a flattening, or **platymeria**, of the upper part of the shaft. The meric index (AP diameter × 100/mediolateral diameter), taken at the level of the spiral line, can vary from 56 to 128 with 75 or less being considered platymeric (Hepburn, 1896; Parsons, 1914; Holtby, 1918; Schofield, 1959). In the anthropological literature, platymeria has usually been attributed to biomechanical causes including excessive use of the vasti, but both Buxton (1938) and Townsley (1946) proposed that platymeria was a pathological condition. Buxton found platymeria correlated with flattening of other bones and associated it with a possible nutritional deficiency and Townsley described it as a mechanical adaptation to support body weight, as he claimed that platymeria usually existed together with an abnormally declined femoral neck.

The posterior middle third of the shaft is occupied by the **linea aspera,** which is a roughened area for muscular attachment. To its medial lip are attached the vastus medialis muscle and the adductores longus et magnus and the medial intermuscular septum. The lateral lip receives the vasti lateralis et intermedius, the short head of biceps femoris and the lateral intermuscular septum. Robust development of the lips of the linea aspera must be distinguished from the condition of **pilastry,** where a strong bar of bone runs down the posterior surface of the shaft (Hepburn, 1896; Hrdlička, 1934a). A pilaster, which starts to develop in late childhood and reaches maximum development by early adult life (Hrdlička, 1934a), is thought to strengthen the shaft, especially where there is a greater degree of anterior curvature. The pilasteric (pilastric) index is calculated from the same measurements as the platymeric index but recorded at the midshaft level and a femur is said to be pilastered if the index is greater than about 115 (Holtby, 1918). The degree of anterior curvature varies in different populations and has been utilized in attempts to establish race (Stewart, 1962; Walensky, 1965; Gilbert, 1976). In North American populations, the Native American femur has the greatest degree of curvature and the Black femur the least, with Americans of European ancestry falling between the two. However, Indians from South America have relatively straight femora (Gilbert, 1976).

Often AP radiographs of the adult femur, and less commonly, adolescents, show two parallel lines enclosing an area of increased radiodensity in the middle of the shaft. The appearance is known radiologically as the 'track sign' and represents the linea aspera-pilaster complex (Pitt, 1982).

The blood supply to the femoral shaft is extremely profuse and fractures often result in massive loss of blood, which can lead to hypovolaemic shock. The arteries of the shaft, which usually arise from perforating branches of the profunda femoris artery, enter along the linea aspera but can be variable in both number and position (Hepburn, 1896; Lütken, 1950; Laing, 1953; MacLaughlin and Bruce, 1985). Mysorekar (1967) reported that 51% of femora had more than one foramen, of which 90% lay in the middle third of the bone and over half between the lips of the linea aspera. The entrances slope towards the proximal end. Sendemir and Çimen (1991) found 86% of nutrient foramina on the linea aspera, or its lips, but the proximodistal position was very variable. When a single artery enters in the middle segment of the medullary cavity, it immediately bifurcates to supply the upper and lower regions of the shaft (Crock, 1967, 1996). Bridgeman and Brookes (1996) and Brookes and Revell (1998) found that the number and distribution of arteries to the femoral diaphysis varied both with sex and side but admitted that it is difficult to relate this bilateral asymmetry to functional differences.

The narrowest shaft breadth lies between 64% and 60% along the shaft, measured from the condylar plane (Kennedy, 1983) and the maximum anteroposterior diameter lies somewhat below the midshaft point (MacLaughlin and Bruce, 1985). Variation in shape of the shaft has been reported by Hrdlička (1934b) and Dokládal (1971). Atkinson and Weatherell (1967), investigating the variation in density of the cortical bone, reported that the spiral pattern of trabeculae seen in the head and neck was repeated in a density spiral in the shaft. The normal osteoporotic changes that occur with age accentuate the spiral pattern by increasing the contrast between more and less dense bone.

The lower third of the femoral shaft is delineated posteriorly by the division of the linea aspera into **medial** and **lateral supracondylar ridges** that enclose a flat area, the popliteal surface. A smooth gap can usually be felt in the medial ridge, which provides for the posterior passage of the femoral vessels through the adductor hiatus onto the popliteal surface. The distal end of the bone consists of two large, ellipsoidal, cartilage-covered knuckles, which articulate with the superior surface of the tibial plateau (Figs. 11.1b and 11.2). The medial and lateral condyles extend posteriorly beyond the popliteal surface and enclose a deep midline **intercondylar fossa** (notch) between them, delimited above by the **intercondylar line** (ridge) to which the capsule of the knee joint and the oblique popliteal ligament are attached. The condyles form about half of a flattened sphere but each has a different radius of curvature. In a lateral

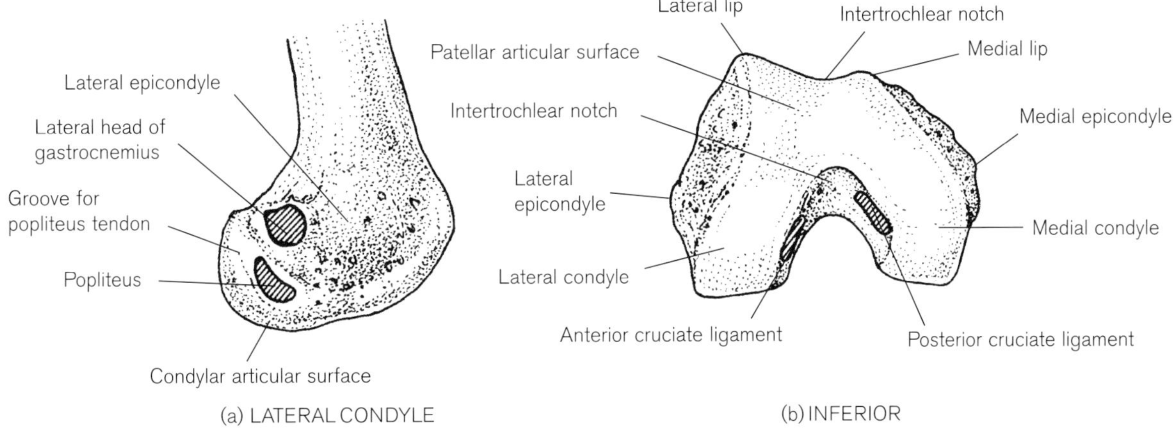

Figure 11.2 Right adult femur.

knee radiograph where the images overlap, the lateral condyle can be distinguished by its more flattened contour. The **lateral condyle** is more in line with the shaft and supports the direct weight of the body. On its lateral surface (Fig. 11.2a) it bears the protruding **lateral epicondyle** for the fibular (lateral) collateral ligament of the knee joint. Above this is an impression for the lateral head of the gastrocnemius muscle and further superiorly the plantaris muscle continues onto the supracondylar ridge. The popliteus is attached in a pit below the epicondyle and its tendon is accommodated during flexion of the knee, in a contiguous groove extending to the articular surface. The medial side of the condyle forms the lateral wall of the intercondylar fossa and bears a smooth surface for the anterior cruciate ligament. The larger circumference of the **medial condyle** is taken up when the 'screw home' mechanism operates in full extension of the knee joint. The medial surface bears an equivalent **medial epicondyle** for the attachment of the tibial (medial) collateral ligament. Directly superior to this is the prominent adductor tubercle to which the hamstring portion of the adductor magnus muscle is attached, while between it and the epicondyle, the medial head of the gastrocnemius muscle takes its origin. The lateral side of the condyle forms the medial wall of the intercondylar fossa and provides an attachment for the posterior cruciate ligament. Either or both heads of the gastrocnemius muscles may contain a sesamoid bone known as the fabella (Latin, diminutive of faba meaning, a 'bean'). They are much more common on the lateral side (Parsons and Keith, 1897) and occasionally may be fractured and cause nerve injury (Levowitz and Kletschka, 1955; Mangieri, 1973).

Anteriorly, the articular surface for the patella has an asymmetrical trochlear shape as the lateral lip is more prominent and projects further superiorly and sideways than the medial lip (Fig. 11.2b). This shape is considered to be the main factor preventing the patella from dislocating laterally which, especially in females, has a high bicondylar angle. However, Wanner (1977) suggested that other factors were responsible as there was considerable variation in the individual components that comprise the groove and no direct correlation between its lateral lip and the bicondylar angle (see 'Patella'). The medial lip is shallower but extends further posteromedially towards the intertrochlear notch to provide extra-articular surface for the most medial facet on the patella when the knee is fully flexed. There are usually two faint grooves separating the trochlear (patellar) from the meniscal articular surfaces, the edges of which, on axial (sunrise) projection radiographs and CT scans, may simulate compression fractures or osteochondritis dissecans (Harrison *et al.*, 1976; Patel *et al.*, 1983).

The blood supply of the lower end of the femur is via radiate arteries, which penetrate the condyles from the circumference. They arise from the descending medial and lateral genicular arteries, which are branches of the femoral and popliteal arteries (Crock, 1962, 1967, 1996). Rogers and Gladstone (1950) identified groups of anterior and posterior supracondylar, medial and lateral condylar and central (foveal) and peripheral intercondylar vascular foramina. This generous supply of the lower end of the femur contrasts with that of the upper end and explains the relative lack of ischaemic necrosis after fractures of the distal end.

There are a variety of minor anomalies at the lower end of the femur, some of which appear to be of such common occurrence that they could be regarded as normal. Parsons (1914), Stopford (1914), Nadgir (1917) and Frazer (1948) described supracondyloid tubercles on the popliteal surface superior to the condyles and just lateral to the epicondylar lines. They were much more common on the medial side and were interpreted as attachments for the medial head of gastrocnemius. However, Kostick (1963) described a 'tibial imprint' in the same position, which he proposed could either accommodate a fabella (gastrocnemius sesamoid) during flexion of the knee or the posterior border of the tibial condyle, which bears a 'tuberculum quadratum tendonis' (Cave and Porteous, 1958, 1959) for the semimembranosus muscle. On the medial side, Charles' facet (Charles, 1893; Kostick, 1963) is a small cartilage-covered facet continuous with the medial condylar surface above and behind the medial epicondyle, which may reach the adductor tubercle. Martin's facet (Martin, 1932; Kostick, 1963) is a crescentic extension of the trochlear surface onto the lateral aspect of the lateral condyle. Peritrochlear grooves occur when the medial trochlear margin is raised to form a gutter extending from the supratrochlear surface to a notch, which demarcates the trochlea from the condylar surface (Kostick, 1963). These extend on the medial and sometimes the lateral side down to the notch separating the trochlear from the condylar surface. Meyer (1924b) described supracondylar fossae on the anterior surface of the femur, which were ascribed to pressure exerted by the osteophytic edges of patellae deformed by arthritis. Martin (1932) and Siddiqi (1934) also described a variant of the normal horizontal intercondylar line, which had a distinct upward convexity crossed by a groove. Martin (1932) ascribed this to a mark made by the posterior cruciate ligament when the knee was in a hyperflexed position. The incidence of anomalies at the lower end of the femur appears to be higher in populations whose postural habits involve long periods with flexed knees, either seated on very low stools, or squatting with buttocks on heels, knees apart and toes turned outwards (Charles, 1893;[3] Siddiqi, 1934; Kostick, 1963). However, Trinkaus (1975), discussing squatting in Neandertals, argued that conclusions drawn from the presence of variations in skeletal morphology alone, should be viewed with caution.

There have been many studies on sexual dimorphism of the femur (Dwight, 1905; Parsons, 1915; Thieme and Schull, 1957; Singh and Singh, 1972b; Dibennardo and Taylor, 1982, 1983; Işcan and Miller-Shaivitz. 1984a; Dittrick and Suchey, 1986; Becker, 1987; MacLaughlin, 1987) and levels of accuracy vary between 76% (Dibennardo and Taylor, 1982) to 95% (Işcan and Miller-Shaivitz, 1984a). However, some of the studies have been carried out on undocumented material, where sex was determined from morphological or archaeological evidence and they therefore inevitably involve circular reasoning (see Chapter 2). Methods of determination of sex from fragmentary remains can be found in Black (1978b), MacLaughlin and Bruce (1985) and Seidemann *et al.* (1998).

Stature estimation from the femur has the highest accuracy of all the long bones as it contributes to a major part of body height. However, as the femur/height ratio varies in different races, it is important to use tables or regression equations specific to the population under investigation (Stevenson, 1929; Breitinger, 1937; Telkkä, 1950; Dupertuis and Hadden, 1951; Trotter and Gleser, 1952, 1958; Genovés, 1967; Farrally and Moore, 1975; Dibennardo and Taylor, 1983; Jantz, 1992). Feldesman *et al.* (1990) and Feldesman and Fountain (1996) have discussed the problem of estimation of height, both in fossil genera and in skeletal remains of unknown 'racial' origin. They considered that, if race is definitely known, then race-specific ratios are more accurate but, if race is unknown, a generic femur/stature equation gives better results. For fragmentary remains, Simmons *et al.* (1990) reported on a revision of the Steele (1970) method and Prasad *et al.* (1996a) calculated regression equations for reconstruction of femoral length from markers at the proximal end. Craig (1995) found that there is a consistent and statistically significant difference between American Blacks and Whites in the intercondylar shelf angle (between the roof of the intercondylar fossa and the posterior surface of the shaft).

Early development of the femur

The early development of the femur has been much studied and details may be found in Bardeen and Lewis (1901), Bardeen (1905), Gardner and Gray (1950), Gray and Gardner (1950), Haines (1953), Gardner and O'Rahilly (1968) and O'Rahilly and Gardner (1975). The mesenchymal femur is visible at stage 17 (about 11–14 mm CRL/41 days). The cartilaginous femur begins to form during stages 18 and 19 (about 13–18 mm/44–47 days) and is complete by the end of the embryonic period. At 48 days, the head begins to chondrify and by 52 days the neck, both trochanters and the condyles, are well formed in cartilage (Gardner and O'Rahilly, 1968; O'Rahilly and Gardner, 1975). At the eighth week of embryonic life the femur is about 3.5 mm in length (Felts, 1954).

Ossification

Primary centre

Two detailed studies of the later development of the femur, from the end of the embryonic period, are by Felts (1954) and Gardner and Gray (1970). A bony collar appears in the midshaft at Stage 22 (weeks 7–8 – Gardner and Gray, 1970; O'Rahilly and Gardner, 1975) and about a week later, endochondral ossification can be identified histologically in the centre of the shaft, although it is not apparent radiologically until about 2 weeks later. At first, periosteal bone occupies more of the length of the diaphysis, but after about 32 weeks, periosteal and endochondral bone formation are co-extensive. Burkus and Ogden (1984) made a detailed histological study of growth in the distal femur from 9 fetal weeks to 16 postnatal years. Burkus and Ogden (1982) also report a very rare case of bipartite primary ossification in an embryo of about 7 weeks (CRL 30 mm). They suggest that this could be a possible mechanism for congenital deformity of the femur, as has been postulated in the clavicle (Chapter 8), although in the latter, a dual ossification centre is the rule rather than the exception. A nutrient canal is first seen at about week 11. This does not necessarily coincide with the definitive later canal(s) and, as in the adult, the number and site of canals is very variable. Skawina and Miaskiewicz (1982) found that in fetuses between the ages of 13 and 28 weeks, over half had two nutrient foramina in the region of the linea aspera. The nutrient arteries are essential

[3]Ralph Havelock Charles, Professor of Anatomy in Lahore, Surgeon Captain Bengal Medical Service and Surgeon to the Mayo Hospital, Lahore described the facet which bears his name. In a description of the squatting posture adopted by both sexes, he remarks that squatting is easy for the 'Panjabi Falstaff' (i.e. a corpulent individual) whereas 'in the European it often happens that increasing corpulence deprives the individual of the power of tying his shoe latchet'.

vessels for cortical development, as in the fetus there is no supply to the cortex from periosteal vessels (Skawina *et al.*, 1994; Brookes and Revell, 1998). If the main nutrient artery is ligated in experimental animals, there is insufficient collateral circulation and the bone on the operated side is significantly shorter than controls (Brookes, 1957).

By about 12–13 weeks, ossification in the shaft has reached almost to the neck region proximally and to the lower epiphysis distally. The fovea in the head becomes obvious at about this time and the linea aspera and the gluteal tuberosity, which are not preformed in cartilage, develop by an increase in thickness of the periosteal bone. The growth zone at the greater trochanter is co-extensive with that in the neck, while that for the lesser trochanter is at right angles to the shaft (Felts, 1954; Gardner and Gray, 1970). From the beginning of the second trimester, the presence of osteoclasts external to the compacta signifies remodelling, which begins proximally, at the level of the lesser trochanter and distally, around the medial supracondylar line. Resorption and apposition then lead to enlargement in length and width but subsequent growth proceeds rather more slowly. At about this time, the morphology of the femoral diaphysis is sufficiently distinct to permit identification.

During the second part of the prenatal period, there is an increase in robusticity and an alteration in the morphology of the extremities of the ossified part of the shaft (Felts, 1954). By the seventh prenatal month, the proximal end changes from a convex dome shape to become angulated into two planes which lie under the cartilaginous head and greater trochanter. In the last prenatal month, to coincide with the appearance of the secondary centre (see below), the distal end of the ossified shaft usually develops a central depression. Torsion appears to occur throughout the length of the shaft, unlike the humerus, where it is thought to be restricted to the junction of the shaft and proximal epiphysis. It is initially negative but increases markedly to reach a circumnatal value of 30–40° (Elftman, 1945). Both inclination (neck-shaft angle) and obliquity are difficult to determine as they are affected by torsion, but apparent inclination increases slightly throughout the prenatal period and obliquity decreases, so that by term, it is less than in the adult (Felts, 1954). After the first trimester, total increase in shaft length is about 0.1–0.3 mm for every millimetre increase in CRL. At term, 75–80% of the overall length of the bone is occupied by ossified shaft (Felts, 1954; Gardner and Gray, 1970).

When the perinatal bone (Fig. 11.3) is placed horizontally, resting on the lower metaphysis and epiphyseal surface of the lesser trochanter, the anterior surface is flat and the posterior surface is curved concavely upwards along the long axis of the bone. The shaft is rounded in the upper two-thirds and flattened anteroposteriorly in the lower third. It widens towards the proximal end, curving medially towards the head, which inclines anteriorly. Posteriorly, the linea aspera is usually visible, with a prominent lateral lip that either fades out centrally, or is continued into the lateral supracondylar line. By contrast, on the medial side, the lip is smooth and the supracondylar line is rounded. There are usually two nutrient foramina in the upper and middle thirds of the linea aspera whose entrances slope distally. The proximal epiphyseal surface (Fig. 11.3c) is roughly oval in circumference and raised centrally, sloping away on either side to the capital and greater trochanteric surfaces. The surface is continuous at right angles with the epiphyseal surface for the lesser trochanter, which lies laterally on the posterior surface. There is often a large nutrient foramen anteriorly at the proximal end of the shaft beneath the articular surface. The distal epiphyseal surface (Fig. 11.3d) is oval in circumference, with a flat posterior border and a slightly hollowed anterior border. Most bones have a central depression (see above) dividing the surface into a circular lateral, and an oval medial portion.

The morphology and angulation of the femoral shaft alters considerably during infancy, childhood and adolescence. The initially more vertical neck is formed by early growth of the medial part of the proximal growth plate. As the hip abductors develop in response to walking, there is a marked lessening of the angle (Morgan and Somerville, 1960). By the age of 2 years, the neck divides the original single growth plate into two separate metaphyseal growth surfaces for the head and greater trochanter (Fig. 11.4 and 11.5). The neck/shaft angle can be as high as 141° during fetal life but declines up to term and continues to do so during childhood to an average of about 127° (Humphry, 1889). Walmsley (1933) noted that from birth until about the age of 3 years, the load axis (a perpendicular line from the centre of the femoral head at right angles to the bicondylar plane) passes medial to the axis of the shaft of the bone. After this time, the change in the angle of the neck causes the load axis to intersect the axis of the femoral shaft and brings the knee closer to the midline relative to the hip. This is usually quantified as an increase in the bicondylar angle and coincides with the adoption of efficient walking at the beginning of childhood (Aiello and Dean, 1990). Tardieu and Trinkaus (1994) have charted the ontogeny of the bicondylar angle from birth to adolescence in both living humans and skeletal samples. In the skeletal sample, low adult values were seen

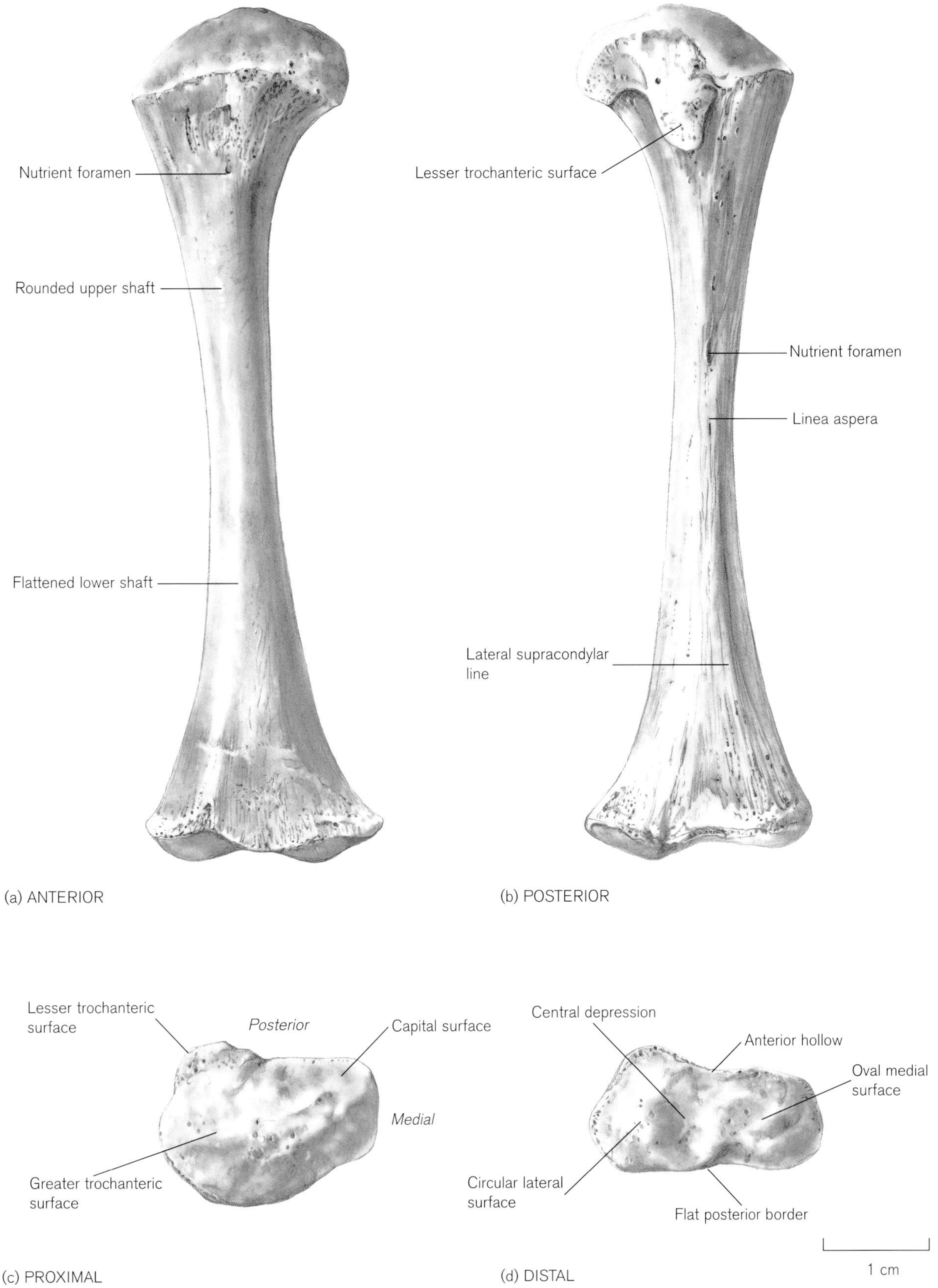

Nutrient foramen
Rounded upper shaft
Flattened lower shaft
Lesser trochanteric surface
Nutrient foramen
Linea aspera
Lateral supracondylar line
(a) ANTERIOR
(b) POSTERIOR
Lesser trochanteric surface
Posterior
Capital surface
Medial
Greater trochanteric surface
Central depression
Anterior hollow
Oval medial surface
Circular lateral surface
Flat posterior border
1 cm
(c) PROXIMAL
(d) DISTAL

Figure 11.3 Right perinatal femur.

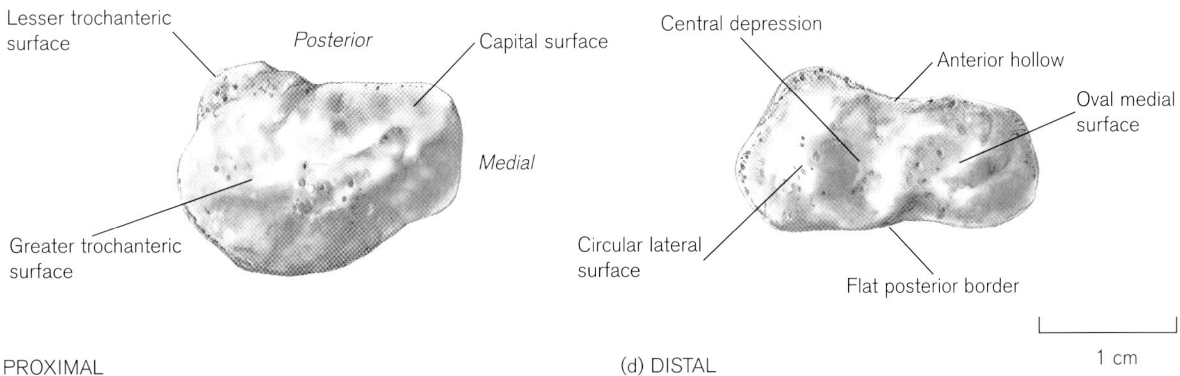

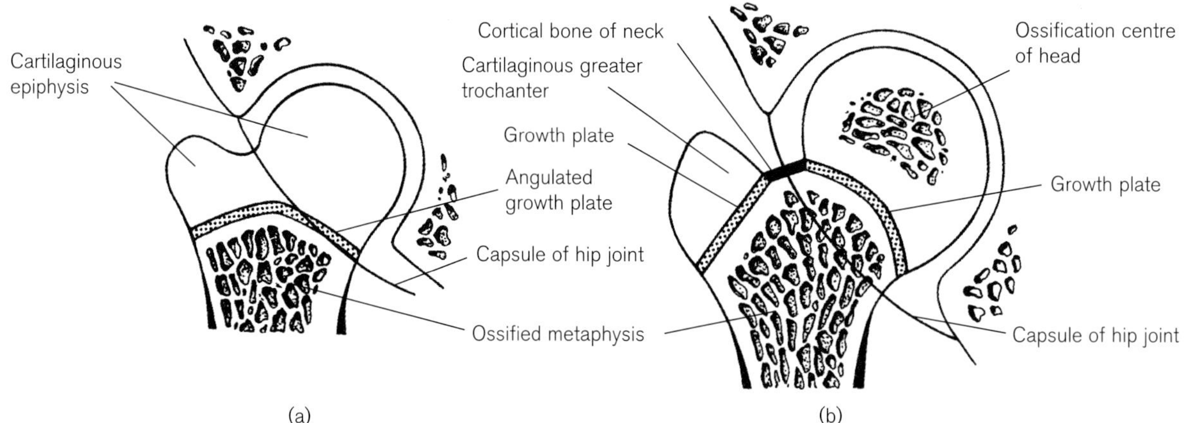

Figure 11.4 Development of the proximal end of the femur. (a) At birth; (b) 3–4 years.

by about 4 years of age whilst two patients, one with minimum walking ability and the other non-ambulatory, showed little and no development, respectively. Tardieu (1998) charted the change in angle of obliquity of the shaft and attributed angular remodelling to increased apposition on the medial surface of the distal end of the metaphysis. While this undoubtedly contributes to angulation of the shaft, the change in the morphology and angulation of the femoral neck in infancy is also an important factor.

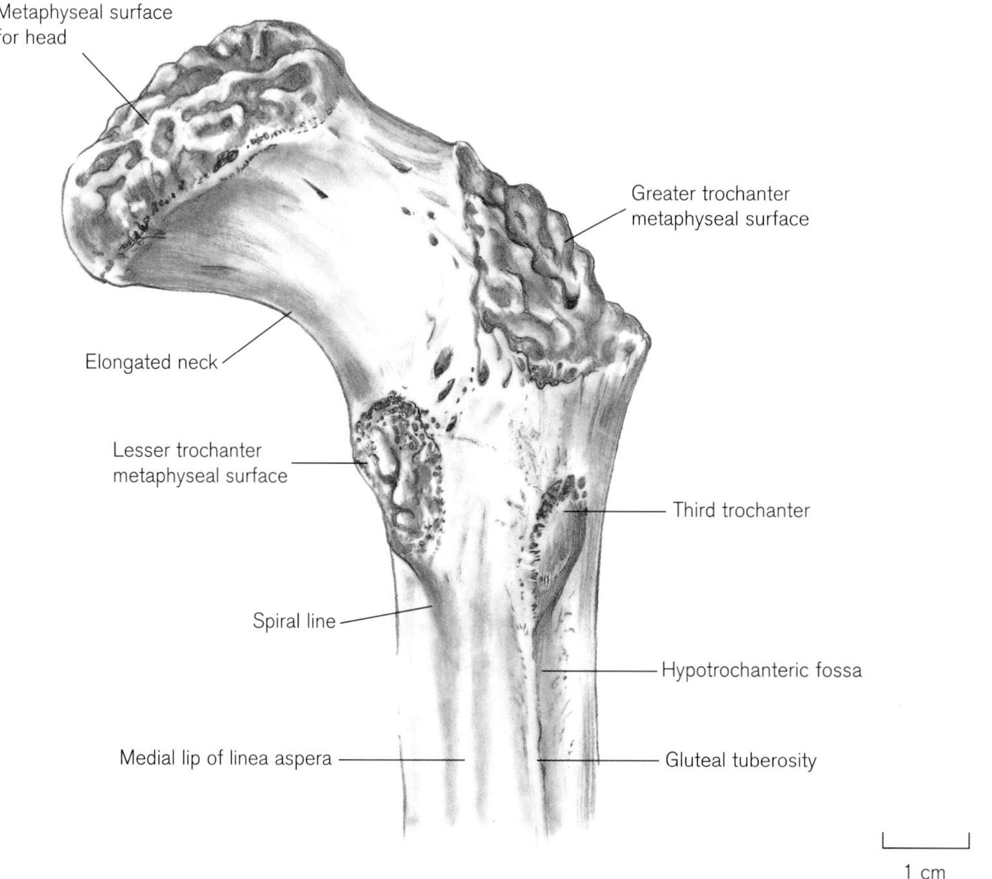

Figure 11.5 Posterior view of proximal fragment of right femur. This is a damaged archaeological fragment of about 11–12 years skeletal age. It has a third trochanter and a hypotrochanteric fossa.

The trabecular architecture of the neck and shaft also changes during the early years, as remodelling occurs in response to weight bearing as the child begins to stand and then to walk (Townsley, 1948). Osborne *et al.* (1980) and Osborne and Effmann (1981) evaluated the radiological changes from birth to adolescence. During the first year, trabeculae are orientated along the long axis of the shaft but during the second year, as the neck starts to form, principal medial and lateral groups become visible and by 5 years, secondary trabeculae become obvious. Tobin (1955) showed slab cuts of the proximal femur at this age in which there was no clear-cut triangular area of weak trabeculation, as is apparent in the adult. Ozonoff and Ziter (1985, 1987) described notch-like defects both in the subfoveal area of the femoral head, and in the cortex on the medial side of the neck, which are asymptomatic and occur as normal variants.

Hrdlička (1934a) studied the development of the linea aspera and the pilaster during ontogeny and found that the time of appearance of the linea was very variable. It may appear in the form of a simple ridge in mid-uterine life, but its development is often delayed until after birth, and its distinctive form is sometimes not attained until adolescence. The pilaster is rarely seen as early as late childhood but develops after puberty and is maximal by middle age. A strong linea and pilastry appear to be unrelated. Anterior curvature also shows a progressive increase with age. Walensky (1965), in a series of 45 subadults, reported that between 3 and 6 years the femur was relatively straight and a significant curvature developed between 7 and 13 years.

In our series of juvenile femora, by about 7–8 years of age, the lateral lip of the linea aspera is usually obvious and the spiral line and the gluteal tuberosity become evident. There is a visible anterior curvature at about the age of 18 months, which would coincide with weight-bearing and walking.

Normal shaft torsion decreases throughout postnatal life from its circumnatal value of about 35°. Fabry *et al.* (1973) reported a decrease from a mean of 31.13° at 1 year to 15.35° at 16 years. Engel and Staheli (1974) and Staheli (1977) noticed an accelerated decrease between 1 and 2 years, and another between 14 and 16 years, which correlates with initial walking and then possible modification of walking style caused by adolescent changes in pelvic proportions. They found that increases beyond the normal range of anteversion are a significant factor in intoeing gait and in many pathological hip conditions of childhood. Upadhyay *et al.* (1990) used ultrasound to measure femoral anteversion in 219 healthy children between the ages of 1 and 15 years. They reported a decrease in torsion from 40° at birth to about 12° in adult life. There appeared to be no sexual dimorphism, but a significant correlation between siblings, which suggested a genetic explanation. Children with a value of more than two standard deviations from the mean showed orthopaedic symptoms and signs.

The metaphyseal surface of the lower end of the shaft develops changes to mirror the shape of the developing epiphysis. By about 6 months of age, the anterior border develops a hollow which is co-extensive with the trochlear surface of the epiphysis and the posterior border becomes notched as the intercondylar fossa ossifies. By 3 years, the lateral surface projects more anteriorly than the medial surface, as the asymmetry of the trochlea develops. By about 4–5 years, condylar and trochlear areas can be distinguished on the metaphyseal surface (Fig. 11.6).

70% of fractures of the shaft of the femur are in the midshaft region and transverse, oblique or spiral, but rarely comminuted. Child abuse is the most common cause in the first 2 years of life (Staheli, 1984).

Secondary centres

The **distal end** of the femur has the largest and fastest growing epiphysis in the body. It normally develops from a single ossific nucleus, which is the first of the long bone epiphyses to appear and one of the last to fuse. Its ossification is an important marker, both of fetal maturity, and for forensic identification of legal term status (Knight, 1996). The centre normally

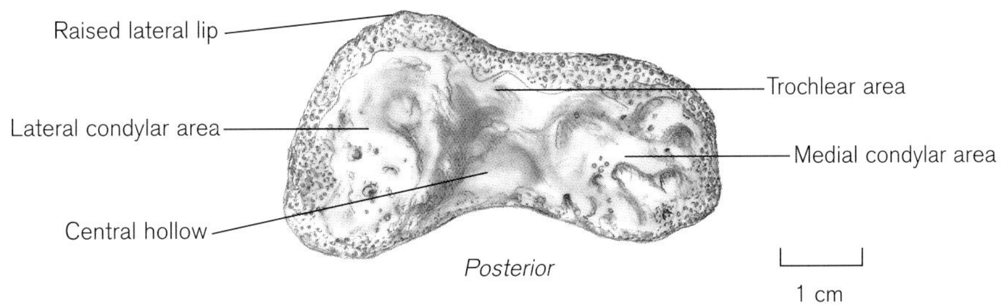

Figure 11.6 Right distal metaphyseal surface – 4 years, female.

appears in the month before birth and is therefore sometimes absent in premature infants (Flecker, 1932b). Kuhns and Finnstrom (1976) reported that in North American and Swedish populations, the epiphysis was radiographically visible in fetal weeks 31 and 39 for the 5th and 95th percentiles, respectively. It is present in over 98% of cases at birth (Puyhaubert, 1913; Davies and Parsons, 1927; Paterson, 1929; Flecker, 1932b; Menees and Holly, 1932; Francis *et al.*, 1939; Elgenmark, 1946; Kelly and Reynolds, 1947; Christie, 1949; Hansman, 1962) and is always obvious by 3 *postpartum* months. Ossification starts in the proximal half of the cartilaginous epiphysis, as illustrated by Crock (1967) and Gardner and Gray (1970).

The detailed radiological appearance of the distal femoral epiphysis is shown by Pyle and Hoerr (1955) and Scheller (1960). Even at birth, the standard for girls is about 2 weeks in advance of that for boys and this discrepancy in developmental timing increases with age so that by puberty, girls are some 2 years in advance of boys. At birth, the epiphysis is an oval nodule of bone lying inferior to the depression in the metaphysis (see above) with its long axis at right angles to the long axis of the bone. For the first 2 weeks, the femoral epiphysis has a larger vertical and horizontal diameter than the tibial epiphysis. In the second half of the first year, the epiphyseal plate begins to develop and the epiphysis becomes ovoid, the lateral side being larger than the medial side. By 2 years, the mediolateral diameter is 18–24 mm and the vertical and AP diameter 8–12 mm (Puyhaubert, 1913). Between 1 and 3 years, the epiphysis grows rapidly in width as ossification spreads into the condylar areas of the cartilage. It takes on a 'wooden shoe' (sabot) appearance radiologically, because of the greater vertical diameter of the lateral condyle (Pyle and Hoerr, 1955). The bony epiphysis becomes recognizable during the second year. It is roughly kidney-shaped with a flat anterior border and an indented posterior border forming the shallow intercondylar fossa. The articular surface is gently rounded and pitted with nutrient foramina which are numerous within the fossa. On the metaphyseal side, the anterior trochlear third is separated by a faint transverse ridge from the posterior condylar two-thirds, which is itself divided by a central rounded elevation into circular lateral and oval medial areas (Fig. 11.7a).

By the age of 7 years in girls and 9 years in boys, the epiphysis is as wide as the metaphysis (Pyle and Hoerr, 1955). The condyles and intercondylar fossa have now assumed their distinctive shape and the latter is the main site for nutrient foramina. The anterior (trochlear) border has an asymmetrical, sinuous curve, with the lateral lip projecting anteriorly. Tardieu (1998) reported these changes at a later age as an adolescent phenomenon. The trochlear area occupies rather more of the metaphyseal surface than before and this mirrors the distal end of the diaphysis (Fig. 11.7b). Smith (1962a) viewed the transverse ridge separating the two areas of the epiphysis as reflecting the division between weight-bearing compressive forces acting on the condyles and tensile forces pulling downwards on the cruciate ligaments. The adductor tubercle is visible on radiographs at about 8 years in girls and 11 years in boys (Pyle and Hoerr, 1955), by which time it is sometimes also identifiable on the bony epiphysis. Between 8 and 12 years, the epiphysis starts to cap the end of the shaft. The condyles are covered with smooth, cortical bone and the lateral lip of the intercondylar groove projects anterosuperiorly. They are themselves divided into condylar and trochlear areas. The metaphyseal surface is deeply hollowed and grooved and the adductor tubercle is prominent on the posteromedial border (Fig. 11.7c). From this time until fusion, the distal epiphysis resembles the adult bone.

It is not uncommon to find accessory ossification centres around the periphery of the developing epiphysis at any time during childhood and on some radiological views a groove for the popliteus tendon can be seen that may contain a cyamella sesamoid (Scheller, 1960). Sesamoid bones in the lateral heads of the gastrocnemius muscle (fabellae) were identified in their cartilaginous phase in 14-week fetuses (Gray and Gardner, 1950).

Fracture separation of the lower femoral epiphysis is relatively uncommon. Infantile separation is associated with breech birth or child abuse, whereas that occurring later is usually related to hyperextension force caused by road traffic accidents or sports injuries. Because of the proximity of the large vessels and nerves in the popliteal fossa, there may be acute vascular or neural compromise (Beaty and Kumar, 1994).

Fusion of the lower end of the femur coincides with cessation of growth in height as the epiphyses around the knee are the growing ends of the lower limb bones. The distal epiphysis is responsible for about 70% of growth in length of the bone (Digby, 1915; Gill and Abbott, 1942; Anderson *et al.*, 1963; Ogden, 1984d). Most radiographic observations state that this occurs between the ages of 14–18 years in females and 16–19 years in males (Davies and Parsons, 1927; Paterson, 1929; Flecker, 1932b; Hansman, 1962). On the Pyle and Hoerr (1955) radiographic standards, there is definite fusion in the centre of the epiphyseal plate at 14.5 years in females and 17 years in males and the growth plates are replaced by lines of fusion by 15.5 years in females and 18 years in males.

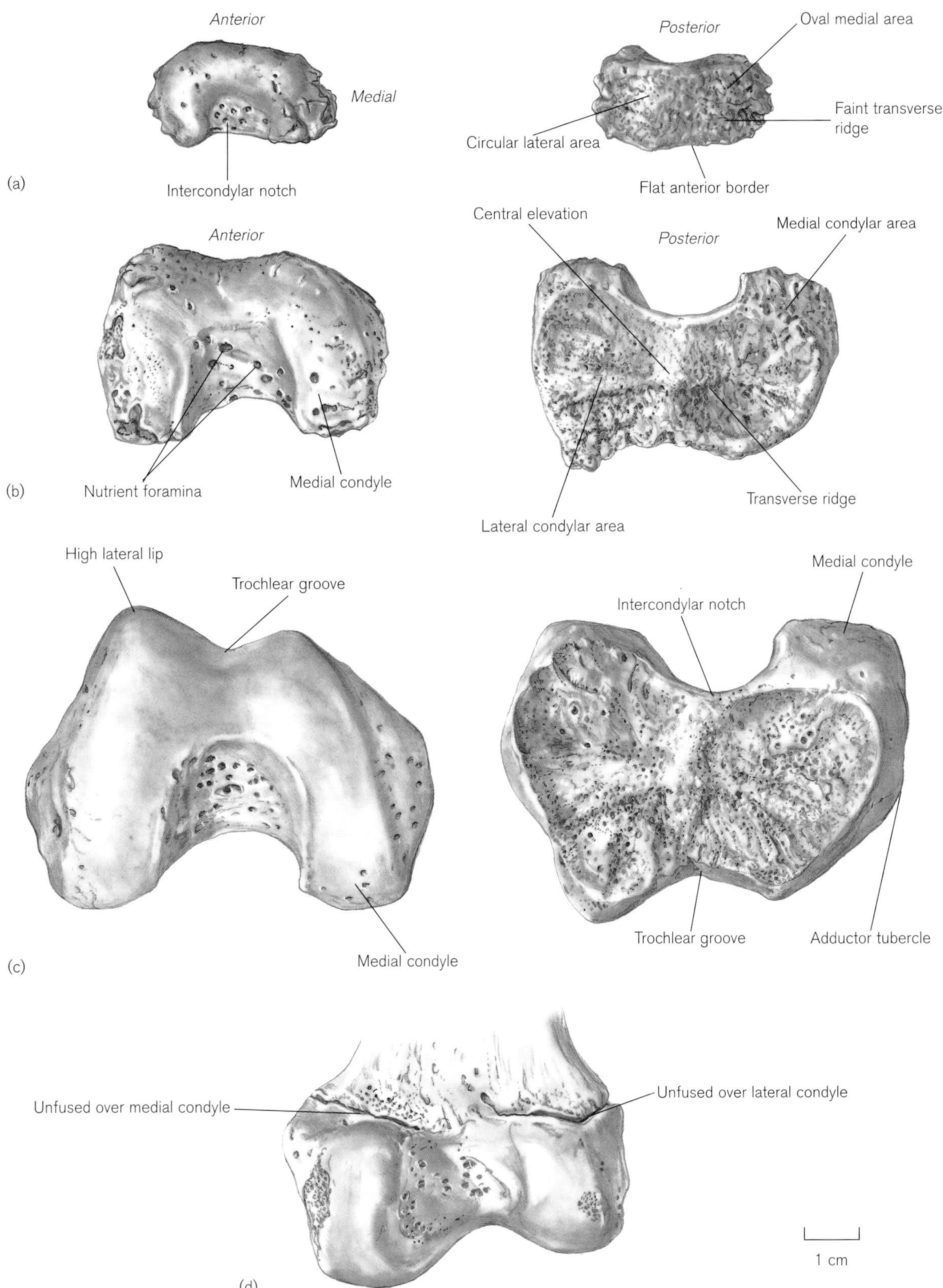

Figure 11.7 Development of the distal right femoral epiphysis. (a) 2 years, female; (b) 8 years, male; (c) 12 years, male. Left row – articular surfaces. Right row – metaphyseal surfaces; (d) posterior surface of distal right femur from an undocumented adolescent.

However, McKern and Stewart (1957), from observations on dry bone, place the lower end of the femur in their Group II of delayed union and stated that the early stage of union in males can be as late as 20 years and that fusion was not 100% complete in their specimens until 22 years. They describe the last sites for fusion on the posteromedial side of the epiphysis above the medial condyle. In our series of juvenile skeletons, fusion at the periphery always occurred first over the medial and lateral aspects of the epiphysis. It then proceeded across the anterior border and the intercondylar fossa part of the posterior border, leaving the last sites posteriorly over the condyles (Fig. 11.7d).

The **proximal end of the femur** has three, and sometimes four separate secondary centres of ossification but, in contrast to those of the humerus, they do not form a compound epiphysis but develop and fuse independently with the neck or shaft of the bone. At birth, although the whole of the proximal end of the bone is composed of cartilage,[4] the head and both trochanters are well defined. At this stage, the single growth plate can be divided into a medial, subcapital section and a lateral subtrochanteric portion. Only a small area of the medial edge of the growth plate is intra-articular, but gradually the neck begins to form by medial extension of the osseous shaft and so more of the growth plate becomes intracapsular. Observations in pigs injected with tetracycline indicated that the capital section of the plate contributes significantly to the metaphyseal growth of the neck and little to the appositional growth of the femoral head, whereas the trochanteric part forms more of the epiphysis and contributes less to the metaphyseal growth (Edgren, 1965). By the age of about 2 years, the growth of the neck has divided the original combined epiphyseal surface into separate areas for the head and greater trochanter (Fig. 11.4). A similar process also separates the epiphyseal surface for the lesser trochanter so that it comes to lie below and medial to the combined epiphyseal surface. Each secondary ossification centre then develops in its own separate cartilaginous territory. It is difficult, therefore, to understand the statement by Trueta (1957) that 'even at puberty, the infantile unity of the epiphyseal plate of the upper end still persists where a single epiphyseal cartilage covers the whole of the neck under the epiphysis of head and greater trochanter'. Edgren (1965) described and illustrated a rare case of a bony bridge that developed between the capital epiphysis and that of the greater trochanter after a congenital hip subluxation.

[4]Walmsley (1915b) called this the tri-epiphyseal cartilage, a confusing term, fortunately not subsequently adopted, as the term is more usually given to the growth cartilage of the acetabulum.

The **centre for the head** is very rarely seen at birth but is present in 60–90% of infants at 6 months and is nearly always visible by the age of 1 year (Puyhaubert, 1913; Walmsley, 1915b; Davies and Parsons, 1927; Paterson, 1929; Flecker, 1932b; Menees and Holly, 1932; Francis *et al.*, 1939; Elgenmark, 1946; Ryder and Mellin, 1966). Hansman (1962) reported the median for girls as 5 months (range – birth to 1 year) and that for boys as 6 months (range – 2 months to 1 year) and Garn *et al.* (1967b) gave the 50th percentile as a little earlier than this. Ossification begins above and medial to the centre point of the whole head and at first, may sometimes be composed of a number of osseous granules (Walmsley, 1915b; Trueta, 1957) or a double centre (Keats, 1992).

The ossified part of the epiphysis is spherical for about the first year-and-a-half and then becomes flattened inferiorly as it accommodates itself to the medial section of the proximal end of the shaft and the growth plate is established. At about 3 years of age, it is almost hemispherical in shape, with the lateral side slightly flattened (Fig. 11.8a). The articular surface is rounded and pitted with numerous vascular foramina. The metaphyseal surface is almost flat except for a blunt, beak-like projection that is in line with the posterior surface of the neck. By 6–8 years (Fig. 11.8b), the fovea can be distinguished on the inferomedial side of the articular surface. The almost circular circumference has a sharp edge, which extends down over the neck, except for a small flattened section on the lateral side contiguous with the superior surface of the neck. Smith (1962a) emphasized that the major part of the circumference conforms to the articular margin, while this superior flattened section has large foramina through which the main blood vessels enter the head. The metaphyseal surface is roughened and the beak-like projection is now more obvious at the posterior end of the flattened border. It fits into a reciprocal hollow in the metaphyseal surface of the capital area of the shaft and could possibly act as a locking mechanism to counteract slipping of the epiphysis. By puberty, the articular surface is smooth except for the fovea and consists of about two-thirds of a sphere (Fig. 11.8c). The metaphyseal surface is a shallow cup-shape with sharp edges, as ossification has spread down round the circumference except at the juxtacervical surface. This has an anterior angle, which juts laterally over the anterosuperior margin of the neck and a more rounded posterior angle, which is in line with the posterosuperior margin. The flat lateral margin is still pitted with nutrient foramina.

The major part of the arterial supply to the epiphysis of the head comes from epiphyseal branches of

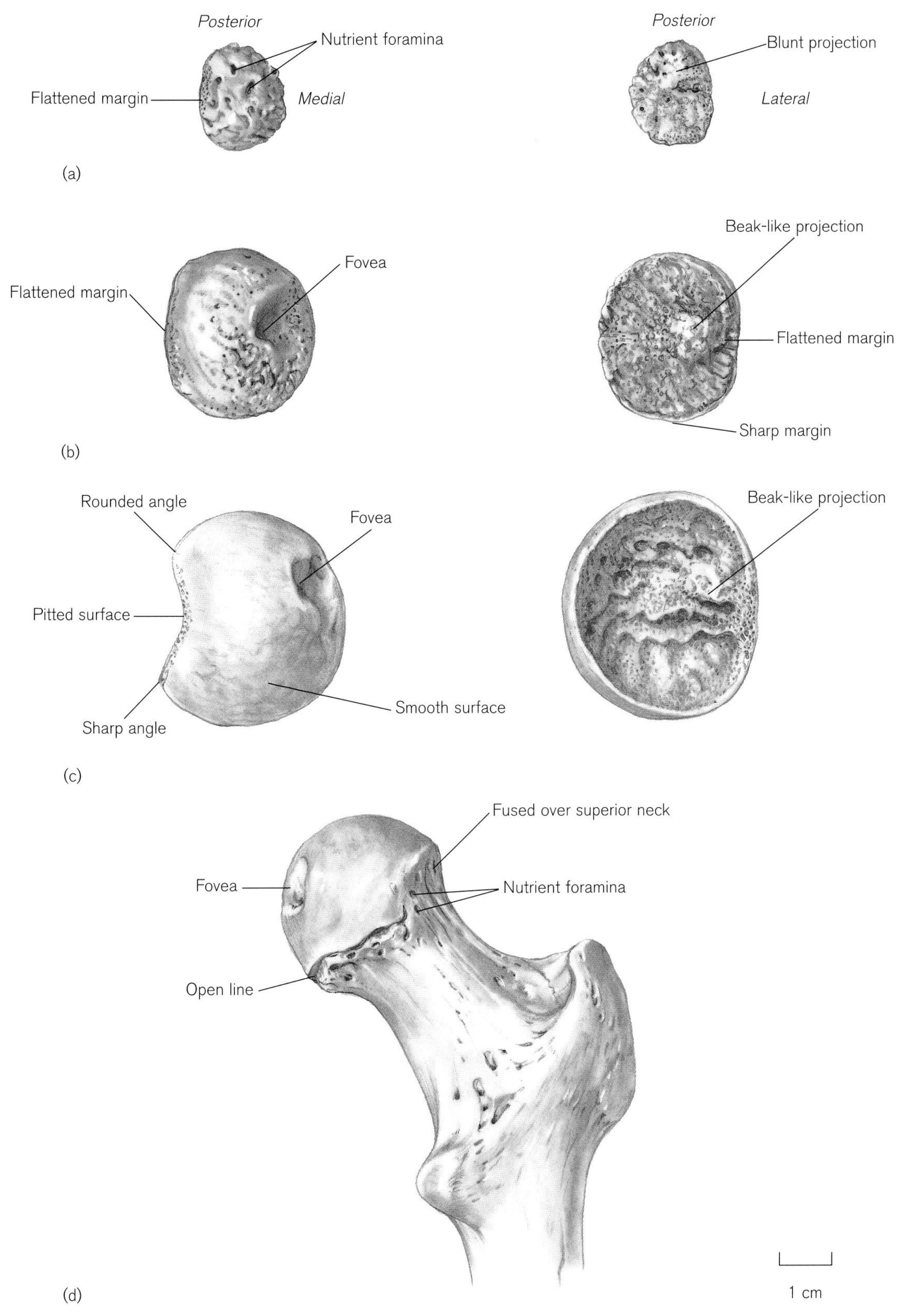

Figure 11.8 Development of the right capital femoral epiphysis. (a) 3 years, male; (b) 8 years, male; (c) undocumented early adolescent. Left row – articular surfaces. Right row – metaphyseal surfaces; (d) posterior surface of right proximal femur from an undocumented late adolescent.

ascending cervical branches, which in turn arise from the arterial ring of the neck (Crock, 1965, 1967, 1996). There is also a vital supply to a limited area around the fovea, via vessels accompanying the ligament of the head from branches of the obturator or medial circumflex femoral artery (Tucker, 1949). Ogden (1974a) found that at birth, the anterior and posterior halves of the growth plate were supplied equally by the lateral and medial circumflex arteries, respectively. Subsequent vascular changes caused regression of the supply from the lateral artery so that during the transition phase, the capital epiphysis is susceptible to ischaemic necrosis in the event of injury.

Hughes and Beaty (1994) have reviewed fracture sites of the head, neck and subtrochanteric region in children and related them to the anatomy and blood supply. They are comparatively rare in children compared to adults and account for fewer than 1% of all paediatric fractures. However, epiphysiolysis (slipped epiphysis) and Perthes' disease (Legg-Calvé-Perthes disease/coxa plana) are conditions that result from the particular morphological development of the proximal femur and its vulnerable blood supply. Slipped epiphysis is rarely seen in young children under the age of 3 years, except as a birth injury (Michail *et al.*, 1958), in battered child syndrome or other forms of severe trauma. Early diagnosis and treatment is essential to prevent serious deformity (Ratliff, 1968; Lindseth and Rosene, 1971; Milgram and Lyne, 1975). As the neck/shaft angle alters throughout childhood (see above), it is accompanied by a change in direction of the plane of the epiphyseal growth plate to a more varus and posterior direction. This reaches its maximum between the ages of 10 years and puberty when there is the greatest risk of slipped epiphysis. The previously perpendicular force on the growth plate is altered and it is temporarily placed in a position more susceptible to shear stress as increasing body weight is transmitted down the femur (Ogden *et al.*, 1975a). Interestingly, this coincides with the appearance of 'juvenile beaking' in the triradiate region of the acetabulum (see Chapter 10). The vulnerability of the blood supply may lead to non-union, varus deformity or premature closure of the growth plate. The highest risk is of avascular necrosis, which is directly related to the amount of displacement. Perthes' disease is also an avascular necrosis of the femoral head of unknown origin. It usually causes flattening of the head, sometimes fragmentation of the epiphysis and thickening of the neck. It occurs uni- or bilaterally, at a peak age of 4 years and more often in boys than girls in a ratio of about 4:1 (Hunt, 1995). Again, it can lead to premature closure of the growth plate and subsequent delay in skeletal development.

Ages for **fusion of the femoral head** as observed on radiographs are given by Davies and Parsons (1927), Paterson (1929), Flecker (1932b) and Hasselwander (1938). Hansman (1962) reported the mean for girls as 14 years and 2 months (range 11–16 years) and for boys as 16 years and 3 months (range 14–19 years). Stevenson (1924) and McKern and Stewart (1957) reported observations on dry bone. Stevenson does not distinguish between the sexes and his 'beginning' to 'complete' stages extend from 17 to 18.5 years. McKern and Stewart, reporting on the Korean War dead, are only able to give figures for the latter part of the range in males, as the proximal femoral epiphyses form part of their Group I, early union. They found 88% fused at 17–18 years and 100% fusion by 20 years and note that fusion begins anterolaterally and proceeds to the posteromedial part of the head. Haines *et al.* (1967) and Dvonch and Bunch (1983) described initiation of fusion in the superior aspect of the head which proceeded inferiorly. This was confirmed in our series of adolescent skeletons, where the head was undergoing union. The flattened section of the epiphyseal edge across the superior surface of the neck always fused first, with the inferomedial aspect being the last part to remain open (Fig. 11.8d).

The centre of ossification appears in the cartilaginous mass of the **greater trochanter** between 2 and 5 years of age, with girls being several months in advance of boys (Puyhaubert, 1913; Davies and Parsons, 1927; Paterson, 1929; Flecker, 1932b; Francis *et al.*, 1939; Elgenmark, 1946; Garn *et al.*, 1967b). Hansman (1962) reported the median for girls as 2 years 10 months (range 18 months to 4 years) and for boys as 4 years (range 2–6 years). By the time that the centre for the trochanter begins to ossify, the growth of the femoral neck has removed it from the vicinity of the head and the two centres subsequently maintain separate development. Ossification begins in the base of the epiphysis next to the growth plate and by about the age of 5–6 years it is a boomerang-shaped ossicle with the anterior limb slightly larger than the posterior limb. It is finely pitted on both surfaces (Fig. 11.9a). By 8–9 years, ossification spreads upwards from the base, it assumes a semilunar shape and the trochanteric fossa is usually obvious (Fig. 11.9b). By puberty, the trochanter has assumed its adult morphology (Fig. 11.9c). It is a large, pyramidal-shaped knob of bone with a base and three unequal sides. The original smaller posterior section is now much larger than the anterior part and is attached obliquely at the junction of the neck and shaft. The flat anterior surface is small and reaches further medially onto the neck than the curved posterolateral surface, which is larger. This projects superiorly to form the apex of the

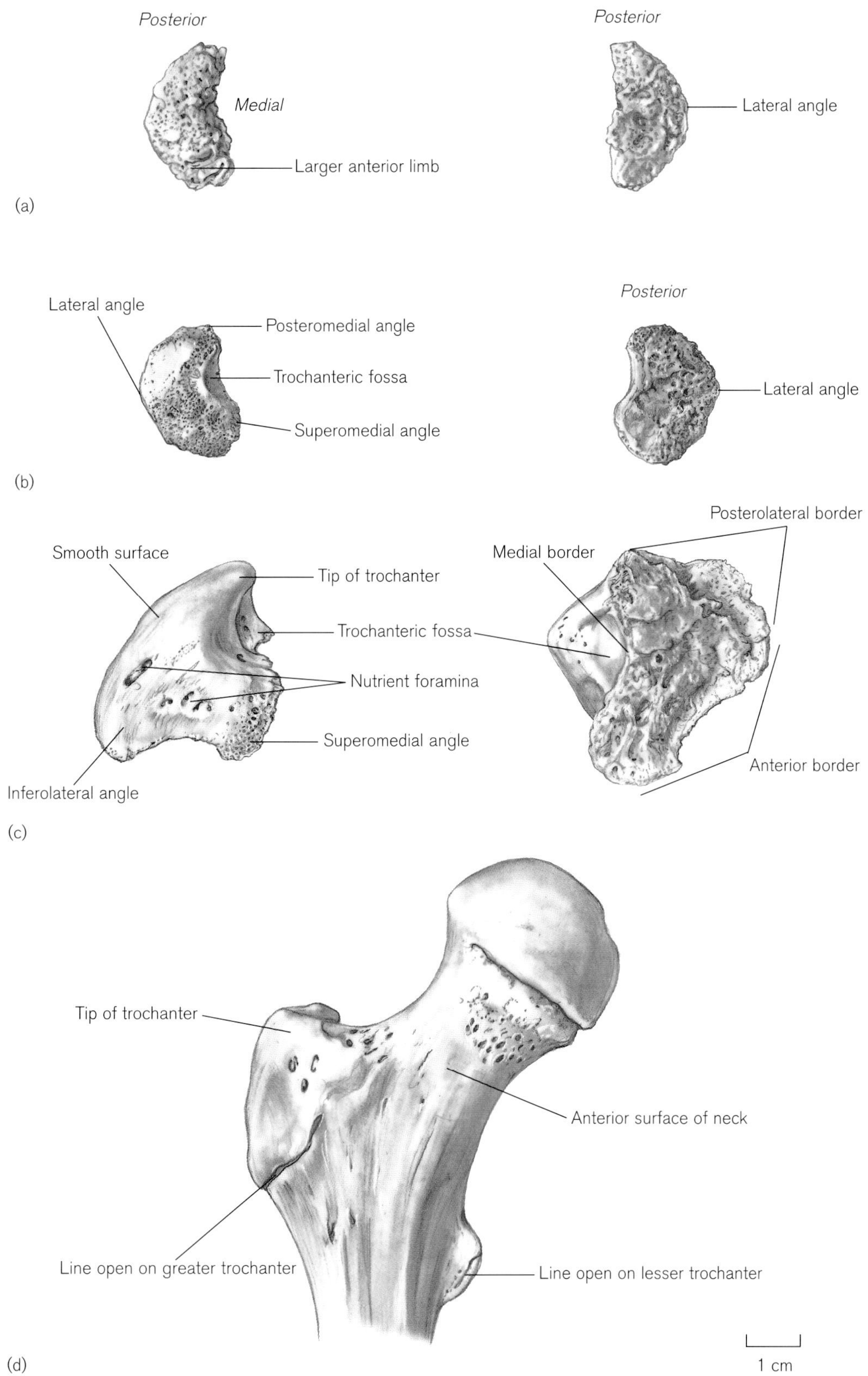

Figure 11.9 Development of the right greater trochanteric epiphysis. (a) Skeletal age 7–8 years; (b) 6 years, female; (c) undocumented early adolescent. Left row – superior surfaces. Right row – metaphyseal surfaces. Note that the documented 6-year-old trochanter is more mature than that of the 7–8 year old; (d) anterior surface of right proximal femur from an undocumented late adolescent.

trochanter, which overhangs the medial surface where the well-formed trochanteric fossa lies posteriorly. The surface is covered with smooth cortical bone but is still pitted with numerous nutrient foramina, some of them large. The roughened metaphyseal surface is triangular with a long anterior border, a shorter posterolateral border and a curved medial border.

Age ranges for **fusion** of the greater trochanter are wide, but with girls again being in advance of boys. It occurs about 14–16 years in females and 16–18 years in males. Haines *et al.* (1967) found that the first site of union was in the region of the trochanteric fossa and McKern and Stewart (1957) illustrated the last area of fusion posteromedially. In our series of juvenile skeletons, the greater trochanter always fused around the superior, posterior and anterior borders first with the inferior border being the last to complete union. In any one individual, its maturity was always slightly in advance of the epiphysis for the head.

Descriptions of the ossification centre of the **lesser trochanter** are extremely variable, times of appearance ranging from 7–11 years and of fusion from 16–17 years. Some anatomical accounts even throw doubt on its existence as a separate centre and both Paterson (1929) and Flecker (1932b, 1936b) state that it is not always present, the latter suggesting that it might be more common in males than in females. Puyhaubert (1913) and Paterson (1929) describe it as small and flake-like, which is similar to the epiphysis of the anterior inferior iliac spine (Chapter 10) or the radial tuberosity (Chapter 9). However, the lesser trochanteric epiphysis is commonly referred to in the clinical literature, usually in connection with avulsion injuries in adolescence (Dimon, 1972; Fernbach and Wilkinson, 1981). Haines *et al.* (1967) illustrated a substantial epiphysis fusing at its upper and lower borders, displaying an open line in the centre. In our series of juvenile skeletons, the younger specimens usually had an obvious billowed surface on the posterior part of the shaft and the older specimens showed a partially fused epiphysis. Union always began on the lateral border and remained open longer medially (Fig. 11.9d). The only completely separate epiphysis observed was 2 cm long and 1.2 cm in breadth and depth. The fact that an individual epiphysis is rarely seen probably reflects its short existence as a separate entity. McKern and Stewart (1957) reported that 100% fusion did not take place until the age of 20 years. They illustrated a lesser trochanteric epiphysis partially fused with an open line inferiorly.

From accounts in the literature it appears that the upper end of the gluteal ridge may ossify separately as a flake at the same time as the lesser trochanter. If this does occur, it could be viewed as the **epiphysis of the third trochanter**. Dixon (1896) described

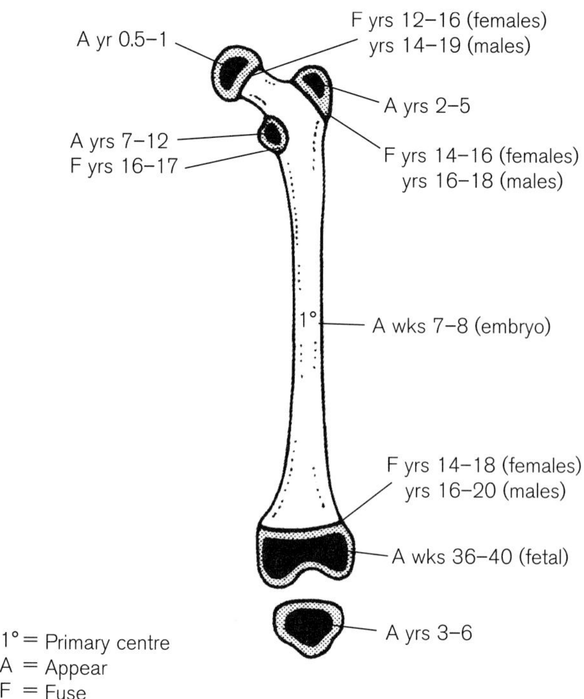

Figure 11.10 Appearance and fusion times of the femoral and patellar ossification centres.

such an epiphysis as a flat, narrow scale of bone, in line with the long axis of the shaft, at the same level as the lowest part of the lesser trochanter. There appears to be no account of its time of fusion.

The appearance and fusion of the femoral centres of ossification are summarised in Fig. 11.10.

Practical notes

Sideing

Diaphysis – sideing the perinatal or early infant femoral diaphysis relies on identifying the medial curve of the shaft towards the head and the surface for the lesser trochanter on the posterior surface (Fig. 11.3). Once the neck of the femur has started to develop at about 2 years of age, the sideing of the diaphysis becomes obvious (Fig. 11.5).

Distal epiphysis – sideing of the epiphysis is possible from about 2 years of age. It depends on identifying the intercondylar fossa posteriorly and the lateral circular and medial oval areas on the metaphyseal surface (Fig. 11.7). After this time, the distal epiphysis rapidly assumes its adult morphology.

Capital epiphysis – from about the age of 3–4 years it is possible to side the epiphysis for the head by recognizing the flattened lateral margin of the circumference and the blunt raised projection at its posterior edge on the metaphyseal surface (Fig. 11.8).

Table 11.1 Means and ranges for lengths of diaphyses of major long bones at 10 lunar months

	Mean (mm)	Range (mm)
Humerus	64.9	61.6–70.0
Radius	51.8	47.5–58.0
Ulna	59.3	55.0–65.5
Femur	74.3	69.0–78.7
Tibia	65.1	60.0–71.5
Fibula	62.3	58.0–68.5

Adapted from Fazekas and Kósa (1978).

Greater trochanteric epiphysis – sideing of this bony epiphysis at the 'boomerang' stage of development relies on identifying the lateral angle and larger anterior segment. After this time, the superior part of the epiphysis develops and the trochanteric fossa can be seen at the posterior end of the medial surface (Fig. 11.9).

Bones of a similar morphology

Perinatal diaphyses – the six major long bones of the limbs can be divided into two groups: the femur, humerus and tibia are larger and more robust than the radius, ulna and fibula. In the first group, the femur is always bigger than the humerus and tibia which are almost equal in length (Table 11.1). From birth onwards the femur increases in size rapidly and always remains the longest and largest of the long bones.

Proximal femoral fragment – this may be confused with a proximal humeral fragment (see Humerus – Practical notes).

Distal femoral fragment – this is flattened like a distal humerus but can be distinguished from it by the presence of the olecranon fossa in the humerus (Figs. 9.6b, d and 11.3b, d). It is oval like the proximal tibia, but the latter is distinguished by the tuberosity anteriorly (Fig. 11.17a, c).

Proximal femoral and humeral epiphyses – see Humerus (Practical notes, Fig. 9.11).

Morphological summary (Fig. 11.10)

Fetal

Wk 7–8	Primary ossification centre appears in shaft
Wks 36–40	Secondary centre for distal epiphysis appears
Birth	Represented by shaft and distal epiphysis
By yr 1	Secondary centre for head appears
2–5 yrs	Secondary centre for greater trochanter appears
3–6 yrs	Ossification appears in the patella
By yrs 3–4	Epiphysis of head hemispherical and recognizable
By yrs 3–5	Distal epiphysis recognizable by characteristic shape
6–8 yrs	Greater trochanter becomes recognizable
7–12 yrs	Secondary centre for lesser trochanter appears
12–16 yrs	Head fuses in females
14–19 yrs	Head fuses in males
14–16 yrs	Greater trochanter fuses in females
16–18 yrs	Greater trochanter fuses in males
16–17 yrs	Lesser trochanter fuses
14–18 yrs	Distal epiphysis fuses in females
16–20 yrs	Distal epiphysis fuses in males

Metrics

Fazekas and Kósa (1978) measured the length and distal width of the fetal femoral diaphysis on dry bones (Table 11.2) and Mehta and Singh (1972) also measured the lengths of the ossified shafts of fetuses from about 12–36 weeks. It is difficult to make direct comparisons of these two sets of data as the bone lengths, are given against age in lunar months and CR lengths, respectively. The Fazekas and Kósa data are much closer to those measured by ultrasound (Jeanty, 1983), especially at the beginning and end of the age range (Table 11.3). However, the Fazekas and Kósa data reflects a linear growth, whereas the ultrasound data produce a curved growth graph. Trotter and Peterson (1969) recorded the length and weight of the perinatal femoral diaphysis (Table 11.4).

Table 11.2 Length and width of the fetal femoral diaphysis

Age (weeks)	Length (mm)	Distal width (mm)
12	8.5	1.9
14	12.4	2.2
16	20.7	4.7
18	26.4	6.2
20	32.6	8.0
22	35.7	8.8
24	40.3	9.8
26	41.9	10.6
28	47.1	11.7
30	48.7	12.3
32	55.5	14.3
34	59.8	15.3
36	62.5	16.4
38	69.0	18.7
40	74.4	19.9

Length: maximum length.
Width: maximum mediolateral width at distal end.
Adapted from Fazekas and Kósa (1978).

Table 11.3 Length of the fetal femur as measured by ultrasound

	Length (mm)		
	Percentile		
Age (weeks)	5th	50th	95th
12	–	9	–
14	5	15	19
16	13	22	24
18	19	28	31
20	22	33	39
22	29	39	44
24	34	44	49
26	39	49	53
28	45	53	57
30	49	58	62
32	53	62	67
34	57	65	70
36	61	69	74
38	62	72	79
40	66	75	81

Adapted from Jeanty (1983).

Table 11.4 Length and weight of the perinatal femur

	Length (mm)	Weight (g)
White male	75.4	4.49
White female	70.7	3.41
Black male	70.2	3.27
Black female	75.3	3.63
Mean	72.9	3.70

Adapted from Trotter and Peterson (1969).

Table 11.5 Regression equations of age on maximum femoral length (mm)

Linear

Age (weeks) = $(0.3303 \times \text{femur}) + 13.5583 \pm 2.08$

Logarithmic

Age (weeks) = $(19.727\log_e \times \text{femur}) - 47.1909 \pm 2.04$

Adapted from Scheuer *et al.* (1980).

Table 11.6 Femoral length (mm) – 2 months–18 years

	Male			Female		
Age (years)	*n*	Mean	SD	*n*	Mean	SD
Diaphyseal length						
0.125	59	86.0	5.4	68	87.2	4.3
0.25	59	100.7	4.8	65	100.8	3.6
0.50	67	112.2	5.0	78	111.1	4.6
1.00	72	136.6	5.8	81	134.6	4.9
1.5	68	155.4	6.8	84	153.9	6.4
2.0	68	172.4	7.3	84	170.8	7.1
2.5	72	187.2	7.8	82	185.2	7.7
3.0	71	200.3	8.5	79	198.4	8.7
3.5	73	212.1	11.4	78	211.1	10.0
4.0	72	224.1	9.9	80	223.2	10.1
4.5	71	235.7	10.5	78	235.5	11.4
5.0	77	247.5	11.1	80	247.0	11.5
5.5	73	258.2	11.7	74	257.0	12.2
6.0	71	269.7	12.0	75	268.9	13.5
6.5	72	280.3	12.6	81	279.0	13.8
7.0	71	291.1	13.3	86	288.8	13.6
7.5	76	301.2	13.5	83	299.8	15.2
8.0	70	312.1	14.6	85	309.8	15.6
8.5	72	321.0	14.6	82	318.9	15.8
9.0	76	330.4	14.6	83	328.7	16.8
9.5	78	340.0	15.8	83	338.8	18.6
10.0	77	349.3	15.7	84	347.9	19.1
10.5	76	357.4	16.2	75	356.5	21.4
11.0	75	367.0	16.5	76	367.0	22.4
11.5	76	375.8	18.1	75	378.0	23.4
12.0	74	386.1	19.0	71	387.6	22.9
Total length including epiphyses						
10.0	76	385.1	17.0	83	382.8	21.1
10.5	76	394.2	17.9	75	392.6	23.7
11.0	75	405.2	17.9	76	403.5	24.8
11.5	77	414.8	19.4	75	415.4	25.2
12.0	77	425.6	20.6	74	427.9	25.2
12.5	71	437.1	19.6	67	437.9	23.9
13.0	73	447.4	21.5	69	447.2	24.1
13.5	73	458.4	24.0	63	453.1	22.0
14.0	75	470.8	24.1	64	459.9	22.5
14.5	69	478.9	25.2	41	464.5	20.8
15.0	61	489.0	23.5	57	464.4	21.4
15.5	52	498.5	23.4	12	471.5	26.0
16.0	60	502.8	22.8	40	466.7	24.0
16.5	38	504.5	24.9	3	–	–
17.0	50	508.9	23.2	18	462.9	26.2
18.0	28	511.7	24.4	4	–	–

Adapted from Maresh (1970).

Scheuer *et al.* (1980) gave linear and logarithmic regression equations for age on femoral diaphyseal length as measured on radiographs from 24 fetal weeks to 6 weeks postnatal (Table 11.5). Data showing the length of the femur at 6-monthly intervals (2-monthly for the first half year) in males and females from birth to the cessation of growth are shown in Table 11.6. These data from Maresh (1970) are from the University of Colorado longitudinal study and are of bony diaphyses except between ages 10 and 12, when double sets of figures give lengths with and without epiphyses. Measurements from radiographs at the Harvard School of Public Health by Anderson *et al.* (1964) are of total femoral length, including epiphyses at yearly intervals in males and females (Table 11.7). Pritchett (1992), using the Colorado data, charted growth and predictions of growth from the lower limb bones. The contribution of the distal femoral growth plate varies from 60% at 7 years to 90% at 14 years in females and 55% at 7 years to 90% at 16 years in males. Because of the difference of timing of the adolescent growth spurt, Feldesman (1992) recommended the use of separate male and female femur/stature ratios to estimate height between the ages of 12 and 18 years (femur = 27.16% body height in females and 27.44% body height in males).

Diaphyseal length data for some archaeological populations from Africa, Europe and North America are given in Appendix 3. Most of the age at death estimates are based on dental development.

Table 11.7 Femoral length (mm) – 1–18 years

	Male			Female		
Age (years)	*n*	Mean	SD	*n*	Mean	SD
1	21	144.8	6.28	30	148.1	6.73
2	57	181.5	8.74	52	182.3	8.88
3	65	210.9	10.31	63	212.9	11.00
4	66	236.5	11.97	66	239.2	13.39
5	66	259.2	13.42	66	263.2	14.37
6	67	280.0	15.06	66	285.2	16.16
7	67	302.5	16.82	67	306.0	18.27
8	67	322.8	18.07	67	327.2	19.36
9	67	343.6	19.33	67	347.1	21.17
10	67	362.9	20.57	67	367.2	23.00
11	67	381.6	22.37	67	388.1	24.68
12	67	401.2	24.47	67	407.4	25.07
13	67	421.7	27.65	67	423.1	24.28
14	67	441.8	28.09	67	431.4	22.69
15	67	456.9	25.12	67	434.7	21.97
16	67	466.6	22.44	67	435.8	21.93
17	67	470.7	20.51	67	436.0	21.92
18	67	472.3	19.58	67	436.3	21.95

Adapted from Anderson *et al.* (1964).

II. THE PATELLA

The adult patella

The patella[5] is the largest sesamoid[6] bone in the body. It is contained within the tendon of the quadriceps femoris muscle at the front of the knee and is separated from the skin by the pre-patellar bursa. It articulates with the lower end of the femur at the patellofemoral joint.

The normal anatomical position of the patella is not easy to measure under clinical conditions (Insall and Salvati, 1971; Blackburne and Peel, 1977). The distance from the lower pole to the insertion of the tendon at the tibial tuberosity is about equal to the midsagittal height of the patella. More than 20% higher or lower than this is known as patella alta or patella infera (baja), respectively and probably indicates an abnormal position and is associated with orthopaedic pathology at the knee joint (Lancourt and Cristini, 1975; Ogden, 1984e). As the position of the tibial tuberosity may vary, Blackburne and Peel (1977) compared the height of the patella from the tibial plateau to its articular length. In normal knees, the ratio was 0.8 and again, deviation from this figure was associated with clinical problems (Blackburne and Peel, 1977; Jakob *et al.*, 1981).

Experimental work on cadavers and clinical tests have shown that the presence of the patella improves the biomechanical efficiency of knee extension, especially towards the end of the range, by holding the patellar tendon away from the axis of movement and thereby increasing the pull of the quadriceps muscle (Haxton, 1945; Kaufer, 1971). Interestingly, in animals such as marsupials that lack a patella, or possess only a rudimentary one, this function is replaced by an enlarged tibial tuberosity (Haxton, 1944) and in man, tibial tubercleplasty after patellectomy produces the same effect (Kaufer, 1971).

Sixty per cent of patellae are roughly triangular in outline, but Corner (1900) also distinguished oblique, elliptical and circular shapes. The normal bone has a superior base and an inferior apex, the latter lying just proximal to the line of the knee joint in the anatomical position. It is compressed anteroposteriorly and has anterior and articular (posterior) surfaces (Fig. 11.11).

The **basis patellae** (superior border) slopes antero-inferiorly from behind, and is the site of attachment of the quadriceps femoris muscle arranged in three

[5] *Patella* (Latin meaning 'small pan, dish or plate'). In some of the older anatomical texts, e.g. Quain (1915) the patella is referred to as the 'kneepan'.

[6] *Sesamum indicum* is a East Indian plant with flat, oval seeds that were used as purgatives by Greek physicians. The bones are said to have been first named sesamoid by Galen (Hubay, 1949).

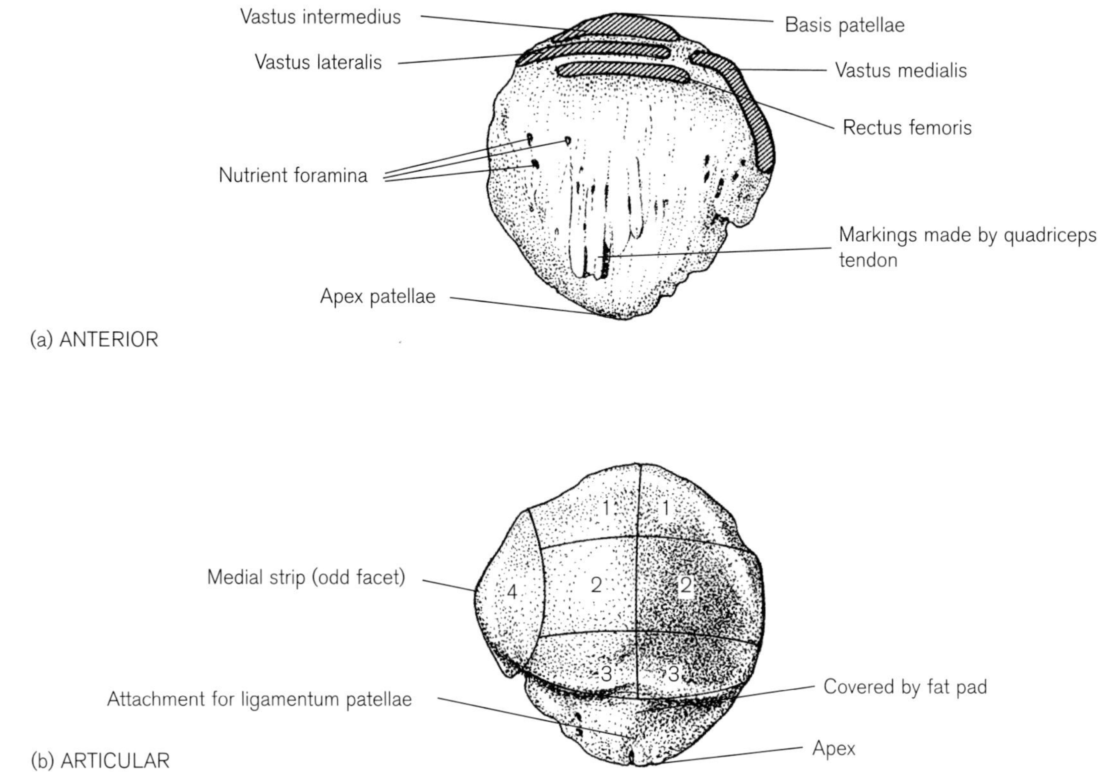

Figure 11.11 Right adult patella. 1 articulates with femur in flexion; 2 articulates with femur in extension; 3 covered by fat pad; 4 articulates with femur in full flexion.

planes (Ehrenborg and Engfeldt, 1961a). The tendon of rectus femoris lies anteriorly, with some of its fibres continuing inferiorly onto the anterior surface and vastus intermedius is attached posteriorly. In the plane between these two layers the vastus lateralis muscle occupies most of the upper border, leaving a small section for vastus medialis, whose main attachment is to the medial border, where the lowest fibres run almost horizontally. Some accounts of the muscle differentiate this section, visible in the living as a separate bulge on the medial side of the patella, as the vastus medialis obliquus, which also has contributions originating from the tendon of adductor magnus. Its nerve supply is via a separate filament of the femoral nerve and the muscle is particularly vulnerable to wasting in malfunctions of the knee joint. It provides an active mechanism which, together with the high lateral lip of the patellar groove of the femur, counteracts the tendency of the patella to dislocate laterally. Basmajian *et al.* (1972) found that, although the vastus medialis was active throughout the whole range of extension, its activity increased rapidly towards the end of the movement.

Recurrent dislocation (subluxation) of the patella is a common phenomenon, said to be especially prevalent in adolescent females. However, Hughston (1968) believed it to be an often unrecognized condition that occurs commonly in adolescent and young adult athletes of both sexes. The aetiology is probably due to a variety of causes. Cross and Waldrop (1975) found that, although there was no significant difference in width of the whole patella, difference in the size between the medial and lateral patellar facets was exaggerated in patients with patellofemoral instability. It is also likely that this condition is exacerbated by a congenital anomalous condition, where there is a failure of full development of the lateral condyle of the femur (Thompson and Bosworth, 1947; Green and Waugh, 1968). Subluxation is thought to be associated with a high-riding patella (patella alta; Lancourt and Cristini, 1975) and a significant increase in lateral tibial torsion (Turner and Smillie, 1981).

The medial and lateral borders are thinner than the superior border and have the aponeuroses of the vasti medialis et lateralis attached to them. These so-called patellar retinacula are lined by synovial membrane and blend with the capsule to form part of the anterior surface of the knee joint, the lateral retinaculum receiving a contribution from the iliotibial tract. The **apex patellae** is a sloping triangular area, which has the infrapatellar fat pad related to it above and the **ligamentum patellae** attached below.

The **anterior surface**, which is covered by the aponeurosis of the quadriceps tendon, bears 10–12 nutrient foramina lying between longitudinal fissures (Scapinelli, 1967). The **articular surface** is covered with hyaline cartilage and consists of three separate areas: a smooth, vertical ridge lying in the centre divides a larger, lateral concave half and a medial part, which is itself divided again by a ridge separating off a narrow, vertical facet on the medial border called the odd facet. Both the main medial and lateral sides have been described as being each subdivided horizontally into three facets, but these are often difficult to distinguish (Goodsir,[7] 1855; Fig. 11.11b). When the knee is in full extension, the lowest pair of facets ③ is separated from the femoral surface by the folds of the infrapatellar fat pad. As the knee flexes, the middle pair of facets ② and then the highest pair ① come into contact with the femur. Between 90° and 135° the patella rotates slightly and the odd facet ④ engages with the femur (Goodfellow *et al.*, 1976a). The ridge between the medial and the odd facet is subject to high loading, which it is believed sometimes leads to a small area of cartilage undergoing degeneration (Goodfellow *et al.*, 1976b). In populations whose squatting postural habits involve extreme flexion for considerable periods of time (see ‘Femur’), the articular surface becomes modified and it is not possible to distinguish the usual facets (Lamont,[8] 1910). Mann *et al.* (1991b) also noticed altered patellar surfaces in early twentieth century individuals whose medical history described pathological flexion contractures of the knees.

The blood supply of the patella comes from superior and inferior genicular vessels that derive from the femoral, popliteal and anterior tibial arteries, which form an anastomosis around the front of the knee joint. Two main groups of arteries enter the bone (Scapinelli, 1967). First, midpatellar vessels from the anastomosis enter the vascular foramina on the middle third of the anterior surface but send few branches to the superior border or margins. The second group arises from the inferior genicular and anterior tibial arteries, which anastomose behind the patellar ligament and pierce the deep surface or the lower pole to supply the lower third (Crock, 1996). In cases of transverse fracture, this often leaves the upper fragment liable to ischaemic necrosis because of damage to the inadequate supply of the superior pole.

Emargination of the upper lateral border of the patella appears so frequently that it could be viewed as a common variant rather than as an anomaly. It presents as a scooped-out depression, which can manifest throughout a range starting from a slight flattening to a deep curve marked by a tubercle at the upper limit and a spinous process below (Kempson, 1902; Wright, 1903; Todd and McCally, 1921; Oetteking, 1922). Kempson (1902) described the attachment of two separate parts of the vastus lateralis muscle onto the patellar borders. The upper fibres form the thin aponeurotic tendon on the upper border posterior to rectus femoris and the lower fibres are inserted via a shorter, flat tendon into the emarginated area. Associated with emargination is the presence of either a separate ossicle filling in the emarginated area, or a partially fused piece (termed a patellula by Oetteking, 1922), joined by an interface of fragmented fibrocartilaginous tissue (Wright, 1903; Holland, 1921; Todd and McCally, 1921; George, 1935). This is known as a bipartite, or multipartite patella. It may present clinically as a painful patella following some minor injury, which separates the ossicle (Salmond, 1919; Devas, 1960; Green, 1975; Ogden *et al.*, 1982), but must be distinguished from a genuine fracture (Salmond, 1919; Adams and Leonard, 1925; Ogden *et al.*, 1982). A true bipartite patella has a separate ossicle, (sometimes on both sides and therefore tripartite) that is most often situated on the upper lateral border. The surface adjacent to the main part of the bone is smooth and consists of cortical bone. It is thought to be a developmental anomaly (see below). Saupe (1943) classified bipartite patellae according to the position of the accessory ossicle and gave their frequency. Type I (5%) is at the inferior pole, Type II (20%) along the length of the lateral margin and Type III (75%) at the superolateral margin.

Dorsal defect of the patella (DDP) is a radiographically recognized benign, lytic, circular lesion, which also occurs on the superolateral aspect of the bone abutting against the articular cartilage. It may be seen at any age, in either sex and may be bilateral. Goergen *et al.* (1979) and Johnson and Brogdon (1982) found that it occurred in 1% of 1192 consecutive patients. The more modern clinical descriptions are similar to the ‘punched out’ depression noted in dry bone by Todd and McCally (1921). Holsbeeck *et al.* (1987) believe this to have a developmental aetiology (see below).

Rare anomalies of the patella vary from absence of the bone to a variety of knee dysplasias. Complete absence without other abnormalities has been reported, but is extremely rare (Kutz, 1949; Bernhang and Levine, 1973). Still uncommon is the hypoplasia of the

[7] Sir John Goodsir, Professor of Anatomy in Edinburgh, first described the facets of the patella in a lecture on the knee at the University. It was reproduced in the first volume of the Edinburgh Medical Journal and the relevant passage on the facets of the patella is in his memoirs (1868) and quoted at length by Oetteking (1922).

[8] J.C. Lamont was a Lt Col. in the Indian Medical Service who, on his retirement from the army, followed Sir Havelock Charles as Professor of Anatomy in Lahore (see femur) and then became a lecturer in histology at the University College, Dundee.

patella seen in 'small patella' syndrome (Scott and Taor, 1979) or as part of the nail-patella syndrome (hereditary onycho-osteodysplasia; Duncan and Soutar, 1963), which is associated with irregular ossification in the elbow and iliac crest (see Chapter 10).

Introna *et al.* (1998) tested sex discrimination based on patellar measurements from skeletons of known age and sex. The highest value of 83.8% was achieved with a function associating maximum width and thickness.

Early development of the patella

Details of the early development of the patella may be found in accounts of the embryology of the femur, the knee joint and the foot (Gray and Gardner, 1950; O'Rahilly *et al.*, 1957; Gardner and O'Rahilly, 1968; O'Rahilly and Gardner, 1975; Finnegan and Uhthoff, 1990). These essentially agree with earlier accounts of the development of the patella by Walmsley (1940) and McDermott (1943). The mesenchymal patella and the patellar retinacula are recognizable at the anterior aspect of the developing knee joint at stages 18 and 19 (seventh week/13–18 mm CRL). Precartilaginous changes can be seen a week later. Chondrification takes place at stages 21 and 22 (7–8 wks/18–26 mm CRL; O'Rahilly *et al.*, 1957). At about 11–12 weeks, the perichondrium on the anterior surface is fused to that of the femur. Cavitation of the joint occurs at the end of the embryonic period and soon after this, the knee joint clearly resembles the adult in form and arrangement (Walmsley, 1940).

By 12–13 weeks, a definite suprapatellar pouch is formed. At this stage, the patella is relatively small compared with the distal surface of the femur but growth is then rapid until about 6 lunar months. From this time until birth, it grows at the same rate as the other bones of the lower limb. At about 7 lunar months, the articular surface becomes divided by a vertical ridge into larger lateral and smaller medial areas. It does not acquire the transverse ridges until after birth, when the limb is in use and full extension of the knee joint becomes possible (Walmsley, 1940). Congenital lateral dislocation of the patella before, or soon after birth, is a rare but serious condition. It prevents full active extension of the knee joint and so may cause fixed contractures (Green and Waugh, 1968). At birth, and for the first few years of life, the patella is entirely cartilaginous. It resembles any other unossified epiphysis and is penetrated by an extensive cartilage canal vascular network and surrounded by perichondrium, which is responsible for the major part of the growth (Haines, 1937; Ogden, 1984e).

Ossification

Ossification may begin as early as 18 months but may not be present until 4 or 5 years. Paterson (1929) noted that the appearance of the centre was the most irregular in the knee joint. Ranges are 1.5–4 years in girls and 2.5–6 years in boys (Flecker, 1932b; Hasselwander, 1938; Francis *et al.*, 1939; Elgenmark, 1946; Garn *et al.*, 1967b; Prakash *et al.*, 1979; Caffey, 1993). Ossification is typically multifocal, but coalescence of separate centres soon takes place. Pyle and Hoerr (1955) describe and illustrate the centre in girls at 2 years 8 months and boys at 3 years 6 months as a vertically elongated nodule in the centre of the knee. It rapidly enlarges and the margins may have a granular or irregular radiographic appearance and by about 4 years in girls and 5 years in boys, it is a biconvex disc. By about the age of 9–10 years, the chondro-osseous margins form a defined subchondral plate, indicating a reduction in rate of growth. On section, about one-third of the diameter is seen to be still unossified (Ogden, 1984e). The vertical part of the posterior surface is slightly concave, the postero-inferior surface is flat and the superolateral margin is usually irregular (Pyle and Hoerr, 1955). Over the next 2 years, there is a slow expansion into the rest of the epiphyseal cartilage and trabecular orientation becomes well defined longitudinally in the anterior third. By early adolescence, it is a slim version of the adult bone. The last part to ossify is the superior part of the lateral border, which often remains flat (Fig. 11.12). The patella assumes essentially adult contours by 14 years in females and 16 years in males (Pyle and Hoerr, 1955).

Additional ossification centres may become apparent in the adolescent period, by far the most common being one at the superolateral border, where the margin remains irregular. It may then fuse with the main centre or remain separated from it to form a bipartite

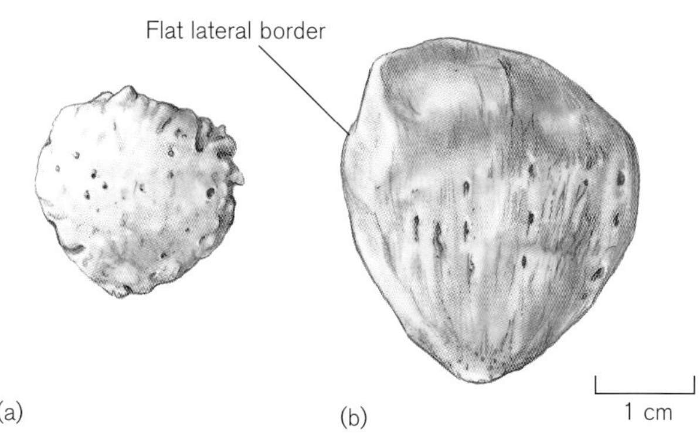

Figure 11.12 Juvenile patellae. (a) skeletal age 7–8 years; (b) 12 years, female.

patella, with the two parts being joined by fibro-cartilaginous tissue. This may be disrupted by minor injury leading to the painful bipartite patella in which excision of the fragment may be the preferred option (Devas, 1960; Smillie, 1962; Green, 1975). Multipartite patellae have been described but are much less common than the bipartite variety (Wright, 1903; Holland, 1921; Holsbeeck *et al.*, 1987). The last authors believe that the dorsal defect of the patella (DDP) and a bipartite or multipartite patella are stress-induced anomalies of ossification. They both occur in the same characteristic location at the superolateral border, typically in patients in the second decade of life. Symptomatic DDP occurred in four of six patients with multipartite patella, three of whom were sporting adolescents. Abnormal muscular traction by the vastus lateralis associated with possible vascular insufficiency was thought to play a part in the condition.

Sinding-Larson-Johanson syndrome is a traction epiphysitis of the lower pole of the patella, which can occur in vigorous adolescent athletes (Medlar and Lyne, 1978). This proximal attachment of the patellar ligament is subject to similar strains as the tibial tuberosity and irregular calcification or separate ossicles at the inferior pole are not uncommon (Ogden, 1984e). The condition could be viewed as the patellar equivalent of Osgood-Schlatter's disease (see Tibia).

Practical notes

Sideing

It is difficult to side a juvenile patella until ossification has spread well into the articular surface, which is not until late childhood. Before that time it is a biconvex disc with a slightly pointed apex. Both surfaces are composed of porous bone. In early adolescence the superior part of the lateral border is often flat (Fig. 11.12b).

Morphological summary

See Femur (Fig. 11.10).

III. THE TIBIA

The adult tibia

The tibia[9] forms the skeleton of the medial part of the leg and articulates proximally with the condyles of the femur at the knee joint, distally with the body of the talus at the ankle joint and both proximally and distally with the fibula at the superior and inferior tibiofibular joints. It is a long bone consisting of a shaft with expanded proximal and distal ends (Fig. 11.13).

The main features of the upper end of the tibia are a horizontal articular plateau proximally, a roughened tibial tuberosity anteriorly and a posterolateral fibular facet. The articular surface (Fig. 11.14) consists of medial and lateral condyles separated by an intercondylar area. Each condyle has a slightly hollow centre and a flattened peripheral area with a fibro-cartilaginous, semilunar meniscus resting on its surface. The menisci slightly decrease the incongruity between the femoral and tibial articular surfaces. They are attached around their outer edges, have a free inner border and usually leave a faint imprint on the bone. The region between the condyles, the **intercondylar eminence**, consists of **medial** and **lateral intercondylar tubercles** (spines), from which lead triangular **anterior** and **posterior intercondylar areas**. The apex of the anterior area lies between the tubercles and its base slopes down to the central anterior margin of the plateau. The anterior horn of the medial meniscus is related to the anteromedial side of the base of the triangle. Its fibres are continuous with the transverse ligament. A smooth area posteriorly provides the tibial attachment for the anterior cruciate ligament. To the lateral side of the area, the anterior horn of the lateral meniscus reaches up to the lateral intercondylar tubercle. The rest of the area, lying anterolaterally, is related to the infrapatellar fat pad and bears several nutrient foramina. The posterior intercondylar area is also triangular, but smaller than the anterior area and slopes steeply backwards. The posterior horn of the lateral meniscus is related to the slope of the lateral tubercle and behind it is a depression for the posterior horn of the medial meniscus. The rest of the area is smooth and provides the tibial attachment of the posterior cruciate ligament. The morphology of the intercondylar area is complex and variable and the details of the attachments of the menisci and cruciate ligaments have been described by Parsons (1906), Jacobsen (1974) and Girgis *et al.* (1975).

The articular surface of the **medial condyle** is oval in shape with its long axis running anteroposteriorly. Part of the inner band of the **tibial collateral ligament** of the knee is attached to the medial meniscus and bridges over the condyle to be inserted into the medial side of the shaft. The posterior surface of the condyle is grooved and at its lateral end bears a tubercle, the 'tuberculum quadratum tendinis' for the main attachment of the semimembranosus

[9]Tibia – (Latin meaning 'the shin bone; pipe or flute'). Musical instruments of long, tubular form were made of a variety of materials, but especially from the straight tibiae of both animals and birds, especially crane.

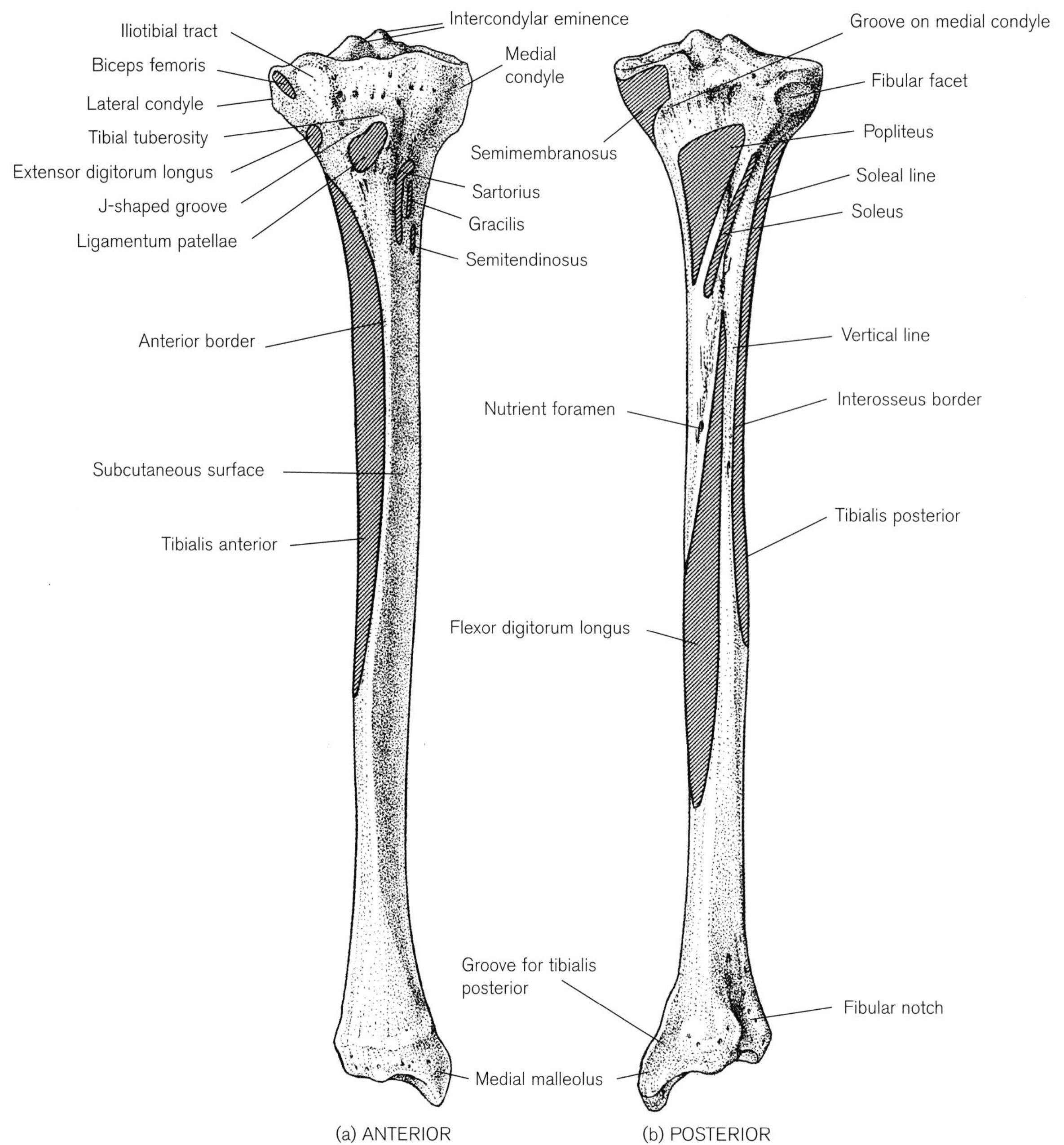

Figure 11.13 Right adult tibia.

muscle (Cave and Porteous, 1958, 1959). The **lateral condyle** is smaller than the medial condyle, more circular in shape and often has a rounded posterior margin. On its anterior surface, a smooth, facet-like area has the anterior part of the iliotibial tract attached to it and from here there is a sharp ridge leading to the lateral side of the tibial tuberosity. On the postero-lateral surface there is a facet for articulation with the fibula, whose shape and exact position varies (Ogden, 1984f). On the lateral side of the condyle below the facets are small tibial attachments for the extensor digitorum longus, peroneus longus and biceps femoris muscles. The outer surfaces of both condyles are liberally supplied with nutrient foramina.

The central part of the articular surface is continuous with a triangular area on the front of the shaft. The upper part of the triangle bears many nutrient foramina and just below this is a smooth area of bone related to the deep infrapatellar bursa. The **tibial tuberosity**, which forms the apex of the triangular area, lies about 2 cm below the anterior edge of the plateau and varies in form from a faint elevation to a prominent boss. It is divided into a smooth, rounded proximal and a rough, distal part, which marks the position of the epiphyseal line. The tuberosity is separated from the rest of the triangular area by an inverted, 'J'-shaped groove, which is frequently expanded to a shallow trough. It begins at the upper medial corner of the tuberosity, extends along its superior border and turns distally to run down the lateral margin of the tuberosity, usually to the junction of the smooth and rough parts. Both the groove and the line demarcating the smooth and rough parts run obliquely inferolaterally (Hughes and Sunderland, 1946). Both anatomical and clinical texts differ as to which part of the tuberosity provides attachment for the ligamentum patellae. Lewis (1958) described two alternative types of attachment, occurring in roughly equal numbers. In the first, the deep part of the tendon is attached to the smooth area, while the more superficial fibres continue down the shaft below the line. The last remaining fibres enter the bone at a stepwise crest or ridge, which usually runs inferolaterally. In the second type, all the fibres of the ligament are attached to the smooth part of the tuberosity, which is often limited below by a rough crest or ridge of diaphyseal origin. The first type of attachment is thus both epiphyseal and diaphyseal, whereas the second type is attached only to the diaphyseal part of the bone. The type of attachment is therefore related to the course of development of the tibial tuberosity (see below).

The blood supply of the upper end of the tibia arises from a profuse arterial network around the knee joint, the main arteries of supply being the medial and lateral inferior genicular and recurrent branches from the anterior tibial artery (Crock, 1962, 1967, 1996). Radiate arteries then enter the whole circumference of the upper end like spokes of a wheel (Nelson *et al.*, 1960) and a number enter the intercondylar area both from in front and behind (Crock, 1967).

Differences in both the morphology and proportions of the upper end of the tibia are found in various ethnic groups (Hrdlička, 1898; Wood, 1920). The Negroid tibia is significantly longer and narrower than the Caucasian tibia. This results in a difference in the force generated in the patellar ligament and possibly in locomotion in the two groups (Farrally and Moore, 1975). The angle the tibial plateau makes with the shaft varies, both throughout life, and in adults of

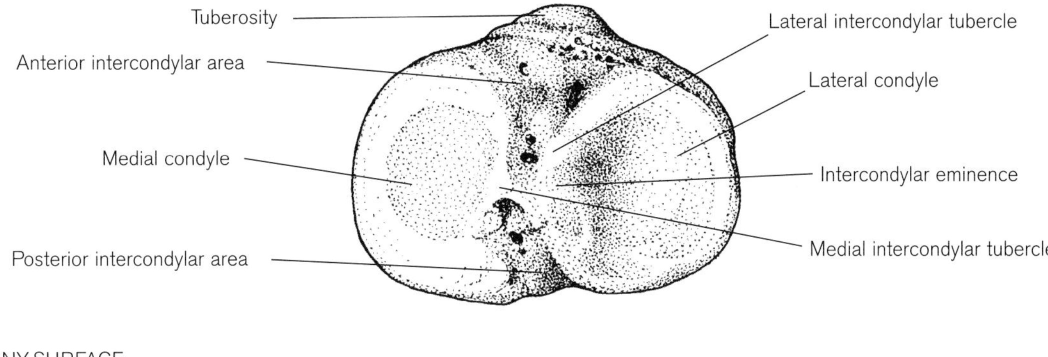

(a) BONY SURFACE

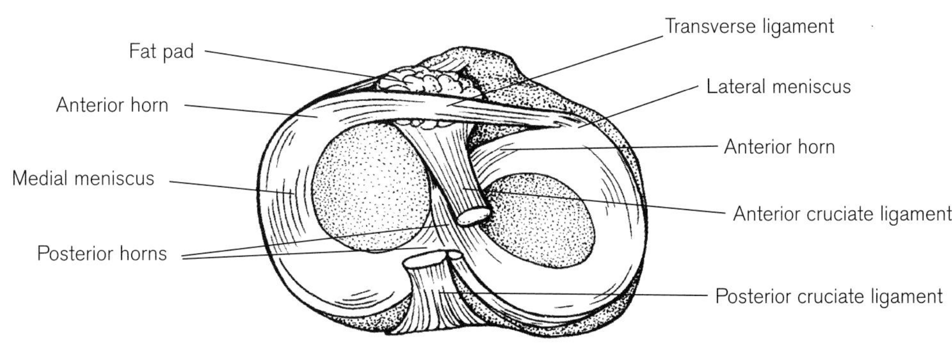

(b) LIGAMENTOUS ATTACHMENTS

Figure 11.14 Proximal articular surface of right adult tibia.

different populations (Thomson, 1889; Derry, 1906; Wood, 1920). It is measured either as the angle of retroversion between the plateau and the long axis of the shaft, or as the angle of inclination between the plateau and the mechanical axis of the shaft. The latter is a line drawn through the centre of the medial condyle and the centre of the distal articular surface (Wood, 1920). High angles of retroversion are seen in human fetuses, newborns and populations who habitually adopt a squatting posture, all of whom have lower limbs in a hyperflexed position for long periods of time (Thomson, 1889; Charles, 1893; Aitken, 1905; Derry, 1906; Wood, 1920; Kate and Robert, 1965). It has been generally assumed that this is a response to the tension of the patellar ligament on the anterior plateau and the compression caused by body weight on the posterior plateau. However, Trinkaus (1975) suggested a more general mechanical explanation for retroversion. It allows the main force to pass through the partially flexed knee at right angles to the tibial plateau and thereby minimize the anteroposterior shear stress at the joint. This is the position when there is least congruity between the femoral and tibial condyles (Barnett, 1954a) and also the point at which there is maximum force during locomotion and other high activity levels.

A further modification of the upper end of the tibia that appears to be related to the squatting posture is the presence of a vertical groove with a prominent lateral lip deep to the course of the ligamentum patellae (Kate and Robert, 1965). It extends proximally from the top of the J-shaped groove of the tuberosity and can be seen on the bone as an indentation on the anteromedial side of the lateral condyle when viewed from above. The presence of the groove, which never appeared in non-squatters, was confirmed both from dissections and from radiographs of living subjects.

The **shaft** of the tibia is roughly triangular in cross-section, although there is great variability in its shape

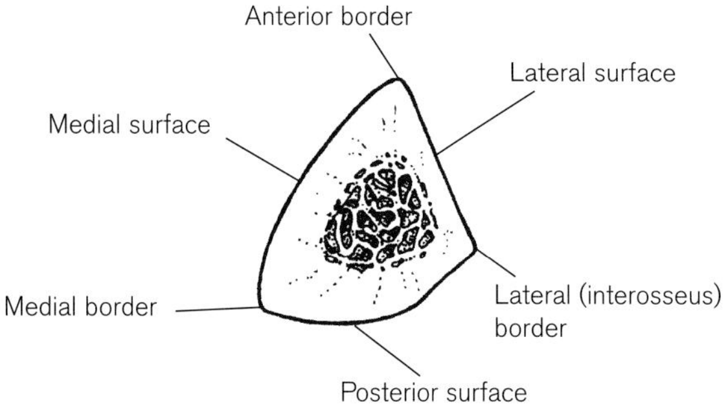

Figure 11.15 Cross-section of adult tibia in middle third of shaft.

(Hrdlička, 1898; Dokládal, 1973). It is narrowest at the junction of the middle and distal thirds and fractures most often occur here (Adams and Hamblen, 1992). It has three borders and three surfaces throughout most of its length (Figs. 11.13 and 11.15). The anterior border extends from the medial side of the impression for the iliotibial tract to the anterior edge of the medial malleolus and is subcutaneous throughout its length. It is a sharp lateral crest and as it passes the tuberosity it swings into an anterior position, where it remains for two-thirds of its length. In the distal third, it becomes more rounded and passes medially across the front of the bone. It provides attachment for the deep fascia of the leg, which is thickened at the lower end to form the extensor retinaculum above the malleolus. The interosseous (lateral) border arises anterior to the fibular facet and runs down the bone to the anterior lip of the fibular notch. It is sharp throughout its length except for a small, indistinct proximal section. Attached to most of its length is the interosseous membrane passing across to the fibula except for a small gap proximally, which allows passage of the anterior tibial vessels and nerves. Distally, it merges with the anterior tibiofibular ligament. The medial border begins beneath the groove on the medial condyle and passes to the posterior margin of the medial malleolus. Its proximal quarter is rounded and has attached to it the popliteal fascia, the posterior fibres of the tibial collateral ligament and slips from the semimembranosus muscle. The middle two-quarters are sharp and the distal quarter rounded and it provides attachment for the fascia covering the deep muscles of the calf. At its distal end it continues into the medial lip of the groove for the tibialis posterior tendon.

The medial surface of the tibia lies between the anterior and medial borders and actually faces anteromedially. It is the broad, smooth surface of the shin whose periosteum is covered only by skin throughout most of its length, except at the proximal and distal ends. Just below the medial condyle it has attached to it the anterior part of the tibial collateral ligament and some of the numerous extensive tendinous slips from the semimembranosus muscle. Between these attachments and the side of the tuberosity is an area known as the 'pes anserinus' (Latin, goose's foot) consisting of the long slim insertions of the three 'guy-ropes' of the thigh, the sartorius, gracilis and semitendinosus muscles (Last, 1973). At the distal end of the surface, just in front of the medial malleolus, the great saphenous vein crosses the bone. The lateral surface lies between the anterior and interosseous borders and faces laterally for about two-thirds of its length. It then comes to lie anteriorly at the distal end as the anterior and interosseous borders swing medially. The lateral facing part has attached at its proximal end some fibres of the extensor digitorum longus muscle, but most of its surface gives origin to the tibialis anterior muscle. Both these muscles become tendinous towards the lower third of the bone where they cross to the medial malleolus, together with the anterior tibial nerves and vessels. The posterior surface lies between the interosseous and medial borders and is wide above, where it lies below the posterior surface of the condyles, and narrows towards the back of the ankle. The most obvious feature of the surface is the roughened soleal line, which runs across the proximal third of the bone inferomedially. It separates off a triangular surface of bone from which the popliteus muscle arises and itself gives origin to part of the soleus muscle. The line does not reach the interosseous border but just inferior to the fibular facet there is a tubercle, often faintly marked, to which a tendinous aponeurotic arch of the soleus crosses to the fibula to continue its attachment. From the centre of the soleal line a vertical line marks a division between the territories of flexor digitorum longus medially and tibialis posterior laterally, which occupy the middle two-quarters of the surface. The line varies considerably in length and prominence. It may continue straight down or approach the interosseous border (Derry, 1906). The distal quarter of the surface is crossed by the flexor tendons passing towards the medial malleolus.

The main blood supply to the medullary cavity is usually from a single nutrient artery, which arises from the anterior surface of the posterior tibial artery near its origin. Once in the medullary canal it divides and the descending branch continues down in the line of the main vessel, while the ascending branch turns abruptly upwards (Crock, 1967). There is nearly always a single large nutrient foramen whose entrance slopes distally (Mysorekar, 1967; Sendemir and Çimen, 1991). 77% of foramina are in the upper third and the rest in the middle third of the posterior surface of the bone. 74% are lateral to the vertical line and 11% on the line. The periosteal supply is mainly from the anterior tibial artery, which descends on the interosseous membrane and sends out ring arteries to the posterior and medial surfaces (Crock, 1967). If the endosteal supply becomes compromised in fractures of the tibial shaft, the periosteal supply assumes a prime role but there is often a problem in healing of the distal section (Macnab, 1957).

Tibial shafts that have surfaces of approximately equal size are known as eurycnemic, whereas a mediolaterally flattened tibial shaft is known as platycnemic (Greek – *platy* meaning flat, *cneme* meaning knee). The cnemic index is usually calculated as (mediolateral diameter × 100/AP diameter) measured at the level of the nutrient foramen. However, both Thomson (1889) and Andermann (1975) criticized the concept of the index being taken at a datum point that is so variable in position. Thomson took measurements at the junction of the soleal (popliteal) line with the medial (internal) border but Andermann suggested that more meaningful data could be obtained if the index were taken at the junction of the proximal and middle thirds of the bone. A cnemic index between 55.0 and 62.9 is usually regarded as platycnemic and an index of above 70 as eurycnemic (Thomson, 1889; Derry, 1906; Lovejoy *et al.* 1976; Bass, 1987). Eurycnemic tibiae are common in Blacks and Caucasians, whereas most platycnemic tibiae are found in Native Americans, Indians and the Ainu of Japan (Martin and Saller, 1959). Platycnemic tibiae may have a bony pilaster on the posterior surface in the region of the vertical line (see above). Lovejoy *et al.* (1976) calculated that this made the bone more able to withstand anteroposterior bending and torsional strains, but eurycnemic tibiae were stronger in the mediolateral plane. Buxton (1938) regarded both platymeria and platycnemia as pathological conditions, probably due to a dietary insufficiency.

The shaft of the tibia is twisted about its long axis so that a line drawn across the most posterior points of the plateau lies at an angle to a line joining the distal tip of the medial malleolus to the midpoint of the fibular notch. Torsion is regarded as positive when the distal end is externally (laterally) rotated with respect to the proximal end, which is the condition in about 95% of adults (Hutter and Scott, 1949). This lateral torsion of the tibia is necessary to prevent a pigeon-toed gait (Aiello and Dean, 1990). The foot is modelled around the subtalar axis, which is orientated medial to the sagittal plane (Lewis, 1980, 1981) so that lateral torsion, which occurs in most individuals, allows the feet to lie parallel or turn slightly outwards. Rosen and Sandick (1955) pointed out that true torsion is a twisting about the axis of an individual bone and this must be distinguished during measurement from rotation between two units, which is the turning of one bone in relation to another at a joint. Using various methods of measurement and different populations, mean reported tibial torsion varies between 20° and 40° (Elftman, 1945; Hutter and Scott, 1949; Ritter *et al.*, 1976; Malekafzali and Wood, 1979; Jakob *et al.*, 1980; Clementz, 1989; Eckhoff *et al.*, 1994b). The different methods involved a variety of fixed points, some of which included the fibula, and this probably accounts for the large reported range (Jakob *et al.*, 1980). Torsion increases with age from birth onwards (see development) but there appears to be no association

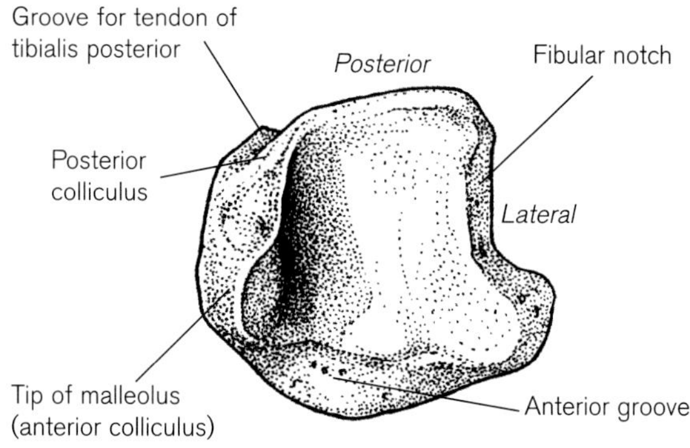

Figure 11.16 Distal articular surface of right adult tibia.

with sex or adult age. Some investigations found a significant but unexplained limb asymmetry with more torsion on the right than the left. Tibial torsion *in vivo* is obviously more difficult to measure than in the dry bone and a review of four different methods of measurement of *in vivo* torsion suggested that, because of lack of repeatability, new methods need to be developed (Milner and Soames, 1998).

The tibia expands to a quadrilateral shape towards its **distal end** and projects inferiorly at the medial malleolus (Fig. 11.16) The lateral surface of the shaft turns in its distal third to become the anterior, smooth and slightly bulging surface. It ends at a narrow groove to which is attached the capsule of the ankle joint. In some populations that adopt squatting as an habitual posture, there may be modifications of this border both on the medial and lateral sides to form so-called squatting facets (Thomson, 1889; Aitken, 1905; Wood, 1920; Barnett, 1954b; Singh, 1959b; Rao, 1966). The lateral facet articulates with a reciprocal facet on the talus when the foot is in a position of extreme dorsiflexion, but there appears to be some doubt about the causation of the medial facet, which is much rarer (Barnett, 1954b; Rao, 1966; see also 'Talus'). The medial surface of the shaft continues onto the smooth, projecting, subcutaneous surface of the medial malleolus. The posterior surface of the shaft divides to produce posterior and lateral surfaces distally. The tendon of tibialis posterior in its synovial sheath passes in a well-defined, oblique groove at the medial end of the posterior surface. The flexor retinaculum is attached to the anterior edge of the groove. The lateral surface of the distal end is formed by the triangular fibular notch, which has a roughened floor proximally but may be covered by articular cartilage distally. Wood (1920) described a peg-shaped ('praefibular') process, which is common in Native Australian tibiae. It lies at the anterior border of the fibular notch and the articular surface extends onto its lateral aspect. The anterior and posterior edges of the notch converge towards the interosseous border and here the fibula and tibia are bound together by tibiofibular ligaments in a syndesmotic joint that forms the upper part of the strong 'mortice' of the ankle (talocrural) joint. The distal articular surface of the tibia consists of two parts set at right angles to each other, both of which articulate with the body of the talus. The main part, roughly quadrilateral, articulates with the trochlear surface of the talus and reflects its shape, being wider anteriorly than posteriorly. It is slightly sellar, being concave sagittally and slightly convex transversely. The articular surface continues onto the lateral surface of the medial malleolus, where it articulates with the comma-shaped medial surface of the talar body.

The blood supply of the lower end of the tibia is derived from an arterial network that is supplied from branches of the anterior and posterior tibial and the peroneal arteries. Radiate epiphyseal arteries are given off, which penetrate the distal end down to the subchondral capillary bed (Crock, 1967).

The **medial malleolus** is a stout, thick buttress projecting from the distal medial tibial shaft. The outer surface gives attachment to the proximal end of the medial collateral (deltoid) ligament of the ankle joint. The inferior border is divided by a groove into a larger anterior and a smaller posterior colliculus, which are clearly visible on a lateral ankle radiograph. On an anteroposterior projection, the outline of the posterior colliculus can be seen through the shadow of the anterior colliculus (Coral, 1987). An occasional accessory bone, the os subtibiale, is related to the medial malleolus. There is confusion about the terminology of this bone but Coral (1987) believes the term should be reserved for the rare, genuine accessory bone related to the posterior colliculus.

Fractures of the medial malleolus are common. A shearing fracture of the whole malleolus is caused by an adductor force and an avulsion fracture of the tip by abduction or lateral rotation (Adams and Hamblen, 1992).

Sexual dimorphism of the tibia has been studied in a variety of populations (Telkkä, 1950; Steel, 1962; Singh *et al.*, 1975; Işcan and Miller-Shaivitz, 1984b,c; Holland, 1991; Işcan *et al.*,1994). Methods for estimation of stature from whole tibiae can be found in Breitinger (1937), Trotter and Gleser (1952, 1958), Allbrook (1961), Genovés (1967), Krogman and Işcan (1986), Jantz (1992) and Jantz *et al.* (1995) and from fragmentary tibiae in Steele and McKern (1969), Steele (1970) and Holland (1992). The crural index (total tibial length × 100/total femoral length) varies in different populations and may provide indications of racial origin (Krogman and Işcan, 1986).

Early development of the tibia

Details of the early development of the tibia may be found in Gray and Gardner (1950), Haines, (1953), Gardner and O'Rahilly (1968) and O'Rahilly and Gardner (1975). The mesenchymal tibia is visible at stage 17 (11–14 mm CRL/about 41 days). Chondrification begins at stage 18 and between stages 19 and 21, the condyles are clearly visible, although the lower end may still be at the blastemal stage (O'Rahilly *et al.*, 1957). By stage 23, both menisci, collateral ligaments, cruciate ligaments, the ligamentum patellae and the tendon of popliteus are evident.

Ossification

Primary centre

Ossification of the tibia begins at stages 22–23 (23–31 mm CRL/week 8), when a bony collar can be seen and about a week later, endochondral ossification commences in the centre of the shaft and spreads quickly both proximally and distally (O'Rahilly *et al.*, 1957). Vascular canals start to invade at about week 12 and by week 14 the growth plates become established. By week 20, all morphological structures around the knee and ankle are easily recognizable (Finnegan and Uhthoff, 1990). At birth, 80% of the overall length of the bone is occupied by ossified shaft (Puyhaubert, 1913).

The shaft of the perinatal tibia (Fig. 11.17) is arched somewhat posteriorly in the proximal third and straight in the distal two-thirds. It is widely flared at its proximal end, especially on the medial side. The proximal metaphyseal surface is smoothly convex and roughly oval in outline, with rounded lateral and more pointed medial ends. The outline is straight posteriorly and slopes down anteriorly towards the tuberosity. The anterior border is a sharp ridge turning medially at its distal end. The interosseous and medial borders are rounded in their proximal thirds but become more defined in their distal two-thirds. At the proximal end of the medial surface the area of the tibial tuberosity forms a triangular area of porous bone. Posteriorly, the triangular surface covered by the popliteus muscle is distinguished as an area of porous-looking bone from the cortical surface distal to it. The inferolateral border of the triangle is formed by the soleal line, which is flat at this stage and rarely obvious as a raised ridge before the age of 6–8 years. In over 90% of fetuses there is normally an extremely large, single nutrient foramen below and usually lateral to the popliteal area, whose entrance slopes distally (Skawina and Miaskiewicz, 1982). It is by far the largest vascular foramen found in any of the juvenile long bones and appears out of proportion to the size of the bone. The distal metaphyseal surface is flat. Its outline is either quadrangular with rounded corners or oval. The lateral border is flatter than the other three sides and a faint notch can sometimes be seen in its centre.

By the age of about 6 months, the proximal metaphyseal surface has flattened and by the end of the first year, a depressed area on the anterior surface of the metaphysis can be seen on lateral radiographs. This is deep to the tongue of the epiphysis that will be involved with the formation of the tuberosity. The anterior border of the distal end soon becomes scalloped in the centre. By 4–5 years, both the proximal and distal metaphyseal surfaces are ridged and billowed and reflect the markings of their respective epiphyses (Fig. 11.18). The proximal surface has a groove formed by the posterior cruciate attachment, which runs from the centre to the posterior border and partly divides the surface into a larger, flatter medial and smaller, more sloping lateral section. The anterior intercondylar area slopes forwards on its lateral side to become continuous with the growth area of the tuberosity. The distal surface has a definite D-shaped outline and the medial half of the surface is hollowed out.

Prenatal torsion is in a medial direction and at birth, it may still be medial or neutral but this changes rapidly in the first year of life, even before attempts at walking are made (Elftman, 1945). Staheli and Engel (1972) reported that there was an external rotation of 5° during the first year, another 10° by mid-childhood and in older children and adults torsion reached 14°. These figures are lower than those previously reported, as the measurements were taken on patients with knees flexed at 90°, thus already involving some medial rotation. Turner and Smillie (1981) reported that adult torsion had usually developed by the age of 5 years. A significant proportion of individuals do not undergo the full range of postnatal lateral torsion and, as a consequence, walk in a 'twine-toed' manner. Hutter and Scott (1949) found that in 50 normal 2 year olds, 30% had not developed any external torsion and walked with toes turned in. Between the ages of 5 and 7 years, 8–10% of children still had an intoeing walk, with 5% having quite severe deformity. There appeared to be little correction of an internally rotated tibia after the age of 7 years. In a survey of 800 adults, 8% of males and 9% of females showed internal tibial torsion. The retroversion of the upper end of the shaft that is present at birth gradually decreases throughout childhood, although the amount varies between populations (see adult).

The tibia is reported to grow at a fairly uniform rate throughout childhood, while the femur grows more

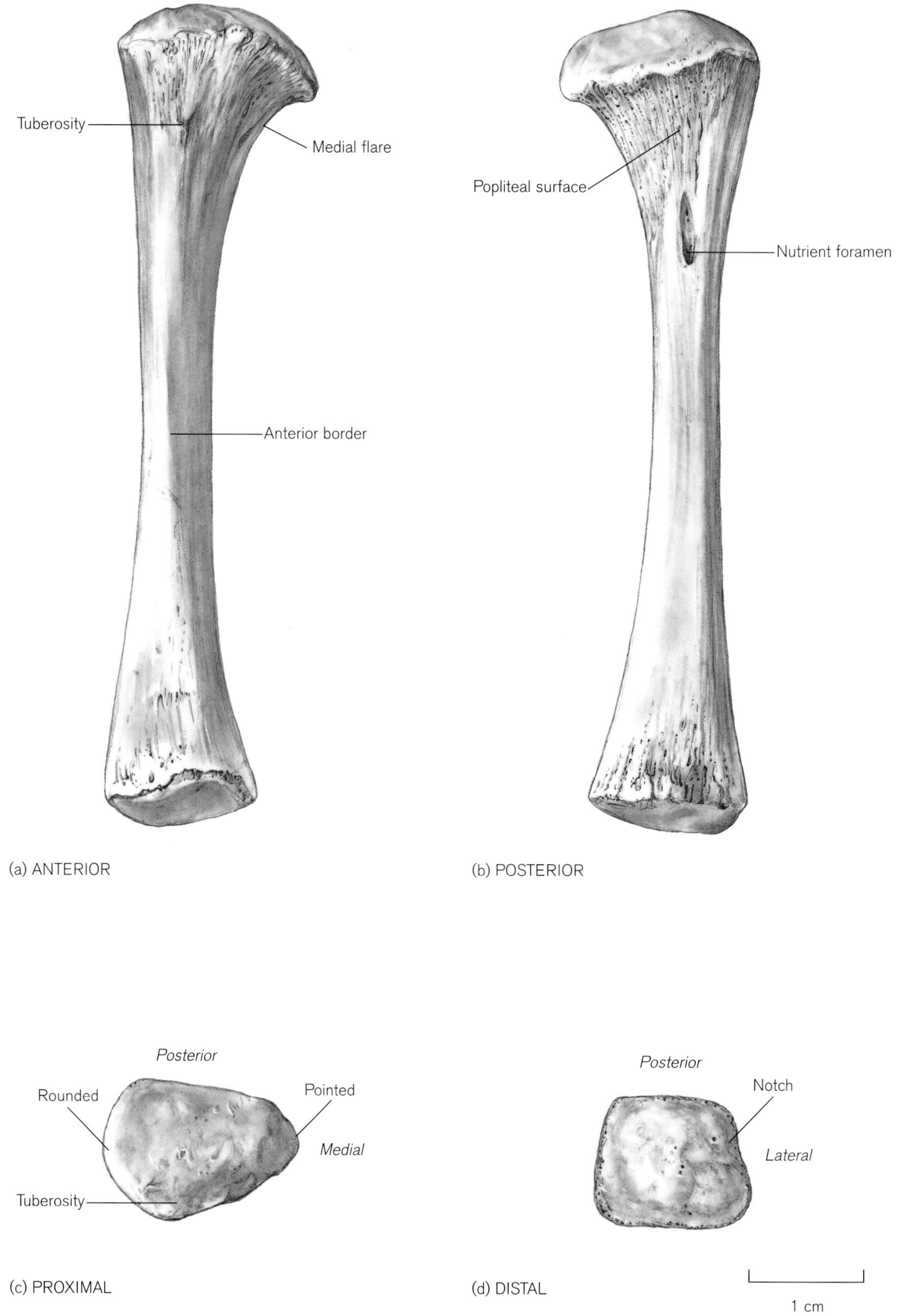

Tuberosity
Medial flare
Anterior border
Popliteal surface
Nutrient foramen
(a) ANTERIOR
(b) POSTERIOR
Posterior
Rounded
Pointed
Medial
Tuberosity
Posterior
Notch
Lateral
(c) PROXIMAL
(d) DISTAL
1 cm

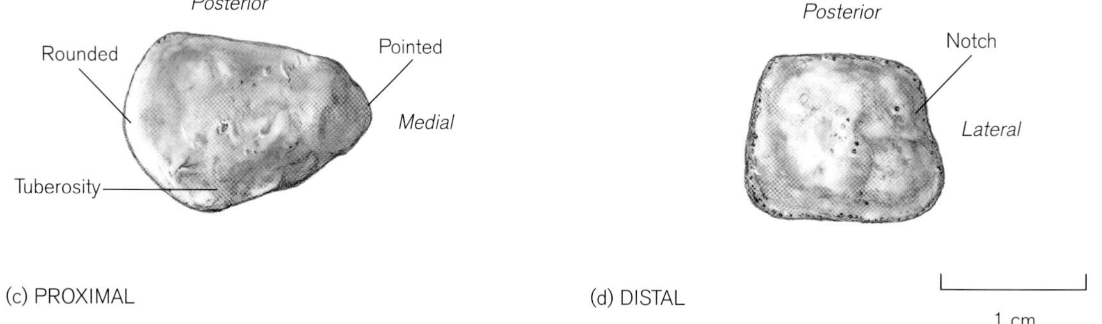

Figure 11.17 Right perinatal tibia.

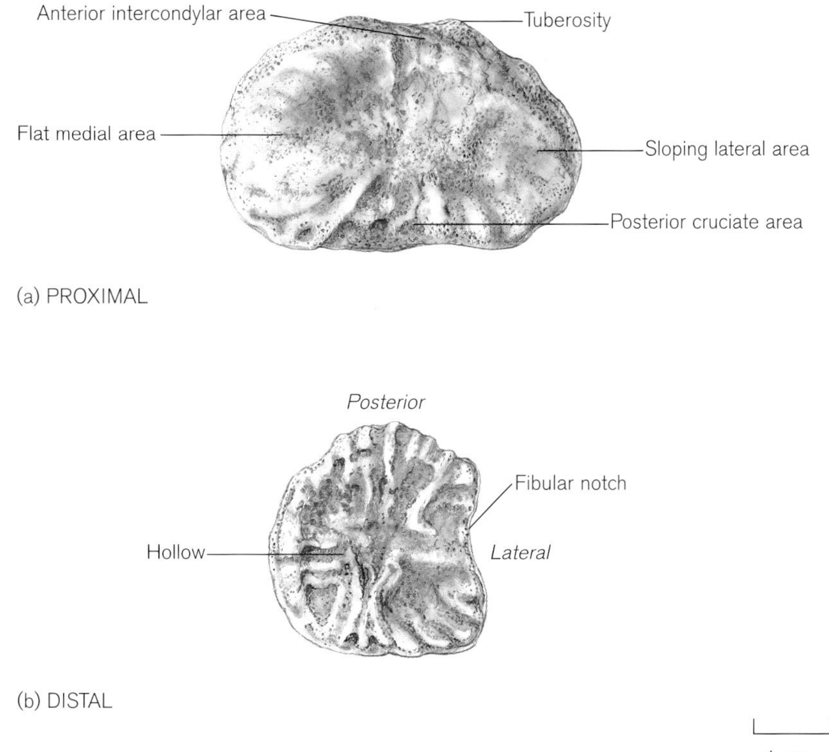

Figure 11.18 Proximal and distal metaphyseal surfaces of right juvenile tibia, 8 years, male.

slowly up to puberty and then increases rapidly with the pubertal growth spurt. This means that the crural index (total tibial length × 100/total femoral length) increases from about 6 years to puberty and then decreases after that time (Davenport, 1933). By puberty, the borders and surfaces of the tibial shaft are more clearly defined. The lower end of the metaphysis is distinctly quadrangular, with the lateral border showing the concavity of the fibular notch.

At the distal end of the tibial shaft it is common to find Harris lines, which are laid down in infancy and childhood and may persist into adult life (Garn and Schwager, 1967). This makes it possible to calculate the age of formation of Harris lines (Maat, 1984). The hypothesis that lines of increased density are growth arrest lines that cause ultimate retardation in growth was discounted by Gindhart (1969) as no difference in finally attained adult stature was found between heavily and lightly lined individuals (see Chapter 3).

Fractures of the tibial shaft in children are amongst the most common injuries to the lower limb and usually caused by a rotational force produced whilst the foot is stationary, or by direct violence, such as falls or road traffic accidents. They normally heal readily and delayed union or non-union hardly ever occurs (Dias, 1984).

Secondary centres

The ossification of the **proximal epiphysis** of the tibia, like that of the distal femur, is an important marker for the estimation of fetal maturity in forensic cases, as it is present in about 80% of full-term infants (Knight, 1996). The centre appears in the majority of fetuses just before birth and is therefore sometimes absent in premature infants (Flecker, 1932b). Kuhns and Finnstrom (1976) reported that in North American and Swedish populations, the epiphysis was radiographically visible in fetal week 35 for the 5th percentile and between 2 and 5 postnatal weeks for the 95th percentile. It is always present by the third month *postpartum* (Puyhaubert, 1913; Davies and Parsons, 1927; Paterson, 1929; Hasselwander, 1938; Francis *et al.*, 1939; Christie, 1949; Pyle and Hoerr, 1955; Hansman, 1962).

Girls are in advance of boys during the whole of postnatal development of the proximal epiphysis and this difference increases from a few weeks at birth to 2–3 years at adolescence. At birth the tibial ossification centre is an oval nodule aligned vertically below that of the distal femoral epiphysis. Its transverse diameter is less than that of the femoral centre but within 2 weeks the two bony nodules are equal in size (Pyle and Hoerr, 1955). The basic morphology of the whole epiphysis reflects that of the mature shape, but there is a 10–15° posterior tilt of the articular surface (Ogden, 1984f). During the second year, the osseous expansion causes inferior flattening and the growth plate becomes established, while superiorly there is an extension towards the tibial spines.

By 3–4 years of age, the proximal epiphysis is an elongated nodule of bone with a rounded, pitted superior surface, a flattened metaphyseal surface, a scalloped posterior margin and a roughly oval outline (Fig. 11.19a). Growth is rapid and there may be disseminated calcification round the edges of the epiphysis and accessory ossification centres are sometimes seen around the medial and lateral condyles (Scheller, 1960). By 6–7 years, the growth of the centre has stabilized to within 1–3 mm of the periphery of the cartilaginous edge and the margins are smooth (Ogden, 1984f). Ossification has extended into the intercondylar region and the tubercles. The articular surface is smooth and the condyles have reached their characteristic adult shape, the lateral being circular and the medial elongated anteroposteriorly. The triangular anterior intercondylar area and the groove for the posterior cruciate ligament are obvious (Fig. 11.19b). By 7 years in girls and 9 years in boys, the epiphyseal and metaphyseal diameters are equal in width (Pyle and Hoerr, 1955). By 11–13 years, the epiphysis is very substantial (Fig. 11.19c). Both the medial and lateral sides of the epiphysis cap the metaphysis. The medial margin is grooved and pitted with nutrient foramina. The lateral margin has a smooth facet for the attachment of the iliotibial tract at its anterior end and the articular facet for the fibula at its posterior end. The facet is variable in orientation and Ogden (1984f) distinguished two types of joints, each of which had associated clinical sequelae (Ogden, 1974b,c). The posterior margin has a characteristically scalloped appearance in the centre at the attachment of the posterior cruciate ligament. The proximal ossified part of the tibial tuberosity protrudes inferolaterally from the centre of the anterior margin and its length depends on whether fusion has taken place with the distal centre (see below). Prior to fusion, the distal section of the tuberosity is sometimes found as a separate ossicle and can be recognized as an almond-shaped, smooth nodule attached to pitted, porous bone on it superolateral aspect (Fig. 11.19d).

Fracture of the proximal tibial epiphysis accounts for only about 3% of physeal injuries as it is well protected by muscles and ligaments. As with injuries to the distal femoral epiphysis, the proximity of the popliteal artery and sciatic and common peroneal nerves carries a potential risk of serious neurovascular complications (Beaty and Kumar, 1994). Roberts (1984) stated that fractures of the intercondylar eminence in children are often related to bicycle accidents.

Fusion coincides with cessation of growth in height as the epiphyses around the knee are the growing end of the lower limb bones. The proximal epiphysis is responsible for about 57% of growth in length of the bone (Digby, 1915; Gill and Abbott, 1942; Anderson *et al.*, 1963; Ogden and McCarthy, 1983). In the radiographic knee atlas, the standard for commencement of fusion is 13 years in females and 15.5 years in males, with completion about 1.5 years later (Pyle and Hoerr, 1955). Other observations have rather later times for complete fusion extending to 17 years in females and 19.5 years in males.

McKern and Stewart (1957) reporting on dry bone found that, in males, there were still 10% and 2% of epiphyses at early stages of union at 17 and 19 years, respectively and that 100% complete fusion did not occur until 23 years. The last site of union was on the posteromedial side of the epiphysis, where there could still be a persistent groove at 24 years. In our series of juvenile skeletons, fusion started on the medial and lateral sides of the condyles and the last open lines were posterior, especially under the fibular facet (Fig. 11.19e).

The **tibial tuberosity** has a unique development as part of, yet distinct from, the main part of the proximal epiphysis (Hughes and Sunderland, 1946; Lewis, 1958; Ehrenborg and Engfeldt, 1961a; Smith, 1962a, Ogden *et al.*, 1975b; Ogden 1984e). During the fourth month of fetal life, there is an outgrowth of the proximal epiphysis on the anterior part of the shaft of the bone at the level of the proximal growth plate. This forerunner of the tuberosity gradually becomes partially separated from the main shaft by an area of fibrovascular tissue that grows into it from the zone of Ranvier. During the first few months after birth, the tuberosity is slightly distal to the main proximal tibial growth plate, which has bent anterodistally onto the front of the metaphysis. In this area, the proximal part of the growth plate has the typical structure of an endochondral ossification process, except that the cartilage cell columns are shorter than normal. Distal to this is a fibrocartilaginous zone where fibrocartilage forms bone by intramembranous ossification and yet further distally, there is transition from hyaline cartilage to fibrous tissue and subsequent formation of bone. The fibrovascular region contributes to the intramembranous remodelling of the anterior metaphysis (Ogden *et al.*, 1975b). It is postulated that this specialized cellular arrangement, which is also found in other mammals (Badi, 1972a, b), is a response to the very strong tensile stresses imposed on the tissues by the pull of the patellar tendon (Lewis, 1958; Smith, 1962a, 1962b; Ogden *et al.*, 1975b;

Ogden 1984e). Radiographically, the proximal part of the tuberosity can be seen as a separate tongue, which projects over the anterior surface of the metaphysis as early as 4.5 years in girls and 6 years in boys (Pyle and Hoerr, 1955). In archaeological specimens however, the central anterior part of the main epiphysis to which the tongue is attached nearly always appears eroded and the tongue is not seen on dry bone until it has reached a more substantial size. Between 8–12 years in girls and 9–14 years in boys, one or more additional centres for the tuberosity appear in the tip of the cartilaginous tongue and ossification gradually spreads proximally. At adolescence, the proximal tongue is still separated from the distal centre by a cartilaginous bridge, but by the time they eventually coalesce, the fibrous zone occupies only the most distal part of the growth plate. The line of separation of this combined epiphysis with the diaphysis is gradually obliterated as the oblique and vertical parts of the tuberosity unite with the diaphyseal ledge. The pattern of fusion is variable. Hughes (1948a) states that the tip of the beak remains unfused and the Pyle and Hoerr (1955) atlas shows the fusion of the tuberosity occurring a little later than the main part of the proximal epiphysis at 14 years in females and 16.5 years in males.

Haines *et al.* (1967) show the tip of the tuberosity fusing first and in our series of juvenile skeletons the sides of the tuberosity were more advanced in fusion than the principal proximal epiphysis, but there was often an open line at the inferior tip (Fig. 11.19e).

This specialized structure and late development of the tuberosity is thought to be a predisposing factor in the aetiology of Osgood-Schlatter's disease. Onset of the condition is seen typically after minor trauma in late childhood or adolescence, when there is maximum activity in the growth plate of the tuberosity (Uhry, 1944; Hughes, 1948a; Ogden and Southwick, 1976; Ogden *et al.*, 1980). In spite of the addition of fibrous tissue, there appears to be an inability in some individuals to withstand the large tensile forces that develop in the tendon of the quadriceps muscle and this results in avulsion of segments of the growth plate. It usually occurs when most of the ligamentum patellae is inserted into cartilage, which has a relatively low tensile strength and lacks pain receptors, so that the injury is at first silent (Ehrenborg and Engfeldt, 1961a). Extra bones are sometimes formed in the intervening fibrous tissue and there is often marked nodular irregularity of the tibial tuberosity. Detailed radiological and histological descriptions of the progression of the lesion can be found in Ehrenborg and Lagergren (1961) and Ehrenborg and Engfeldt (1961b). Reactive bony spurs in the region of the tuberosity have been diagnosed as Osgood-Schlatter's disease in archaeological material (Wells, 1968; Ortner and Putschar, 1985; Stirland, 1991). A related but separate clinical entity, Sinding–Larson–Johansson syndrome, is described under the section on the Patella.

The **distal epiphysis** of the tibia starts to ossify during the first year of life. The centre may be seen at 3–4 months of age but often is not obvious until 7–8 months. At first, it is a rounded nodule related to the anterior part of the metaphysis and lying directly above the trochlea of the talus (Hoerr *et al.*, 1962). It rapidly becomes oval in shape, with its long axis lying mediolaterally. By 14 months in girls and 18 months in boys, the centre accommodates itself to the metaphysis and the growth plate becomes established.

The epiphysis first becomes recognizable between 3–4 years of age. It is a flattish, oval disc, thicker on the medial side with a projecting beak on the anteromedial aspect of the metaphyseal surface. About a year later, the epiphysis becomes rectangular and the thicker, medial border develops an inferior flange as ossification begins to spread into the base of the medial malleolus. The articular surface is smooth and slightly concave on the medial side. The billowed metaphyseal surface has a raised ridge running anteroposteriorly across the medial side (Fig. 11.20a). Growth is rapid, in keeping with that of the foot and by 5 years in girls and 6.5 years in boys the epiphyseal and metaphyseal widths are equal. By about 6 years, ossification around the medial side may become irregular as it spreads towards the cartilaginous medial malleolus (Ogden and McCarthy, 1983).

Between 8 and 10 years, the epiphysis starts to cap the shaft and the medial malleolar ossification can be seen below the joint surface on radiographs (Hoerr *et al.*, 1962). At this stage, the epiphysis is rhomboidal in outline and the malleolus is obvious on the rounded medial side. The posterior border is flat and joined to the lateral border at a rounded right angle. The anterior border is longer than the posterior border as it slopes medially back to the malleolus, which now extends inferomedially beyond the width of the metaphysis. The metaphyseal surface has a thick, protruding ridge, more obvious anteriorly, under the base of the medial malleolus (Fig. 11.20b).

By puberty, the anterior border is grooved and pitted with numerous nutrient foramina and the lateral border bears the concavity for the fibular notch. The groove for the tendon of tibialis posterior is obvious at the medial end of the posterior surface. The medial malleolus has anterior and posterior colliculi, separated by a notch. The articular surface has assumed its adult sellar shape, being concave sagittally and convex mediolaterally. The metaphyseal surface has furrows

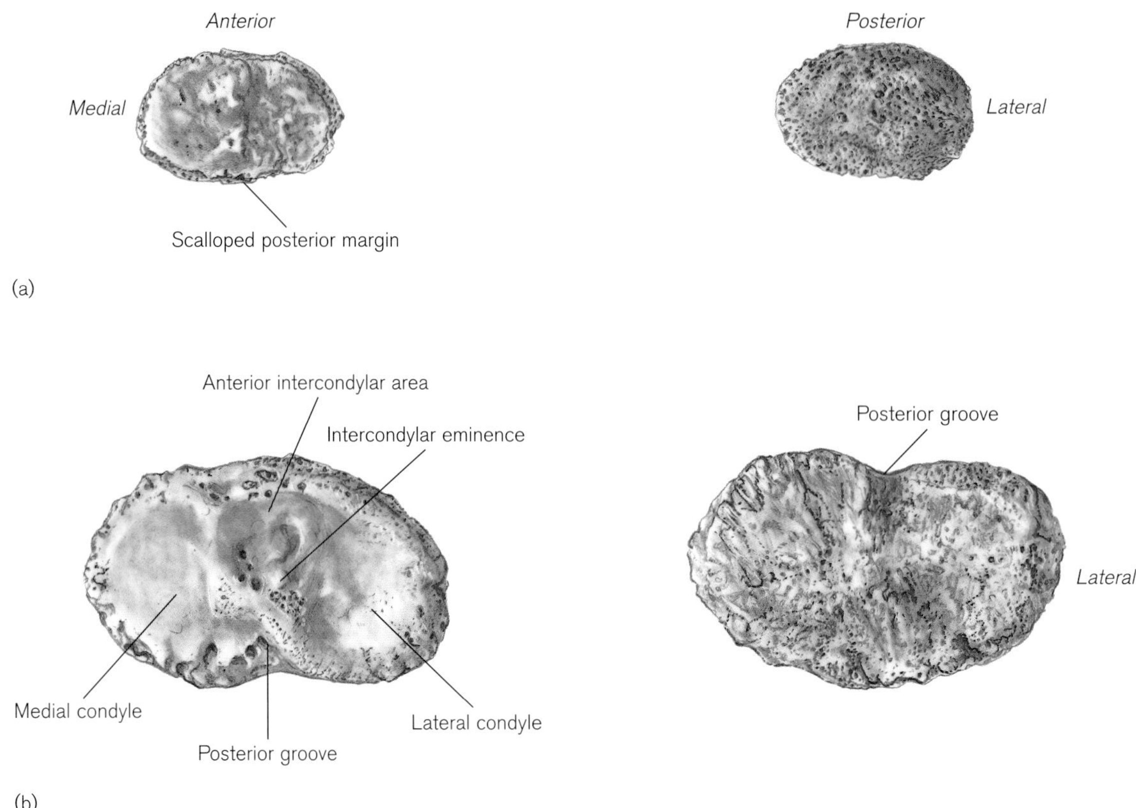

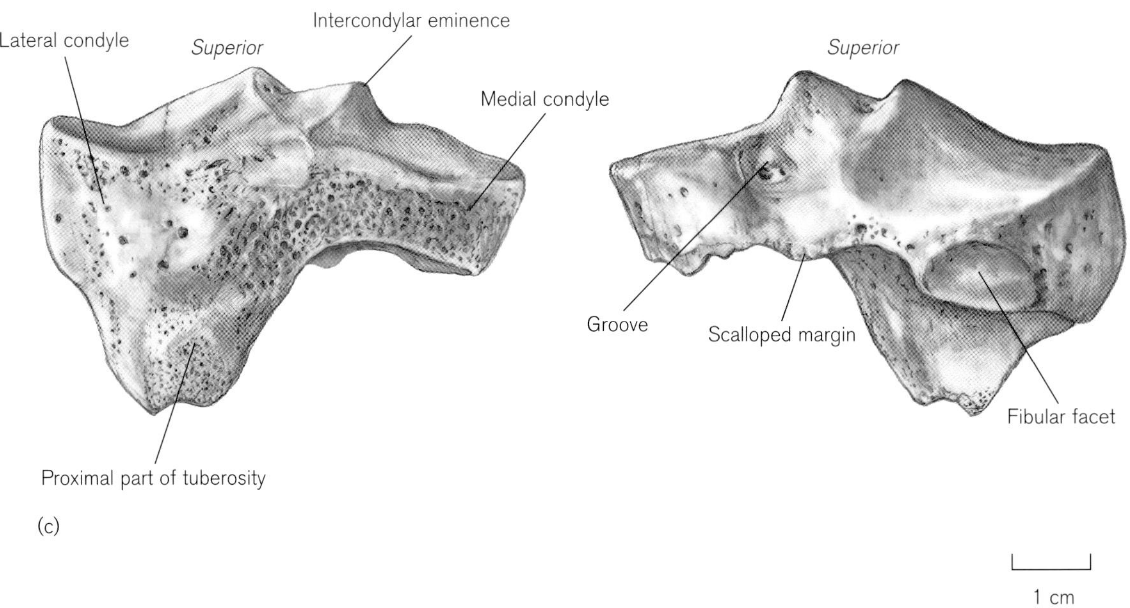

Figure 11.19 Development of the right proximal tibial epiphysis. (a) 3 years 4 months, male; (b) 8 years, male. Left row – articular surfaces. Right row – metaphyseal surfaces; (c) 14 years, female. Left – anterior; right – posterior of right·epiphysis.

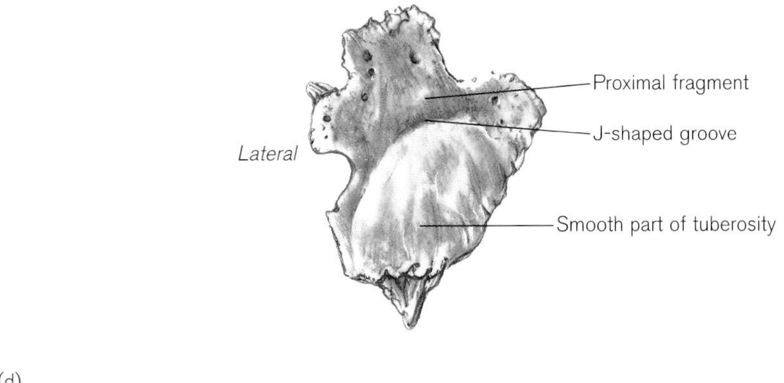

(d)

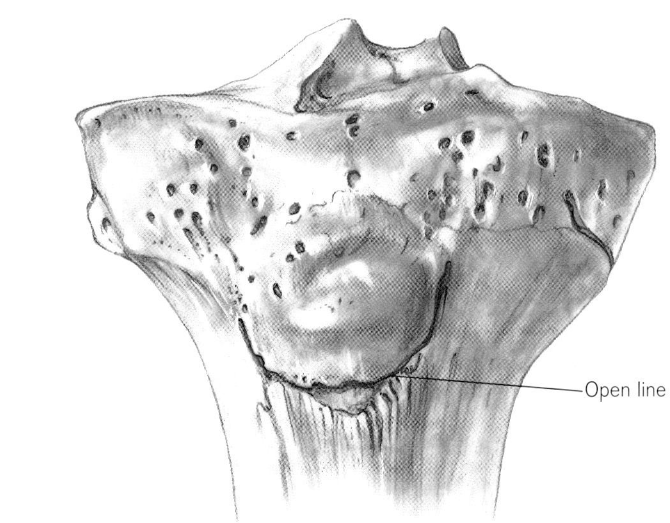

(e)

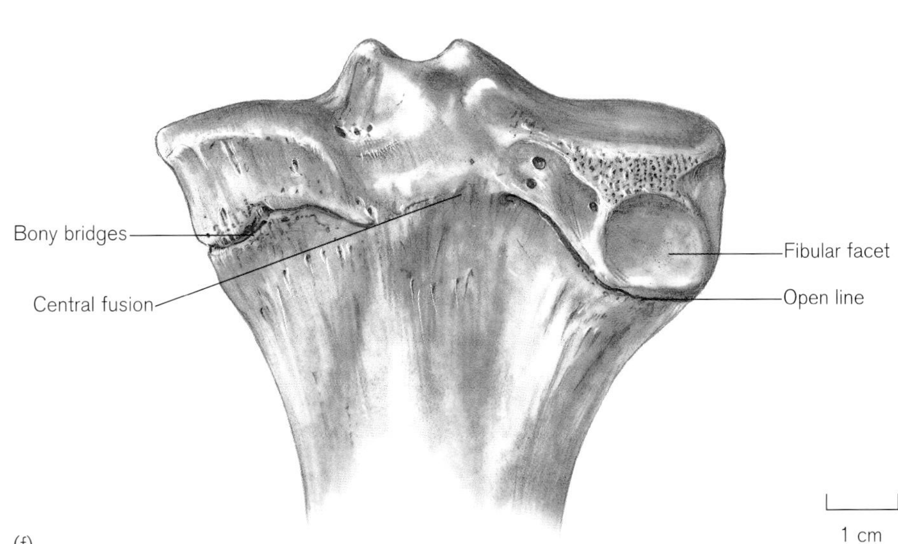

(f)

Figure 11.19 *(Continued)* (d) fragment of tibial tuberosity from an archaeological specimen; (e) anterior surface and (f) posterior surface, 17 years, male.

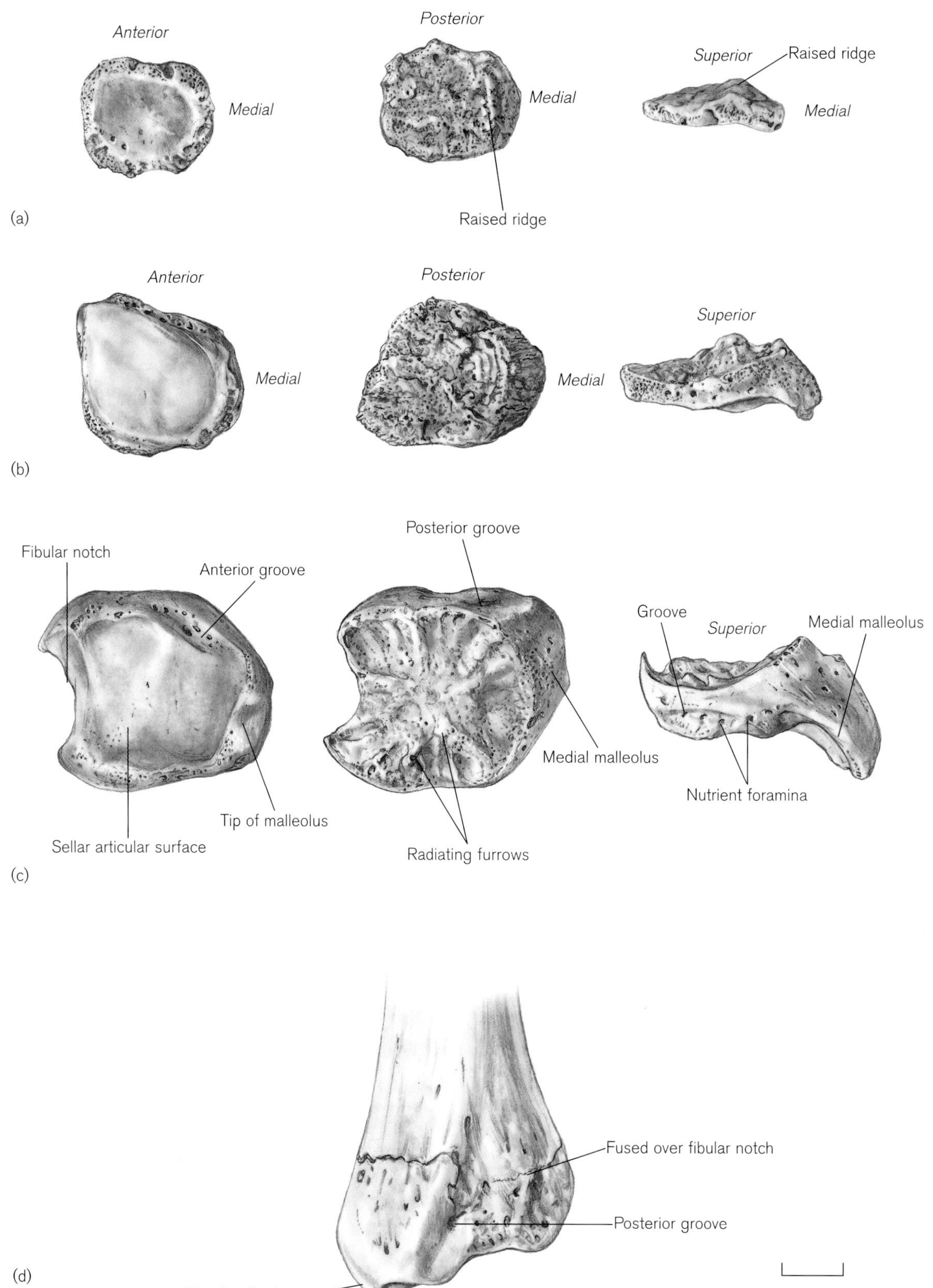

Figure 11.20 Development of the right distal tibial epiphysis. (a) Skeletal age 4–5 years; (b) 8 years, male; (c) 14 years, female. Left row – articular surfaces. Middle row – metaphyseal surfaces. Right row – anterior surfaces; (d) posterior surface undocumented adolescent.

radiating from the centre (Fig. 11.20c). Epiphyseal clefts, which normally close spontaneously, have been reported as normal variants in the medial margin of the epiphysis (Harrison and Keats, 1980). Fractures of the distal tibial epiphysis are not common but can lead to asymmetrical growth, shortening of the limb or angular deformity (Dias, 1984).

It is not unusual for the tip of the medial malleolus to develop from a separate centre of ossification (Den Hoed, 1925; Lapidus, 1933; Powell, 1961; Selby, 1961; Coral, 1987; Ogden and Lee, 1990). This seems to be more common in girls and centres appear between the ages of 7–8 years in girls and 9–10 in boys. They usually fuse with the main part of the epiphysis within 2 years. They may be avulsed and cause acute or chronic symptoms which, if not treated, can lead to a fibrous union or pseudoarthrosis (Ogden and Lee, 1990; Ishii *et al.*, 1994). Nomenclature in the literature is confusing as many authors call the extra centre an os subtibiale, but Coral (1986, 1987) maintained that this term should be confined to the rare occurrence of a separate bone beneath the medial malleolus persisting after the normal age of fusion. He also stated that the true os subtibiale is related to the posterior colliculus, while an accessory ossification centre occurs distal to the anterior colliculus.

Ages for the initiation of **fusion** of the distal epiphysis are 12–13 years in females and 14–15 years in males and the mean age for completion is 14.5 and 16.5 years, respectively (Hansman, 1962; Hoerr *et al.*, 1962). McKern and Stewart's (1957) observations on dry bone state that there was not 100% union in young males until 20 years of age and this agrees with Hansman's range of 14–20 years in males. Ogden and McCarthy (1983) and Dias (1984) state that fusion always occurs from medial to lateral and McKern and Stewart (1957) state that the last evidence of fusion is at the anterolateral side of the epiphysis. In our series of juvenile skeletons this was not always so, as there was often a conspicuous line open over the medial malleolus when the rest of the epiphysis had fused (Fig. 11.20d).

The appearance and fusion of the tibial centres of ossification are summarized in Fig. 11.21.

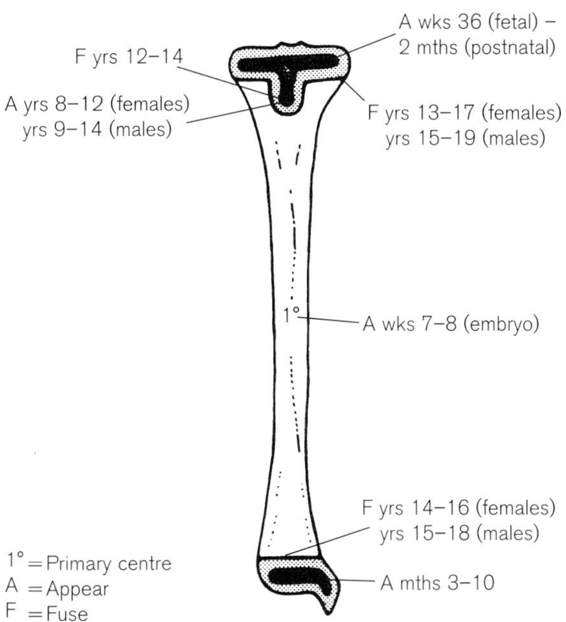

Figure 11.21 Appearance and fusion times of the tibial ossification centres.

Practical notes

Sideing

Diaphysis – sideing the perinatal diaphysis relies on identifying the rounded and more flared proximal end and the flatter, less flared distal end. The anterior surface is marked by the sharp border that curves medially at its distal end. The posterior surface has a very large nutrient foramen. At the proximal end the medial border is more concave, and at the distal metaphyseal surface the lateral side is flat and often marked by a small notch (Fig. 11.17). After the perinatal period, the shaft of the tibia rapidly assumes adult morphology.

Proximal epiphysis – the epiphysis is probably identifiable during the second year as an elongated ossicle, rounded on one side and flat on the other. However, sideing relies on identifying the posterior cruciate groove and lateral and medial condylar areas on the metaphyseal surface, which do not become clear until about 3–4 years of age (Fig. 11.19). An isolated tibial tuberosity, sometimes recovered from an adolescent skeleton, extends inferolaterally from an inverted, 'J'-shaped line (Fig. 11.19d).

Distal epiphysis–this is distinctive from about 3–4 years of age. The medial (malleolar) side of the epiphysis is thicker than the lateral side and has a distinct projection anteriorly on the metaphyseal surface (Fig. 11.20a). From about the age of 6 years the medial malleolus becomes obvious (Fig. 11.20b) The anterior surface has a horizontal groove and from about 11–12 years the oblique groove for the tibialis posterior tendon can be identified on the posterior surface (Fig. 11.20c).

Bones of a similar morphology

Perinatal diaphyses – the six major long bones of the limbs can be divided into two groups: the femur, tibia and humerus are larger and look more robust than the radius, ulna and fibula. The femur is the largest and longest bone in the first group, while the tibia and humerus are very similar in length (Table 11.1). The distal humerus is flattened and has the obvious olecranon fossa posteriorly, whereas the tibial shaft is triangular and flares out both proximally and distally (Figs. 9.6b,d and 11.17). From birth onwards, the tibia increases in length faster than the humerus.

Proximal tibial fragment – is oval like the distal femur but is smaller and distinguished by the presence of the tuberosity anteriorly (Figs. 11.17c and 11.3c).

Distal tibial fragment – the metaphyseal surface is about the same size as the proximal humerus but it is flat, with a D-shaped outline and a straight lateral border. The humerus has a rounded surface with the intertubercular sulcus visible anteriorly (Figs. 11.17d and 9.6c).

Morphological summary (Fig. 11.21)

Fetal

Wks 7–8	Primary ossification centre appears in the shaft
Wks 36–40	Secondary centre for proximal epiphysis appears
Birth	Represented by shaft and usually proximal epiphysis
By 6 wks	Proximal secondary centre present
3–10 mths	Distal secondary centre appears
3–5 yrs	Medial malleolus starts to ossify
8–13 yrs	Distal part of tuberosity starts to ossify from one or more centres
12–14 yrs	Proximal and distal parts of tuberosity unite
14–16 yrs	Distal epiphysis fuses in females
15–18 yrs	Distal epiphysis fuses in males
13–17 yrs	Proximal epiphysis fuses in females
15–19 yrs	Proximal epiphysis fuses in males

Metrics

Fazekas and Kósa (1978) measured the length of the fetal tibial diaphysis on dry bones (Table 11.8) and Jeanty (1983) recorded the lengths, as seen by ultrasound (Table 11.9). Trotter and Peterson (1969) recorded the length and weight of the perinatal tibial diaphysis (Table 11.10).

Scheuer *et al.* (1980) gave linear and logarithmic regression equations for age on tibial diaphyseal length, as measured on radiographs from 24 fetal weeks to 6 weeks postnatal (Table 11.11). Data showing the length of the tibial diaphysis from 1 month to 18 years (3-monthly for the first year) in males and females are shown in Table 11.12. These are recorded from radiographs from the Fels Research Institute by Gindhart (1973). Data showing the length of the tibia at 6-monthly intervals (2-monthly for the first half year) in males and females from birth to cessation of growth are shown in Table 11.13. These data from Maresh (1970) are from the University of Colorado longitudinal study and are of bony diaphyses, except between ages 10–12, when double sets of figures give lengths with and without epiphyses. Measurements from radiographs at the Harvard School of Public Health by Anderson *et al.* (1964) are of total tibial length, including epiphyses at yearly intervals in males and females (Table 11.14). Pritchett (1992), using the Colorado data, charted growth and predictions of growth from the lower limb bones. The contribution

Table 11.8 Length of the fetal tibial diaphysis

Age (weeks)	Length (mm)
12	6.0
14	10.2
16	17.4
18	23.4
20	28.5
22	32.6
24	35.8
26	38.0
28	42.0
30	43.9
32	48.6
34	52.7
36	54.7
38	60.1
40	65.2

Length: maximum length.
Adapted from Fazekas and Kósa (1978).

Table 11.9 Length of the fetal tibia as measured by ultrasound

	Length (mm)		
	Percentile		
Age (weeks)	5th	50th	95th
12	–	7	–
14	2	13	19
16	7	19	25
18	14	24	29
20	19	29	35
22	25	34	39
24	28	39	45
26	33	43	49
28	38	47	52
30	41	51	56
32	46	54	59
34	47	57	64
36	49	60	68
38	54	62	69
40	58	65	69

Adapted from Jeanty (1983).

of the proximal tibial growth plate varies from 50% at 7 years in both boys and girls to 80% at 14 years in females and 16 years in males.

Table 11.10 Length and weight of the perinatal tibia

	Length (mm)	Weight (g)
White male	66.8	2.86
White female	60.8	2.08
Black male	62.0	2.12
Black female	65.9	2.26
Mean	63.9	2.33

Adapted from Trotter and Peterson (1969).

Diaphyseal length data for some archaeological populations from Africa, Europe and North America are given in Appendix 3. Most of the age at death estimates are based on dental development.

Table 11.11 Regression equations of age on tibial length

Linear

Age (weeks) $= (0.4207 \times \text{tibia}) + 11.4724 \pm 2.12$

Logarithmic

Age (weeks) $= (21.207\log_e \times \text{tibia}) - 50.2331 \pm 2.11$

Adapted from Scheuer *et al.* (1980).

Table 11.12 Tibial diaphyseal length (mm) – 1 month–18 years

	Male			Female		
Age	*n*	Mean	SD	*n*	Mean	SD
1 month	156	72.14	4.90	108	71.34	4.53
3 months	118	84.83	4.20	98	84.95	18.14
6 months	176	99.26	5.34	132	97.06	5.01
9 months	116	110.06	5.02	101	109.49	17.32
1.0 years	155	119.57	5.81	122	117.08	5.82
1.5 years	110	135.53	6.87	90	134.24	6.98
2.0 years	133	150.14	7.43	108	148.08	7.49
2.5 years	92	162.74	7.53	84	163.04	19.04
3.0 years	130	174.15	9.31	107	173.07	9.93
3.5 years	83	183.98	9.11	85	183.73	10.47
4.0 years	132	194.00	10.67	115	193.68	11.25
4.5 years	85	203.59	10.29	77	203.62	11.96
5.0 years	125	212.37	11.66	109	213.18	12.54
5.5 years	78	221.89	11.76	71	223.62	13.85
6.0 years	157	232.95	13.09	118	231.15	15.16
6.5 years	98	240.88	14.19	101	241.19	16.61
7.0 years	150	250.42	14.26	113	250.29	16.91
7.5 years	101	258.93	15.37	101	261.01	19.31
8.0 years	147	268.36	15.86	109	270.47	20.15
8.5 years	97	276.88	16.16	96	278.56	20.91
9.0 years	144	287.97	17.43	100	290.74	21.51
9.5 years	83	295.89	16.82	83	298.97	22.07
10.0 years	127	305.60	18.38	98	307.98	20.06
10.5 years	12	315.92	11.67	17	310.20	22.55
11.0 years	98	322.21	19.18	82	323.86	19.24
11.5 years	13	327.64	12.23	10	325.62	25.59
12.0 years	73	336.95	19.33	55	336.24	20.26
13.0 years	53	358.05	27.61	42	246.45	20.21
14.0 years	31	372.41	27.65	33	352.67	19.93
15.0 years	21	386.85	45.57	20	357.75	19.63
16.0 years	19	402.06	28.97	23	366.63	20.67
17.0 years	18	411.72	27.27	15	374.21	24.50
18.0 years	18	404.19	23.85	11	367.05	31.48

Adapted from Gindhart (1973).

Table 11.13 Tibial length (mm) – 2 months–18 years

	Male			Female		
Age (years)	*n*	Mean	SD	*n*	Mean	SD
Diaphyseal length						
0.125	59	70.8	5.4	69	70.3	4.6
0.25	58	81.9	5.3	65	80.8	4.6
0.50	67	91.0	5.2	78	88.9	5.3
1.00	72	110.3	5.2	81	108.5	4.8
1.5	68	126.1	6.0	84	124.0	5.6
2.0	68	140.1	6.5	84	138.2	6.5
2.5	72	152.5	6.8	82	150.1	7.0
3.0	72	163.5	7.7	79	161.1	8.2
3.5	73	172.8	9.8	78	171.2	8.7
4.0	72	182.8	9.0	80	180.8	9.5
4.5	71	191.8	9.2	78	190.9	10.5
5.0	77	201.4	9.9	80	199.9	11.4
5.5	73	210.3	10.7	74	207.9	12.5
6.0	71	218.9	10.0	75	217.4	12.6
6.5	72	227.8	11.6	81	226.3	13.6
7.0	71	236.2	11.8	86	234.1	14.1
7.5	76	244.2	12.4	83	243.2	15.0
8.0	70	253.3	12.9	85	251.7	15.6
8.5	72	260.6	12.3	82	259.1	15.6
9.0	76	268.7	13.4	83	265.5	17.1
9.5	78	276.9	14.4	83	276.6	18.7
10.0	77	284.9	14.2	84	284.3	19.3
10.5	76	292.0	15.1	75	292.4	21.4
11.0	75	298.8	15.0	76	300.8	21.2
11.5	76	306.8	16.5	75	310.5	21.4
12.0	73	315.9	17.0	71	318.2	21.7
Total length including epiphyses						
10.0	76	320.0	15.7	83	321.1	21.7
10.5	76	328.9	17.0	75	330.9	23.7
11.0	75	338.6	17.1	76	340.1	23.1
11.5	77	347.4	18.5	75	350.4	23.2
12.0	76	357.3	19.1	75	360.9	23.8
12.5	67	367.5	18.6	65	367.3	23.0
13.0	69	376.7	20.6	69	374.5	22.2
13.5	69	388.2	22.0	62	379.0	21.8
14.0	69	397.4	21.9	64	384.3	21.4
14.5	64	406.0	23.1	42	386.9	20.5
15.0	60	412.2	21.5	57	385.7	20.8
15.5	52	420.5	22.3	12	390.5	28.5
16.0	60	422.6	21.8	40	386.8	22.6
16.5	38	425.1	24.2	3	–	–
17.0	50	426.5	23.2	18	380.7	23.6
18.0	28	429.5	25.6	4	–	–

Adapted from Maresh (1970).

Table 11.14 Tibial length (mm) – 1–18 years

	Male			Female		
Age (years)	*n*	Mean	SD	*n*	Mean	SD
1	61	116.0	6.20	61	115.7	6.46
2	67	145.4	8.09	67	145.1	7.39
3	67	167.9	9.35	67	168.1	8.93
4	67	186.7	10.91	67	188.6	11.44
5	67	204.6	12.47	67	207.7	13.00
6	67	221.2	14.18	67	225.3	14.58
7	67	237.6	16.32	67	242.2	16.40
8	67	253.8	17.78	67	258.9	17.86
9	67	269.9	19.61	67	275.6	19.93
10	67	285.3	21.13	67	292.8	21.93
11	67	301.0	23.01	67	310.0	23.84
12	67	317.5	25.36	67	326.1	24.24
13	67	334.9	28.33	67	338.3	23.74
14	67	351.8	28.65	67	344.3	22.28
15	67	363.8	26.16	67	345.9	21.73
16	67	370.4	24.12	67	346.3	21.51
17	67	372.2	23.16	67	346.5	21.58
18	67	372.9	22.54	67	346.5	21.61

Adapted from Anderson *et al.* (1964).

IV. THE FIBULA

The adult fibula

The fibula[10] forms the skeleton of the lateral part of the leg and articulates proximally and distally with the tibia at the superior and inferior tibiofibular joints and also distally with the body of the talus at the ankle joint. It is a slender long bone with an expanded proximal head and a distal end forming the lateral malleolus of the ankle.

The **head** of the fibula (Fig. 11.22) is an irregular knob of bone whose main feature is a facet tilted anteromedially towards the tibia, which articulates with the posterolateral surface of the lateral condyle and in about 10% of the joint cavities communicates with the knee joint. Owen (1901) reported a partial septum as a common finding in the joint, which is not generally described in anatomical texts. Ogden (1974b, 1974c, 1984f) described two basic types of

[10]Fibula – (Latin meaning 'buckle, brooch, needle') refers to the pin with which an ornament was fastened to the dress of priestly vestments. The French word for fibula (péroné) is derived from the Greek word *perone* with the same meaning, hence the name for the peroneal muscles. Also related, the Latin *infibulatio*, a silver needle inserted into the prepuce of young boys to prevent premature sexual intercourse.

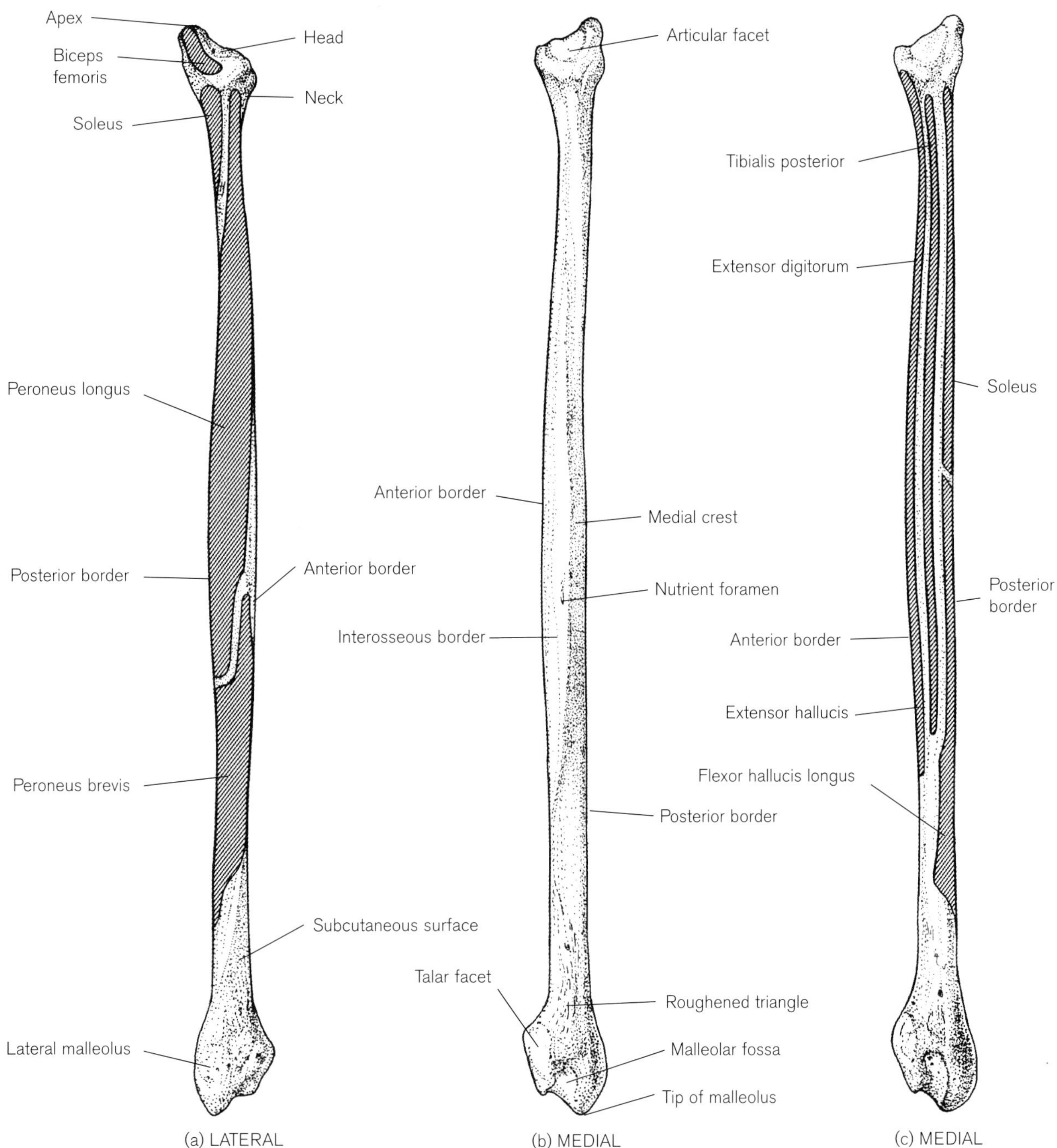

Figure 11.22 Right adult fibula.

articulation between the proximal fibular and tibial epiphyses, which affect the stability of the juvenile joint (see below). The more common is a horizontal joint, usually circular and planar, that lies under and posterior to the projection of the lateral tibial epiphysis. Less commonly, the joint is oblique and the surfaces are more variable in area, configuration and inclination. The **apex** (styloid process) of the head projects superolaterally and provides attachment for the fibular collateral ligament of the knee joint and part of the tendon of the biceps femoris muscle. Most of the muscle fibres from the long head of the biceps femoris muscle surround the ligament on the lateral, posterior and medial sides, while most of those originating from the short head continue onto the lateral tibial condyle (Sneath, 1955). Below the head there is a narrow neck around which the common peroneal nerve runs in contact with the bone. Its subcutaneous position makes it especially vulnerable to damage, often resulting in foot drop. The extensor digitorum longus, peroneus longus and soleus have attachments that extend up from the shaft onto the neck.

The **shaft** of the fibula is long and slender and marked with several crests that are variable in structure and often difficult to identify individually throughout their length as they sometimes merge with one another. Descriptions of the shaft also vary in different texts but usually three borders and three surfaces are described (Fig. 11.23). The anterior border runs distally from the head of the bone for about three-quarters of the length of the shaft, inclining slightly laterally as it descends. It divides in the distal quarter to enclose a triangular, subcutaneous area that lies above the lateral malleolus. The posterior border also runs distally from the head but is more rounded and therefore less distinct in its proximal part. It inclines medially at its distal end, where it forms the medial lip of a groove on the posterior surface of the lateral malleolus. The third described border faces medially towards the tibia and has the interosseous membrane attached to it, but it is often difficult to identify at its extremities. Proximally it may join the anterior border and distally it usually runs into the medial crest (see below). The surface between the anterior and posterior borders faces laterally for most of its length and provides, attachment for the peroneus longus and brevis muscles. At the distal end it turns posteriorly, where the tendons of the muscles lie in a groove on the posterior surface of the malleolus covered by the peroneal retinaculum, which is attached to the lateral border of the groove. The so-called medial surface lies between the anterior and interosseous borders, but because of the variation in position of the interosseous border, it often faces anteromedially or anteriorly and is often not discernible as a separate surface at its upper end. It has part of the extensor digitorum longus and the extensor hallucis longus muscles attached to it. The posterior (in some texts medial) surface lies between the interosseous and posterior borders and is divided longitudinally for part of its length by a **medial crest**, which merges with the interosseous border distally. It divides the surfaces into posteromedial and medially facing surfaces. The tibialis posterior muscle is attached between the crest and the interosseous border and the bone is sometimes deeply hollowed and may be further marked by another small crest for a tendinous septum within the muscle. The surface between the crest and the posterior border has attached to it the soleus muscle proximally and the flexor hallucis muscle distally. The combined medial crest and interosseous border ends distally at a roughened triangle above the articular surface of the lateral malleolus to which the inferior tibiofibular ligament is attached.

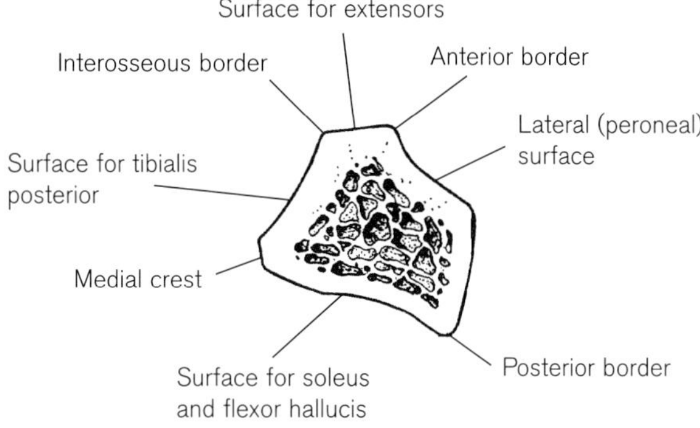

Figure 11.23 Cross-section of adult fibula in middle third of shaft.

The shaft of the fibula is usually supplied by one main nutrient artery, which enters in the middle third of the bone and then divides into ascending and descending branches (Crock, 1996). Between 56% and 88% of nutrient foramina are on the medial crest (Mysorekar, 1967; Sendemir and Çimen, 1991), and in the vast majority, the entrance slopes distally.

Ogden (1974b, 1974c) believed that dislocation at the proximal tibiofibular joint was related to the inclination of the joint surface. The relatively immobile, oblique type of joint (see above) prevented the necessary dorsiflexion at the ankle joint and so increased torsional stress and made the bone more susceptible to fracture or dislocation. Fracture of the fibular shaft resulting from violence seldom occurs without involving the tibia or without simultaneous injury at the ankle. A rotational force normally fractures the bone more proximally than the tibia, the most common place being at the junction of the middle and upper third of the bone. Fatigue or stress fractures normally affect the lower third (Adams and Hamblen, 1992).

The lower end of the fibula forms the slightly expanded **lateral malleolus**, which projects posteriorly and distally. The lateral surface is subcutaneous and the posterior surface is marked by the **malleolar sulcus** (peroneal groove) in which the tendons of peroneus longus and brevis run (Fig. 11.24). Medially there is a triangular, vertical facet that articulates with the lateral side of the trochlea of the talus and above this a small facet for the tibia can sometimes be distinguished. Behind and below the talar facet is

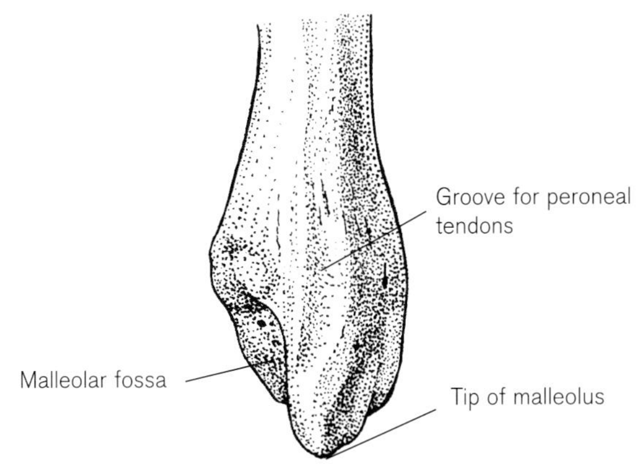

Figure 11.24 Posterior surface of right adult lateral malleolus.

the rough **malleolar fossa**, pitted with nutrient foramina, in which are attached the posterior tibiofibular and talofibular ligaments. The tip of the malleolus, which extends distal to the fossa has the calcaneofibular ligament attached to it.

Fractures of the lateral malleolus are fairly common. A shearing fracture of the whole malleolus is caused by abduction or lateral rotation and an avulsion fracture of the tip by adductor force. Severe violence can cause diastasis (rupture) of the tibiofibular ligament (Adams and Hamblen, 1992).

Attempts to determine the weight-bearing capacity of the fibula have involved experiments with cadaveric material. Lambert (1971), using an indirect method, estimated that it carried about one-sixth of the body weight, but Takebe *et al.* (1984), using a more direct method, found this to be only 6.4%, although it increased somewhat on dorsiflexion of the ankle joint. Apart from some weight-bearing and providing surface for muscle attachments, it had long been generally accepted that the main role of the fibula was relatively passive. However, it has since been demonstrated that the fibula rotates laterally about its long axis during extension (dorsiflexion) at the ankle joint (Barnett and Napier, 1952). Ogden (1974b) observed that patients with arthrodesis of the superior tibiofibular joint displayed ankle symptoms and believed that part of the function of the fibula was to dissipate torsional loading, for which some degree of rotational movement at the joint was essential. Weinert *et al.* (1973) demonstrated on films of normal walking that the fibula actually moves down and laterally during the heel strike phase of gait. This downward movement, when weight-bearing forces are greatest, was thought to dissipate compression forces by converting them to tension in the stretched ligaments and interosseous membrane. In athletes with damaged ankles the surgical removal of a fixed tibiofibular syndesmosis reduced pain, which was thought to have been caused by forcing of the anterior talus into a fixed mortice and possibly by foot flexor muscles going into spasm after repeated isometric contraction against the fixed fibula (Scranton *et al.*, 1976).

Of all the long bones, the fibula is the most commonly congenitally absent (Coventry and Johnson, 1952). Farmer and Laurin (1960) reviewed 24 patients and the associated anomalies. Calculation of stature can be made using the tables of Telkkä (1950), Trotter and Gleser (1952, 1958), Genovés (1967) and those in Krogman and Işcan (1986).

Early development of the fibula

Details of the early development of the fibula may be found in Gray and Gardner (1950), Haines (1953), O'Rahilly *et al.*, (1957), Gardner and O'Rahilly (1968) and O'Rahilly and Gardner (1975). The mesenchymal fibula is visible by stage 17 (41 days) but chondrification lags slightly behind that of the tibia and does not usually begin until stage 19. The femur and fibula are very close at this stage and there was debate in the early literature about a possible fibulofemoral joint (Grünbaum, 1892). O'Rahilly (1951) described a temporary femorofibular interzone at the chondrification stage, but believed that a proper joint never comes to fruition. Haines (1953) interpreted the same tissue differently and did not consider that the condensation of cells was a true interzone, but both authors agree that in a few days the area between the two elements is invaded by tibial tissue. The femur and fibula are, however, joined by condensations for the fibular collateral ligament and the tendon of popliteus is also visible. At stage 20, the distal end of the fibula is still blastemal and is separated from the calcaneus by a dense cellular zone. By stage 23 (about 8 weeks), it is separated from the calcaneus by a small part of the talus. The lateral malleolus extends below that of the medial malleolus by the fifth fetal month and this increases as development proceeds (Wilgress, 1900).

Ossification

Primary centre

Ossification of the fibula may begin at stage 23 (27–31 mm CRL/week 8), but usually a bone collar does not develop until the beginning of the fetal period (O'Rahilly and Gardner, 1975). It thus starts to ossify later than all the other major long bones of the limbs.

Flat metaphyseal surface
Posterior border
Anterior border
Subcutaneous surface
Downward slope
(a) LATERAL
Anterior border
Posterior border
Nutrient foramen
Interosseous border
Rough area for ligament
(b) MEDIAL
Lateral
Anterior
(c) PROXIMAL
Medial
Posterior
Angled lateral surface
(d) DISTAL
1 cm

Figure 11.25 Right perinatal fibula.

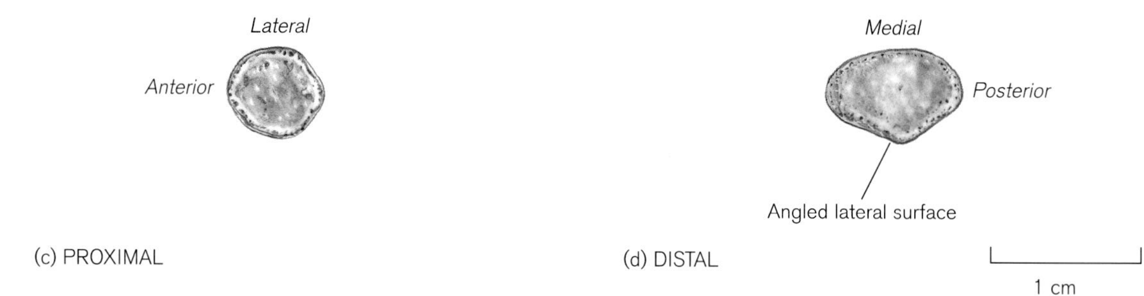

The perinatal fibula (Fig. 11.25) is a slender, straight bone that is rounded or angled in the proximal half and flattened mediolaterally in the distal half. The anterior and posterior borders are sharp especially in the distal part and the interosseous border is usually discernible in the middle third. The anterior border divides distally to enclose the subcutaneous area, which is often covered with porous-looking bone. The shaft flares slightly towards the proximal metaphyseal surface, which is flat and circular. The medial surface at the distal end usually has a roughened triangle for the inferior transverse part of the posterior tibiofibular ligament. The distal metaphyseal surface slopes slightly downwards posteriorly and has a flattened medial border and a rounded or angled lateral border. There is usually one, and sometimes two, nutrient foramina on the medial side in the region of the interosseous border, whose entrances slope distally.

By 2 years of age, the proximal end of the shaft is more flared and consequently the neck also becomes more obvious. The subcutaneous triangle is also more marked and the distal metaphyseal surface is flat. By 6 years, the shaft of the fibula has achieved close to adult morphology and the main borders and surfaces can usually be identified. The distal metaphyseal surface is triangular in outline and the proximal surface is either circular or has a flattened border, which may be dependent on the configuration of the superior tibiofibular joint (Fig. 11.26).

Secondary centres

The order in which the secondary centres of the fibular epiphyses ossify is different from that of other long bones. It is normal for ossification to begin first in those epiphyses at the growing ends of long bones. In the lower limb this takes place around the knee and the distal femur and proximal tibia follow the usual pattern and begin to ossify during the perinatal period. In the fibula, however, the proximal epiphysis does not start to ossify until about 2 years after its distal end, although its union with the diaphysis is in accordance with that of the other knee centres and is considerably later than that of the distal end. Walmsley (1918) thought the late appearance of the proximal end was in accordance with other traction epiphyses and that the delay in fusion may be due to the fact that it was bound to the tibia at the growing end. Although true, this does not explain the earlier development of the distal end. Other authors interpreted the anomalous timing as an early distal development rather than a delayed proximal fusion. Jones (1946) connected the early distal ossification with the rapid growth of the lower end of the fibula during the perinatal period and Le Gros Clark (1958) suggested that the precocious appearance and fusion of the lower end might be related to infant walking. However, a comparative study in different mammals revealed that the pattern peculiar to the fibula is a widespread mammalian feature and is therefore probably not related to any special feature of the human skeleton (Ellis and Joseph, 1954).

The ossification centre of the **distal epiphysis** appears at the end of the first year or beginning of the second year of life at the time when the infant does indeed start to walk (Puyhaubert, 1913; Davies and Parsons, 1927; Paterson, 1929; Flecker, 1932b; Francis *et al.*, 1939; Elgenmark, 1946; Hansman,

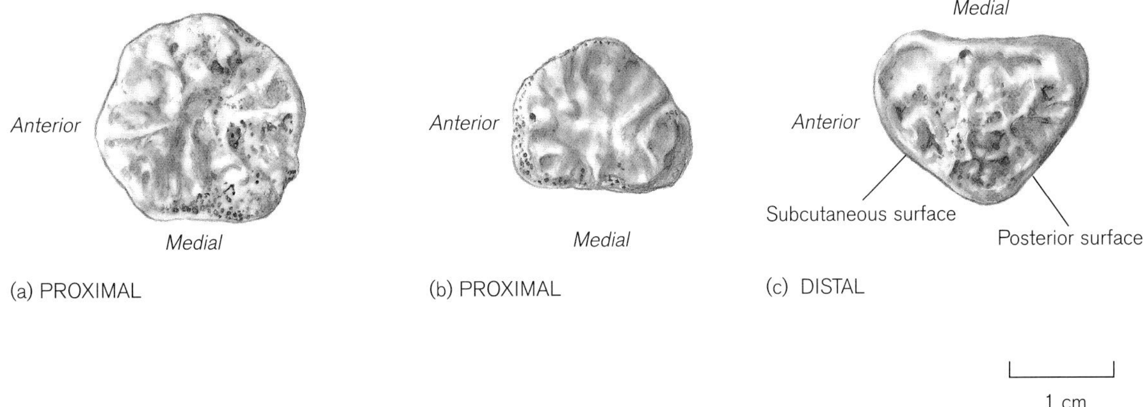

Figure 11.26 Right juvenile fibulae. (a) Proximal metaphyseal surface, 14 years, female; (b) proximal metaphyseal surface, 12 years, female; (c) distal metaphyseal surface, 14 years, female.

1962; Hoerr *et al.*, 1962). Even at this early stage, girls are in advance of boys in their development by about 2 months (Hoerr *et al.*, 1962) and this difference increases throughout development, so that by adolescence there is a 3-year difference. In the perinatal period, the epiphyseal/metaphyseal line is at the same level as the epiphysis of the tibia but as development proceeds, there appears to be a distal migration so that by 3 years of age, the growth plate of the fibular epiphysis is level with the tibiotalar articular surface. This relative change in the level of the growth plate coincides with establishment of walking and failure to do this, as for instance in cerebral palsy, may contribute to the valgus deformity characteristic of the condition (Ogden and McCarthy, 1983; Love *et al.*, 1990). At first, the long axis of the epiphysis is transverse and by 18 months in girls and 2 years in boys, the growth plate is established. At 3–4 years, ossification spreads into the region of the malleolar fossa and the epiphyseal cartilage starts to cap the metaphysis.

The bony epiphysis is usually recognizable by this time and is an irregular nodule of bone with a flat metaphyseal surface. The lateral surface is almost flat and has a straight posterior border and a sloping anterior border. The medial surface is angled but has not yet developed an articular facet (Fig. 11.27a). There is often irregular ossification around the margins and also accessory centres may develop but they soon fuse with the main part of the epiphysis (Ogden and McCarthy, 1983). By about 6 years, bone occupies most of the epiphysis. The malleolar fossa is well formed and contains many large and small nutrient foramina (Fig. 11.27b). By adolescence, the tip of the malleolus extends distal to the fossa, the groove for the peroneal tendons can usually be seen and the metaphyseal surface is billowed and has an undulated margin (Fig. 11.27c). Accessory centres are rarer than at the medial malleolus, especially those that fail to fuse, so forming a true os subfibulare, (Powell, 1961; Ogden and Lee, 1990).

The distal fibular growth plate contributes a greater percentage of distal leg growth than that of the tibia (Beals and Skyhar, 1984). Bridges of bone start to appear at about 12 years in females and 15 years in males and **fusion** is normally complete by 14 years in females and 16.5 years in males (Hoerr *et al.*, 1962). As with other limb bones, fusion, as judged by inspection of dry bone, is reported at a later age than that seen in radiographs. McKern and Stewart (1957) described 90% and 100% fusion at 17 and 20 years, respectively in males, with the last fusion medially over the talar articulation. This was confirmed in our series of juvenile skeletons, where the lateral surface of the malleolus was always the first to fuse, leaving an open line over the medial side (Fig. 11.27d).

Ossification in the **proximal epiphysis** of the fibula commences during the fourth year in girls and the fifth year in boys, but timing is more variable than at the distal end (Puyhaubert, 1913; Davies and Parsons, 1927; Paterson, 1929; Flecker, 1932b; Francis *et al.*, 1939; Elgenmark, 1946; Hansman, 1962; Hoerr *et al.*, 1962). The centre, which may be multinodular, is located distal to that of the tibia. It develops at the same time as ossification is spreading into the intercondylar region of the proximal tibial epiphysis. Ossification spreads slowly and about 2 years later, the ossified epiphysis has a rounded superior border, which is level with the tibial growth plate. The styloid process does not become ossified until about 8 years in girls and 10.5 years in boys (Pyle and Hoerr, 1955). The more common type of circular joint surface lies under and posterior to the tibial condyle. This position provides stability and prevents forward displacement of the fibula, thus making the proximal tibiofibular joint amongst the rarest of epiphyseal childhood injuries. The less common arrangement is for the surfaces to be variable in area and configuration and sometimes a more oblique inclination is associated with subluxation or dislocation (Ogden, 1984f).

The proximal epiphysis is an irregular piece of bone with a rounded superior surface, most of which is occupied by the semilunar tibial facet, which is set at an angle facing anteromedially towards a straight border. The surface slopes away on the other sides. The metaphyseal surface is flat and D-shaped (Fig. 11.28a). Because ossification spreads slowly, it is not until late childhood that the epiphysis shows its distinctive features and even then it can be very variable, having a triangular or rhomboidal shape. The articular facet can be triangular, oval or comma-shaped. The styloid process projects from the posterolateral corner (Fig. 11.28b).

Ages reported for **fusion** of the proximal epiphysis are variable and have a wide range. Flecker (1932b) gave 17 years for females and 19 years for males and the equivalent ranges given by Hansman (1962) are 12–17 years for females and 15–20 years for males. McKern and Stewart (1957) recorded 96% fusion by 19 years and 100% by 22 years in males, the last site of fusion being anterolateral. There did not appear to be a constant pattern of fusion in our series of juvenile skeletons.

The appearance and fusion times of the fibular centres of ossification are summarized in Fig. 11.29.

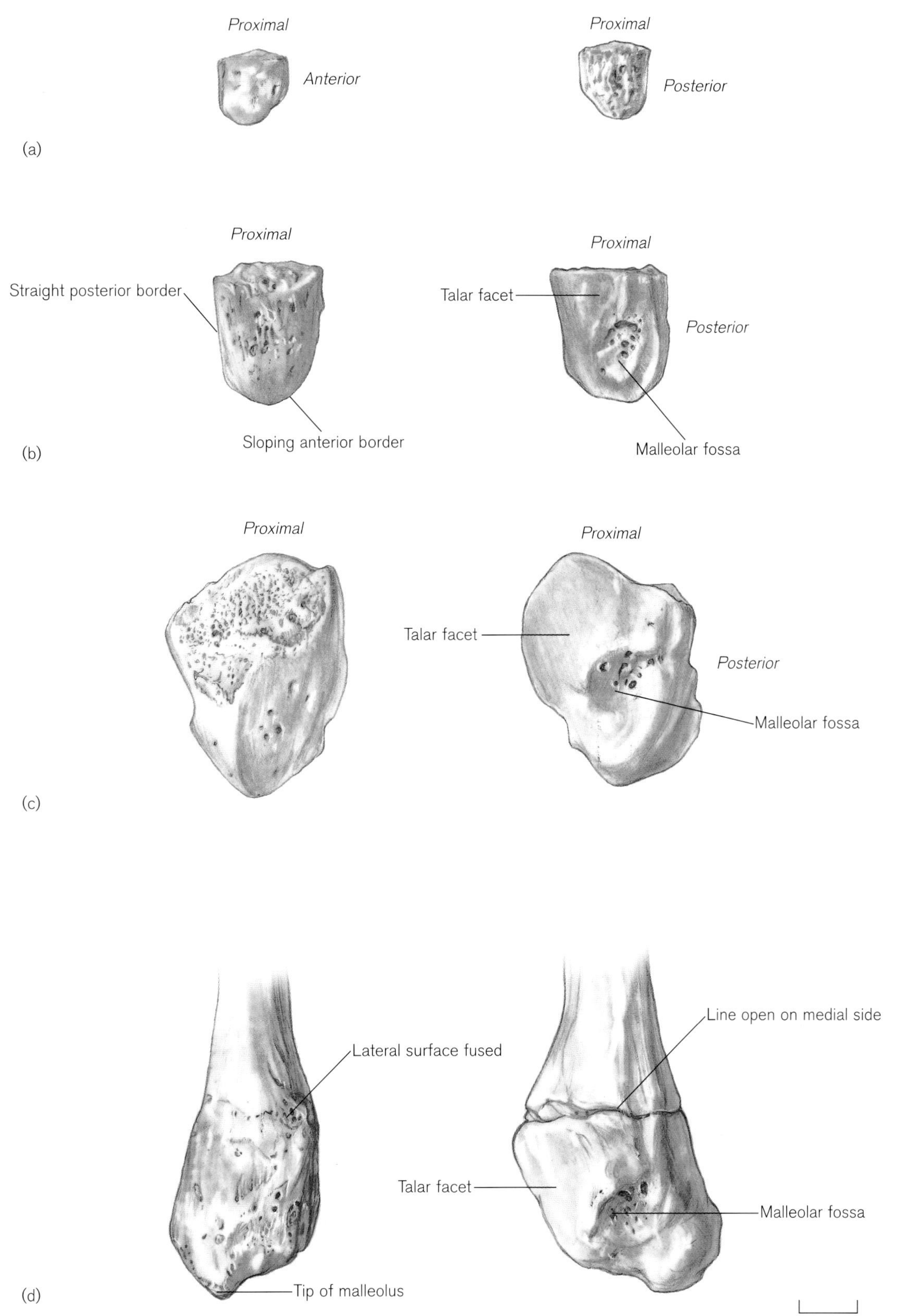

Figure 11.27 Development of the right distal fibular epiphysis. (a) Skeletal age 3 years; (b) 6 years, female; (c) early adolescent; (d) late adolescent. Left row – lateral surfaces. Right row – medial surfaces.

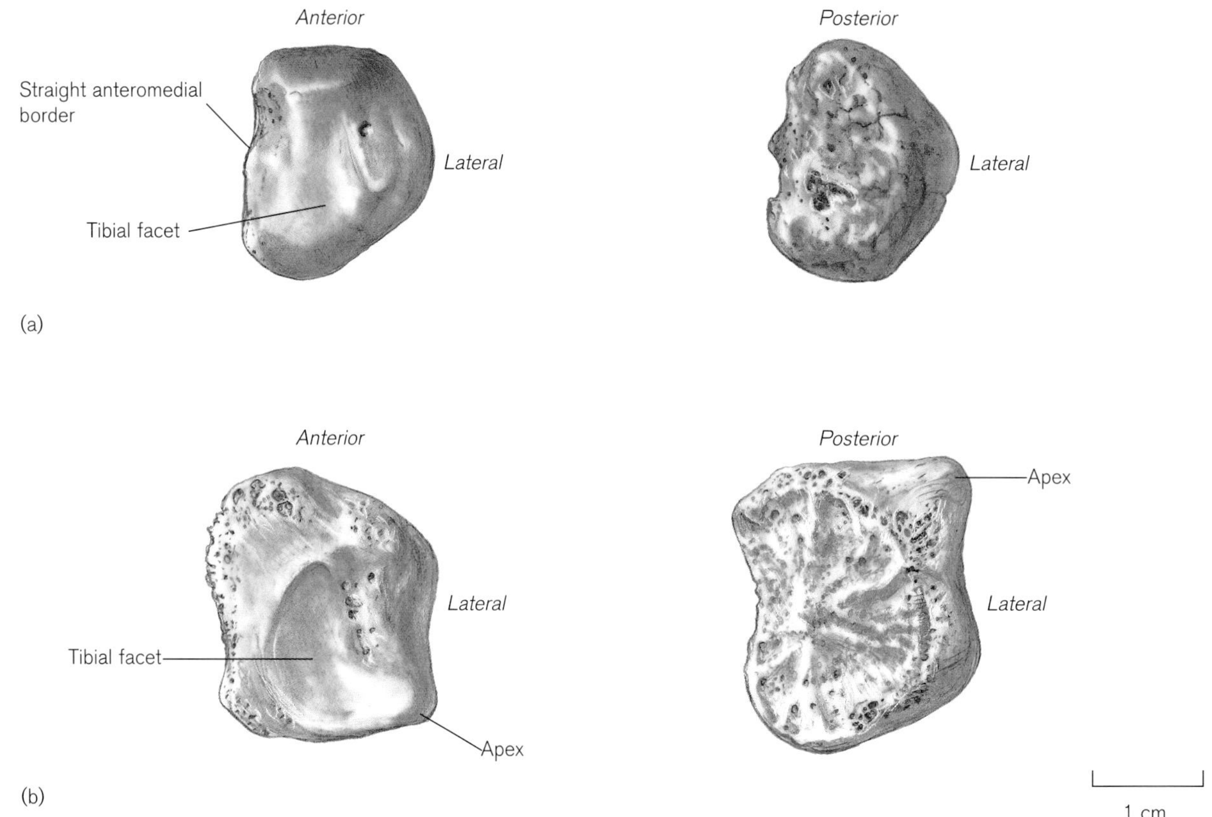

Figure 11.28 Development of the right proximal fibular epiphysis: (a) 12 years, male; (b) late adolescent. Left row – articular surfaces. Right row – metaphyseal surfaces.

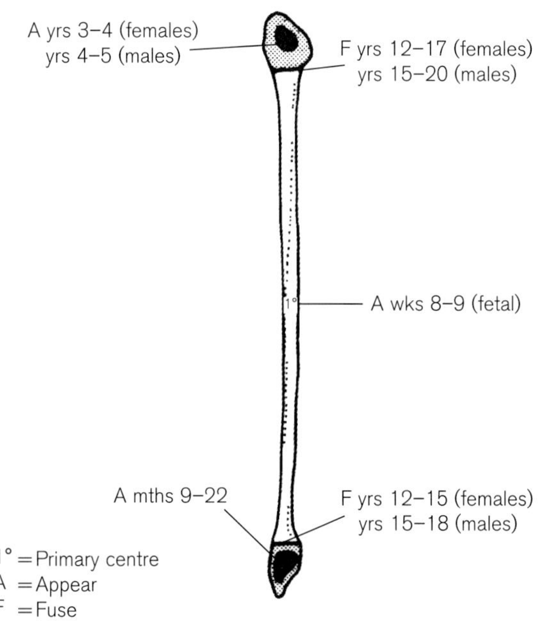

Figure 11.29 Appearance and fusion times of the fibular ossification centres.

Practical notes

Orientation and sideing

Diaphysis – owing to its fragility, the fibula is the least likely long bone to survive inhumation intact. Even if complete, it is the most difficult of the perinatal long bones to side as it is relatively featureless and may be poorly marked. Proximodistal orientation depends on recognizing the slightly flared and comparatively rounded proximal shaft with a circular metaphyseal surface. The distal half of the shaft is flattened, ending in a more oval or triangular metaphyseal surface. Several features may help to distinguish the medial and lateral sides of the bone. Nutrient foramina are nearly always found on the medial side, which may also show an interosseous border in the middle third. The roughened triangle for the inferior part of the posterior tibiofibular ligament runs distally from anterior to posterior on the medial side. The division of the sharp anterior border at the distal end to form the subcutaneous triangle may be seen on the lateral side. The distal metaphyseal surface slopes down posteriorly (Fig. 11.25).

Distal epiphysis – with the metaphyseal surface facing superiorly, the flat surface is medial and the malleolar fossa is posterior (Fig. 11.27b, c).

Proximal epiphysis – this is probably not recognizable until mid-childhood when its distinctive features have developed. The tibial facet and the straight border face anteromedially and the apex projects posterolaterally (Fig. 11.28b).

Bones of a similar morphology

Perinatal diaphyses – of the diaphyses of the six major long bones from any one individual, the radius, ulna and fibula are shorter and look less robust than the femur, humerus and tibia (Table 11.1). The fibula and ulna are of similar length but the ulna, although shorter is more bulky with its characteristic proximal end. The fibula is straight, narrow and relatively featureless.

Proximal and distal fibular fragments – both these can be difficult to distinguish from each other, a distal ulna or possibly a distal radius. The fibular proximal shaft is rounded and the metaphyseal surface is circular. The distal fibular shaft is flattened mediolaterally and triangles can usually be discerned on the medial and lateral surfaces (see above). Both the upper limb bones are more robust than the fibula. The distal ulna is slightly curved anteriorly and has a notch posteriorly. The distal radius is flared, curved anteriorly and has a larger metaphyseal surface than either the fibula or ulna (Fig. 9.17).

Morphological summary (Fig. 11.29)

Fetal

Wk 8	Primary ossification centre appears in the shaft
Birth	Represented by shaft only
9–22 mths	Distal secondary centre appears
During 4th yr	Proximal centre appears in girls
During 5th yr	Proximal centre appears in boys
During 8th yr	Styloid process ossifies in girls
During 11th yr	Styloid process ossifies in boys
12–15 yrs	Distal epiphysis fuses in females
15–18 yrs	Distal epiphysis fuses in males
12–17 yrs	Proximal epiphysis fuses in females
15–20 yrs	Proximal epiphysis fuses in males

Metrics

Lengths of fetal bones were recorded by Fazekas and Kósa (1978 – Table 11.15) and the length of the fetal fibula as measured by ultrasound is taken from Jeanty (1983) (Table 11.16). Data showing the length of the fibula at 6-monthly intervals (2-monthly for the first half year) from birth to the cessation of growth (Table 11.17) are taken from Maresh (1970).

There is a little fibular diaphyseal length data from archaeological populations from Africa, Europe and North America and these are given in Appendix 3. Most of the age at death estimates are based on dental development.

Table 11.15 Length of the fetal fibular diaphysis

Age (weeks)	Length (mm)
12	6.0
14	9.9
16	16.7
18	22.6
20	27.8
22	31.1
24	34.3
26	36.5
28	40.0
30	42.8
32	46.8
34	50.5
36	51.6
38	57.6
40	62.0

Adapted from Fazekas and Kósa (1978).

Table 11.16 Length of the fetal fibula as measured on ultrasound

	Length (mm)		
	Percentile		
Age (weeks)	5th	50th	95th
12	–	5	–
14	6	11	10
16	6	17	22
18	10	22	28
20	18	27	30
22	21	31	37
24	26	35	41
26	32	39	43
28	36	43	47
30	38	47	52
32	40	50	56
34	46	52	56
36	51	55	56
38	54	57	59
40	54	59	62

Adapted from Jeanty (1983).

Table 11.17 Fibular length (mm) – 2 months–18 years

	Male			Female		
Age (years)	*n*	Mean	SD	*n*	Mean	SD
Diaphyseal length						
0.125	59	68.1	5.3	69	66.8	4.4
0.25	58	78.6	4.9	65	77.1	4.1
0.50	67	87.2	4.8	78	84.9	5.2
1.00	72	107.1	5.5	81	105.0	5.1
1.5	68	123.9	6.2	84	121.3	5.9
2.0	68	138.1	6.7	84	136.0	6.8
2.5	72	150.7	7.1	82	147.9	7.1
3.0	72	162.1	7.7	79	159.4	7.9
3.5	73	171.6	9.6	78	169.6	8.3
4.0	72	181.8	8.7	80	179.5	9.1
4.5	71	190.8	8.8	78	189.4	10.2
5.0	77	200.4	9.6	80	198.6	11.1
5.5	73	209.0	10.2	74	206.5	11.7
6.0	71	217.5	9.6	75	216.0	12.2
6.5	72	226.0	10.5	81	224.3	13.4
7.0	71	234.2	11.3	86	232.1	13.4
7.5	76	242.1	11.8	83	240.8	14.5
8.0	70	251.0	12.4	85	248.8	14.8
8.5	72	257.7	11.8	82	256.1	15.2
9.0	76	265.6	13.0	83	263.7	16.3
9.5	78	273.8	13.8	83	272.2	17.6
10.0	77	281.3	13.9	84	279.4	18.3
10.5	76	287.8	14.6	75	287.2	20.4
11.0	75	294.9	14.6	76	294.4	19.8
11.5	76	301.7	16.0	75	303.8	20.7
12.0	73	310.1	16.4	71	311.1	20.8
Total length including epiphyses						
10.0	76	310.4	15.2	83	307.9	19.5
10.5	76	318.0	16.2	75	316.7	21.8
11.0	75	326.2	15.9	76	324.7	21.5
11.5	77	334.0	17.6	74	334.6	22.1
12.0	76	342.8	18.0	75	344.6	22.7
12.5	67	351.9	16.8	65	351.0	22.2
13.0	69	360.2	19.8	69	358.5	21.9
13.5	69	371.1	21.4	62	363.4	21.4
14.0	69	380.3	21.3	64	367.9	20.6
14.5	64	388.5	22.5	42	368.9	21.5
15.0	60	395.3	21.5	57	370.2	20.0
15.5	52	404.4	22.1	12	375.7	25.8
16.0	60	406.3	21.7	40	372.4	21.5
16.5	38	408.6	22.8	3	–	–
17.0	50	410.4	22.6	18	366.8	24.2
18.0	28	412.8	24.2	4	–	–

Adapted from Maresh (1970).

V. THE FOOT

It is not clear where the origin of the word 'foot' lies, although it may be derived from Old English via a Germanic source (Fuss). The Latin equivalent is *pes*, hence the derivation of words such as pedal, pedestrian and pedicure and the Greek equivalent is *podos*, hence words such as podium, chiropody and podiatry.[11] However, there is some confusion over the origin of words such as pedicle, pediculus and peduncle, which do not mean 'little foot' but seem to take their origin from the Latin *pedis* which pertains to a louse, and so the imagery is somewhat obscure. Holden (1882) described the foot as *pes altera manus*, which translates as 'the other hand'.[12] It is clear, however, that the integral design of the foot is not as a dextrous appendage, but rather as a stable means of support and locomotion (Hall, 1994). Yet, it is obvious from the pedal abilities of thalidomide victims in particular, that a considerable degree of dexterity can be achieved when it is necessary.

The foot is often given but slight attention in anthropological investigations and is even considered to be the 'Cinderella' of orthopaedics (Helal and Wilson, 1988), but Jones (1946) accredited its value as being beyond that of any other component of the human skeleton for the elucidation of what is truly 'man'.

> *Man's foot is all his own. It is unlike any other foot. It is the most distinctly human part of his anatomical make-up. It is a human specialisation and whether he be proud of it or not, it is his hallmark and so long as Man has been Man and so long as he remains Man, it is by his feet that he will be known from all other members of the animal kingdom.*

Perhaps this is somewhat of an overexuberant viewpoint, but it is certainly true that the skeletal components of the foot play a vital role in the characterization of what is considered to be anthropologically 'human'.

It is not only the foot itself but also the prints that it leaves behind, that has been studied extensively[13] and they may be used as an indirect means to examine posture, gait and prehensility in extinct forms

[11]The term 'Oedipus' literally means 'swollen foot'. His father (Laius) attempted to kill the infant Oedipus by piercing his feet with a spike. He was subsequently abandoned and survived only to have his feet crushed by the wheels of a carriage driven by Laius. Noted for his swollen and deformed feet, Oedipus unwittingly killed his father and married his mother thereby leading to Freud's classical description of the Oedipus complex.

[12]A whimsical condition has been allegedly attributed to HRH Duke of Edinburgh, who is reported to have said that he suffers from dentopedology – the art of putting one's foot in one's mouth!

[13]Incredibly, there is an 'International Footprint Association'!

(Blanc, 1952; Molleson *et al.*, 1972; White, 1980; Behrensmeyer and Laporte, 1981; Day and Wickens, 1981; Leakey and Hay, 1987; Day, 1991). However, footprints can also prove to be an essential source of evidence in medicolegal investigations (Robbins, 1976, 1985; Barker, 1991; Barker and Scheuer, 1998).

The individual bones of the foot cannot be examined in detail without some understanding of the functional involvement of the structure as a whole. The foot is said to subserve two main functions – to support the weight of the body while standing, and to act as a mechanism of propulsion in locomotion (Tachdjian, 1972). Because of its dual action, the structure of the foot requires to be able to dissipate forces and act as a strong lever, yet maintain pliability. This is primarily achieved through:

- segmentation of the structure of the foot
- the presence of arches, which facilitate both support and elasticity
- the presence of tie and beam connections via ligaments and muscles.

However, the foot not only operates in the plane of plantar and dorsiflexion (flexion and extension) but must also maintain the ability to evert and invert to allow the foot to mould to uneven surfaces. Although the foot does maintain some mobility, it has been greatly sacrificed for the stability of the structure, as through evolution it has altered its principal function from a grasping to a supportive role. All primates except the Tupaiidae and the Hominidae possess opposable big toes and apart from the tree shrews, man is the only primate who does not possess a divergent big toe (Napier, 1957). To transfer a grasping organ into a supportive one requires the great toe to be brought into line with the long axis of the foot (it should be borne in mind that the axis of the foot passes along the line of the second toe). Due to its propulsive role the first toe becomes more robust, while the others, which serve only in a supportive role, tend to regress. This almost accessory role of the lesser toes can be clearly seen following amputation. Amputation of a single toe (other than the first) results in little disturbance to either stance or gait. Amputation of all the toes is a radical surgical procedure that is adopted only when absolutely necessary and tends to occur following severe trauma, an attempt to limit gangrenous damage or to counteract progressive painful deformities of the toes (Andrews, 1988). However, it should be said that following recovery from surgery, the patient often experiences little impairment when either standing or walking, but it is only in hurried movement that limping and an awkwardness of gait becomes appreciable (Andrews, 1988; Thomas *et al.*, 1988).[14]

The foot is separated into three segments, which are more radiologically than functionally derived, although they correspond closely to favoured amputation lines (Figs. 11.30–11.33). The 'hindfoot' comprises the talus, calcaneus and navicular, the 'midfoot' comprises the cuneiforms and cuboid and the 'forefoot' comprises the metatarsals and phalanges. Segmentation bestows considerable flexibility on the structure as a whole and allows it to withstand proportionally greater forces than if it were a rigid structure. While standing, the arches sink, the bones lock together and the ligaments are at maximum strength so that the foot becomes an immobile pedestal. When walking commences, weight is released from the arches, which then unlock, transforming the foot into a mobile system of levers (Ellis, 1992). The arching system of the foot is unique to man and is visible even from a very early developmental stage. Although the immature footprint appears to be flat, with no evidence of arches, it is in fact only because the concavity is filled with fatty connective tissue that will eventually disappear around 2 years of age. It has often been said that the shape of the arches is only maintained by the ligaments and the shape of the bones but it is clear from clinical studies that the most common cause of flat footedness is muscle weakness. Therefore, maintenance of the arches is via a complex ligamentous musculoskeletal mechanism and it is advised that more specific texts be examined if further details are required (Jones 1946; Frazer, 1948; Hicks, 1953, 1954; Smith, 1954; Sarrafian, 1983; Williams *et al.*, 1995).

The **medial arch** consists of the calcaneus, talus, navicular, medial cuneiform and medial three metatarsals (Fig. 11.33). It is responsible for transmitting the full thrust from the tibia and transferring it backwards to the calcaneus and forwards through the navicular and medial cuneiform to the metatarsals. The **lateral arch** consists of the calcaneus, cuboid and lateral two metatarsals (Fig. 11.32). As it is lower and less mobile than the medial arch, its primary function is to transmit weight and thrust and so provide a steady base. The so-called **transverse arch** does not really exist as a true supportive structure as half the arch is formed from each foot by the respective cuboid and cuneiforms and therefore only becomes an arch when the two feet are placed side-by-side during standing.

[14]This surgical procedure has become known as the 'Pobble amputation', after the character in Edward Lear's (1812–1888) classical humorous poem of the same name, which carries the line 'It's a fact the whole world knows, That Pobbles are happier without their toes'.

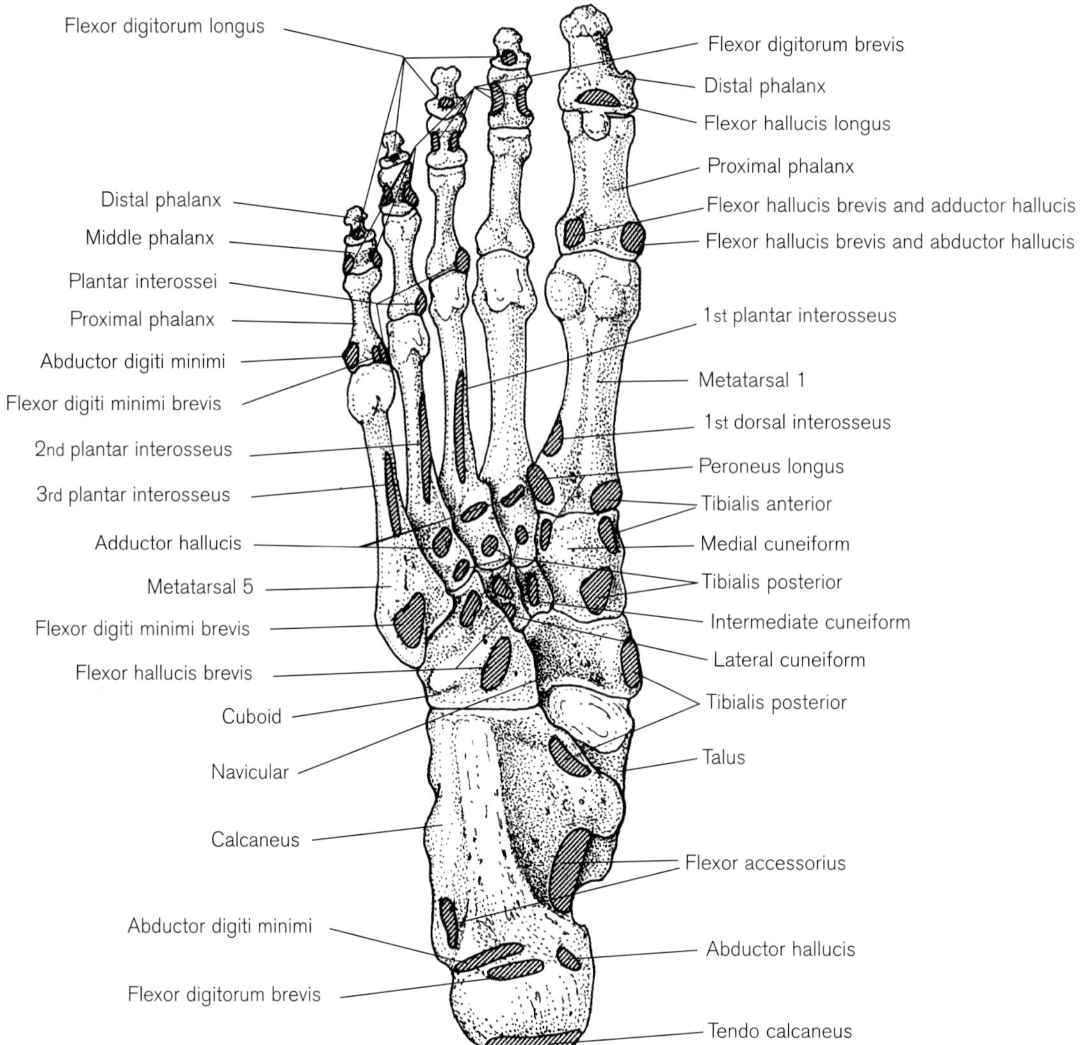

Figure 11.30 The plantar surface of the right adult foot showing sites of muscle attachment.

The adult foot

The foot articulates with the leg at the ankle (talocrural) joint and is formed from 28 constant bones – seven tarsals, five metatarsals, fourteen phalanges and two sesamoids (Figs. 11.30–11.33).

Tarsals

The **tarsals** are essentially grouped into proximal and distal rows.[15] The proximal row comprises the talus and calcaneus, while the distal row comprises the three cuneiforms and the cuboid, with the navicular as an additional intermediate element.

The **talocrural** (ankle) **joint** is effectively a uni-axial synovial hinge joint between the talus and the lower end of the tibia and its medial malleolus medially and the lateral malleolus of the fibula laterally. Although the joint is considered to be uni-axial for the sake of simplicity, there is also some degree of dynamic movement in a rotational plane (Sammarco, 1977; Lundberg *et al.*, 1989). Active movements of the joint include dorsiflexion of approximately 10° and plantar flexion of approximately 20°. The strong ligaments and the close-packed nature of the joint ensure that it rarely dislocates, but if it does, then in the adult it normally involves an associated malleolar fracture (Detenbeck and Kelly, 1969). The most usual pattern

[15]The origin of the term 'tarsus' is somewhat obscure. It is thought to be derived from the Greek meaning a frame of wickerwork or flat basket used for drying cheeses. It is unlikely to have any origin from the ancient city of the same name in Cilicia made famous by Anthony and Cleopatra, although the city was built on a flat and open plain. The term became synonymous with any object that was flattened or expanded and so was first used by Galen (*c.* AD 180) to refer to the flat part of the foot or hand (Field and Harrison, 1957).

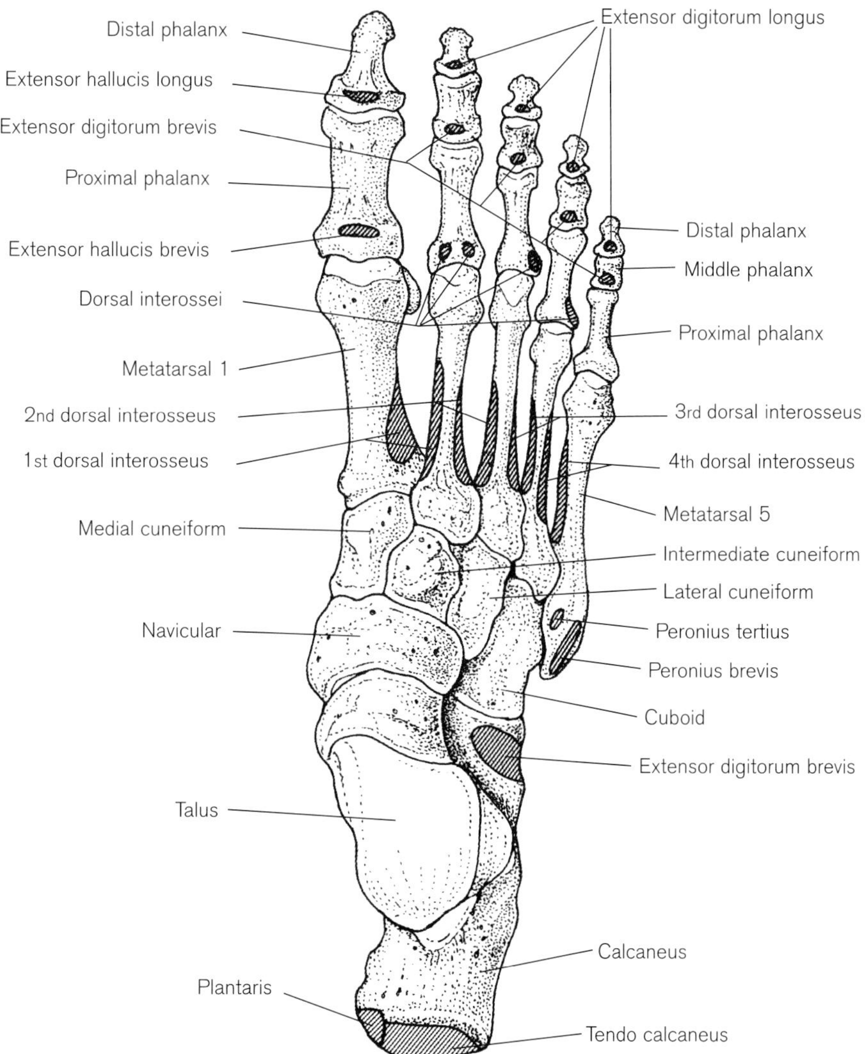

Figure 11.31 The dorsal surface of the right adult foot showing sites of muscle attachment.

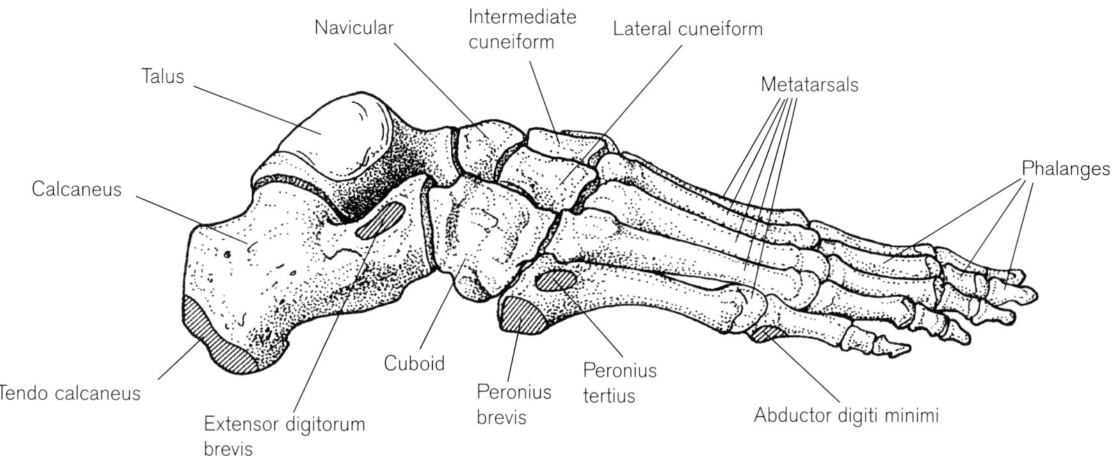

Figure 11.32 The lateral aspect of the right adult foot showing sites of muscle attachment.

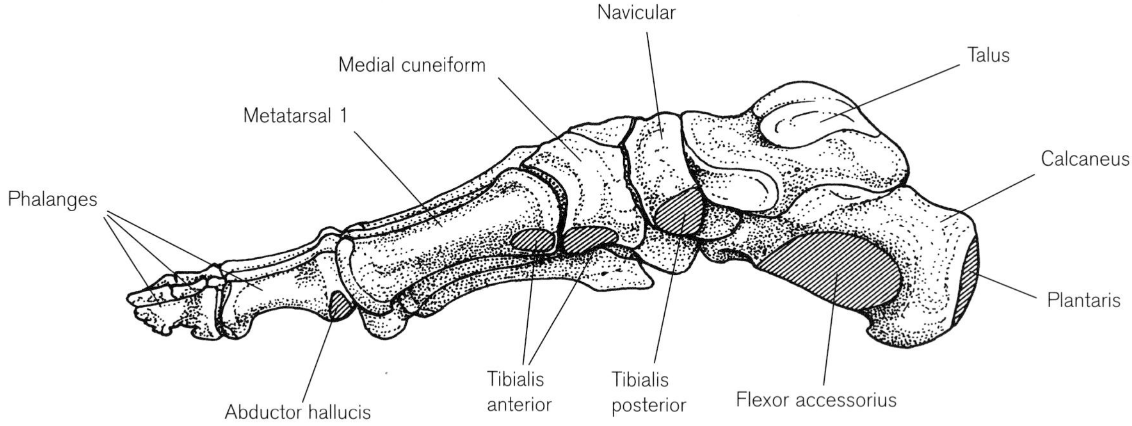

Figure 11.33 The medial aspect of the right adult foot showing sites of muscle attachment.

of fracture in the ankle follows an abduction–extension rotation injury (e.g. foot in a rabbit hole), where there is a torsional fracture of the lateral malleolus, avulsion of the medial collateral ligaments, possible avulsion of a small part of the medial malleolus and shearing of the lower end of the tibia against the talus resulting in a Pott's fracture (Ellis, 1992).

Of the intertarsal joints, the **subtalar joint** (talocalcaneal) is probably the most important as this is the principal site of movement during inversion and eversion of the foot (Manter, 1941; Shepard, 1951). Movement at the joint occurs in a screw-like fashion around an axis of rotation (Brantigan *et al.*, 1977). A rigid subtalar joint is a relatively common clinical condition, which can often occur as a result of osteoarthritis. The inability to effectively evert and invert the foot dramatically affects the efficiency of locomotion (Bower *et al.*, 1989). Dislocation of this joint is not common, but tends to occur following violent trauma to the region of the ankle and hindfoot (El-Khoury *et al.*, 1982). The joint is firmly bound by strong interosseous ligaments and if they tear, then avascular necrosis of the talus can result, as its blood supply runs with the ligaments (Haliburton *et al.*, 1958; Gelberman and Mortensen, 1983; Kanagasuntheram *et al.*, 1987; Goldie, 1988). Avascular necrosis can also arise as a direct result of fracture through the neck of the talus. In earlier times this was called an 'aviator's fracture', as it tends to arise following a fall from a great height. (It should be said that this term was only of any diagnostic value when the accident was not fatal!)

Although the tarsal bones are said to be homologous with the carpals and it is agreed that there is a fundamental unity of plan, the differences are such that we will consider each tarsal bone separately and refrain from discussing similarities or differences with individual carpal bones (Baur, 1885; Bardeleben, 1894; Broom, 1904; Lewis, 1964).

The **talus** is the site of the articular link between the foot and the lower leg. As such, it is required to bear the entire body weight during walking and standing and it has been calculated that the compressive forces that pass across the joint can in fact reach as much as five times body weight (Stauffer *et al.*, 1977). Interest has therefore been expressed in the lines of stress within the cancellous bone that represent the dissipation of compressive forces and the centre of the talus has been recognized as a junctional region for force distribution (Manter, 1946; Bacon *et al.*, 1984; Sinha, 1985; Pal and Routal, 1998).

The term 'talus' is derived from the Latin for 'ankle bone' and was often referred to as the 'astragalus' (see Chapter 6).[16] It is the only bone in the lower limb that has no muscular attachments (Detenbeck and Kelly, 1969), although it does have extensive ligamentous attachments. It serves a pivotal role in the foot, being involved in many articulations and it consists of a body, neck and head (Sewell 1904a, 1904b, 1905).

The **body** bears a concavo-convex (trochlear) articular facet on its superior surface for articulation with the inferior aspect of the tibia. It is strongly convex in the anteroposterior direction, gently concave in the mediolateral plane and wider distally than proximally. The superior articular surface is continuous medially with that for the medial malleolus of the tibia and laterally with that for the lateral malleolus of the fibula. The medial articulation for the tibia is said to be comma-shaped, wider distally than proximally and

[16]The astragalus was a rounded piece of bone used as a gambling die. The game was played with four tali and the best cast was a 'Venus', which offered different numbers on all four tali. The worst cast was a 'canis', with the number 1 only on each talus (Goldie, 1988).

gently concave. The lateral articulation for the fibular malleolus is larger than that on the medial aspect and is roughly triangular in outline and vertically concave. This articular surface extends inferiorly towards the apex or lateral process to which is attached the lateral talocalcaneal ligament. The posterior surface of the body is small and ends in two processes or tubercles (medial and lateral) between which is an oblique groove formed by the flexor hallucis longus tendon. If the lateral tubercle becomes particularly well developed it is often referred to as 'Stieda's process' (Wakeley *et al.*, 1996). The plantar surface of the body articulates with the calcaneus via an obliquely orientated concave facet and is separated from the plantar surface of the head by a deep groove (sulcus tali), which forms the roof of the **sinus tarsi**. The interosseous talocalcaneal and cervical ligaments occupy this space.

The **head** of the talus bears articular facets distally for the navicular and inferiorly and medially for the calcaneus. The distal articular surface is oval and convex with its long axis directed inferomedially to articulate with the navicular. The head of the talus rests on the **sustentaculum tali** (Latin meaning 'prop or support'), which is a shelf-like medially orientated projection from the distal part of the upper surface of the calcaneus. Some anatomical texts state that there are three distinct articular surfaces between the head of the talus and the calcaneus (Frazer, 1948; Williams *et al.*, 1995). However in reality, they are often very difficult to differentiate and the most common pattern is for the facet to form a continuous elongated oval shape, which is convex and orientated anteromedially (Gupta *et al.*, 1977).

The **neck** of the talus is the narrow region of bone between the body and the head. Its axis is inclined distally and medially and allegedly makes an angle of approximately 150° with the body. The angle is reported to be only between 130–140° in the new born, which is thought to account in part for the inverted appearance of the neonatal foot. The increasing angle of the neck is then associated with the change in the shape of the foot as it comes into contact with the ground in preparation for walking at about 10–12 months. So-called accessory 'squatting facets' have been reported in the dorsolateral region of the neck and are thought to indicate sites of articulation with the anterior tibial margin in extreme dorsiflexion of the ankle joint (Aitken, 1905). Facets can occur on either the medial or lateral sides of the dorsal surface of the neck of the talus, although those on the lateral side are more common (Thomson, 1889; Trinkaus, 1975; Finnegan, 1978; Oygucu *et al.*, 1998). Squatting facets occur more frequently in Asian and native Australian populations than in either Europeans or Americans (Barnett, 1954b; Singh, 1959b; Rao, 1966), although in Europeans there appears to be a higher frequency in fetuses than in adults (Barnett, 1954b; Bunning and Barnett, 1965).

The **calcaneus** (os calcis) is the largest of the tarsal bones.[17] It is an irregularly shaped, six-sided bone that articulates superiorly with the talus and anteriorly and laterally with the cuboid (Laidlaw, 1904, 1905). It has proved to be of some value in the identification of sex and race (Singh and Singh, 1975; Steele, 1976; Holland, 1995; Riepert et al, 1996). Interestingly, it has also been used as a predictor of limb dominance. Webber and Garnett (1976) showed that the trabecular structure was greatest in the calcaneus on the side of the dominant hand and they found this dominance to be present before birth. Other authors state, however, that side dominance in the upper limb does not usually correspond with side dominance in the lower limb (Pande and Singh, 1971). The trabecular structure of the calcaneus has also been used to assess bone mineral loss in osteoporotic conditions, as part of the bone is readily accessible to radiographic and densitometric assessment (Ahl *et al.*, 1988; Baran *et al.*, 1988). The calcaneus is also susceptible to microfractures (also known as stress or march fractures), particularly in service men and athletes, where the cancellous struts can be broken by the force of pounding feet on a hard surface (Devas, 1988; Woolf and Dixon, 1988). These microfractures tend to be temporary and will usually repair with time and adequate rest. Actual clinical fracture of the calcaneus is rare (incidence of between 2 and 2.5%), tends not to be well managed and as a result, the prognosis is poor (Fisk, 1988).[18] The patterns of calcaneal fracture are many and varied but tend to result from a fall onto the heel from a height and so are predominantly industrial and therefore male-related injuries.

The **superior surface** can be separated into three distinct regions – the area behind the ankle joint, the facets of the talocrural joint and the area distal and lateral to them, which is partly articular and partly traversed by the **sinus calcanei,** which forms the floor of the sinus tarsi (Smith, 1958; Bunning, 1964). The area posterior to the ankle joint projects backwards as the heel of the foot and is covered by fibro-adipose tissue. This area acts as a strong, short lever for the attachment of the plantar flexor muscles of the calf

[17]The term 'calcaneus' is derived either from the Latin 'calx' meaning a 'heel', 'calceo' meaning a 'shoe' or 'calcar' meaning a 'spur'.
[18]In fact it has been said that 'The man who breaks his heel is done for as far as his industrial future is concerned' Cotton and Henderson (1916) *Am J Ortho Surg* 14: 290.

(gastrocnemius and soleus – also known collectively as the triceps surae) via the tendo calcaneus. This is both the thickest and strongest tendon in the human body and the spiral arrangement of its fibres permits some storage of energy that can be released during the appropriate phase of locomotion (White, 1943; Alexander and Vernon, 1975). The inconstant plantaris muscle (from the Latin 'planta' meaning a shoot or a twig) may also attach to the calcaneus via the common tendon or it may have a separate attachment to the more medial aspect of the posterior surface (Daseler and Anson, 1943). The middle third of the superior surface bears the oval, convex articular facet for the talus, which is set at an oblique angle and is directed inferolaterally. Distal and medial to the sinus calcanei is an elongated, raised strip of articular bone that sits on the sustentaculum tali and articulates with the long facet on the plantar surface of the anterior aspect of the talus (Bunning and Barnett, 1965). This articular surface may be continuous or separated into two or even three distinct articular areas (Bunning and Barnett, 1963; Forriol Campos and Gomez Pellico, 1989).

The **anterior surface** is the smallest of the calcaneal surfaces and is represented by a concavo-convex articular facet for the cuboid (Bojsen-Møller, 1979). The lateral aspect of this facet is wider than the medial, which passes deep to the sustentaculum tali to articulate with the so-called calcaneal process of the cuboid. The **posterior surface** is separated into three distinct transverse regions and is narrower above than below. The superior region is smooth and separated from the tendo calcaneus by a bursa and fibro-adipose tissue. The middle area, which is also smooth, is limited above and below by obvious horizontal ridges, and is the site of attachment of the tendo calcaneus.[19] Calcification of the tendon (calcaneal spurring) is one of the common diagnostic criteria found in DISH (diffuse idiopathic skeletal hyperostosis or Forestier's disease). Although most standard anatomical texts state that the middle area is the site of tendon attachment, there is some evidence to suggest that it extends more proximally (Protheroe, 1969). The inferior section, which is rough and vertically striated, is the subcutaneous weight-bearing region and extends onto the plantar surface.

[19]The tendo calcaneus is, of course, also known as the Achilles tendon. Achilles was a Greek hero and the son of Peleus and Thetis. The legend states that to render her son's body invincible, Thetis dipped the infant Achilles into the river Styx holding him by the right heel. The sacred water therefore did not reach this part and so when injured in the heel by an arrow (fired by Paris but supposedly guided by Apollo) he subsequently died from his wounds during the storming of the city of Troy. The term was first used in anatomy by Verheyen in 1693, who was the infamous surgeon that dissected his own amputated leg. The name 'Achilles' actually means 'lipless'.

The **plantar surface** is rough but relatively featureless, apart from the medial and lateral processes of the calcaneal tuberosity, which are more distally located and separated by a notch. While standing, the calcaneus rests solely on the tubercles with the anterior part of the bone raised off the ground. Weidenreich (1940) proposed that erect posture forces the heel down onto the ground and so the tuberosity of the calcaneus and the medial and lateral tubercles take on the role of supporting body weight. The medial tubercle is always larger than the lateral and Weidenreich suggested that, in the more primitive anthropoids, the lateral tubercle is more distally located and further removed from the calcaneal tuberosity. However, as the anthropoids became more highly developed and bipedal locomotion predominated, so the two moved closer together. He explained this change in position in accordance with the shift in the centre of gravity that occurs with upright posture. The medial tubercle gives rise to the abductor hallucis and flexor digitorum brevis muscles, the plantar aponeurosis and the superficial part of the flexor retinaculum. The abductor digiti minimi muscle is attached to both the medial and lateral tubercles. Tibialis posterior is partly attached to the distal region of the plantar surface of the sustentaculum tali.

About half way along the **lateral surface** is the peroneal tubercle, which has an oblique inferior groove for the peroneus longus tendon and a shallower more proximal one for the peroneus brevis tendon. This tubercle is variable both in size and location and may in fact be absent (Edwards, 1928). Above and behind this tubercle is the retrotrochlear eminence for the attachment of the calcaneofibular ligament. This protuberance is often larger than the peroneal tubercle and more constant in appearance (Meyer and O'Rahilly, 1976). The extensor digitorum brevis muscle originates in front of the groove for the peroneus brevis tendon and can be palpated in the living as a small elevation, just distal to the lateral malleolus when the toes are dorsiflexed.

The **medial surface** is characterized by a concavity that is accentuated by the presence of the sustentaculum tali, which can be palpated in the living, immediately distal to the tip of the medial malleolus. The plantar surface of the sustentaculum tali is grooved by the passage of the tendon of the flexor hallucis longus and the margins of the groove give attachment to the flexor retinaculum. Below and behind this groove is the site of attachment of the medial head of the flexor accessorius (quadratus plantae) muscle. Numerous vascular foramina are to be found on this surface and it is said that they are predominantly arterial in origin, while those on the lateral surface are mainly venous in nature (Frazer, 1948).

The **navicular** (scaphoid) derives its name from the Latin meaning a 'little ship' in reference to the scooped-out appearance of its proximal articular surface, which has also been referred to as the acetabulum pedis. It is interposed between the head of the talus proximally and the three cuneiforms distally. The **proximal articular surface** is oval and concave with its long axis facing downwards and medially. The diameter of the surface is wider in its upper lateral aspect than in its lower medial area, where it tapers to an apex. The **distal articular surface** is convex in the transverse plane and separated into three virtually triangular regions for articulation with each of the cuneiforms. The facet for the medial cuneiform is usually the largest. The **dorsal surface** is roughened for ligamentous attachments and convex both proximodistally and mediolaterally. The **medial surface** is also rough in appearance and terminates in a tuberosity that can be palpated in the living and is the principal site of attachment for the tibialis posterior tendon. The tuberosity is a common site for avulsion fracture (Hooper and Hughes, 1988), which should not be confused with the accessory 'os tibiale externum' (see below). The **plantar surface** is also rough in appearance and is separated from the tuberosity by a groove through which passes part of the tibialis posterior tendon to attach to the distal bones of the foot. The surface can on occasion bear a small articular facet for the calcaneus. The **lateral surface** is irregular in appearance and often bears an articular facet for the cuboid. Fractures of the navicular become more common with age and are particularly prevalent in golf players, where the foot is in equinus and body weight placed on the dorsiflexed forefoot (Main and Jowett, 1975). In this position, the navicular is compressed against the cuneiforms and the head of the talus and fractures vertically along the shearing planes in line with one of the intercuneiform joints (Main and Jowett, 1975; Devas, 1988).

The **medial cuneiform** (Latin meaning 'wedge-shaped') is the largest of the cuneiforms and articulates proximally with the medial facet on the distal extremity of the navicular, distally with the base of the first metatarsal and laterally with the intermediate cuneiform. The **proximal surface** bears a concave, triangular articular facet that is wider below than above. The **distal surface** has a convex, roughly kidney-shaped articular surface (hilum), which faces laterally, with the larger of the surfaces being dorsal and the smaller, plantar. It has a rough, narrow, triangular **dorsal surface** for ligamentous attachment and a subcutaneous vertically convex **medial surface** whose distal plantar angle bears an impression caused by the tendon of tibialis anterior, which has an attachment to both the medial and plantar surfaces. This smooth oval facet is partly for the insertion of the tendon and partly for a bursa that sits under a sesamoid cartilage in the fibres that are passing over it to reach their insertion into the first metatarsal. The **plantar surface** receives tendinous slips from both the tibialis posterior and peroneus longus muscles. The **lateral surface** has both articular and non-articular regions. A virtually right-angled articular strip is present along the proximal and dorsal margins for the intermediate cuneiform that is separated from a small square area at the dorsodistal corner for articulation with the medial surface of the second metatarsal base. The remainder of this surface is rough for the attachment of interosseous ligaments.

The **intermediate cuneiform** is the smallest of the three and articulates with the base of the second metatarsal distally, the navicular proximally, the lateral cuneiform laterally and the medial cuneiform medially. Both the **distal** and **proximal surfaces** are triangular with their bases along the dorsal surface and a slight concavity facing laterally. While the distal articular surface is virtually planar, the proximal tends to be slightly concave. The **lateral surface** has a concave L-shaped articular strip along the proximal and dorsal borders, with the remainder being rough for attachment of strong interosseous ligaments. The **medial surface** also has an L-shaped articular strip (which may be separated into two distinct areas) along the proximal and dorsal margins, for articulation with the medial cuneiform. Again, the remainder of the surface is given over to the attachment of the strong interosseous ligaments. The **dorsal surface** is roughly square in outline and rough for ligamentous attachment and the **plantar surface** is very narrow and simply receives a tendinous slip from the tibialis posterior muscle. The medial and lateral cuneiforms project distally beyond the intermediate, thereby forming a recess for the base of the second metatarsal (see below). The intermediate cuneiform is therefore the only one of the three to articulate with a single metatarsal.

The **lateral cuneiform** articulates with the second, third and fourth metatarsals distally, the navicular proximally, the intermediate cuneiform medially and the cuboid laterally. The **distal surface** is essentially triangular, with its base along the dorsal margin and its apex pointing in a plantar direction. There is a curved notch along the lateral border so that in truth the surface is more comma-shaped. The plantar aspect of the **proximal surface** is sharpened and rough for ligamentous attachment, while the dorsal aspect has an oval articular facet medially for the navicular and a ridge laterally, which separates it from the lateral surface of the bone. This articular surface is continuous with that on the **medial surface** for articulation with the intermediate cuneiform, which forms a roughly triangular surface on the proximal and dorsal margins. The remainder of this surface is roughened for interosseous ligamentous attachment except for a small articular notch in the dorsodistal corner for the second metatarsal. The **lateral surface** has a large oval concave facet in the proximal dorsal corner for articulation with the cuboid and a small concave facet in the dorsodistal corner for articulation with the base of the fourth metatarsal. The remainder of this surface is roughened for ligamentous attachment. The **dorsal surface** is rectangular in shape and the **plantar surface** is a narrow strip that receives a tendinous slip from the tibialis posterior and sometimes the flexor hallucis brevis muscles.

The **cuboid**, so-called because of its supposed cuboidal shape, is the largest and most lateral bone in the distal tarsal row. It articulates with the calcaneus proximally, the fourth and fifth metatarsals distally and with the lateral cuneiform (and occasionally the navicular) medially. The **distal surface** is divided vertically into a virtually rectangular surface medially for the base of the fourth metatarsal and a more triangular lateral area for the base of the fifth metatarsal. The **proximal surface** has a large, irregular concavo-convex articular surface for the calcaneus. The medial plantar angle of this surface projects proximally and inferior to the projecting distal end of the calcaneus (calcaneal process) to which is attached the expansion from the tibialis posterior muscle. Flexor hallucis brevis takes its origin from this expansion and from the surrounding bone. The **medial surface** is mostly non-articular but bears an oval facet for the lateral cuneiform and occasionally a small facet for the navicular. The **lateral surface** is a small, roughened area with a notch on its plantar edge, which is continuous with the oblique groove on the **plantar surface** for the tendon of peroneus longus. The groove ends laterally in a small tuberosity that may bear a facet for articulation with a sesamoid in the peroneal tendon. The **dorsal surface** really faces dorsolaterally and is roughened for ligamentous attachments.

Fracture of the cuboid is not common, but so-called 'nutcracker' fractures can occur following compression between the calcaneus and the bases of the fourth and fifth metatarsals (Hermel and Gershon-Cohen, 1953; Simonian *et al.*, 1995). This generally occurs when the front of the foot is fixed and the weight of the body is transmitted through the foot in plantar flexion. In adults, this tends to be a more common fracture pattern seen in females associated with a stumble or trip when wearing high-heeled shoes (Dewar and Evans, 1968).

Metatarsals

With the exception of the first, the metatarsals are long and slender, with robust bases and small heads. They all articulate proximally with the distal tarsal row via the tarsometatarsal synovial joints and distally with the bases of the proximal phalanges at the synovial metatarsophalangeal joints. Each is classified as a long bone and consists of a three-sided shaft, a large, relatively square proximal base and a small, laterally compressed distal head. The shaft is prismatic in cross-section and tapers gradually from the base to the head with a slight longitudinal curve so that the plantar aspect is concave and the dorsal surface is convex. Being a long bone, it is not surprising that the metatarsals have been utilized in both the determination of sex and stature (Byers *et al.*, 1989; Smith, 1997).

The first metatarsal is considerably more robust than the lateral four bones and this is as a direct result of its involvement in the toe-off phase of walking, where it is responsible for the thrust of forward propulsion and weight support. The remainder of the metatarsals offer a supportive role only, by preserving the balance of the body. There is therefore a tendency for the bones to reduce in size from medial to lateral. As such, the common length formula for the metatarsals is that metatarsal two is the longest, followed in decreasing order of size by the third, fourth, fifth and finally the first, which is the shortest (but most robust) (Aiello and Dean, 1990).

The arterial supply to the metatarsus has received quite a considerable amount of attention due the involvement of these bones in autonomic neuropathies such as leprosy (Brand, 1966; Jopling and McDougall, 1988). The position and direction of the nutrient foramina have been studied in an attempt to elucidate the origin of the arterial vessels supplying the bone (Huber, 1941; Jaworek, 1973; Shereff, 1991). This process is often undertaken via perfusion, using various substances such as acrylics, gelatin dyes, radio-opaque barium and polyester resins (Shereff *et al.*, 1987; Barker, 1993; Crock, 1996). Patake and Mysorekar (1977) concluded that each metatarsal normally possesses a single nutrient foramen in the middle third of the shaft, which is directed towards the head of the first metatarsal and the bases of the other four metatarsals. Ali (1991) found that the foramen is normally sited on the medial surface of the fifth metatarsal and on the lateral surfaces of the first and second bones. The position of the foramen in the third and fourth metatarsals was reported to be very variable.

The **first metatarsal** is the shortest but most robust of the metatarsals with a particularly wide diameter in the dorsoplantar plane, which enables the bone to resist the not inconsiderable bending stresses that occur during 'toe-off'. It articulates proximally with the medial cuneiform and distally with the first proximal phalanx. Although the proximal region of its lateral surface frequently comes into contact with the second metatarsal, it rarely forms an articular facet. The **shaft** is said to be prismatic in form with three surfaces that are separated by rounded borders. The dorsal surface is gently convex and generally unremarkable in appearance. The plantar (medial) surface is deeply concave in its proximal region and bounded laterally by a strong ridge that arches between the head and the base. The lateral surface is relatively flat distally and gently concave proximally and is the site of attachment of the medial head of the first dorsal interosseous muscle. The **base** of the first metatarsal is large and characteristically reniform in shape for articulation with the medial cuneiform. The convexity of the surface is along the medial border, and the concavity along the lateral border with the indentation (hilum) occurring closer to the plantar surface so that two articular facets are formed, with the plantar tending to be the smaller. A transverse ridge can often be seen traversing the articular surface so that two quite distinct concave articular facets are formed for the articulation with the medial cuneiform (Singh, 1960). Tibialis anterior attaches to the medial/plantar aspect of the base and peroneus longus attaches to a roughened oval prominence on the lateral aspect. The **head** is large and expanded in a mediolateral direction. The articular surface extends for some distance onto the dorsal aspect to permit a greater degree of dorsiflexion, which is important in the 'toe-off' phase of walking (Joseph, 1954). Ubelaker (1979) identified articular facets on the dorsal aspect of the metatarsal shafts in prehistoric remains from Ecuador and he considered these to be evidence of frequent kneeling, as such an occupation might involve extended periods of hyperdorsiflexion of the toes.

The distal articular surface extends even further onto the plantar surface and exhibits paired parallel deep grooves for the medial (tibial) and lateral (fibular) **sesamoid bones**, which are separated by an intersesamoidal ridge. The medial groove is invariably wider and deeper than the lateral groove. These are constant pedal sesamoids and after the patella, are the largest in the body (Pfitzner, 1892; Bizzaro, 1921). The medial sesamoid occurs in the combined tendon of the abductor hallucis and the medial head of the flexor hallucis brevis muscles, while the lateral is present in the combined tendon of the adductor hallucis and lateral head of the flexor hallucis brevis muscles. The medial sesamoid is typically larger than the more rounded and smaller lateral sesamoid and they are both concave on their dorsal aspect and convex on the plantar surface.[20] They are intracapsular and stabilized by a connecting thick fibrous intersesamoidal ligament, which forms a groove for the passage of the flexor hallucis longus tendon (Orr, 1918). In this location, the sesamoids serve to protect the long hallucial flexor tendon by forming a tunnel so that in weight-bearing, the tendon is spared and the forces are absorbed by the small sesamoids. The medial sesamoid tends to act as a shock absorber as it is located directly under the metatarsophalangeal joint and is therefore more likely to fracture, as it lies directly in the line of maximum weight transfer (Freiberg, 1920; Inge and Ferguson, 1933). Fractures tend to occur as a result of acute impact trauma or chronic weight-bearing stresses and are most common in athletes and new conscripts to the services (Potter *et al.*, 1992; Heim, *et al.*, 1997). The symptoms are disabling pain on walking, especially at the end of each step, when the toes are in dorsiflexion and body weight is transferred to the region of the ball of the foot (Powers, 1934). Congenital absence of the hallucial sesamoids is very rare and variation is more likely to be seen in the number of osseous components that make up the sesamoid structure (bipartite, tripartite or quadripartite). Repeated trauma to the sesamoids is most frequently seen in females who habitually wear high heels and spend prolonged periods standing or walking (Hubay, 1949).

The **second metatarsal** is the longest and articulates proximally with the three cuneiforms and the third metatarsal and distally with the proximal phalanx of the second toe. The **shaft** is roughly triangular in outline, being slightly flattened on its dorsal aspect, and gives attachment to the lateral head of the first dorsal interosseous on its medial aspect and to the medial head of the second dorsal interosseous on its lateral aspect. The **base** of this metatarsal projects

[20]The medial sesamoid has adopted mythical connotations and was referred to as the 'Luz' or 'Lus', a repository for the soul after death, by Rabbi Uschaia in the third century A.D. Casper Bauhimus wrote in the seventeenth century that this bone 'cannot be destroyed by fire, water or any other element, nor be broken or bruised by any force; this bone God shall, in his exceeding wisdom, water with the celestial dew, whence the other members shall be joined to it, coalescing to form the body, which, breathed upon by the Divine Spirit, shall be raised up alive' (Inge and Ferguson, 1933). This sesamoid is also called the 'albadaran' by Arabs with reference to its similarity to the small gold coins scattered to the assembly by a bride's mother to celebrate the wedding of her daughter (Helal, 1988)

further proximally than any of the others and so is wedged into a space bounded proximally by the intermediate cuneiform and mortised between the medial and lateral cuneiforms. This arrangement promotes stability and renders the second ray the stiffest and most stable in the foot (Manter, 1946; Sammarco, 1988). The articular facet for the intermediate cuneiform is triangular and slightly concave, with a constriction on the lateral aspect. The articular surface for the medial cuneiform tends to be restricted to a small area on the dorsomedial angle but it can be quite variable in size (Singh, 1960). The articular area for the lateral cuneiform may be single or paired and is usually continuous with the articular surfaces for the third metatarsal, although sometimes separated by a small ridge. The oblique head of the adductor hallucis attaches to the plantar surface of the base, as does a slip of the tibialis posterior tendon. The **head** is longer in its dorsoplantar than in its mediolateral plane and projects further onto the plantar surface via a lateral condyle. An inconstant sesamoid can occur at the second metatarsophalangeal (MTP) joint and tends to be located on the medial aspect of the head (Bizzaro, 1921; Holland, 1928; Burman and Lapidus, 1931; Lapidus, 1940). Bizzaro (1921) reported an incidence of 1–1.6% for this sesamoid. The lateral aspect of the head generally shows a well-developed site of attachment for the transverse metatarsal ligaments and the corresponding site is often not well marked on the medial side. Dorsal tubercles are present for the attachment of the strong collateral ligaments and generally the medial is the larger and more proximally located, to guide the ligament onto the first metatarsal.

The **third metatarsal** articulates distally with the proximal phalanx of the third toe and proximally with the lateral cuneiform and second and fourth metatarsals. The **shaft** is twisted along its long axis so that the articular surface of the head is not in the same plane as the more medial metatarsals, with the dorsal aspect being deflected medially and the plantar aspect laterally (Singh, 1960). As a result, the dorsal surface is not flattened as in the first two metatarsals but presents a longitudinal ridge that marks the boundary of a slight hollow on the lateral aspect. The lateral head of the second dorsal interosseous muscle is attached to its medial surface and the first plantar and medial head of the third dorsal interossei are attached to its lateral aspect. The flat **base** is roughly triangular in outline, although the plantar margin may be longer than that found in the second metatarsal, which is usually more pointed in profile. An indentation is usually found on the lateral border towards the plantar aspect, which is formed by the attachment of the strong intermetatarsal ligament connecting to the fourth metatarsal. There are normally two separate facets for articulation with the second metatarsal, with the more dorsally located generally being the larger, although it is not uncommon for the plantar facet to be absent (Singh, 1960). There is a single, large arched facet at the dorsal margin of the lateral surface for articulation with the fourth metatarsal. The oblique head of the adductor hallucis and a tendinous slip from the tibialis posterior attach to the plantar aspect of the base. The **head** is smaller than that of the second metatarsal, both in the dorsoplantar and mediolateral planes. The lateral plantar condyle is larger than the medial and the medial dorsal tubercle is more distally located and more strongly developed than its lateral counterpart. An inconstant sesamoid of the third MTP joint has been reported (Burman and Lapidus, 1931; Lapidus, 1940).

The **fourth metatarsal** is smaller than the third and articulates distally with the proximal phalanx of the fourth toe and proximally with the cuboid, lateral cuneiform and third and fifth metatarsals. As with the third metatarsal, the axis of the **shaft** is twisted so that the dorsal surface presents a longitudinal ridge, which marks a distinct lateral concavity along the length of the shaft. The lateral head of the third dorsal interosseous and the second plantar interosseous muscles are attached to the medial aspect, while the medial head of the fourth dorsal interosseous is attached to the lateral surface. The **base** has an obliquely orientated quadrilateral facet for articulation with the cuboid. The medial aspect shows a large arched facet along its dorsal margin, which is frequently grooved in a dorsoplantar direction so that the distal part articulates with the third metatarsal and the proximal part articulates with the lateral cuneiform. There is a single facet on the lateral aspect for articulation with the fifth metatarsal, which is bounded by a deep groove for the strong intermetatarsal ligament. The oblique head of the adductor hallucis and a tendinous slip from the tibialis posterior attach to the plantar aspect of the base. The **head** is similar in both shape and size to that of the third metatarsal. The lateral plantar condyle is larger than the medial and again a rare inconstant sesamoid has been reported on the medial aspect (Burman and Lapidus, 1931; Lapidus, 1940). The medial dorsal tubercle is more distally located and more strongly developed than its lateral counterpart.

The **fifth metatarsal** articulates distally with the proximal phalanx of the fifth toe and proximally with the cuboid and the fourth metatarsal. The **shaft** shows a well-defined dorsal ridge, which slopes gradually down to a lateral border that is markedly concave. The fourth dorsal interosseous and the third plantar interosseous are attached to the medial surface of the shaft. The **base** has a well-defined tubercle (styloid process) on its lateral aspect that is readily palpated in the living and to which is attached the peroneus brevis muscle. The proximal surface of the base articulates with the cuboid via an oblique triangular facet, which is continuous onto the medial surface with the articulation for the fourth metatarsal. The peroneus tertius is attached to the medial aspect of the dorsal surface of the base and it may extend distally onto the medial border of the shaft. The tendon of abductor digiti minimi grooves the plantar aspect of the base and the flexor digiti minimi brevis is attached to the plantar aspect of the tubercle. The **head** is the smallest of all the metatarsals and is obliquely set. The lateral plantar condyle is located more distal than the medial but they are equally well developed. Inconstant sesamoids occur at this joint and they are just as likely to be paired as single with an occurrence of approximately 5–10% (Pfitzner, 1896; Bizzaro, 1921; Holland, 1928). The shaft of the fifth metatarsal is also a recognized location for chronic stress (fatigue) fractures in new conscripts.

Phalanges

In the normal situation, the great toe possesses only two phalanges (proximal and distal), while the remaining toes each have three (proximal, middle and distal). However, in reality, the number of separate phalanges is extremely variable, as it is not uncommon for phalangeal fusion to occur, particularly in the lateral toes. It is thought that biphalangeal toes arise from the lack of differentiation of the distal interphalangeal joint (see below) and not necessarily from fusion of the middle and proximal phalanges (concrescentia phalangum) or indeed absence of the middle phalanx, as has been proposed in the past (Pfitzner, 1896; Venning, 1954, 1956; Garn *et al.*, 1965d; Asin, 1966; Ellis *et al.*, 1968; Sandström and Hedman, 1971; McKusick, 1990; Le Minor, 1995). Within the primates, biphalangia of the toes is strictly a human condition and is considered by some authors to be evidence of an adaptation to bipedalism (Le Minor, 1995). Distal symphalangism in the hand is considered to be a congenital defect but it occurs with such a high frequency in the foot that it must be considered as a normal variant. For example, a biphalangeal fifth toe may occur in 36–43% of European feet and by as much as 72–80% in Japanese, where it is most common (Morita *et al.*, 1971). It is interesting to note that the incidence of biphalangia of a given toe is not independent of the condition in the other toes. It is most common in the fifth toe, less common in the fourth and is rare in the third and second. However, it has been shown that all toes that lie lateral to the first biphalangeal digit will display this condition, thereby suggesting a developmental gradient effect (Le Minor, 1995). This is, however, a normal developmental variation and should not be confused with many of the pedal disfigurements that can arise from the effect of shoe wearing (Straus, 1942; Napier, 1957; Sim-Fook and Hodgson, 1958; Barnett, 1962a).

Unlike the fingers, which have all been assigned a specific name, the toes are simply numbered from 1–5, passing from medial to lateral. This numbering can lead to some confusion if the observer is unsure of whether toe 1 is the most medial or the most lateral (Heyes, 1992). Only the great/big toe or hallux (from the Greek meaning to leap) and the small/little toe have been assigned a name.[21] The first toe is normally the longest (54% of cases), although it is as common for the second toe to be the longest as it is for the first and second toes to be of equal length (23%) (Skinner, 1931). The third, fourth and fifth toes always decrease in size to the point at which Wood Jones (1918) described the fifth toe as being 'but a poor thing'.

Next to clubfoot, polydactyly is probably the most frequently reported congenital abnormality of the foot, with a frequency of approximately one in every 2000 births (Harrower, 1925).[22] It is frequently the fifth toe that is affected and often there is no bony component, with the additional appendage being composed of only soft tissue (Smith and Boulgakoff, 1923). Oligodactyly (absence of a normal digit) is less common than polydactyly, with a reported incidence of approximately one in every 3000 births (Lewin, 1917; Viladot, 1988).

For the same reasons as have been given for the phalanges of the hand, we will only describe typical proximal, middle and distal pedal phalanges and not attempt to assign morphology to individual digital rays, other than the first.

Each phalanx can be described as having a shaft, base and head, although it may become difficult to discern this basic morphology in the middle and distal phalanges of the lateral toes. The **first proximal phalanx** is the largest and most robust of the phalanges.

[21] An American medical student, with clearly too much time on his hands, decided this was a discriminatory act against the toes and, like the fingers, they too deserved their own individual names. He suggested the following, passing from medial to lateral – Porcellus fori, Porcellus domi, Porcellus carnivorus, Porcellus non voratus and Porcellus plorare domi (bearing in mind that Porcellus is the Latin for 'small pig')!

[22] Interestingly, 'Seisdedos' (six digits) is not an uncommon surname in the Barcelona telephone directory! Six digits in the hand are probably more common than in the foot and many condemned Queen Anne Boleyn as a witch, as she was reported to have six fingers on one hand.

It articulates proximally with the head of the first metatarsal and distally with the terminal phalanx at the interphalangeal joint. The **shaft** is short in comparison to the overall robusticity of the bone, giving it a somewhat stunted appearance. The shaft is flat on the plantar surface and convex across the dorsal surface from medial to lateral. The expanded **base** has a deeply concave ellipsoidal surface for articulation with the head of the first metatarsal. The surface is wider transversely than in the dorsoplantar plane and is surrounded by a distinct rim. The extensor hallucis brevis muscle attaches to the dorsal aspect of the base. The adductor hallucis and flexor hallucis brevis muscles attach to the lateral plantar aspect of the base and the abductor hallucis and the second head of the flexor hallucis brevis attach to the corresponding medial aspect of the plantar surface of the base, with each combined tendon carrying a sesamoid. The **head** of the first proximal phalanx is trochlear in shape for articulation with the corresponding base of the first distal phalanx. The central area is grooved by the passage of the tendon of the flexor hallucis longus, which can possess a sesamoid in this location (with an incidence of approximately 50%). The head is frequently deflected somewhat laterally, so that the lateral border of the shaft is often more obviously concave than the medial. The normal hallux valgus angle (between the axis of the first metatarsal and that of the proximal phalanx) is in the range of 0–36° with a mean of 16° (Hardy and Clapham, 1951). This lateral deviation of the first toe is a characteristically human condition and it is thought to dissipate the forces of the 'toe-off' phase to prevent buckling of the bone (Griffiths, 1902; Wilkinson, 1954; Barnett, 1962b). In the pathological condition of hallux valgus, there is an increased lateral deviation of the phalanges of the first toe in relation to the metatarsal (Haines and McDougall, 1954). The skin over the medially displaced metatarsal head often becomes compressed against footwear and a bursal swelling (bunion) is formed. There is a strong correlation between the development of hallux valgus and the wearing of shoes (Sim-Fook and Hodgson, 1958; Shine, 1965). However, Gottschalk *et al.* (1980) and Noakes (1981) concluded that the condition was due to some basic early developmental abnormality and not to shoe wearing.

In general, the proximal phalanges reduce in size from the longest in the great toe to the smallest in the fifth toe (Aiello and Dean, 1990). The **shaft** is gracile and slightly constricted in the middle region, expanding proximally and distally towards the extremities. The dorsal aspect is convex from side to side but generally flat and straight along its long axis and tends to flatten out proximal to the head. The plantar surface is slightly convex from side to side but concave along its length, displaying a groove for the flexor tendons. The medial and lateral sides may be exaggerated into ridges (as are found in the hand) for the attachment of the flexor tendon sheath. The **base** is relatively broad and elliptical in shape, with a uniformly concave articular facet that has a distinct raised rim. The base is convex along the dorsal margin but is straighter and more flattened along the plantar margin, although it can be grooved by the passage of the flexor tendons. The plantar interossei attach to the medial aspects of the bases of proximal phalanges 3–5, while the dorsal interossei attach to the medial and lateral aspects of the bases of proximal phalanx 2 and only to the lateral surface of 3 and 4. The lumbricals pass distally on the medial sides of the four lateral toes to the proximal phalangeal attachments of the dorsal digital expansions. The long extensor tendon is bound firmly to the plantar surfaces of the base of the proximal phalanges and metatarsophalangeal joints by an aponeurotic sling. Therefore, pull on the extensor digitorum tendon results in hyperextension of the proximal phalanx, with no extensor action on the interphalangeal joints. The tendon only becomes an extensor of the interphalangeal joints when the proximal phalanx is held in flexion at the metatarsophalangeal joint (Sarrafian and Topouzian, 1969). The plantar aspect of the base of the fifth toe receives the tendons of the third plantar interosseous and the flexor digiti minimi brevis muscles medially and the abductor digiti minimi laterally. The plantar surface of the **head** of the proximal phalanx is grooved in the centre and elevated on either side to form a trochlea or pulley-shaped articular surface. The head is wider in the transverse plane and shorter in the dorsoplantar plane, so that it appears somewhat compressed from above to below. Sesamoids can occur in the long tendons at both the proximal and distal articulations of the second metatarsal (2% and 1% incidence respectively), in the distal articulation of the third metatarsal (1%), in the proximal articulation of the fourth metatarsal (2%) and in both the proximal and distal articulations of the fifth metatarsal (incidence of 10% in both locations). The phenomenon of paired sesamoids seems to be restricted to the metatarsophalangeal joints of the first and last toes and probably occurs as a protective mechanism to spare the long tendons from weight-bearing pressures (Helal, 1988).

The **middle phalanges** are short in length and as broad as they are long. That of the second toe is normally the longest, with that of the fifth toe generally being the shortest and frequently being represented by little more than an irregular bony nodule, even in the adult. The **shaft** is short and slightly concave on both its plantar and dorsal surfaces. Ridges may be present along the medial and lateral borders of the plantar aspect for the attachment of the flexor sheath and a groove may run along the axis of the shaft caused by the passage of the long flexor tendon. The flexor digitorum brevis muscle attaches to the plantar aspects of the shafts of the middle phalanges by paired points of insertion. The **base** is slightly expanded compared to the shaft and bears two concave facets separated by a raised midline keel that corresponds with the reciprocal pulley shape on the distal facet of the proximal phalanx. The dorsal surface of the base is convex, while the plantar margin is straighter and often slightly concave for the passage of the long flexor tendon. The tendons of extensor digitorum brevis attach to the dorsal aspect of the base of the middle phalanges.

The **distal phalanx** of the first digit is the largest, with that of the fifth toe being the smallest and most amorphous. The **shaft** is short, smooth dorsally and roughened on the plantar aspect for the attachment of the long digital flexor. The **base** is elliptical in shape, being flattened in the dorsoplantar plane. The articular surface is concave in both the mediolateral and dorsoplantar planes and often presents a small midline projection on both the plantar and dorsal surfaces to fit the central concavity of the middle phalangeal head. The extensor hallucis longus tendon is attached to the dorsal aspect of the base. The **head** is distinctly convex distally at its free end and less 'harpoon-like' than the distal phalanges of the hand (see Chapter 9). The dorsal surface is smooth for the support of the soft tissues of the nail bed and the plantar surface is roughened for the attachment of the fibrous pulp of the toe pads. These serve to anchor the toe pads and effectively distribute loads during weight-bearing, particularly in the final stages of stance (Sammarco, 1988).

Early development of the foot

Given the nature of the pentadactyl limb, it is not surprising that much of the early development of the foot follows the pattern that has already been described in the section on the early development of the hand (Chapter 9). Therefore, it is advised that this section is read in advance, to prevent unnecessary repetition. However, as a direct result of the proximodistal organization of the human embryo, the development of the foot lags behind that of the hand by approximately 5–6 days from the very earliest embryonic stages (O'Rahilly *et al.*, 1957).

Around day 37 of intrauterine life, the **footplate** becomes visible on the caudal end of the lower limb bud (Fig. 11.34) (O'Rahilly and Müller, 1987). It is slightly tilted so that the pre-axial border is more laterally situated than the postaxial border, i.e. the sole faces cranially and medially (O'Rahilly and Gardner, 1975). Even at this early stage in the development of the foot, the tibial nerve has entered the region of the footplate.

By day 41, the tarsal region can be recognized as mesenchymal condensations with three or four digital prolongations (digital plate) extending distally from the caudal extremity of the footplate (Gardner *et al.*, 1959; O'Rahilly and Gardner, 1975). The margin of this **digital plate** is rounded and set off at a slight angle from the crurotarsal region. A slight ventral prominence in the margin indicates the position of the developing first pedal ray (O'Rahilly, 1973). By this stage, the tibial nerve has reached the plantar surface of the developing foot. By day 44, there is a common cellular condensation for the developing tarsal region with distinct **digital rays**, although the rim of the digital plate may not yet be crenulated (Streeter, 1948; O'Rahilly *et al.*, 1957; Gardner *et al.*, 1959; Larsen, 1993).

Week 7 (days 43–49) is the time of active chondrification of the proximal mesenchymal pedal template. Chondrification generally commences in the centre of a blastemal mass and will continue to develop

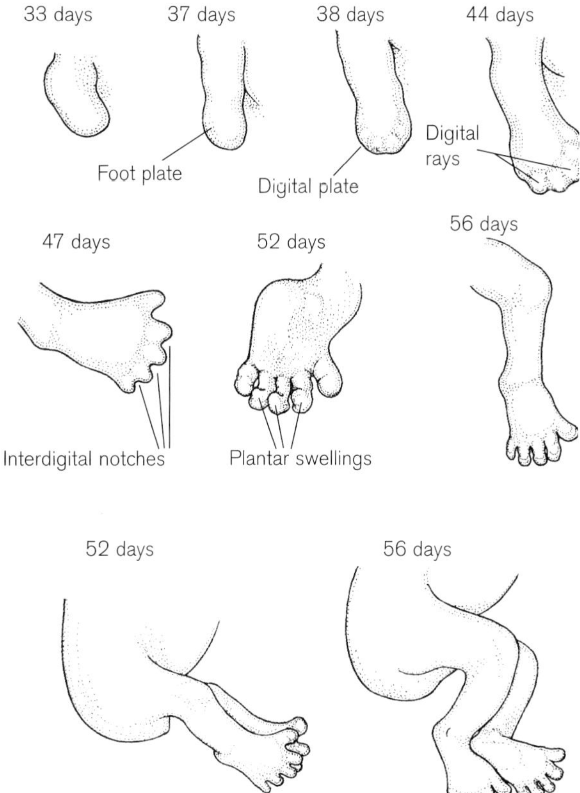

Figure 11.34 The development of the lower limb between 5 and 8 fetal weeks (redrawn after Larsen, 1993).

throughout the embryonic period proper (Gardner *et al.*, 1959; O'Rahilly *et al.*, 1960). There is essentially a proximodistal sequence of chondrification within the digits of the foot, although the pattern in the more proximal segments is a little more irregular. Chondrification is first evident in the region of metatarsals 2–4 followed in order by the cuboid, metatarsal 5, calcaneus, talus, medial cuneiform, intermediate cuneiform, lateral cuneiform, metatarsal 1, navicular, proximal phalanges, middle phalanges and finally by the distal phalanges (Senior, 1929; O'Rahilly *et al.*, 1957; O'Rahilly, 1973). By the end of week 7, each tarsal and metatarsal will have commenced chondrification. The process is simplest in the cuboid and the lateral two cuneiforms as each develops from only a single central nucleus of chondrification. The calcaneus is said to chondrify from two separate centres, with the distal nucleus appearing before the more proximal one. These will ultimately fuse into a single cartilaginous mass by day 48 (Cihák, 1972). The talus reportedly chondrifies from three separate regions, with the largest being the first to appear, while the two later centres are considerably smaller. The first centre forms the head and the body of the talus while the second is said to form the lateral process and the third forms the posterior process (Cihák, 1972). The developing medial cuneiform is separated into plantar and dorsal regions by a horizontal strip of non-cartilaginous tissue. This is a constant embryological condition and may explain the divided facets that are sometimes seen on the adult bone (Cihák, 1972) and the incidence of bipartite medial cuneiforms (see below). The navicular is the last of the tarsal bones to commence chondrification and it may not in fact begin until well into week 8. It forms from two distinct nuclei, with the most distal and medial forming in advance of that which is more proximal and lateral. Chondrification develops separately in the navicular tuberosity but does eventually fuse with the principal mass (Cihák, 1972). By the end of the seventh week, the lower limb begins to flex towards a parasagittal plane so that the pre-axial (tibial) border is rostral in position and the postaxial (fibular) border is caudal (O'Rahilly *et al.*, 1957; Larsen, 1993).

Week 8 (days 50–56) is the time of active chondrification in the more distal mesenchymal pedal template. Around day 51, the proximal phalanges commence chondrification and interzones (see Chapter 9) are visible in the metatarsophalangeal joints (Gardner *et al.*, 1959; O'Rahilly and Gardner, 1975). The digital plate becomes crenulated and a fan-like arrangement of the toes is evident. When five radiating mesodermal columns have been formed, selective cell necrosis (apoptosis) will occur in the interdigital zones of ectoderm and underlying mesoderm to form the separate toes (Kelley, 1970, 1973; O'Rahilly, 1973; Hurle and Colvee, 1982). As with the fingers, if a teratogenic agent is introduced at this time or there is some other upset in the normal process of development, then syndactyly of the digits may ensue (Menkes and Deleanu, 1964; Christ *et al.*, 1986). At this time, the tuberosity of the calcaneus is represented by only a mesenchymal condensation and chondrification has not yet commenced in this region (O'Rahilly and Gardner, 1975).

By day 52, chondrification is now evident in the middle phalanges and in the region of the tuberosity of the calcaneus (O'Rahilly *et al.*, 1957; Gardner *et al.*, 1959). Cellular condensations can be seen in the region between the talus and calcaneus at the site of the future sustentaculum tali and also in the tuberosity of the fifth metatarsal (O'Rahilly *et al.*, 1957; Kawashima and Uhthoff, 1990). Homogenous interzones are present in the ankle and most of the intertarsal joints (Gardner *et al.*, 1959; O'Rahilly and Gardner, 1975).

By day 54, chondrification has commenced in the sustentaculum tali and this separate centre soon joins with the main mass of the calcaneus (Kawashima and Uhthoff, 1990). The sustentaculum tali is the last of the tarsal elements to commence chondrification but maturation is rapid and development has generally caught up with the main body of the calcaneus by the ninth week. Concurrent with chondrification of the sustentaculum tali, the blastemal tissue at the posterior portion of the future joint between the talus and calcaneus develops into an undifferentiated mesenchymal mass, which by the end of week 8 forms a homogenous cellular interzone (Kawashima and Uhthoff, 1990). In some cases however, the mesenchymal mass may differentiate into a fibrous structure at the site of the future joint capsule, forming a talocalcaneal bridge (Harris, 1955; Kawashima and Uhthoff, 1990). In the early fetal period the incidence of talocalcaneal bridging is high, but talocalcaneal fusion in the adult is low and it has been suggested that the breakdown of the bridge arises due to the drastic changes that occur in the biomechanical environment after birth and especially following standing and walking (Gardner *et al.*, 1959). Talocalcaneal bridging is a common anomaly associated with peroneal spastic flat foot and although total fusion of the two bones is rare, it has been reported in the literature (Hirschtick, 1951).

As in the carpal region, the pathomechanism of tarsal coalition has been attributed either to a failure of joint formation, or fusion of an accessory ossicle to contiguous tarsal bones (Harris and Beath, 1948; Outland and Murphy, 1953; Ruano-Gil *et al.*, 1978;

Buccholz, 1987). It is within week 8 that cavitation of most of the intertarsal joints will commence and so it is at this stage that future congenital tarsal coalitions may form. Coalitions can theoretically occur between any two contiguous tarsal bones, but it is more common in some than in others (Sloane, 1946; Austin, 1951; Geelhoed *et al.*, 1969; Heiple and Lovejoy, 1969; de Lima and Mishkiu, 1996). For example, calcaneonavicular synostosis is not uncommon and generally results in a painful spasmodic foot, which can be treated by arthrodesis (Slomann, 1926; Seddon, 1932; Chambers, 1950; Mitchell and Gibson, 1967; Oestreich *et al.*, 1987). It is thought to arise via a specific gene mutation as an autosomal dominant with reduced penetration (Wray and Herndon, 1963). Talocalcaneal and calcaneonavicular coalitions are probably the most common, but fusions do occur, albeit less frequently, in the other tarsals, e.g. talonavicular coalition (Lapidus, 1932; O'Donoghue and Sell, 1943; Boyd, 1944; Weitzner, 1946), naviculocuneiform coalition (Lusby, 1959; Gregersen, 1977) and cubonavicular coalition (del Sel and Grand, 1959).

In addition to the tarsal coalitions, the presence of accessoria adds considerably to the variation that is encountered in the pedal skeleton (O'Rahilly *et al.*, 1960). There are over 50 reported accessoria or supernumerary bones that have been identified in the foot (O'Rahilly, 1953a, 1956/57). They are reported to be more common in the fetus than in the adult and it is likely that during development they either disappear or alternatively fuse with other centres to form the tubercles or prominences of the constant tarsal bones (Biermann, 1922; Hauch, 1946). They are also reported to have a relatively high incidence in males between 10 and 15 years and in females between 8 and 12 years (Hoerr *et al.*, 1962). They have the potential to persist into adulthood as small supernumerary bones and in many cases there are no clinical symptoms to forewarn their presence but, if necessary, most can be excised with relative ease. In many instances, it is difficult to make a satisfactory distinction between what is truly a supernumerary bone or an inconstant sesamoid and as a result, the naming of these structures is often inaccurate and confusing. As with the carpal bones, it is best to use terms that describe the position of the structure and where possible avoid eponyms such as 'os Vesalii'. Much has been written in the clinical literature on these relatively inconsequential structures and readers are directed to the following texts with regards to specific tarsal associations – Calcaneus (Krida, 1923; Mercer, 1931; Kassianenko, 1935; Milliken, 1937; Anderson, 1988b; Mann, 1990; Bencardino *et al.*, 1997); Talus (McDougall, 1955; Wakeley *et al.*, 1996); Navicular (Zadek, 1926; Kidner, 1929; Zadek and Gold, 1948; Lawson *et al.*, 1984; Sella *et al.*, 1986; Chen *et al.*, 1997) and Cuboid (Dwight, 1910). An overview of the supernumerary pedal bones can be found in many texts, including Geist (1914), Kleinberg (1917), Bizzaro (1921), Holland (1921), Pirie (1921), Burman and Lapidus (1931), Trolle (1948), O'Rahilly (1953a, 1956/57) and Helal (1988).

The first and arguably the most common supernumerary element develops around day 54, when an accessory anlage can be identified at the tarsometatarsal border between the primordia of the first and second metatarsals. This dense region of mesenchyme assumes characteristics of a prochondral primordium and may start to commence chondrification but will rapidly de-differentiate and disappear after day 57. It is said that if this structure persists and subsequently ossifies, then it will form an os intermetatarseum, which generally persists as a free ossicle but can fuse to either the medial cuneiform or to either of the adjacent metatarsal bases (Delano, 1941; Cihák, 1972; O'Rahilly, 1973; Case *et al.*, 1997).

By day 57 of intra-uterine life, the foot has reached the end of its embryonic development and all elements have commenced chondrification including the distal phalanges, the sustentaculum tali and the tuberosity of the fifth metatarsal (O'Rahilly *et al.*, 1957). All interzones are present by this stage and cavitation has commenced in the ankle and metatarsophalangeal joints. Therefore, by the end of the embryonic period proper, tarsal coalitions and symphalangism can often be predicted (Gardner *et al.*, 1959). At this time, the soles of the feet face medially and dorsally and the toes of one side are generally in contact with those on the other side (praying feet). The foot is in line with the leg and angulation of the ankle has not really begun, so the foot is in an equinus position. The development of the individual arches of the foot can be detected by the end of the embryonic period (O'Rahilly, 1973).

Talipes equinovarus (clubfoot) is probably one of the most studied congenital abnormalities of the foot and certainly the literature devoted to this condition is voluminous. It is said to occur in one in every 1000 live Caucasian births, to be more frequent in twins and to have a male to female ratio of 2:1 (Böhm, 1929; Stewart, 1951; Wiley, 1959; Waisbrod, 1973; Bates and Chung, 1988). However, its true aetiology is still unknown, although there are several theories as to how this condition arises. Ruano-Gil (1988) reported that in the embryo, the talus and calcaneus sit next to each other in a forced equinus position and that this classical embryological alignment is achieved through the influence of growth at the distal end of the fibula. However, in week 9, the position of the talus relative to the calcaneus alters through the influence of growth at the distal end of the tibia. The talus is said to gradually shift until it finally adopts the characteristic position on top of the calcaneus (Victoria-Diaz, 1979). If this latter phase of growth is halted, then the foot remains in the embryological position, thereby producing talipes equinovarus (clubfoot) where the patient walks on the outer aspect of the talus. Although attractive, arguments against this theory are numerous and it is more likely that 'clubfoot' is really 'a collection of various pathological entities of different aetiology that manifest in a commonly identifiable foot deformity' (Bates and Chung, 1988).

Ossification

If one ignores the accessoria and the sesamoids, there are potentially 46 separate centres of ossification in the foot. Of these, 26 are primary and 20 (but often less) are secondary. Unlike many other areas of the body (except the hand of course) many of the primary centres arise in the early fetal period and the remainder do not develop until after birth, while the appearance of the secondary centres are interspersed between the sequential appearance of the primary centres. Therefore, for the sake of both clarity and conformity with the other chapters, we will still examine these centres under the headings of primary and secondary, but the reader should be aware that there is no direct line of time continuity between these two sections. It should also be appreciated that there has been a considerable amount of research dedicated to the radiographic identification of appearance and fusion times in the foot and this has resulted in many slightly conflicting reports of the time of a specific event. It is certain that much of this interest has resulted not only from the ready availability of the foot for radiography, but also the large number of centres of ossification provides a substantial volume of information regarding growth and maturity over an extended period of time. There is certainly a considerable degree of individual variability in the timing of events in the foot and when this is coupled with racial variation and environmental factors, it is clear that it is impossible to arrive at a universal time for either the appearance of a specific centre or its subsequent fusion. Therefore, we have attempted to summarize much of the information that is available, so that a relatively broad time spectrum of events is presented. These timings should not, of course, be considered definitive, as variations will inevitably occur.

Primary centres

Within the fetal period, ossification commences first in the metatarsals, followed closely by the distal phalanges, proximal and finally the middle phalanges (Noback and Robertson, 1951; Kjar, 1974; MacLaughlin-Black and Gunstone, 1995). It should be noted that this is a different order from that found in the hand, where the distal phalanges are the first to commence ossification (see Chapter 9).

The primary centres for the shafts of the **metatarsals** appear between 8–10 fetal weeks, which is at a similar time to that for the metacarpals (Frazer, 1948; Jit, 1957; Gardner *et al.*, 1959; Hoerr *et al.*, 1962; Birkner, 1978; Fazekas and Kósa, 1978). Metatarsals 2–4 tend to appear before metatarsal 5, while the first metatarsal may not appear until 12 fetal weeks (Tachdjian, 1985). This order of appearance is fundamentally in agreement with the pattern of metacarpal appearance found in the hand. As with the first metacarpal, in all aspects of ossification and fusion, the first metatarsal behaves more like a proximal phalanx than a true metatarsal (Jit, 1957; Kjar, 1974; MacLaughlin-Black and Gunstone, 1995).

The **distal phalanges** appear around the end of the second and throughout the third month of intra-uterine life and so may appear before the shaft of the first metatarsal (Frazer, 1948). The distal phalanx of the first toe appears in advance of the others around 7 weeks according to O'Rahilly *et al.* (1960) or week 9 according to Birkner (1978). Ossification of the distal phalanges of the more lateral toes occurs between 11 and 12 fetal weeks (Garn *et al.*, 1967b), while that of the fifth toe may not occur until the fifth or sixth fetal month (MacLaughlin-Black and Gunstone, 1995). As with the distal phalanges of the hand, ossification commences at the tip and not in the centre, as is found with all other primary centres of long bones. Therefore, ossification can only progress in a proximal direction. A shell of subperiosteal bone is deposited rather like a thimble over the cartilaginous phalanx, while the ungual tuberosity forms by intramembranous ossification on the exterior of the subperiosteal cap (Dixey, 1881; Schuscik, 1918; O'Rahilly *et al.*, 1960). In general, ossification of the distal phalanges of the foot lags behind those of the hand by approximately 3–5 weeks (Gardner *et al.*, 1959).

The primary centres of ossification for the **proximal phalanges** appear in the fourth fetal month, around 14–16 fetal weeks (Frazer, 1948; Garn *et al.*, 1967b). The centres for the first to the third toes tend to appear in advance of those for the fourth and fifth toe (MacLaughlin-Black and Gunstone, 1995).

As with the hand, the **middle phalanges** of the foot are the last of the long bones to commence ossification. It is well documented that their appearance is somewhat erratic and in the cases of the fourth and fifth toes in particular, ossification may not be detected until after birth (Frazer, 1948; MacLaughlin-Black and Gunstone, 1995). The middle phalanx of the second toe may appear in the fourth fetal month and that of the third in the fifth fetal month but in truth, the time of appearance cannot be stated with any degree of certainty. It is thought that this somewhat unpredictable behaviour of the middle phalanges of the most lateral toes may go some way towards explaining the reduction in the number of phalanges (biphalangism) that can be seen in these toes in particular (see above).

In summary therefore, the primary centres of ossification for the metatarsals and phalanges are all present (with the probable exception of the middle phalanges of the lateral toes) by the end of the fifth fetal month.

The second group of primary centres of ossification in the foot give rise to the tarsal bones and while most

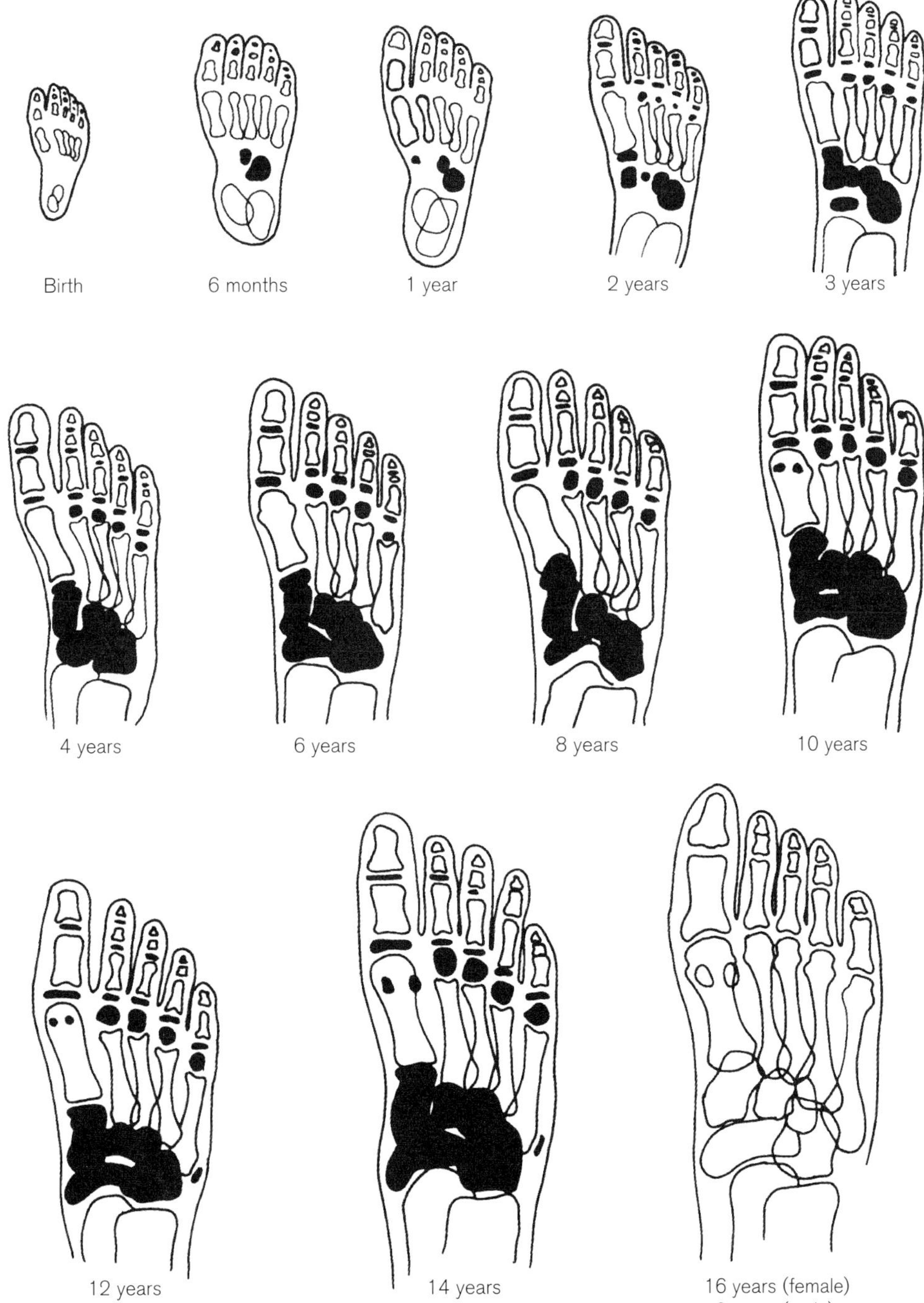

Figure 11.35 Various stages of osseous development in the foot from birth to adolescence (redrawn after Birkner, 1978).

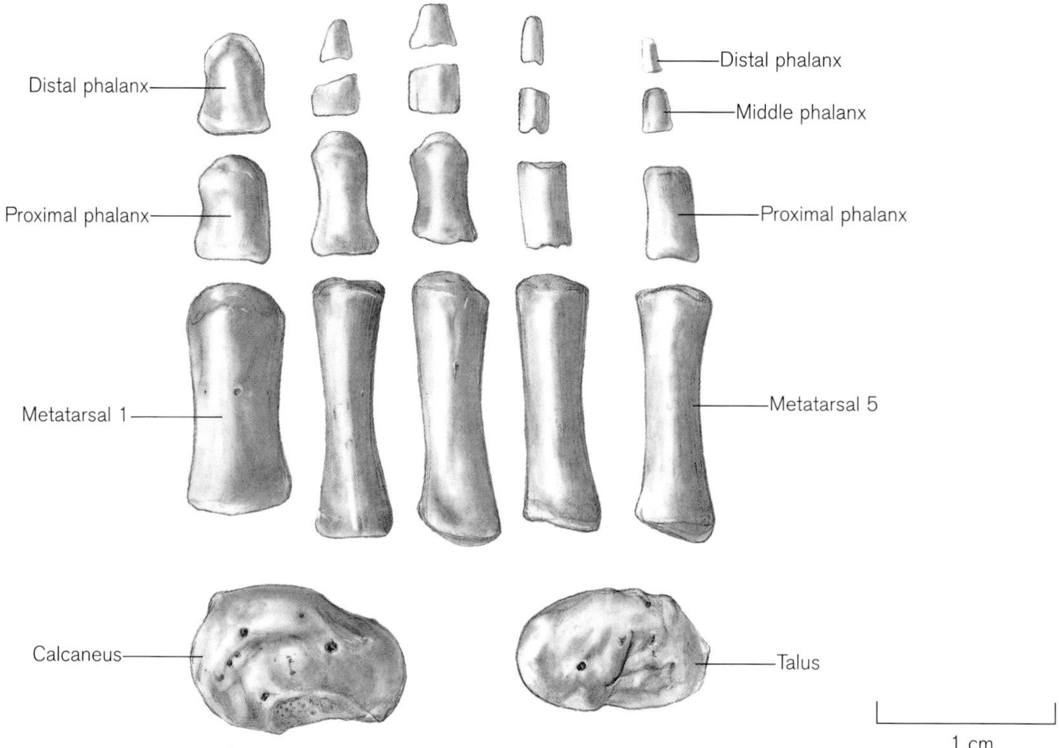

Figure 11.36 The right perinatal foot.

develop in the postnatal years, certainly two and often three, appear before birth (Figs. 11.35 and 11.36). The normal sequence of appearance for the tarsal bones is relatively constant and well documented. The calcaneus appears first, followed closely by the talus and then the cuboid. The remainder of the tarsal bones always appear after birth and the sequence begins with the lateral cuneiform and is followed by the medial and then the intermediate cuneiform, with the navicular being the last to commence ossification.

The **calcaneus** is the first of the tarsal bones to commence ossification and frequently does so from two separate centres (Gardner *et al.*, 1959; O'Rahilly *et al.*, 1960; Szaboky *et al.*, 1970; Meyer and O'Rahilly, 1976; Birkner, 1978; Goldstein *et al.*, 1988; Stripp and Reynolds, 1988). The lateral centre is not constant but when present, it always precedes the formation of the constant medial centre. The former has been described as an osseous shell that develops on the fibular side of the bone and is perichondral in origin. It is located posterior to the site of the future peroneal trochlea and between the lateral process and the retrotrochlear eminence (Meyer and O'Rahilly, 1976). Texts vary on the time of appearance of this centre but it seems to occur around the fourth and fifth fetal months. The second centre appears somewhat later, around 5–6 fetal months and is said to be endochondral in nature, as it appears in the centre of the anterior third of the cartilaginous mass of the calcaneus (Meyer and O'Rahilly, 1976). The two centres will fuse over the next month, although it can occur, but rarely, after birth (Birkner, 1978). A bifid os calcis arises when the two centres fail to fuse and this is characterized by a deep cleft that separates the anterior third of the bone from the posterior two-thirds (Szaboky *et al.*, 1970). This condition is asymptomatic and so does not tend to require any surgical intervention.

As with the bones of the hand, most of the descriptions of changes in the shape of the tarsals has been derived from radiographic texts and not from actual bone specimens. Unlike the carpals however, we have found that the tarsals adopt a more recognizable form at a younger age and so many can be positively identified at an earlier stage of development.

By around birth, or certainly within the first month *postpartum*, the calcaneus can be identified as a pyriform shaped nodule with a shallow indentation just distal to the centre of the dorsal surface (Fig. 11.37). This is the forerunner of the calcaneal groove that forms the floor of the sinus tarsi and at this early stage of development it displays a large nutrient foramen.

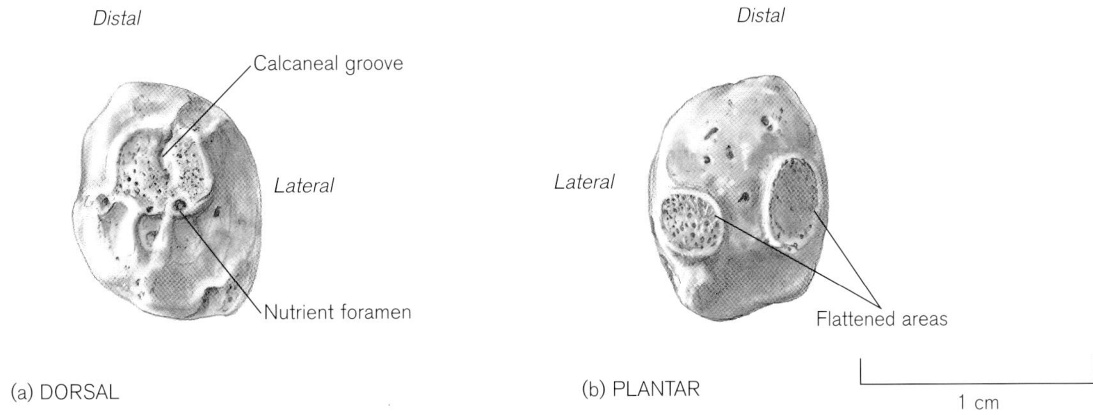

Figure 11.37 The right perinatal calcaneus.

The proximal end of the bony nodule is broader than the distal end and is drawn downwards so that the greatest vertical dimension is in the proximal segment of the bone (Hoerr *et al.*, 1962).

The surface of the perinatal calcaneal nodule displays not only flattened regions that do not appear to bear any relevance to future anatomical structures but also various pits, foramina and spiky projections. We have studied this stage extensively and can only offer the following as a tentative explanation for the morphology of the perinatal calcaneus. The uneven surface of the developing nodule is consistent with endochondral bone formation that is occurring in a centrifugal fashion within a cartilaginous precursor. Therefore, the flattened regions may represent the point at which the endochondral ossification has made contact with the perichondrium and so the future flat, subperiosteal surface of the bone is developing. Two constant flat areas are present on every perinatal calcaneus we have examined – one on the medial surface of the bone and one on the lateral aspect of the plantar surface.

This classical perinatal appearance disappears within the first few months of birth as the bone starts to elongate and develop its characteristic morphology (Fig. 11.38). The distal segment becomes wider, producing a medial shelf that will go on to form the sustentaculum tali. The area of subperiosteal bone below this is fully formed at this stage and corresponds in position with the flattened region seen on the perinatal bone. The lateral surface of the calcaneus is relatively featureless in the first few months and the presence of fully formed subperiosteal bone coincides with the location of the lateral flattening seen in the perinatal bone. Only the proximal posterior segment (tuberosity) of the bone and the region around the developing sustentaculum tali are clearly metaphyseal in nature, displaying characteristic ridges and furrows.

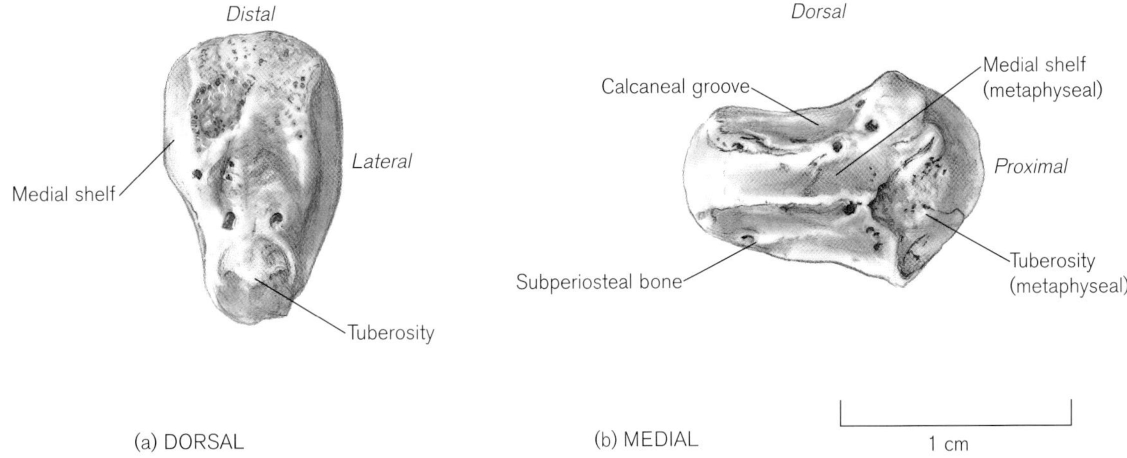

Figure 11.38 The right calcaneus from a child of approximately 3 months *postpartum*.

At around 2.5–3 months, the anterior surface of the calcaneus begins to flatten as it assumes a reciprocal shape to the cuboid. By 4–6 months, the plantar tubercles are quite distinct and by 6–7 months the bone has increased considerably in length. Flattening of the talar facets and recognizable development of the sustentaculum tali begins around the end of the first year, which coincides with the onset of unassisted walking. By 3–4 years, the proximal segment displays the characteristic ridge-and-furrow system of an active metaphysis (Fig. 11.39). By 5–6 years of age the delimitation around the articular facets is clearly defined and the bone is close to its final form (Fig. 11.40).

The calcaneus can be readily identified at birth but its characteristic morphology is not readily perceived until at least the end of the first year, when it is modified by the influences of locomotion. The bone alters considerably both in shape and size within the first 2 years, but from then until puberty the changes are gradual and small. Further development of the calcaneus is discussed below in the section on secondary centres.

While the calcaneus may be the first tarsal bone to show ossification, the **talus** is reported to be the first to show evidence of vascular invasion (Gardner *et al.*, 1959). Interestingly, Waisbrod (1973) found that in fetuses with clubfoot, the vascular channels within the talus were less well organized and fewer in number and the ossification centre tended to be smaller. Therefore, he suggested that the aetiology of clubfoot might be blastemal in origin. Ossification of the talus commences in the sixth fetal month in females and the seventh in males (Hill, 1939; Flecker, 1942; Frazer, 1948; Fazekas and Kósa, 1978; Stripp and Reynolds, 1988). Goldstein *et al.* (1988) found that the centre was present in 16% of fetuses at 16 weeks and in all fetuses by 23 weeks. However, cases have been reported of the talar centre being absent at birth (Vogt and Vickers, 1938; Gardner *et al.*, 1959; O'Rahilly *et al.*,

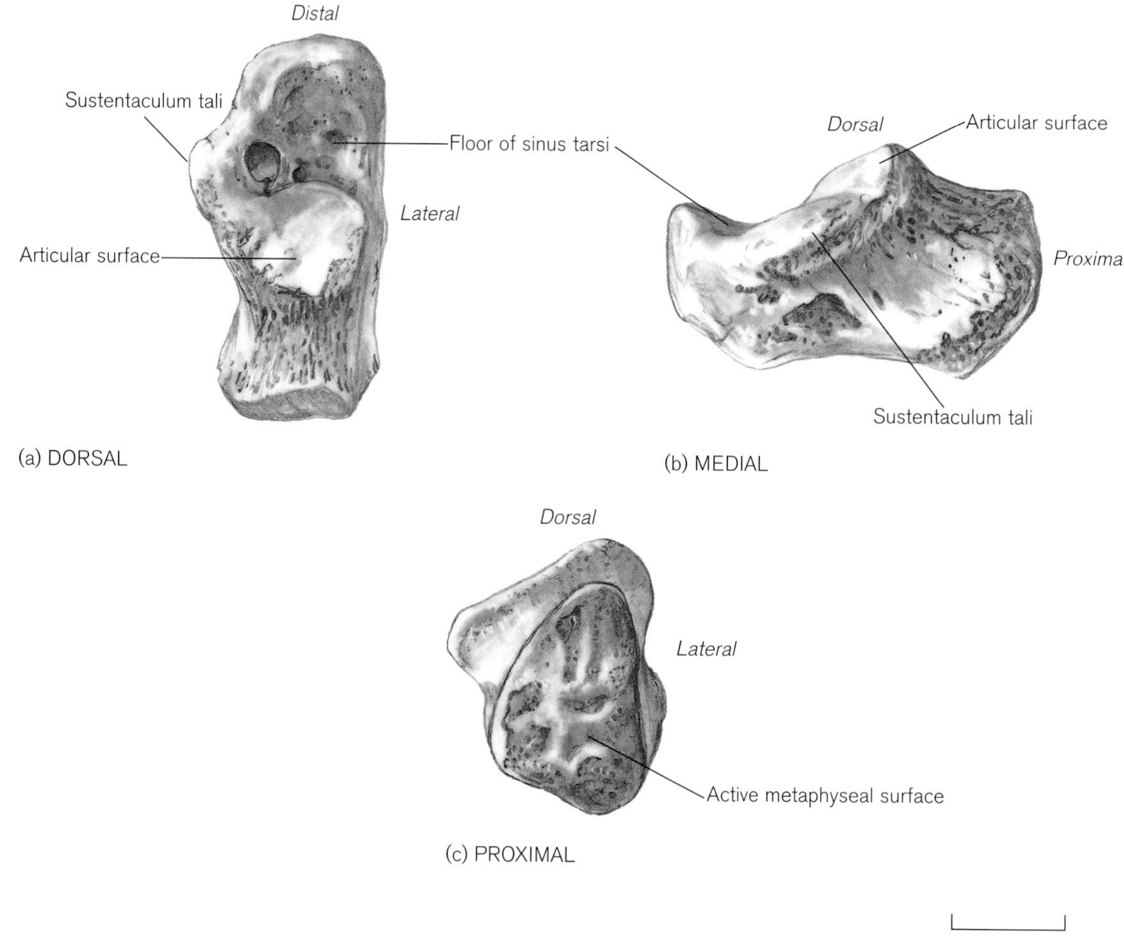

Figure 11.39 The right calcaneus from a child of approximately 3–4 years of age.

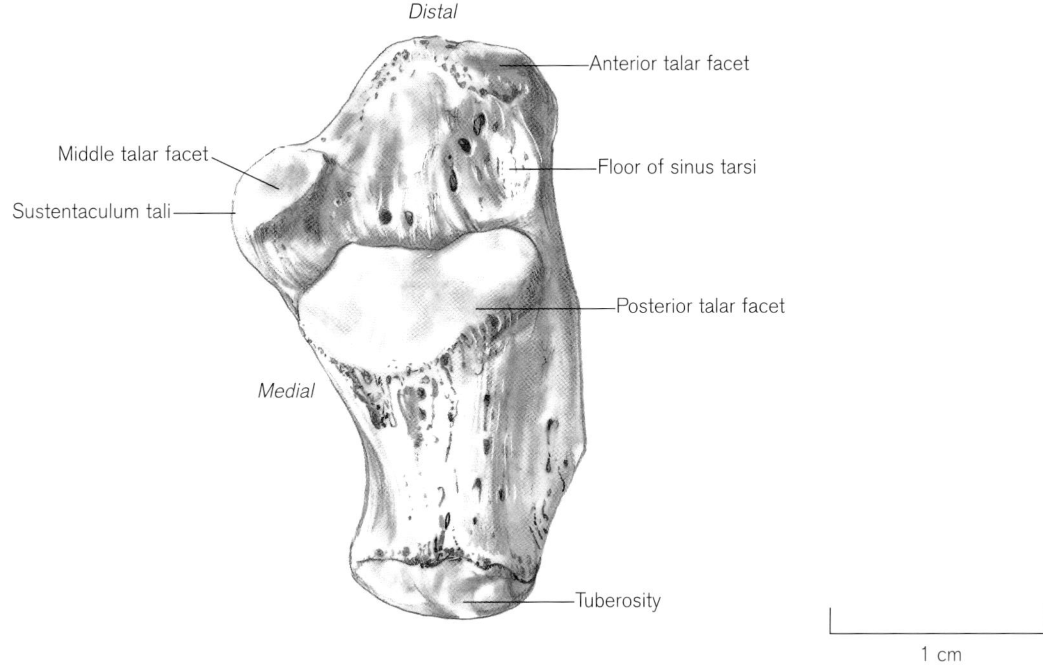

Figure 11.40 The right calcaneus from a girl aged 6 years.

1960) but appearing shortly afterwards. Ossification may arise from more than one nucleus, but they will rapidly coalesce to form a single centre (Gardner *et al.*, 1959).

The perinatal talus is oval in shape and its radiographic image is said to resemble a 'stubby peanut', with its long axis lying horizontally along the proximodistal plane (Hoerr *et al.*, 1962). Just distal to the centre of the dorsal surface there is a small indentation, which is angled in a distomedial direction. The indentation on the dorsal surface coincides in position with a similar depression on the plantar surface. These two mark the position of the future talar neck and are separated on the lateral surface by a thin dividing bony strip (Fig. 11.41). The indentation on the dorsal surface separates the future articular portion proximally from the head distally, while the indentation on the plantar surface separates the future anterior and posterior talocalcaneal facets and coincides with the position of the groove for the roof of the sinus tarsi. By 2.5–3 months *postpartum*, the neck of the talus is well defined.

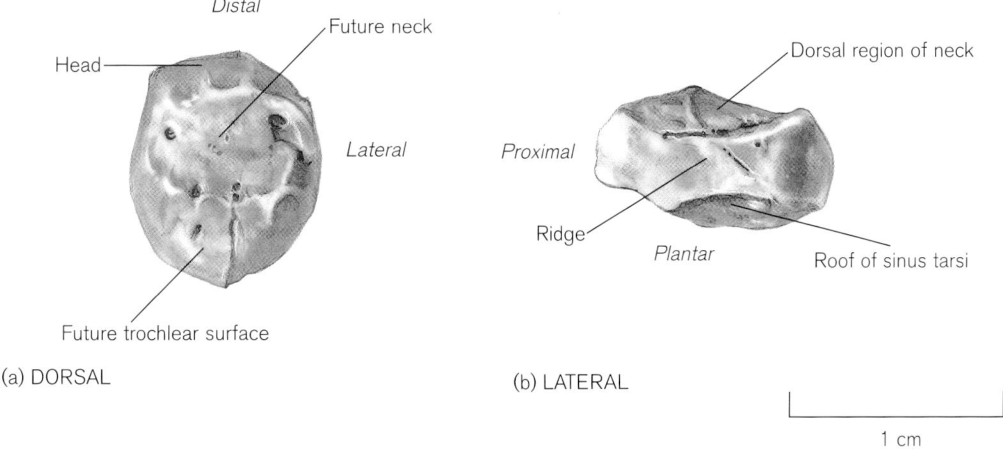

Figure 11.41 The right perinatal talus.

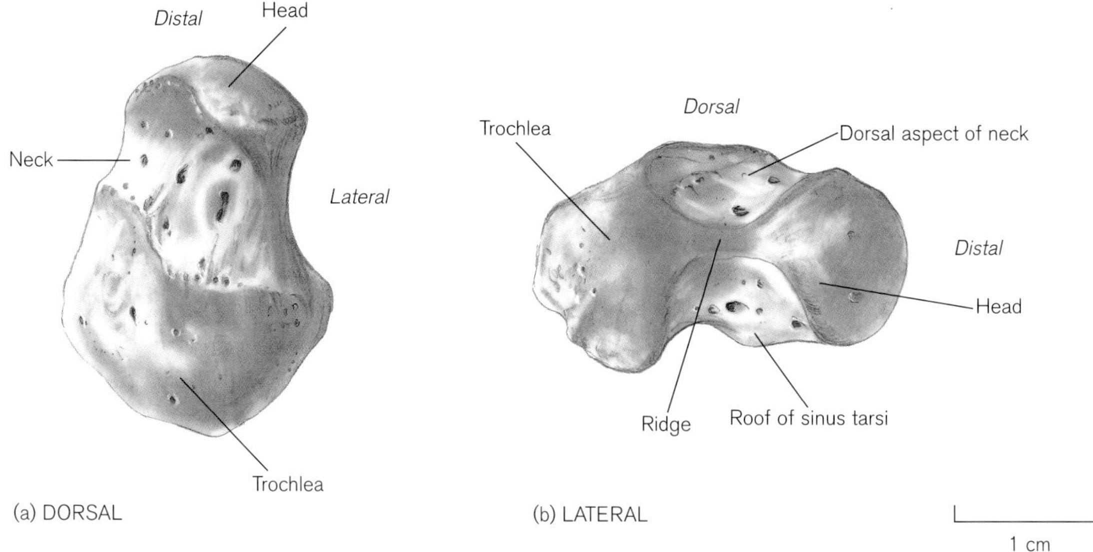

Figure 11.42 The right talus from a girl aged 2 years.

Ossification of the lateral process of the talus begins around 5 months, as does the development of the sinus tarsi and by 7 months the neck region is clearly defined and covered by a smooth layer of subperiosteal bone. Around 2 years of age, the posterolateral wall of the sinus tarsi starts to develop as a downward-projecting triangular process. The roundness of the trochlear surface also begins to develop at this age and the bone adopts an identifiable adult morphology (Fig. 11.42). By around 6 years of age, the articular facets are clearly delimited and only the area around the posterior tubercle shows evidence of continued metaphyseal activity (Fig. 11.43). The posterior tubercle begins to develop by 7–8 years in girls and 9–10 years in boys, but this will be discussed below in the section on secondary centres.

One of the most frequently discussed congenital conditions of the foot involves the talus and is extremely rare (Duncan and Fixsen, 1999). This is the condition of congenital vertical talus (congenital convex pes valgus or rocker-bottom foot) and its aetiology is unknown, although some authors consider it to be caused by a delay in development early in the first trimester of pregnancy (Lamy and Weissman, 1939). One of the characteristic features of this condition is a hypoplastic sustentaculum tali on the calcaneus, so there is no support for the head of the talus, which subsequently becomes displaced (Drennan, 1995). Diagnosis can be made at birth by the rocker-bottom appearance of the foot, which is caused by the head of the vertical talus being palpable in the sole. The condition presents with a valgus deviation of the heel, a talar displacement down, forward and medially (hence the 'vertical' talus) and a subsequent dorsal dislocation of the navicular onto the neck of the talus (Clark *et al.*, 1977; Dodge *et al.*, 1987; Fixsen, 1998). The abnormal position of the navicular may not be appreciated radiologically until the child is in excess of 3 years of age, as the navicular does not ossify until this time (Eyre-Brook, 1967). Congenital vertical talus is idiopathic, but it does show a higher incidence in patients suffering from other conditions, such as cere-

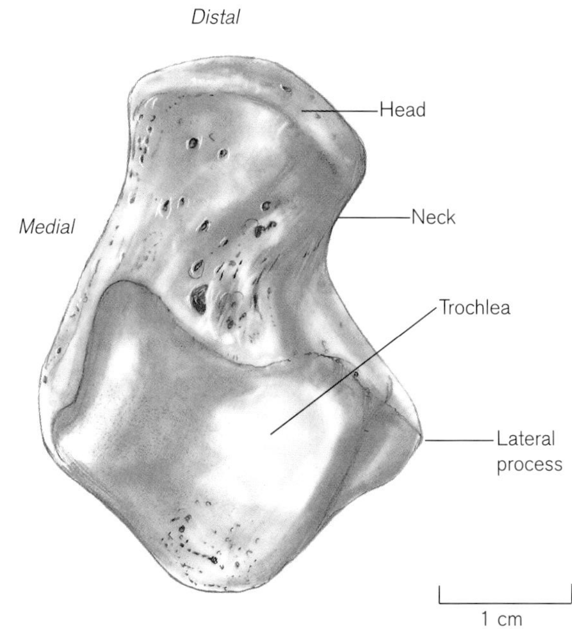

Figure 11.43 The right talus from a girl aged 6 years.

bral palsy, spina bifida and Down's syndrome (Harrold, 1967). In this clinical condition, the talus is longer than usual, possesses a shorter neck and has a rounded or pointed head. It also displays uncharacteristic articulation facets with both the calcaneus and the navicular. An extremely rare condition of congenital vertical talus in association with talocalcaneal coalition has been reported (Klein *et al.*, 1996).

It is well documented in the literature that the neck of the talus changes in direction with the growth of the foot (Goldie, 1988). Gardner (1956) reported that the neck of the talus points towards the medial side of the foot in the young fetus and that the angle between the head and the body increases throughout the fetal period from 16 weeks onwards. Paturet (1951) called this the 'declination angle' and reported it to be between 150–160° in the adult. Waisbrod (1973), however, disagreed with this, as he found the angle to be around 150° even in the fetus. He did, however, find that fetuses with clubfoot displayed markedly reduced angles of declination of between 124 and 154°.

The **cuboid** often commences ossification prior to birth but it is not uncommon for it to occur as late as 3 months *postpartum* in females and 6 months in males (Puyhaubert, 1913; Francis *et al.*, 1939; Hill, 1939; Flecker, 1942; Pyle and Sontag, 1943; Elgenmark, 1946; Harding, 1952a; O'Rahilly *et al.*, 1960; Hoerr *et al.*, 1962; Acheson, 1966; Garn *et al.*, 1967b). Menees and Holly (1932) found the cuboid to be present at birth in 35% of males and 56.5% of females. Christie *et al.* (1941) found that is was more commonly present at birth in Negro babies, girls, neonates of a greater maturity and in the offspring of mothers with no recorded pregnancy complications. In addition, they found that the centre was further advanced in the offspring of older (20+ years) and multiparous mothers. For example, the centre was present in 80% of Negro baby girls of high birth weight and only 16% of Negro baby boys of low birth weight.

What is clear is that the presence or absence of the cuboid centre of ossification is not a reliable indicator of a full term fetus (Birkner, 1978). In fact, the cuboid may originate from a cluster of ossific nodules (aligned with the long axis of the calcaneus), which will fuse within the first few months after birth to form a single round homogenous nodule (Hoerr *et al.*, 1962; Birkner, 1978). Between 6 months *postpartum* and 1 year, the medial surface that will articulate with the lateral cuneiform begins to flatten. By the end of the second year, the posterior surface that articulates with the calcaneus begins to flatten. Between 3 and 4 years, blunt-angled corners develop so that the characteristic triangular appearance of the bone is achieved (Fig. 11.44). The distal surface is flat and slopes laterally, the medial surface is virtually straight, the proximal surface is rounded and the lateral surface is clearly non-articular. Also at this stage, the groove for the peroneus longus tendon is evident on the plantar surface. By the end of the fourth year the definition between the articular and non-articular areas of the medial surface are clearly defined and by 8 years of age the bone appears as a miniature of its adult form (Fig. 11.45). Therefore, the cuboid can be identified in isolation from approximately 3–4 years and develops only in terms of size and definition with advancing age.

The **lateral cuneiform** generally ossifies within the first year but in the male, it can apparently be delayed until as late as the third year (Stripp and Reynolds, 1988). During the fourth year, a second and even a third nucleus has been reported, lying above and distal to the primary ossific nucleus (Stripp and Reynolds, 1988) – this, however, does not seem to be

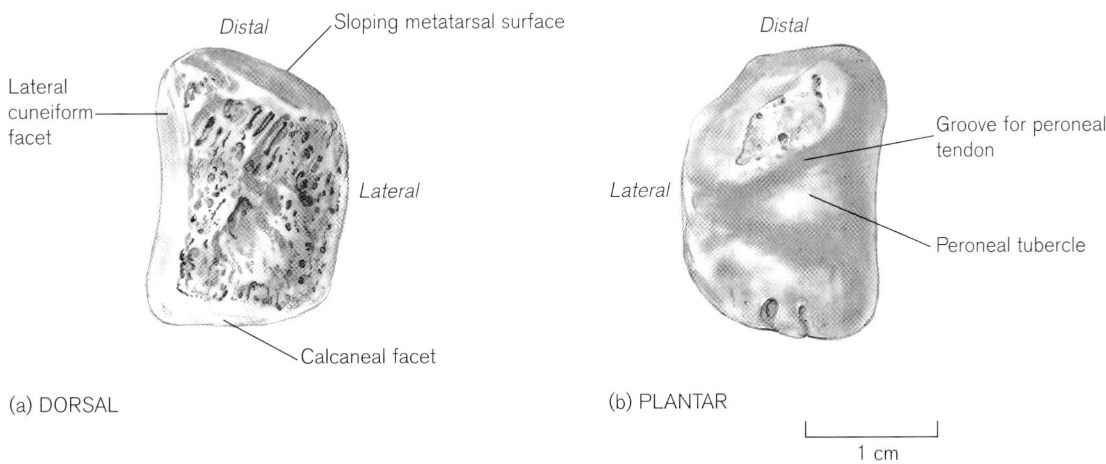

Figure 11.44 The right cuboid from a child of approximately 3–4 years.

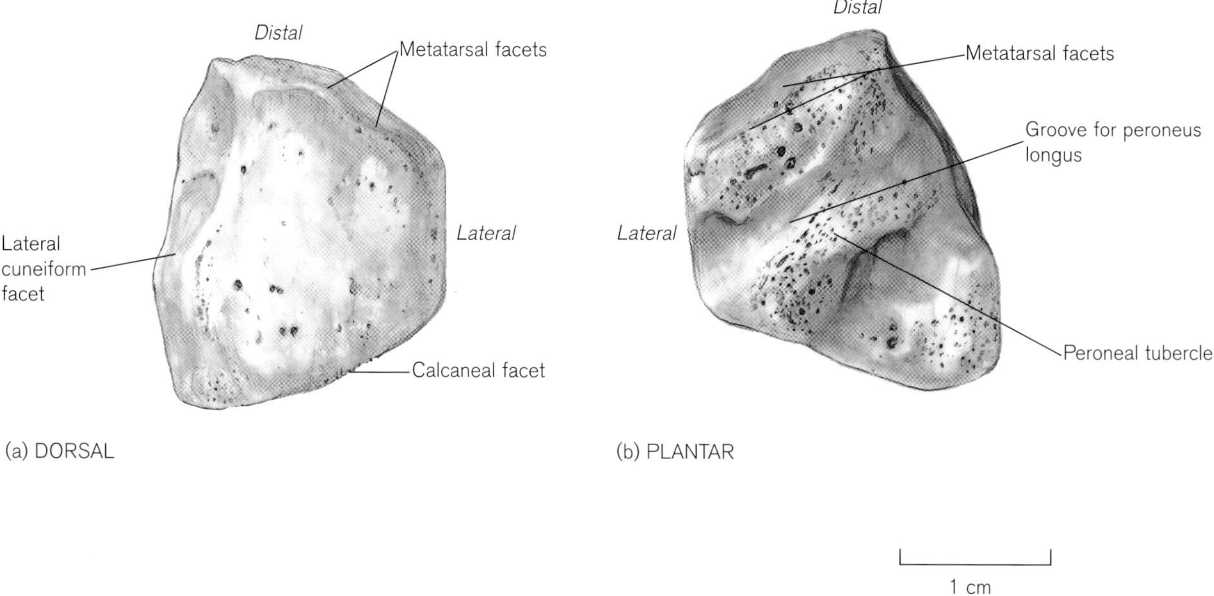

Figure 11.45 The right cuboid from a boy aged 8 years.

confirmed in any other literature. Menees and Holly (1932) found that the centre was present at birth in 3.8% of females and 0.3% of males and this was fundamentally confirmed by Hill (1939). Francis *et al.* (1939) found that in females, the centre was present in 60% of cases by 3 months, 85% by 6 months and 100% by 24 months. They found that in males, the centre was present in 50% of cases by 3 months *post-partum*, 75% by 6 months, 90% by 12 months and 100% by 18 months. Elgenmark (1946) concluded that the centre was always present by 9 months *post-partum* in females and 20 months in males. In summary, the appearance of the ossification centre for the lateral cuneiform is variable but it is likely that it will be present in many females by 3–4 months and many males by 5–6 months (Flecker, 1942; Pyle and Sontag, 1943; O'Rahilly *et al.*, 1960; Acheson, 1966; Garn *et al.*, 1967b; Birkner, 1978; Fazekas and Kósa, 1978). Until the end of the first year, when the margins of the bone begin to flatten, the lateral cuneiform appears as either a rounded or oval nodule. It becomes recognizable in isolation around the fourth year, when the individual surfaces can be identified (Fig. 11.46). The dorsal surface is non-articular, broad and slightly con-

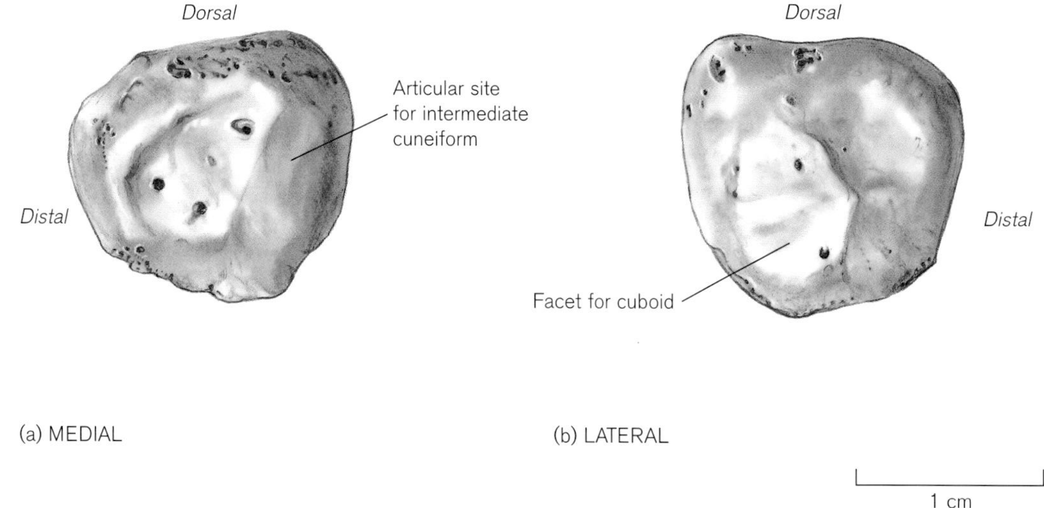

Figure 11.46 The right lateral cuneiform from a girl aged 4 years.

vex from side to side and from proximal to distal. The proximal and distal articular surfaces are convex and not clearly defined. The lateral surface bears a well-defined articular facet proximally and a non-articular region distally. The medial surface shows a well-defined central area of flat subperiosteal bone with numerous nutrient foramina. Between 4 and 6 years of age, the bone gradually adopts its basic adult form.

The **medial cuneiform** commences ossification within the second year in females and often into the third year in males (Puyhaubert, 1913; Frazer, 1948; Harding, 1952a; O'Rahilly *et al.*, 1960; Hoerr *et al.*, 1962; Acheson, 1966; Garn *et al.*, 1967b; Fazekas and Kósa, 1978; Stripp and Reynolds, 1988). Elgenmark (1946) reported that the centre was always present in girls by 2 years 11 months and in boys by 4 years 3 months. Francis *et al.* (1939) found that the centre was present in 1% of girls by 6 months *postpartum*, 69% by 18 months and 100% by 2 years 6 months. They found that the centre was present in 2% of boys by 6 months *postpartum*, 38% by 18 months and 100% by 3 years. Ossification may commence as a single nodule, but it is more likely to arise from a compound centre that may be double or multiple in origin. It is common for the bone to arise from double centres of ossification, one dorsal and one plantar, so that in the absence of synostosis, bipartition (os cuneiforme 1 bipartitum) may occur (Smith, 1886; Jones, 1946; O'Rahilly, 1953a; Birkner, 1978; Anderson, 1988c). It has been reported that the bipartite medial cuneiform is generally larger than its non-bipartite counterpart (Barlow, 1942). The division between the two elements may not be strictly horizontal, but more obliquely placed so that the two bone parts are more correctly labelled as dorsolateral and plantomedial (Barclay, 1932).

Despite its relatively late time of formation, the bone is still identifiable in isolation by between 3–4 years of age, when it appears as a roughly piriform-shaped bone with a pointed dorsolateral aspect and a more rounded and thicker plantomedial area (Fig. 11.47). By approximately 5 years of age, the bone still shows a clearly pointed dorsolateral region and a small patch of smooth subperiosteal bone can be identified on the lateral aspect, indicating the site of the future interosseous ligament connecting to the intermediate cuneiform. By around 6 years of age, this bone has also reached close to its adult morphology.

The **intermediate cuneiform** commences ossification around 2.5 years in females and 3.5 years in males (Puyhaubert, 1913; Frazer, 1948; Harding, 1952a; O'Rahilly *et al.*, 1960; Hoerr *et al.*, 1962; Acheson, 1966; Birkner, 1978), although it may be delayed in the male until the fourth or even the fifth

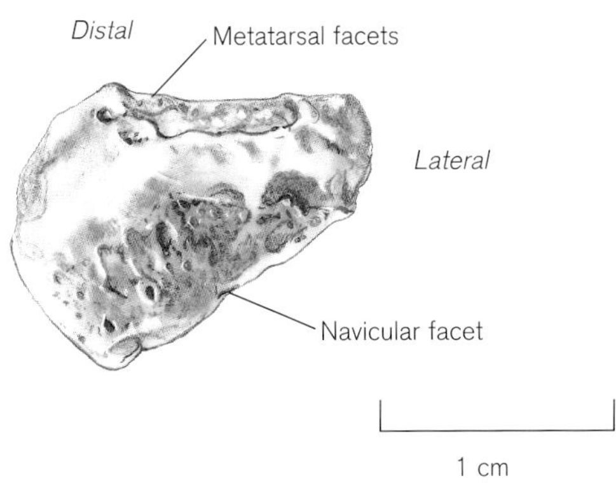

Figure 11.47 The right medial cuneiform from a child of approximately 3–4 years.

year (Stripp and Reynolds, 1988). Elgenmark (1946) reported that the centre was always present in girls by 2 years 8 months and in boys by 4 years 3 months. Francis *et al.* (1939) reported that the centre was present in 2% of girls by 9 months *postpartum*, 72% by 2 years and 100% by 3 years of age. They found the centre to be present in 1% of boys by 6 months *postpartum*, 59% by 2 years and 100% by 4 years 6 months. The intermediate cuneiform normally arises as a single centre of ossification, although multiple centres have been reported (Hoerr *et al.*, 1962). The intermediate cuneiform cannot be reliably identified in isolation until it has assumed close to adult morphology by around 6 years of age (Fig. 11.48).

The **navicular** is the last of the tarsal bones to commence ossification and does not tend to do so until the end of the second year in girls and the beginning of the fourth year in boys (Puyhaubert, 1913; Frazer, 1948; Harding, 1952a; Hoerr *et al.*, 1962; Acheson, 1966; Stripp and Reynolds, 1988). There is, however, considerable variation in the reported times of appearance and they range between 2 and 6 years (Pyle and Sontag, 1943; Garn *et al.*, 1967b; Birkner, 1978; Fazekas and Kósa, 1978). Elgenmark (1946) reported that the centre was always present in both girls and boys by 4 years 3 months. Ossification may commence from a single nucleus, two nuclei or multiple foci (Hoerr *et al.*, 1962; Birkner, 1978). By around 5 years of age, the bone has a domed distal surface and a flat proximal articular region (Fig. 11.49) but by 7–8 years the curved arc of the talar surface is well defined and the bone can be readily identified in isolation (Fig. 11.50). The tuberosity of the navicular does not develop until later and will be described under the section on secondary centres.

Avascular necrosis of the navicular (Köhler's disease) is thought to arise from a combination of mechanical and vascular vulnerability and has a male

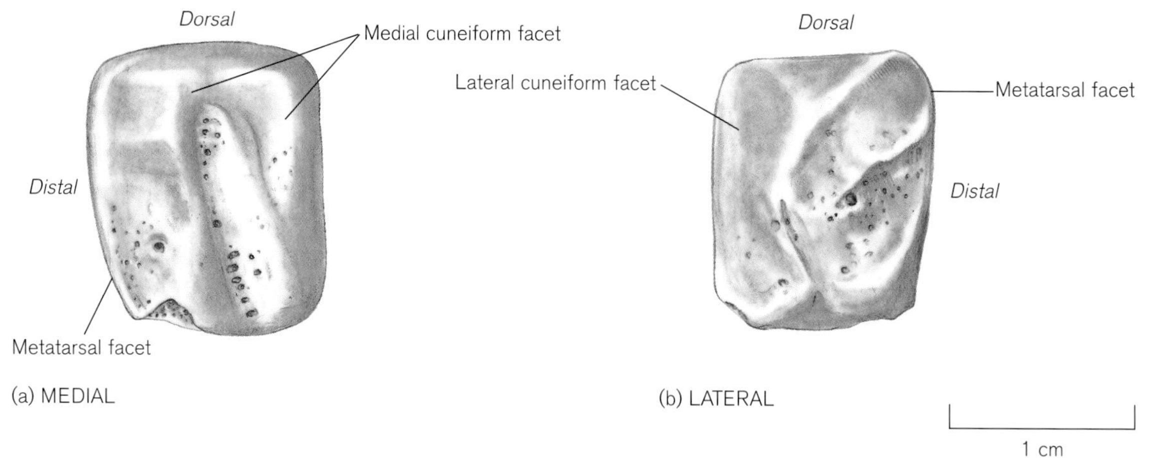

Figure 11.48 The right intermediate cuneiform from a girl aged 6 years.

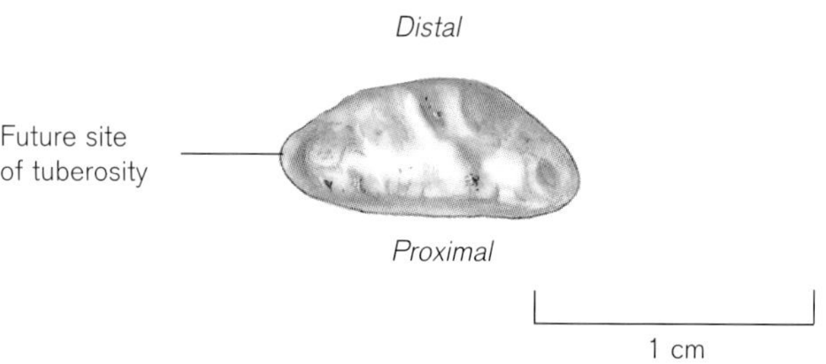

Figure 11.49 The dorsal surface of the right navicular from a child of approximately 5 years.

to female ratio of 6:1 respectively. It has been suggested that because the navicular is the last to commence ossification, it might be more susceptible to the arch compression forces of weight bearing and this, coupled with an inherent vascular insufficiency, may give rise to stress fractures, which leads to subsequent necrosis (Williams and Cowell, 1981; Scranton, 1988). This osteochondrosis of the navicular is normally detectable between 4 and 8 years (Aufderheide and Rodriguez-Martin, 1998).

The time of ossification of the **sesamoids** associated with the great toe is well documented. It is generally recognized that the lateral (fibular) sesamoid appears before the medial (tibial) sesamoid (by about 2 months) and that they ossify in girls before boys (Inge and Ferguson, 1933). The sesamoids commence ossification around 9 years in girls and 11–12 years in boys (Puyhaubert, 1913; Orr, 1918; O'Rahilly *et al.*, 1960; Hoerr *et al.*, 1962; Feldman *et al.*, 1970; Birkner, 1978), although they can appear as early as 8 years or as late as 15 years (Tachdjian, 1985).

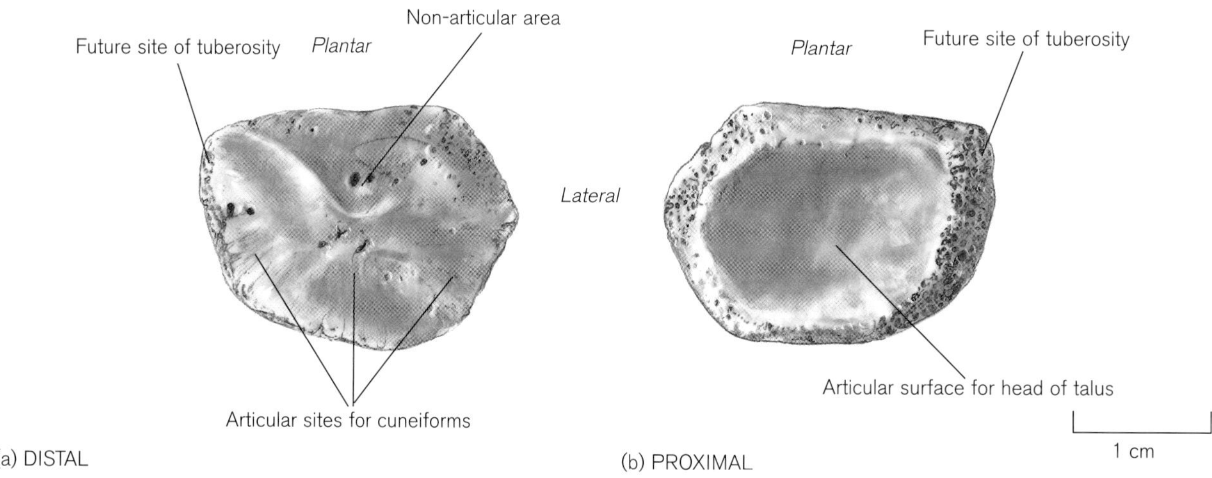

Figure 11.50 The right navicular from a boy aged 8 years.

Ossification occurs most commonly from a single focus, but it is not unusual for it to arise from double or multiple centres (Inge and Ferguson, 1933; Walling and Ogden, 1991; Potter *et al.*, 1992). Non-union of multiple centres can lead to partite sesamoids, which surprisingly do not necessarily predispose towards pain but are commonly misidentified as fractures (Powers, 1934). Partition is more common in the medial sesamoid and more likely to affect females (Potter *et al.*, 1992).

Congenital absence (aplasia) of the sesamoids of the great toe is rare, but when it does occur it is more commonly the medial that is affected (Inge, 1936; Lapidus, 1939; Zinsmeister and Edelman, 1985; Dennis and McKinney, 1990; Goez and De Lauro, 1995). While aplasia of the lateral sesamoid is considered to be exceedingly rare (Jahss, 1981; Jeng *et al.*, 1998), bilateral absence is even less common (Helal, 1981; Wright, 1998). Congenital absence of the hallucial sesamoids must be distinguished from resorption following disease (Conway *et al.*, 1989). It is interesting that both unilateral and bilateral absence is normally encountered by accident as they rarely display clinical symptoms. Le Minor (1988) reported that bilateral hallucial sesamoids are the norm in most mammalian orders and relatively constant in most of the primate groups. However, they were found to be inconstant in both gorillas and orang-utans and it was suggested that aplasia in the human might be related to a general decline in sesamoids within hominoid primates.

Ossification of the remaining sesamoids in the foot (see above) tends to occur around or after 15 years of age (Tachdjian, 1985).

Secondary centres

Appearance

The secondary centres of ossification in the foot appear, with at least one and possibly as many as four exceptions, in the cartilaginous extremities of the long bones. There are six morphologically distinct groups of epiphyses in the foot – the heads of the lateral four metatarsals, the base of the first metatarsal, proximal, middle and distal phalanges and the cap-like epiphysis of the calcaneus. Inconstant and perhaps somewhat questionable epiphyses are associated with the talus, navicular and fifth metatarsal (see below). Unlike the situation found in other long bones, where epiphyses arise in both the proximal and distal poles, in the foot, as in the hand, they tend to be restricted to one end of the bone, although in rare circumstances, supernumerary epiphyses have been documented. It is a general rule that, with the exception of the first metatarsal, the heads of all other metatarsals ossify from a separate secondary centre of ossification. The first metatarsal behaves more like a proximal phalanx, as all phalanges ossify from a single centre, which forms the shaft and the distal articular surface, while the base of the bone, at its proximal extremity, develops from a separate secondary centre of ossification.

It is well recognized that many of the epiphyses of the long bones of the foot may commence ossification from more than one locus. Roche and Sunderland (1959) showed that multiple foci (up to eight in some circumstances) are the norm for the development of the epiphyses of the first metatarsal and first proximal phalanx. As a general rule, all metatarsal epiphyses may develop from more than one centre, as indeed may all the epiphyses of the proximal phalanges, although in the female it may be restricted to only the first and fifth proximal phalanges. Multiple foci are not common in either the middle or distal phalanges, although they have been recorded in the second middle phalanx and the first distal phalanx in males only (Roche and Sunderland, 1959). However, by about 4 years of age, the multiple centres will start to consolidate rather like a string of pearls, so that after this date, only a single secondary centre can be detected in these locations.

There are several reports in the literature that state the **order of appearance** of the secondary centres and, of course, few of these agree. Therefore, we have summarized the views of the following papers and presented the most frequently reported pattern for secondary centre ossification (Francis *et al.*, 1939; Pyle and Sontag, 1943; Elgenmark, 1946; Harding, 1952a; Hoerr *et al.*, 1962; Acheson, 1966; Garn *et al.*, 1967b). As a general rule, the secondary centre for the first distal phalanx is usually the first to form, followed loosely in order by the secondary centres for middle phalanges 2–4, all proximal phalanges and the base of the first metatarsal. The appearance of the secondary centres for the metatarsals and distal phalanges of digits 2–4 then follow. The secondary centres for the bases of both the middle and distal phalanges of the fifth digit are very variable with regards to their time of appearance, if in fact they will form at all.

The secondary centre for the base of the first distal phalanx appears at approximately 9 months *post-partum* in females and 14 months in males. At this stage, the foot is already represented by the shafts of all the long bones, the calcaneus, talus, cuboid and lateral cuneiform. Few authors have published detailed information on the appearance of the secondary centres for the middle phalanges and this may simply be explained by the fact that they can be masked in many radiographic views of the foot due to the curled nature of the toes and so difficult to identify with any degree of certainty. The epiphyses of the middle phalanges of digits 2–4 are said to appear between 11 and 14 months in females and 14 and 24 months in boys. There does not appear to be any specific order with relation to the epiphysis of a specific digit appearing first. Some authors state that the epiphyses for the proximal phalanges develop in advance of those for the middle phalanges (Francis *et al.*, 1939; Elgenmark, 1946), while others state the opposite (Garn *et al.*, 1967b). The epiphyses for the proximal phalanges appear between 11 and 20 months in females and 18 months to 2 years 4 months in males, by which stage the medial cuneiform has commenced ossification. There does seem to be some evidence to suggest that ossification is first detected in the third proximal phalanx, followed in sequence by the fourth, second, first and finally by the fifth. There is some discrepancy in the literature concerning the time of ossification in the epiphysis of the base of the first metatarsal. Francis *et al.* (1939) report it to be 14 months in females and 22 months in males, whereas most other reports place the time at somewhat later between 18 and 20 months in females and 26 and 31 months in males (Pyle and Sontag, 1943; Elgenmark, 1946; Hoerr *et al.*, 1962; Garn *et al.*, 1967b). It is at this stage that the intermediate cuneiform commences ossification. The epiphysis for the head of the second metatarsal commences ossification between 19 months and 2 years in females and between 2 years 3 months and 2 years 10 months in males. The epiphysis for the head of the third metatarsal commences ossification somewhat later at approximately 2 years 5 months in females and 3 years 5 months in males. The epiphysis for the head of the fourth metatarsal commences ossification a little later at 2 years 8 months in females and 4 years in males. By the stage at which all epiphyses of the medial four metatarsals are represented, the navicular has commenced formation.

The epiphyseal centres for the distal phalanges of digits 2–4 appear in the female between 2 years 6 months and 3 years and in males between 4 years and 4 years 7 months. There is some evidence to suggest that if the epiphysis for the distal phalanx of the fifth digit is to develop, then it does so in advance of the other distal phalangeal epiphyses. The epiphysis of the distal phalanx of digit 5 appears at approximately 2 years 3 months in girls and 3 years 11 months in boys (Garn *et al.*, 1967b). For the remainder of these epiphyses, there is a clear pattern that the fourth digit appears before that of the third, with that for the second being the last to form. The epiphysis for the head of the fifth metatarsal is the last of the constant epiphyses to form and does so almost concomitant with the distal phalangeal epiphyses between 2 years 11 months and 3 years 2 months in females and between 4 years and 4 years 5 months in males.

The epiphysis for the middle phalanx of digit 5 behaves in a similar fashion to the epiphysis for the distal phalanx of the same digit. It may not develop at all, but if it does, then it can appear around 2 years in females and 2 years 11 months in males (Elgenmark, 1946). However, it has also been reported to appear as late as 5 years of age in both sexes (Francis *et al.*, 1939).

The **metatarsal heads** appear as small undifferentiated nodules of bone until approximately 4–5 years of age. From this time, they become recognizable, with rounded convex articular distal surfaces, flattened proximal metaphyseal surfaces and elongated oval outlines. After this, they continue to approach the adult morphology. It is interesting to note that according to Roche (1964b, 1965) between 20 and 30% of shaft growth in the metatarsals occurs at the non-epiphyseal ends. Identification of individual metatarsal heads is difficult and confidence will be greatest when only one individual is present and the individual is close to puberty so that an appropriate head can be fitted to a shaft. The head of the second metatarsal can be readily separated from the others, due to its larger size, while the fifth is the most distinctive due to the difference in angulation. When the articular surfaces are viewed from above, the head of the second metatarsal is somewhat stellate in appearance, displaying prolongations from each corner, with the plantolateral corner being particularly well developed (Fig. 11.51). The plantar border shows a particularly well developed notch for the passage of the long flexor tendon. The heads of metatarsals 3 and 4 are very similar in morphology and probably require the presence of a shaft to permit identification via best-fit procedures. When the distal articular surface of the fifth metatarsal head is viewed from above, it is obvious that the entire surface is skewed towards the medial aspect. The medial surface of the head is almost vertical, while the lateral surface has a distinct shallow slope. The anterior border displays the characteristic notch for the passage of the long flexor tendon and the medial tubercle is considerably smaller than the lateral.

The proximal metaphyseal surfaces are quite distinctive in appearance and can be readily differentiated from the corresponding metacarpal heads (see Chapter 9). This surface bears a centrally located raised region that is generally concave, more obviously raised at the plantar border and traversed from medial to lateral by a depression, which corresponds with a ridge on the metaphyseal surface of the metatarsal shaft (Fig. 11.51). This ridge-and-groove mechanism, together with the raised plantar border that locks into a depression on the metatarsal shaft, probably acts as a stop, to prevent both plantar and medial dislocation of the surfaces during locomotion.

Freiberg's infraction is characterized by an osteochondrosis of the second metatarsal head and tends to arise between 10 and 18 years of age (Freiberg, 1914). Females are three times more likely to be affected than males and the cause may be attributed to trauma, arterial insufficiency, developmental anomalies, or perhaps a combination of these (Braddock, 1959; Anderson and Carter, 1993; Aufderheide and Rodriguez-Martin, 1998) although the theory of avascular necrosis tends to be favoured in the clinical literature (Scranton, 1988; Thomas *et al.*, 1988). In general, the metatarsal is shorter than normal and the head has collapsed (hence infraction) and in

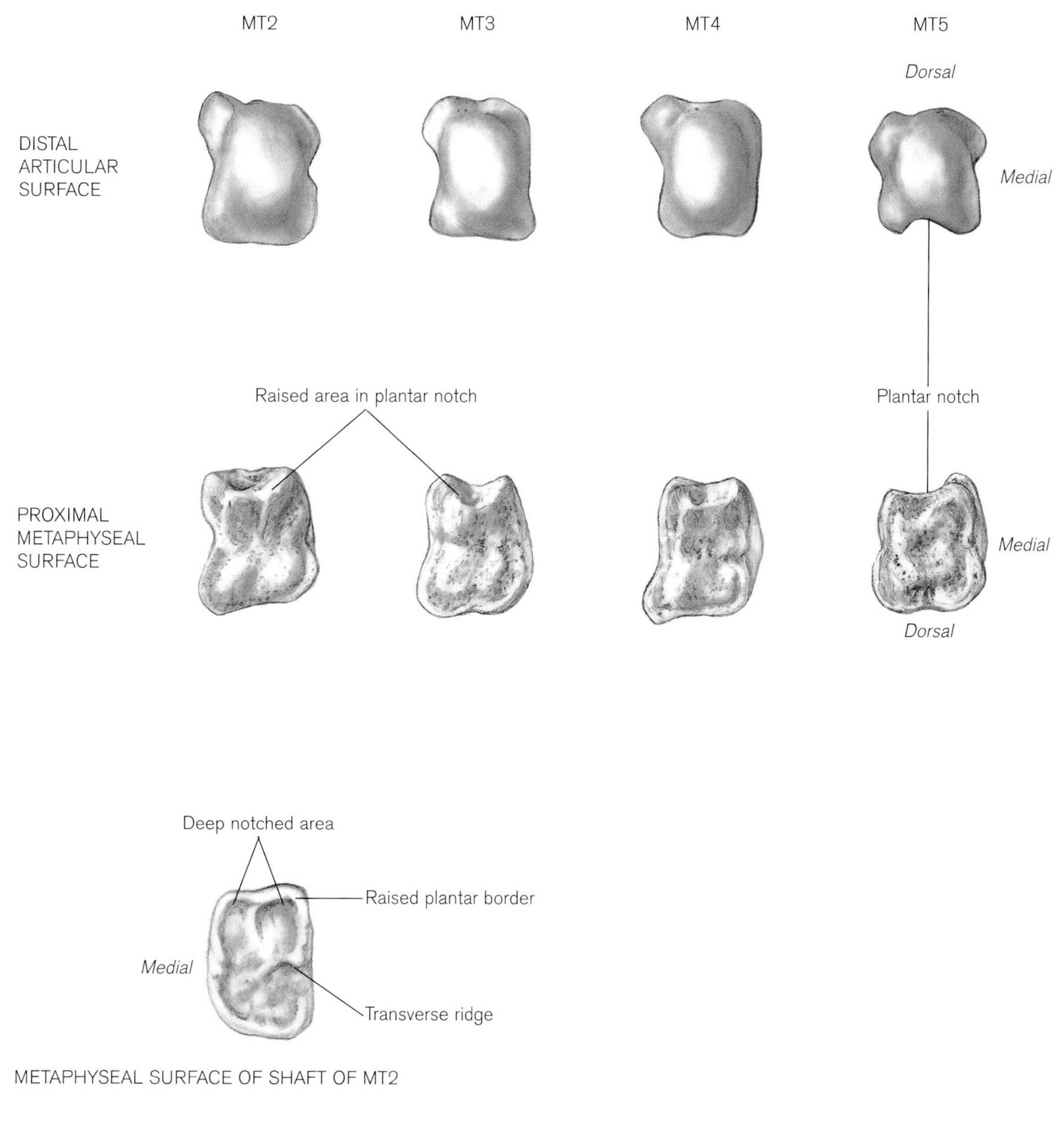

Figure 11.51 The distal and proximal surfaces of the right metatarsal (2–5) head epiphyses (approx. 12 years).

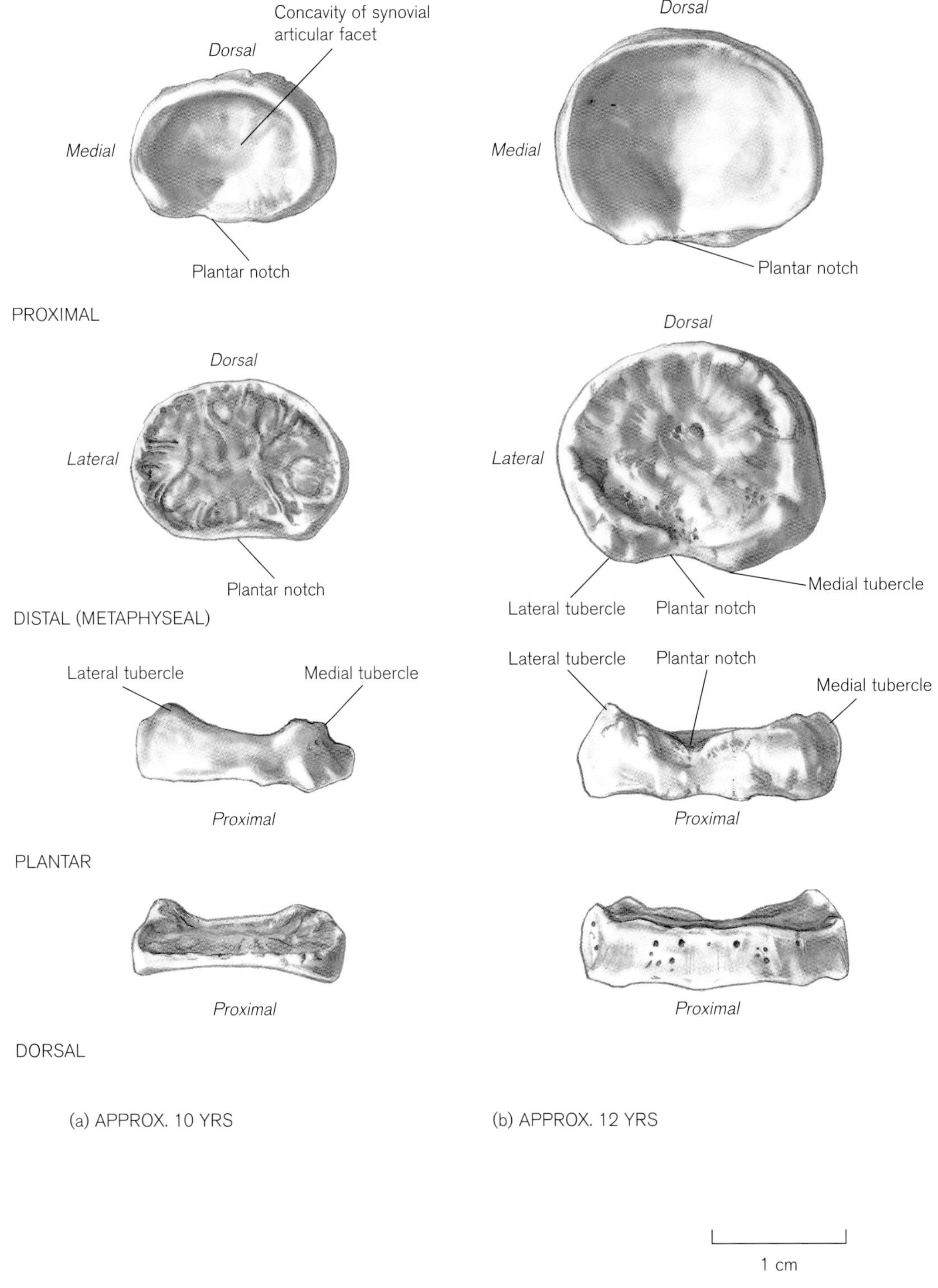

Figure 11.52 The epiphysis at the base of the right hallucial proximal phalanx.

severe cases it may even be separate from the shaft (Ortner and Putschar, 1985).

The epiphyses of the **proximal phalanges** can generally be described as flattened discs that are convex and uneven on their distal surface and smooth and concave on their proximal surface. The hallucial epiphysis is obviously larger and more robust than any of its more lateral counterparts. The articular surface is deeply concave and wider in the transverse than in the dorsoplantar plane. The dorsal, medial and lateral border form an almost uniform disc, while the plantar border is raised into medial and lateral tubercles, with an intervening notch for the passage of the flexor hallucis longus tendon. Until approximately 6–8 years of age, the epiphysis of the proximal hallucial phalanx is disc shaped and not readily recognizable. But as the epiphysis begins to conform to the shape of the diaphysis by about 7–10 years, its contours become more characteristic (Fig. 11.52). Epiphyseal clefts or fragmentation are most commonly observed in the basal epiphysis of the proximal phalanx of the great toe (Harrison and Keats, 1980; Lyritis, 1983). Although their aetiology is unknown, it is thought that they may only appear around the time of puberty and may not be related to multiple foci of ossification, as was originally considered. On a radiographic image, this epiphysis tends to be sclerotic in appearance, which is similar to that seen in the calcaneal epiphysis (see below) and considered to be a normal reaction to the stresses imposed on these structures. It is interesting to note that a sclerotic appearance does not occur in children who never walk (Harrison and Keats, 1980).

The remainder of the proximal phalangeal epiphyses are fairly constant in appearance and tend to vary only in size. Assigning a particular epiphysis to a specific proximal phalanx can only be achieved with any degree of accuracy when only one individual is represented and the epiphyses have formed a true cap over the diaphysis to allow a best-fit scenario to be adopted. The proximal articular surface is smooth and concave and slightly wider in the transverse than in the dorsoplantar direction. The plantar margin is straight or slightly concave, while the dorsal margin is gently rounded. The distal (metaphyseal) surface is roughened with a central elevated region that displays at least one, and often two, tooth-like structures close to the region of the plantar notch. These distally directed prolongations probably act as a type of locking mechanism to increase the stability of the joint and so prevent dislocation during locomotion (Fig. 11.53). As with the shafts of the metatarsals, so the shafts of the proximal phalanges also display a deep recess on the plantar border to accommodate the projections from the epiphysis. This phenomenon probably equates with the radiological condition of 'cone-shaped epiphyses'. While this morphology may be more obvious in certain clinical conditions, the frequency of occurrence in normal developing feet, renders them more likely to have a functional, rather than a pathological, aetiology. So-called conic epiphyses have also been likened in appearance to the indentation on the base of a wine bottle and are reported to be more common in females and fuse at an earlier age than non-conic epiphyses (Venning, 1961). Interestingly, a similar formation has been described in both the reptilian and avian literature (Fell, 1925; Haines,

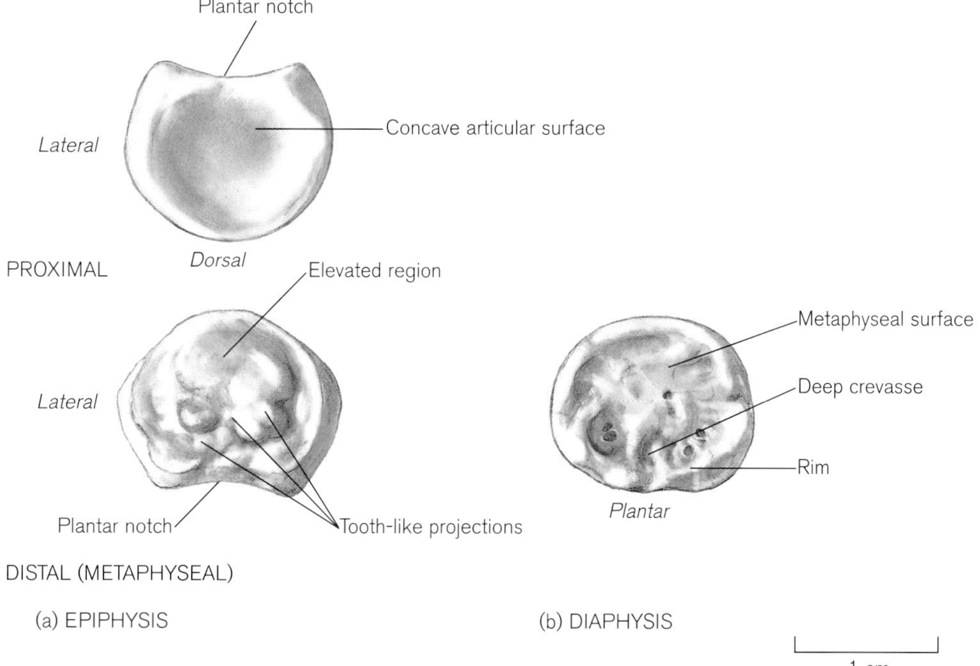

Figure 11.53 The right proximal phalangeal epiphysis from a child of approximately 7 years.

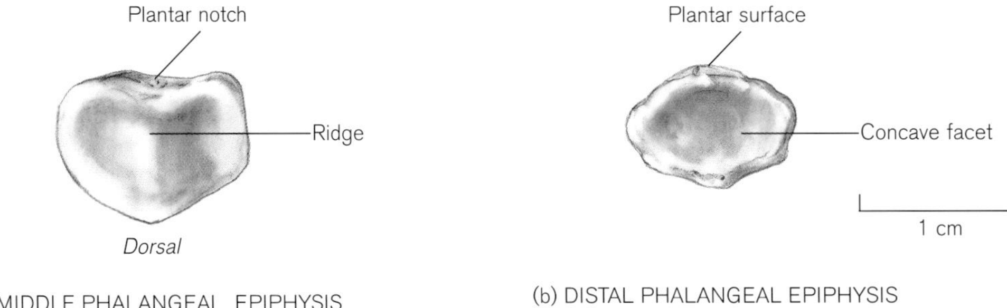

Figure 11.54 The right middle and distal phalangeal epiphyses.

1938, 1942), where a long cone or peg of cartilage is described that projects from the epiphysis into the diaphysis (Venning, 1960). While de Iturriza and Tanner (1969) admit that the aetiology of cone epiphyses is unknown, they do suggest that it may be related to circulation during fetal life. If not circulatory, then they also suggest that it may be related to some tissue metabolic gradient resulting in a difference in cell proliferation and maturation between central and peripheral parts of the epiphysis.

The epiphyses of the **middle phalanges** are often very difficult to identify and assign to a specific digit. These are disc-like structures with a biconcave facet located proximally for articulation with the head of the proximal phalanx (Fig. 11.54). The two facets are separated by a weak ridge that runs from the plantar to the dorsal rim of the surface. The plantar border is indented to accommodate the passage of the long flexor tendon and the dorsal border is gently rounded. The epiphysis is essentially oval in outline being longer in its transverse than in its dorsoplantar plane.

The epiphyses of the **distal phalanges** are equally difficult to identify and assign to a specific digit, with the obvious exception of the first digit. The epiphysis of the hallucial distal phalanx is larger and more robust than any of its more lateral counterparts. The concave proximal synovial surface is considerably wider in its transverse than in its dorsoplantar plane, with a wide plantar notch and a gently rounded dorsal border (Fig. 11.55). The medial aspect of the epiphysis is considerably larger than the lateral aspect, presumably due to the influence of the attachment of the flexor hallucis longus tendon. The remainder of the distal phalangeal epiphyses can best be described as small, oval discs (Fig. 11.54). The proximal synovial articular surfaces are concave both from plantar to dorsal and medial to lateral. Given the size and unpredictability of these epiphyses, we have not been able to assign an epiphysis to a specific distal phalangeal diaphysis with any degree of reliability.

The epiphysis for the **base of the first metatarsal** is sufficiently different from all the other pedal epiphyses to merit a separate description (Fig. 11.56). It is well developed and recognizable by 6–7 years of age. At this age the proximal articular surface is oval in shape and slightly thicker at the plantar margin. The lateral border is straighter than the more rounded medial

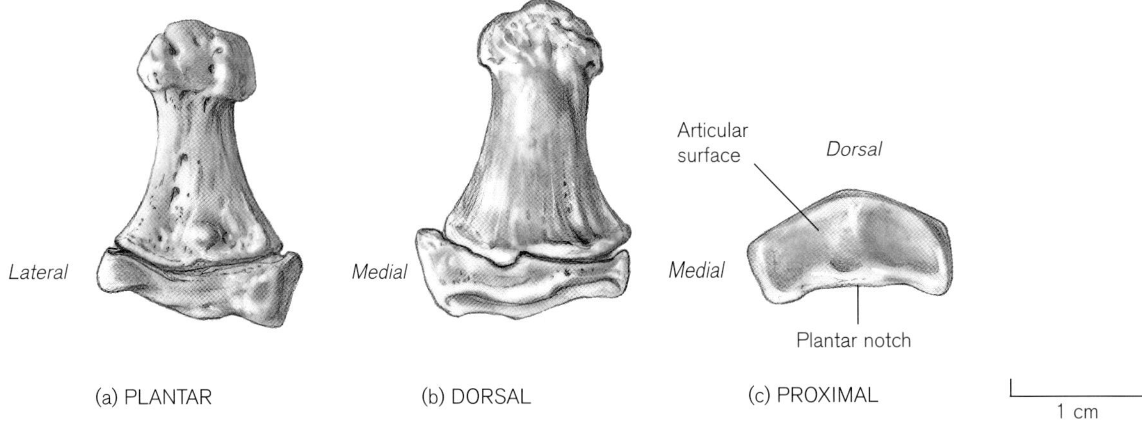

Figure 11.55 The right distal hallucial phalanx from a child of approximately 10 years.

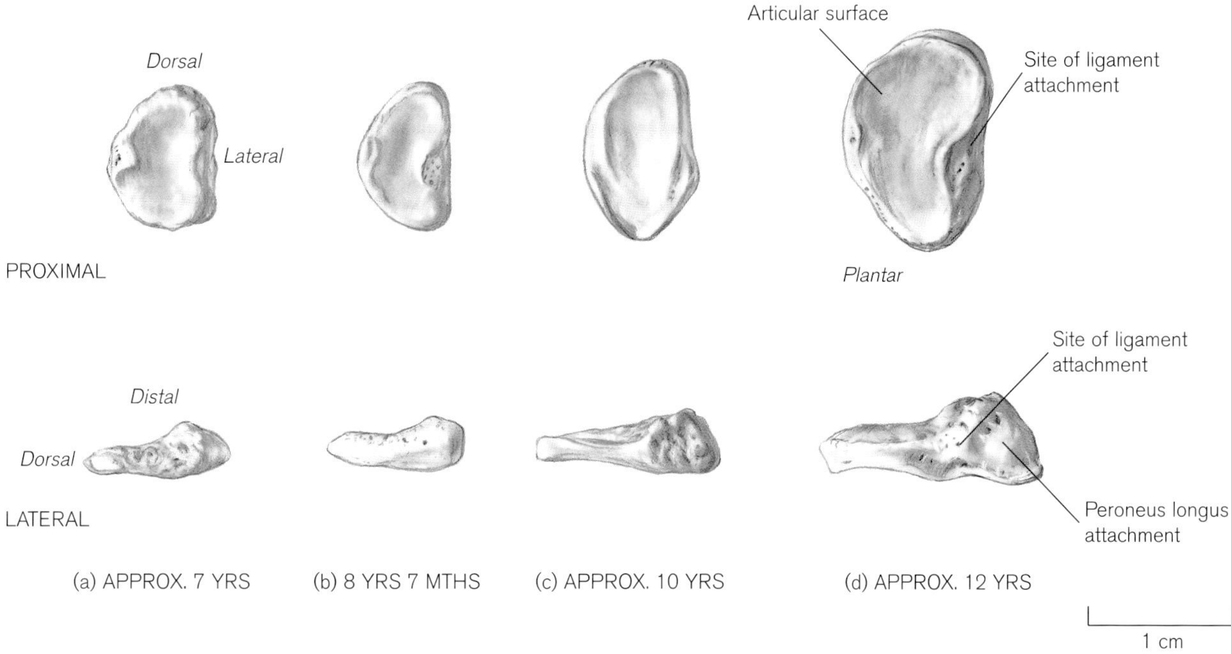

Figure 11.56 The development of the epiphysis of the base of the right first metatarsal.

border and there is a suggestion of a constriction separating the plantar from the dorsal articular area. By 8 years of age, the readily recognizable form of the epiphysis has developed with its characteristic reniform shape. By approximately 10 years of age, the articular margins of the epiphysis have become clearly defined and the site of attachment of the peroneus longus muscle is identifiable. By approximately 12 years of age, the epiphysis has adopted close to adult morphology and it is interesting to note that a deep crater can be detected in the central region of the distal metaphyseal surface of the epiphysis. This corresponds in position with a centrally located raised mound on the metaphyseal surface of the diaphysis and it is likely that they act as a mortice to lock the two developing centres together and prevent movement under the immense forces imposed by locomotion (Fig. 11.57).

So called 'pseudo-epiphyses' (Fig. 11.58) are commonly reported at the distal end of the first metatarsal (Burman and Pomeranz, 1932). As with those seen in the metacarpals, they tend to appear as notches or clefts in the normally non-epiphyseal end of the bone (see Chapter 9). While true epiphyses have been reported in this location (Posener *et al.*, 1939), these phenomena generally represent a normal stage in the physeal invasion of the primary centre into the region of the head of the metatarsal and normally appear between the ages of 4–5 years (Ogden *et al.*, 1994).

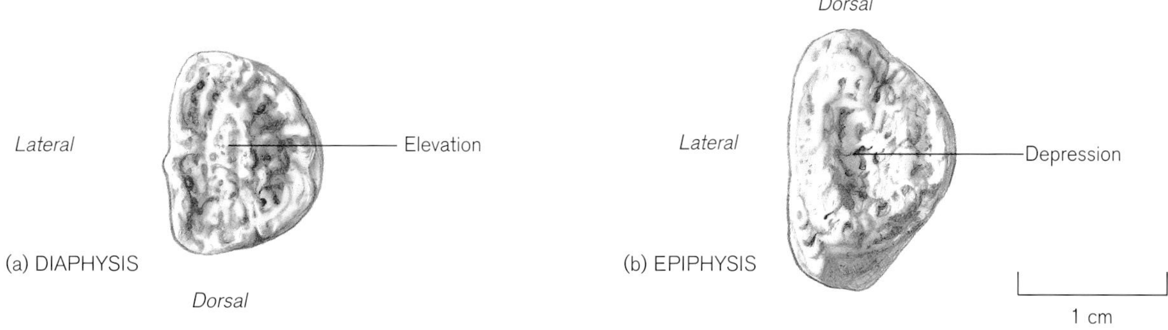

Figure 11.57 The metaphyseal surfaces of the diaphysis and epiphysis of the right first metatarsal from a child of approximately 12 years.

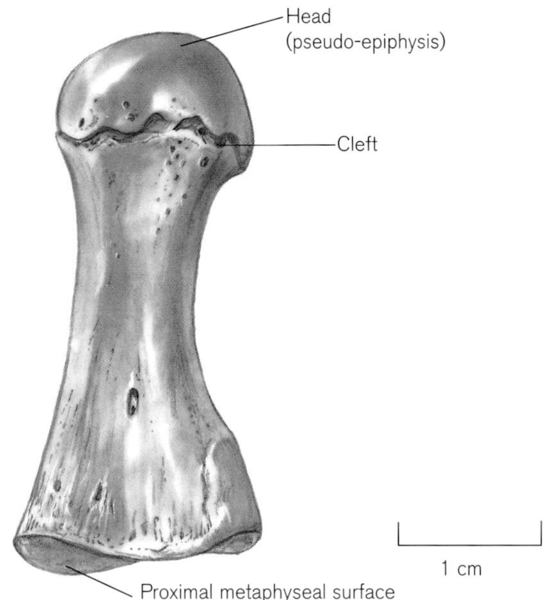

Figure 11.58 Pseudo-epiphysis at the distal end of the right first metatarsal in a girl aged 8 years 7 months.

While there is no controversy over the fact that the calcaneus is associated with a true secondary centre of ossification, most anatomical texts state that it is the exception within the tarsal bones. However, there is a considerable volume of evidence that shows that epiphyses may also be associated with the talus, navicular and the fifth metatarsal.

The epiphysis of the **calcaneus** is considered to be a traction epiphysis associated with the attachment of the tendo calcaneus and has, confusingly, been likened to the pisiform of the hand (Frazer, 1948). Ossification commences in this epiphysis via multiple centres which appear between 5–6 years in girls and 7–8 years in boys, although it has been reported as early as 4 years in girls and as late as 10 years in boys (Lurie *et al.*, 1943; Pyle and Sontag, 1943; Frazer, 1948; Ferguson and Gingrich, 1959; Hoerr *et al.*, 1962; Acheson, 1966; Garn *et al.*, 1967b; Birkner, 1978; Fazekas and Kósa, 1978; Tachdjian, 1985; Scranton, 1988). The centres usually appear below the middle of the posterior border of the calcaneus and spread both proximally and distally until they finally unite to form a cap-like covering around 8 years in girls and 10 years in boys (Hughes, 1948b; Hoerr *et al.*, 1962). This cap initially covers the lower two-thirds of the posterior aspect of the calcaneus, while the upper third will form either from a plate-like projection of this epiphysis or from a separate centre (Hughes, 1948b; Harding, 1952b). This accessory epiphysis may commence ossification between 10 and 12 years in girls and 11 and 14 years in boys. Fusion may occur directly with the body of the calcaneus or inferiorly with the superior border of the principal calcaneal epiphysis.

Painful heels are a relatively common complaint in children between the ages of 9 and 12, especially if they are involved in athletic pursuits. This condition was previously misinterpreted as avascular necrosis of the calcaneal epiphysis or so-called 'Sever's disease' (comparable to Osgood–Schlatter's disease), but is now recognized as stress fractures in the epiphysis following repeated pounding activities (Ferguson and Gingrich, 1959; Scranton, 1988). When viewed on a radiograph, the calcaneal epiphysis normally appears more dense than the body of the calcaneus and this is recognized as normal and is not attributed to any pathological condition (Hughes, 1948b; Fisk, 1988; Scranton, 1988).

It is unlikely that the calcaneal epiphyses could be identified in isolation prior to 8 years in girls and 10 years in boys. Certainly by 10 years of age, the epiphysis has formed a well-defined cap that sits over the lower two-thirds of the posterior surface of the calcaneal metaphysis and may extend down into the region of the lateral tubercle (Figs 11.59 and 11.60). The epiphysis is convex on its posterior aspect, concave on its metaphyseal surface, thicker in the lower plantar region and more scale-like in its upper extension.

The epiphysis of the **talus** is unlikely to be identified successfully as a separate structure due to its small size and indeed it may not always be present. The fact that this structure does exist is borne out by two facts. First, an active metaphyseal surface can be identified on many specimens (Fig. 11.61) and second, if the structure persists then it becomes known as the os trigonum, which is a well-recognized accessory bone with an incidence of approximately 5% in the general population (Turner, 1882; McDougall, 1955; Schreiber *et al.*, 1985; Helal, 1988; Grogan *et al.*, 1990; Wakeley *et al.*, 1996). When present, this epiphysis is located on the posterior aspect of the talus, in the region of the lateral tubercle. Ossification commences around 8 years in girls and 11 years in boys and fuses within a year or so of appearance (O'Rahilly *et al.*, 1960; Hoerr *et al.*, 1962; Tachdjian, 1985; Wakeley *et al.*, 1996). Persistence of the os trigonum can give rise to pain during activities that involve forced plantar flexion (ballet dancers, javelin throwers, footballers, etc.). This os trigonum syndrome or posterior triangle pain can often only be alleviated by removal of the offending ossicle (Martin, 1989; Wredmark *et al.*, 1991; Marrotta and Michelie, 1992).

The presence of an epiphysis in the **navicular** is more contentious. The region of the tuberosity of the navicular may show evidence of metaphyseal activity (Fig. 11.62). This is the site of attachment of the tibialis posterior tendon and in approximately 5–10% of

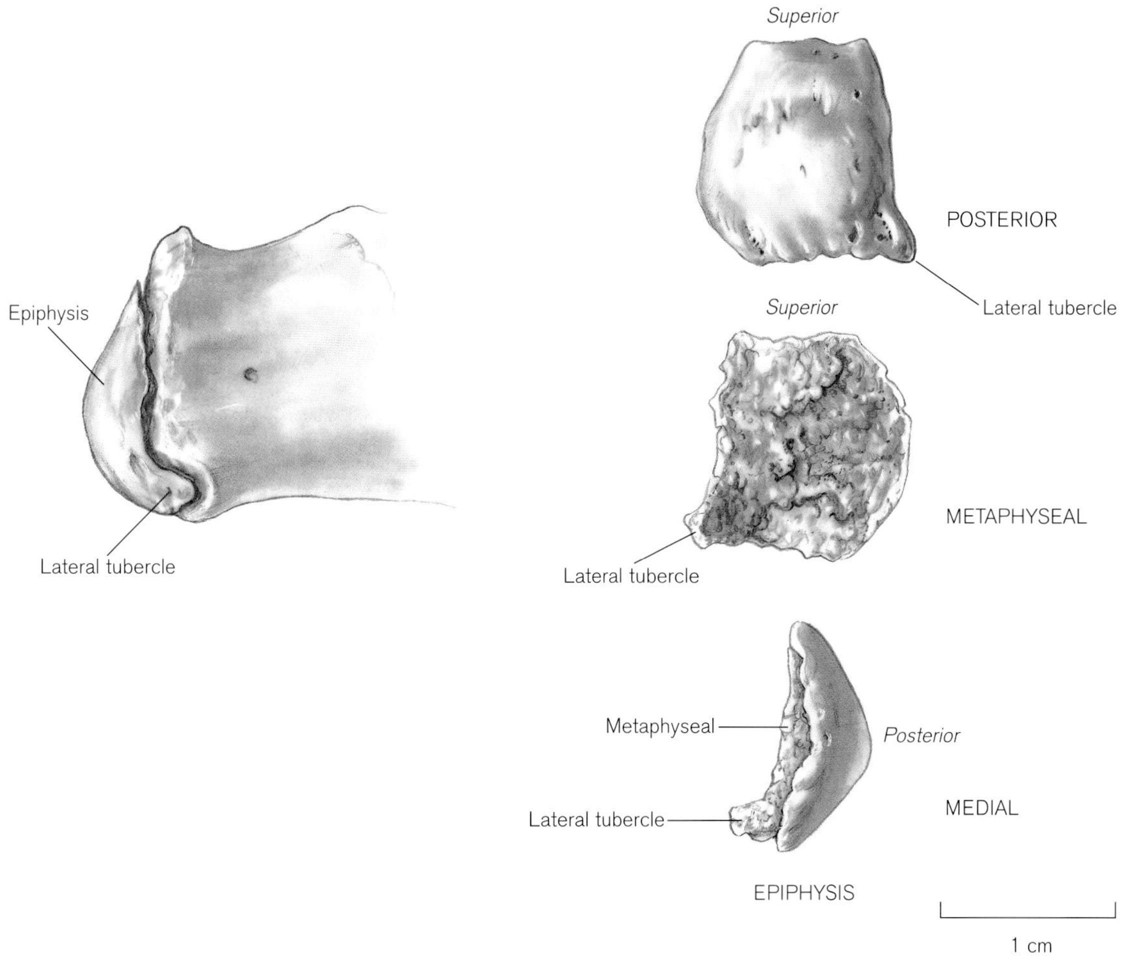

Figure 11.59 The right calcaneal epiphysis from a child of approximately 10 years.

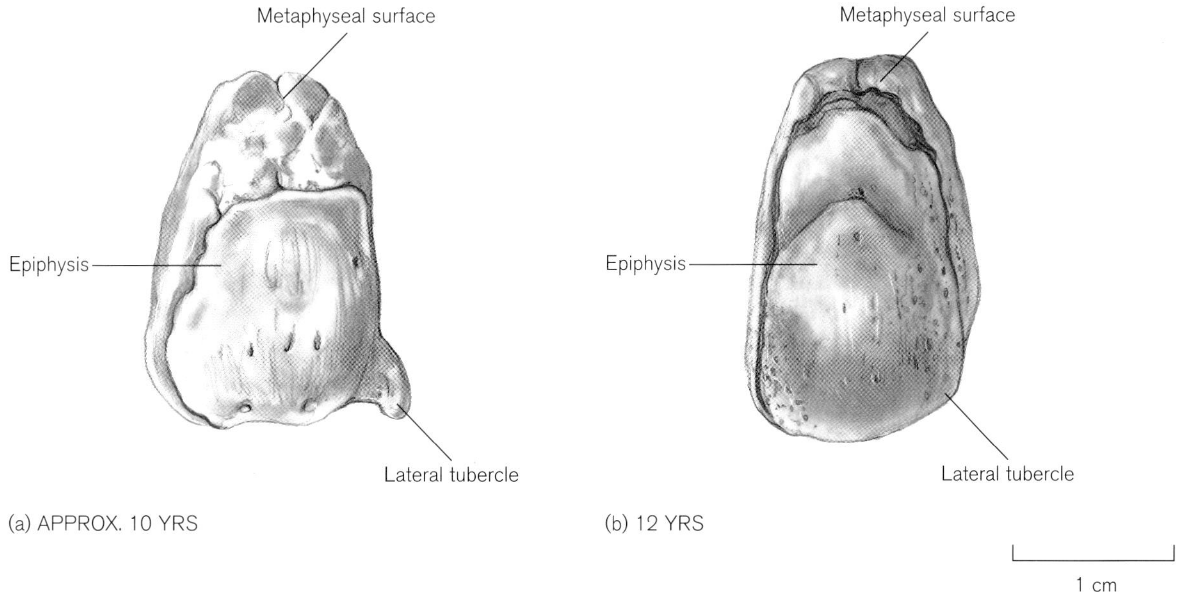

Figure 11.60 Fusion of the right calcaneal epiphysis.

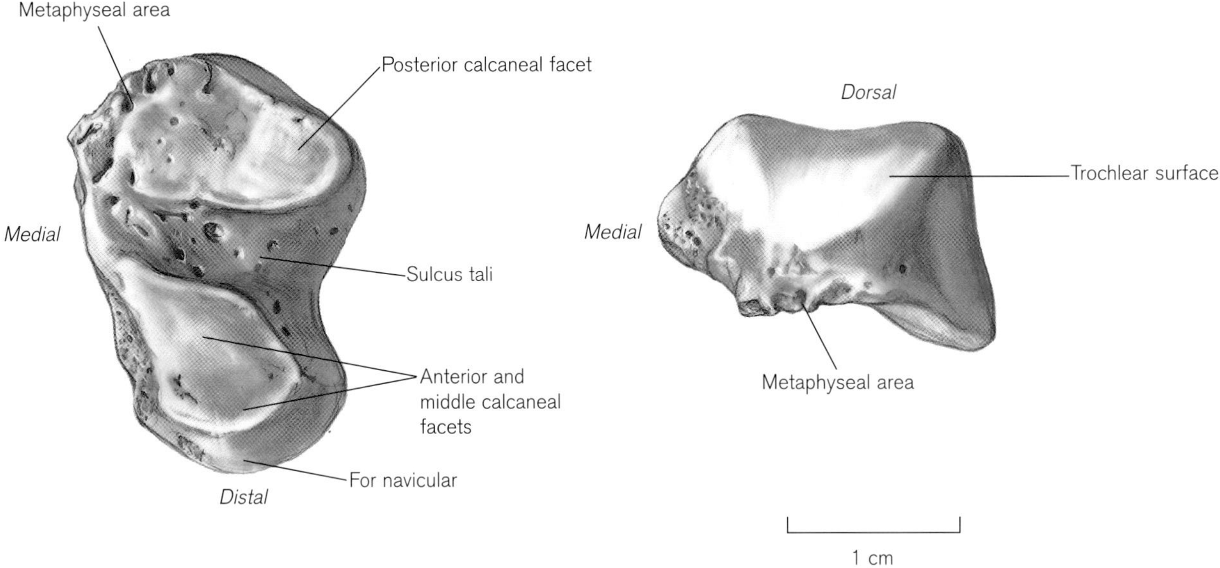

Figure 11.61 The site of the right talar epiphysis in a girl aged 8 years 7 months.

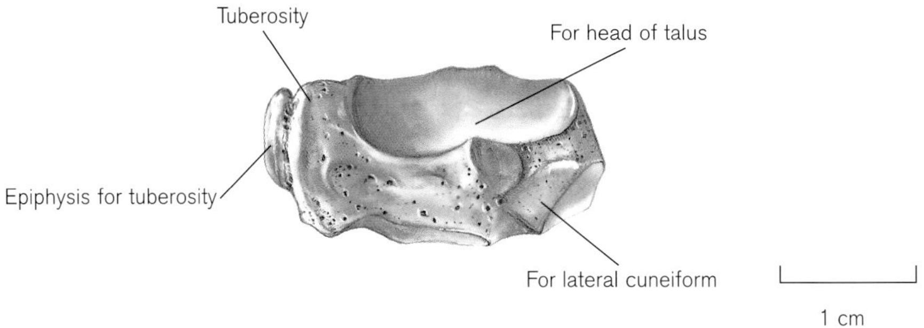

Figure 11.62 The plantar surface of the right navicular from a girl aged 12 years.

the general population it may remain as a separate accessory ossicle (os tibiale externum or prehallux). Persistence of a separate bone usually leads to inflammation of the overlying skin due to shoe pressure and excision is the normal course of action, although care must be taken not to damage the tibialis posterior tendon (Kidner, 1929; Zadek and Gold, 1948; Helal, 1988). The epiphysis is said to commence ossification around 9–10 years in girls and 12–13 years in boys, with fusion occuring shortly thereafter (Hoerr *et al.*, 1962; Acheson, 1966; Tachdjian, 1985).

The presence of an epiphysis for the tubercle at the base of the **fifth metatarsal** is even more contentious than that for the navicular and is not synonymous with either the os peroneum (a sesamoid in the tendon of peroneus longus) or the os Vesalii (Dameron, 1975). The epiphysis is said to commence ossification around 9–10 years in girls and 12 years in boys and fuses within the next 24 months (O'Rahilly *et al.*, 1960; Hoerr *et al.*, 1962; Dameron, 1975). It is unlikely that the epiphysis could ever be identified in isolation (Fig. 11.63).

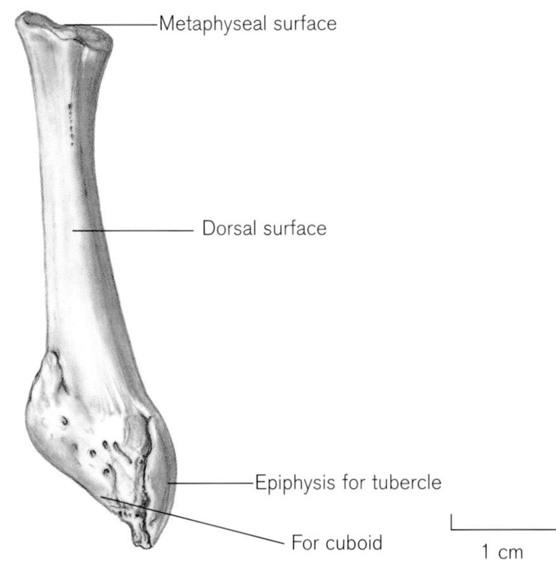

Figure 11.63 The epiphysis on the tubercle of the right fifth metatarsal from a child of approximately 10 years.

Fusion

It is not surprising that the order of appearance of the secondary centres of ossification does not mirror their order of fusion to the primary centre. While Birkner (1978) claimed that fusion occurs in a distoproximal sequence, commencing with the fusion of the epiphyses of the distal phalanges and ending with the closure of the metatarsal heads, this is perhaps too simplistic. It is probably true that fusion first commences in the distal phalanges, followed very closely by the middle phalanges and this occurs between 11–12 years of age in females and 14–15 years in males. The heads of metatarsals 2–5 fuse to the diaphyses between 11–13 years in females and 14–16 years in males, while the proximal phalanges and the base of the first metatarsal are a little later at 13–15 years in females and 16–18 years in males (Paterson, 1929; Lurie *et al.*, 1943; Pyle and Sontag, 1943; Hoerr *et al.*, 1962; Tachdjian, 1985). With the exception of the calcaneal epiphysis, it has been reported that 75% of all females will have completed epiphyseal fusion by 15 years of age and 75% of all males by 17 years of age. It is probably safe to say that epiphyseal fusion is usually always completed by 16 years in females and 18 years in males (Paterson, 1929).

Fusion of the calcaneal epiphysis occurs between 12 and 15 years, but obliteration of the diaphyseo-epiphyseal junction will not be completed until 15–16 years in females and 18–20 years in males (Pyle and Sontag, 1943; Acheson, 1966; Tachdjian, 1985). Fusion generally commences in the region of the lateral tubercle, while the final area to close is usually across the margin of the upper border (Fig. 11. 64).

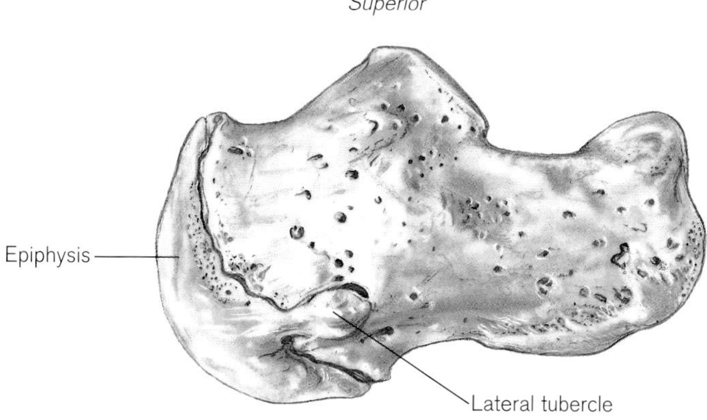

(a) LATERAL SURFACE – APPROX. 14 YRS

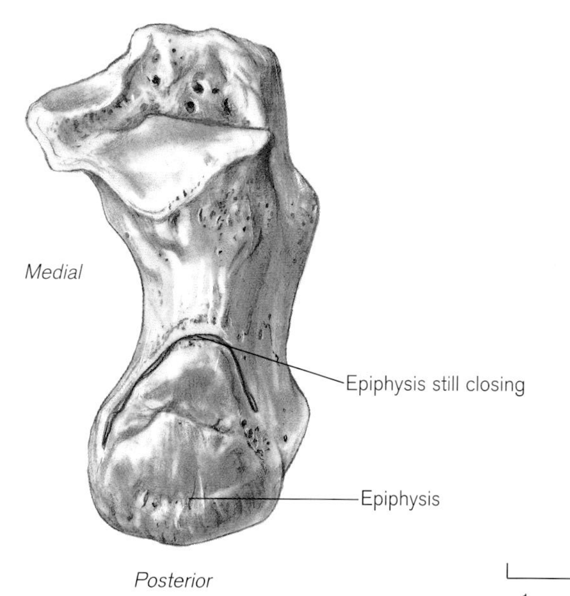

(b) SUPERIOR SURFACE – APPROX. 17 YRS

Figure 11.64 Closure of the right calcaneal epiphysis.

Growth of the foot

A sound understanding of growth of the foot as a whole is of considerable clinical importance. The length of the fetal foot has been used to predict gestational age and has also been of some value in neonatal anthropology in the study of congenital abnormalities and even to monitor neonates at risk (Streeter, 1920; Scammon and Calkins, 1929; Davenport, 1932; Blais *et al.*, 1956; Jordaan, 1982; Mathur *et al.*, 1982; Ramachandran, 1986; Mercer *et al.*, 1987; Barr and Hayashi, 1988; Campbell *et al.*, 1988; Daga *et al.*, 1988; Platt *et al.*, 1988; de Vasconcellos *et al.*, 1992; Gunstone, 1992). It is vital that due consideration be given to the longitudinal growth of the foot prior to pediatric pedal surgery (Tachdjian, 1985). In fact, the relative growth of different parts of the foot has also been interpreted in terms of its evolutionary significance (Straus, 1927b; Schultz, 1963).

The developing foot is strongly inverted by 2 fetal months and gradual eversion will occur over the next 7 months, although the foot will remain in an inverted talipes varus position at birth. The neonate has a considerable degree of dorsiflexion at the ankle joint but plantar flexion is limited due to the shortness of the extensor muscles (Crelin, 1973). The foot of the newborn is long and thin in appearance, with no external evidence of longitudinal arches. The average length of the neonatal foot is approximately 8 cms, which is in fact longer than the average length of either the femur or the tibia at this stage (Meredith, 1944; Anderson *et al.*, 1956). At birth, the foot is approximately 34% of its final adult size. By approximately 1 year of age in females and 1.5 years in males the foot has reached half of its mature length and by 2 years of age the longitudinal arches have descended to reach the adult form (Hoerr *et al.*, 1962). This precocious development of the foot tends, to protect it from future insults (whether they be nutritional, mechanical, metabolic, etc.), so that even if growth in stature is interrupted, there is little effect on foot size. There is a sharp decrease in the rate of growth of the foot from infancy to 5 years of age and from 5–12 years in females and 5–14 years in males there is an increase of only 0.9 cm per year in foot length (Hill, 1958; Tachdjian, 1985). The rate of growth decreases rapidly after 12 years in females and 14 years in males, so that 95% of mature length is achieved by 12–13 years in females and 15 years in males (Meredith, 1944). Mature length is generally achieved by 14 years in females and 16 years in males, which naturally coincides with the cessation of epiphyseal growth. There is a small adolescent growth spurt in foot length, which tends to start and finish earlier than that seen either in stature or overall length of the lower limb and precedes normal peak growth spurt by approximately 6–18 months (Anderson *et al.*, 1956).

Practical notes

Sideing

The bones of the foot tend to mature at an earlier age than their counterparts in the hand and so positive identification can occur at an earlier age (certainly by 6 years).

Tarsals

It is possible to correctly side the neonatal **calcaneus**, although it is much easier to do so by the end of the first year. At birth, the indentation that will form the calcaneal groove is located on the distal aspect of the superior surface and the larger of the two flattened regions is located on the medial aspect of the plantar surface. Within the first few months after birth, the medial projection of the sustentaculum tali begins to form and so the identification of side is apparent.

The **talus** can also be identified and assigned to the correct side of the body by full term, if not slightly before. The position of the talar neck is established early in fetal development and can be seen as depressions on both the dorsal and plantar surfaces that are situated closer to the distal extremity. These two indentations are separated on the lateral aspect by a clearly defined ridge of bone, while on the medial aspect they are separated by a considerable expanse of bone with no distinguishing characteristics.

Although the **navicular** can probably be recognized at around 5 years of age, assigning the specimen to the correct side of the body probably cannot be achieved until closer to 7 or 8 years of age, when the site of the tuberosity can be established. The concavity of the proximal talar surface and the convexity of the distal cuneiform surface are established at an early age, but until the tuberosity develops on the plantomedial aspect of the bone, orientation is extremely difficult.

The **medial cuneiform** is recognizable at 3–4 years of age and can also be assigned to the correct side at this age. It is represented by a thick, rounded plantomedial area and a thin, pointed dorsolateral projection with a relatively flat dorsal surface and a slightly concave plantar surface. The articular region is larger on the distal surface than that on the proximal for articulation with the navicular.

The **intermediate cuneiform** can be readily identified in isolation by around 6 years of age, when it can also be correctly attributed to a specific side of the body. The dorsal surface is flat, the plantar surface is represented by a blunt ridge and the distal surface is generally longer than the proximal. The lateral aspect bears an articulation for the lateral cuneiform along the distal and proximal margins, while the medial aspect bears an articulation for the medial cuneiform that runs almost the entire length of both the dorsal and proximal margins.

The **lateral cuneiform** is recognizable in isolation by around 4 years and at this stage it can successfully be attributed to the correct side of the body. The dorsal surface is flat and the plantar surface ends in a blunt ridge. The medial surface displays a flattened area of subperiosteal bone, with an articulation for the intermediate cuneiform lying proximal to it. The lateral surface bears a rounded articular facet for the cuboid, which is located on the proximal margin of this surface closer to the dorsal surface. This is important to identify, as often it is very difficult to differentiate between the distal articular surface for the third metatarsal and the proximal articulation with the navicular.

The **cuboid** can be identified in isolation and assigned to the correct side by approximately 3–4 years of age, when the nodule starts to develop some of the mature characteristics of the bone. The groove caused by the tendon of peroneus longus can be recognized on the plantar surface, while the dorsal aspect is flattened and clearly non-articular. The distal surface is flat and relatively short compared to the longer and more concave proximal aspect. The lateral border is short with no distinguishing characteristics, while the medial border is longer and bears a well-defined articular facet for the lateral cuneiform.

Metatarsals

Until the metatarsals begin to adopt the adult form of articulations at their bases, it is very difficult to correctly identify both side and specific digit to all except the first. Even at the neonatal stage, the first metatarsal can be separated from all others due to its size and robusticity. The dorsal surface of the shaft is relatively flat, while the plantar surface displays a gentle concavity along its length. The base of the shaft is convex along its medial border and concave along its lateral border. The medial aspect of the head is generally larger than the lateral. The heads of the metatarsals are very difficult to assign to the correct side of the body and can probably only be achieved with any degree of reliability in the second and fifth bones at around 4–5 years of age. The second metatarsal head displays a prominent tubercle at the junction of the plantar and lateral surfaces, while that of the fifth is distinctly skewed towards the medial surface. The epiphysis at the base of the first metatarsal is well developed by 6 years of age and can be readily assigned to a specific side of the body. The medial border tends to be straighter than the lateral border, which displays a slight constriction around the middle of its length. Due to the site of attachment of the peroneus longus tendon on the plantar aspect of the base, this region of the epiphysis tends to be thicker than the dorsal aspect.

Phalanges

Other than the components of the first digit, it is virtually impossible to assign a phalanx to a specific digital ray (let alone side of the body) in the adult, and so there is little value in attempting to do so in the juvenile. The proximal phalanx of the big toe can be easily attributed to the correct side, as the medial border is always longer than the lateral border. The same is true for the terminal phalanx of this digit and reflects the normal hallux deviation that is present from an early age (Griffiths, 1902).

The only other epiphysis that can be attributed to the correct side of the body is that for the distal hallucial phalanx. Correct sideing relies on being able to identify a relatively larger tubercle on the medial aspect of the epiphysis than occurs on the lateral aspect.

Bones of a similar morphology

Whilst it is true that before 3–4 years of age several tarsals could be mistaken for many developing bones as they appear as relatively undifferentiated nodules, beyond this age, each develops its own characteristic morphology so that close attention to detail should prevent misidentification. The similarities between the metatarsals and the metacarpals and the manual and pedal phalanges ensure that they are the bones that are most likely to be incorrectly identified. Metatarsals are usually longer than metacarpals, with straighter shafts that are compressed in the mediolateral direction. In addition, the heads of the metatarsals are also compressed in the mediolateral plane. Further, the heads of the metatarsals are relatively smaller compared to their bases than is found in the metacarpals and obviously the arrangement of articular facets on the base will differ from those found in the hand bones. The pedal phalanges are consistently shorter and more slender than those found in the hand and their morphology can be quite irregular. The proximal pedal phalanges have relatively large bases and heads but slender, mediolaterally compressed shafts, whereas those of the hand tend to be longer and more robust. The middle and distal pedal phalanges are very short and have shafts that are concave on both the dorsal and the plantar surfaces, whereas those of the hand are longer and convex on the posterior surface. The distal pedal phalanges tend to have more pronounced ungual tuberosities than the manual distal phalanges, to support the end of the digit.

Morphological summary

Fetal	
8–10 wks	Primary ossification centres appear for metatarsals 2–5
9–12 wks	Primary ossification centres appear for distal phalanges
12 wks	Primary ossification centre appears for base of metatarsal 1
14–16 wks	Primary ossification centres appear for proximal phalanges
16–20 wks	Primary ossification centres appear for middle phalanges
5–6 mths	Ossification centre appears for calcaneus
6–7 mths	Ossification centre appears for talus
Birth	At least 16 of the primary centres of ossification for the long bones of the foot are present (middle phalanges of the lateral toes may appear after birth). In addition, both the calcaneus and talus are present and can be identified in isolation (cuboid centre of ossification may be present)
1–3 mths	Ossification centre appears for cuboid
3–6 mths	Ossification centre appears for lateral cuneiform
9 mths (female) 14 mths (male)	Epiphysis for base of distal phalanx 1 appears
11–14 mths (female) 14–24 mths (male)	Epiphyses for middle phalanges 2–4 appear
11–20 mths (female) 18–28 mths (male)	Epiphyses for proximal phalanges appear
12–24 mths (female) 24–36 mths (male)	Ossification centre appears for medial cuneiform
18–20 mths (female) 26–31 mths (male)	Epiphysis for base of metatarsal 1 appears
19–24 mths (female) 27–34 mths (male)	Epiphysis for head of metatarsal 2 appears
24–36 mths (female) 36–48 mths (male)	Ossification centre appears for intermediate cuneiform
2 yrs 5mths (female) 3 yrs 5mths (male)	Epiphysis for head of metatarsal 3 appears
2 yrs 8 mths (female) 4 yrs (male)	Epiphysis for head of metatarsal 4 appears
2–3 yrs (female) 4–5 yrs (male)	Ossification centre appears for navicular as do epiphyses for distal phalanges 2–4 and epiphysis for head of metatarsal 5
3–5 yrs (female) 5–7 yrs (male)	By this stage, the cuboid, navicular, cuneiforms and metatarsal heads are all identifiable in isolation
5–6 yrs (female) 7–8 yrs (male)	Epiphysis for calcaneus appears
8 yrs (female) 11 yrs (male)	Epiphysis for talus appears
9 yrs (female) 12 yrs (male)	Sesamoids of great toe appear and fusion of talar epiphysis occurs
9–10 yrs (female) 12–13 yrs (male)	Epiphysis for navicular may appear (and fuse shortly after). Epiphysis at base of metatarsal 5 may appear and will also fuse within the next 24 months
10–12 yrs (female) 11–14 yrs (male)	Calcaneal epiphysis commences fusion
11–13 yrs (female) 14–16 yrs (male)	Epiphyseal fusion in distal phalanges, middle phalanges and metatarsal heads 2–5
13–15 yrs (female) 16–18 yrs (male)	Epiphyseal fusion in proximal phalanges and base of metatarsal 1
15–16 yrs (female) 18–20 yrs (male)	Completion of fusion at the calcaneal epiphysis

Metrics

There is very little information on age-related growth in individual bones of the foot. Fazekas and Kósa (1978) give measurements on the fetal first metatarsal from 16 fetal weeks to term and this is summarized in Table 11.18. De Vasconcellos and Ferreira (1998) reported on metatarsal growth in 78 Brazilian fetuses from the second trimester (Table 11.19).

Table 11.18 Diaphyseal length of fetal metatarsal 1, from 16–40 weeks

Age (weeks)	Diaphyseal length (mm)
16	2.4
18	3.2
20	4.0
22	5.0
24	5.8
26	6.3
28	7.3
30	8.2
32	9.1
34	10.7
36	11.5
38	12.3
40	13.2

Length: maximum length of the diaphysis (in mm).
Adapted from Fazekas and Kósa (1978).

Table 11.19 Diaphyseal length of metatarsals 1–5 from 14–23 weeks gestation

	Metatarsal maximum diaphyseal length (mm)				
Gestational age (weeks)	1	2	3	4	5
14	2.04	2.80	2.34	2.34	2.02
15	2.88	3.87	3.61	3.57	3.33
16	3.35	4.45	4.43	4.18	–
17	4.00	5.40	4.94	4.55	4.30
18	4.29	5.68	5.56	5.20	4.88
19	4.45	6.02	5.73	5.35	5.06
20	5.26	7.24	6.87	6.30	5.96
21	5.20	7.27	6.84	6.43	5.97
22	6.06	7.96	7.70	7.38	–
23	6.20	8.23	7.86	7.39	6.87

Adapted from de Vasconcellos and Ferreira (1998).

Appendix 1

Historically, there have been many different ways of designating the lifespan of an individual. Aristotle distinguished three major phases: growth, perfection and decline. Shakespeare famously described the 'The Seven Ages of Man' as infancy, boyhood, puberty, youth, manhood, old age and decrepitude.[1] In his lectures on Medical Jurisprudence[2] given at the new London University, A.T. Thomson (1836) quoted Aristotle's three phases but preferred five divisions: infancy, boyhood, youth, manhood and old age. These categories, together with his lectures beginning, 'Gentlemen,' obviously ignore the entire female sex!

At the present time terminology varies, both in different countries and as used by clinicians, auxologists and evolutionary and skeletal biologists and this can lead to confusion.

The accepted definitions used by paediatricians, of the time periods from the beginning of life through the childhood years are shown below:

Prenatal	up to the time of birth; expressed clinically from last menstrual period (LMP) in terms of days (280), weeks (40) or lunar months (10) or embryologically in days (266) or lunar months (9.5) from fertilization
Embryo	the first 8 weeks (2 lunar months) of intra-uterine life
Fetus	from week 9 to birth
Trimester	one-third of the time of normal pregnancy, thus first, second and third trimesters
Preterm	from < 37 weeks (258 days) gestation
Fullterm	from 37–42 weeks (259–293 days) gestation
Post-term	> 42 weeks (294 days) gestation
Stillbirth	infant born after gestational period of 24 weeks who shows no signs of life (in UK reduced from 28 weeks in 1992 – Forfar, 1998)
Perinatal	literally around the time of birth – from 24 weeks gestation to 7 postnatal days
Neonatal	from birth to 28 days
Infant	from birth to the age of 1 year
Childhood	from 1 year to puberty/adolescence. Sometimes arbitrarily divided into: *early childhood* – preschool years; *late childhood* – about 6 to about 12 years, although some paediatricians (e.g. Forfar, 1998) give the childhood range as 1–15 years.

After this stage, usage varies. *Puberty* is generally taken to be a physiological term describing the beginning of secondary sexual change, usually ranging from 10–14 years in girls and 12–16 years in boys. *Adolescence* is used by some authors interchangeably with *puberty* but by others as referring to the behavioural and psychological changes at puberty. Some paediatricians describe adolescence as from 13 to 19 years of age (Forfar, 1998).

Two schemes commonly used by **skeletal biologists** vary in the terms that are applied to the period between the end of childhood (14–15 years) and adult life, which is defined as the time of closure of the spheno-occipital synchondrosis. Acsádi and Nemeskéri (1970) use the term *juvenile* and the WEA (1980) call the same period *adolescence*. However, the age ranges of between 17 and 25 years quoted in most standard anatomical texts for the closure of the spheno-occipital synchondrosis are almost certainly too late. Recourse to the original literature describing the inspection of dry skulls, cadavers and histological and radiological observations report this as occurring

[1] Jacques in *As You Like It* – Act II, Scene 7.
[2] Thomson, A.T. (1836). *Lancet* **1**: 281–286.

between 11 and 15 years (see 'Occipital bone', Chapter 5, Table 5.1). The whole of the juvenile or adolescent time period as defined by the two schemes would thus be eliminated.

In some continental European countries (Knussmann, 1988) skeletal biologists divide the period of childhood into:

Infans I birth to 7 years (i.e. until emergence of first permanent molar teeth)
Sometimes divided into:
Infans Ia birth to 2 years
Infans Ib 2–7 years

Infans II 7–14 years (i.e. between emergence of first and second permanent molars)

Juvenil until closure of spheno-occipital synchondrosis (about year 22)

Adult onset of suture closure.

The second molars emerge earlier than this (11–13 years) and again, the time for the closure of the skull base is too late.

Behavioural biologists (e.g. Bogin, 1997) have yet another set of definitions:

Infancy the time when the young is dependent on the mother for nourishment via lactation. The duration may vary from few months to about 3 years, depending on the society.

Childhood the period following weaning when the child is still dependent on adults for feeding and protection. It also coincides with the period of rapid brain growth, a relatively small digestive system and an immature dentition (for discussion on the brain to body size/gut size relationship see Aiello and Wheeler, 1995).

Juvenility is the period at completion of brain growth and the beginning of the eruption of the permanent dentition at about 7 years.

Adolescence beginning with puberty at about 10 years in girls and 12 years in boys and including the adolescent growth spurt.

Adulthood from the end of the growth spurt, the attainment of adult stature, the completion of dental maturity and the achievement of full reproductive maturity.

In the UK and North America, the 'umbrella' terms *immature*, *sub-adult* and *non-adult* are also used for any age that is not truly adult. However, in more recent publications, the term *juvenile* is replacing these terms (Hoppa, 1992; Saunders, 1992; Molleson and Cox, 1993; Saunders and Hoppa, 1993; Saunders *et al.*, 1993; Huda and Bowman, 1995; Scheuer and Bowman, 1995; Lampl and Johnston, 1996; Steyn and Henneberg, 1996; Scheuer, 1998)

In the present text the accepted paediatric definitions are used for the early stages of the lifespan and *juvenile* is used in the general sense, as described above, to include any stage previous to the adult. *Puberty* and *adolescence* are used interchangeably to describe a period of about 10–13 years in girls and 12–16 years in boys. *Young adult* is used from the time of cessation of growth in height (fusion of long bone epiphyses) until the final fusion of all other epiphyses, such as the vertebrae, sacrum, scapula, pelvis and jugular growth plate (see under individual bones for details).

Appendix 2

Table 1 Time-scale of embryonic period proper (8 postovulatory weeks)

Pairs of somites	Carnegie stage	Crown–rump length (mm)	Age (postovulatory)	
			Days	Weeks
	6	–	15	
	7	–	16	3
	8	–	18	
1–3	9	1.5–2.5	20	
4–12	10	2.0–3.5	22	
13–20	11	2.5–4.5	24	4
21–29	12	3.0–5.0	26	
30+	13	4.0–6.0	28	
	14	5.0–7.0	32	5
	15	7.0–9.0	33	
	16	8.0–11.0	37	6
	17	11.0–14.0	41	
	18	13.0–17.0	44	7
	19	16.0–18.0	47	
	20	18.0–22.0	50	
	21	22.0–24.0	52	8
	22	23.0–28.0	54	
	23	27.0–31.0	56	

Table 2 Time-scale of the prenatal period

Days	Weeks	Months	CRL (mm)		
1–28	1–4	1	See Table 1	Embryo	
29–56	5–8	2	See Table 1	Embryo	
57–84	9–12	3	34–85	Fetus	
85–112	13–16	4	86–140	Fetus	
113–140	17–20	5	141–190	Fetus	
141–168	21–24	6	191–250	Fetus	
169–196	25–28	7	251–290	Fetus	
197–224	29–32	8	291–328	Fetus	Perinate
225–252	33–36	9	329–349	Fetus	Perinate
253–280	37–40	10	350–360	Fetus	Perinate

Appendix 3: Metrics from Archaeological Material

	Upper limb			Lower limb			Other
	Humerus	Radius	Ulna	Femur	Tibia	Fibula	
Johnston (1962)	✓	✓	✓	✓	✓	✓	–
Walker (1969)	✓	✓	✓	✓	✓	✓	–
Armelagos *et al.* (1972)	✓	✓	✓	✓	✓	–	Clavicle
Y'Edynak (1976)	✓	✓	✓	✓	✓	✓	–
Merchant & Ubelaker (1977)	✓	✓	✓	✓	✓	✓	Ilium
Stloukal & Hanáková (1978)	✓	✓	✓	✓	✓	✓	–
Sundick (1978)	✓	✓	✓	✓	✓	✓	–
Hummert & van Gerven (1983)	✓	✓	✓	✓	✓	–	–
Owsley & Bradtmiller (1983)	–	–	–	✓	–	–	–
Cook (1984)	–	–	–	✓	–	–	–
Jantz & Owsley (1984)	✓	✓	–	✓	✓	–	–
Mays (1985)	–	–	–	✓	–	–	–
Mensforth (1985)	–	–	–	–	✓	–	–
Owsley & Jantz (1985)	✓	✓	✓	✓	✓	–	–
Storey (1986)	✓	✓	✓	✓	✓	–	Ilium
Molleson (1989)	✓	✓	–	✓	✓	–	–
Lovejoy *et al.* (1990)	✓	✓	✓	✓	✓	✓	–
Saunders & Melbye (1990)	–	✓	–	✓	–	–	Mandible
Wall (1991)	✓	✓	✓	✓	✓	✓	–
Hoppa (1992)	✓	✓	✓	✓	✓	✓	Ilium
Saunders *et al.* (1993a)	✓	✓	✓	✓	✓	✓	Ilium Scapula
Miles & Bulman (1994)	✓	✓	✓	✓	✓	✓	–
Mays (1995)	✓	✓	✓	✓	✓	✓	–
Ribot & Roberts (1996)	✓	–	–	✓	✓	–	–
Steyn & Henneberg (1996)	✓	✓	✓	✓	✓	✓	–

	Sample	Age range
Johnston (1962)	Indian Knoll, Kentucky, USA Eastern Archaic, 5000 yrs BP	Fetal–5.5 yrs
Walker (1969)	Late Woodland, Illinois, USA AD 1208 ± 90 yrs	Birth–12 yrs
Armelagos *et al.* (1972)	Nubia, Sudan Meroitic 350 BC–350 AD X-Group 350 AD–550 AD Christian 550 AD–1400 AD	6 mths–31 yrs
Y'Edynak (1976)	Aleut & W. Eskimo, pre-nineteenth cent. Canada	Birth–19.9 yrs
Merchant & Ubelaker (1977)	Arikara, Mobridge, S. Dakota, USA Protohistoric, eighteenth century	Birth–18.5 yrs
Stloukal & Hanáková (1978)	Old Slavic, Czechoslovakia seventh–ninth cent. AD	Birth–15 yrs
Sundick (1978)	Alternerding, Munich, Germany sixth–seventh cent. AD	Birth–18 yrs
Hummert & van Gerven (1983)	Kulubnarti, Nubia, Sudan 550–1450 AD	Birth–16 yrs
Owsley & Bradtmiller (1983)	Arikara, four sites S. Dakota, USA 1600–1832 AD	Perinatal
Cook (1984)	Lower Illinois Valley, USA Woodland & Mississippian, 800–1100 AD	Birth–6 yrs
Jantz & Owsley (1984)	Arikara, several sites S. Dakota, USA 1600–1832 AD	6 mths–11.9 yrs
Mays (1985)	Poundbury Camp, Dorset, England Romano–British, first–fifth cent. AD	2–18 yrs
Mensforth (1985)	Libben, Ohio & Bt-5, Kentucky, USA Late Woodland 800–1100 AD Late Archaic 2655–3992 BC	Birth–10 yrs
Owsley & Jantz (1985)	Arikara, several sites S. Dakota, USA 1600–1832 AD	Perinatal
Storey (1986)	Teotihuacan, Central Mexico Pre-Columbian 150 BC–750 AD	Perinatal
Molleson (1989)	Poundbury Camp, Dorset, England Romano–British, fourth and fifth cent. AD	Fetal–1 yr
Lovejoy *et al.* (1990)	Libben, Ohio, USA Late Woodland 800–1100 AD	Birth–12 yrs
Saunders & Melbye (1990)	Iroquois Ontario, Canada Late Ontario 1580–1600	Birth–15 yrs
Wall (1991)	Central California, USA Amerindian 4250–300 BP	Birth–5 yrs
Hoppa (1992)	Raunds, Northamptonshire, England Anglo-Saxon, tenth cent.	Birth–18 yrs
Saunders *et al.* (1993)	Belleville, Ontario, Canada	Birth–12 yrs
Miles & Bulman (1994)	Ensay, W. Isles, Scotland 1500–1850 AD	Birth–20 yrs
Mays (1995)	Wharram Percy, N. Yorkshire, England Mediaeval eleventh–sixteenth cent.	2–17 yrs
Ribot & Roberts (1996)	Raunds, Northamptonshire, England Chichester, Hampshire, England	Fetal–18 yrs Fetal–18 yrs
Steyn & Henneberg (1996)	N. Transvaal, South Africa Iron Age	Birth–17.5 yrs

Bibliography

Abbot, L.C. and Lucas, D.B. (1954). The functions of the clavicle. *Annals of Surgery* **140**: 583–597.

Abel, M.S. (1985). Jogger's fracture and other stress fractures of the lumbo-sacral spine. *Skeletal Radiology* **13**: 221–227.

Abitbol, M.M. (1987). Obstetrics and posture in pelvic anatomy. *Journal of Human Evolution* **16**: 243–255.

Abitbol, M.M. (1988a). Evolution of the ischial spine and of the pelvic floor in the Hominoidea. *American Journal of Physical Anthropology* **75**: 53–67.

Abitbol, M.M. (1988b). Effect of posture and locomotion on energy expenditure. *American Journal of Physical Anthropology* **77**: 191–199.

Abitbol, M.M. (1989). Sacral curvature and supine posture. *American Journal of Physical Anthropology* **80**: 379–389.

Abramowitz, I. (1959). Triphalangeal thumb in a Bantu family. *Journal of Bone and Joint Surgery* **41B**: 766–771.

Acheson, R.M. (1954). A method of assessing skeletal maturity from radiographs: a report from the Oxford Child Health Survey. *Journal of Anatomy* **88**: 498–508.

Acheson, R.M. (1957). The Oxford method of assessing skeletal maturity. *Clinical Orthopaedics and Related Research* **10**: 19–39.

Acheson, R.M. (1966). Maturation of the Skeleton. In: F. Falkner (editor). *Human Development.* Philadelphia, PA: W.B. Saunders.

Acheson, R.M. and Archer, M. (1959). Radiological studies of the growth of the pituitary fossa in man. *Journal of Anatomy* **93**: 52–67.

Acheson, R.M. and Hewitt, D. (1954). Oxford Child Health Survey. Stature and skeletal maturation in the pre-school child. *British Journal of Preventive and Social Medicine* **8**: 59–65.

Acsádi G. and Nemeskéri, J. (1970). *History of Human Life Span and Mortality*. Budapest: Akadémiai Kiadó.

Ada, J.R. and Miller, M.E. (1991). Scapular fractures. Analysis of 113 cases. *Clinical Orthopaedics and Related Research* **269**: 174–180.

Adair, F.L. (1918). The ossification centers of the fetal pelvis. *American Journal of Obstetrics and Diseases of Women and Children* **78**: 175–199.

Adair, F.L. and Scammon, R.E. (1927). Observations on the parietal fontanelle in the newborn and in young infants. *American Journal of Obstetrics and Gynecology* **14**: 149–159.

Adams, J.L. (1934). The supracondyloid variation in the human embryo. *Anatomical Record* **59**: 315–333.

Adams, J.C. (1948). Recurrent dislocation of the shoulder. *Journal of Bone and Joint Surgery* **30B**: 26–38.

Adams, J.C. (1950). The humeral head defect in recurrent anterior dislocation of the shoulder. *British Journal of Radiology* **23**: 151–156.

Adams, W.S. (1951). The aetiology of swimmer's exostoses of the external auditory canals and of associated changes in hearing. *Journal of Laryngology and Otology* **65**: 133–153.

Adams, J.C. and Hamblen, D.L. (1992). *An Outline of Fractures*, 10th edition. Edinburgh: Churchill Livingstone.

Adams, M.A. and Hutton, W.C. (1980). The effect of posture on the role of the apophysial joints in resisting compressive force. *Journal of Bone and Joint Surgery* **49A**: 713–720.

Adams, J.D. and Leonard, R.D. (1925). A developmental anomaly of the patella frequently diagnosed as fracture. *Surgery, Gynecology and Obstetrics* **41**: 601–604.

Adson, A.W. and Coffey, J.R. (1927). Cervical rib. *Annals of Surgery* **85**: 839–857.

Aeby, C. (1885). Uber die symphyse ossium pubis des Menschens nebst Beiträgen zur Lehre vom hyalinen Knorpel und seiner Verknocherungen. *Zeitschrift für Rationelle Medicine Reihe* **3**: 1–77.

Agarwal, S.K., Malhotra, V.K. and Tewari, S.P. (1979). Incidence of metopic suture in adult Indian crania. *Acta Anatomica* **105**: 469–474.

Ahl, T., Sjoberg, H.E. and Dalen, N. (1988). Bone mineral content in the calcaneus after ankle fracture. *Acta Orthopedica Scandinavica* **59**: 173–176.

Ahlqvist, J. and Damsten, O. (1969). A modification of Kerley's method for the microscopic determination of age in human bone. *Journal of Forensic Sciences* **14**: 205–212.

Aiello, L. and Dean, C. (1990). *An Introduction to Human Evolutionary Anatomy.* London: Academic Press.

Aiello, L.C. and Molleson, T. (1993). Are microscopic ageing techniques more accurate that macroscopic ageing techniques? *Journal of Archaeological Science* **20**: 689–704.

Aiello, L.C. and Wheeler, P. (1995). The expensive-tissue hypothesis. *Current Anthropology* **36**: 199–221.

Aitken, D.M. (1905). A note on the variations of the tibia and astragalus. *Journal of Anatomy and Physiology* **39**: 489–491.

Ajmani, M.L. (1990). A metrical study of the laryngeal skeleton in adult Nigerians. *Journal of Anatomy* **171**: 187–191.

Ajmani, M.L. (1994). Anatomical variation in position of the greater palatine foramen in the adult human skull. *Journal of Anatomy* **184**: 635–637.

Ajmani, M.L., Jain, S.P. and Saxena, S.K. (1980). A metrical study of laryngeal cartilages and their ossification. *Anatomischer Anzeiger* **148**: 42–48.

Ajmani, M.L., Mittal, R.K. and Jain, S.P. (1983). Incidence of metopic suture in adult Nigerian skulls. *Journal of Anatomy* **137**: 177–183.

Akabori, E. (1934). Septal apertures in the humerus in Japanese, Ainu and Koreans. *American Journal of Physical Anthropology* **18**: 395–400.

Akisaka, T., Nakayama, M., Yoshida, H. and Inoue, M. (1998). Ultrastructural modifications of the extracellular matrix upon calcification of growth plate cartilage as revealed by quick-freeze deep etching technique. *Calcified Tissue International* **63**: 47–56.

Alberch, P. and Kollar, E. (1988). Strategies of head development: workshop report. *Development* **103**(Suppl.): 25–30.

Albert, A.M. (1998). The use of vertebral ring epiphyseal union for age estimation in two cases of unknown identity. *Forensic Science International* **97**: 11–20.

Albert, A.M. and Maples, W.R. (1995). Stages of epiphyseal union for thoracic and lumbar vertebral centra as a method of age determination for teenage and young adult skeletons. *Journal of Forensic Sciences* **40**: 623–633.

Albinus, B.S. (1737). *Icones ossium foetus humani.* Leidae Batavorum.

Alexander, C. (1965). The aetiology of primary protrusio acetabuli. *British Journal of Radiology* **38**: 567–580.

Alexander, R.M. and Vernon, A. (1975). The mechanics and hopping by kangaroos. *Journal of Zoology* **177**: 265–303.

Ali, R.S. (1989). The influence of sex, body size and age on the auricular surface and the post-auricular area of the adult human ilium. Unpublished BSc dissertation, University of London.

Ali, R.S. (1991). The arterial supply of the human metatarsus. Unpublished clinical dissertation, University of London.

Ali, S.Y. and Evans, L. (1973). The uptake of [^{45}Ca] calcium ions by matrix vesicles isolated from calcifying cartilage. *Biochemistry Journal* **134**: 647–650.

Ali, R.S. and MacLaughlin, S.M. (1991). Sex identification from the auricular surface of the adult human ilium. *International Journal of Osteoarchaeology* **1**: 57–61.

Allbrook, D.B. (1955). The East African vertebral column: a study in racial variability. *American Journal of Physical Anthropology* **13**: 489–511.

Allbrook, D.B. (1961). The estimation of stature in British and East African males based on tibial and ulnar bone lengths. *Journal of Forensic Medicine* **8**: 15–28.

Alldred, A.J. (1963). Congenital pseudoarthrosis of the clavicle. *Journal of Bone and Joint Surgery* **45B**: 312–319.

Allen, J.C., Bruce, M.F. and MacLaughlin, S.M. (1987). Sex determination from the radius in humans. *Human Evolution* **2**: 373–378.

Alley, R.G. (1936). Enlarged parietal foramina. *Radiology* **27**: 233–235.

Allman, F.L. (1967). Fractures and ligamentous injuries of the clavicle and its articulations. *Journal of Bone and Joint Surgery* **49A**: 774–784.

Altmann, F. (1955). Congenital atresia of the ear in man and animals. *Annals of Otology, Rhinology and Laryngology* **64**: 824–858.

Alvesalo, L. (1997). Sex chromosomes and human growth. A dental approach. *Human Genetics* **101**: 1–5.

Alvesalo, L., Mayhall, J.T. and Varrela, J. (1996). Torus mandibularis in 45, X females (Turner's syndrome). *American Journal of Physical Anthropology* **101**: 145–149.

Amjad, A.H., Scheer, A.A. and Rosenthal, J. (1969). Human internal auditory meatus. *Archives of Otolaryngology* **89:** 709–714.

Amonoo-Kuofi H.S. (1995). Age related variations in the horizontal and vertical diameters of the pedicles of the lumbar spine. *Journal of Anatomy* **186**: 321–328.

Amprino, R. (1948). A contribution to the functional meaning of the substitution of primary by secondary bone tissue. *Acta Anatomica* **5**: 291–300.

Amprino, R. (1984). The development of the vertebrate limb. *Clinical Orthopaedics and Related Research* **188**: 263–284.

Amstutz, H.C. and Sissons, H.A. (1969). The structure of vertebral spongiosa. *Journal of Bone and Joint Surgery* **51B**: 540–550.

Anagnostopoulou, S., Venieratos, D. and Spyropoulos, N. (1991). Classification of human maxillar sinuses according to their geometric features. *Anatomischer Anzeiger* **173**: 121–130.

Andermann, S. (1975). The cnemic index: a critique. *American Journal of Physical Anthropology* **44**: 369–370.

Andersen, H. (1962). Histochemical studies of the development of the human hip joint. *Acta Anatomica* **48**: 258–292.

Andersen, H. (1963). Histochemistry and development of the human shoulder and acromio-clavicular joints with particular reference to the early development of the clavicle. *Acta Anatomica* **55**: 124–165.

Andersen, E. (1971). Comparison of Tanner–Whitehouse and Greulich–Pyle methods in a large scale Danish survey. *American Journal of Physical Anthropology* **35**: 373–376.

Andersen, B.C. (1988). Pelvic scarring analysis: parturition or excess motion? *American Journal of Physical Anthropology* **75**: 181.

Andersen, H. and Matthiessen, M. (1967). Histochemistry of the early development of the human central face and nasal cavity with special reference to the movements and fusion of the palatine process. *Acta Anatomica* **68**: 473–508.

Anderson, J. (1884). The transverse measurements of human ribs. *Journal of Anatomy and Physiology* **18**: 171–173.

Anderson, W. (1891). Comment in the Proceedings of the Anatomical Society of Great Britain and Ireland. Feb. *Journal of Anatomy and Physiology* **25**: v.

Anderson, J.E. (1960). The development of the tympanic plate. *National Museum of Canada Bulletin* **180**: 143–153.

Anderson, H.C. (1969). Vesicles associated with calcification in the matrix of epiphyseal cartilage. *Journal of Cell Biology* **41**: 59–72.

Anderson, T. (1988a). A medieval hypoplastic dens: a note on its discovery and a review of the previous literature. *Ossa* **13**: 13–37.

Anderson, T. (1988b). Calcaneus secundarius: an osteoarchaeological note. *American Journal of Physical Anthropology* **77**: 529–531.

Anderson, T. (1988c). A Medieval bipartite cuneiform I with attempted unilateral fusion. *Ossa* **13**: 39–48.

Anderson, H.C. (1990). The role of cells versus matrix in bone induction. *Connective Tissue Research* **24**: 3–12.

Anderson, T. (1993). Processus paramastoideus or processus paracondylaris, manifestation of an occipital vertebra. *Paleopathological Newsletter* **81**: 13–15.

Anderson, T. (1995). An anomalous medieval parietal bone. *Journal of Paleopathology* **7**: 223–226.

Anderson, T. (1996). Paracondylar process: manifestation of an occipital vertebra. *International Journal of Osteoarchaeology* **6**: 195–201.

Anderson, T. and Carter, A.R. (1993). The first archaeological example of Freiberg's infraction. *International Journal of Osteoarchaeology* **3**: 219–221.

Anderson, T. and Carter, A.R. (1994). Periosteal reaction in a new born child from Sheppey, Kent. *International Journal of Osteoarchaeology* **4**: 47–48.

Anderson, H.C. and Morris, D.C. (1993). Mineralization. In: *Physiology and Pharmacology of Bone* (G.R. Mundy, and T.J. Martin, Eds.), pp. 267–298. Berlin: Springer.

Anderson, D.L. and Popovich, F. (1981). Association of relatively delayed emergence of mandibular molars with molar reduction and molar position. *American Journal of Physical Anthropology* **54**: 369–376.

Anderson, J.Y. and Trinkaus, E. (1998). Patterns of sexual, bilateral and interpopulational variation in human femoral neck-shaft angles. *Journal of Anatomy* **192**: 279–285.

Anderson, M., Blais, M. and Green, W.T. (1956). Growth of the normal foot during childhood and adolescence. Length of the foot and interrelations of foot, stature and lower extremity as seen in serial records of children between 1–18 years of age. *American Journal of Physical Anthropology* **14**: 287–308.

Anderson, M., Green, W.T. and Messner, M.B. (1963). Growth and the predictions of growth in the lower extremities. *Journal of Bone and Joint Surgery* **45A**: 1–14.

Anderson, M., Messner, M.B. and Green, W.T. (1964). Distribution of lengths of the normal femur and tibia from one to eighteen years of age. *Journal of Bone and Joint Surgery* **46A**: 1197–1202.

Anderson, D.L., Anderson, G.W. and Popovich, F. (1976). Age of attainment of mineralization stages of the permanent dentition. *Journal of Forensic Sciences* **21**: 191–200.

Andrews, B.G. (1988). *Amputations* (B. Helal and D. Wilson, Eds.), pp. 1245–1252. Edinburgh: Churchill Livingstone.

Anetzberger, H. and Putz, R. (1996). The scapula: princples of construction and stress. *Acta Anatomica* **156**: 70–80.

Angel, J.L. (1964). The reaction of the femoral neck. *Clinical Orthopaedics and Related Research* **32**: 130–142.

Angel, J.L. (1974). Bones can fool people. *FBI Law Enforcement Bulletin* **43**: 16–20.

Angel, J.L. and Kelley, J.O. (1986). Posterior ramus edge inversion: a new racial trait. *American Journal of Physical Anthropology* **69**: 172.

Annett, M. (1985). *Left, Right, Hand and Brain: The Right Shift Theory*. London: Erlbaum.

Anson, B.J. and Bast, T.H. (1958). Anatomical structure of the stapes and the relation of the stapedial footplate to vital parts of the otic labyrinth. *Annals of Otology, Rhinology and Laryngology* **67**: 389–399.

Anson, B.J., Bast, T.H. and Cauldwell, E.W. (1948). The development of the auditory ossicles, the otic capsule and the extracapsular tissues. *Annals of Otology, Rhinology and Laryngology* **57**: 603–632.

Anson, B.J., Bast, T.H. and Richany, S.F. (1955). The fetal and early postnatal development of the tympanic ring and related structures in man. *Annals of Otology, Rhinology and Laryngology* **64**: 802–822.

Anson, B.J., Hanson, J.S. and Richany, S.F. (1960). Early embryology of the auditory ossicles and associated structures in relation to certain anomalies observed clinically. *Annals of Otology, Rhinology and Laryngology* **69**: 427–447.

Anson, B.J., Harper, D.G. and Warpeha, R.L. (1963). Surgical anatomy of the facial canal and facial nerve. *Annals of Otology, Rhinology and Laryngology* **72**: 713–734.

Antonov, A.N. (1947). Children born during the siege of Leningrad in 1942. *Journal of Pediatrics* **30**: 250–259.

Aoki, J., Yamamoto, I., Hino, M., Kitamura, N., Sone, T., Itoh, H. and Torizuka, K. (1987). Reactive endosteal bone formation. *Skeletal Radiology* **16**: 545–551.

Applbaum, Y., Gerard, P. and Bry, K.D. (1983). Elongation of the anterior tubercle of a cervical vertebral transverse process: an unusual variant. *Skeletal Radiology* **10**: 265–267.

Appleton, A.B. (1922). On the hypotrochanteric fossa and accessory adductor groove of the primate femur. *Journal of Anatomy* **56**: 295–306.

Apuzzio, J.J., Adhate, A., Ganesh, V., Leo, M.V. and Holland, B.K. (1992). Prenatal ultrasonographic fetal iliac bone measurement. Correlation with gestational age. *Journal of Reproductive Medicine* **37**: 348–350.

Arensburg, B. and Nathan, H. (1971). Observations on a notch in the short (superior or posterior) process of the incus. *Acta Anatomica* **78**: 84–90.

Arensburg, B. and Nathan, H. (1972). A propos de deux osselets de l'oreille moyenne s'un Néandertaloïd trouvés à Qafzeh (Israel). *L'Anthropologie* **76**: 301–307.

Arensburg, B. and Nathan, H. (1979). Anatomical observations on the mylohyoid groove, and the course of the mylohyoid nerve and vessels. *Journal of Oral Surgery* **37**: 93–96.

Arensburg, B. and Tillier, A-M. (1983). A new Mousterian child from Qafzeh (Israel): Qafzeh 4a. *Bulletin et Mémoirs de la Société d'Anthropologie de Paris* **10**: 61–69.

Arensburg, B., Nathan, H. and Ziv, M. (1977). Malleus fixed (ossified) to the tegmen tympani in an ancient skeleton from Israel. *Annals of Otology, Rhinology and Laryngology* **86**: 75–79.

Arensburg, B., Harell, M. and Nathan, H. (1981). The human middle ear ossicles: morphometry and taxonomic implications. *Journal of Human Evolution* **10**: 199–205.

Arensburg, B., Tillier, A.M., Vandermeersch, B., Duday, H., Schepartz, L.A. and Rak, Y. (1989). A Middle Palaeolithic human hyoid bone. *Nature* **338**: 758–760.

Arensburg, B., Pap, I., Tillier, A-M. and Chech, M. (1996). The Subalyuk 2 middle ear stapes. *International Journal of Osteoarchaeology* **6**: 185–188.

Arey, L.B. (1950). The craniopharyngeal canal reviewed and reinterpreted. *Anatomical Record* **106**: 1–16.

Arias-Cazorla, S. and Rodriguez-Larralde, A. (1987). Metacarpophalangeal pattern profiles in Venezuelan and Northern Caucasoid samples compared. *American Journal of Physical Anthropology* **73**: 71–80.

Arkless, R. and Graham, C.B. (1967). An unusual case of brachydactyly-peripheral dysostosis? Pseudo-pseudo hypoparathyroidism? Cone epiphysis? *American Journal of Roentgenology* **99**: 724–725.

Armelagos, G.J., Mielke, J.H., Owen, K.H., Van Gerven, D.P., Dewey, J.R. and Mahler, P.E. (1972). Bone growth and development in prehistoric populations from Sudanese Nubia. *Journal of Human Evolution* **1**: 89–119.

Ars, B. (1989). Organogenesis of the middle ear structures. *Journal of Laryngology and Otology* **103**: 16–21.

Arsenault, A.L. (1989). A comparative electron microscopic study of apatite crystals in collagen fibrils of rat bone, dentin and calcified turkey leg tendons. *Bone and Mineral* **6**: 165–177.

Ascenzi, A. and Bonucci, E. (1967). The tensile properties of single osteons. *Anatomical Record* **158**: 375–386.

Ashley, G.T. (1954). The morphological and pathological significance of synostosis at the manubrio-sternal joint. *Thorax* **9**: 159–166.

Ashley, G.T. (1956a). The relationship between the pattern of ossification and the definitive shape of the mesosternum in man. *Journal of Anatomy* **90**: 87–105.

Ashley, G.T. (1956b). A comparison of human and anthropoid mesosterna. *American Journal of Physical Anthropology* **14**: 449–462.

Ashley, G.T. (1956c). The human sternum: the influence of sex and age in its measurement. *Journal of Forensic Medicine* **3**: 27–43.

Ashley-Montagu, M.F. (1935). The premaxilla in primates. *Quarterly Review of Biology* **10**: 32–59, 181–208.

Ashley-Montagu, M.F. (1937). The medio-frontal suture and the problem of metopism in the primates. *Journal of the Royal Anthropological Institute of Great Britain and Ireland* **67**: 157–201.

Ashley-Montagu, M.F. (1940). Medio-palatine bones. *American Journal of Physical Anthropology* **27**: 139–150.

Ashley-Montagu, M.F. (1954). The direction and position of the mental foramen in the great apes and man. *American Journal of Physical Anthropology* **12**: 503–518.

Ashworth, J.T., Allison, M.J., Gerszten, E. and Pezzia, A. (1976). The pubic scars of gestation and parturition in a group of Pre-Columbian and colonial Peruvian mummies. *American Journal of Physical Anthropology* **45**: 85–91.

Asin, H.M. (1966). Symphalangism of the fifth toes. *Journal of the American Podiatry Association* **56**: 411–413.

Atchley, W.R. and Hall, B.K. (1991). A model for development and evolution of complex morphological structures. *Biological Reviews* **66**: 101–157.

Atkinson, W.B. and Elftman, H. (1945). The carrying angle of the human arm as a secondary sex character. *Anatomical Record* **91**: 49–52.

Atkinson, P.J. and Weatherell, J.A. (1967). Variation in the density of the femoral diaphysis with age. *Journal of Bone and Joint Surgery* **49B**: 781–788.

Aubin, J.E., Lemieux, M., Tremblay, M., Behringer, R.R. and Jeannotte, L. (1998). Transcriptional interferences at the Hoxa 4/Hoxa 5 locus: importance of correct Hoxa 5 expression for the proper specification of the axial skeleton. *Developmental Dynamics* **212**: 141–156.

Aufderheide, A.C. and Rodriguez-Martin, C. (1998). *The Cambridge Encyclopedia of Human Paleopathology.* Cambridge: Cambridge University Press.

Augier, M. (1931). Squelette céphalique. *In: Traité d'Anatomie Humaine* (P. Poirier, and A. Charpy, Eds.). Paris: Masson.

Austin, F.H. (1951). Symphalangism and related fusions of tarsal bones. *Radiology* **56**: 882–885.

Axelsson, G. and Hedegård, B. (1981). Torus mandibularis among Icelanders. *American Journal of Physical Anthropology* **54**: 383–389.

Axelsson, G. and Hedegaard, B. (1985). Torus palatinus in Icelandic schoolchildren. *American Journal of Physical Anthropology* **67**: 105–112.

Aymard, J.L. (1917). Some new points in the anatomy of the nasal septum and their surgical significance. *Journal of Anatomy* **51**: 293–303.

Azaz, B. and Lustmann, J. (1973). Anatomical configurations in dry mandibles. *British Journal of Oral Surgery* **11**: 1–9.

Bach-Petersen, S. and Kjær, I. (1993). Ossification of lateral components in the human prenatal cranial base. *Journal of Craniofacial Genetics and Developmental Biology* **13**: 76–82.

Backman, S. (1957). The proximal end of the femur: investigations with special reference to the etiology of femoral neck fractures. *Acta Radiologica Supplement* **146**: 1–166.

Bacon, G.E., Bacon, P.J. and Griffiths, R.K. (1984). A neutron diffraction study of the bones of the foot. *Journal of Anatomy* **139**: 265–273.

Badgley, C.E. (1941). The articular facets in relation to low-back pain and sciatic radiation. *Journal of Bone and Joint Surgery* **23**: 481–496.

Badgley, C.E. (1949). Etiology of congenital dislocation of the hip. *Journal of Bone and Joint Surgery* **31A**: 341–356.

Badi, M.H. (1972a). Ossification in the fibrous growth plate at the proximal end of the tibia in the rat. *Journal of Anatomy* **111**: 201–219.

Badi, M.H. (1972b). Calcification and ossification of fibrocartilage in the attachment of the patellar ligament in the rat. *Journal of Anatomy* **112**: 415–421.

Baer, M.J. and Durkatz, J. (1957). Bilateral asymmetry in skeletal maturation of the hand and wrist. A roentgenographic analysis. *American Journal of Physical Anthropology* **15**: 181–196.

Bagnall, K.M., Jones, P.R.M. and Harris, P.F. (1975). Estimating the age of the human foetus from crown-rump measurements. *Annals of Human Biology* **2**: 387–390.

Bagnall, K.M., Harris, P.F. and Jones, P.R.M. (1977a). A radiographic study of the human fetal spine. 1. The development of the secondary cervical curvature. *Journal of Anatomy* **123**: 777–782.

Bagnall, K.M., Harris, P.F. and Jones, P.R.M. (1977b). A radiographic study of the human fetal spine. 2. The sequence of development of ossification centres in the vertebral column. *Journal of Anatomy* **124**: 791–802.

Bagnall, K.M., Harris, P.F. and Jones, P.R.M. (1982). Radiographic study of the longitudinal growth of primary ossification centers in limb long bones of the human fetus. *Anatomical Record* **203**: 293–299.

Bagnall, K.M., Higgins, S.J. and Saunders, E.J. (1988). The contribution made by a single somite to the vertebral column; resegmentation using the chick-quail chimera model. *Development* **103**: 69–85.

Bailit, H. and Hunt, E.E. (1964). The sexing of children's skeletons from teeth alone and its genetic implications. *American Journal of Physical Anthropology* **22**: 171–174.

Bainbridge, D. and Tarazaga, S. (1956). A study of sex differences in the scapula. *Journal of the Royal Anthropological Institute* **86**: 109–134.

Balthazard, V. and Dervieux. (1921). Études anthropologiques sur le foetus humain. *Annales de Médicine Legales* **1**: 37–42.

Bambach, M., Saracci, R. and Young, H.B. (1973). Emergence of teeth in Tunisian children in relation to sex and social class. *Human Biology* **45**: 435–444.

Bankart, A.S.B. (1938). Recurrent or habitual dislocation of the shoulder joint. *British Journal of Surgery* **26**: 23–29.

Banta, J.V. and Nichols, O. (1969). Sacral agenesis. *Journal of Bone and Joint Surgery* **51A**: 693–703.

Baran, D.T., Kelley, A.M., Karellas, A., Giaret, M., Price, M., Leahey, D., Steuterman, S., McSherry, B. and Roche, J. (1988). Ultrasound attenuation of the os calcis in women with osteoporosis and hip fractures. *Calcified Tissue International* **43**: 138–143.

Barber, G., Shepstone, L. and Rogers, J. (1995). A methodology for estimating age at death using arachnoid granulation counts. *American Journal of Physical Anthropology* **20**(Suppl.): 61.

Barclay, M. (1932). A case of duplication of the internal cuneiform bone of the foot (cuneiforme bipartitum). *Journal of Anatomy* **67**: 175–177.

Barclay-Smith, E. (1897). Bipartite zygomatic bone. *Journal of Anatomy and Physiology* **32**: xi.

Barclay-Smith, E. (1909). Two cases of Wormian bones in the bregmatic fontanelle. *Journal of Anatomy and Physiology* **44**: 312–314.

Barclay-Smith, E. (1911). Multiple anomaly in a vertebral column. *Journal of Anatomy and Physiology* **45**: 144–171.

Bardeen, C.R. (1900). Costo-vertebral variation in man. *Anatomischer Anzeiger* **XVlll**: 377.

Bardeen, C.R. (1904). Vertebral variation in the human adult and embryo. *Anatomischer Anzeiger* **25**: 497–519.

Bardeen, C.R. (1905). Studies on the development of the human skeleton. *American Journal of Anatomy* **4**: 265–302.

Bardeen, C.R. and Lewis, W.H. (1901). The development of the limbs, body-wall and back in man. *American Journal of Anatomy* **1**: 1–36.

Bardeleben, K. (1894). On the bones and muscles of the mammalian hand and foot. *Proceedings of the Zoological Society of London* 354–376.

Bareggi, R., Grill, V., Sandrucci, M.A., Baldini, G., DePol, A., Forabosco, A. and Narducci, P. (1993). Developmental pathways of vertebral centra and neural arches in human embryos and fetuses. *Anatomy and Embryology* **187**: 139–144.

Bareggi, R., Grill, V., Zweyer, M., Sandrucci, M.A., Narducci, P. and Forabosco, A. (1994a). The growth of long bones in human embryological and fetal upper limbs and its relationship to other developmental patterns. *Anatomy and Embryology* **189**: 19–24.

Bareggi, R., Grill, V., Zweyer, M., Narducci, P. and Forabosco, A. (1994b). A quantitative study on the spatial and temporal ossification patterns of vertebral centra and neural arches and their relationship to the fetal age. *Annals of Anatomy* **176**: 311–317.

Bareggi, R., Grill, V., Zweyer, M., Sandrucci, M.A., Martelli, A.M., Narducci, P., and Forabosco, A. (1996). On the assessment of the growth patterns in human fetal limbs: longitudinal measurements and allometric analysis. *Early Human Development* **45**: 11–25.

Barker, S.L. (1991). An investigation into the value of footprints in a forensic context. Unpublished BSc dissertation, University of London.

Barker, S.L. (1993). An investigation into the blood supply to the metatarsals. Unpublished clinical dissertation, University of London.

Barker, S.L. and Scheuer, J.L. (1998). Predictive value of human footprints in a forensic context. *Medicine, Science and the Law* **38**: 341–346.

Barker, D.J.P., Osmond, C., Simmonds, S.J. and Wield, G.A. (1993). The relation of small head circumference and thinness at birth to death from cardiovascular disease in adult life. *British Medical Journal* **306**: 422–426.

Barlow, T. (1883). Congenital absence of both clavicles and malformation of the cranium. *British Medical Journal* **1**: 909.

Barlow, T.E. (1942). Os cuneiforme I bipartitum. *American Journal of Physical Anthropology* **29**: 95–111.

Barnard, L.B. and McCoy, S.M. (1946). The supracondyloid process of the humerus. *Journal of Bone and Joint Surgery* **28**: 845–850.

Barnes, E. (1994). *Developmental Defects of the Axial Skeleton in Palaeopathology.* Colorado: University Press of Colorado.

Barnett, C.H. (1954a). A comparison of the human knee and avian ankle. *Journal of Anatomy* **88**: 59–70.

Barnett, C.H. (1954b). Squatting facets on the European talus. *Journal of Anatomy* **88**: 509–513.

Barnett, C.H. (1956). The phases of human gait. *The Lancet* **2**: 617–621.

Barnett, C.H. (1962a). The normal orientation of the human hallux and the effect of footwear. *Journal of Anatomy* **96**: 489–494.

Barnett, C.H. (1962b). Valgus deviation of the distal phalanx of the great toe. *Journal of Anatomy* **96**: 171–177.

Barnett, C.H. and Lewis, O.J. (1958). The evolution of some traction epiphyses in birds and mammals. *Journal of Anatomy* **92**: 593–607.

Barnett, C.H. and Napier, J.R. (1952). The axis of rotation at the ankle joint in man. Its influence upon the form of the talus and the mobility of the fibula. *Journal of Anatomy* **86**: 1–9.

Barnett, C.H., Bowden, R.E.M. and Napier, J.R. (1956). Shoe wear as a means of analysing abnormal gait in males. *Annals of Physical Medicine* **3**: 121–142.

Barr, M. and Hayashi, R.H. (1988). Fetal foot length as a predictor of fetal age. *American Journal of Obstetrics and Gynecology* **158**: 218–219.

Barr, J.S., Elliston, W.A., Musnick, H., Delarme, T.L., Hanelin, J. and Thibodeau, A.A. (1953). Fracture of the carpal navicular (scaphoid) bone. *Journal of Bone and Joint Surgery* **35A**: 609–625.

Barrett, M.J., Brown, T. and Cellier, K.M. (1964). Tooth eruption sequence in a tribe of central Australian Aborigines. *American Journal of Physical Anthropology* **22**: 79–89.

Barson, A.J. (1970). The vertebral level of termination of the spinal cord during normal and abnormal development. *Journal of Anatomy* **106**: 489–497.

Basmajian, J.V. (1974). *Muscles Alive – Their Functions Revealed By Electromyography.* Baltimore, MD: Williams and Wilkins.

Basmajian, J.V. and Slonecker, C.E. (1989). *Grant's Method of Anatomy. A Clinical Problem-solving Approach.* Baltimore, MD: Williams and Wilkins.

Basmajian, J.V., Harden, T.P. and Regenos, E.M. (1972). Integrated actions of the four heads of quadriceps femoris: an electromyographic study. *Anatomical Record* **172**: 15–20.

Bass, W.M. (1987). *Human Osteology: A Laboratory and Field Manual.* Missouri: Missouri Archaeological Society.

Bassoe, E. and Bassoe, H.H. (1955). The styloid bone and Carpe Bossu disease. *American Journal of Roentgenology* **74**: 886–888.

Bast, T.H. (1930). Ossification of the otic capsule in human fetuses. *Contributions to Embryology* **21**: 53–82.

Bast, T.H. and Anson, B.J. (1950). Postnatal growth and adult structure of the otic (endolymphatic) sac. *Annals of Otology, Rhinology and Laryngology* **59**: 1088–1101.

Bast, T.H. and Forester, H.B. (1939). Origin and distribution of air cells in the temporal bone. *Archives of Otolaryngology* **30**: 183–205.

Bast, T.H., Anson, B.J. and Gardner, W.D. (1947). The developmental course of the human auditory vesicle. *Anatomical Record* **99**: 55–74.

Bateman, J.E. (1968). Neurovascular syndromes related to the clavicle. *Clinical Orthopedics and Related Research* **58**: 75–82.

Bates, E.H. and Chung, W.K. (1988). Congenital talipes equinovarus. In: *The Foot* (B. Helal, and D. Wilson, Eds.), pp. 219–234. Edinburgh: Churchill Livingstone.

Baughan, B. and Demirjian, A. (1978). Sexual dimorphism in the growth of the cranium. *American Journal of Physical Anthropology* **49**: 383–390.

Baur, G. (1885). On the morphology of the carpus and tarsus of vertebrates. *American Naturalist* **19**: 718–720.

Baur, R. (1969). Zum Problem der Neugliederung der Wirbelsäule. *Acta Anatomica* **72**: 321–356.

Baxter, A. (1971). Dehiscence of the Fallopian canal. An anatomical study. *Journal of Laryngology and Otology* **85**: 587–594.

Beal, M.C. (1982). The sacro-iliac problem: review of anatomy, mechanics and diagnosis. *Journal of the American Osteopath Association* **81**: 667–679.

Beals, R.K. (1976). The normal carrying angle of the elbow – a radiographic study of 422 patients. *Clinical Orthopaedics and Related Research* **119**: 194–196.

Beals, R.K. and Eckhardt, A.L. (1969). Hereditary onycho-osteodysplasia (nail-patella syndrome). *Journal of Bone and Joint Surgery* **51A**: 505–516.

Beals, R.K. and Skyhar, M. (1984). Growth and development of the tibia, fibula and ankle joint. *Clinical Orthopaedics and Related Research* **182**: 289–292.

Beaty, J.H. and Kumar, A. (1994). Fractures about the knee in children. Current concepts review. *Journal of Bone and Joint Surgery* **76A**: 1870–1880.

Beck, F.W. (1963). Paraseptal cartilage in some mammals including man. *Laryngoscope* **73**: 288–305.

Beck, W.C. and Berkheiser, S. (1954). Prominent costal cartilages (Tietze's Syndrome). *Surgery* **35**: 762–765.

Becker, M.J. (1986). Mandibular symphysis (medial suture) closure in modern *Homo sapiens*: preliminary evidence from archaeological populations. *American Journal of Physical Anthropology* **69**: 499–501.

Becker, M.J. (1987). Gender determination of the Iron Age population from Gabii, near Rome, using discriminant function analysis of the femur. *American Journal of Physical Anthropology* **72**: 177.

Beddard, D. and Saunders, W.H. (1962). Congenital defects in the Fallopian canal. *Laryngoscope* **72**: 112–115.

Behrensmeyer, A.K. and Laporte, L.F. (1981). Footprints of a Pleistocene hominid in Northern Kenya. *Nature* **289**: 167–169.

Behrents, R.G. and Harris, E.F. (1991). The premaxillary–maxillary suture and orthodontic mecanotherapy. *American Journal of Orthodontics and Dentofacial Orthopedics* **99**: 1–6.

Behringer, B.R. and Wilson, F.C. (1972). Congenital pseudoarthrosis of the clavicle. *American Journal of Diseases of Children* **123**: 511–517.

Behrman, R.E. (1992). *Nelson Text Book of Pediatrics*, 14th edition. Philadelphia, PA: W.B. Saunders.

Bell, L.S. (1990). Palaeopathology and diagenesis: An SEM evaluation of structural changes using back scattered electron imaging. *Journal of Archaeological Science* **17**: 85–102.

Bell, L.S., Skinner, M.F. and Jones, S.J. (1996). The speed of post mortem change to the human skeleton and its taphonomic significance. *Forensic Science International* **82**: 129–140.

Bellairs, A. d'A. (1951). Observations on the incisive canaliculi and nasopalatine ducts. *British Dental Journal* **91**: 281–291.

Bellamy, P., Park, W. and Rooney, P.J. (1983). What do we know about the sacro-iliac joint? *Seminars in Arthritis and Rheumatism* **12**: 282–313.

Bencardino, J., Rosenberg, Z.S., Beltran, J. and Sheskier, S. (1997). Os sustentaculi: depiction on MR images. *Skeletal Radiology* **26**: 505–506.

Benfer, R.A. and McKern, T.W. (1966). The correlation of bone robusticity with the perforation of the coronoid-olecranon septum in the humerus of man. *American Journal of Physical Anthropology* **24**: 247–252.

Benfer, R.A. and Tappen, N.C. (1968). The occurrence of septal perforation of the humerus in three non-human primate species. *American Journal of Physical Anthropology* **29**: 19–28.

Bennett, K.A. (1965). The etiology and genetics of Wormian bones. *American Journal of Physical Anthropology* **23**: 255–260.

Bérard, A. (1835). Mémoire sur le rapport qui existe entre la direction des conduits nourriciers des os longs et l'ordre suivant lequel les épiphyses see soudent au corps de l'os. *Archives Générales de Médicine* **7**: 176–183.

Beresowski, A. and Lundie, J.K. (1952). Sequence in the time of ossification of the carpal bones of 705 African children from birth to 6 years of age. *South African Journal of Medical Sciences* **17**: 25–31.

Bergfelder, T. and Herrmann, B. (1980). Estimating fertility on the basis of birth – traumatic changes in the pubic bone. *Journal of Human Evolution* **9**: 611–613.

Bergkamp, A.B.M. and Verhaar, J.A.N. (1995). Dislocation of the coccyx. *Journal of Bone and Joint Surgery* **77B**: 831–832.

Bergot, C. and Bocquet-Appel, J-P. (1976). Étude systématique en fonction de l'âge de l'os spongieux et de l'os cortical de l'humérus et du fémur. *Bulletin et Mémoirs de la Sociétié d'Anthropologie de Paris* **3**: 215–242.

Berkovitz, B.K.B., Holland G.R. and Moxham, B.J. (1978). *A Colour Atlas and Textbook of Oral Anatomy*. London: Wolfe.

Berlis, A., Putz, R. and Schumacher, M. (1992). Direct and CT measurements of canals and foramina of the skull base. *British Journal of Radiology* **65**: 653–661.

Bermúdez de Castro, J.M. (1989). Third molar agenesis in human prehistoric populations of the Canary Islands. *American Journal of Physical Anthropology* **79**: 207–215.

Bernard, G.W. and Pease, D.C. (1969). An electron microscopic study of initial intramembranous osteogenesis. *American Journal of Anatomy* **125**: 271–290.

Bernhang, A.M. and Levine, S.A. (1973). Familial absence of the patella. *Journal of Bone and Joint Surgery* **55A**: 1088–1090.

Bernstein, P.E. and Peterson, R.R. (1966). Numerical variation of the pre-sacral vertebral column in three population groups in North America. *American Journal of Physical Anthropology* **25**: 139–146.

Berrizbeitia, E.L. (1989). Sex determination with the head of the radius. *Journal of Forensic Sciences* **34**: 1206–1213.

Berry, R.J.A. (1909). A case of os parietale bipartum in an Australian aboriginal skull. *Journal of Anatomy and Physiology* **44**: 73–82.

Berry, A.C. (1975). Factors affecting the incidence of non-metrical skeletal variants. *Journal of Anatomy* **120**: 519–535.

Berry, A.C. and Berry, R.J. (1967). Epigenetic variation in the human cranium. *Journal of Anatomy* **101**: 361–379.

Bertino, E., Di Battista, E., Bossi, A., Pagliano, M., Fabris, C., Aicardi, G. and Milani, S. (1996). Fetal growth velocity: kinetic, clinical and biological aspects. *Archives of Disease in Childhood* **74**: F10–F15.

Bezirdjian, D.R. and Szucs, R. (1989). Sickle-shaped scapulae in a patient with Pierre Robin syndrome. *British Journal of Radiology* **62**: 171–173.

Bhargava, K.N., Garg, T.C. and Bhargava, S.N. (1960). Incidence of the os Japonicum (bipartite zygomatic bone) in Madhya Pradesh skulls. *Journal of the Anatomical Society of India* **9**: 21–23.

Bhaskar, S.N. (1953). Growth pattern of the rat mandible from 13 days insemination age to 30 days after birth. *American Journal of Anatomy* **92**: 1–53.

Bhaskar, S.N. (1980). *Orban's Oral Histology and Embryology*. 9th edition, St Louis, MD: Mosby Yearbook.

Bhaskar, S.N., Weinmann, J.P. and Schour, I. (1953). Role of Meckel's cartilage in the development of the rat mandible. *Journal of Dental Research* **32**: 398–410.

Bick, E.M. and Copel, J.W. (1950). Longitudinal growth of the human vertebra: a contribution to human osteogeny. *Journal of Bone and Joint Surgery* **32A**: 803–814.

Bick, E.M. and Copel, J.W. (1951). The ring apophysis of the human vertebra. *Journal of Bone and Joint Surgery* **33A**: 783–787.

Biermann, M.I. (1922). The supernumerary pedal bones. *American Journal of Roentgenology* **9**: 404–411.

Birch, R. and Brooks, D. (1984). *The Hand*. London: Butterworth.

Birkbeck, J.A. (1976). Metrical growth and skeletal development of the human fetus. In: *The Biology of Human Fetal Growth* (D.F. Roberts and A.M. Thomson, Eds.). pp. 39–68. London: Taylor and Francis.

Birkby, W.H. and Gregg, J.B. (1975). Otosclerotic stapedial footplate fixation in an eighteenth century burial. *American Journal of Physical Anthropology* **42**: 81–84.

Birkner, R. (1978). *Normal Radiographic Patterns and Variances of the Human Skeleton – An X-ray Atlas of Adults and Children*. Baltimore (Munich): Urban and Schwarzenberg.

Bisaria, K.K. (1984). Grooves on the free edge of the dorsum sellae. *Journal of Anatomy* **138**: 365–369.

Bisaria, K.K., Saxena, R.C., Bisaria, S.D., Lakhtakia, P.K., Agarwal, A.K. and Presagar, I.C. (1989). The lacrimal fossa in Indians. *Journal of Anatomy* **166**: 265–268.

Bisaria, K.K., Kumar, N., Jaiswal, A.K., Sharma, P.K., Mittal, M. and Bisaria, S.D. (1996a). An accessory foramen deep in the infraorbital fissure. *Journal of Anatomy* **189**: 461–462.

Bisaria, K.K., Kumar, N., Prakesh, M., Sharma, P.K., Agarwal, P.P., Bisaria, S.D., Lakhtakia, P.K. and Premesagar, I.C. (1996b). The lateral rectus spine of the superior orbital fissure. *Journal of Anatomy* **189**: 243–245.

Bisgard, J.D. and Bisgard, M.E. (1935). Longitudinal growth of long bones. *Archives of Surgery* **31**: 568–578.

Bizzaro, A.H. (1921). On sesamoid and supernumerary bones of the limbs. *Journal of Anatomy* **55**: 256–268.

Björk, A. (1963). Variations in the growth pattern of the human mandible: longitudinal radiographic study by the implant method. *Journal of Dental Research* **42**: 400–411.

Björk, A. and Skieller, V. (1977). Growth of the maxilla in three dimensions as revealed radiographically by the implant method. *British Journal of Orthodontics* **4**: 53–64.

Black, T.K. (1978a). Sexual dimorphism in the tooth-crown diameters of the deciduous teeth. *American Journal of Physical Anthropology* **48**: 77–82.

Black, T.K. (1978b). A new method for assessing the sex of fragmentary skeletal remains. *American Journal of Physical Anthropology* **48**: 227–232.

Black, S.M. and Scheuer, J.L. (1996a). A report on occipitalisation of the atlas with reference to its embryological development. *International Journal of Osteoarchaeology* **6**: 189–194.

Black, S.M. and Scheuer, J.L. (1996b). Age changes in the clavicle: from the early neonatal period to skeletal maturity. *International Journal of Osteoarchaeology* **6**: 425–434.

Black, S.M. and Scheuer, J.L. (1997). The ontogenetic development of the cervical rib. *International Journal of Osteoarchaeology* **7**: 2–10.

Blackburne, J.S. and Peel, T.E. (1977). A new method of measuring patellar height. *Journal of Bone and Joint Surgery* **59B**: 241–242.

Blackwood, H.J.J. (1957). The double-headed mandibular condyle. *American Journal of Physical Anthropology* **15**: 1–8.

Blackwood, H.J.J. (1965). The vascularization of the condylar cartilage of the human mandible. *Journal of Anatomy* **99**: 551–563.

Blair, W. and Hanson, C. (1979). Traumatic closure of the triradiate cartilage. Report of a case. *Journal of Bone and Joint Surgery* **61A**: 144–145.

Blais, M.M., Green, W.T. and Anderson, M. (1956). Lengths of the growing foot. *Journal of Bone and Joint Surgery* **38A**: 998–1000.

Blanc, A.C. (1952). The Oldest Human Footprints. *London News*, 1 March, pp. 377–379.

Blanco, R.A., Acheson, R.M., Canosa, C. and Salomón, J.B. (1972). Retardation in appearance of ossification centres in deprived Guatemalan children. *Human Biology* **44**: 525–536.

Blanco, R., Habicht, J., Salomon, J.B. and Canosa, C. (1973). Prevalence of brachymesophalangia-5 in Guatemalan rural children. *Human Biology* **45**: 571–581.

Blankenstein, R., Cleaton-Jones, P.E., Maistry, P.K., Luk, K.M. and Fatti, L.P. (1990). The onset of eruption of permanent teeth amongst South African Indian children. *Annals of Human Biology* **17**: 515–521.

Blauth, W. and Schneider-Sickert, F. (1981). *Congenital Deformities of the Hand: An Atlas of their Surgical Treatment*. Berlin: Springer.

Blechschmidt, E. (1969). The early stages of human limb development. In: *Limb Development and Deformity*, (C.A. Swinyard, Ed.). Springfield, IL: C.C. Thomas.

Blincoe, H. (1962). Significant hand types in women according to relative lengths of fingers. *American Journal of Physical Anthropology* **20**: 45–49.

Blondiaux, G., Blondiaux, J., Secousse, F., Cotten, A., Danze, P.M. and Ripo, R.M. (1998). Rickets and child abuse: the case of a fourth-century girl from Normandy. *Papers on Paleopathology*, 26–29 August 1998: 4.

Blumel, J., Evans, E.B. and Eggers, G.N.N. (1958). Partial and complete agenesis or malformation of the sacrum with associated anomalies. *Journal of Bone and Joint Surgery* **41A**: 497–518.

Bocquet-Apel, J-P and Masset, C. (1982). Farewell to palaeodemography. *Journal of Human Evolution* **11**: 321–333.

Bocquet-Apel, J-P. and Masset, C. (1985). Matters of moment. *Journal of Human Evolution* **14**: 107–111.

Boddington, A. (1987). Chaos, disturbance and decay in an Anglo-Saxon cemetery. In: *Death, Decay and Reconstruction* (A. Boddington, A.N. Garland and R.C. Janaway, Eds.), pp.27–42. Manchester: Manchester University Press.

Bogin, B. (1997). Evolutionary hypotheses for human childhood. *Yearbook of Physical Anthropology* **40**: 63–89.

Böhm, M. (1929). The embryonic origin of club foot. *Journal of Bone and Joint Surgery* **11**: 229–259.

Bojsen-Møller, F. (1979). The calcaneocuboid joint and stability of the longitudinal arch at high and low gear push off. *Journal of Anatomy* **129**: 165–176.

Bolk, L. (1917). On metopism. *American Journal of Anatomy* **22**: 27–47.

Boller, R. (1964). Fetal morphogenesis of the human dentition. *Journal of Dentistry for Children* **31**: 67–97.

Bollobás, E. (1984a). Fissures, canals and syndesmoses in the fetal maxilla. *Acta Morphologica Hungarica* **32**: 231–243.

Bollobás, E. (1984b). The body and processes of the fetal maxilla. *Acta Morphologica Hungarica* **32**: 217–230.

Bollow, M., Braun, J., Kannenberg, J., Biedermann, T., Schauer-Petrowskaja, C., Paris, S., Mutze, S. and Hamm, B. (1997). Normal morphology of the sacroiliac joints in children: magnetic resonance studies related to age and sex. *Skeletal Radiology* **26**: 697–704.

Bonaldi, L.V., De Angelis, M.A. and Smith, R.L. (1997). Developmental study of the round window region. *Acta Anatomica* **159**: 25–29.

Bonucci, E. (1967). Fine structure of early cartilage calcification. *Journal of Ultrastructural Research* **20**: 33–50.

Bonucci, E. (1971). The locus of initial calcification in cartilage and bone. *Clinical Orthopaedics and Related Research* **78**: 108–139.

Bonucci, E. (1992). Role of collagen fibrils in calcification. In: *Calcification in Biological Systems* (Bonucci, E. Ed.), pp. 20–39. Boca Raton: CRC Press.

Boocock, P., Roberts, C.A. and Manchester, K. (1995). Maxillary sinusitis in medieval Chichester, England. *American Journal of Physical Anthropology* **98**: 483–495.

Boreadis, A.G. and Gershon-Cohen, J. (1956). Luschka joints of the cervical spine. *Radiology* **66**: 181–187.

Bosley, R.C. (1991). Total acromionectomy: A 20-year review. *Journal of Bone and Joint Surgery* **73A**: 961–968.

Bossy, J. and Gaillard, L. (1963). Les vestiges ligamentaires du cartilage de Meckel. *Acta Anatomica* **52**: 282–290.

Botella Lopez, M.C. and De Linares von Schmiterlow, C.G. (1975). Estudio de los huesos del oido medio en craneos Argaricos de Granada. *Anales des Desarrollo* **19**: 25–33.

Boucher, B.J. (1955). Sex differences in the foetal sciatic notch. *Journal of Forensic Medicine* **2**: 51–54.

Boucher, B.J. (1957). Sex differences in the foetal pelvis. *American Journal of Physical Anthropology* **15**: 581–600.

Bouvier, M. and Ubelaker, D. (1977). A comparison of two methods for the microscopic determination of age at death. *American Journal of Physical Anthropology* **46**: 391–394.

Bowden, R.E.M. (1967). The functional anatomy of the foot. *Physiotherapy* **53**: 120–126.

Bowdler, J.D. (1971). Persistence of the so-called craniopharyngeal canal. *Journal of Anatomy* **110**: 509.

Bowen, V. and Cassidy, J.D. (1981). Macroscopic and microscopic anatomy of the sacro-iliac joint from embryonic life until the eighth decade. *Spine* **6**: 620–628.

Bower, B.L., Keyser, C.K. and Gilula, L.A. (1989). Rigid subtalar joint–a radiographic spectrum. *Skeletal Radiology* **17**: 583–588.

Bowman, J.E., MacLaughlin, S.M. and Scheuer, J.L. (1992). The relationship between biological and chronological age in the juveniles from St Bride's Church, Fleet Street. *Annals of Human Biology* **19**: 216.

Boyan, B.D., Schwartz, Z. and Swain, L.D. (1990). Matrix vesicles as a marker of endochondral ossification. *Connective Tissue Research* **24**: 67–75.

Boyd, G.I. (1930). The emissary foramina of the cranium in man and the anthropoids. *Journal of Anatomy* **65**: 108–121.

Boyd, G.I. (1933). Bipartite carpal navicular bone. *British Journal of Surgery* **20**: 455–458.

Boyd, H.B. (1944). Congenital talonavicular synostosis. *Journal of Bone and Joint Surgery* **26**: 682–686.

Boyde, A. (1963). Estimation of age at death of young human skeletal remains from incremental lines in dental enamel. *Third International Meeting in Forensic Immunology, Medicine, Pathology and Toxicology.* London, 16–24 April, 1963. In: *Primate Life History and Evolution* (C. Jean de Rousseau, Ed.). New York: Wiley-Liss.

Boyer, D.W. (1975). Trapshooter's shoulder: stress fractures of the coracoid process. *Journal of Bone and Joint Surgery* **57A**: 862.

Braddock, G.T.F. (1959). Experimental epiphyseal injury and Freiberg's disease. *Journal of Bone and Joint Surgery* **41B**: 154–159.

Bradley, O.C. (1906). A contribution to the development of the interphalangeal sesamoid bone. *Anatomischer Anzeiger* **28**: 528–536.

Bradshaw, P. and McQuaid, P. (1963). The syndrome of vertebro-basilar insufficiency. *Quarterly Journal of Medicine* **32**: 279–296.

Braga, J., Crubézy, E. and Elyaktine, M. (1998). The posterior border of the sphenoid greater wing and its phylogenetic usefulness in human evolution. *American Journal of Physical Anthropology* **107**: 387–399.

Brailsford, J.F. (1929). Deformities of the lumbosacral region of the spine. *British Journal of Surgery* **16**: 562–627.

Brailsford, J.F. (1943). Variations in the ossification of the bones of the hand. *Journal of Anatomy* **77**: 170–175.

Brailsford, J.F. (1953). *The Radiology of Bones and Joints*, 5th edition. Baltimore, MD: Williams and Wilkins.

Brand, P. (1966). *Insensitive Feet: A Practical Handbook on Foot Problems in Leprosy.* London: The Leprosy Mission.

Brandner, M.E. (1970). Normal values of vertebral body and inter-vertebral disc index during growth. *American Journal of Roentgenology* **110**: 618–627.

Brantigan, J.W., Pedegave, L.R. and Lippert, F.G. (1977). Instability of the subtalar joint. *Journal of Bone and Joint Surgery* **59A**: 321–324.

Brash, J.C. (1915). Vertebral column with six and a half cervical and thirteen true thoracic vertebrae, with associated abnormalities of the cervical spinal cord and nerves. *Journal of Anatomy and Physiology* **49**: 243–273.

Bray, T.J., Swafford, A.R. and Brown, R.L. (1985). Bilateral fracture of the hook of the hamate. *Journal of Trauma* **25**: 174–175.

Breitinger, E. (1937). Zur Berechnung der Körperhöhe aus den langen Gliedermassenknochen. *Anatomischer Anzeiger* **14**: 249–274.

Bridgeman, G. and Brookes, M. (1996). Blood supply to the human femoral diaphysis in youth and senescence. *Journal of Anatomy* **188**: 611–621.

Briscoe, C. (1925). The interchondral joints of the human thorax. *Journal of Anatomy* **59**: 432–437.

Brodeur, A.E., Silberstein, M.J. and Graviss, E.R. (1981). *Radiology of the Pediatric Elbow.* Boston, MA: G.K. Hall.

Brodie, A.G. (1941). On the growth pattern of the human head from the third month to the eighth year of life. *American Journal of Anatomy* **68**: 209–262.

Broker, F.H.L. and Burbach, T. (1990). Ultrasonic diagnosis of separation of the proximal humeral epiphysis in the newborn. *Journal of Bone and Joint Surgery* **72A**: 187–191.

Bromage, T.G. and Dean, M.C. (1985). Re-evaluation of the age at death of immature fossil hominids. *Nature* **317**: 525–527.

Broman, G.E. (1957). Precondylar tubercles in American Whites and Negroes. *American Journal of Physical Anthropology* **15**: 125–135.

Brook, A.H. and Barker, D.K. (1972). Eruption of teeth among the racial groups of eastern New Guinea: a correlation of tooth eruption with calendar age. *Archives of Oral Biology* **17**: 751–759.

Brooke, R. (1924). The sacro-iliac joint. *Journal of Anatomy* **59**: 299–305.

Brookes, M. (1957). Femoral growth after occlusion of the principal nutrient canal in day old rabbits. *Journal of Bone and Joint Surgery* **39B**: 563–571.

Brookes, M. (1958). The vascularization of long bones in the human fetus. *Journal of Anatomy* **92**: 261–267.

Brookes, M. (1963). Cortical vascularisation and growth in foetal tubular bones. *Journal of Anatomy* **97**: 597–609.

Brookes, M. (1971). *The Blood Supply of Bone: An Approach to Bone Biology.* London: Butterworth.

Brookes, M. and Harrison, R.G. (1957). The vascularization of the rabbit femur and tibiofibula. *Journal of Anatomy* **91**: 61–72.

Brookes, M. and Revell, W.J. (1998). *Blood Supply of Bone–Scientific Aspects*, 2nd edition. London: Springer.

Brooks, S. (1955). Skeletal age at death: the reliability of cranial and pubic age indicators. *American Journal of Physical Anthropology* **13**: 567–598.

Brooks, S. and Suchey, J.M. (1990). Skeletal age determination based on the os pubis: A comparison of the Acsadi-Nemeskeri and Suchey-Brooks methods. *Human Evolution* **5**: 227–238.

Broom, R. (1897). On the existence of a sterno-coracoidal articulation in a foetal marsupial. *Journal of Anatomy and Physiology* **31**: 513–515.

Broom, R. (1904). The origin of the mammalian carpus and tarsus. *Transactions of the South African Philosophical Society* **15**: 89–96.

Broom, R. (1906). On the arrangement of the epiphyses of the mammalian metacarpals and metatarsals. *Anatomischer Anzeiger* **28**: 106–108.

Brothwell, D.R. (1981). *Digging up Bones. The excavation, treatment and study of human skeletal remains*, 3rd edition. Oxford: Oxford University Press.

Brown, L.T. (1937). The mechanics of the lumbosacral and sacro-iliac joints. *Journal of Bone and Joint Surgery* **19**: 770–775.

Brown, T. (1978). Tooth emergence in Australian aboriginals. *Annals of Human Biology* **5**: 41–54.

Brown, W.A.B. (1985). *Identification of Human Teeth.* Bulletin **21/22**. London: Institute of Archaeology.

Brown, W.A.B., Molleson, T.I. and Chinn, S. (1984). Enlargement of the frontal sinus. *Annals of Human Biology* **11**: 221–226.

Browning, H. (1953). The confluence of dural venous sinuses. *American Journal of Anatomy* **93**: 307–329.

Bruce, H.E., Harvey, J.P. and Wilson, J.C. (1963). Monteggia fractures. *Journal of Bone and Joint Surgery* **56A**: 1563–1576.

Bruder, S.P. and Caplan, A.I. (1989). Cellular and molecular events during embryonic bone development. *Connective Tissue Research* **20**: 65–71.

Bruintjes, Tj.D., Panhuysen, R.G.A.M. and Van Maurik, W.A.M. (1997). An unusual stapes from medieval Maastricht. *International Journal of Osteoarchaeology* **7**: 641–642.

Bruneton, J.N., Drouillard, J.P., Sabatier, J.C., Elie, G.P. and Tavernier, J.F. (1979). Normal variants of the sella turcica. *Radiology* **131**: 99–104.

Bruyn, G.W. and Bots, G.Th.A.M. (1977). Biparietal osteodystrophy. *Clinical Neurology and Neurosurgery* **80**: 125–148.

Bruzek, J. and Soustal, K. (1981). Contribution to ontogenesis of human bony pelvis. *Acta Universitatis Carolinae – Biologica* **12**: 37–45.

Bryce, T.H. (1915). Osteology. In: *Quain's Elements of Anatomy*, Vol. IV, Pt 1 (E.A. Schäfer, J. Symington and T.H. Bryce, Eds.), p. 184. London: Longmans, Green and Co.

Bryce, T.H. and Young, M. (1917). Observations on metopism. *Journal of Anatomy* **51**: 153–166.

Buccholz, J.M. (1987). Peroneal spastic flat foot. In: *Fundamentals of Foot Surgery* (E.D. McGlamry, Ed.), pp. 337–344. Baltimore, MD: Williams and Wilkins.

Bucholz, R.W., Ezaki, M. and Ogden, J.A. (1982). Injury to the acetabular triradiate physeal cartilage. *Journal of Bone and Joint Surgery* **64A**: 600–609.

Budinoff, L.C. and Tague, R.G. (1990). Anatomical and developmental bases for the ventral arc of the human pubis. *American Journal of Physical Anthropology* **82**: 73–79.

Budorick, N.E., Pretorius, D., Grafe, M.R. and Lou, K.V. (1991). Ossification of the fetal spine. *Radiology* **181**: 561–565.

Buehl, C.C. and Pyle, S.I. (1942). The use of age at first appearance of three ossification centres in determining the skeletal status of children. *Journal of Pediatrics* **21**: 335–342.

Buikstra, J.E., Gordon, C.C. and St. Hoyme, L. (1984). The case of the severed skull. Individuation in forensic anthropology. In: *Human Identification. Case Studies in Forensic Anthropology* (T.A. Rathbun, and J.E. Buikstra, Eds.), pp. 121–135. Springfield, IL: C.C. Thomas.

Bunnell, S. (1938). Opposition of the thumb. *Journal of Bone and Joint Surgery* **20B**: 269–284.

Bunning, P.S.C. (1964). Some observations on the West African calcaneus and the associated talo-calcaneal inter-osseous ligamentous apparatus. *American Journal of Physical Anthropology* **22**: 467–472.

Bunning, P.S.C. and Barnett, C.H. (1963). Variations in the talocalcaneal articulation. *Journal of Anatomy* **97**: 643.

Bunning, P.S.C. and Barnett, C.H. (1965). A comparison of adult and foetal talocalcaneal articulations. *Journal of Anatomy* **99**: 71–76.

Burdi, A.R. (1965). Sagittal growth of the nasomaxillary complex during the second trimester of human prenatal development. *Journal of Dental Research* **44**: 112–125.

Burdi, A.R. (1968). Morphogenesis of mandibular arch shape in human embryos. *Journal of Dental Research* **47**: 50–58.

Burdi, A.R. and Silvey, R.G. (1969a). Sexual differences in the closure of the human palatal shelves. *Cleft Palate Journal* **6**: 1–7.

Burdi, A.R. and Silvey, R.G. (1969b). The relation of sex-associated facial profile reversal and stages of human palatal closure. *Teratology* **2**: 297–304.

Burdi, A.R., Garn, S.M. and Miller, R.L. (1970a). Developmental advancement of the male dentition in the first trimester. *Journal of Dental Research* **49**: 889.

Burdi, A.R., Garn, S.M. and Miller, R.L. (1970b). Mesiodistal gradient of mandibular precedence in the developing dentition. *Journal of Dental Research* **49**: 644.

Burdi, A.R., Garn, S.M. and Superstine, J.N. (1975). Mandibular precedence in the prenatal development of four permanent teeth. *American Journal of Physical Anthropology* **43**: 363–366.

Burke, F.D. (1989). *Principles of Hand Surgery*. Edinburgh: Churchill Livingstone.

Burke, J.T. and Harris, J.H. (1989). Acute injuries of the axis vertebra. *Skeletal Radiology* **18**: 335–346.

Burke, A.C., Nelson, C.E., Morgan, A. and Tabin, C. (1995). Hox genes and the evolution of vertebrate axial morphology. *Development* **121**: 333–346.

Burkitt, A.N. and Lightoller, G.H.S. (1923). Preliminary observations on the nose of the Australian aboriginal, with a table of aboriginal head measurements. *Journal of Anatomy* **57**: 295–312.

Burkus, J.K. and Ogden, J.A. (1982). Bipartite primary ossification in the developing femur. *Journal of Pediatric Orthopedics* **2**: 63–65.

Burkus, J.K. and Ogden, J.A. (1984). Development of the distal femoral epiphysis: a microscopic morphological investigation of the zone of Ranvier. *Journal of Pediatric Orthopedics* **4**: 661–668.

Burman, M.S. and Lapidus, P.W. (1931). The functional disturbances caused by the inconstant bones and sesamoids of the foot. *Archives of Surgery* **22**: 936–975.

Burman, M.S. and Pomeranz, M. (1932). Epiphysitis of the proximal epiphysis of the first metatarsal and of the first phalanx of the big toe; coincidental presence of proximal or pseudometatarsal epiphyses. *Journal of Bone and Joint Surgery* **14**: 177–180.

Burton, P., Nyssen-Behets, C. and Dhem, A. (1989). Haversian remodelling in human fetus. *Acta Anatomica* **135**: 171–175.

Buschang, P.H. and Malina, R.M. (1980). Brachymesophalangia-5 in five samples of children: a descriptive and methodological study. *American Journal of Physical Anthropology* **53**: 189–195.

Buschang, P.H., Baume, R.M. and Nass, G.G. (1983). A craniofacial growth maturity gradient for males and females between 4 and 16 years of age. *American Journal of Physical Anthropology* **61**: 373–381.

Buschang, P.H., Tanguay, R., Demirjian, A., La Palme, L. and Goldstein, H. (1986). Sexual dimorphism in mandibular growth of French–Canadian children 6 to 10 years of age. *American Journal of Physical Anthropology* **71**: 33–37.

Butler, P.M. (1967a). Comparison of the development of the second deciduous molar and first permanent molar in man. *Archives of Oral Biology* **12**: 1245–1260.

Butler, P.M. (1967b). Relative growth within the human first upper permanent molar during the prenatal period. *Archives of Oral Biology* **12**: 983–992.

Butler, P.M. (1968). Growth of the human second lower deciduous molar. *Archives of Oral Biology* **13**: 671–682.

Buxton, L.H.D. (1938). Platymeria and platycnemia. *Journal of Anatomy* **73**: 31–36.

Byers, S. (1991). Technical note: calculation of age at formation of radiopaque transverse lines. *American Journal of Physical Anthropology* **85**: 339–343.

Byers, S., Akoshima, K. and Curran, B. (1989). Determination of adult stature from metatarsal length. *American Journal of Physical Anthropology* **79**: 275–279.

Byers, S.N., Churchill, S.E. and Curran, B. (1997). Identification of Euro-Americans, African Americans and Amerindians from palatal dimensions. *Journal of Forensic Sciences* **42**: 3–9.

Caffey, J. (1953). On the accessory ossicles of the supraoccipital bone. *American Journal of Roentgenology* **70**: 401–412.

Caffey, J. (1993). Caffey's *Pediatric X-ray Diagnosis*, 9th edition (F.N. Silverman and J.P. Kuhns, Eds.), St Louis, MO: Mosby Yearbook.

Caffey, J. and Madell, S.H. (1956). Ossification of the pubic bones at birth. *Radiology* **67**: 346–350.

Caffey, J. and Ross, S.E. (1956). The ischio-pubic synchondrosis in healthy children: some normal roentgenologic finds. *American Journal of Roentgenology* **76**: 488–494.

Caffey, J. and Silverman, W.A. (1945). Infantile cortical hyperostoses. Preliminary report on a new syndrome. *American Journal of Roentgenology* **54**: 1–16.

Cahill, B.R. (1992). Atraumatic osteolysis of the distal clavicle. *Sports Medicine* **13**: 214–222.

Calcagno, J.M. (1981). On the applicability of sexing human skeletal material by discriminant function analysis. *Journal of Human Evolution* **10**: 189–198.

Calder, J. and Chessell, G. (1988). *An Atlas of Radiological Interpretation: The Bones.* London: Wolfe.

Caldwell, W.F. and Moloy, H.C. (1933). Anatomical variations in the female pelvis and their effect in labor with a suggested classification. *American Journal of Obstetrics and Gynaecology* **26**: 479–504.

Caldwell, W.E., Moloy, H.C. and D'Esopo, D.A. (1940). The more recent conceptions of the pelvic architecture. *American Journal of Obstetrics and Gynaecology* **40**: 558–565.

Callender, G.W. (1869). The formation and early growth of the bones of the human face. *Philosophical Transactions of the Royal Society of London* **159**: 163–172.

Calonius, P.E.B., Lunin, M. and Stout, F. (1970). Histological criteria for age estimation of the developing human dentition. *Oral Surgery, Oral Medicine and Oral Pathology* **29**: 869–876.

Camacho, F.J.F., Pellico, L.G. and Rodriguez, R.F.V. (1993). Osteometry of the human iliac crest: Patterns of normality and its utility in sexing human remains. *Journal of Forensic Sciences* **38**: 779–787.

Camarda, A.J., Deschamps, C. and Forest, D. (1989a). I. Stylohyoid chain ossification: a discussion of etiology. *Oral Surgery, Oral Medicine and Oral Pathology* **67**: 508–514.

Camarda, A.J., Deschamps, C. and Forest, D. (1989b). II. Stylohyoid chain ossification: a discussion of etiology. *Oral Surgery, Oral Medicine and Oral Pathology* **67**: 515–520.

Cameron, J. (1930). Craniometric studies – numbers 25–27. *American Journal of Physical Anthropology* **14**: 273–304.

Cameron, J. and McCredie, J. (1982). Innervation of the undifferentiated limb bud in rabbit embryo. *Journal of Anatomy* **134**: 795–808.

Camp, J.D. and Cilley, E.I.L. (1931). Diagrammatic chart showing time of appearance of the various centres of ossification and period of union. *American Journal of Roentgenology* **26**: 905.

Camp, J.D. and Cilley, E.I.L. (1939). The significance of asymmetry of the pori acustici as an aid in diagnosis of VIII nerve tumors. *American Journal of Roentgenology* **41**: 713–718.

Camp, J.D. and Nash, L.A. (1944). Developmental thinness of parietal bones. *Radiology* **42**: 42–47.

Campbell, C.J., Grisolia, A. and Zanconato, G. (1959). The effects produced in the cartilaginous epiphyseal plate of immature dogs by experimental surgical traumata. *Journal of Bone and Joint Surgery* **41A**: 1221–1242.

Campbell, L.R., Dayton, D.H. and Sohal, G.S. (1986). Neural tube defects: a review of human and animal studies on the etiology of neural tube defects. *Teratology* **34**: 171–178.

Campbell, J., Henderson, A. and Campbell, S. (1988). The fetal femur foot length ratio: a new parameter to assess dysplastic limb reduction. *Obstetrics and Gynecology* **72**: 181–184.

Carels, C.E.L., Kuipers-Jagtman, A.M., Van der Linden, F.P.G.M. and Van't Hof, M.A. (1991). Age reference charts of tooth formation in Dutch children. *Journal de Biologie Buccale* **19**: 297–303.

Carlson, D.H. (1981). Coalition of the carpal bones. *Skeletal Radiology* **7**: 125–127.

Caro, P.A. and Borden, S. (1988). Plastic bowing of the ribs in children. *Skeletal Radiology* **17**: 255–258.

Carola, R., Harley, J.P. and Noback, C.R. (1992). *Human Anatomy*. London: McGraw-Hill.

Carpenter, G. (1899). A case of absence of the clavicles. *Lancet* **7**: 13–17.

Carroll, S.E. (1963). A study of the nutrient foramina of the humeral diaphysis. *Journal of Bone and Joint Surgery* **45B**: 176–181.

Carter, R.M. (1941). Carpal boss: a commonly overlooked deformity of the carpus. *Journal of Bone and Joint Surgery* **23A**: 935–940.

Carter, R.B. and Keen, E.N. (1971). The intramandibular course of the inferior alveolar nerve. *Journal of Anatomy* **108**: 433–440.

Carwardine, T. (1893). The suprasternal bones in man. *Journal of Anatomy and Physiology* **27**: 232–234.

Case, D.T., Ossenberg, N.S. and Burnett, S.E. (1997). The os intermetatarseum: a heritable accessory bone of the foot. *Papers on Palaeopathology*, **5**.

Castellana, C. and Kósa, F. (1999). Morphology of the cervical vertebrae in the fetal and neonatal human skeleton. *Journal of Anatomy* **194**: 147–152.

Castellvi, A.E., Goldstein, L.A. and Chan, D.P.K. (1984). Lumbo-sacral transitional vertebrae and their association with lumbar extradural defects. *Spine* **9**: 493–495.

Cattell, H.S. and Filtzer, D.L. (1965). Pseudoluxation and other normal variations in the cervical spine in children. *Journal of Bone and Joint Surgery* **47A**: 1295–1309.

Caughell, K.A., Martin, A.H. and Uhthoff, H.K. (1990). The development of the wrist and hand. In: *The Embryology of the Human Locomotor System* (H.K. Uhthoff, Ed.), pp. 95–106. Berlin: Springer.

Cauna, N. (1963). Concerning the nature and evolution of limbs. *Journal of Anatomy* **97**: 23–34.

Cave, A.J.E. (1926). Fusion of carpal elements. *Journal of Anatomy* **60**: 460–461.

Cave, A.J.E. (1927). Bilateral and unilateral thinning of parietal bone. *Journal of Anatomy* **61**: 486–487.

Cave, A.J.E. (1928). Two cases of congenitally enlarged parietal foramina. *Journal of Anatomy* **63**: 172–174.

Cave, A.J.E. (1929). The distribution of the first intercostal nerve and its relation to the first rib. *Journal of Anatomy* **63**: 367–379.

Cave, A.J.E. (1930). On fusion of the atlas and axis vertebrae. *Journal of Anatomy* **64**: 337–343.

Cave, A.J.E. (1931). The craniopharyngeal canal in man and anthropoids. *Journal of Anatomy* **65**: 363–367.

Cave, A.J.E. (1934). Cervical intercostal articulations. *Journal of Anatomy* **68**: 521–524.

Cave, A.J.E. (1936). The morphology of the last thoracic transverse process. *Journal of Anatomy* **70**: 275–277.

Cave, A.J.E. (1937). The vertebra critica. *Journal of Anatomy* **72**: 319.

Cave, A.J.E. (1961). The nature and morphology of the costoclavicular ligament. *Journal of Anatomy* **95**: 170–179.

Cave, A.J.E. (1975). The morphology of the mammalian cervical pleurapophysis. *Journal of Zoology* **177**: 377–393.

Cave, A.J.E. and Brown, R.W. (1952). On the tendon of the subclavius muscle. *Journal of Bone and Joint Surgery* **34B**: 466–469.

Cave, A.J.E. and Porteous, C.J. (1958). The attachments of the m.semimembranosus. *Journal of Anatomy* **92**: 638.

Cave, A.J.E. and Porteous, C.J. (1959). A note on the semimembranosus muscle. *Annals of the Royal College of Surgeons of England* **24**: 251–256.

Cave, A.J.E., Griffiths, J.U. and Whiteley, M.M. (1955). Osteo-arthritis deformans of Luschka joints. *Lancet* **1**: 176–179.

Cavendish, M.E. (1972). Congenital elevation of the scapula. *Journal of Bone and Joint Surgery* **54B**: 395–408.

Cerný, M. (1983). Our experience with estimation of an individual's age from skeletal remains of the degree of thyroid cartilage ossification. *Acta Universitatis Palackianae Olomucensisi* **3**: 121–144.

Chagula, W.K. (1960). The age at eruption of third permanent molars in male East Africans. *American Journal of Physical Anthropology* **18**: 77–82.

Chambers, C.H. (1950). Congenital anomalies of the tarsal navicular with particular reference to calcaneo-navicular coalition. *British Journal of Radiology* **23**: 580–586.

Chandler, S.B. and Derezinski, C.F. (1935). The variations of the middle meningeal artery within the middle cranial fossa. *Anatomical Record* **62**: 309–319.

Chandraraj, S. and Briggs, C.A. (1991). Multiple growth cartilages in the neural arch. *Anatomical Record* **230**: 114–120.

Chandraraj, S., Briggs, C.A. and Opeskin, K. (1998). Disc herniation in the young and end plate vascularity. *Clinical Anatomy* **11**: 171–176.

Chang, C.H. and Davis, W.C. (1961). Congenital bifid sternum with partial ectopia cordis. *American Journal of Roentgenology* **86**: 513–516.

Chang, H.H., Tse, Y. and Kaufman, M.H. (1998). Analysis of interdigital spaces during mouse limb development at intervals following amniotic sac puncture. *Journal of Anatomy* **192**: 59–72.

Charles, R.H. (1893). The influence of function as exemplified in the morphology of the lower extremity of the Panjabi. *Journal of Anatomy and Physiology* **28**: 1–18.

Charles, S.W. (1925). The temporo-mandibular joint and its influence on the growth of the mandible. *British Dental Journal* **46**: 845–855.

Charles, D.K., Condon, K., Cheverud, J.M. and Buikstra, J.E. (1986). Cementum annulation and age determination in *Homo sapiens*. I. Tooth variability and observer error. *American Journal of Physical Anthropology* **71**: 311–320.

Chase, S.W. (1942). The early development of the human premaxilla. *Journal of the American Dental Association* **29**: 1991–2001.

Chemke, J. and Robinson, A. (1969). The third fontanelle. *Journal of Pediatrics* **75**: 617–622.

Chen, J.M. (1952a). Studies on the morphogenesis of the mouse sternum. I. Normal embryonic development. *Journal of Anatomy* **86**: 373–386.

Chen, J.M. (1952b). Studies on the morphogenesis of the mouse sternum. II. Experiments on the origin of the sternum and its capacity for self differentiation in vitro. *Journal of Anatomy* **86**: 387–401.

Chen, J.M. (1953). Studies on the morphogenesis of the mouse sternum. III. Experiments on the closure and segmentation of the sternal bands. *Journal of Anatomy* **87**: 130–149.

Chen, Y.M. and Bohrer, S.P. (1990). Coracoclavicular and coraco-acromial ligament calcification and ossification. *Skeletal Radiology* **19**: 263–266.

Chen, Y.J., Hsu, R.W-W., and Liang, S-C. (1997). Degeneration of the accessory navicular synchondrosis presenting as rupture of the posterior tibial tendon. *Journal of Bone and Joint Surgery* **79A**: 1791–1798.

Chigra, M. and Shimizu, T. (1989). Computed tomographic appearances of sternocostoclavicular hyperostosis. *Skeletal Radiology* **18**: 347–353.

Chilton, L.A., Dorst, J.P. and Garn, S.M. (1983). The volume of the sella turcica in children: new standards. *American Journal of Roentgenology* **140**: 797–801.

Cho, B.P. and Kang, H.S. (1998). Articular facets of the coracoclavicular joint in Koreans. *Acta Anatomica* **163**: 56–62.

Choi, S.C. and Trotter, M. (1970). A statistical study of the multivariate structure and race-sex differences of American White and Negro fetal skeletons. *American Journal of Physical Anthropology* **33**: 307–312.

Choi, D., Carroll, N. and Abrahams, P. (1996). Spinal cord diameters in cadaveric specimens and magnetic resonance scans, to assess embalming artefacts. *Surgical Radiology and Anatomy* **18**: 133–135.

Chole, R.A. (1985). Petrous appicitis: surgical anatomy. *Annals of Otology, Rhinology and Laryngology* **94**: 251–257.

Chole, R.A. (1993). Differential osteoclast activation in endochondral and intramembranous bone. *Annals of Otology, Rhinology and Laryngology* **102**: 616–619.

Chouké, K.S. (1946). On the incidence of the foramen of Civinini and the porus crotaphitico-buccinatorius in American Whites and Negroes. I. Observations on 1544 skulls. *American Journal of Physical Anthropology* **4**: 203–225.

Chouké, K.S. (1947). On the incidence of the foramen of Civinini and the porus crotophitico-buccinatorius in American Whites and Negroes. II. Observations on 2745 additional skulls. *American Journal of Physical Anthropology* **5**: 79–86.

Chouké, K.S. (1949). Injection of mandibular nerve and Gasserian ganglion. *American Journal of Surgery* **78**: 80–85.

Chouké, K.S. and Hodes, P.J. (1951). The pterygo-alar bar and its recognition by roentgen methods in trigeminal neuralgia. *American Journal of Roentgenology* **65**: 180–182.

Christ, B. and Wilting, J. (1992). From somites to vertebral column. *Annals of Anatomy* **174**: 23–32.

Christ, B., Jacob, H.J. and Brand, B. (1986). Principles of hand ontogenesis in man. *Acta Morphologica Neerlando-Scandinavica* **24**: 249–268.

Christensen, G.J. and Kraus, B.S. (1965). Initial calcification of the human permanent first molar. *Journal of Dental Research* **44**: 1338–1342.

Christie, A. (1949). Prevalence and distribution of ossification centers in the newborn infant. *American Journal of Diseases of Children* **77**: 355–361.

Christie, A.U., Dunham, E.C., Jenss, R.M. and Dippel, A.L. (1941). Development of the center for the cuboid bone in newborn infants: a roentgenographic study. *American Journal of Diseases of Children* **61**: 471–482.

Chung, S.M.K. and Nissenbaum, M.M. (1975). Congenital and developmental defects of the shoulder. *Orthopedic Clinics of North America* **6**: 381–392.

Chung, M.S., Kim, J.J., Kang, H.S. and Chung, I.H. (1995). Locational relationship of the supraorbital notch or foramen and infraorbital and mental foramina in Koreans. *Acta Anatomica* **154**: 162–166.

Churchill, S.E. and Morris, A.G. (1998). Muscle marking morphology and labour intensity in prehistoric Khoisan foragers. *International Journal of Osteoarchaeology* **8**: 390–411.

Cihák, R. (1972). *Ontogenesis of the Skeleton and Intrinsic Muscles of the Human Hand and Foot.* New York: Springer.

Ciochon, R.L. and Corruccini, R.S. (1977). The coraco-acromial ligament and projection index in man and other anthropoid apes. *Journal of Anatomy* **124**: 627–632.

Clark, M.W., D'ambrosia, R.D. and Ferguson, A.B. (1977). Congenital vertical talus: Treatment by open reduction and navicular excision. *Journal of Bone and Joint Surgery* **59A**: 816–824.

Clark, G.A., Hall, N.R., Armelagos, G.J., Borkan, G.A., Panjabi, M.M. and Wetzel, F.T. (1986). Poor growth prior to early childhood: decreased health and life-span in the adult. *American Journal of Physical Anthropology* **70**: 145–160.

Clark, D.I., Chell, J. and Davis, T.R.C. (1998). Pollicisation of the index finger. *Journal of Bone and Joint Surgery* **80B**: 631–635.

Cleaver, F. (1937–8). A contribution to the biometric study of the human mandible. *Biometrika* **29**: 80–112.

Cleaves, E.N. (1937). Adolescent sacro-iliac joints: their normal development and their appearance in epiphysitis. *American Journal of Roentgenology* **38**: 450–456.

Cleland, J. (1862). On the relations of the vomer, ethmoid and intermaxillary bones. *Philosophical Transactions of the Royal Society of London* **152**: 289–321.

Cleland, J. (1889). On certain distinctions of form hitherto unnoticed in the human pelvis characteristic of sex, age and race. *Memoirs and Memoranda in Anatomy* **1**: 95–103.

Clementz, B.-G. (1989). Assessment of tibial torsion and rotational deformity with a new fluoroscopic technique. *Clinical Orthopaedics and Related Research* **245**: 199–209.

Cobb, W.M. (1937). The ossa suprasternalia in Whites and American Negroes and the form of the superior border of the manubrium sterni. *Journal of Anatomy* **71**: 245–291.

Cocchi, U. (1950). Zur Frage der Epiphysenossifikation des Humeruskopfes: Das Tuberculum minus. *Radiologica Clinica* **19**: 18–23.

Cockshott, W.P. (1963). Carpal fusions. *American Journal of Roentgenology* **89**: 1260–1271.

Cockshott, W.P. (1992). The geography of coracoclavicular joints. *Skeletal Radiology* **21**: 225–227.

Cockshott, W.P. and Park, W.M. (1983). Observer variation in skeletal radiology. *Skeletal Radiology* **10**: 86–90.

Cohen, J. and Harris, W.H. (1958). The three dimensional anatomy of Haversian systems. *Journal of Bone and Joint Surgery* **40A**: 419–434.

Cohen, J., Currarino, G. and Neuhauser, E.B.D. (1956). A significant variant in the ossification centres of the vertebral bodies. *American Journal of Roentgenology* **76**: 469–475.

Cohn, I. (1921a). Observations on the normally developing shoulder. *American Journal of Roentgenology* **8**: 721–729.

Cohn, I. (1921b). Observations on the normally developing elbow. *Archives of Surgery* **2**: 455–492.

Cohn, I. (1924). Normal bones and joints. *Annals of Roentgenology* **IV**. New York: P.B. Hoeber.

Coleman, W.H. (1969). Sex differences in the growth of the human bony pelvis. *American Journal of Physical Anthropology* **31**: 125–152.

Collins, H.B. (1926). The temporo-frontal articulation in man. *American Journal of Physical Anthropology* **9**: 343–348.

Collins, H.B. (1928). Frequency and distribution of the fossa pharyngea in human crania. *American Journal of Physical Anthropology* **11**: 101–106.

Collins, H.B. (1930). Notes on the pterion. *American Journal of Physical Anthropology* **14**: 41–44.

Colwell, H.A. (1927). Case showing abnormal epiphyses of metatarsals and first metacarpals. *Journal of Anatomy* **62**: 183.

Condon, K., Charles, D.K., Cheverud, J.M. and Buikstra, J.E. (1986). Cementum annulation and age determination in *Homo sapiens*. II. Estimates and accuracy. *American Journal of Physical Anthropology* **71**: 321–330.

Cone, R.O., Flournoy, J. and MacPherson, R.I. (1981). The cranio-cervical junction. *Radiographics* **1**: 1–3.

Conforty, B. (1979). Anomaly of the scapula associated with Sprengel's deformity. *Journal of Bone and Joint Surgery* **61A**: 1243–1244.

Congdon, E.D. (1920). The distribution and mode of origin of septa and walls of the sphenoid sinus. *Anatomical Record* **18**: 97–123.

Conolly, W.B. and Kilgore, E.S. (1975). *Hand Injuries and Infections: An Illustrated Guide.* London: Arnold.

Conway, W.F., Hayes, C.W. and Murphy, W.A. (1989). Total resorption of the lateral sesamoid secondary to Pseudomonas aeruginosa osteomyelitis. *Skeletal Radiology* **18**: 483–484.

Cook, D.C. (1984). Subsistence and health in Lower Illinois valley: osteological evidence. In: *Paleopathology at the Origins of Agriculture* (M.N. Cohen and G.J. Armelagos, Eds.), pp. 235–269. Orlando, FL: Academic Press.

Cool, S.M., Hendrikz, J.K. and Wood, W.B. (1995). Microscopic age changes in the human occipital bone. *Journal of Forensic Sciences* **40**: 789–796.

Coonrad, R.W. and Goldner, J.L. (1968). A study of the pathological findings and treatment in soft tissue injury of the thumb metacarpophalangeal joint. *Journal of Bone and Joint Surgery* **50A**: 439–451.

Cooper, R.R., Milgram, J.W. and Robinson, R.A. (1966). Morphology of the osteon: An electron microscopic study. *Journal of Bone and Joint Surgery* **48A**: 1239–1271.

Cooper, P.D., Stewart, J.H. and McCormick, W.F. (1988). Development and morphology of the sternal foramen. *American Journal of Forensic Medicine and Pathology* **9**: 342–347.

Coote, H. (1861). Exostosis of the left transverse process of the seventh cervical vertebra surrounded by blood vessels and nerves; successful removal. *Lancet* **1**: 360.

Cope, V.Z. (1917). The internal structure of the sphenoidal sinus. *Journal of Anatomy* **51**: 127–136.

Cope, V.Z. (1920). Fusion lines of bones. *Journal of Anatomy* **55**: 36–37.

Copland, S.M. (1946). Total resection of the clavicle. *American Journal of Surgery* **72**: 280–281.

Coral, A. (1986). Os subtibiale mistaken for a recent fracture. *British Medical Journal* **292**: 1571–1572.

Coral, A. (1987). The radiology of skeletal elements in the subtibial region: incidence and significance. *Skeletal Radiology* **16**: 298–303.

Coren, S. and Porac, C. (1977). Fifty centuries of right handedness. The historical record. *Science* **198**: 631–632.

Corner, E.M. (1896a). The processes of the occipital and temporal regions of the skull. *Journal of Anatomy and Physiology* **30**: 386–389.

Corner, E.M. (1896b). On the temporal fossa. *Journal of Anatomy and Physiology* **30**: 377–385.

Corner, E.M. (1900). The varieties and structure of the patella in man. *Journal of Anatomy and Physiology* **34**: xxvii–xxviii.

Corrigan, G.E. (1960a). The neonatal clavicle. *Biologia Neonatorum* **2**: 79–92.

Corrigan, G.E. (1960b). The neonatal scapula. *Biologia Neonatorum* **2**: 159–167.

Costa, R.L. (1986). Asymmetry of the mandibular condyle in Haida Indians. *American Journal of Physical Anthropology* **70**: 119–123.

Cotteril, P.C., Kostuik, J.P., D'Angelo, G., Fernie, G.R. and Maki, B.E. (1986). An anatomical comparison of the human and bovine thoracolumbar spine. *Journal of Orthopedic Research* **4**: 298.

Couly, G.F., Coltey, P.M. and Le Douarin, N.M. (1992). The developmental fate of the cephalic mesoderm in quail-chick chimeras. *Development* **114**: 1–15.

Couly, G.F., Coltey, P.M. and Le Douarin, N.M. (1993). The triple origin of skull in higher vertebrates: a study in quail-chick chimeras. *Development* **117**: 409–429.

Covell, W.P. (1927). Growth of the human prenatal hypophysis and the hypophyseal fossa. *American Journal of Anatomy* **38**: 379–422.

Coventry, M.B. and Johnson, E.W. (1952). Congenital absence of the fibula. *Journal of Bone and Joint Surgery* **34A**: 941–955.

Cox, M. (1995). A dangerous assumption: anyone can be a historian! The lessons from Christchurch, Spitalfields. In: *Grave Reflections: Portraying the Past through Cemetery Studies* (S.R. Saunders and A. Herring, Eds.), pp.19–29. Toronto: Canadian Scholars' Press.

Cox, M. (1996). *Life and Death in Spitalfields 1700–1850.* York: Council for British Archaeology.

Cox, M. and Scott, A. (1992). Evaluation of the obstetric significance of some pelvic characters in an eighteenth-century British sample of known parity status. *American Journal of Physical Anthropology* **89**: 431–440.

Craig, E.A. (1995). Intercondylar shelf angle: a new method to determine race from the distal femur. *Journal of Forensic Sciences* **40**: 777–782.

Crelin, E.S. (1954). The effects of estrogen and relaxin on the pubic symphysis and transplanted ribs in mice. *Anatomical Record* **120**: 23–31.

Crelin, E.S. (1969). Interpubic ligament: elasticity in pregnant free-tailed bat. *Science* **164**: 81–82.

Crelin, E.S. (1973). *Functional Anatomy of the Newborn.* New Haven, CT: Yale University Press.

Crelin, E.S., Wood, P.B. and Honeyman, M.S. (1957). Flexibility changes of pelvic joints in pregnant and hormonally injected mice. *Anatomical Record* **127**: 408.

Crock, H.V. (1962). The arterial supply and venous drainage of the bones of the human knee joint. *Anatomical Record* **144**: 199–218.

Crock, H.V. (1965). A revision of the anatomy of the arteries supplying the upper end of the human femur. *Journal of Anatomy* **99**: 77–88.

Crock, H.V. (1967). *The Blood Supply of the Lower Limbs in Man.* Edinburgh: Churchill Livingstone.

Crock, H.V. (1996). *An Atlas of Vascular Anatomy of the Skeleton and Spinal Cord.* London: Dunitz.

Crock, H.V., Yoshizawa, H. and Kame, S.K. (1973). Observations on the venous drainage of the human vertebral body. *Journal of Bone and Joint Surgery* **55B**: 528–533.

Crock, H.V., Chari, P.R. and Crock, M.C. (1981). *The blood supply of the wrist and hand bones in man.* In: *The Hand* (R. Tubiana, Ed.). Philadelphia, PA: W.B. Saunders.

Croft, M.S., Desai, G., Seed, P.T., Pollard, J.I. and Perry, M.E. (1999). Application of obstetric ultrasound to determine the most suitable parameters for the aging of formalin-fixed human fetuses using manual measurements. *Clinical Anatomy* **12**: 84–93.

Cross, M.J. and Waldrop, J. (1975). The patellar index as a guide to the understanding and diagnosis of patellofemoral instability. *Clinical Orthopaedics and Related Research* **110**: 174–176.

Crossner, C.G. and Mansfield, L. (1983). Determination of dental age in adopted non-European children. *Swedish Dental Journal* **7**: 1–10.

Cullen, R.L. and Vidić, B. (1972). The dimensions and shape of the human maxillary sinus in the perinatal period. *Acta Anatomica* **83**: 411–415.

Cummins, C.A., Anderson, K., Bowen, M., Nuber, G. and Roth, S.I. (1998). Anatomy and histological characteristics of the spinoglenoid ligament. *Journal of Bone and Joint Surgery* **80A**: 1622–1625.

Cundy, P., Paterson, D., Morris, L. and Foster, B. (1988). Skeletal age estimation in leg length discrepancy. *Journal of Pediatric Orthopaedics* **8**: 513–515.

Cunha, E. (1995). Testing identification records: evidence from the Coimbra identified skeletal collections (nineteenth and twentieth centuries). In: *Grave Reflections: Portraying the Past through Cemetery Studies* (S.R. Saunders and A. Herring, Eds.). Toronto: Canadian Scholars' Press.

Cunningham, D.J. (1890). The occasional eighth true rib in man and its relation to right handedness. *Journal of Anatomy and Physiology* **24**: 127–129.

Curr, J.F. (1946/47). Congenital fusion of the lunate and triquetrum. *British Journal of Surgery* **34**: 99–100.

Curran, B.K. and Weaver, D.S. (1982). The use of the coefficient of agreement and likelihood ratio test to examine the development of the tympanic plate using a known age sample of fetal and infant skeletons. *American Journal of Physical Anthropology* **58**: 343–346.

Currarino, G. (1976). Normal variants and congenital anomalies in the region of the obelion. *American Journal of Roentgenology* **127**: 487–494.

Currarino, G. and Silverman, F.N. (1958). Premature obliteration of sternal sutures and pigeon-breast deformity. *Radiology* **70**: 532–540.

Currarino, G. and Swanson, G.E. (1964). Developmental variant of ossification of the manubrium sterni in Mongolism. *Radiology* **82**: 916.

Currarino, G. and Weinberg, A. (1974). Os supra petrosum of Meckel. *American Journal of Roentgenology* **121**: 139–142.

Currarino, G., Maravilla, K.R. and Salyer, K.E. (1985). Transsphenoidal canal (large craniopharyngeal canal) and its pathologic implications. *American Journal of Neuroradiology* **6**: 39–43.

Curtis, D.J., Allman, R.M., Brion, J., Holborow, G.S. and Brahman, S.L. (1985). Calcification and ossification in the arytenoid cartilage: incidence and patterns. *Journal of Forensic Sciences* **30**: 1113–1118.

Curtiss, P.H. (1961). The hunchback carpal bone. *Journal of Bone and Joint Surgery* **43A**: 392–394.

Cybulski, J.S. (1988). Brachydactyly – a possible inherited anomaly at prehistoric Prince Rupert Harbour. *American Journal of Physical Anthropology* **76**: 363–376.

Cyriax, E.F. (1919). A brief note on 'floating clavicle'. *Anatomical Record* **16**: 379–380.

Daga, S.R., Daga, A.S., Patole, S., Kadam, S. and Mukadam, Y. (1988). Foot length measurement from foot print for identifying a newborn at risk. *Journal of Tropical Pediatrics* **34**: 16–19.

Dahlberg, A.A. and Menegaz-Bock, R.M. (1958). Emergence of the permanent teeth in Pima Indian children. *Journal of Dental Research* **37**: 1123–1140.

Dahm, M.C., Shepherd, R.K. and Clark, G.M. (1993). The postnatal growth of the temporal bone and its implications for cochlear implantation in children. *Acta Oto-Laryngologica (Stockh.)* **505**(Suppl.): 1–27.

Dalby, G., Manchester, K. and Roberts, C.A. (1993). Otosclerosis and stapedial footplate fixation in archaeological material. *International Journal of Osteoarchaeology* **3**: 207–212.

Dalgleish, A.E. (1985). A study of the development of thoracic vertebrae in the mouse assisted by autoradiography. *Acta Anatomica* **122**: 91–98.

Dalinka, M.K., Rosenbaum, A.E. and Van Houten, F. (1972). Congenital absence of the posterior arch of the atlas. *Radiology* **103**: 581–583.

Dameron, T.B. (1975). Fractures and anatomical variations of the proximal portions of the fifth metatarsal. *Journal of Bone and Joint Surgery* **57A**: 788–792.

Dameron, T.B. and Rockwood, C.A. (1984). Fractures and dislocation of the shoulder. In: *Fractures in Children* (C.A. Rockwood, K.E. Wilkins and R.E. King, Eds.), pp. 577–682. Philadelphia, PA: Lippincott.

D'Amico-Martell, A. (1982). Temporal patterns of neurogenesis in avian cranial sensory and autonomic ganglia. *American Journal of Anatomy* **163**: 351–372.

D'Amico-Martell, A. and Noden, D.M. (1983). Contributions of placodal and neural crest cells to avian peripheral ganglia. *American Journal of Anatomy* **166**: 445–468.

Danforth, C.H. (1930). Numerical variation and homologies in vertebrae. *American Journal of Physical Anthropology* **14**: 463–481.

Das, A.C. and Hasan, M. (1970). The occipital sinus. *Journal of Neurosurgery* **33**: 307–311.

Das, A.C., Saxena, R.C. and Beg, M.A.Q. (1973). Incidence of metopic suture in U.P. subjects. *Journal of the Anatomical Society of India* **22**: 140–143.

Daseler, E.H. and Anson, B.J. (1943). The plantaris muscle. An anatomical study of 780 specimens. *Journal of Bone and Joint Surgery* **25**: 822–827.

Dass, R. and Makhni, S.S. (1966). Ossification of ear ossicles. The stapes. *Archives of Otolaryngology* **84**: 306–312.

Dass, R., Grewal, B.S. and Thapar, S.P. (1966a). Human stapes and its variations. I. General features. *Journal of Laryngology and Otology* **80**: 11–25.

Dass, R., Grewal, B.S. and Thapar, S.P. (1966b). Human stapes and its variations. II. Footplate. *Journal of Laryngology and Otology* **80**: 471–480.

Dass, R., Thapar, S.P. and Makhni, S.S. (1969). Foetal stapes. I. General features. *Journal of Laryngology and Otology* **83**: 101–117.

Davenport, C.B. (1932). The growth of the human foot. *American Journal of Physical Anthropology* **17**: 167–212.

Davenport, C.B. (1933). The crural index. *American Journal of Physical Anthropology* **17**: 333–353.

David, K.M., McLachlan, J.C., Aiton, J.F., Whiten, S.C., Smart, S.D., Thorogood, P.V. and Crockard, H.A. (1998). Cartilaginous development of the human craniovertebral junction as visualised by a new three-dimensional computer reconstruction technique. *Journal of Anatomy* **192**: 269–277.

Davidoff, L.M. (1936). Convolutional digitations seen in roentgenograms of immature human skulls. *Bulletin of the Neurological Institute of New York* **5**: 61–71.

Davies, A. (1932). A re-survey on the morphology of the nose in relation to climate. *Journal of the Royal Anthropological Institute* **62**: 337–359.

Davies, J.W. (1955). Man's assumption of the erect posture – its effect on the position of the pelvis. *American Journal of Obstetrics and Gynaecology* **70**: 1012–1020.

Davies, D.A. and Parsons, F.G. (1927). The age order of the appearance and union of the normal epiphyses as seen by X-rays. *Journal of Anatomy* **62**: 58–71.

Davis, P.R. (1955). The thoraco-lumbar mortice joint. *Journal of Anatomy* **89**: 370–377.

Davis, P.J. and Hägg, U. (1994). The accuracy and precision of the 'Demirjian system' when used for age determination in Chinese children. *Swedish Dental Journal* **18**: 113–116.

Davis, D.B. and King, J.C. (1938). Cervical rib in early life. *American Journal of Diseases of Children* **56**: 744–755.

Davis, P.R. and Rowland, H.A.K. (1965). Vertebral fractures in West Africans suffering from Tetanus. *Journal of Bone and Joint Surgery* **47B**: 61–71.

Davis, R.A., Anson, B.J., Budinger, J.M. and Kurth, LeR.E. (1956). Surgical anatomy of the facial nerve and parotid gland based upon a study of 350 cervicofacial halves. *Surgery, Gynecology and Obstetrics* **102**: 385–412.

Davivongs, V. (1963). The femur of the Australian aborigine. *American Journal of Physical Anthropology* **21**: 457–467.

Dawson, A.B. (1925). The ossicle at the sternal end of the clavicle in the albino rat: the homologue of the sternal epiphysis of the clavicle in man. *Anatomical Record* **30**: 205–210.

Dawson, A.B. (1929). A histological study of the persisting cartilaginous plates in retarded or lapsed epiphyseal union in the albino rat. *Anatomical Record* **43**: 109–129.

Day, M.H. (1991). Bipedalism and prehistoric footprints. *Origine de la Bipédie chez les Hominidés*, pp. 199–213. Paris: Cahiers de Paléoanthropologie, Editions du CNRS.

Day, M.H. and Napier, J.R. (1961). The two heads of flexor pollicis brevis. *Journal of Anatomy* **95**: 123–130.

Day, M.H. and Pitcher-Wilmott, R.W. (1975). Sexual differentiation in the innominate bone studied by multivariate analysis. *Annals of Human Biology* **2**: 143–151.

Day, M.H. and Wickens, E.H. (1981). Laetoli hominid footprints and bipedalism. *Nature* **286**: 385–387.

Dean, M.C. and Beynon, A.D. (1991). Histological reconstruction of crown formation times and initial root formation times in a modern human child. *American Journal of Physical Anthropology* **86**: 215–228.

Dean, R.F.A. and Jones, P.R.M. (1959). Fusion of the triquetral and lunate bones shown in serial radiographs. *American Journal of Physical Anthropology* **17**: 279–288.

Dean, M.C., Stringer, C.B. and Bromage, T.G. (1986). Age at death of the Neanderthal child from Devil's Tower, Gibraltar and its implications for studies of general growth and development in Neanderthals. *American Journal of Physical Anthropology* **70**: 301–309.

Dean, M.C., Beynon, A.D., Thackeray, J.F. and Macho, G.A. (1993). Histological reconstruction of dental development and age at death of a juvenile *Paranthropus robustus* specimen, SK 63, from Swartkrans, South Africa. *American Journal of Physical Anthropology* **91**: 401–419.

de Beer, G.R. (1937). *The Development of the Vertebrate Skull*. Oxford: Clarendon Press.

Debrunner, H.V. (1985). *Biomechanik des Fusses*. Stuttgart: Enke.

de Campo, J.F. and Boldt, D.W. (1986). Computed tomography of partial growth plate arrest: initial experience. *Skeletal Radiology* **15**: 526–529.

de Carle, D.W. (1957). Pregnancy associated with severe angular deformities of the spine. *American Journal of Obstetrics and Gynaecology* **73**: 296–300.

Decker, H.R. (1915). Report of the anomalies in a subject with a supernumerary lumbar vertebra. *Anatomical Record* **9**: 181–189.

Dedick, A.P. and Caffey, J. (1953). Roentgen findings in the skull and chest on 1030 newborn infants. *Radiology* **61**: 13–20.

Dee, P.M. (1981). The pre-auricular sulcus. *Radiology* **140**: 354.

de Iturriza, J.R. and Tanner, J.M. (1969). Cone shaped epiphyses and other minor anomalies in the hands of normal British children. *Journal of Pediatrics* **75**: 265–272.

De Jager, L.T. and Hoffman, E.B. (1991). Fracture separation of the distal humeral epiphysis. *Journal of Bone and Joint Surgery* **73B**: 143–146.

de La Cruz, A., Linthicum, F.H. and Luxford, W.M. (1985). Congenital atresia of the external auditory canal. *Laryngoscope* **95**: 421–427.

Delaere, O., Kok, V., Nyssen-Behets, C. and Dhem, A. (1992). Ossification of the human fetal ilium. *Acta Anatomica* **143**: 330–334.

Delano, P.J. (1941). Os intermetatarseum: unusual variant. *Radiology* **37**: 102–103.

de Lima, R.T. and Mishkiu, F.S. (1996). The bone scan in tarsal coalition: a case report. *Pediatric Radiology* **26**: 754–756.

Del Sel, J.M. and Grand, N.E. (1959). Cubo-navicular synostosis. A rare tarsal anomaly. *Journal of Bone and Joint Surgery* **41B**: 149.

de Melo e Freitas, M.J. and Salzano, F.M. (1975). Eruption of permanent teeth in Brazilian whites and blacks. *American Journal of Physical Anthropology* **42**: 145–150.

Demirjian, A. (1986). Dentition. In: *Human Growth*, 2nd edition, Vol. 2. *Postnatal Growth* (F. Falkner and J.M. Tanner, Eds.), pp 269–298. New York: Plenum Press.

Demirjian, A. and Goldstein, H. (1976). New systems for dental maturity based on seven and four teeth. *Annals of Human Biology* **3**: 411–421.

Demirjian, A. and Levesque, G.-Y. (1980). Sexual differences in dental development and predictions of emergence. *Journal of Dental Research* **59**: 1110–1122.

Demirjian, A., Goldstein, H. and Tanner, J.M. (1973). A new system of dental age assessment. *Human Biology* **45**: 211–227.

Demisch, A. and Wartmann, P. (1956). Calcification of the mandibular third molar and its relation to skeletal and chronological development. *Child Development* **27**: 459–472.

Denham, R.H. and Dingley, A.F. (1967). Epiphyseal separation of the medial end of the clavicle. *Journal of Bone and Joint Surgery* **49A**: 1179–1183.

Den Hoed, D. (1925). Separate centres of ossification of the tip of the internal malleolus. *British Journal of Radiology* **30**: 67–68.

Denninger, H.S. (1931). Cervical ribs: a prehistoric example. *American Journal of Physical Anthropology* **26:** 211–214.

Dennis, K.J. and McKinney, S. (1990). Sesamoids and accessory bones of the foot. *Clinics in Podiatric Medicine and Surgery* **7**: 717–722.

Dennis, D.A., Ferlic, D.C. and Clayton, M.L. (1986). Acromial stress fractures associated with cuff tear arthropathy. *Journal of Bone and Joint Surgery* **68A**: 937–940.

Denyer, S.E. (1904). Description of an ossicle occurring in the ilium. *Journal of Anatomy and Physiology* **38**: 24–25.

de Palma, A.F. (1957). *Degenerative Changes in the Sternoclavicular and Acromioclavicular Joints in Various Decades.* Springfield, IL: C.C. Thomas.

de Roo, T. and Schröder, H.J. (1976). *Pocket Atlas of Skeletal Age.* The Hague: Martinus Nijhoff.

Derry, D.E. (1906). Notes on predynastic Egyptian tibiae. *Journal of Anatomy and Physiology* **41**: 123–130.

Derry, D.E. (1908). Note on the innominate bone as a factor in the determination of sex: with special reference to the sulcus preauricularis. *Journal of Anatomy and Physiology* **43**: 266–276.

Derry, D.E. (1910). Note on accessory articular facets between the sacrum and ilium and their significance. *Journal of Anatomy and Physiology* **45**: 202–210.

Derry, D.E. (1911). The significance of the sulcus preauricularis. *Anatomischer Anzeiger* **39**: 13–20.

Derry, D.E. (1938). Two skulls with absence of the premaxilla. *Journal of Anatomy* **72**: 295–298.

Detenbeck, L.C. and Kelly, P.J. (1969). Total dislocation of the talus. *Journal of Bone and Joint Surgery* **51A**: 283–288.

Deutsch, D., Goultschin, J. and Anteby, S. (1981). Determination of fetal age from the length of femur, mandible and maxillary incisor. *Growth* **45**: 232–238.

Deutsch, D., Pe'er, E. and Gedalia, I. (1984). Changes in size, morphology and weight of human anterior teeth during the fetal period. *Growth* **48**: 74–85.

Deutsch, D., Tam, O. and Stack, M.V. (1985). Postnatal changes in size, morphology and weight of developing postnatal deciduous anterior teeth. *Growth* **49**: 202–217.

Devas, M. (1960). Stress fracture of the patella. *Journal of Bone and Joint Surgery* **42B**: 71–74.

Devas, M. (1988). Stress Fractures. In: *The Foot* (B. Helal, and D. Wilson, Eds.), pp. 967–993. Edinburgh: Churchill Livingstone.

de Vasconcellos, H.A. and Ferreira, E. (1998). Metatarsal growth during the second trimester: a predictor of gestational age? *Journal of Anatomy* **193**: 145–149.

de Vasconcellos, H.A., Prates, J.C. and de Moraes, L.G.B. (1992). A study of human foot length growth in the early fetal period. *Annals of Anatomy* **174**: 473–474.

DeVito, C. and Saunders, S.R. (1990). A discriminant function analysis of deciduous teeth to determine sex. *Journal of Forensic Sciences* **35**: 845–858.

Dewar, F.P. and Evans, D.F. (1968). Occult fracture-subluxation of the mid tarsal joint. *Journal of Bone and Joint Surgery* **50B**: 386–388.

Diamond, M.K. (1992). Homology and evolution of the orbitotemporal sinuses of humans. *American Journal of Physical Anthropology* **88**: 211–244.

Dias, L.S. (1984). Fractures of the tibia and fibula. In: *Fractures in Children* (C.A. Rockwood, K.E. Wilkins and R.E. King, Eds.), pp. 983–1042. Philadelphia, PA: Lippincott.

DiBartolomeo, J.R. (1979). Exostoses of the external auditory canal. *Annals of Otology, Rhinology and Laryngology* **88**(Suppl. **61**): 1–20.

Dibennardo, R. and Taylor, J.V. (1982). Classification and misclassification in sexing the black femur by discriminant function analysis. *American Journal of Physical Anthropology* **58**: 145–151.

Dibennardo, R. and Taylor, J.V. (1983). Multiple discriminant function analysis of sex and race in the postcranial skeleton. *American Journal of Physical Anthropology* **61**: 305–314.

Di Chiro, G. and Nelson, K.B. (1962). The volume of the sella turcica. *American Journal of Roentgenology* **87**: 989–1008.

Di Chiro, G., Fisher, R.L. and Nelson, K.B. (1964). The jugular foramen. *Journal of Neurosurgery* **21**: 447–460.

Diewert, V.M. (1985). Development of human craniofacial morphology during the embryonic and early fetal periods. *American Journal of Orthodontics* **88**: 64–76.

Digby, K.H. (1915). The measurement of diaphysial growth in proximal and distal directions. *Journal of Anatomy* **50**: 187–188.

Dillaman, R.M. (1984). Movement of ferritin in the 2 day old chick femur. *Anatomical Record* **209**: 445–453.

Dimon, J.H. (1972). Isolated fractures of the lesser trochanter of the femur. *Clinical Orthopaedics and Related Research* **82**: 144–148.

Ditch, L.E. and Rose, J.C. (1972). A multivariate dental sexing technique. *American Journal of Physical Anthropology* **37**: 61–64.

Dittrick, J. and Suchey, J.M. (1986). Sex determination of prehistoric central California skeletal remains using discriminant analysis of the femur and humerus. *American Journal of Physical Anthropology* **70**: 3–9.

Dixey, F.A. (1881). On the ossification of the terminal phalanges of the digits. *Royal Society of London Proceedings* **31**: 63–71.

Dixon, A.F. (1896). Ossification of the third trochanter in man. *Journal of Anatomy and Physiology* **30**: 502–504.

Dixon, A.F. (1904). On certain markings, due to nerves and blood vessels, upon the cranial vault; their significance and the relative frequency of their occurrence in the different races of mankind. *Journal of Anatomy and Physiology* **38**: 377–398.

Dixon, A.F. (1910). The architecture of the cancellous tissue forming the upper end of the femur. *Journal of Anatomy and Physiology* **44**: 223–230.

Dixon, A.F. (1920). Note on the vertebral epiphyseal discs. *Journal of Anatomy* **55**: 38–39.

Dixon, A.D. (1953). The early development of the maxilla. *Dental Practitioner* **3**: 331–336.

Dixon, A.D. (1958). The development of the jaws. *Dental Practitioner* **9**: 10–18.

Doane, C.P. (1936). Fractures of the supracondylar process of the humerus. *Journal of Bone and Joint Surgery* **18**: 757–759.

Dodge, L.D., Ashler, R.K. and Gilbert, R.J. (1987). Treatment of the congenital vertical talus: a retrospective view of 36 feet with long term follow up. *Foot and Ankle* **7**: 326.

Dodo, Y. (1980). Appearance of bony bridging of the hypoglossal canal during the fetal period. *Journal of the Anthropological Society of Nippon* **88**: 229–238.

Dodo, Y. (1986a). Observations on the bony bridging of the jugular foramen in man. *Journal of Anatomy* **144**: 153–165.

Dodo, Y. (1986b). A population study of the jugular foramen bridging of the human cranium. *American Journal of Physical Anthropology* **69**: 15–19.

Doherty, B.J. and Heggeness, M.H. (1994). The quantitative anatomy of the atlas. *Spine* **19**: 2497–2500.

Doig, T.N., McDonald, S.W. and McGregor, I.A. (1998). Possible routes of spread of carcinoma of the maxillary sinus to the oral cavity. *Clinical Anatomy* **11**: 149–156.

Dokládal, M. (1970). Die Morpholgie der symphysealen Gelenkfläche des os pubis bei den Primaten. *Proceedings of the Third International Congress on Primatology, Zurich* **1**: 163–168.

Dokládal, M. (1971). Variability in the shape of the shaft in the human femur. *Scripta Medica* **44**: 419–428.

Dokládal, M. (1973). Variability in the shape of the shaft of the human tibia. *Scripta Medica* **46**: 305–316.

Dokládal, M. (1977). Variability of the cross-section shape of the shaft of the humerus and its practical significance. *Folia Morphologica* **25**: 343–349.

Dokládal, M. (1978). Variability in the shape of the shaft in the human humerus. *Scripta Medica* **51**: 19–30.

Dollé, P., Izpisua-Belmonte, J.C., Falkenstein, H., Renucci, A. and Duboule, D. (1989). Co ordinate expression of the murine *Hox*-5 complex homeobox-containing genes during limb pattern formation. *Nature* **342**: 767–772.

Doménech-Mateu, J.M. and Sañudo, J.R. (1990). Chondrification of laryngeal cartilages. *Proceedings XIV World Congress September 1989, Otorhinolaryngology, Head and Neck Surgery* **2**: 2095–2097.

Dommisse, G.F. (1959). Lumbo-sacral inter-body spinal fusion. *Journal of Bone and Joint Surgery* **41B**: 87–95.

Donaldson, J.A., Lambert, P.M., Duckert, L.G. and Rubel, E.W. (1992). *Surgical Anatomy of the Temporal Bone and Ear*, 4th edition. New York: Raven Press.

Donisch, E.W. and Trapp, W. (1971). The cartilage end plates of the human vertebral column (some considerations of postnatal development). *Anatomical Record* **169**: 705–715.

Dore, D.D., MacEwen, G.D. and Boulos, M.I. (1987). Cleidocranial dysostosis and syringomyelia: review of literature and case report. *Clinical Orthopaedics and Related Research* **214**: 229–234.

Dorosin, N. and Davis, J.G. (1956). Carpal boss. *Radiology* **66**: 234–236.

Dory, M.A. and Francois, R.J. (1978). Cranio-caudal axial views of the sacro-iliac joint. *American Journal of Roentgenology* **130**: 1125–1131.

Doub, H.P. and Danzer, J.T. (1934). Lükenschädel of the newborn. *Radiology* **22**: 532–538.

Downie, I.P., Evans, B.T. and Mitchell, B. (1995). The middle ethmoidal foramen and its contents. *Clinical Anatomy* **8**: 149.

Dreizen, S., Snodgrasse, R.M., Webb-Peploe, H. and Spies, T.D. (1958). The retarding effect of protracted undernutrition on the appearance of the postnatal ossification centres in the hand and wrist. *Human Biology* **30**: 253–264.

Dreizen, S., Spirakis, C.N. and Stone, R.E. (1965). The distribution and disposition of anomalous notches in the non-epiphyseal ends of human metacarpal shafts. *American Journal of Physical Anthropology* **23**: 181–187.

Drennan, M.R. (1937). The torus mandibularis in the Bushman. *Journal of Anatomy* **72**: 66–70.

Drennan, J.C. (1995). Congenital vertical talus. *Journal of Bone and Joint Surgery* **77A**: 1916–1923.

Drinkwater, H. (1916). Hereditary abnormal segmentation of the index and middle fingers. *Journal of Anatomy and Physiology* **50**: 177–186.

du Boulay, G. (1956). The significance of digital impressions in children's skulls. *Acta Radiologica* **46**: 112–122.

Dubowitz, L.M.S. and Dubowitz, V. (1977). *Gestational Age of the Newborn.* Reading, MA: Addison-Wesley.

Dubowitz, L.M.S., Dubowitz, V. and Goldberg, C. (1970). Clinical assessment of gestational age in the newborn infant. *Journal of Pediatrics* **77**: 1–10.

Duc, G. and Largo, R.H. (1986). Anterior fontanel: size and closure in term and preterm infants. *Pediatrics* **78**: 904–908.

Duckworth, W.L.H. (1902). On an unusual form of nasal bone in a human skull. *Journal of Anatomy and Physiology* **36**: 257–259.

Dudar, J.C. (1993). Identification of rib number and assessment of intercostal variation at the sternal end. *Journal of Forensic Sciences* **38**: 788–797.

Duff, C. (1954). *A New Handbook of Hanging.* London: Melrose.

Duhamel, B. (1961). From the mermaid to anal imperfection: the syndrome of caudal regression. *Archives of Diseases of Children* **36**: 152–155.

Dunaway, C.L., Williams, J.P. and Brogdon, B.G. (1983). Case report 222. Sacral and coccygeal supernumerary ribs (pelvic ribs). *Skeletal Radiology* **9**: 212–214.

Duncan, R.D.D. and Fixsen, J.A. (1999). Congenital convex pes valgus. *Journal of Bone and Joint Surgery* **81B**: 250–254.

Duncan, G. and Soutar, W.A. (1963). Hereditary onycho-osteodysplasia, the nail-patella syndrome. *Journal of Bone and Joint Surgery* **45B**: 242–258.

Dunlap, S.S. (1982). The preauricular sulcus in a cadaveric population. *American Journal of Physical Anthropology* **57**: 182.

Dunn, A.W. and Morris, H.D. (1968). Fractures and dislocations of the pelvis. *Journal of Bone and Joint Surgery* **50A**: 1639–1648.

Dupertuis, C.W. and Hadden, J.A. (1951). On the reconstruction of stature from long bones. *American Journal of Physical Anthropology* **9**: 15–53.

Durward, A. (1929). A note on symmetrical thinning of the parietal bone. *Journal of Anatomy* **63:** 356–362.

Duthie, R.A., Bruce, M.F. and Hutchison, J.D. (1998). Changing proximal femoral geometry in north east Scotland: an osteometric study. *British Medical Journal* **316**: 1498.

Dvonch, V.M. and Bunch, W.H. (1983). Pattern of closure of the proximal femoral and tibial epiphyses in man. *Journal of Pediatric Orthopedics* **3**: 498–501.

Dvorak, J. and Panjabi, M.M. (1987). Functional anatomy of the alar ligaments. *Spine* **12**: 183–190.

Dwight, T. (1887). Account of the two spines with cervical ribs, one of which has a vertebra suppressed and absence of the anterior arch of the atlas. *Journal of Anatomy and Physiology* **21**: 539–550.

Dwight, T. (1904). A separate subcapitatum in both hands. *Anatomischer Anzeiger* **24**: 253–255.

Dwight, T. (1905). The size of the articular surfaces of the long bones as characteristics of sex as an anthropological study. *American Journal of Physical Anthropology* **4**: 19–31.

Dwight, T. (1907a). Stylo-hyoid ossification. *Annals of Surgery* **46**: 721–735.

Dwight, T. (1907b). *A Clinical Atlas. Variations in the Bones of the Hands and Feet.* Philadelphia, PA: Lippincott.

Dwight, T. (1909). A criticism of Pfitzner's theory of the carpus and tarsus. *Anatomischer Anzeiger* **35**: 366–370.

Dwight, T. (1910). Description of a free cuboides secundarium with remarks on that element and on the calcaneus secundarius. *Anatomischer Anzeiger* **37**: 218–224.

Dyck, P. (1978). Os odontoideum in children: neurological manifestations and surgical management. *Neurosurgery* **8**: 93–99.

Eagle, W. (1937). Elongated styloid process: report of two cases. *Archives of Otolaryngology* **25**: 584–587.

Eagle, W. (1948). Elongated styloid process: further observations and a new syndrome. *Archives of Otolaryngology* **47**: 630–640.

Eanes, E. and Hailer, A.W. (1985). Liposome-mediated calcium phosphate formation in metastable solutions. *Calcified Tissue International* **37**: 390–394.

Eberhart, H.D., Inman, V.T. and Bresler, B. (1954). The principal elements in human locomotion. In: *Human Limbs and their Substitutes* (P.E. Klopsteg and P.D. Wilson, Eds.), pp. 437–471. New York: McGraw-Hill.

Eby, T.L. and Nadol, J.B. (1986). Postnatal growth of the human temporal bone. Implications for cochlear implants in children. *Annals of Otology, Rhinology and Laryngology* **95**: 356–364.

Eckel, H.E., Sittel, C., Zorowka, P. and Jerke, A. (1994). Dimensions of the laryngeal framework in adults. *Surgical and Radiologic Anatomy* **16**: 31–36.

Eckhoff, D.G., Kramer, R.C., Watkins, J.J., Alongi, C.A. and Van Gerven, D.P. (1994a). Variation in femoral anteversion. *Clinical Anatomy* **7**: 72–75.

Eckhoff, D.G., Kramer, R.C., Watkins, J.J., Burke, B.J., Alongi, C.A., Stamm, E.R. and Van Gerven, D.P. (1994b). Variation in tibial torsion. *Clinical Anatomy* **7**: 76–79.

Edelson, J.G. (1995a). Bony bridges and other variations of the suprascapular notch. *Journal of Bone and Joint Surgery* **77B**: 505–506.

Edelson, J.G. (1995b). The 'hooked' acromion revisited. *Journal of Bone and Joint Surgery* **77B**: 284–287.

Edelson, J.G., Zuckerman, J. and Hershkovitz, I. (1993). Os acromiale: anatomy and surgical implications. *Journal of Bone and Joint Surgery* **75B**: 551–555.

Edgren, W. (1965). Coxa plana. A clinical and radiological investigation with particular reference to the importance of the metaphyseal changes for the final shape of the proximal part of the femur. *Acta Orthopaedica Scandinavica*, **84**(Suppl.).

Edmonds, S.E.F. (1990). An investigation into the errors involved in recording measurements from radiographs of the second metacarpal. Unpublished BSc dissertation, University of London.

Edwards, M.E. (1928). The relations of the peroneal tendons to the fibula, calcaneus and cuboideum. *American Journal of Anatomy* **42**: 213–242.

Ehrenborg, G. and Engfeldt, B. (1961a). The insertion of the ligamentum patellae on the tibial tuberosity. Some views in connection with the Osgood-Schlatter lesion. *Acta Chirurgica Scandinavica* **121**: 491–499.

Ehrenborg, G. and Engfeldt, B. (1961b). Histologic changes in the Osgood-Schlatter lesion. *Acta Chirurgica Scandinavica* **121**: 328–337.

Ehrenborg, G. and Lagergren, C. (1961). Roentgenologic changes in the Osgood-Schlatter lesion. *Acta Chirurgica Scandinavica* **121**: 315–327.

Eijgelaar, A. and Bijtel, J.H. (1970). Congenital cleft sternum. *Thorax* **25**: 490–498.

Einy, S., Smith, P. and Becker, A. (1984). On the measurement of cranial thickness at nasion on cephalographs. *American Journal of Physical Anthropology* **65**: 313–314.

Elftman, H.O. (1932). The evolution of the pelvic floor in Primates. *American Journal of Anatomy* **51**: 307–346.

Elftman, H. (1945). Torsion of the lower extremity. *American Journal of Physical Anthropology* **3**: 255–265.

Elftman, H. and Manter, J. (1935). Chimpanzee and human feet in bipedal walking. *American Journal of Physical Anthropology* **20**: 69–79.

Elgenmark, O. (1946). The normal development of the ossific centres during infancy and childhood. *Acta Paediatrica Scandinavica* **33**(Suppl. **1**).

Eliot, M.M., Souther, S.P. and Park, E.A. (1927). Transverse lines in X-ray plates of the long bones of children. *Bulletin of the Johns Hopkins Hospital* **41**: 364–388.

El-Khoury, G.Y., Yousefzadeh, D.K., Mulligan, G.M. and Moore, T.E. (1982). Subtalar dislocation. *Skeletal Radiology* **8**: 99–103.

Elkington, N.M. (1989). Sex determination from the metacarpals and first digit phalanges. Unpublished BSc dissertation, University of London.

Elkington, S.G. and Huntsman, R.G. (1967). The Talbot fingers: a study of symphalangism. *British Medical Journal* **1**: 407–411.

Elliot, J.M., Rogers, L.F., Wissinger, J.P. and Fletcher-Lee, J. (1972). The hangman's fracture. *Radiology* **104**: 303–307.

Ellis, T. (1889). *The Human Foot.* London: Churchill.

Ellis, H. (1992). *Clinical Anatomy*, 8th edition. London: Blackwells.

Ellis, H. and Feldman, S. (1993). *Anatomy for Anaesthetists.* Oxford: Blackwells.

Ellis, F.G. and Joseph, J. (1954). Time of appearance of the centres of ossification of the fibular epiphyses. *Journal of Anatomy* **88**: 533–536.

Ellis, R., Short, J.G. and Knepley, D.W. (1968). The two phalanged fifth toe. *Journal of the American Medical Association* **206**: 2526.

El-Najjar, M.Y. and Dawson, G.L. (1977). The effect of artificial cranial deformation on the incidence of Wormian bones in the lambdoidal suture. *American Journal of Physical Anthropology* **46**: 155–160.

Eloff, F.C. (1952). On the relations of the human vomer to the anterior paraseptal cartilages. *Journal of Anatomy* **86**: 16–19.

Elson, R. (1965). Costal chondritis. *Journal of Bone and Joint Surgery* **47B**: 94–99.

Elster, A.D. (1989). Bertolotti's syndrome revisited – transitional vertebrae of the lumbar spine. *Spine* **14**: 1373–1377.

Elwany, S., Yacout, Y.M., Talaat, M., El-Hahass, M., Gunied, A. and Talaat, M. (1983). Surgical anatomy of the sphenoid sinus. *Journal of Laryngology and Otology* **97**: 227–241.

Engel, D. (1943). The etiology of the undescended scapula and related syndromes. *Journal of Bone and Joint Surgery* **25**: 613–625.

Engel, G.M. and Staheli, L.T. (1974). The natural history of torsion and other factors influencing gait in childhood. *Clinical Orthopaedics and Related Research* **99**: 12–17.

Engfeldt, B. and Reinholt, F.P. (1992). Structure and calcification of epiphyseal growth cartilage. In: *Calcification in Biological Systems* (Bonucci, E., Ed.), pp. 217–241. Boca Raton, FL: CRC Press.

England, M.A. (1990). *A Colour Atlas of Life Before Birth.* London: Wolfe.

Enlow, D.H. (1963). *Principles of Bone Remodelling.* Springfield, IL: C.C. Thomas.

Enlow, D.H. and Bang, S. (1965). Growth and remodelling of the human maxilla. *American Journal of Orthodontics* **51**: 446–464.

Enlow, D.H. and Hans, M.G. (1996). *Essentials of Facial Growth.* Philadelphia, PA: W.B. Saunders.

Enlow, D.H. and Harris, D.B. (1964). A study of the postnatal growth of the human mandible. *American Journal of Orthodontics* **50**: 25–50.

Epstein, J.A. and Epstein, B.S. (1967). Deformities of the skull surface in infancy and childhood. *Journal of Pediatrics* **70**: 636–647.

Ericksen, M.F. (1991). Histologic estimation of age at death using the anterior cortex of the femur. *American Journal of Physical Anthropology* **84**: 171–179.

Etter, L.E. (1963). Opacification studies of normal and abnormal paranasal sinuses. *American Journal of Roentgenology* **89**: 1137–1146.

Evans, E.M. (1951). Fractures of the radius and ulna. *Journal of Bone and Joint Surgery* **33B**: 548–561.

Evans, K.T. and Knight, B. (1981). *Forensic Radiology.* Oxford: Blackwells.

Evans, F.G. and Krahl, V.E. (1945). The torsion of the humerus: a phylogenetic survey from fish to man. *American Journal of Anatomy* **76**: 303–337.

Evans, F.G., Alfaro, A. and Alfaro, S. (1950). An unusual anomaly of the superior extremities in a Tarascan Indian girl. *Anatomical Record* **106**: 37–48.

Evans, R.A., McDonnell, G.D. and Schieb, M. (1978). Metacarpal cortical area as an index of bone mass. *British Journal of Radiology* **51**: 428–431.

Eveleth, P.B. and Tanner, J.M. (1990). *Worldwide Variation in Human Growth*, 2nd edition. Cambridge: Cambridge University Press.

Ewers, S.R. (1968). A study of prenatal growth of the human bony palate from 3 to 9 months. *American Journal of Orthodontics* **54**: 3–28.

Eyler, D.L. and Markee, J.E. (1954). The anatomy and function of the intrinsic musculature of the fingers. *Journal of Bone and Joint Surgery* **36A**: 1–9.

Eyre-Brook, A.L. (1967). Congenital vertical talus. *Journal of Bone and Joint Surgery* **49B**: 618–627.

Fabry, G., MacEwen, G.D. and Shands, A.R. (1973). Torsion of the femur. *Journal of Bone and Joint Surgery* **55A**: 1726–1738.

Failla, J. (1993). Hook of hamate vascularity: vulnerability to osteonecrosis and non-union. *Journal of Hand Surgery* **18A**: 1075–1079.

Fairbank, H.A.T. (1914). Congenital elevation of the scapula: a series of 18 cases with a detailed description of a dissected specimen. *British Journal of Surgery* **1**: 553–572.

Fairbank, H.A.T. (1930). Congenital dislocation of the hip: with special reference to the anatomy. *British Journal of Surgery* **17**: 380–416.

Fairbank, H.A.T. (1949). Cranio-cleido-dysostosis. *Journal of Bone and Joint Surgery* **31B**: 608–617.

Falkner, F. (1971). Skeletal maturity indicators in infancy. *American Journal of Physical Anthropology* **35**: 393–394.

Fanning, E.A. (1961). A longitudinal study of tooth formation and root resorption. *New Zealand Dental Journal* **57**: 202–217.

Fanning, E.A. (1962). Effect of extraction of deciduous molars on the formation and eruption of their successors. *Angle Orthodontist* **32**: 44–53.

Fanning, E.A. and Brown, T. (1971). Primary and permanent tooth development. *Australian Dental Journal* **16**: 41–43.

Farmer, A.W. and Laurin, C.A. (1960). Congenital absence of the fibula. *Journal of Bone and Joint Surgery* **42A**: 1–12.

Farrally, M.R. and Moore, W.J. (1975). Anatomical differences in the femur and tibia between negroids and caucasoids and their effects upon locomotion. *American Journal of Physical Anthropology* **43**: 63–70.

Faruqi, N.A. and Hasan, S.A. (1984). A dimensional study of the internal auditory meatus in Indian skulls. *Journal of the Anatomical Society of India* **33**: 181–185.

Fawcett, E. (1895). The structure of the inferior maxilla with special reference to the position of the inferior dental canal. *Journal of Anatomy and Physiology* **29**: 355–366.

Fawcett, E. (1897). On the sesamoid bones of the hand: A skiographic confirmation of the work done by Pfitzner. *Journal of Anatomy and Physiology* **31**: 157–161.

Fawcett, E. (1904). The presence of two centres of ossification in the olecranon process of the ulna. *Journal of Anatomy and Physiology* **38**: xxvii.

Fawcett, E. (1905a). On the early stages in the ossification of the pterygoid plates of the sphenoid bone in man. *Anatomischer Anzeiger* **26**: 280–286.

Fawcett, E. (1905b). Abstract of paper on the ossification of the lower jaw of man. *Journal of Anatomy and Physiology* **39**: 494–495.

Fawcett, E. (1905c). Ossification of the lower jaw in man. *Journal of the American Medical Association* **45**: 696–705.

Fawcett, E. (1906). On the development, ossification and growth of the palate bone in man. *Journal of Anatomy and Physiology* **40**: 400–406.

Fawcett, E. (1907). On the completion of ossification of the human sacrum. *Anatomischer Anzeiger* **30**: 414–421.

Fawcett, E. (1910a). Description of a reconstruction of the head of a thirty millimetre embryo. *Journal of Anatomy and Physiology* **44**: 303–311.

Fawcett, E. (1910b). Notes on the development of the human sphenoid bone. *Journal of Anatomy and Physiology* **44**: 207–222.

Fawcett, E. (1910c). Anatomical notes (on a fetal clavicle and scapula). *Journal of Anatomy and Physiology* **44**: 204–205.

Fawcett, E. (1911a). The development of the human maxilla, vomer and paraseptal cartilages. *Journal of Anatomy and Physiology* **45**: 378–405.

Fawcett, E. (1911b). Some notes on the epiphyses of ribs. *Journal of Anatomy and Physiology* **45**: 172–178.

Fawcett, E. (1913). The development and ossification of the human clavicle. *Journal of Anatomy and Physiology* **47**: 225–234.

Fawcett, E. (1923). Some observations on the roof of the primordial human cranium. *Journal of Anatomy* **57**: 245–250.

Fawcett, E. (1930). A model of the left half of the human mandible at the 17mm C.R. stage. *Journal of Anatomy* **64**: 369–370.

Fawcett, E. (1932). A note on the identification of the lumbar vertebrae of man. *Journal of Anatomy* **66**: 384–386.

Fazekas, I.Gy. and Kósa, F. (1978). *Forensic Fetal Osteology*. Budapest: Akadémiai Kiadó.

FDI–Fédération Dentaire International (1971). Two-digit system of designating teeth. *International Dental Journal* **21**: 104–106.

Feik, S.A. and Storey, E. (1983). Remodelling of bone and bones: Growth of normal and abnormal transplanted caudal vertebrae. *Journal of Anatomy* **136**: 1–14.

Fein, J.M. and Brinker, R.A. (1972). Evolution and significance of giant parietal foramina. *Journal of Neurosurgery* **37**: 487–492.

Felber, P. (1919). Anlage und Entwicklung des Maxillare und Praemaxillare beim Menschen. *Gegenbaurs Morphologisches Jahrbuch* **50**: 451. [Abstract in English under Schultz, A.H. (1920) *American Journal of Physical Anthropology* **3**: 269–270.]

Feldesman, M.R. (1992). Femur/stature ratio and estimates of stature in children. *American Journal of Physical Anthropology* **87**: 447–459.

Feldesman, M.R. and Fountain, R.L. (1996). 'Race' specificity and the femur/stature ratio. *American Journal of Physical Anthropology* **100**: 207–224.

Feldesman, M.R., Kleckner, J.G. and Lundy, J.K. (1990). The femur/stature ratio and estimates of stature in mid- and late-Pleistocene fossil hominids. *American Journal of Physical Anthropology* **83**: 359–372.

Feldman, F., Pochaczevsky, R. and Hecht, H. (1970). The case of the wandering sesamoid and other sesamoid afflictions. *Radiology* **96**: 275–283.

Fell, H.B. (1925). The histogenesis of cartilage and bone in the long bones of the embryonic fowl. *Journal of Morphology* **40**: 417–460.

Felts, W.J.L. (1954). The prenatal development of the human femur. *American Journal of Anatomy* **94**: 1–44.

Ferembach, D., Schwidetsky, I. and Stloukal, M. (1980). Recommendations for age and sex diagnoses of skeletons. Report of the Workshop of European Anthropologists (WEA). *Journal of Human Evolution* **9**: 517–549.

Ferguson, W.R. (1950). Some observations on the circulation in foetal and infant spines. *Journal of Bone and Joint Surgery* **32A**: 640–648.

Ferguson, A. and Gingrich, R. (1959). The normal and abnormal calcaneal apophysis and tarsal navicular. *Clinical Orthopaedics* **10**: 87–95.

Fernbach, S.K. and Wilkinson, R.H. (1981). Avulsion injuries of the pelvis and proximal femur. *American Journal of Roentgenology* **137**: 581–584.

Ferner, H. and Staubesand, J. (1983). *Sobotta's Atlas of Human Anatomy*, 10th English edition, Vol. 1. Baltimore, MD: Urban and Schwarzenberg.

Ferrario, V.F., Sforza, C., Guazzi, M. and Serrao, G. (1996). Elliptic Fourier analysis of mandibular shape. *Journal of Craniofacial Genetics and Developmental Biology* **16**: 208–217.

Ferris, B.D., Kennedy, C., Bhamra, M. and Muirhead-Allwood, W. (1989). Morphology of the femur in proximal femoral fractures. *Journal of Bone and Joint Surgery* **71B**: 475–477.

Field, G.P. (1878). On the aetiology of aural exostoses: osseous tumour following extraction of polypus. *British Medical Journal* **1**: 152–153.

Field, E.J. and Harrison, R.J. (1957). *Anatomical Terms: Their Origin and Derivation.* Cambridge: Heffer.

Field, J.H. and Krag, D.O. (1973). Congenital constricting bands and congenital amputation of the fingers: placenta studies. *Journal of Bone and Joint Surgery* **55A**: 1035–1041.

Fielding, J.W. (1965). Disappearance of the central portion of the odontoid process. *Journal of Bone and Joint Surgery* **47A**: 1228–1230.

Fielding, J.W. and Griffin, P.P. (1974). Os odontoideum: an acquired lesion. *Journal of Bone and Joint Surgery* **56A**: 187–190.

Fielding, J.W., Hensinger, R.N. and Hawkins, R.J. (1980). Os odontoideum. *Journal of Bone and Joint Surgery* **62**: 376–383.

Fileti, A. (1927). Embriologia e morfologia del canale ottico. *Annali di Ottalmologia e Clinica Oculistica* **55**: 493–554.

Filipsson, R. (1975). A new method for assessment of dental maturity using the individual curve of number of erupted permanent teeth. *Annals of Human Biology* **2**: 13–24.

Filly, R.A. and Golbus, M.S. (1982). Ultrasonography of the normal and pathologic fetal skeleton. *Radiologic Clinics of North America* **20**: 311–323.

Finder, J.G, (1936). Congenital anomaly of the coracoid: os coracosternale vestigiale. *Journal of Bone and Joint Surgery* **18**: 148–152.

Finnegan, M. (1978). Non-metric variation of the infracranial skeleton. *Journal of Anatomy* **125**: 23–37.

Finnegan, M.A. and Uhthoff, H.K. (1990). The development of the knee. In: *The Embryology of the Human Locomotor System* (H.K. Uhthoff, Ed.), p. 130. Berlin: Springer.

Fischer, K.C., White, R.I., Jordan, C.E., Dorst, J.P. and Neill, C.A. (1973). Sternal abnormalities in patients with congenital heart disease. *American Journal of Roentgenology* **119**: 530–538.

Fisk, G.R. (1988). Calcaneal fractures. In: *The Foot* (B. Helal and D. Wilson, Eds.), pp. 894–915. Edinburgh: Churchill Livingstone.

FitzGerald, C.M. (1998). Do dental microstructures have a regular time dependency? Conclusions from the literature and a large-scale survey. *Journal of Human Evolution* **35**: 371–386.

FitzGerald, C., Foley, R.A. and Dean, M.C. (1996). Variation of circaseptan cross striations in the tooth enamel of three modern human populations. *American Journal of Physical Anthropology*, **22**(Suppl.): 104.

Fitzwilliams, D.C.L. (1910). Hereditary cranio-cleido-dysostosis. *Lancet* **2**: 1466–1475.

Fixsen, J.A. (1998). Problem feet in children. *Journal of the Royal Society of Medicine* **91**: 18–22.

Flander, L.B. and Corruccini, R.S. (1980). Shape differences in the sacral alae. *American Journal of Physical Anthropology* **52**: 399–403.

Flecker, H. (1913). Observations on absence of lacrimal bones and of existence of perilacrimal ossicles. *Journal of Anatomy and Physiology* **48**: 52–72.

Flecker, H. (1932a). Roentgenographic observations of the human skeleton prior to birth. *Medical Journal of Australia* **19**: 640–643.

Flecker, H. (1932b). Roentgenographic observations of the times of appearance of epiphyses and their fusion with the diaphyses. *Journal of Anatomy* **67**: 118–164.

Flecker, H. (1936a). Epiphysis for symphysis pubis. *American Journal of Roentgenology* **35**: 541.

Flecker, H. (1936b). Epiphysis for the lesser trochanter. *American Journal of Roentgenology* **35**: 540.

Flecker, H. (1942). Time of appearance and fusion of ossification centres as observed by roentgenographic methods. *American Journal of Roentgenology* **47**: 97–159.

Fleege, M.A., Jebson, P.J., Renfrew, D.L., Steyers, C.M. and El-Khoury, G.Y. (1991). Pisiform fractures. *Skeletal Radiology* **20**: 169–172.

Flickinger, R.A. (1974). Muscle and cartilage differentiation in small and large explants from the chick limb bud. *Developmental Biology* **41**: 202–208.

Floud, R., Wachter, K. and Gregory, A. (1990). *Height, Health and History. Nutritional Status in the United Kingdom; 1750–1980.* Cambridge: Cambridge University Press.

Flower, W.H. (1879). On the scapular index as a race character in man. *Journal of Anatomy and Physiology* **14**: 13–17.

Folliason, A. (1933). Un cas d'os acromial. *Revue* **20**: 533–535.

Fong, E.E. (1946). 'Iliac horns' (symmetrical bilateral central posterior iliac processes). *Radiology* **47**: 517–518.

Ford, E.H.R. (1956). The growth of the foetal skull. *Journal of Anatomy* **90**: 63–72.

Ford, E.H.R. (1958). Growth of the human cranial base. *American Journal of Orthodontics* **44**: 498–506.

Ford, D., McFadden, K.D. and Bagnall, K.M. (1982). Sequence of ossification in human vertebral neural arch. *Anatomical Record* **203**: 175–178.

Forest, M. (1998). Osteoma and bone island. In: *Orthopedic Surgical Pathology* (M. Forest, B. Tomeno and D. Vanel, Eds.), pp. 71–77. Edinburgh: Churchill Livingstone.

Forfar, J.O. (1998). Demography, vital statistics and the pattern of disease in childhood. In: *Forfar and Arneil's Textbook of Pediatrics*, 5th edition (A.G.M. Campbell and N. McIntosh, Eds.), pp. 1–15. Edinburgh: Churchill Livingstone.

Forland, M. (1962). Cleidocranial dysostosis. *American Journal of Medicine* **33**: 792–799.

Forman, G.H. and Smith, N.J.D. (1984). Bifid mandibular condyle. *Oral Surgery, Oral Medicine and Oral Pathology* **57**: 371–373.

Formicola, V., Frayer, D.W. and Heller, J.A. (1990). Bilateral absence of the lesser trochanter in a late Epigravettian skeleton from Arene Candide (Italy). *American Journal of Physical Anthropology* **83**: 425–437.

Forrest, W.J. and Basmajian, J.V. (1965). Functions of human thenar and hypothenar muscles: An electromyographic study of 25 hands. *Journal of Bone and Joint Surgery* **47A**: 1585–1594.

Forriol Campos, F. and Gomez Pellico, L.G. (1989). Talar articular facets (Facies articulares talares) in human calcanei. *Acta Anatomica* **134**: 124–127.

Foster, T.D., Grundy, M.C. and Lavelle, C.L.B. (1977). A longitudinal study of dental arch growth. *American Journal of Orthodontics* **72**: 309–314.

Foucher, G., Schund, F., Merle, M. and Brunelli, F. (1985). Fractures of the hook of the hamate. *Journal of Hand Surgery* **10B**: 205–210.

Fowler, A.W. (1957). Flexion compression injury of the sternum. *Journal of Bone and Joint Surgery* **39B**: 487–497.

Fowler, E.P. (1961). Variations in the temporal bone course of the facial nerve. *Laryngoscope* **71**: 937–946.

Fowler, E.P. and Osmun, P.M. (1942). New bone growth due to cold water in the ears. *Archives of Otolaryngology* **36**: 455–466.

France, D. (1983). Sex determination of the humerus using single variables from different positions on the bone. In: *Human Osteology*, 3rd edition (W.M. Bass, Ed.). Columbia, MO: Missouri Archaeological Society.

France, D.L. (1988). Osteometry at muscle origin and insertion in sex determination. *American Journal of Physical Anthropology* **76**: 515–526.

Francis, C.C. (1940), The appearance of centres of ossification from 6–15 years. *American Journal of Physical Anthropology* **27**: 127–138.

Francis, C.C. (1951). Appearance of centres of ossification in human pelvis before birth. *American Journal of Roentgenology* **65**: 778–783.

Francis, C.C. (1955a). Variations in the articular facets of the cervical vertebrae. *Anatomical Record* **122**: 589–602.

Francis, C.C. (1955b). Dimensions of the cervical vertebrae. *Anatomical Record* **122**: 603–609.

Francis, C.C., Werle, P.P. and Behm, A. (1939). The appearance of centers of ossification from birth to 5 years. *American Journal of Physical Anthropology* **24**: 273–299.

Francois, R.J. and Dhem, A. (1974). Microradiographic study of the normal human vertebral body. *Acta Anatomica* **89**: 251–265.

Frantz, C.H. and Aitken, G.T. (1967). Complete absence of the lumbar spine and sacrum. *Journal of Bone and Joint Surgery* **49A**: 1531–1540.

Frantz, C.H. and O'Rahilly, R. (1961). Congenital limb deficiencies. *Journal of Bone and Joint Surgery* **43A**: 1202–1224.

Frazer, J.E. (1908). The derivation of the human hypothenar muscles. *Journal of Anatomy and Physiology* **42**: 326–334.

Frazer, J.E. (1910a). The early development of the Eustachian tube and nasopharynx. *British Medical Journal* **2**: 1148–1150.

Frazer, J.E. (1910b). The development of the larynx. *Journal of Anatomy and Physiology* **44**: 156–191.

Frazer. J.E. (1914). The second visceral arch and groove in the tubo-tympanic region. *Journal of Anatomy and Physiology* **48**: 391–408.

Frazer, J.E. (1922). The early formation of the middle ear and Eustachian tube: a criticism. *Journal of Anatomy* **57**: 18–30.

Frazer, J.E. (1948). *The Anatomy of the Human Skeleton*, 4th edition. London: Churchill.

Freedman, E. (1934). Os acetabuli. *American Journal of Roentgenology* **31**: 492–495.

Freeman, E., Ten Cate, A.R. and Dickinson, J. (1975). Development of a gomphosis by toothgerm implants in the parietal bone of mice. *Archives of Oral Biology* **20**: 139–140.

Freiband, B. (1937). Growth of the palate in the human fetus. *Journal of Dental Research* **16**: 103–122.

Freiberg, A.M. (1914). Infraction of second metatarsal bone. *Surgical Gynecology and Obstetrics* **19**: 191–193.

Freiberg, A.M. (1920). Injuries to the sesamoid bones of the great toe. *Journal of Orthopaedic Surgery* **2**: 453–465.

Freiberger, R.H. (1991). The unilateral wavy clavicle. *Skeletal Radiology* **20**: 192.

Freiberger, R.H., Wilson, P.D. and Nicholas, J.A. (1965). Acquired absence of the odontoid process. *Journal of Bone and Joint Surgery* **47A**: 1231–1236.

Freud, P. and Slobody, L.B. (1943). Symphalangism. A familial malformation. *American Journal of Diseases of Children* **65**: 550–557.

Friant, M. (1960). L'evolution du cartilage de Meckel humain, jusqu'a la fin du sixième mois de la vie foetale. *Acta Anatomica* **41**: 228–239.

Friedlander, J.S. and Bailit, H.L. (1969). Eruption times of the deciduous and permanent teeth of natives on Bougainville Island, Territory of New Guinea: a study of racial variation. *Human Biology* **41**: 51–65.

Frisancho, A.R., Garn, S.M. and Ascoli, W. (1970). Childhood retardation resulting in reduction of adult body size due to lesser adolescent skeletal delay. *American Journal of Physical Anthropology* **33**: 325–336.

Frommer, J. and Margolies, M.R. (1971). Contribution of Meckel's cartilage to the ossification of the mandible in mice. *Journal of Dental Research* **50**: 1260–1267.

Frootko, N., Maconnachie, E. and Boyde, A. (1984). The functional state of human incus bone surfaces. *Journal of Dental Research* **63**: 499.

Fujioka, M. and Young, L.W. (1978). The sphenoidal sinuses: radiographic patterns of normal development and abnormal findings in infants and children. *Radiology* **129**: 133–136.

Fullenlove, T.M. (1954). Congenital absence of the odontoid process. Report of a case. *Radiology* **63**: 72–73.

Gabriel, A.C. (1958). Some anatomical features of the mandible. *Journal of Anatomy* **92**: 580–586.

Gadow, H.F. (1933). *The Evolution of the Vertebral Column. A Contribution to the Study of Vertebrate Phylogeny* (J.F. Gaskell and H.L.L.H. Green, Eds.). Cambridge: Cambridge University Press.

Gaillard, J. (1961). Valeur de l'indice ischio-pubien pour la determination sexuelle de l'os coxal. *Bulletins et Memoires de la Société d'Anthropologie de Paris* **2**: 92–108.

Galindo, S. de L. and Galindo, M.E. de C. (1975). Semimicroscopical observations on the crista stapedis. *Acta Anatomica* **92**: 615–629.

Galstaun, G. (1930). Some notes on the union of epiphyses in Indian girls. *Indian Medical Gazette* **65**: 191–192.

Galstaun, G. (1937). A study of ossification as observed in Indian subjects. *Indian Journal of Medical Research* **25**: 267–324.

Ganguly, D.N. and Roy, K.K.S. (1964). A study on the craniovertebral joint in man. *Anatomischer Anzeiger* **114**: 433–452.

Gannon, P.J., Eden, A.R. and Laitman, J.T. (1988). The subarcuate fossa and cerebellum of extant Primates: comparative study of a skull–brain interface. *American Journal of Physical Anthropology* **77**: 143–164.

Gans, C. and Northcutt, R.G. (1983). Neural crest and the origin of vertebrates: a new head. *Science* **220**: 268–274.

Ganzhorn, R.W., Hocker, J.T., Horowitz, M. and Switzer, H.E. (1981). Suprascapular nerve entrapment. *Journal of Bone and Joint Surgery* **63A**: 492–494.

Garcia, G. and McQueen, D. (1981). Bilateral suprascapular nerve entrapment syndrome. *Journal of Bone and Joint Surgery* **63A**: 491–492.

Garden, R.S. (1961). The structure and function of the upper end of the femur. *Journal of Bone and Joint Surgery* **43B**: 576–589.

Gardner, E. (1956). Osteogenesis in the human embryo and foetus. Chapter 13. In: *The Biochemistry and Physiology of Bone* (G. Bourne, Ed.). New York: Academic Press.

Gardner, E. (1963). The development and growth of bone and joints. *Journal of Bone and Joint Surgery* **45A**: 856–862.

Gardner, E. (1968). The embryology of the clavicle. *Clinical Orthopedics and Related Research* **58**: 9–16.

Gardner, E. (1973). The early development of the shoulder joint in staged human embryos. *Anatomical Record* **175**: 503–519.

Gardner, E. and Gray, D.J. (1950). Prenatal development of the human hip joint. *American Journal of Anatomy* **87**: 163–211.

Gardner, E. and Gray, D.J. (1953). Prenatal development of the human shoulder and acromio-clavicular joints. *American Journal of Anatomy* **92**: 219–276.

Gardner, E. and Gray, D.J. (1970). The prenatal development of the human femur. *American Journal of Anatomy* **129**: 121–140.

Gardner, E. and O'Rahilly, R. (1968). The early development of the knee joint in staged human embryos. *Journal of Anatomy* **102**: 289–299.

Gardner, E. and O'Rahilly, R. (1972). The early development of the hip joint in staged human embryos. *Anatomical Record* **172**: 451–452.

Gardner, E. and O'Rahilly, R. (1976). Neural crest, limb development and thalidomide embryopathy. *Lancet* **1**: 635–637.

Gardner, E., Gray, D.J. and O'Rahilly, R. (1959). Prenatal development of the skeleton and joints of the human foot. *Journal of Bone and Joint Surgery* **41A**: 847–876.

Garmus, A. (1993). *Pelvic Bones in Forensic Medicine.* Vilnius: Baltic Medicolegal Association.

Garn, S.M. (1962). X-linked inheritance of developmental timing in man. *Nature* **196**: 695–696.

Garn, S.M. (1970). *The Earlier Gain and Later Loss of Cortical Bone in Nutritional Perspective.* Springfield, IL: C.C. Thomas.

Garn, S.M. and Burdi, A.R. (1971). Prenatal ordering and postnatal sequence in dental development. *Journal of Dental Research* **50**: 1407–1414.

Garn, S.M. and Lewis, A.B. (1957). Relationship between the sequence of calcification and the sequence of eruption of the mandibular molar and premolar teeth. *Journal of Dental Research* **36**: 992–995.

Garn, S.M. and McCreery, L.D. (1970). Variability of postnatal ossification timing and evidence for a 'dosage' effect. *American Journal of Physical Anthropology* **32**: 139–144.

Garn, S.M. and Rohmann, C.G. (1960). Variability in the order of ossification of the bony centres of the hand and wrist. *American Journal of Physical Anthropology* **18**: 219–230.

Garn, S.M. and Rohmann, C.G. (1962a). Parent–child similarities in hand-wrist ossification. *American Journal of Diseases of Children* **103**: 603–607.

Garn, S.M. and Rohmann, C.G. (1962b). The adductor sesamoid of the thumb. *American Journal of Physical Anthropology* **20**: 297–302.

Garn, S.M. and Rohmann, C.G. (1963). On the prevalence of skewness in incremental data. *American Journal of Physical Anthropology* **21**: 235–236.

Garn, S.M. and Schwager, P.M. (1967). Age dynamics of persistent transverse lines in the tibia. *American Journal of Physical Anthropology* **27**: 375–378.

Garn, S.M. and Smith, B.H. (1980). Developmental communalities in tooth emergence timing. *Journal of Dental Research* **59**: 1178.

Garn, S.M., Lewis, A.B. and Shoemaker, D.W. (1956). The sequence of calcification of the mandibular molar and premolar teeth. *Journal of Dental Research* **35**: 555–561.

Garn, S.M., Lewis, A.B., Koski, K. and Polacheck, D.L. (1958). The sex difference in tooth calcification. *Journal of Dental Research* **37**: 561–567.

Garn, S.M., Lewis, A.B. and Polacheck, D.L. (1959). Variability of tooth formation. *Journal of Dental Research* **38**: 135–148.

Garn, S.M., Lewis, A.B. and Bonné, B. (1961a). Third molar polymorphism and the timing of tooth formation. *Nature* **192**: 989.

Garn, S.M., Rohmann, C.G. and Apfelbaum, B. (1961b). Complete epiphyseal fusion of the hand. *American Journal of Physical Anthropology* **19**: 365–371.

Garn, S.M., Lewis, A.B. and Bonné, B. (1962). Third molar formation and its developmental course. *Angle Orthodontist* **32**: 270–279.

Garn, S.M., Rohmann, C.G. and Davis, A.A. (1963). Genetics of hand wrist ossification. *American Journal of Physical Anthropology* **21**: 33–40.

Garn, S.M., Lewis, A.B. and Kerewsky, R.S. (1964). Sex differences in tooth size. *Journal of Dental Research* **43**: 306.

Garn, S.M., Blumenthal, T. and Rohmann, C.G. (1965a). On skewness in the ossification centers of the elbow. *American Journal of Physical Anthropology* **23**: 303–304.

Garn, S.M., Lewis, A.B. and Blizzard, R.M. (1965b). Endocrine factors in dental development. *Journal of Dental Research* **44**: 243–258.

Garn, S.M., Lewis, A.B. and Kerewsky, R.S. (1965c). Genetic, nutritional and maturational correlates of dental development. *Journal of Dental Research* **44**: 228–242.

Garn, S.M., Rohmann, C.G. and Silverman, F.N. (1965d). Missing secondary ossification centres of the foot. Inheritance and developmental meaning. *Annals of Radiology* **8**: 629–644.

Garn, S.M., Rohmann, C.G. and Blumenthal, T. (1966a). Ossification sequence polymorphism in skeletal development. *American Journal of Physical Anthropology* **24**: 101–116.

Garn, S.M., Lewis, A.B. and Kerewsky, R.S. (1966b). Sexual dimorphism in buccolingual tooth diameter. *Journal of Dental Research* **45**: 1819.

Garn, S.M., Lewis, A.B. and Kerewsky, R.S. (1967a). Sex differences in tooth size. *Journal of Dental Research* **46**: 1470.

Garn, S.M., Rohmann, C.G. and Silverman, F.N. (1967b). Radiographic standards for postnatal ossification and tooth calcification. *Medical Radiography and Photography* **43**: 45–66.

Garn, S.M., Fels, S.L. and Israel, H. (1967c). Brachymesophalangia of digit 5 in 10 populations. *American Journal of Physical Anthropology* **27**: 205–210.

Garn, S.M., Silverman, F.N., Hertzog, K.P. and Rohmann, C.B. (1968). Lines and bands of increased density. *Medical Radiography and Photography* **44**: 58–89.

Garn, S.M., Rohmann, C.G. and Hertzog, K.P. (1969). Apparent influence of the x-chromosome on timing of 73 ossification centres. *American Journal of Physical Anthropology* **30**: 123–128.

Garn, S.M., Frisancho, A., Poznanski, A.K., Schweitzer, J. and McCann, M.B. (1971). Analysis of triquetral-lunate fusion. *American Journal of Physical Anthropology* **34**: 431–433.

Garn, S.M., Gall, J.E. and Nagy, J.M. (1972a). Brachymesophalangia-5 without cone epiphysis mid-5 in Down's Syndrome. *American Journal of Physical Anthropology* **36**: 253–256.

Garn, S.M., Poznanski, A.K., Nagy, J.M. and McCann, M.B. (1972b). Independence of brachymesophalangia-5 from brachymesophalania-5 with cone mid-5. *American Journal of Physical Anthropology* **36**: 295–298.

Garn, S.M., Sandusky, S.T., Rosen, N.N. and Trowbridge, F. (1973a). Economic impact on postnatal ossification. *American Journal of Physical Anthropology* **38**: 1–3.

Garn, S.M., Nagy, J.M., Sandusky, S.T. and Trowbridge, F. (1973b). Economic impact on tooth emergence. *American Journal of Physical Anthropology* **39**: 233–238.

Garn, S.M., Sandusky, S.T., Nagy, J.M. and Trowbridge, F. (1973c). Negro-Caucasoid differences in permanent tooth emergence at a constant income level. *Archives of Oral Biology* **18**: 609–615.

Garn, S.M., Burdi, A.R. and Babler, W.J. (1974). Male advancement in prenatal hand development. *American Journal of Physical Anthropology* **41**: 353–360.

Garn, S.M., Burdi, A.R., Babler, W.J. and Stinson, S. (1975a). Early prenatal attainment of adult metacarpal-phalangeal rankings and proportions. *American Journal of Physical Anthropology* **43**: 327–332.

Garn, S.M., Poznanski, A.K., and Larson, K.E. (1975b). Magnitude of sex differences in dichotomous ossification sequences of the hand and wrist. *American Journal of Physical Anthropology* **42**: 85–90.

Garn, S.M., Burdi, A.R. and Babler, W.J. (1976a). Prenatal origins of carpal fusions. *American Journal of Physical Anthropology* **45**: 203–208.

Garn, S.M., Babler, W.J. and Burdi, A.R. (1976b). Prenatal origins of brachymesophalangia-5. *American Journal of Physical Anthropology* **44**: 413–416.

Garn, S.M., Cole, P.E. and Van Alstine, W.L. (1979). Sex discriminatory effectiveness using combinations of root lengths and crown diameters. *American Journal of Physical Anthropology* **50**: 115–118.

Garson, J.G. (1881). Pelvimetry. *Journal of Anatomy and Physiology* **16**: 106–134.

Gasser, H. (1965). Delayed union and pseudoarthrosis of the carpal navicular: Treatment by compression screw osteosynthesis. *Journal of Bone and Joint Surgery* **47A**: 249–266.

Gebbie, D.A.M. (1981). *Reproductive Anthropology – Descent Through Woman.* Chichester: Wiley.

Geddes, A.C. (1912). The ribs in the second month of development. *Journal of Anatomy and Physiology* **47**: 18–30.

Geelhoed, G.W., Neel, J.V. and Davidson, R.T. (1969). Symphalangism and tarsal coalitions: hereditary syndromes; A report on two families. *Journal of Bone and Joint Surgery* **51B**: 278–289.

Geist, E.S. (1914). Supernumerary bones of the foot – A röentgen study of the feet of 100 normal individuals. *American Journal of Orthopaedic Surgery* **12**: 403–414.

Gelberman, R.H. and Menon, J. (1980). The vascularity of the scaphoid bone. *Journal of Hand Surgery* **5**: 508–513.

Gelberman, R.H. and Mortensen, W.W. (1983). The arterial anatomy of the talus. *Foot and Ankle* **4**: 64–72.

Gelberman, R.H., Bauman, T.D., Menon, J. and Akeson, W.H. (1980). The vascularity of the lunate bone and Kienbock's disease. *Journal of Hand Surgery* **5**: 272–278.

Genez, B.M., Ford, M.L. and Day, R.H. (1989). Ossified styloid complex with pseudoarthroses. *Skeletal Radiology* **18**: 623–625.

Genovés, S. (1956). A study of sex differences in the innominate bone (os coxae). Unpublished PhD dissertation, University of Cambridge.

Genovés, S. (1967). Proportionality of the long bones and their relation to stature among Mesoamericans. *American Journal of Physical Anthropology* **26**: 67–78.

George, R. (1935). Bilateral bipartite patellae. *British Journal of Surgery* **22**: 555–560.

Gepstein, R., Weiss, R.E. and Hallel, T. (1984). Acetabular dysplasia and hip dislocation after selective premature fusion of the triradiate cartilage. *Journal of Bone and Joint Surgery* **64B**: 334–336.

Gerscovich, E.O. and Greenspan, A. (1990). Case report 598: Os centrale carpi. *Skeletal Radiology* **19**: 143–145.

Gershenson, A., Nathan, H. and Luchansky, E. (1986). Mental foramen and mental nerve: changes with age. *Acta Anatomica* **126**: 21–28.

Ghantus, M.K. (1951). Growth of the shaft of the human radius and ulna during the first two years of life. *American Journal of Roentgenology* **65**: 784–786.

Ghorayeb, B.Y. and Graham, M.D. (1978). Human incus long process. Depressions in the surface of the normal ossicle. *Laryngoscope* **88**: 1184–1189.

Ghormley, R.K., Black, J.R. and Cherry, J.H. (1941). Ununited fractures of the clavicle. *American Journal of Surgery* **51**: 343–349.

Gibson, D.A. and Carroll, N. (1970). Congenital pseudoarthrosis of the clavicle. *Journal of Bone and Joint Surgery* **52B**: 629–643.

Giedion, A. (1965). Cone shaped epiphyses. *Annals of Radiology* **8**: 135–145.

Gilad, I. and Nissan, M. (1985). Sagittal radiographic measurements of the cervical and lumbar vertebrae in normal adults. *British Journal of Radiology* **58**: 1031–1034.

Gilbert, B.M. (1973). Misapplication to females of the standard for ageing the male os pubis. *American Journal of Physical Anthropology* **38**: 39–40.

Gilbert, B.M. (1976). Anterior femoral curvature: its probable basis and utility as a criterion of racial assessment. *American Journal of Physical Anthropology* **45**: 601–604.

Gilbert, B.M. and McKern, T.W. (1973). A method for aging the female os pubis. *American Journal of Physical Anthropology* **38**: 31–38.

Giles, E. (1964). Sex determination by discriminant function analysis of the mandible. *American Journal of Physical Anthropology* **22**: 129–136.

Gill, N.W. (1969). Congenital atresia of the ear. *Journal of Laryngology and Otology* **83**: 551–587.

Gill, G.G. and Abbott, L.C. (1942). Practical method of predicting the growth of the femur and tibia in the child. *Archives of Surgery* **45**: 286–315.

Gindhart, P.S. (1969). The frequency of appearance of transverse lines in the tibia in relation to childhood illness. *American Journal of Physical Anthropology* **31**: 17–22.

Gindhart, P.S. (1973). Growth standards for the tibia and radius in children aged one month through eighteen years. *American Journal of Physical Anthropology* **39**: 41–48.

Ginsberg, L.E., Pruett, S.W., Chen, M.Y.M. and Elster, A.D. (1994). Skull-base foramina of the middle cranial fossa: reassessment of normal variation with high resolution CT. *American Journal of Neuroradiology* **15**: 283–291.

Giraud-Guille, M.M. (1988). Twisted plywood architecture of collagen fibrils on human compact bone osteons. *Calcified Tissue International* **42**: 167–180.

Girdany, B.R. and Blank, E. (1965). Anterior fontanel bones. *American Journal of Roentgenology* **95**: 148–153.

Girdany, B.R. and Golden, R. (1952). Centres of ossification of the skeleton. *American Journal of Roentgenology* **68**: 922–924.

Girgis, F.G., Marshall, J.L. and al Monajem, A.R.S. (1975). The cruciate ligaments of the knee joint. Anatomical, functional and experimental analysis. *Clinical Orthopaedics and Related Research* **106**: 216–231.

Gladstone, R.J. (1897). A case of an additional presacral vertebra. *Journal of Anatomy and Physiology* **31**: 530–538.

Gladstone, R.J. and Erichsen Powell, W. (1915). Manifestation of occipital vertebrae and fusion of the atlas with the occipital bone. *Journal of Anatomy and Physiology* **49**: 190–209.

Gladstone, R.J. and Wakeley, C.P.G. (1924). Variations of the occipito-atlantal joint in relation to the metameric structure of the craniovertebral region. *Journal of Anatomy* **59**: 195–216.

Gladstone, R.J. and Wakeley, C.P.G. (1932a). Cervical ribs and rudimentary first thoracic ribs considered from the clinical and etiological standpoint. *Journal of Anatomy* **66**: 334–370.

Gladstone, R.J. and Wakeley, C.P.G. (1932b). The morphology of the sternum and its relation to the ribs. *Journal of Anatomy* **66**: 508–564.

Glanville, E.V. (1967). Perforation of the coronoid-olecranon septum – humero-ulnar relationships in Netherlands and African populations. *American Journal of Physical Anthropology* **26**: 85–92.

Glanville, E.V. (1969). Nasal shape, prognathism and adaptation in man. *American Journal of Physical Anthropology* **30**: 29–37.

Glaser, K.L. (1949). Double contours, cupping and spurring in roentgenograms of long bones in infants. *American Journal of Roentgenology* **61**: 482–492.

Glassman, D.M. and Bass, W.M. (1986). Bilateral asymmetry of long arm bones and jugular foramen: implications for handedness. *Journal of Forensic Sciences* **31**: 589–595.

Glassman, D.M. and Dana, S.E. (1992). Handedness and bilateral asymmetry of the jugular foramen. *Journal of Forensic Sciences* **37**: 140–146.

Gleiser, I. and Hunt, E.E. (1955). The permanent mandibular first molar: its calcification, eruption and decay. *American Journal of Physical Anthropology* **13**: 253–284.

Glenister, T.W. (1976). An embryological view of cartilage. *Journal of Anatomy* **122**: 323–330.

Glessner, J.R. (1963). Spontaneous intra-uterine amputations. *Journal of Bone and Joint Surgery* **45A**: 351–355.

Godycki, M. (1957). Sur la certitude de détermination du sexe d'après le fémur, le cubitus, et l'humérus. *Bulletin et Mémoirs de la Sociétié d'Anthropologie de Paris* **8**: 405–410.

Goergen, T.G., Resnick, G. and Saltzstein, S.L. (1979). Dorsal defect of the patella: a characteristic radiographic lesion. *Radiology* **130**: 333–336.

Goez, J. and De Lauro, T. (1995). Congenital absence of the tibial sesamoid. *Journal of the American Podiatric Association* **85**: 509–510.

Goldberg, S. (1970). The origin of the lumbrical muscles in the hand of the South African native. *The Hand* **2**: 168–171.

Goldbloom, R.B. and Scott Dunbar, J. (1960). Calcification of cartilage in the trachea and larynx in infancy associated with congenital stridor. *Pediatrics* **26**: 669–673.

Goldie, I. (1988). Talar and peritalar injuries. In: *The Foot* (B. Helal, and D. Wilson, Eds.), pp. 916–936. Edinburgh: Churchill Livingstone.

Goldsmith, W.M. (1922). The Catlin mark: the inheritance of an unusual opening in the parietal bones. *Journal of Heredity* **13**: 69–71.

Goldstein, H. (1986). Sampling for growth studies. In: *Human Growth, A Comprehensive Treatise*, Vol. 3, 3rd edition (F. Falkner and J.M. Tanner, Eds.), pp. 59–78. New York: Plenum Press.

Goldstein, R.S. and Kalcheim, C. (1992). Determination of epithelial half-somites in skeletal morphogenesis. *Development* **116**: 441–445.

Goldstein, I., Reece, E.A. and Hobbins, J.C. (1988). Sonographic appearance of the fetal heel ossification centers and foot length measurements provide independent markers for gestational age estimation. *American Journal of Obstetrics and Gynaecology* **159**: 923–926.

Golthamer, C.R. (1957). Duplication of the clavicle (os subclaviculare). *Radiology* **68**: 576–578.

Goode, H., Waldron, T. and Rogers, J. (1993). Bone growth in juveniles: a methodological note. *International Journal of Osteoarchaeology* **3**: 321–323.

Goodfellow, J., Hungerford, D.S. and Zindel, M. (1976a). Patello-femoral joint mechanics and pathology. 1. Functional anatomy of the patello-femoral joint. *Journal of Bone and Joint Surgery* **58B**: 287–290.

Goodfellow, J., Hungerford, D.S. and Woods, C. (1976b). Patello-femoral joint mechanics and pathology. 2. Chondromalacia patellae. *Journal of Bone and Joint Surgery* **58B**: 291–299.

Gooding, C.A. and Neuhauser, E.B.D. (1965). Growth and development of the vertebral body in the presence and absence of normal stress. *American Journal of Roentgenology* **93**: 388–394.

Goodman, R.M., Adam, A. and Sheba, C. (1965). A genetic study of stub thumbs among various ethnic groups in Israel. *Journal of Medical Genetics* **2**: 116–121.

Goodrich, E.S. (1930). *Studies on the Structure and Development of Vertebrates.* London: MacMillan.

Goodshall, R.W. and Hansen, C.A. (1973). Incomplete avulsion of a portion of the iliac epiphysis. *Journal of Bone and Joint Surgery* **55**: 1301–1302.

Goodsir, J. (1855). On the horizontal curvature of the internal femoral condyle: on the movements and relations of the patella; semilunar cartilages; and synovial pads of the human knee joint. *Edinburgh Medical Journal* **1**: 91–95.

Gopinathan, K. (1992). A rare anomaly of 5 ossicles in the pre-interparietal part of the squamous occipital bone in north Indians. *Journal of Anatomy* **180**: 201–202.

Gordon, C.L., Halton, J.M., Atkinson, S.A. and Webber, C.E. (1991). The contributions of growth and puberty to peak bone mass. *Growth, Development and Aging* **55**: 257–262.

Goret-Nicaise, M. and Dhem, A. (1982). Presence of chondroid tissue in the symphyseal region of the growing human mandible. *Acta Anatomica* **113**: 189–195.

Goret-Nicaise, M. and Dhem, A. (1984). The mandibular body of the human fetus. *Anatomy and Embryology* **169**: 231–236.

Gossman, J.R. and Tarsitano, J.J. (1977). The styloid-stylohyoid syndrome. *Journal of Oral Surgery* **35**: 555–560.

Gottlieb, K. (1978). Artificial cranial deformation and the increased complexity of the lambdoid suture. *American Journal of Physical Anthropology* **48**: 213–214.

Gottschalk, F.A.B., Sallis, J.G., Beighton, P.H. and Solomon, L. (1980). A comparison of the prevalence of hallux valgus in three South African populations. *South African Medical Journal* **57**: 355–357.

Gower, C.D. (1923). A contribution to the morphology of the apertura piriformis. *American Journal of Physical Anthropology* **6**: 27–36.

Gowland, W.P. (1915). Preliminary note on a diarthrodial articulation between the clavicle and the coracoid. *Journal of Anatomy and Physiology* **49**: 187–189.

Gradoyevitch, B. (1939). Coracoclavicular joint. *Journal of Bone and Joint Surgery* **21**: 918–920.

Granieri, G.F. and Bacarini, L. (1996). The pelvic digit: five new examples of an unusual anomaly. *Skeletal Radiology* **25**: 723–726.

Grant, J.C.B. (1948). *A Method of Anatomy*, 4th edition. London: Baillière, Tindall and Cox.

Graves, W.W. (1921). The types of scapula: A comparative study of some correlated characters in human scapulae. *American Journal of Physical Anthropology* **4**: 111–128.

Graves, W.W. (1922). Observations on age changes in the scapula. *American Journal of Physical Anthropology* **5**: 21–33.

Gray, D.J. (1942). Variations in human scapulae. *American Journal of Physical Anthropology* **29**: 57–72.

Gray, D.J. and Gardner, E. (1950). Prenatal development of the human knee and superior tibiofibular joints. *American Journal of Anatomy* **86**: 235–287.

Gray, D.J. and Gardner, E. (1951). Prenatal development of the human elbow joint. *American Journal of Anatomy* **88**: 429–470.

Gray, D.J. and Gardner, E. (1969). The prenatal development of the human humerus. *American Journal of Anatomy* **124**: 431–445.

Gray, D.J., Gardner, E. and O'Rahilly, R. (1957). The prenatal development of the skeleton and joints of the human hand. *American Journal of Anatomy* **101**: 169–224.

Green, H.L.H.H. (1930). An unusual case of atlanto-occipital fusion. *Journal of Anatomy* **65**: 140–144.

Green, E.L. (1939). The inheritance of a rib variation in the rabbit. *Anatomical Record* **74**: 47–60.

Green, W.T. (1975). Painful bipartite patella. *Clinical Orthopaedics and Related Research* **110**: 197–200.

Green, R.M. (1987). The position of the mental foramen: a comparison between the southern (Hong Kong) Chinese and other ethnic and racial groups. *Oral Surgery, Oral Medicine and Oral Pathology* **63**: 287–290.

Green, R.M. and Darvell, B.W. (1988). Tooth wear and the position of the mental foramen. *American Journal of Physical Anthropology* **77**: 69–75.

Green, J.P. and Waugh, W. (1968). Congenital lateral dislocation of the patella. *Journal of Bone and Joint Surgery* **50B**: 285–289.

Greenspan, A. (1995). Bone island (enostosis): current concept–a review. *Skeletal Radiology* **24**: 111–115.

Greenspan, A. and Norman, A. (1982). The 'pelvic digit'. An unusual developmental anomaly. *Skeletal Radiology* **9**: 118–122.

Gregersen, H.N. (1977). Naviculocuneiform coalition. *Journal of Bone and Joint Surgery* **59A**: 128–130.

Gregg, J.B. and Bass, W.M. (1970). Exostoses in the external auditory canals. *Annals of Otology, Rhinology and Laryngology* **74**: 834–839.

Gregg, J.B. and McGrew, R.N. (1970). Hrdlička revisited (external auditory canal exostoses). *American Journal of Physical Anthropology* **33**: 37–40.

Gregg, J.B., Steele, J.P. and Holzheuter, A. (1965). Roentgenographic evaluation of temporal bones from South Dakota Indian burials. *American Journal of Physical Anthropology* **23**: 51–62.

Greig, D.M. (1892). Congenital and symmetrical perforation of both parietal bones. *Journal of Anatomy and Physiology* **26**: 187–191.

Greig, D.M. (1917). Two cases of congenital symmetrical perforation of the parietal bones. *Edinburgh Medical Journal* **18**: 205–209.

Greig, D.M. (1926). On symmetrical thinness of the parietal bones. *Edinburgh Medical Journal* **33**: 645–671.

Greig, D.M. (1927a). Congenital absence of the tympanic element of both temporal bones. *Journal of Laryngology and Otology* **42**: 309–314.

Greig, D.M. (1927b). Abnormally large parietal foramina. *Edinburgh Medical Journal* **34**: 629–648.

Greig, D.M. (1929). Congenital anomalies of the foramen spinosum. *Edinburgh Medical Journal* **36**: 363–371.

Greulich, W.W. (1960). Skeletal features visible on roentgenogram of hand and wrist which can be used for establishing individual identification. *American Journal of Roentgenology* **83**: 756–764.

Greulich, W.W. (1973). A comparison of the dysplastic middle phalanx of the fifth finger in mentally normal Caucasians, Mongoloids and Negroes with that of individuals of the same racial groups who have Down's Syndrome. *American Journal of Roentgenology* **118**: 259–281.

Greulich, W.W. and Pyle, S.I. (1959). *Radiographic Atlas of Skeletal Development of the Hand and Wrist*. Stanford, CA: Stanford University Press.

Greulich, W.W. and Thoms, H. (1938). The dimensions of the pelvic inlet of 789 white females. *Anatomical Record* **72**: 45–52.

Greulich, W.W. and Thoms, H. (1944). The growth and development of the pelvis of individual girls before, during and after puberty. *Yale Journal of Biology and Medicine* **17**: 91–97.

Greyling, L.M., Le Grange, F. and Meiring, J.H. (1997). Mandibular spine: a case report. *Clinical Anatomy* **10**: 416–418.

Griffith, T.W. (1896). Fusion of the occipital bone and atlas. *Journal of Anatomy and Physiology* **30**: 17–19.

Griffiths, J. (1902). The normal position of the big toe. *Journal of Anatomy and Physiology* **36**: 344–355.

Grogan, D.P., Walling, A.K. and Ogden, J.A. (1990). Anatomy of the os trigonum. *Journal of Pediatric Orthopedics* **10**:618–622.

Grøn, A.-M. (1962). Prediction of tooth emergence. *Journal of Dental Research* **41**: 573–585.

Gross, A., Gross, P. and Langer, B. (1989). *Surgery: A Complete Guide for Patients and their Families.* Toronto: HarperCollins.

Grossman, J.W. (1945). The triticeous cartilages. A roentgen-anatomic study. *American Journal of Roentgenology* **53**: 166–170.

Grube, D. and Reinbach, W. (1976). Das Cranium eines menschlichen Embryo von 80mm Sch.-St.-Länge. *Anatomy and Embryology* **149**: 183–208.

Grünbaum, A.S. (1892). Embryonic relation of the fibula to the femur. *Journal of Anatomy and Physiology* **26**.

Grüneberg, H. (1963). *The Pathology of Development: A Study of Inherited Skeletal Disorders in Animals.* Oxford: Blackwell Scientific.

Gruspier, K.L. and Mullen, G.J. (1991). Maxillary suture obliteration: a test of the Mann method. *Journal of Forensic Sciences* **36**: 512–519.

Guida, G., Cigala, F. and Riccio, V. (1969). The vascularization of the vertebral body in the human fetus at term. *Clinical Orthopaedics and Related Research* **65**: 229–234.

Guild, S.R. (1949). Natural absence of part of the bony wall of the facial canal. *Laryngoscope* **59**: 668–673.

Gumpel-Pinot, M. (1984). Muscle and skeleton of limbs and body wall. pp281–310. In: *Chimeras in Developmental Biology* (N.A. Le Douarin and A. McLaren, Eds.). London: Academic Press.

Gunderson, C.H., Greenspan, R.H., Glaser, G.H. and Lubs, H.A. (1967). The Klippel- Feil syndrome, genetic and clinical re-evaluation of cervical fusion. *Medicine* **46**: 491–512.

Gunn, G. (1928). Patella cubiti. *British Journal of Surgery* **15**: 612–615.

Gunsel, E. (1951). Das os coracoideum. *Fortschritte auf dem Gebiete der Röentgenstrahlen* **74**: 112–115.

Gunstone, A.E.B. (1992). An investigation into the relationship between size and maturity of the skeleton through the early perinatal period. Unpublished BSc dissertation, University of London.

Gupta, S.C., Gupta, C.D. and Arora, A.K. (1977). Pattern of talar articular facets in Indian calcanei. *Journal of Anatomy* **124**: 651–655.

Gupta, R., Sher, J., Williams, G.R. and Iannotti, J.P. (1998). Non-union of the scapular body: a case report. *Journal of Bone and Joint Surgery* **80A**: 428–430.

Gurd, F.B. (1941). The treatment of complete dislocation of the outer end of the clavicle: An hitherto undescribed operation. *Annals of Surgery* **113**: 1094–1098.

Gurd, F.B. (1947). Surplus parts of the skeleton. *American Journal of Surgery* **74**: 705–720.

Gurdon, J.B., Mohun, T.J., Sharpe, C.R. and Taylor, M.V. (1989). Embryonic induction and muscle gene activation. *Trends in Genetics* **5**: 51–56.

Gusis, S.E., Babini, J.C., Garay, S.M., Garcia Morteo, O. and Maldonado Cocco, J.A. (1990). Evaluation of the measurement methods for protrusio acetabuli in normal children. *Skeletal Radiology* **19**: 279–282.

Gustafson, G. (1950). Age determinations on teeth. *Journal of the American Dental Association* **41**: 45–54.

Gustafson, G. and Koch, G. (1974). Age estimation up to 16 years of age based on dental development. *Odontologisk Revy* **25**: 297–306.

Guy, H., Masset, C. and Baud, C.-A. (1997). Infant taphonomy. *International Journal of Osteoarchaeology* **7**: 221–229.

Gwinn, J.L. and Smith, J.L. (1962). Acquired and congenital absence of the odontoid process. *American Journal of Roentgenology* **88**: 424–431.

Haas, S.L. (1939). Growth in length of the vertebrae. *Archives of Surgery* **38**: 245–249.

Haas, J.D., Hunt, E.E. and Buskirk, E.R. (1971). Skeletal development of non-institutionalized children with low intelligence quotients. *American Journal of Physical Anthropology* **35**: 455–466.

Haataja, J. (1965). Development of the mandibular permanent teeth of Helsinki children. *Proceedings of the Finnish Dental Society* **61**: 43–53.

Haavikko, K. (1970). The formation and the alveolar and clinical eruption of the permanent teeth. An orthopantographic study. *Proceedings of the Finnish Dental Society* **66**: 101–170.

Haavikko, K. (1973). The physiological resorption of the roots of deciduous teeth in Helsinki children. *Proceedings of the Finnish Dental Society* **69**: 93–98.

Haavikko, K. (1974). Tooth formation age estimated on a few selected teeth: a simple method for clinical use. *Proceedings of the Finnish Dental Society* **70**: 15–19.

Hadley, L.A. (1948). Atlanto-occipital fusion, ossiculum terminale and occipital vertebra as related to basilar impression with neurological symptoms. *American Journal of Roentgenology* **59**: 511–524.

Hadley, L.A. (1952). Accessory sacro-iliac articulations. *Journal of Bone and Joint Surgery* **34A**: 149–155.

Hadley, L.A. (1958). Tortuosity and deflection of the vertebral artery. *American Journal of Roentgenology* **80**: 306–312.

Haffajee, M.R. (1997). A contribution by the ascending pharyngeal artery to the arterial supply of the odontoid process of the axis vertebra. *Clinical Anatomy* **10**: 14–18.

Hagelberg, E. and Clegg, J.B. (1991). Isolation and characterisation of DNA from archaeological bone. *Proceedings of the Royal Society of London (Biol.)* **244**: 45–50.

Hagelberg, E., Sykes, B. and Hedges, R. (1989). Ancient bone DNA amplified. *Nature* **342**: 485.

Hägg, U. and Matsson, L. (1985). Dental maturity as an indicator of chronological age: the accuracy and precision of three methods. *European Journal of Orthodontics* **7**: 24–34.

Haher, T.R., O'Brien, M., Dryer, J.W., Nocci, R., Zipnic, R. and Leone, D.J. (1994). The role of the lumbar facet joints in spinal stability–identification of alternate paths of loading. *Spine* **19**: 2667–2671.

Haines, R.W. (1933). Cartilage canals. *Journal of Anatomy* **68**: 45–64.

Haines, R.W. (1937). Growth of cartilage canals in the patella. *Journal of Anatomy* **71**: 471–479.

Haines, R.W. (1938). The primitive form of epiphysis in the long bones of tetrapods. *Journal of Anatomy* **72**: 323–343.

Haines, R.W. (1940). Note on the independence of sesamoid and epiphyseal centres of ossification. *Journal of Anatomy* **75**: 101–105.

Haines, R.W. (1942). The evolution of epiphyses and of endochondral bone. *Biological Reviews* **17**: 267–291.

Haines, R.W. (1944). The mechanism of rotation at the first carpometacarpal joint. *Journal of Anatomy* **78**: 44–46.

Haines, R.W. (1951). The extensor apparatus of the finger. *Journal of Anatomy* **85**: 251–259.

Haines, R.W. (1953). The early development of the femoro-tibial and tibio-fibular joints. *Journal of Anatomy* **87**: 192–206.

Haines, R.W. (1974). The pseudoepiphysis of the first metacarpal of man. *Journal of Anatomy* **117**: 145–158.

Haines, R.W. (1975). The histology of epiphyseal union in mammals. *Journal of Anatomy* **120**: 1–25.

Haines, R.W. (1976). Destruction of hyaline cartilage in the sigmoid notch of the ulna. *Journal of Anatomy* **122**: 331–334.

Haines, R.W. and McDougall, A. (1954). The anatomy of hallux valgus. *Journal of Bone and Joint Surgery* **36B**: 272–293.

Haines, R.W. and Mohuiddin, A. (1962). Epiphyseal growth and union in the pigeon. *Journal of the Faculty of Medicine – Baghdad* **4**: 4–21.

Haines, R.W., Mohuiddin, A., Okpa, F.I. and Viega-Pires, J.A. (1967). The sites of early epiphysial union in the limb girdles and major long bones of man. *Journal of Anatomy* **101**: 823–831.

Halaby, F.A. and DiSalvo, E.I. (1965). Osteolysis: a complication of trauma. *American Journal of Roentgenology* **94**: 591–594.

Hale, J.E. and Wuthier, R.E. (1987). The mechanism of matrix vesicle formation: studies on the composition of chondrocyte microvilli and on the effects of microfilament-perturbing agents on cellular vesiculation. *Journal of Biological Chemistry* **262**: 1916–1925.

Hales, S. (1727). *Statical essays. Vol. 1. Vegetable staticks*. London: W. Innys.

Haliburton, R.A., Sullivan, C.R., Kelley, P.J. and Peterson, L.F.A. (1958). The extraosseous and intraosseous blood supply of the talus. *Journal of Bone and Joint Surgery* **40A**: 1115–1120.

Hall, F.J.S. (1950a). Coracoclavicular joint: a rare condition treated successfully by operation. *British Medical Journal* **1**: 766–768.

Hall, K. (1950b). The effect of oestrone and progesterone on the histological structure of the symphysis pubis of the castrated female mouse. *Journal of Endocrinology* **7**: 54–63.

Hall, M.C. (1961). The trabecular patterns of the neck of the femur with particular reference to changes in osteoporosis. *Canadian Medical Association Journal* **85**: 1141–1144.

Hall, B.K. (1967). The formation of adventitious cartilage by membrane bones under the influence of mechanical stimulation *in vitro*. *Life Sciences* **6**: 663–667.

Hall, B.K. (1983). *Cartilage Vol. 2. Development, Differentiation and Growth.* New York: Academic Press.

Hall, B.K. (1984). Developmental mechanisms underlying the formation of atavisms. *Biology Reviews* **59**: 89–124.

Hall, B.K. (1988). The embryonic development of bone. *American Science* **76**: 174–181.

Hall, B.K. (1994). *Homology: The Hierarchical Basis of Comparative Biology.* San Diego, CA: Academic Press.

Hall, B.K. and Miyake, T. (1992). The membranous skeleton: the role of cell condensations in vertebrate skeletogenesis. *Anatomy and Embryology* **186**: 107–124.

Hallel, T. and Salvati, E.A. (1977). Premature closure of the triradiate cartilage: a case report and animal experiment. *Clinical Orthopedics and Related Research* **124**: 278–281.

Halloran, W. (1960). Report of sacral ribs. *Quarterly Bulletin of Northwestern University Medical School* **34**: 304.

Hamilton, W.J. and Mossman, H.W. (1972). *Hamilton, Boyd and Mossman's Human Embryology – Prenatal Development of Form and Function.* London: Williams and Wilkins.

Hammer, G. and Rådberg, C. (1961). The sphenoidal sinus. An anatomical and roentgenologic study with reference to transsphenoid hypophysectomy. *Acta Radiologica* **56**: 401–422.

Hancox, N.M., Hay, J.D., Holden, W.S., Moss, P.D. and Whitehead, A.S. (1951). The radiological 'double contour' effect in the long bones of newly born infants. *Archives of Disease in Childhood* **26**: 534–548.

Hanihara, K. (1952). Age changes in the male Japanese pubic bone. *Journal of the Anthropological Society of Nippon* **62**: 245–260.

Hanihara, K. (1959). Sex diagnosis of Japanese skulls and scapulae by means of discriminant functions. *Journal of the Anthropological Society of Nippon* **67**: 21–27.

Hanihara, K. and Suzuki, T. (1978). Estimation of age from the pubic symphysis by means of multiple regression analysis. *American Journal of Physical Anthropology* **48**: 233–241.

Hanihara, T., Ishida, H. and Dodo, Y. (1998). Os zygomaticum bipartitum: frequency distribution in major human populations. *Journal of Anatomy* **192**: 539–555.

Hansen, E.S. (1993). Microvascularization, osteogenesis and myelopoiesis in normal and pathological conditions. In: *Bone Circulation and Vascularization in Normal and Pathological Conditions* (A. Shoutens, J.W.M. Gardiniers, and S.P.F. Hughes, Eds.), pp. 29–41. New York: Plenum Press.

Hansman, C.F. (1962). Appearance and fusion of ossification centres in the human skeleton. *American Journal of Roentgenology* **88**: 476–482.

Hanson, F.B. (1920a). The history of the earliest stages in the human clavicle. *Anatomical Record* **19**: 309–325.

Hanson, F.B. (1920b). The problem of the coracoid. *Anatomical Record* **19**: 327–345.

Hanson, J.R., Anson, B.J. and Strickland, E.M. (1962). Branchial sources of the auditory ossicles in man – Part II. *Archives of Otolaryngology* **76**: 200–215.

Haraldsson, S. (1959). On osteochondrosis deformans juvenilis capituli humeri including investigation of intraosseous vasculature in distal humerus. *Acta Orthopaedica Scandinavica* **38**(Suppl.).

Haraldsson, S. (1962). The vascular pattern of a growing and full-grown human epiphysis. *Acta Anatomica* **48**: 156–167.

Haramati, N., Cook, R.A., Raphael, B., McNamara, T.S., Staron, R.B. and Feldman, F. (1994). Coraco-clavicular joint: Normal variant in humans: a radiographic demonstration in the human and non-human primate. *Skeletal Radiology* **23**: 117–119.

Harding, V.S.V. (1952a). A method of evaluating osseous development from birth to 14 years. *Child Development* **23**: 247–271.

Harding, V.S.V. (1952b). Time schedule for the appearance and fusion of a second accessory center of ossification of the calcaneus. *Child Development* **23**: 181–184.

Hardman, T.G. and Wigoder, S.B. (1928). An unusual development of the carpal scaphoid. *British Journal of Radiology* **1**: 155–158.

Hardy, R.H. and Clapham, J.C.R. (1951). Observations on hallux valgus. *Journal of Bone and Joint Surgery* **33B**: 376–391.

Harjeet and Jit, I. (1992). Dimensions of the thyroid cartilage in neonates, children and adults in northwest Indian subjects. *Journal of the Anatomical Society of India* **41**: 81–92.

Harle, T.S. and Stevenson, J.R. (1967). Hereditary symphalangism associated with carpal and tarsal fusions. *Radiology* **89**: 91–94.

Harris, H.A. (1926a). The growth of the long bones in childhood: with special reference to certain bony striations of the metaphysis and to the role of the vitamins. *Archives of International Medicine* **38**: 785–806.

Harris, H.A. (1926b). Congenital absence of the middle turbinate bone associated with precocious ossification of the limb bones in a stillborn female. *Journal of Anatomy* **60**: 148–151.

Harris, H.A. (1933). *Bone Growth in Health and Disease.* London: Oxford University Press.

Harris, B.J. (1955). Anomalous structures in the developing human foot. *Anatomical Record* **121**: 399.

Harris, N.H. (1974). Lesions of the symphysis pubis in women. *British Medical Journal* **4**: 209–211.

Harris, R.I. and Beath, T. (1948). Etiology of peroneal spastic flat foot. *Journal of Bone and Joint Surgery* **30B**: 624–634.

Harris, R.S. and Jones, D.M. (1956). The arterial supply to the adult cervical vertebral bodies. *Journal of Bone and Joint Surgery* **38B**: 922–927.

Harris, H. and Joseph, J.J. (1949). Variation in extension of the metacarpo-phalangeal and interphalangeal joints of the thumb. *Journal of Bone and Joint Surgery* **31B**: 547–559.

Harris, R.I. and MacNab, I. (1954). Structural changes in the lumbar intervertebral discs. Their relationship to low back pain and sciatica. *Journal of Bone and Joint Surgery* **36B**: 304–322.

Harris, N.H. and Murray, R.O. (1974). Lesions of the symphysis in athletes. *British Medical Journal* **4**: 211–214.

Harris, A.M.P., Wood, R.E., Nortjé, C.J. and Thomas, C.J. (1987). Gender and ethnic differences of radiographic image of the frontal region. *Journal of Forensic Odonto-Stomatology* **5**: 51–57.

Harrison, R.G. (1901). On the occurrence of tails in man, with a description of the Case reported by Dr Watson. *John Hopkins Hospital Bulletin* **12**: 96–101.

Harrison, D.F.N. (1951). Exostoses of the external auditory meatus. *Journal of Otology and Laryngology* **65**: 704–714.

Harrison, T.J. (1957). Pelvic growth. PhD dissertation, University of Belfast.

Harrison, T.J. (1958). The growth of the pelvis in the rat – a mensural and morphological study. *Journal of Anatomy* **92**: 236–260.

Harrison, T.J. (1961). The influence of the femoral head on pelvic growth and acetabular formation in the rat. *Journal of Anatomy* **95**: 12–24.

Harrison, T.J. (1965). The growth of the ischio-pubic part of the pelvis in the rat. *Journal of Anatomy* **99**: 206.

Harrison, T.J. (1968). The growth of the caudal half of the pelvis in the rat. *Journal of Anatomy* **103**: 155–170.

Harrison, D.F.N. and Denny, S. (1983). Ossification in the primate larynx. *Acta Otolaryngologica* **95**: 440–446.

Harrison, R.B. and Keats, T.E. (1980). Epiphyseal clefts. *Skeletal Radiology* **5**: 23–27.

Harrison, R.B., Wood, M.B. and Keats, T.E. (1976). The grooves of the distal articular surface of the femur – a normal variant. *American Journal of Roentgenology* **126**: 751–754.

Harrold, J.J. (1967). Congenital vertical talus in infancy. *Journal of Bone and Joint Surgery* **49B**: 634–643.

Harrower, G. (1925). A septdigitate foot in man. *Journal of Anatomy* **60**: 106–109.

Harrower, G. (1928). A biometric study of one hundred and ten Asiatic mandibles. *Biometrika* **20B**: 279–293.

Hartley, J.B. and Burnett, C.W.F. (1943a). A study of craniolacunia. *Journal of Obstetrics and Gynaecology of the British Empire* **50**: 1–12.

Hartley, J.B. and Burnett, C.W.F. (1943b). The radiological diagnosis of craniolacunia. *British Journal of Radiology* **16**: 99–108.

Hartley, J.B. and Burnett, C.W.F. (1944). New light on the origin of craniolacunia. *British Journal of Radiology* **17**: 110–114.

Harty, M. (1957). The calcar femorale and the femoral neck. *Journal of Bone and Joint Surgery* **39A**: 625–630.

Hasselwander, A. (1910). Untersuchungen über die Ossifikation des menschlichen Fussskelets. *Zeitschrift für Morphologie und Anthropologie* **12**: 1–140.

Hasselwander, A. (1938). Die obere Extremität and Die untere Extremität. In: *Handbuch der Anatomie des Kindes*, Vol. 2 (K. Peter, G. Wetzel and F. Heiderich, Eds.), pp. 512–525, 550–565. Munich: Bergmann.

Hast, M.H. (1970). The developmental anatomy of the larynx. *Otolaryngologic Clinics of North America* **3**: 413–438.

Hately, W., Evison, G. and Samuel, E. (1965). The pattern of ossification in the laryngeal cartilages: a radiological study. *British Journal of Radiology* **38**: 585–591.

Hatfield, M.K., Gross, B.H., Glazer, G.M. and Martel, W. (1984). Computed tomography of the sternum and its articulations. *Skeletal Radiology* **11**: 197–203.

Hattner, R. and Frost, H.M. (1963). Mean skeletal age: its calculation and theoretical effects on skeletal tracer physiology and on the physical characteristics of bone. *Henry Ford Hospital Medical Bulletin* **11**: 201–216.

Hauch, P.P. (1946). The fate of an accessory ossicle. *British Journal of Radiology* **19**: 518–519.

Hauser, G. and De Stefano, G.F. (1985). Variations in form of the hypoglossal canal. *American Journal of Physical Anthropology* **67**: 7–11.

Havers, C. (1691). *Osteologia Nova*, 2nd edition. London: Smith.

Hawkins, R.J., Fielding, J.W. and Thompson, W.J. (1976). Os odontoideum: congenital or acquired? *Journal of Bone and Joint Surgery* **58A**: 413–414.

Haxton, H. (1944). The patellar index in mammals. *Journal of Anatomy* **78**: 106–107.

Haxton, H. (1945). The function of the patella and the effects of its excision. *Surgery, Gynecology and Obstetrics* **80**: 389–395.

Hayner, J.C. (1949). Variations of the torcular Herophili and transverse sinuses. *Anatomical Record* **103**: 542.

Healy, M.J.R. (1986). Statistics of growth standards. In: *Human Growth, A Comprehensive Treatise*, Vol. 3, 2nd edition (F. Falkner and J.M. Tanner, Eds.), pp. 47–58. New York: Plenum Press.

Heeg, M. (1988). Injuries of the acetabular triradiate cartilage and sacro-iliac joint. *Journal of Bone and Joint Surgery* **70B**: 34–37.

Heim, J.L. (1982). *Les enfants Néandertaliens de la Ferrassie*. Paris: Masson.

Heim, M., Sieu-Ner, Y., Nadvorna, H., Marcovich, C., Engelberg, S. and Azaria, M. (1997). Metatarsal-phalangeal sesamoid bones. *Current Orthopaedics* **11**: 267–270.

Heindon, C.N. (1951). Cleidocranial dysostosis. *American Journal of Human Genetics* **3**: 314–324.

Heiple, K.G. and Lovejoy, C.O. (1969). The antiquity of tarsal coalition. *Journal of Bone and Joint Surgery* **51A**: 979–983.

Helal, B. (1964). Fracture of the manubrium sterni. *Journal of Bone and Joint Surgery* **46B**: 602–607.

Helal, B. (1981). The great toe sesamoid bones: the Lus or lost souls of Uschaia. *Clinical Orthopaedics and Related Research* **157**: 82–87.

Helal, B. (1988). The accessory ossicles and sesamoids. In: *The Foot* (B. Helal and D. Wilson, Eds.), pp. 567–580. Edinburgh: Churchill Livingstone.

Helal, B. and Wilson, D. (1988). *The Foot*. Edinburgh: Churchill Livingstone.

Hellman, M. (1928). Ossification of epiphyseal cartilages in the hand. *American Journal of Physical Anthropology* **11**: 223–258.

Helm, S. (1969). Secular trends in tooth eruption. A comparative study of Danish school children of 1913 and 1965. *Archives of Oral Biology* **14**: 1177–1191.

Helm, S. and Seidler, B. (1974). Timing of tooth emergence in Danish children. *Community Dentistry and Oral Epidemiology* **2**: 122–129.

Henderson, J. (1987). Factors determining the state of preservation of human remains. In: *Death, Decay and Reconstruction* (A. Boddington, A.N. Garland and R.C. Janaway, Eds.), pp. 43–54. Manchester: Manchester University Press.

Hensinger, R.N. and MacEwan, C. (1975). Congenital anomalies of the spine. In: *The Spine*. Philadelphia, PA: W.B. Saunders.

Hepburn, D. (1896). The platymeric, pilastric and popliteal indices of the race collection of femora in the anatomical museum of the University of Edinburgh. *Journal of Anatomy and Physiology* **31**: 116–156.

Hepburn, D. (1907). Anomalies in the supra-inial portion of the occipital bone, resulting from irregularities of its ossification with consequent variations of the interparietal bone. *Journal of Anatomy and Physiology* **42**: 88–92.

Herman, S. (1973). Congenital bilateral pseudoarthroses of the clavicle. *Clinical Orthopedics and Related Research* **91**: 162–163.

Hermel, M.B. and Gershon-Cohen, J. (1953). Nutcracker fracture of the cuboid by indirect violence. *Radiology* **60**: 850–854.

Heron, I.C. (1923). Measurements and observations upon the human auditory ossicles. *American Journal of Physical Anthropology* **6**: 11–26.

Herrera, M. and Puchades-Orts, A. (1998). Morphology of the articular processes of the sixth cervical vertebra in humans. *Journal of Anatomy* **192**: 309–311.

Hershkovitz, I., Latimer, B., Dutour, O., Jellema, L.M., Wish-Baratz, S., Rothschild, C. and Rothschild, B. (1997). The elusive petroexoccipital articulation. *American Journal of Physical Anthropology* **103**: 365–373.

Hertzog, K.P. (1967). Shortened fifth medial phalanges. *American Journal of Physical Anthropology* **27**: 113–118.

Hertzog, K.P., Garn, S.M. and Church, S.F. (1968). Cone shape epiphyses in the hand. Population frequencies, anatomic distribution and developmental stages. *Investigative Radiology* **3**: 433–441.

Hesdorffer, M.B. and Scammon, R.E. (1928). Growth of long-bones of human fetus as illustrated by the tibia. *Proceedings of the Society for Experimental Biology and Medicine* **25**: 638–641.

Hess, J.H. (1917). The diagnosis of the age of the fetus by the use of roentgenograms. *American Journal of Diseases of Children* **14**: 397–423.

Hess, L. (1945). The metopic suture and the metopic syndrome. *Human Biology* **17**: 107–136.

Hess, A.F. and Weinstock, M. (1925). A comparison of the evolution of carpal centres in White and Negro new born infants. *American Journal of Diseases of Children* **29**: 347–354.

Hess, A.F., Lewis, J.M. and Roman, B. (1932). A radiographic study of crowns of the teeth from birth to adolescence. *Dental Cosmos* **74**: 1053–1061.

Hewitt, D., Westropp, C.K. and Acheson, R.M. (1955). Oxford Child Health Survey. Effect of childish ailments on skeletal development. *British Journal of Preventive and Social Medicine* **9**: 179–186.

Heyes, F.L.P. (1992). On the naming of toes – porcine nomenclature. *Journal of the Medical Defence Union* **4**: 94.

Heyman, J. and Lundqvist, A. (1932). The symphysis pubis in pregnancy and parturition. *Acta Obstetrica Gynaecolgia Scandinavica* **12**: 191–226.

Heyse-Moore, G.H. and Stoker, D.J. (1982). Avulsion fractures of the scapula. *Skeletal Radiology* **9**: 27–32.

Hicks, J.H. (1953). The mechanics of the foot. I. The joints. *Journal of Anatomy* **87**: 345–357.

Hicks, J.H. (1954). The mechanics of the foot. II. The plantar aponeurosis and the arch. *Journal of Anatomy* **88**: 25–30.

Hicks, J.H. (1955). The foot as a support. *Acta Anatomica* **25**: 34–45.

Hicks, R.E. and Kinsbourne, M. (1976). Human handedness: a partial cross-fostering study. *Science* **192**: 908–910.

Hilali, A.S., Saleh, H.A. and Hickey, S.A. (1997). Clicking hyoid. *Journal of the Royal Society of Medicine* **90**: 689–690.

Hildebrand, M. (1988). *Analysis of Vertebrate Structure.* London: Wiley.

Hill, A.H. (1939). Fetal age assessment by centres of ossification. *American Journal of Physical Anthropology* **24**: 251–272.

Hill, L.M. (1958). Changes in the proportions of the female foot during growth. *American Journal of Physical Anthropology* **16**: 349–366.

Hill, A. (1992). Development of tone and reflexes in the fetus and newborn. In: *Fetal and Neonatal Physiology* (R.A. Polin and W.W. Fox, Eds.), pp. 1578–1587. Philadelphia, PA: W.B. Saunders.

Hill, H.A. and Sachs, M.D. (1940). The grooved defect of the humeral head. *Radiology* **35**: 690–700.

Hillson, S. (1996). *Dental Anthropology*. Cambridge: Cambridge University Press.

Himes, J.H. (1984). An early hand-wrist atlas and its implications for secular change in bone age. *Annals of Human Biology* **11**: 71–75.

Himes, J.H. and Malina, R.M. (1977). Sexual dimorphism in metacarpal dimensions and body size of Mexican school children. *Acta Anatomica* **99**: 15–20.

Himes, J.H., Malina, R.M. and Stepick, C.D. (1976). Relationships between body size and second metacarpal dimensions in Oaxaca (Mexico) school children 6 to 14 years of age. *Human Biology* **48**: 677–692.

Himes, J.H., Yarbrough, C. and Martorell, R. (1977). Estimation of stature in children from radiographically determined metacarpal length. *Journal of Forensic Sciences* **22**: 452–456.

Hinck, V.C., Hopkins, C.E. and Sauara, B.S. (1962). The size of the atlantal spinal canal: a sex difference. *Human Biology* **34**: 197–205.

Hinck, V.C., Hopkins, C.E. and Clark, W.M. (1965). Sagittal diameter of the lumbar spinal canal in children and adults. *Radiology* **85**: 929–937.

Hinck, V.C., Clark, W.M. and Hopkins, C.E. (1966). Normal interpediculate distances (min and max) in children and adults. *American Journal of Roentgenology* **97**: 141–153.

Hindman, B.W. and Poole, C.A. (1970). Early appearance of the secondary vertebral ossification centres. *Radiology* **95**: 359–361.

Hirschtick, A.B. (1951). An anomalous tarsal bone. *Journal of Bone and Joint Surgery* **33A**: 907–910.

Hodges, P.C. (1933). An epiphyseal chart. *American Journal of Roentgenology* **30**: 809–810.

Hodges, D.C., Harker, L.A. and Schermer, S.J. (1990). Atresia of the external acoustic meatuses in prehistoric populations. *American Journal of Physical Anthropology* **83**: 77–81.

Hoerr, N.L., Pyle, S.I. and Francis, C.C. (1962). *Radiographic Atlas of Skeletal Development of the Foot and Ankle: A Standard of Reference.* Springfield, IL: C.C. Thomas.

Högberg, P. (1952). Length of stride, stride frequency, 'flight' period and the maximum distance between the feet during running with different speeds. *Arbeitsphysiologie* **14**: 431–436.

Holcomb, S.M.C. and Konigsberg, L.W. (1995). Statistical study of sexual dimorphism in the human fetal sciatic notch. *American Journal of Physical Anthropology* **97**: 113–125.

Holcomb, G.R., Irving, T.E. and Smith, R.D. (1958). Coronal deviation and tilt in the proximal interphalangeal joint of man. *American Journal of Physical Anthropology* **16**: 429–440.

Holden, L. (1882). *Human Osteology*, 6th edition. London: Churchill.

Holland, C.T. (1921). On rarer ossifications seen during X-ray examinations. *Journal of Anatomy* **55**: 235–248.

Holland, C.T. (1928). The accessory bones of the foot. *The Robert Jones Birthday Volume: A Collection of Surgical Essays*, pp. 157–182. London: Oxford Medical Publications.

Holland, P.W.H. (1988). Homeobox genes and the vertebrate head. *Development* **103**(Suppl.): 17–24.

Holland, T.D. (1991). Sex assessment using the proximal tibia. *Journal of Physical Anthropology* **85**: 221–227.

Holland, T.D. (1992). Estimation of adult stature from fragmentary tibias. *Journal of Forensic Sciences* **37**: 1223–1229.

Holland, T.D. (1995). Brief communication: estimation of adult stature from the calcaneus and talus. *American Journal of Physical Anthropology* **96**: 315–320.

Holland, P.W.H. and Hogan, B.L.M. (1988). Spatially restricted patterns of expression of the homeobox-containing gene *Hox2.1* during mouse embryogenesis. *Development* **102**: 159–174.

Hollender, L. (1967). Enlarged parietal foramina. *Oral Surgery, Oral Medicine and Oral Pathology* **23**: 447–453.

Hollinshead, W.H. (1965). Anatomy of the spine: points of interest to orthopaedic surgeons. *Journal of Bone and Joint Surgery* **47A**: 209–215.

Hollinshead, W.H. (1982). *Anatomy for Surgeons*, 3rd edition. Philadelphia, PA: Harper and Row.

Holman, D.J. and Bennett, K.A. (1991). Determination of sex from arm bone measurements. *American Journal of Physical Anthropology* **84**: 421–426.

Holsbeeck, M. van, Vandamme, B., Marchal, G., Martens, M., Victor, J. and Baert, A.L. (1987). Dorsal defect of the patella: concept of its origin and relationship with bipartite and multipartite patella. *Skeletal Radiology* **16**: 304–311.

Holt, C.A. (1978). A re-examination of parturition scars on the human female pelvis. *American Journal of Physical Anthropology* **49**: 91–94.

Holtby, J.R.D. (1918). Some indices and measurements of the modern femur. *Journal of Anatomy* **52**: 363–382.

Holzhueter, A.M., Gregg, J.B. and Clifford, S. (1965). A search for stapes footplate fixation in an Indian population, prehistoric and historic. *American Journal of Physical Anthropology* **23**: 35–40.

Honeij, J.A. (1920). Cervical ribs. *Surgery, Gynaecology and Obstetrics* **30**: 481–493.

Hooper, G. and Hughes, S. (1988). Midfoot and navicular injuries. In: *The Foot* (B. Helal and D. Wilson, Eds.), pp. 932–943. Edinburgh: Churchill Livingstone.

Hooton, E.A. (1918). On certain Eskimoid characters in Icelandic skulls. *American Journal of Physical Anthropology* **1**: 53–76.

Hooton, E.A. (1960). *Up from the Ape*. New York: Macmillan.

Hoppa, R.D. (1992). Evaluating human skeletal growth: an Anglo-Saxon example. *International Journal of Osteoarchaeology* **2**: 275–288.

Hoppa, R.D. and Garlie, T.N. (1998). Secular trend on the growth of Toronto children during the last century. *Annals of Human Biology* **25**: 553–561.

Hoppa, R.D. and Gruspier, K.L. (1996). Estimating diaphyseal length from fragmentary subadult skeletal remains: implications for paleodemographic reconstructions of southern Ontario ossuary. *American Journal of Physical Anthropology* **100**: 341–345.

Horsman, A., Simpson, M. and Armes, F. (1981). A left/right comparison of sequential bone loss from the metacarpals of postmenopausal women. *American Journal of Physical Anthropology* **54**: 457–460.

Horst, M. and Brinckmann, P. (1981). Measurement of the distribution of axial stress on the endplate of the vertebral body. *Spine* **6**: 217–232.

Horswell, B.B., Holmes, A.D., Barnett, J.S. and Levant, B.A. (1987). Maxillonasal dysplasia (Binder's syndrome): a critical review and case study. *Journal of Oral and Maxillofacial Surgery* **45**: 114–122.

Hotson, S. and Carty, H. (1982). Lumbosacral agenesis: A report of three new cases and a review of the literature. *British Journal of Radiology* **55**: 629–633.

Hough, J.V.D. (1958). Malformations and anatomical variations seen in the middle ear during operation for mobilization of the stapes. *Laryngoscope* **68**: 1337–1379.

Houghton, P. (1974). The relationship of the pre-auricular groove of the ilium to pregnancy. *American Journal of Physical Anthropology* **41**: 381–390.

Houghton, P. (1977). Rocker jaws. *American Journal of Physical Anthropology* **47**: 365–369.

Houghton, P. (1978). Polynesian mandibles. *Journal of Anatomy* **127**: 251–260.

Howard, F.M. (1965). Injuries to the clavicle with neurovascular complications. *Journal of Bone and Joint Surgery* **47A**: 1335–1346.

Hrdlička, A. (1898). Study of the normal tibia. *American Anthropologist* **11**: 307–312.

Hrdlička, A. (1902). New instances of complete division of the malar bone, with notes on incomplete division. *The American Naturalist* **36**: 273–294.

Hrdlička, A. (1904). Further instances of malar division. *The American Naturalist* **38**: 361–366.

Hrdlička, A. (1923). Incidence of the supracondylar process in whites and other races. *American Journal of Physical Anthropology* **6**: 405–412.

Hrdlička, A. (1932). The humerus: Septal apertures. *Anthropologie Prague* **10**: 31–96.

Hrdlička, A. (1934a). Contributions to the study of the femur: the crista aspera and the pilaster. *American Journal of Physical Anthropology* **19**: 17–37.

Hrdlička, A. (1934b). The human femur: shape of shaft. *Anthropologie (Praha)* **12**(Suppl.): 129–163.

Hrdlička, A. (1935). Ear exostoses. *Smithsonian Miscellaneous Collections* **93**: 1–100. Summary in *American Journal of Physical Anthropology* (1935) **20**: 489–490.

Hrdlička, A. (1937). Gluteal ridge and gluteal tuberosities. *American Journal of Physical Anthropology* **23**: 127–198.

Hrdlička, A. (1938). The femur of the old Peruvians. *American Journal of Physical Anthropology* **23**: 421–462.

Hrdlička, A. (1940a). Mandibular and maxillary hyperostoses. *American Journal of Physical Anthropology* **27**: 1–55.

Hrdlička, A. (1940b). Lower jaw. I The gonial angle. II The bigonial breadth. *American Journal of Physical Anthropology* **27**: 281–308.

Hrdlička, A. (1940c). Lower jaw. Further studies. *American Journal of Physical Anthropology* **27**: 383–467.

Hrdlička, A. (1941). Lower jaw: Double condyles. *American Journal of Physical Anthropology* **28**: 75–89.

Hrdlička, A. (1942a). The adult scapula: additional observations and measurements. *American Journal of Physical Anthropology* **29**: 363–415.

Hrdlička, A. (1942b). The Scapula: visual observations. *American Journal of Physical Anthropology* **29**: 73–94.

Hrdlička, A. (1942c). The juvenile scapula: further observations. *American Journal of Physical Anthropology* **29**: 287–310.

Hromada, J. (1939). Contribution to the study of the growth of the fetal pelvis. *Anthropologie* **18**: 129–170.

Hubay, C.A. (1949). Sesamoid bones of the hands and feet. *American Journal of Roentgenology* **61**: 493–505.

Huber, G.C. (1912). On the relation of the chorda dorsalis to the anlage of the pharyngeal bursa or median pharyngeal recess. *Anatomical Record* **6**: 373–404.

Huber, J.F. (1941). The arterial network supplying the dorsum of the foot. *Anatomical Record* **80**: 373–391.

Huda, T.F.J. and Bowman, J.E. (1994). Variation in cross-striation number between striae in an archaeological population. *International Journal of Osteoarchaeology* **4**: 49–52.

Huda, T.F.J. and Bowman, J.E. (1995). Age determination from dental microstructure in juveniles. *American Journal of Physical Anthropology* **97**: 135–150.

Hughes, E.S.R. (1948a). Osgood-Schlatter's disease. *Surgery, Gynecology and Obstetrics* **86**: 323–328.

Hughes, E.S.R. (1948b). Painful heels in children. *Surgery, Gynecology and Obstetrics* **86**: 64–68.

Hughes, H. (1952). The factors determining the direction of the canal for the nutrient artery in the long bones of mammals and birds. *Acta Anatomica* **15**: 261–280.

Hughes, L.O. and Beaty, J.H. (1994). Fractures of the head and neck of the femur in children. Current concepts review. *Journal of Bone and Joint Surgery* **76A**: 283–292.

Hughes, E.S.R. and Sunderland, S. (1946). The tibial tuberosity and the attachment of the ligamentum patellae. *Anatomical Record* **96**: 439–444.

Hughes, S. and Sweetnam, R. (1980). *The Basis and Practice of Orthopaedics.* London: Heinemann.

Hughes, P.C.R. and Tanner, J.M. (1966). The development of carpal bone fusion as seen in serial radiographs. *British Journal of Radiology* **39**: 943–949.

Hughston, J.C. (1968). Subluxation of the patella. *Journal of Bone and Joint Surgery* **50A**: 1003–1026.

Hukuda, S., Ota, H., Okabe, N. and Tazima, K. (1980). Traumatic atlanto-axial dislocation causing os odontoideum in infants. *Spine* **5**: 207–210.

Hummert, J.R. and Van Gerven, D.P. (1983). Skeletal growth in a medieval population from Sudanese Nubia. *American Journal of Physical Anthropology* **60**: 471–478.

Hummert, J.R and Van Gerven, D.P. (1985). Observation on the formation and persistence of radio-opaque transverse lines. *American Journal of Physical Anthropology* **66**: 297–306.

Humphrey, L.T. (1998). Growth patterns in the modern human skeleton. *American Journal of Physical Anthropology* **105**: 57–72.

Humphry, G.M. (1878). On the growth of the jaws. *Journal of Anatomy and Physiology* **12**: 288–293.

Humphry, G.M. (1889). The angle of the neck with the shaft of the femur at different periods of life and under different circumstances. *Journal of Anatomy and Physiology* **23**: 273–282, 387–389.

Hunt, D.R. (1990). Sex determination in the subadult ilia: an indirect test of Weaver's non-metric sexing method. *Journal of Forensic Sciences* **35**: 881–885.

Hunt, D.M. (1995). The limping child. In: *Postgraduate Textbook of Clinical Orthopaedics*, 2nd edition (N.H. Harris and R. Birch, Eds.), pp. 133–156. Oxford: Blackwells.

Hunt, E.E. and Gleiser, I. (1955). The estimation of age and sex of preadolescent children from bones and teeth. *American Journal of Physical Anthropology* **13**: 479–487.

Hunt, E.E. and Hatch, J.W. (1981). The estimation of age at death and ages of formation of transverse lines from measurements of human long bones. *American Journal of Physical Anthropology* **54**: 461–469.

Hunter, W. (1743). On the structure and diseases of articular cartilage. *Philosophical Transactions* **42**: 514–521.

Hunter, W. (1761a). A singular case of the separation of the ossa pubis. *Medical Observations and Inquiries* **2**: 321–332.

Hunter, W. (1761b). Remarks on the symphysis of the ossa pubis. *Medical Observations and Inquiries* **2**: 333–339.

Hunter, J. (1837). *Collected Works*, Vol. 4. London: Palmer.

Hunter, R.H. (1924). An abnormal atlas. *Journal of Anatomy* **58**: 140–141.

Hunter, G.K. (1987). An ion exchange mechanism of cartilage calcification. *Connective Tissue Research* **16**: 111–120.

Hunter, W.S. and Garn, S.M. (1972). Disproportionate sexual dimorphism in the human face. *American Journal of Physical Anthropology* **36**: 133–138.

Huntington, G.S. (1905). The derivation and significance of certain supernumerary muscles of the pectoral region. *Journal of Anatomy and Physiology* **39**: 1–54.

Hurle, J.M. and Colvee, E. (1982). Surface changes in the embryonic interdigital epithelium during the formation of the free digits: A comparative study in the chick and duck foot. *Journal of Embryology and Experimental Morphology* **69**: 251–263.

Hurrell, D.J. (1934). The vascularisation of cartilage. *Journal of Anatomy* **69**: 47–61.

Hutchinson, D.L., Denise, C.B., Daniel, H.J. and Kalmus, G.W. (1997). A reevaluation of the cold water etiology of external auditory exostoses. *American Journal of Physical Anthropology* **103**: 417–422.

Hutter, C.G. and Scott, W. (1949). Tibial torsion. *Journal of Bone and Joint Surgery* **31A**: 511–518.

Huxley, A.K. and Jimenez, S.B. (1996). Technical note: Error in Olivier and Pineau's regression formulae for calculation of stature and lunar age from radial diaphyseal length in forensic fetal remains. *American Journal of Physical Anthropology* **100**: 435–437.

Hylander, W.L., Picq, P.G. and Johnson, K.R. (1991). Function of the supraorbital region of primates. *Archives of Oral Biology* **36**: 273–281.

Hyrtl, J. (1862). Über den Porus crotophitico-buccinatorius beim Menschen *Sitzungsberichte der Kaiserlich Akademie der Wissenschaften zu Wien* **46**: 111–115.

Imatani, R.J. (1975). Fractures of the scapula: a review of 53 fractures. *Journal of Trauma* **15**: 473–478.

Imrie, J.A. and Wyburn, G.M. (1958). Assessment of age, sex and height from immature human bones. *British Medical Journal* **1**: 128–131.

Ince, H. and Young, M. (1940). The bony pelvis and its influence on labour: A radiological and clinical study of 500 women. *Journal of Obstetrics and Gynaecology (British Commonwealth)* **47**: 130–190.

Indrayana, N.S., Glinka, J. and Mieke, S. (1998). Mandibular ramus flexure in an Indonesian population. *American Journal of Physical Anthropology* **105**: 89–90.

Ingalls, N.W. (1924). Studies on the femur. *American Journal of Physical Anthropology* **3**: 207–255.

Inge, G.A.L. (1936). Congenital absence of medial sesamoid bone of the great toe – report of 2 cases. *Journal of Bone and Joint Surgery* **18**: 188–190.

Inge, G.A.L. and Ferguson, A.B. (1933). Surgery of the sesamoid bones of the great toe. Anatomic and clinical study. *Archives of Surgery* **27**: 466–489.

Ingervall, B. and Thilander, B. (1972). The human spheno-occipital synchondrosis 1. The time of closure observed macroscopically. *Acta Odontologica Scandinavica* **30**: 349–356.

Inman, V.T. and Saunders, J.B. de C.M. (1937). The ossification of the human frontal bone with special reference to its presumed pre- and post-frontal elements. *Journal of Anatomy* **71**: 383–394.

Inman, V.T. and Saunders, J.B. de C.M. (1944). Referred pain from skeletal structures. *Journal of Nervous and Mental Diseases* **99**: 660–667.

Inman, V.T., Saunders, J.B. de C.M. and Abbot, L.C. (1944). Observations on the function of the shoulder joint. *Journal of Bone and Joint Surgery* **26**: 1–30.

Insall, J. and Salvati, E. (1971). Patella position in the normal knee joint. *Radiology* **101**: 101–104.

Introna, F., Di Vella, G. and Campobasso, C.P. (1998). Sex determination by discriminant analysis of patellar measurements. *Forensic Science International* **95**: 39–45.

Inuzuka, N. (1992). Evolution of the shoulder girdle with special reference to the problems of the clavicle. *Journal of the Anthropological Society of Nippon* **100**: 391–404.

Iordanidis, P. (1961). Détermination du sexe par les os du sequelette. *Annales de Médecine Légale* **41**: 280–291.

Ippolito, E., Tovaglia, V. and Caterini, R. (1984). Mechanisms of acetabular growth in the fetus in relation to the pathogenesis and treatment of congenital dislocation of the hip. *Italian Journal of Orthopedics and Traumatology* **10**: 501–510.

Irvine, E.D. and Taylor, F.W. (1936). Hereditary and congenital large parietal foramina. *British Journal of Radiology* **9**: 456–462.

Irwin, G.L. (1960). Roentgen determination of the time of closure of the spheno-occipital synchondrosis. *Radiology* **75**: 450–453.

Isaac, B., Vettivel, S., Prasad, R., Jeyaseelan, L. and Chandi, G. (1997). Prediction of the femoral neck/shaft angle from the length of the femoral neck. *Clinical Anatomy* **10**: 318–323.

Işcan, M.Y. (1985). Osteometric analysis of sexual dimorphism in the sternal end of the rib. *Journal of the Forensic Science Association* **30**: 1090–1099.

Işcan, M.Y. and Miller-Shaivitz, P.M. (1984a). Determination of sex from the femur in blacks and whites. *Collegium Antropologium (Zagreb)* **8**: 169–175.

Işcan, M.Y. and Miller-Shaivitz, P.M. (1984b). Determination of sex from the tibia. *American Journal of Physical Anthropology* **64**: 53–57.

Işcan, M.Y. and Miller-Shaivitz, P.M. (1984c). Discriminant function sexing of the tibia. *Journal of Forensic Sciences* **29**: 1087–1093.

Işcan, M.Y., Loth, S.R. and Wright, R.K. (1984). Age estimation from the rib by phase analysis: White males. *Journal of the Forensic Science Association* **29**: 1094–1104.

Işcan, M.Y., Loth, S.R. and Wright, R.K. (1985). Age estimation from the rib by phase analysis; White females. *Journal of the Forensic Science Association* **30**: 853–863.

Işcan, M.Y., Yoshino, M. and Kato, S. (1994). Sex determination from the tibia: standards for contemporary Japan. *Journal of Forensic Sciences* **39**: 785–792.

Işcan, M.Y., Loth, S.R., King, C.A., Shihai, D., and Yoshino, M. (1998). Sexual Dimorphism in the humerus: a comparative analysis of Chinese, Japanese and Thais. *Forensic Science International* **98**: 17–29.

Ishii, T., Miyagawa, S. and Hayashi, K. (1994). Traction apophysitis of the medial malleolus. *Journal of Bone and Joint Surgery* **76B**: 802–806.

Isobe, M., Murakami, G. and Kataura, A. (1998). Variations of the uncinate process of the lateral nasal wall with clinical implications. *Clinical Anatomy* **11**: 295–303.

Israel, H. and Lewis, A.B. (1971). Radiographically determined linear permanent tooth growth from age 6 years. *Journal of Dental Research* **50**: 334–342.

Izpisua-Belmonte, J.C., Tickle, C., Dollé, P., Wolpert, L. and Duboule, D. (1991). Expression of homeobox *Hox*-4 genes and the specification of position in chick wing development. *Nature* **350**: 585–589.

Jackson, G. (1909). Aetiology of exostoses of the external auditory meatus. *British Medical Journal* **2**: 1137–1138.

Jackson, H. and Burke, J.T. (1984). The sacral foramina. *Skeletal Radiology* **11**: 282–288.

Jacobs, B. and Thompson, T.C. (1960). Opposition of the thumb and its restoration. *Journal of Bone and Joint Surgery* **42A**: 1015–1026.

Jacobsen, K. (1974). Area intercondylaris tibiae: osseous surface structure and its relation to soft tissue structures and applications to radiography. *Journal of Anatomy* **117**: 605–618.

Jacobsen, J., Jørgensen, J.B. and Kjær, I. (1991). Tooth and bone development in a Danish medieval mandible with unilateral absence of the mandibular canal. *American Journal of Physical Anthropology* **85**: 15–23.

Jacobson, A. (1955). Embryological evidence for the non-existence of the premaxilla in man. *Journal of the Dental Association of South Africa* **10**: 189–210.

Jacobson, A.G. and Meier, S. (1984). Morphogenesis of the head of the newt: Mesodermal segments, neuromeres and distribution of neural crest. *Developmental Biology* **106**: 181–193.

Jacobson, A.G. and Sater, A. (1988). Features of embryonic induction. *Development* **104**: 341–359.

Jahss, M.H. (1981). The sesamoids of the hallux. *Clinical Orthopaedics* **157**: 88–97.

Jakob, R.P., Haertel, M. and Stüssi, E. (1980). Tibial torsion calculated by computerised tomography and compared to other methods of measurement. *Journal of Bone and Joint Surgery* **62B**: 238–242.

Jakob, R.P., von Gumppenberg, S. and Engelhardt, P. (1981). Does Osgood-Schlatter disease influence the position of the patella? *Journal of Bone and Joint Surgery* **63B**: 579–582.

James, T.M., Presley, R. and Steel, F.L.D. (1980). The foramen ovale and sphenoidal angle in man. *Anatomy and Embryology* **160**: 93–104.

Jantz, R.L. (1992). Modification of the Trotter and Gleser female stature estimation formulae. *Journal of Forensic Sciences* **37**: 1230–1235.

Jantz, R.L. and Owsley, D.W. (1984). Long bone growth variation among Arikara skeletal populations. *American Journal of Physical Anthropology* **63**: 13–20.

Jantz, R.L., Hunt, D.R. and Meadows, L. (1995). The measure and mismeasure of the tibia: implications for stature estimation. *Journal of Forensic Sciences* **40**: 758–761.

Jarvik, E. (1965). On the origin of girdles and paired limbs. *Israel Journal of Zoology* **14**: 141–172.

Jarvik, E. (1980). *Basic Structure and Evolution of Vertebrates*, Vols 1 and 2. London: Academic Press.

Jarvis, J.L. and Keats, T.E. (1974). Cleidocranial dysostosis: a review of 40 new cases. *American Journal of Roentgenology* **121**: 5–16.

Jaswal, S. (1983). Age and sequence of permanent-tooth emergence among Khasis. *American Journal of Physical Anthropology* **62**: 177–186.

Jaworek, T.E. (1973). The intrinsic vascular supply to the first metatarsal. Surgical considerations. *Journal of the American Podiatry Association* **63**: 189–197.

Jaworski, Z.F.G., Duck, B. and Sekaly, G. (1981). Kinetics of osteoclasts and their nuclei in evolving secondary Haversian systems. *Journal of Anatomy* **133**: 397–405.

Jaworski, Z.F.G., Kimmel, D.B. and Jee, W.S.S. (1983). Cell kinetics underlying skeletal growth and bone tissue turnover. In: *Bone Histomorphometry: Techniques and Interpretation* (R.R. Richer, Ed.), pp. 225–239. Boca Raton, FL: CRC Press.

Jeannopoulos, C.L. (1952). Congenital elevation of the scapula. *Journal of Bone and Joint Surgery* **34A**: 883–892.

Jeanty, P. (1983). Fetal limb biometry. (Letter). *Radiology* **147**: 601–602.

Jeanty, P., Kirkpatrick, C., Dramaix-Wilmet, M. and Struyven, J. (1981). Ultrasonic evaluation of fetal limb growth. *Radiology* **140**: 165–168.

Jeanty, P., Dramaix-Wilmet, M., van Kerkem, J., Petroos, P. and Schwers, J. (1982). Ultrasonic evaluation of fetal limb growth. Part II. *Radiology* **143**: 751–754.

Jeffery, C.C. (1957). A case of pollicisation of the index finger. *Journal of Bone and Joint Surgery* **39B**: 120–123.

Jeng, C.L., Maurer, A. and Mizel, M.S. (1998). Congenital absence of the hallux fibular sesamoid: a case report and review of the literature. *Foot and Ankle International* **19**: 329–331.

Jenkins, F.A. (1969). The evolution and development of the dens of the mammalian axis. *Anatomical Record* **164**: 173–184.

Jenkins, F. (1972). Chimpanzee bipedalism: cineradiographic analysis and implications for the evolution of gait. *Science* **178**: 877–879.

Jenkins, F. (1974). The movement of the shoulder in claviculate and aclaviculate mammals. *Journal of Morphology* **144**: 71–84.

Jenkins, D.B. (1990). *Functional Anatomy of the Limbs and Back.* Philadelphia, PA: W.B. Saunders.

Jensen, E. and Palling, M. (1954). The gonial angle – a survey. *American Journal of Orthodontics* **40**: 120–133.

Jergensen, F.H. (1975). Orthopedics. In: *Current Surgical Diagnosis and Treatment* (J.E. Dunphy and L.W. Way, Eds.). CA: Lange Medical Publications.

Jewett, T.C., Butsch, W.L. and Hug, H.R. (1962). Congenital bifid sternum. *Surgery* **52**: 932–936.

Jeyasingh, P., Gupta, C.D., Arora, A.K. and Saxena, S.K. (1982). Study of Os japonicum in Uttar Pradesh crania. *Anatomica Anzeiger* **152**: 27–30.

Jinkins, W.K. (1969). Congenital pseudoarthrosis of the clavicle. *Clinical Orthopedics and Related Research* **62**: 183–186.

Jit, I. (1957). Observations on prenatal ossification with special references to the bones of the hand and foot. *Journal of the Anatomical Society of India* **6**: 12–23.

Jit, I. and Bakshi, V. (1984). Incidence of foramina in North Indian sterna. *Journal of the Anatomical Society of India* **33**: 77–84.

Jit, I. and Gandhi, O.P. (1966). The value of the pre-auricular sulcus in sexing bony pelves. *Journal of the Anatomical Society of India* **15**: 104–107.

Jit, I. and Kaur, H. (1989). Time of fusion of the human sternebrae with one another in North West India. *American Journal of Physical Anthropology* **80**: 195–202.

Jit, I. and Kulkarni, M. (1976). Times of appearance and fusion of epiphyses at the medial end of the clavicle. *Indian Journal of Medical Research* **64**: 773–782.

Jit, I. and Shah, M.A. (1948). Incidence of frontal or metopic suture amongst Punjabee adults. *Indian Medical Gazette* **83**: 507–508.

Jit, I. and Singh, S. (1956). Estimation of stature from clavicles. *Indian Journal of Medical Research* **44**: 137–155.

Jit, I. and Singh, S. (1966). The sexing of the adult clavicles. *Indian Journal of Medical Research* **54**: 551–571.

Jit, I. and Singh, B. (1971). A radiological study of the time of fusion of certain epiphyses in Punjabees. *Journal of the Anatomical Society of India* **20**: 1–27.

Jit, I., Jhingan, V. and Kulkarni M. (1980). Sexing the human sternum. *American Journal of Physical Anthropology* **53**: 217–224.

Johanson, G. (1971). Age determination from human teeth. A critical evaluation with special consideration of changes after fourteen years of age. *Odontologisk Revy* **22**(Suppl.): 1–126.

Johnson, E.H. (1937). The narial margins in man. *Journal of Anatomy* **71**: 356–361.

Johnson, J.F. and Brogdon, B.G. (1982). Dorsal defect of the patella. *American Journal of Roentgenology* **139**: 339–340.

Johnson, G.F. and Israel, H. (1979). Basioccipital clefts. *Radiology* **133**: 101–103.

Johnson, D.R. and O'Higgins, P. (1996). Is there a link between changes in the vertebral Hox code and the shape of the vertebrae? A quantitative study of shape change in the cervical vertebral column of mice. *Journal of Theoretical Biology* **183**: 89–93.

Johnson, C.C., Gorlin, R.J. and Anderson, V.E. (1965). Torus mandibularis: a genetic study. *American Journal of Human Genetics* **17**: 433–439.

Johnson, D.R., McAndrew, T.M. and Özkan, O. (1999). Shape differences in the cervical and upper thoracic vertebrae in rats (Rattus norvegicus) and bats (Pteropus poiocephalus): can we see shape patterns derived from position in column and species membership? *Journal of Anatomy* **194**: 249–253.

Johnston, H.M. (1906). Epilunar and hypolunar ossicles, division of the scaphoid and other abnormalities in the carpal region. *Journal of Anatomy and Physiology* **41**: 59–65.

Johnston, F.E. (1961). Sequence of epiphyseal union in a prehistoric Kentucky population from Indian Knoll. *Human Biology* **33**: 66–81.

Johnston, F.E. (1962). Growth of the long bones of infants and children at Indian Knoll. *American Journal of Physical Anthropology* **20**: 249–254.

Johnston, F.E. and Jahina, S.B. (1965). The contribution of the carpal bones to the assessment of skeletal age. *American Journal of Physical Anthropology* **23**: 349–354.

Johnston, F.E. and Zimmer, L.O. (1989). Assessment of growth and age in the immature skeleton. In: *Reconstruction of Life from the Skeleton* (M.Y. Işcan and K.A.R. Kennedy, Eds.), pp. 11–21. New York: Liss.

Johnston, F.E., Whitehouse, R.H. and Hertzog, D.P. (1968). Normal variability in the age and first onset of ossification of the triquetral. *American Journal of Physical Anthropology* **28**: 97–100.

Johnstone, W.H., Keats, T.E. and Lee, M.E. (1982). The anatomic basis for the superior acetabular roof notch 'Superior Acetabular Notch'. *Skeletal Radiology* **8**: 25–27.

Jones, F.W. (1910). On the relation of the limb plexuses to the ribs and vertebral column. *Journal of Anatomy and Physiology* **44**: 377–393.

Jones, F.W. (1912). Some nerve markings on lumbar vertebrae. *Journal of Anatomy* **47**: 118–120.

Jones, F.W. (1913). The anatomy of cervical ribs. *Proceedings of the Royal Society of Medicine* **6**: 95–113.

Jones, F.W. (1941). *The Principles of Anatomy as Seen in the Hand*, 2nd edition. Baltimore, MA: Williams and Warwick.

Jones, F.W. (1946). *Structure and Function as seen in the Foot*, 2nd edition. London: Baillière, Tindall and Cox.

Jones, A.R. (1950). Abraham Colles. *Journal of Bone and Joint Surgery* **32B**: 126–130.

Jones, G.B. (1964). Delta phalanx. *Journal of Bone and Joint Surgery* **46B**: 226–228.

Jones, S.J., Glorieux, F.H., Travers, R. and Boyde, A. (1999). The microscopic structure of bone in normal children and patients with osteogenesis imperfecta: a study using back scattered electron imaging. *Calcified Tissue International* **64**: 8–17.

Jonsson, B., Stromqvist, B. and Egund, N. (1989). Anomalous lumbosacral articulations and low back pain. Evaluation and treatment. *Spine* **14**: 831–835.

Jonsson, K., Niklasson, J. and Josefsson, P.O. (1991). Avulsion of the cervical spine ring apophysis: Acute and chronic appearance. *Skeletal Radiology* **20**: 207–210.

Jopling, W.H. and McDougall, A.C. (1988). *Handbook of Leprosy*, 4th edition. Oxford: Heinemann.

Jordaan, H.V.F. (1982). Fetal foot length. *South African Medical Journal* **62**: 473–475.

Joseph, J. (1951a). Further studies of the metacarpophalangeal and interphalangeal joints of the thumb. *Journal of Anatomy* **85**: 221–229.

Joseph, J. (1951b). The sesamoid bones of the hand and the time of fusion of the epiphyses of the thumb. *Journal of Anatomy* **85**: 230–241.

Joseph, J. (1954). Range of movement of the great toe in man. *Journal of Bone and Joint Surgery* **36B**: 450–457.

Juhl, M.D. and Seerup, K.K. (1983). Os odontoideum. A cause of atlanto-axial instability. *Acta Orthopedica Scandinavica* **54**: 113–118.

Jurik, A.G. (1984). Ossification and calcification of the laryngeal skeleton. *Acta Radiologica Diagnosis* **25**: 17–22.

Kahane, J.C. (1978). A morphological study of the human prepubertal and pubertal larynx. *American Journal of Anatomy* **151**: 11–20.

Kajii, T., Kida, M. and Takahashi, K. (1973). The effect of thalidomide intake during 113 human pregnancies. *Teratology* **8**: 163–166.

Kalla, A.K., Khanna, S., Singh, I.P., Sharma, S., Schnobel, R. and Vogel, F. (1989). A genetic and anthropological study of atlanto-occipital fusion. *Human Genetics* **81**: 105–112.

Kallen, B. and Winberg, J. (1974). Caudal mesoderm pattern of anomalies: from renal agenesis to sirenomelia. *Teratology* **9**: 99–103.

Kalmey, J.K. and Rathbun, T.A. (1996). Sex determination by discriminant function analysis of the petrous portion of the temporal bone. *Journal of Forensic Sciences* **41**: 865–867.

Kalmey, J.K., Thewissen, J.G.M. and Dluzen, D.E. (1998). Age-related size reduction of foramina in the cribriform plate. *Anatomical Record* **251**: 326–329.

Kammerer, F. (1901). Cervical ribs. *Annals of Surgery* **34**: 637–648.

Kanagasuntheram, R. (1967). A note on the development of the tubotympanic recess of the human embryo. *Journal of Anatomy* **101**: 731–741.

Kanagasuntheram, R., Sivanandasingham, P. and Krishnamurti, A. (1987). *Anatomy: Regional, Functional and Clinical.* Singapore: PG Publishing.

Kanavel, A.B. (1932). Congenital malformations of the hand. *Archives of Surgery* **25**: 282–320.

Kanis, J.A. (1994). *Osteoporosis.* Oxford: Blackwells.

Kapadia, Y.K. (1991). An investigation into Harris lines in the documented juveniles from St Brides. Unpublished BSc dissertation, University of London.

Kapadia, Y.K., Bowman, J.E., MacLaughlin, S.M. and Scheuer, J.L. (1992). A study of Harris lines in the juvenile skeletons from St Bride's. *Annals of Human Biology* **19**: 328–329.

Kapandji, I.A. (1974). *The Physiology of the Joints, Vol. 3. The Trunk and Vertebral Column.* London: Churchill Livingstone.

Kapandji, I.A. (1987). *The Physiology of the Joints*, Vol. 2. *Lower Limb.* London: Churchill Livingstone.

Kaplan, E.B. (1965). *Functional and Surgical Anatomy of the Hand.* Philadelphia, PA: Lippincott.

Kaplan, H.A., Browder, A. and Browder, J. (1973). Nasal venous drainage and the foramen caecum. *Laryngoscope* **83**: 327–329.

Kaplan, S.L., Tun, C.G. and Sarkarati, M. (1990). Odontoid fracture complicating ankylosing spondylitis – a case report and a review of the literature. *Spine* **15**: 607–610.

Kaplan, S.B., Kemp, S.S. and Oh, K.S. (1991). Radiographic manifestations of congenital anomalies of the skull. *Radiologic Clinics of North America* **29**: 195–218.

Kassianenko, W.V. (1935). Calcaneus secundarius, Talus accessorius und os Trigonum tarsi beim Pferde. *Anatomischer Anzeiger* **80**: 1–10.

Kate, B.R. (1963). The incidence and cause of cervical fossa in Indian femora. *Journal of the Anatomical Society of India* **12**: 69–76.

Kate, B.R. (1976). Anteversion versus torsion of the femoral neck. *Acta Anatomica* **94**: 457–463.

Kate, B.R. and Robert, S.L. (1965). Some observations on the upper end of the tibia in squatters. *Journal of Anatomy* **99**: 137–141.

Kattan, K.R. and Pais, M.J. (1982). Some borderlands of the cervical spine. Part I. The normal (and nearly normal) that may appear pathologic. *Skeletal Radiology* **8**: 1–6.

Katz, D. and Suchey, J.M. (1986). Age determination of the male os pubis. *American Journal of Physical Anthropology* **69**: 427–435.

Kauer, J.M.G. (1974). The interdependence of carpal articulation chains. *Acta Anatomica* **88**: 481–501.

Kaufer, H. (1971). Mechanical function of the patella. *Journal of Bone and Joint Surgery* **53A**: 1551–1560.

Kaufman, P. de B. (1977). The number of vertebrae in the Southern African Negro, the American Negro and the Bushman (San). *American Journal of Physical Anthropology* **47**: 409–414.

Kaufman, S.M., Elzay, R.P. and Irish, E.F. (1970). Styloid process variation. *Archives of Otolaryngology* **91**: 460–463.

Kaufman, M.H., Whitaker, D. and McTavish, J. (1997). Differential diagnosis of holes in the calvarium: application of modern clinical data to palaeopathology. *Journal of Archaeological Science* **24**: 193–218.

Kaul, S.S. and Pathak, R.K. (1984). The mylohyoid bridge in four population samples from India, with observations on its suitability as a genetic marker. *American Journal of Physical Anthropology* **65**: 213–218.

Kaur, H. and Jit, I. (1990). Age estimation from cortical index of the human clavicle in Northwest Indians. *American Journal of Physical Anthropology* **83**: 297–305.

Kaur, H. and Jit, I. (1991). Coracoclavicular joint in Northwest Indians. *American Journal of Physical Anthropology* **85**: 457–460.

Kaushal, S.P. (1977). Sacral ribs. *International Surgery* **62**: 37.

Kawashima, T. and Uhthoff, H.K. (1990). Prenatal development around the sustentaculum tali and its relation to talocalcaneal coalitions. *Journal of Pediatric Orthopaedics* **10**: 238–243.

Keating, D.R. and Amberg, J.R. (1954). A source of potential error in the roentgen diagnosis of cervical ribs. *Radiology* **62**: 688–694.

Keats, T.E. (1967). The inferior accessory ossicle of the anterior arch of the atlas. *American Journal of Roentgenology* **101**: 834–836.

Keats, T.E. (1992). *Atlas of Normal Roentgen Variants that may Simulate Disease*, 5th edition. St Louis, MO: Mosby Yearbook.

Keats, T.E. and Harrison, R.B. (1980). The epiphyseal spur. *Skeletal Radiology* **5**: 175–177.

Keats, T.E. and Johnstone, W.H. (1982). Notching of the lamina of C7: a proposed mechanism. *Skeletal Radiology* **7**: 273–274.

Keats, T.E. and Pope, T.L. (1988). The acromioclavicular joint: normal variation and the diagnosis of dislocation. *Skeletal Radiology* **17**: 159–162.

Keen, J.A. (1950). A study of the differences between male and female skulls. *American Journal of Physical Anthropology* **8**: 65–79.

Keen, J.A. and Wainwright, J. (1958). Ossification of the thyroid, cricoid and arytenoid cartilages. *South African Journal of Laboratory and Clinical Medicine* **4**: 83–108.

Keith, A. (1929). The history of the human foot and its bearing in orthopaedic practice. *Journal of Bone and Joint Surgery* **11**: 10–32.

Keleman, E., Jánossa, M., Calvo, W. and Fliedner, T.M. (1984). Developmental age estimated by bone-length measurement in human fetuses. *Anatomical Record* **209**: 547–552.

Kelikian, H. (1974). *Congenital Deformities of the Hand and Forearm.* Philadelphia, PA: W.B. Saunders.

Keller, T.S., Hansson, T.H., Aram, A.C., Spengler, D.M. and Panjabi, M.M. (1989). Regional variations in the compressive properties of lumbar vertebral trabeculae: effects of disc degeneration. *Spine* **14**: 1012–1020.

Kelley, R.O. (1970). An electron microscopic study of mesenchyme during development of interdigital spaces in man. *Anatomical Record* **168**: 43–53.

Kelley, R.O. (1973). Fine structure of the apical rim mesenchyme complex during limb morphogenesis in man. *Journal of Embryology and Experimental Morphology* **29**: 117–131.

Kelley, M.A. (1979a). Skeletal changes produced by aortic aneurysms. *American Journal of Physical Anthropology* **51**: 35–38.

Kelley, M.A. (1979b). Sex determination with fragmented skeletal remains. *Journal of Forensic Sciences* **24**: 154–158.

Kelley, M.A. (1979c). Parturition and pelvic changes. *American Journal of Physical Anthropology* **51**: 541–546.

Kelly, H.J. and Reynolds, L. (1947). Appearance and growth of ossification centres and increases in the body dimensions of White and Negro infants. *American Journal of Roentgenology* **57**: 479–516.

Kempson, F.C. (1902). Emargination of the patella. *Journal of Anatomy and Physiology* **36**: 419–420.

Kendrick, G.S. and Biggs, N.L. (1963). Incidence of the ponticulus posticus of the first cervical vertebra between ages of six to seventeen. *Anatomical Record* **145**: 449–454.

Kenna, M.A. (1996). Embryology and development of the ear. In: *Pediatric Otolaryngology,* Vol. 1, 3rd edition (C.D. Bluestone, S.E. Stool and M.A. Kenna, Eds.). Philadelphia, PA: W.B. Saunders.

Kennedy, J.C. (1949). Retrosternal dislocation of the clavicle. *Journal of Bone and Joint Surgery* **31B**: 74–75.

Kennedy, G.E. (1983). Some aspects of femoral morphology in *Homo erectus*. *Journal of Human Evolution* **12**: 587–616.

Kennedy, G.E. (1986). The relationship between auditory exostoses and cold water: a latitudinal analysis. *American Journal of Physical Anthropology* **71**: 401–415.

Kenny, M. (1944). The clinically suspect pelvis and its radiographical investigation in 1,000 cases. *Journal of Obstetrics and Gynaecology (British Commonwealth)* **51**: 277–292.

Kent, R.L., Reed, R.B. and Moorrees, C.F.A. (1978). Associations in emergence age among permanent teeth. *American Journal of Physical Anthropology* **48**: 131–142.

Kerckring, T. (1717). *Specilegium Anatomicum Osteogeniam Foetuum.* Leiden.

Kerley, E.R. (1965). The microscopic determination of age in human bone. *American Journal of Physical Anthropology* **23**: 149–164.

Kerley, E.R. (1976). Forensic anthropology and crimes involving children. *Journal of Forensic Sciences* **21**: 333–339.

Kerley, E.R. and Ubelaker, D.H. (1978). Revisions in the microscopic method of estimating age at death in human cortical bone. *American Journal of Physical Anthropology* **49**: 545–546.

Kerr, H.D. (1933). Anomalies of the skull in the new-born with special reference to 'relief' or 'lacuna skull' ('Lückenschädel'). *American Journal of Roentgenology* **30**: 458–463.

Kessel, M. and Gruss, P. (1991). Homeotic transformations of murine prevertebrae and concomitant alteration of Hox codes induced by retinoic acid. *Cell* **67**: 89–104.

Kessel, L. and Rang, M. (1966). Supracondylar spur of the humerus. *Journal of Bone and Joint Surgery* **48B**: 765–769.

Keyes, J.E.L. (1935). Observations on four thousand optic foramina in human skulls of known origin. *Archives of Ophthalmology* **13**: 538–568.

Khoo, F.Y. and Kuo, C.L. (1948). An unusual anomaly of the inferior portion of the scapula. *Journal of Bone and Joint Surgery* **30A**: 1010–1011.

Khoury, M.B., Kirks, D.R., Martinez, S. and Apple J. (1985). Bilateral avulsion fractures of the anterior superior iliac spines in sprinters. *Skeletal Radiology* **13**: 65–67.

Kidner, F.C. (1929). The prehallux (accessory scaphoid) in its relation to flat foot. *Journal of Bone and Joint Surgery* **11**: 831–837.

Kiely, M.L., Sawyer, D.R. and Gowgiel, J.M. (1995). Styloid chain ossification. *Clinical Anatomy* **8**: 359–362.

Kieny, M., Mauger, A. and Sengel, P. (1972). Early regionalization of the somitic mesoderm as studied by the development of the axial skeleton of the chick embryo. *Developmental Biology* **28**: 142–161.

Kier, E.L. (1966). Embryology of the normal optic canal and its anomalies. *Investigative Radiology* **1**: 346–362.

Kier, E.L. (1968). The infantile sella turcica. New roentgenological and anatomic concepts based on a developmental study of the sphenoid bone. *American Journal of Roentgenology* **102**: 747–767.

Kier, E.L. and Rothman, L.G. (1976). Radiologically significant anatomic variations of the developing sphenoid in humans. In: *Symposium on the Development of the Basicranium* (J.F. Bosma, Ed.), pp. 107–140. Bethesda, MD: US Department of Health, Education and Welfare.

Kimura, K. (1976). Growth of the second metacarpal according to chronological age and skeletal maturation. *Anatomical Record* **184**: 147–158.

Kimura, K. (1992). Estimation of stature from second metacarpal length in Japanese children. *Annals of Human Biology* **19**: 267–275.

King, J.B. (1939). Calcification of the costal cartilages. *British Journal of Radiology* **12**: 2–12.

King, T.S. (1963). Ossification and age changes in the laryngeal cartilages. *Journal of Anatomy* **97**: 140.

Kingsmill, V.J. and Boyde, A. (1998a). Variation in the apparent density of human mandibular bone with age and dental status. *Journal of Anatomy* **192**: 233–244.

Kingsmill, V.J. and Boyde, A. (1998b). Mineralisation density of human mandibular bone: quantitative backscattered electron image analysis. *Journal of Anatomy* **192**: 245–256.

Kirby, A., Wallace, W.A., Moulton, A. and Burwell, R.G. (1993). Comparison of four methods for measuring femoral anteversion. *Clinical Anatomy* **6**: 280–288.

Kirdani, M.A. (1967). The normal hypoglossal canal. *American Journal of Roentgenology* **99**: 700–704.

Kirlew, K.A., Hathout, G.M., Reiter, S.D. and Gold, R.H. (1993). Os odontoideum in identical twins: perspectives on aetiology. *Skeletal Radiology* **22**: 525–527.

Kjar, I. (1974). Skeletal maturation of the human fetus assessed radiographically on the basis of ossification sequences in the hand and foot. *American Journal of Physical Anthropology* **40**: 257–276.

Kjær, I. (1975). Histochemical investigations on the symphysis menti in the human fetus related to skeletal maturation in the hand and foot. *Acta Anatomica* **93**: 606–633.

Kjær, I. (1980). Development of deciduous mandibular incisors related to developmental stages in the mandible. *Acta Odontologica Scandinavica* **38**: 257–262.

Kjær, I. (1990a). Ossification of the human fetal basicranium. *Journal of Craniofacial Genetics and Developmental Biology* **10**: 29–38.

Kjær, I. (1990b). Radiographic determination of prenatal basicranial ossification. *Journal of Craniofacial Genetics and Developmental Biology* **10**: 113–123.

Kjær, I. (1990c). Prenatal human cranial development evaluated on coronal plane radiographs. *Journal of Craniofacial Genetics and Developmental Biology* **10**: 339–351.

Kjær, I. (1990d). Correlated appearance of ossification and nerve tissue in human fetal jaws. *Journal of Craniofacial Genetics and Developmental Biology* **10**: 329–336.

Kjær, I. (1997). Mandibular movements during elevation and fusion of the palatal shelves evaluated from the course of Meckel's cartilage. *Journal of Craniofacial Genetics and Developmental Biology* **17**: 80–85.

Kjær, I., Kjær, T.W. and Græm, N. (1993). Ossification sequence of occipital bone and vertebrae in human fetuses. *Journal of Craniofacial Genetics and Developmental Biology* **13**: 83–88.

Klein, D.M., Merola, A.A. and Spero, C.R. (1996). Congenital vertical talus with a talocalcaneal coalition. *Journal of Bone and Joint Surgery* **78B**: 326–327.

Kleinberg, S. (1917). Supernumerary bones of the foot. An X-ray study. *Annals of Surgery* **65**: 499–509.

Klenerman, L. (1966). Fractures of the shaft of the humerus. *Journal of Bone and Joint Surgery* **48B**: 105–111.

Klima, M. (1968). Early development of the human sternum and the problem of homologization of the so called suprasternal ossicles. *Acta Anatomica* **69**: 473–484.

Kline, D.G. (1966). Atlanto-axial dislocation simulating a head injury: hypoplasia of the odontoid. Case report. *Journal of Neurosurgery* **24**: 1013–1016.

Knight, B. (1996). *Forensic Pathology*, 2nd edition. London: Arnold.

Knott, V.B. (1974). Birotundal diameter of the human sphenoid bone from age six years to early adulthood. *American Journal of Physical Anthropology* **41**: 279–284.

Knott, V.B. and Johnson, R. (1970). Height and shape of the palate in girls: a longitudinal study. *Archives of Oral Biology* **15**: 849–860.

Knox, R. (1841). On the occasional presence of a supracondyloid process in the human humerus. *Edinburgh Medical and Surgical Journal* **56**: 125–128.

Knox, R. (1842/3). On some varieties in human structure, with remarks on the doctrine of 'Unity of the Organization'. *London Medical Gazette* **II**: 529–532.

Knudson, C.B. and Toole, B.P. (1987). Hyaluronate-cell interactions during differentiation of chick embryo limb mesoderm. *Developmental Biology* **124**: 82–90.

Knussmann, R. (1988). *Anthropologie. Handbuch der vergleichenden Biologie des Menschen. Band I.* Stuttgart: Gustav Fisher.

Kobayashi, K. (1967). Trend in the length of life based on human skeletons from prehistoric to modern times in Japan. *Journal of the Faculty of Science, University of Tokyo* **3**: 107–162.

Kobayashi, H., Kusakai, Y., Usui, M. and Ishii, S. (1991). Bilateral deficiency of ossification of the lunate bone. *Journal of Bone and Joint Surgery* **73A**: 1255–1256.

Kobyliansky, E., Hershkovitz, I. and Arensburg, B. (1985). Use of radiograms of hand bones in predicting age and stature of Bedouin child populations, past and present. *Homo* **36**: 27–39.

Koch, A.R. (1960). Die Frühentwicklung der Clavicula beim Menschen. *Acta Anatomica* **42**: 177–212.

Kodama, G. (1976a). Developmental studies on the presphenoid of the human sphenoid bone. In: *Symposium on the Development of the Basicranium* (J.F. Bosma, Ed.), pp. 142–154. Bethesda, MD: US Department of Health, Education and Welfare.

Kodama, G. (1976b). Developmental studies on the body of the human sphenoid bone. In: *Symposium on the Development of the Basicranium* (J.F. Bosma, Ed.), pp. 156–165. Bethesda, MD: US Department of Health, Education and Welfare.

Kodama, G. (1976c). Developmental studies on the orbitosphenoid of the human sphenoid bone. In: *Symposium on the Development of the Basicranium* (J.F. Bosma, Ed.), pp. 166–176. Bethesda, MD: US Department of Health, Education and Welfare.

Koebke, J. (1978). Some observations on the development of the human hyoid bone. *Anatomy and Embryology* **153**: 279–286.

Koertvelyessy, T. (1972). Relationships between the frontal sinus and climatic conditions: a skeletal approach to cold adaptation. *American Journal of Physical Anthropology* **37**: 161–172.

Kohler, A., Zimmer, E.F. and Wilk, S.P. (1968). *Borderlands of the Normal and Early Pathologic in Skeletal Radiology*, 3rd edition. New York: Grune and Stratton.

Kolar, J.C. and Salter, E.M. (1997). Preoperative anthropometric dysmorphology in metopic synostosis. *American Journal of Physical Anthropology* **103**: 341–351.

Kolas, S., Halperin, V., Jefferis, K., Huddleston, S. and Robinson, H.B.G. (1953). The occurrence of torus palatinus and torus mandibularis in 2476 dental patients. *Oral Surgery, Oral Medicine and Oral Pathology* **6**: 1134–1141.

Kolb, L.W. and Moore, R.D. (1967). Fractures of the supracondylar process of the humerus. *Journal of Bone and Joint Surgery* **49A**: 532–534.

Kolte, D.T. and Mysorekar, V.R. (1966). Tri-partite interparietal bone. *Journal of the Anatomical Society of India* **15**: 96.

Konie, J.C. (1964). Comparative value of X-rays of the spheno-occipital synchondrosis and of the wrist for skeletal age assessment. *Angle Orthodontist* **34**: 303–313.

Kootstra, G., Huffstadt, A.J.C. and Kauer, J.M.G. (1974). The styloid bone: a clinical and embryological study. *The Hand* **6**: 185–189.

Kornberg, M. (1988). MRI diagnosis of traumatic Schmorl's node: a case report. *Spine* **13**: 934–935.

Kósa, F., Antal, A. and Farkas, I. (1990). Electron probe analysis of human teeth for the determination of age. *Medicine, Science and the Law* **30**: 109–114.

Koshy, S. and Tandon, S. (1998). Dental age assessment: the applicability of Demirjian's method in south Indian children. *Forensic Science International* **94**: 73–85.

Koski, K. (1996). Mandibular ramus flexure – indicative of sexual dimorphism? *American Journal of Physical Anthropology* **101**: 545–546.

Koski, K., Haataja, J., and Lappalainen, M. (1961). Skeletal development of hand and wrist in Finnish children. *American Journal of Physical Anthropology* **19**: 379–382.

Kostic, D. and Capecchi, M.R. (1994). Targeted disruption of the murine Hoxa-4 and Hoxa-6 genes results in homeotic transformations of components of the vertebral column. *Mechanisms of Development* **46**: 231–247.

Kostick, E.L. (1963). Facets and imprints on the upper and lower extremities of femora from a western Nigerian population. *Journal of Anatomy* **97**: 393–402.

Krahl, V.E. (1948). The bicipital groove: a visible record of humeral torsion. *Anatomical Record* **101**: 319–331.

Krahl, V.E. (1949). A familial study of palatine and mandibular tori. *Anatomical Record* **103**: 477.

Krahl, V.E. (1976). The phylogeny and ontogeny of humeral torsion. *American Journal of Physical Anthropology* **45**: 595–600.

Krahl, V.E. and Evans, F.G. (1945). Humeral torsion in man. *American Journal of Physical Anthropology* **3**: 229–253.

Kraus, B.S. (1959a). Calcification of the human deciduous teeth. *Journal of the American Dental Association* **59**: 1128–1136.

Kraus, B.S. (1959b). Differential calcification rates in the human primary dentition. *Archives of Oral Biology* **1**: 133–144.

Kraus, B.S. (1960). Prenatal growth and morphology of the human bony palate. *Journal of Dental Research* **39**: 1177–1199.

Kraus, B.S. and Decker, J.D. (1960). The prenatal inter-relationships of the maxilla and premaxilla in the facial development of man. *Acta Anatomica* **40**: 278–294.

Kraus, B.S. and Jordan, R.E. (1965). *The Human Dentition before Birth*. London: Henry Kimpton.

Krayenbuhl, H.A. and Yasargil, M.G. (1968). *Cerebral Angiography*. London: Butterworth.

Krida, A. (1923). Secondary os calcis. *Journal of the American Medical Association* **80**: 752–753.

Krogman, W.M. (1932). The morphological characters of the Australian skull. *Journal of Anatomy* **66**: 399–413.

Krogman, W.M. (1951). The problem of 'timing' in facial growth, with special reference to the period of the changing dentition. *American Journal of Orthodontics* **37**: 253–276.

Krogman, W.M. (1973). *The Human Skeleton in Forensic Medicine*, 1st edition. Springfield, IL: C.C. Thomas.

Krogman, W.M. and Işcan, M.Y. (1986). *The Human Skeleton in Forensic Medicine*, 2nd edition. Springfield, IL: C.C. Thomas.

Kronfeld, R. (1935). First permanent molar: its condition at birth and its postnatal development. *Journal of the American Dental Association* **22**: 1131–1155.

Kronfeld, R. and Schour, I. (1939). Neonatal dental hypoplasia. *Journal of the American Dental Association* **26**: 18–32.

Krukierek, S. (1955). Lowering of pelvic inlet index in the ontogeny and phylogeny of man. *American Journal of Physical Anthropology* **13**: 421–428.

Kruyff, E. (1967). Transverse cleft in the basi-occiput. *Acta Radiologica* **6**: 41–48.

Kuczynski, K. (1968). The proximal interphalangeal joint: anatomy and causes of stiffness in the fingers. *Journal of Bone and Joint Surgery* **50B**: 656–663.

Kuczynski, K. (1974). Carpometacarpal joint of the human thumb. *Journal of Anatomy* **118**: 119–126.

Kuettner, K.E. and Pauli, B.U. (1983). Vascularity of cartilage. In: *Cartilage Vol. 1. Structure, Function and Biochemistry* (B.K. Hall, Ed.), pp. 281–312. New York: Academic Press.

Kuhns, L.R. and Finnstrom, O. (1976). New standards of ossification of the newborn. *Radiology* **119**: 655–660.

Kuhns, L.R., Sherman, M.P. and Poznanski, A.K. (1972). Determination of neonatal maturation on the chest radiograph. *Radiology* **102**: 597–603.

Kuhns, L.R., Sherman, M.P., Poznanski, A.K. and Holt, J.F. (1973a). Humeral head and coracoid ossification in the newborn. *Radiology* **107**: 145–149.

Kuhns, L.R., Poznanski, A.K., Harper, H.A.S. and Garn, S.M. (1973b). Ivory epiphyses of the hand. *Radiology* **109**: 643–648.

Kullman, L., Eklund, B. and Grundin, R. (1990). The value of the frontal sinus in identification of unknown persons. *Journal of Forensic Odonto-Stomatology* **8**: 3–10.

Kusec, V., Simic, D., Chaventre, A., Tobin, J.D., Plato, C.C. and Rudan, P. (1988). Age, sex and bone measurements of the second, third and fourth metacarpals (Island of Pag, SR Croatia, Yugoslavia). *Collegium Anthropologium* **2**: 309–322.

Kusiak, J.F., Zins, J.E. and Whitaker, L.A. (1985). The early revascularization of membranous bone. *Plastic and Reconstructive Surgery* **76**: 510–514.

Kutz, E.R. (1949). Congenital absence of the patellae. *Journal of Pediatrics* **34**: 760–762.

Kvinnsland, S. (1969a). Observations on the early ossification of the upper jaw. *Acta Odontologica Scandinavica* **27**: 649–654.

Kvinnsland, S. (1969b). Observations on the early ossification process of the mandible as seen in plastic embedded human embryos. *Acta Odontologica Scandinavica* **27**: 642–648.

Kyrkanides, S., Kjær, I. and Fischer-Hansen, B. (1993). Development of the basilar part of the occipital bone in normal human fetuses. *Journal of Craniofacial Genetics and Developmental Biology* **13**: 184–192.

Lachman, E. (1953). Pseudoepiphyses in hand and foot. *American Journal of Roentgenology* **70**: 149–151.

Lacroix, P. (1951). *The Organization of Bones.* London: Churchill Livingstone.

Laidlaw, P. (1904). The varieties of the os calcis. Part 1. The carpus. *Journal of Anatomy and Physiology* **38**: 133–143.

Laidlaw, P. (1905). The os calcis. Part II. The processus posterior. *Journal of Anatomy and Physiology* **39**: 161–178.

Laing, P.G. (1953). The blood supply of the femoral shaft. An anatomical study. *Journal of Bone and Joint Surgery* **35B**: 462–466.

Laing, P.G. (1956). The arterial supply of the humerus. *Journal of Bone and Joint Surgery* **38A**: 1105–1116.

Lake, N.C. (1943). *The Foot.* London: Baillière, Tindall and Cox.

Lakhtakia, P.K., Premsagar, I.C., Bisaria, K.K. and Bisaria, S.D. (1991). A tubercle at the anterior margin of the foramen magnum. *Journal of Anatomy* **117**: 209–210.

Lambert, K.L. (1971). The weight-bearing function of the fibula. A strain gauge study. *Journal of Bone and Joint Surgery* **53A**: 507–513.

Lame, E.L. (1977). Iliac rib (developmental anomaly). A case report. *Skeletal Radiology* **2**: 47–49.

Lamont, J.C. (1910). Note of the influence of posture on the facets of the patella. *Journal of Anatomy and Physiology* **44**: 149–150.

Lampl, M. and Johnston, F.E. (1996). Problems in the aging of skeletal juveniles: perspectives from maturation assessments of living children. *American Journal of Physical Anthropology* **101**: 345–355.

Lamy, L. and Weissman, L. (1939). Congenital convex pes valgus. *Journal of Bone and Joint Surgery* **21**: 79–91.

Lancourt, J.E. and Cristini, J.A. (1975). Patella alta and patella infera. *Journal of Bone and Joint Surgery* **57A**: 1112–1115.

Landis, W.J. (1995). The strength of a calcified tissue depends in part on the molecular structure and organization of its constituent mineral crystals in their organic matrix. *Bone* **16**: 533–544.

Landsmeer, J.M.F. (1955). Anatomical and functional investigations on the articulation of the human fingers. *Acta Anatomica* **24**(Suppl.): 5–69.

Landsmeer, J.M.F. (1976). *Atlas of Anatomy of the Hand.* London: Churchill Livingstone.

Lane, W.A. (1886). A coracoclavicular sternal muscle. *Journal of Anatomy and Physiology* **21**: 673–674.

Lane, W.A. (1888). The anatomy and physiology of the shoemaker. *Journal of Anatomy and Physiology* **22**: 593–628.

Lang, J. (1977). Structure and postnatal organization of heretofore uninvestigated and infrequent ossifications of the sella turcica region. *Acta Anatomica* **99**: 121–139.

Lang, J. (1989). *Clinical Anatomy of the Nose, Nasal Cavity and Paranasal Sinuses*, trans. P.M. Stell. New York: Thieme.

Lang, J. (1995). *Skull Base and Related Structures – Atlas of Clinical Anatomy.* Stuttgart: Schattauer.

Lang, J., and Baumeister, R. (1982). Über das Postnatale Wachstum der Nasenhöhle. *Gegenbaurs Morphologisches Jahrbuch* **128**: 354–393.

Lang, F.J. and Haslhofer, L. (1932). Changes in the symphysis pubis and sacro-iliac articulations as a result of pregnancy and childbirth. *Archives of Surgery* **25**: 870–879.

Langman, J. (1975). *Medical Embryology.* London: Williams and Wilkins.

Lanier, R.R. (1939). The presacral vertebrae of American White and Negro males. *American Journal of Physical Anthropology* **25**: 341–420.

Lanier, R.R. (1944). Length of first, twelfth and accessory ribs in American Whites and Negroes; Their relationship to certain vertebral anomalies. *American Journal of Physical Anthropology* **2**: 137–146.

Lannigan, F.J., O'Higgins, P. and McPhie, P. (1993). The vascular supply of the lenticular and long process of the incus. *Clinical Otolaryngology* **18**: 387–389.

Lannigan, F.J., O'Higgins, P., Oxnard, C.E. and McPhie, P. (1995). Age related bone resorption in the normal incus: a case of maladaptive remodelling? *Journal of Anatomy* **186:** 651–655.

Lanz, T. and Wachsmut, W. (1982). *Praktische Anatomie. Zweiter Band, siebter Teil: Rücken.* Berlin: Springer.

Lanzieri, C.F., Duchesneau, P.M., Rosenbloom, S.A., Smith, A.S. and Rosenbaum, A.E. (1988). The significance of asymmetry of the Foramen of Vesalius. *American Journal of Neuroradiology* **9**: 1201–1204.

Lapayowker, M.S. (1960). An unusual variant of the cervical spine. *American Journal of Roentgenology* **83:** 656–659.

Lapidus, P.W. (1932). Congenital fusion of the bones of the foot: with a report of a case of congenital astragaloscaphoid fusion. *Journal of Bone and Joint Surgery* **14A**: 888–894.

Lapidus, P.W. (1933). Os subtibiale. Inconstant bone over the tip of the medial malleolus. *Journal of Bone and Joint Surgery* **15**: 766–771.

Lapidus, P.W. (1939). Congenital unilateral absence of medial sesamoid of the great toe. *Journal of Bone and Joint Surgery* **21A**: 208–209.

Lapidus, P.W. (1940). Sesamoids beneath all the metatarsal heads of both feet; report of a case. *Journal of Bone and Joint Surgery* **22A**: 1059–1062.

Lapidus, P.W., Guidotti, F.P. and Coletti, C.J. (1943). Triphalangeal thumb. Report of six cases. *Surgery, Gynaecology and Obstetrics* **77**: 178–186.

Larsen, W.J. (1993). *Human Embryology*. Edinburgh: Churchill Livingstone.

Larsen, W.J. (1994). *Study Guide for Human Embryology*. Edinburgh: Churchill Livingstone.

Larson, S.G. (1988). Subscapularis function in gibbons and chimpanzees: implications for interpretation of humeral head torsion in hominoids. *American Journal of Physical Anthropology* **76**: 449–462.

Larson, R.L. and McMahan, R.O. (1966). The epiphyses and the childhood athlete. *Journal of the American Medical Association* **196**: 607–612.

Lasker, G.W. (1946). The inheritance of cleidocranial dysostosis. *Human Biology* **18**: 104–126.

Last, R.J. (1973). *Anatomy, Regional and Applied*, 5th edition. Edinburgh: Churchill Livingstone.

Latham, R.A. (1966). Observations on the growth of the cranial base in the human skull. *Journal of Anatomy* **100**: 435.

Latham, R.A. (1970). Maxillary development and growth: the septomaxillary ligament. *Journal of Anatomy* **107**: 471–478.

Latham, R.A. (1971). The development, structure and growth pattern of the human mid-palatal suture. *Journal of Anatomy* **108**: 31–41.

Latham, R.A. (1972). The sella point and postnatal growth of the human cranial base. *American Journal of Orthodontics* **61**: 156–162.

Lau, E.C., Mohandas, T.K., Shapiro, L.J., Slavkin, H.C. and Snead, M.L. (1988). Human amelogenin gene loci are on the X and Y chromosomes. *American Journal of Human Genetics* **43**: A149.

Laughlin, W.S. and Jørgensen, J.B. (1956). Isolate variation in Greenlandic Eskimo crania. *Acta Genetica et Statistica Medica* **6**: 3–12.

Laurenson, R.D. (1963). The chondrification and primary ossification of the human ilium. MD thesis, University of Aberdeen.

Laurenson, R.D. (1964a). The primary ossification of the human ilium. *Anatomical Record* **148**: 209–217.

Laurenson, R.D. (1964b). The chondrification of the human ilium. *Anatomical Record* **148**: 197–202.

Laurenson, R.D. (1965). Development of the acetabular roof in the fetal hip. A histological study. *Journal of Bone and Joint Surgery* **47A**: 975–983.

LaVelle, M. (1995). Natural selection and developmental sexual variation in the human pelvis. *American Journal of Physical Anthropology* **98**: 59–72.

Lavelle, C.L.B. (1974). An analysis of the human femur. *American Journal of Anatomy* **141**: 415–426.

Lavelle, C.L.B. and Moore, W.J. (1970). Proportionate growth of the human jaws between the fourth and seventh months of intrauterine life. *Archives of Oral Biology* **15**: 453–459.

Lawrence, T.W.P. (1894). Position of the optic commissure. *Journal of Anatomy and Physiology* **28**: xviii–xx.

Lawson, J.O.N. (1974). Pelvic anatomy. I. Pelvic floor muscles. *Annals of the Royal College of Surgeons* **54**: 244–252.

Lawson, J.P., Ogden, J.A., Sella, E. and Barwick, K.W. (1984). The painful accessory navicular. *Skeletal Radiology* **12**: 250–262.

Lazar, G. and Schulter-Ellis, F.P. (1980). Intramedullary structure of human metacarpals. *Journal of Hand Surgery* **5**: 477–481.

Lazenby, R.A. (1984). Inherent deficiencies in cortical bone microstructural age estimation techniques. *Ossa* **9**: 95–103.

Leach, R.E. and Bolton, P.E. (1968). Arthritis of the carpometacarpal joint of the thumb. Results of arthrodesis. *Journal of Bone and Joint Surgery* **50A**: 1171–1177.

Leakey, M.D. and Hay, R.L. (1987). Pliocene footprints in the Laetolil beds at Laetoli, Northern Tanzania. *Nature* **287**: 317–323.

Lebret, L. (1962). Growth changes in the palate. *Journal of Dental Research* **41**: 1391–1404.

Lechtig, A., Delgado, H., Lasky, R.E., Klein, R.E., Engle, P.L., Yarbrough, C. and Habicht, J.-P. (1975). Maternal nutrition and fetal growth in developing societies. *American Journal of Diseases of Childhood* **129**: 434–437.

Ledley, R.S., Huang, H.K. and Pence, R.G. (1971). Quantitative study of normal growth and eruption of teeth. *Computers in Biology and Medicine* **1**: 231–241.

LeDouble, A.F. (1903). *Traité des Variations des Os du Crâne de l'Homme*, Vol. 1. Paris: Vigot Frères.

Lee, M.M.C. and Garn, S.M. (1967). Pseudoepiphyses or notches in the non-epiphyseal end of metacarpal bones in healthy children. *Anatomical Record* **159**: 263–272.

Lee, M., Rohmann, C.G. and Wiggins, P. (1966). Skeletal maturity and total number of ossification centres present in hand and wrist radiographs of Chinese children. *American Journal of Physical Anthropology* **25**: 202.

Lee, J., Jaruis, J., Uhthoff, H.K. and Avroch, L. (1992). The fetal acetabulum. A histomorphometric study of acetabular anteversion and femoral head coverage. *Clinical Orthopedics and Related Research* **281**: 48–55.

Lees, R.F. and Caldicott, W.J.H. (1975). Sternal anomalies in congenital heart disease. *American Journal of Roentgenology* **124**: 423–427.

Lees, S. and Prostak, K. (1988). The locus of mineral crystallites in bone. *Connective Tissue Research* **18**: 41–54.

Leet, A.I., MacKenzie, W.G., Szoke, G. and Harcke, H.T. (1999). Injury to the growth plate after Pemberton osteotomy. *Journal of Bone and Joint Surgery* **81A**: 169–176.

Leffmann, R. (1959). Congenital dysplasia of the hip with special reference to congenital subluxation or 'pre-luxation'. *Journal of Bone and Joint Surgery* **41B**: 689–701.

Le Gros Clark, W.E. (1958). *The Tissues of the Body*, 4th edition. Oxford: Clarendon Press.

Le Minor, J.M. (1988). The ventral metacarpo- and metatarsophalangeal sesamoid bones: comparative anatomy and evolutionary aspects. *Morphologisches Jahrbuch* **134**: 693–731.

Le Minor, J.M. (1995). Biphalangeal and triphalangeal toes in the evolution of the human foot. *Acta Anatomica* **154**: 237–242.

Le Minor, J.M. (1997). The retrotransverse foramen of the human atlas vertebra: a distinctive variant within primates. *Acta Anatomica* **160**: 208–212.

Lemons, J.A., Kuhns, L.R. and Poznanski, A.K. (1972). Calcification of the fetal teeth as an index of fetal maturation. *American Journal of Obstetrics and Gynecology* **114**: 628–630.

Le Mouellic, H., Lellemand, Y. and Brulet, P. (1992). Homeosis in the mouse induced by a null mutation in the Hox-3.1 gene. *Cell* **69**: 251–264.

Lemperg, R. and Liliequist, B. (1972). Appearance of the ossification centre in the proximal humeral epiphysis of newborn children. *Acta Radiologica Scandinavica – Diagnosis* **12**: 76–80.

Lempert, J. and Wolff, D. (1945). Histopathology of the incus and the head of the malleus in cases of stapedial ankylosis. *Archives of Otolaryngology* **42**: 339–367.

Lengelé, B.G. and Dhem, A.J. (1988). Length of the styloid process of the temporal bone. *Archives of Otolaryngology and Head and Neck Surgery* **114**: 1003–1006.

Lengelé, B.G. and Dhem, A.J. (1989). Microradiographic and histological study of the styloid process of the temporal bone. *Acta Anatomica* **135**: 193–199.

Lenz, W. (1988). A short history of thalidomide embryopathy. *Teratology* **38**: 203–216.

Lenz, W. and Knapp, K. (1962). Foetal malformation due to thalidomide. *German Medical Monthly* **7**: 253–256.

León, X., Maranillo, E., Mirapeix, R.M., Quer, M. and Sañudo, J.R. (1997). Foramen thyroideum: a comparative study in embryos, fetuses and adults. *Laryngoscope* **107**: 1146–1150.

Letts, M., Smallman, T., Afanasiou, R. and Gouw, G. (1986). Fracture of the pars interarticularis in adolescent athletes: a clinical biometrical analysis. *Journal of Pediatric Orthopaedics* **6**: 40–46.

Leutenegger, W. (1972). Functional aspects of pelvic morphology in simian Primates. *Journal of Human Evolution* **3**: 207–222.

Levesque, G.-Y., Demirjian, A. and Tanguay, R. (1981). Sexual dimorphism in the development, emergence and agenesis of the mandibular third molar. *Journal of Dental Research* **60**: 1735–1741.

Levin, B. (1990). The unilateral wavy clavicle. *Skeletal Radiology* **19**: 519–520.

Levine, M.A. (1950). Patella cubiti. *Journal of Bone and Joint Surgery* **32A**: 686–687.

Levine, E. (1972a). Carpal fusions in children of four South African populations. *American Journal of Physical Anthropology* **37**: 75–83.

Levine, E. (1972b). Notches in the non-epiphyseal ends of the metacarpals and phalanges in children of 4 South African populations. *American Journal of Physical Anthropology* **36**: 407–416.

Levowitz, B.S. and Kletschka, H.D. (1955). Fracture of the fabella. *Journal of Bone and Joint Surgery* **37A**: 876–877.

Lewin, P. (1917). Congenital absence or defects of bones of the extremities. *American Journal of Roentgenology* **4**: 431–448.

Lewin, P. (1929). Epiphyses: their growth, development, injuries and diseases. *American Journal of Diseases of Children* **37**: 141–178.

Lewis, W.H. (1901). The development of the arm in man. *American Journal of Anatomy* **1**: 145–183.

Lewis, W.H. (1920). The cartilaginous skull of a human embryo, twenty-one millimeters in length. *Contributions to Embryology* **9**: 301–324.

Lewis, O.J. (1956). The blood supply of developing long bones with special reference to the metaphysis. *Journal of Bone and Joint Surgery* **38B**: 928–933.

Lewis, O.J. (1958). The tubercle of the tibia. *Journal of Anatomy* **92**: 587–592.

Lewis, O.J. (1959). The coraco-clavicular joint. *Journal of Anatomy* **93**: 296–303.

Lewis, O.J. (1964). The homologies of the mammalian tarsal bones. *Journal of Anatomy* **98**: 195–208.

Lewis, O.J. (1965). The evolution of the muscles interossei in the primate hand. *Anatomical Record* **153**: 275–288.

Lewis, O.J. (1974). The wrist articulation of the anthropoidea. In: *Primate Locomotion* (F.A. Jenkins, Ed.). New York: Academic Press.

Lewis, O.J. (1977). Joint remodelling and the evolution of the human hand. *Journal of Anatomy* **123**: 157–201.

Lewis, O.J. (1980). The joints of the evolving foot. Part II. The intrinsic joints. *Journal of Anatomy* **130**: 833–857.

Lewis, O.J. (1981). Functional morphology of the joints of the evolving foot. *Symposia of the Zoological Society of London* **46**: 169–188.

Lewis, O.J. (1983). The evolutionary emergence and refinement of the mammalian pattern of foot architecture. *Journal of Anatomy* **137**: 21–45.

Lewis, A.B. and Garn, S.M. (1960). The relationship between tooth formation and other maturational factors. *Angle Orthodontist* **30**: 70–77.

Lewis, M. and Roberts, C.A. (1997). Growing pains: the interpretation of stress indicators. *International Journal of Osteoarchaeology* **7**: 581–586.

Lewis, O.J., Hamshere, R.J. and Bucknill, T.M. (1970). The anatomy of the wrist joint. *Journal of Anatomy* **106**: 539–552.

Lewis, M.E., Roberts, C.A. and Manchester, K. (1995). Comparative study of the prevalence of maxillary sinusitis in later medieval urban and rural populations in northern England. *American Journal of Physical Anthropology* **98**: 497–506.

Liberson, F. (1937). Os acromiale – a contested anomaly. *Journal of Bone and Joint Surgery* **19**: 683–689.

Liebman, C. and Freedman, N.B. (1938). Anomalies of the clavicle with a previously unreported variation. *Radiology* **31**: 345–347.

Liliequist, B. and Lundberg, M. (1971). Skeletal and tooth development. A methodologic investigation. *Acta Radiologica* **11**: 97–112.

Lilley, J.M., Stroud, G., Brothwell, D.R. and Williamson, M.H. (1994). *The Jewish Burial Ground at Jewbury.* York: Council for British Archaeology.

Lillie, R.D. (1917). Variations of the canalis hypoglossi. *Anatomical Record* **13**: 131–144.

Limson, M. (1924). Metopism as found in Filipino skulls. *American Journal of Physical Anthropology* **7**: 317–324.

Limson, M. (1932). Observations on the bones of the skull in White and Negro fetuses and infants. *Contributions to Embryology* **23**: 205–222.

Lin, M. (1991). The phylogenetic and ontogenetic development of the clavicle: A review of the literature. Unpublished BSc dissertation, University of London.

Linde, A. (1998). Odontogenesis and Craniofacial Development. *European Journal of Oral Sciences* **106**: Suppl. **1**.

Lindseth, R.E. and Rosene, H.A. (1971). Traumatic separation of the upper femoral epiphysis in a newborn infant. *Journal of Bone and Joint Surgery* **53A**: 1641–1644.

Lindsey, R.W., Peipmeier, J. and Burkus, J.K. (1985). Tortuosity of the vertebral artery: an adventitious finding after cervical trauma. *Journal of Bone and Joint Surgery* **67A**: 806–808.

Lister, G. (1993). *The Hand: Diagnosis and Indications,* 3rd edition. Edinburgh: Churchill Livingstone.

Liversidge, H.M. (1994). Accuracy of age estimation from developing teeth of a population of known age (0–5.4 years). *International Journal of Osteoarchaeology* **4**: 37–45.

Liversidge, H.M. (1995a). Growth standards of human deciduous teeth. *Proceedings of the Tenth International Symposium on Dental* Morphology (R.J. Radlanski and H. Renz, Eds.), pp. 184–189. Berlin: 'M' Marketing Services, C&M Brünne.

Liversidge, H.M. (1995b). Crown formation times of the permanent dentition and root extension rate in humans. In: *Aspects of Dental Biology: Palaeontology, Anthropology and Evolution* (J. Moggi-Cecchi, Ed.), pp. 267–275. Florence: International Institute for the Study of Man.

Liversidge, H.M. and Molleson, T.I. (1999). Developing permanent tooth length as an estimate of age. *Journal of Forensic Sciences* **44**: 917–920.

Liversidge, H.M., Dean, M.C. and Molleson, T.I. (1993). Increasing human tooth length between birth and 5.4 years. *American Journal of Physical Anthropology* **90**: 307–313.

Liversidge, H.M., Herdeg, B. and Rösing, F.W. (1998). Dental age estimation of non-adults. A review of methods and principles. In: *Dental Anthropology, Fundamentals, Limits and Prospects* (K.W. Alt, F.W. Rösing and M.Teschler-Nicola, Eds.), pp. 419–442. Vienna: Springer.

Livingstone, S.K. (1937). Sprengel's deformity. *Journal of Bone and Joint Surgery* **19**: 539–540.

Ljunggren, A.E. (1979). Clavicular function. *Acta Orthopedica Scandinavica* **50**: 261–268.

Lloyd-Roberts, G.C., Williams, D.I. and Braddock, G.T.F. (1959). Pelvic osteotomy in the treatment of ectopia vesicae. *Journal of Bone and Joint Surgery* **41B**: 754–757.

Lloyd-Roberts, G.C., Apley, A.G. and Owen, R. (1975). Reflections upon the aetiology of congenital pseudoarthrosis of the clavicle. *Journal of Bone and Joint Surgery* **57B**: 24–29.

Locke, G.R., Gardner, J.I. and Van Epps, E.F. (1966). Atlas-dens interval (ADI) in children. *American Journal of Roentgenology* **97**: 135–140.

Loevy, H. (1983). Maturation of permanent teeth in Black and Latino children. *Acta de Odontologica Pediatrica* **4**: 59–62.

Logan, W.H.G. and Kronfeld, R. (1933). Development of the human jaws and surrounding structures from birth to the age of fifteen years. *Journal of the American Dental Association* **20**: 379–427.

Lombardi, G. (1961). The occipital vertebra. *American Journal of Roentgenology* **86**: 260–269.

Long, C. (1968). Intrinsic-extrinsic muscle control of the fingers. Electromyographic studies. *Journal of Bone and Joint Surgery* **50A**: 973–984.

Long, C. and Brown, M.E. (1964). Electromyographic kinesiology of the hand: muscles moving the long finger. *Journal of Bone and Joint Surgery* **46A**: 1683–1706.

Longia, G.S., Agarwal, A.K., Thomas, R.J., Jain, P.N. and Saxena, S.K. (1982). Metrical study of rhomboid fossa of clavicle. *Anthropologia Anzeiger* **40**: 101–110.

Lorenzo, R.L., Hungerford, G.D., Blumenthal, B.I., Bradford, B., Sanchez, F. and Haranath, B.S. (1983). Congenital kyphosis and subluxation of the thoraco-lumbar spine due to vertebral aplasia. *Skeletal Radiology* **10**: 255–257.

Loth, S.R. (1995). Age assessment of the Spitalfields cemetery population by rib phase analysis. *American Journal of Human Biology* **7**: 465–471.

Loth, S.R. and Henneberg, M. (1996). Mandibular ramus flexure: a new morphologic indicator of sexual dimorphism in the human skeleton. *American Journal of Physical Anthropology* **99**: 473–485.

Loth, S.R. and Henneberg, M. (1998). Mandibular ramus flexure *is* a good indicator of sexual dimorphism. *American Journal of Physical Anthropology* **105**: 91–92.

Love, S.M., Ganey, T. and Ogden, J.A. (1990). Postnatal epiphyseal development: the distal tibia and fibula. *Journal of Pediatric Orthopaedics* **10**: 298–305.

Lovejoy, C.O. (1988). Evolution of human walking. *Scientific American* **259**: 82–89.

Lovejoy, C.O., Burstein, A.H. and Heiple, K.G. (1976). The biomechanical analysis of bone strength: a method and its application to platycnemia. *American Journal of Physical Anthropology* **44**: 489–505.

Lovejoy, C.O., Meindl, R.S., Mensforth, R.P. and Barton, T.J. (1985a). Multifactorial determination of skeletal age at death: a method and blind tests of its accuracy. *American Journal of Physical Anthropology* **68**: 1–14.

Lovejoy, C.O., Meindl, R.S., Pryzbeck, T.R. and Mensforth, R.P. (1985b). Chronological metamorphosis of the auricular surface of the ilium: a new method for the determination of adult skeletal age at death. *American Journal of Physical Anthropology* **68**: 15–28.

Lovejoy, C.O., Russell, K.F., and Harrison, M.L. (1990). Long bone growth velocity in the Libben population. *American Journal of Human Biology* **2**: 533–541.

Low, A. (1905). Abstract in Proceedings of the Anatomical Society. *Journal of Anatomy and Physiology* **39**: xxvi–xxix.

Low, A. (1909). Further observations on the ossification of the human lower jaw. *Journal of Anatomy and Physiology* **44**: 83–95.

Lowman, R.M., Robinson, F. and McAllister, W.B. (1966). The craniopharyngeal canal. *Acta Radiologica* **5**: 41–54.

Lozanoff, S., Sciulli, P.W. and Schneider, K.N. (1985). Third trochanter incidence and metric trait covariation in the human femur. *Journal of Anatomy* **143**: 149–159.

Lucy, D. and Pollard, A.M. (1995). Further comments on the estimation of error associated with the Gustafson dental age estimation method. *Journal of Forensic Sciences* **40**: 222–227.

Lucy, D., Pollard, A.M. and Roberts, C.A. (1994). A comparison of three dental techniques for estimating age at death in humans. *Journal of Archaeological Science* **22**: 151–156.

Lufti, A.M. (1970). Mode of growth, fate and functions of cartilage canals. *Journal of Anatomy* **106**: 135–145.

Luger, E.J., Nissan, M., Karpf, A., Steinberg, E.L. and Dekel, S. (1999). Patterns of weight distribution under the metatarsal heads. *Journal of Bone and Joint Surgery* **81B**: 199–202.

Luke, D.A. (1976). Development of the secondary palate in man. *Acta Anatomica* **94**: 596–608.

Luke, D.A., Stack, M.V. and Hey, E.N. (1978). A comparison of morphological and gravimetric methods of estimating human foetal age from the dentition. In: *Development, Function and Evolution of Teeth* (P.M. Butler and K.A. Joysey, Eds.), pp. 511–518. London: Academic Press.

Lumley, J.S.P. (1990). *Surface Anatomy: The Anatomical Basis of Clinical Examination.* Edinburgh: Churchill Livingstone.

Lumsden, A.G.S. (1988). Spatial organization of the epithelium and the role of neural crest cells in the initiation of the mammalian tooth germ. *Development* **103-** (Suppl.): 155–169.

Lumsden, A.G.S. and Buchanan, J.A.G. (1986). An experimental study of timing and topography of early tooth development in the mouse embryo with an analysis of the role of innervation. *Archives of Oral Biology* **31**: 301–311.

Lundberg, A., Nemeth, G., Svensson, O.K. and Selvik, G. (1989). The axis of rotation of the ankle joint. *Journal of Bone and Joint Surgery* **71B**: 94–99.

Lundy, J.K. (1980). The mylohyoid bridge in the Khoisan of Southern Africa and its unsuitability as a Mongaloid genetic marker. *American Journal of Physical Anthropology* **53**: 43–48.

Lunt, R.C. and Law, D.B. (1974). A review of the chronology of calcification of deciduous teeth. *Journal of the American Dental Association* **89**: 599–606.

Lurie, L.A., Levy, S. and Lurie, M.L. (1943). Determination of bone age in children. *Journal of Pediatrics* **23**: 131–140.

Lusby, H.L.J. (1959). Naviculo-cuneiform synostosis. *Journal of Bone and Joint Surgery* **41B**: 150.

Lütken, P. (1950). Investigation into the position of the nutrient foramen and the direction of the vessel canals in the shafts of the humerus and femur in man. *Acta Anatomica* **9**: 57–68.

Lykaki, G. and Papadopoulos, N. (1988). The ossified hyoid apparatus–morphology, interpretation, clinical and function significance. *Anatomischer Anzeiger* **166**: 187–193.

Lyritis, G. (1983). Developmental disorders of the proximal epiphysis of the hallux. *Skeletal Radiology* **10**: 250–254.

Lysell, L., Magnusson, B. and Thilander, B. (1962). Time and order of eruption of the primary teeth: a longitudinal study. *Odontologisk Revy* **13**: 217–234.

Maat, G.J.R. (1984). Dating and rating of Harris lines. *American Journal of Physical Anthropology* **63**: 291–299.

Maat, G.J.R. and Mastwijk, R.W. (1995). Ossification status of the jugular growth plate. An aid for age at death determination. *International Journal of Osteoarchaeology* **5**: 163–168.

Maat, G.J.R., Matricali, B. and Van Meerten, E.L. (1996). Postnatal development and structure of the neurocentral junction. Its relevance for spinal surgery. *Spine* **21**: 661–666.

Maat, G.J.R., Mastwijk, R.W. and Van der Velde, E.A. (1997). On the reliability of non-metrical morphological sex determination of the skull compared with that of the pelvis in The Low Countries. *International Journal of Osteoarchaeology* **7**: 575–580.

Macalister, A. (1868). Notes on the homologies and comparative anatomy of the atlas and axis. *Journal of Anatomy and Physiology* **3**: 54–64.

Macalister, A. (1884). Notes on the varieties and morphology of the human lachrymal bone and its accessory ossicles. *Proceedings of the Royal Society of London* **37**: 229–250.

Macalister, A. (1893a). Notes on the development and variations of the atlas. *Journal of Anatomy and Physiology* **27**: 519–542.

Macalister, A. (1893b). Notes on the acromion. *Journal of Anatomy and Physiology* **27**: 245–251.

Macalister, A. (1898). The apertura pyriformis. *Journal of Anatomy and Physiology* **32**: 223–230.

Macauly, D. (1951). Digital markings in radiographs of the skull in children. *British Journal of Radiology* **24**: 647–652.

MacCleod, S. and Lewin, P. (1929). Avulsion of the tuberosity of the ischium. *Journal of the American Medical Association* **92**: 1597.

MacConaill, M.A. (1941). The mechanical anatomy of the carpus and its bearings on some surgical problems. *Journal of Anatomy* **75**: 166–175.

MacConaill, M.A. and Basmajian, J.V. (1969). *Muscles and Movements – A Basis of Human Kinesiology.* Baltimore, MD: Williams and Wilkins.

MacConaill, M.A. and Basmajian, J.V. (1977). *Muscles and Movement.* New York: Krieger.

MacDonald, A., Chatrath, P., Spector, T. and Ellis, H. (1999). Level of termination of the spinal cord and the dural sac: a magnetic resonance study. *Clinical Anatomy* **12**: 149–152.

MacKay, D.H. (1952). Skeletal maturation in the hand: a study of development in East African children. *Transactions of the Royal Society of Tropical Medicine and Hygiene* **46**: 135–151.

MacKay, D.H. and Martin, W.J. (1952). Dentition and physique of Bantu children. *Journal of Tropical Medicine and Hygiene* **55**: 265–275.

Macklin, C.C. (1914). The skull of a human fetus of 40 mm. *American Journal of Anatomy* **16**: 317–385 and 387–426.

Macklin, C.C. (1921). The skull of a human fetus of 43 millimeters greatest length. *Contributions to Embryology* **10**: 57–103.

MacLaughlin, S.M. (1987). An evaluation of current techniques for age and sex determination from adult human skeletal remains. Unpublished PhD dissertation, University of Aberdeen.

MacLaughlin, S.M. (1990a). Epiphyseal fusion at the sternal end of the clavicle in a modern Portuguese skeletal sample. *Antropologia Portuguesa* **8**: 59–68.

MacLaughlin, S.M. (1990b). Manubrio-sternal and manubrio-costal synostosis. Pathological? *Papers on Palaeopathology*, p. 5. Pathological Association Publication. P5.

MacLaughlin, S.M. and Bruce, M.F. (1985). A simple univariate technique for determining sex from fragmentary femora: its application to a Scottish short cist population. *American Journal of Physical Anthropology* **67**: 413–417.

MacLaughlin, S.M. and Bruce, M.F. (1986). The sciatic notch/acetabular index as a discriminator of sex in European skeletal remains. *Journal of Forensic Sciences* **31**: 1380–1390.

MacLaughlin, S.M. and Bruce, M.F. (1987). What is the ventral arc? *Journal of Anatomy* **152**: 231.

MacLaughlin, S.M. and Bruce, M.F. (1990a). The accuracy of sex identification in European skeletal remains using the Phenice characters. *Journal of Forensic Sciences* **35**: 1384–1393.

MacLaughlin, S.M. and Bruce, M.F. (1990b). Morphological sexing of the os pubis. An anatomical approach. *American Journal of Physical Anthropology* **81**: 260–261.

MacLaughlin, S.M. and Cox, M. (1989). The relationship between body size and parturition scars. *Journal of Anatomy* **164**: 256–257.

MacLaughlin, S.M. and Oldale, K.N.M. (1992). Vertebral body diameters and sex prediction. *Annals of Human Biology* **19(3)**: 285–292.

MacLaughlin, S.M. and Watts, B.L. (1992). Manubrio-sternal fusion – radiographic investigation. *Annals of Human Biology* **19**: 216.

MacLaughlin-Black, S.M. and Gunstone, A. (1995). Early fetal maturity assessed from patterns of ossification in the hand and foot. *International Journal of Osteoarchaeology* **5**: 51–59.

MacLennan, W.J. and Caird, F.I. (1973). Measurements of bone thickness from radiographs of a metacarpal bone. *Gerontologia Clinica* **15**: 32–36.

Macnab, I. (1957). Blood supply of the tibia. *Journal of Bone and Joint Surgery* **39B**: 799.

Maderson, P.F. (1967). A comment on the evolutionary origin of vertebrate appendages. *American Naturalist* **101**: 71–78.

Madsen, B. (1963). Osteolysis of acromial end of clavicle following trauma. *British Journal of Radiology* **36**: 822–828.

Magriples, U. and Laitman, J.T. (1987). Developmental changes in the position of the fetal human larynx. *American Journal of Physical Anthropology* **72**: 463–472.

Maier, R.J. (1934). Prenatal diagnosis of lacuna skull (Lükenschädel). *Radiology* **23**: 615–619.

Main, B.J. and Jowett, R.L. (1975). Injuries of the mid tarsal joint. *Journal of Bone and Joint Surgery* **57B**: 89–97.

Mainland, D. (1953). Evaluation of the skeletal age method of estimating children's development. I. Systematic errors in the assessment of roentgenograms. *Pediatrics* **12**: 114–129.

Mainland, D. (1954). Evaluation of the skeletal age method of estimating children's development. II. Variable errors in the assessment of roentgenograms. *Pediatrics* **13**: 165–173.

Mainland, D. (1957). Evaluation of the skeletal age method of estimating children's development. III. Comparison of methods and inspection in the assessment of roentgenograms. *Pediatrics* **20**: 979–992.

Maj, G., Bassani, S., Menini, G. and Zannini, O. (1964). Studies on the eruption of permanent teeth in children with normal occlusion and malocclusion. *Transactions of the European Orthodontic Society* **40**: 107–130.

Malekafzali, S. and Wood, M.B. (1979). Tibial torsion – a simple clinical apparatus for its measurement and its application to a normal adult population. *Clinical Orthopedics and Related Research* **145**: 154–157.

Malhotra, V. and Leeds, N.E. (1984). Case report 277. Occipitalization of the atlas with severe cord compression. *Skeletal Radiology* **12**: 55–58.

Mall, F.P. (1905). On the angle of the elbow. *American Journal of Anatomy* **4**: 391–404.

Mall, F.P. (1906). On ossification centres in human embryos less than one hundred days old. *American Journal of Anatomy* **5**: 433–458.

Malmberg, N. (1944). Occurrence and significance of early periosteal proliferation in the diaphyses of premature infants. *Acta Paediatrica Scandinavica* **32**: 626–633.

Mangieri, J.V. (1973). Peroneal nerve injury from an enlarged fabella. *Journal of Bone and Joint Surgery* **55A**: 395–397.

Mann, R.W. (1990). Calcaneus secundarius: Description and frequency in six skeletal samples. *American Journal of Physical Anthropology* **81**: 17–25.

Mann, R.W. (1993). A method of siding and sequencing human ribs. *Journal of Forensic Sciences* **38**: 151–155.

Mann, R.W. and Murphy, S.P. (1990). *Regional Atlas of Bone Disease. A Guide to Pathologic and Normal Variation in the Human Skeleton.* Springfield, IL: C.C. Thomas.

Mann, R.W., Symes, S.A. and Bass, W.M. (1987). Maxillary suture obliteration: aging the human skeleton based on intact or fragmentary maxilla. *Journal of Forensic Sciences* **32**: 148–157.

Mann, R.W., Jantz, R.L., Bass, W.M. and Willey, P.S. (1991a). Maxillary suture obliteration: a visual method for estimating skeletal age. *Journal of Forensic Sciences* **36**: 781–791.

Mann, R.W., Roberts, C.A., Thomas, M.D. and Davy, D.T. (1991b). Pressure erosion of the femoral trochlea, patella baja and altered patellar surfaces. *American Journal of Physical Anthropology* **85**: 321–327.

Mann, R.W., Thomas, M.D. and Adams, B.J. (1998). Congenital absence of the ulna with humeroradial synostosis in a prehistoric skeleton from Moundville, Alabama. *International Journal of Osteoarchaeology* **8**: 295–299.

Manter, J.T. (1941). Movements of the subtalar and transverse tarsal joints. *Anatomical Record* **80**: 397–410.

Manter, J.T. (1946). Distribution of compression forces in the joints of the human foot. *Anatomical Record* **96**: 313–321.

Manzanares, M.C., Goret-Nicaise, M. and Dehm, A. (1988). Metopic sutural closure in the human skull. *Journal of Anatomy* **161**: 203–215.

Manzi, G., Sperduti, A. and Passarello, P. (1991). Behavior induced auditory exostoses in Imperial Roman society: evidence from coeval urban and rural communities near Rome. *American Journal of Physical Anthropology* **85**: 253–260.

Maples, W.R. and Rice, P.M. (1979). Some difficulties with the Gustafson dental age estimations. *Journal of Forensic Sciences* **24**: 168–172.

March, H.C. (1944). A vertebral anomaly: Probable persistent neurocentral synchondrosis. *American Journal of Roentgenology* **52**: 408–411.

Maresh, M.M. (1940). Paranasal sinuses from birth to late adolescence. I. Size of the paranasal sinuses as observed in routine postero-anterior roentgenograms. *American Journal of Diseases of Children* **60**: 55–78.

Maresh, M.M. (1943). Growth of major long bones in healthy children. *American Journal of Diseases of Children* **66**: 227–257.

Maresh, M.M. (1955). Linear growth of long bones of extremities from infancy through adolescence. *American Journal of Diseases of Children* **89**: 725–742.

Maresh, M.M. (1970). Measurements from roentgenograms. In: *Human Growth and Development* (R.W. McCammon, Ed.), pp. 157–200. Springfield, IL: C.C. Thomas.

Maresh, M.M. (1972). A forty-five year investigation for secular changes in physical maturation. *American Journal of Physical Anthropology* **36**: 103–109.

Marie, P. and Sainton, P. (1968). On hereditary cleido-cranial dysostosis. *Clinical Orthopedics and Related Research* **58**: 5–7.

Marino, E.A. (1995). Sex estimation using the first cervical vertebra. *American Journal of Physical Anthropology* **97**: 127–133.

Marrotta, J.J. and Michelie, L.J. (1992). Os trigonum impingement in dancers. *American Journal of Sports Medicine* **20**: 533–536.

Marshall, J.J. (1888). Judicial executions. *British Medical Journal* **2**: 779–782.

Marshall, D.S. (1955). Precondylar tubercle incidence rates. *American Journal of Physical Anthropology* **13**: 147–151.

Martin, R. (1928). *Lehrbuch der Anthropologie*, 2nd edition, Band 2. Jena: Fischer.

Martin, C.P. (1932). Some variations in the lower end of the femur which are especially prevalent in the bones of primitive people. *Journal of Anatomy* **66**: 371–383.

Martin, C.P. (1933). The cause of torsion of the humerus and of the notch on the anterior edge of the glenoid cavity of the scapula. *Journal of Anatomy* **67**: 573–582.

Martin, E.S. (1936). A study of an Egyptian series of mandibles, with special reference to mathematical methods of sexing. *Biometrika* **28**: 149–178.

Martin, B.F. (1958). The annular ligament of the superior radio-ulnar joint. *Journal of Anatomy* **92**: 473–481.

Martin, E.J. (1960). Incidence of bifidity and related rib abnormalities in Samoa. *American Journal of Physical Anthropology* **18**: 179–187.

Martin, B.F. (1989). Posterior triangle pain: the os trigonum. *Journal of Foot Surgery* **28**: 312–318.

Martin, R. and Saller, K. (1959). *Lehrbuch der Anthropologie*, Vol. 2, 3rd edition. Stuttgart: Fischer.

Martin, R.B., Burr, D.B. and Sharkey, N.A. (1998). *Skeletal Tissue Mechanics.* New York: Springer.

Marubini, E. and Milani, S. (1986). Approaches to the analysis of longitudinal data. In: *Human Growth, A Comprehensive Treatise*, Vol. 3, 2nd edition (F. Falkner and J.M. Tanner, Eds.), pp. 79–94. New York: Plenum Press.

Marvaso, V. and Bernard, G.W. (1977). Initial intramembranous osteogenesis in vitro. *American Journal of Anatomy* **149**: 453–468.

Marzke, M.W. (1971). Origin of the human hand. *American Journal of Physical Anthropology* **34**: 61–84.

Marzke, M.W. and Marzke, R.F. (1987). The third metacarpal styloid process in humans: origin and functions. *American Journal of Physical Anthropology* **73**: 415–431.

Masali, M. (1964). Dati sulla variabilita morfometrica e ponderale degli ossicini dell'udito nell'uomo. *Archivio Italiano e di Embriologia* **69**: 435–446.

Massé, G. and Hunt, E.E. (1963). Skeletal maturation of the hand and wrist in West African children. *Human Biology* **35**: 3–25.

Mathur, A., Tak, S.K. and Kothari, P. (1982). 'Foot length' – A newer approach in neonatal anthropology. *Journal of Tropical Pediatrics* **30**: 333–336.

Matsumo, T., Hasegawa, I. and Masuda, T. (1987). Chondroblastoma arising in the triradiate cartilage. A report of two cases with review of the literature. *Skeletal Radiology* **16**: 216–222.

Matsumura, G., Uchiumi, T., Kida, K., Ichikawa, R. and Kodama, G. (1993). Developmental studies on the interparietal part of the human occipital squama. *Journal of Anatomy* **182**: 197–204.

Matsumura, G., England, M.A., Uchiumi, T. and Kodama, G. (1994). The fusion of ossification centres in the cartilaginous and membranous parts of the occipital squama in human fetuses. *Journal of Anatomy* **185**: 295–300.

Mayfield, J.K., Johnson, R.P. and Kilcoyne, R.F. (1976). The ligaments of the human wrist and their functional significance. *Anatomical Record* **186**: 417–428.

Mayhall, J.T. (1992). Techniques for the study of dental morphology. In: *Skeletal Biology of Past Peoples: Research Methods* (S.R. Saunders and M.A. Katzenberg, Eds.), pp. 59–78. New York: Wiley-Liss.

Mayhall, J.T. and Mayhall, M.F. (1971). Torus mandibularis in two Northwest Territories villages. *American Journal of Physical Anthropology* **34**: 143–148.

Mayhall, J.T., Dahlberg, A.A. and Owen, D.G. (1970). Torus mandibularis in an Alaskan Eskimo population. *American Journal of Physical Anthropology* **33**: 57–60.

Mayordomo, R., Rodriguez-Gallardo, L. and Alvarez, I.S. (1998). Morphological and quantitative studies in the otic region of the neural tube in chick embryos suggest a neuroectodermal origin for the otic placode. *Journal of Anatomy* **193**: 35–48.

Mays, S.A. (1985). The relationship between Harris line formation and bone growth and development. *Journal of Archaeological Science* **12**: 207–220.

Mays, S. (1995). The relationship between Harris lines and other aspects of skeletal development in adults and juveniles. *Journal of Archaeological Science* **22**: 511–520.

Mays, S., de la Rua, C. and Molleson, T.I. (1995). Molar crown height as a means of evaluating dental wear scales for estimating age at death in human skeletal remains. *Journal of Archaeological Science* **22**: 659–670.

Mays, S., Steele, J. and Ford, M. (1999). Directional asymmetry in the human clavicle. *International Journal of Osteoarchaeology* **9**: 18–28.

McAuley, J.P. and Uhthoff, H.K. (1990). The development of the pelvis. In: *The Embryology of the Human Locomotor System* (H.K. Uhthoff, Ed.), pp. 107–116. Berlin: Springer.

McCarthy, S.M. and Ogden, J.A. (1982a). Radiology of postnatal skeletal development. V. Distal humerus. *Skeletal Radiology* **7**: 239–249.

McCarthy, S.M. and Ogden, J.A. (1982b). Radiology of postnatal development. VI. Elbow joint. *Skeletal Radiology* **9**: 17–26.

McCleery, R.S., Kesterson, J.E., Kirtley, J.A. and Love, R.B. (1951). Subclavius and anterior scalene muscle compression as a cause of intermittent obstruction of the subclavian vein. *Annals of Surgery* **133**: 588–602.

McClure, J.G. and Raney, R.B. (1974). Double acromion and coracoid processes: Case report of an anomaly of the scapula. *Journal of Bone and Joint Surgery* **56A**: 830–832.

McClure, J.G. and Raney, R.B. (1975). Anomalies of the scapula. *Clinical Orthopedics and Related Research* **110**: 22–31.

McConnell, A.A. (1906/07). A case of fusion of the semilunar and cuneiform bones. *Journal of Anatomy and Physiology* **41**: 302–303.

McCormick, W.F. (1980). Mineralisation of the costal cartilages as an indicator of age: Preliminary observations. *Journal of Forensic Sciences* **25**: 736–741.

McCormick, W.F. (1981). Sternal foramina in man. *American Journal of Forensic Medicine and Pathology* **2**: 249–252.

McCormick, W.F. (1983). Ossification patterns of costal cartilages as an indicator of sex. *Archives of Pathology and Laboratory Medicine* **107**: 206–210.

McCormick, W.F. and Stewart, J.H. (1988). Age related changes in the human plastron: A roentgenographic and morphologic study. *Journal of Forensic Sciences* **33**: 100–120.

McCormick, W.F., Stewart, J.H. and Langford, L.A. (1985). Sex determination from chest plate roentgenograms. *American Journal of Physical Anthropology* **68**: 173–195.

McCredie, J. (1975). Congenital fusion of bones: radiology, embryology and pathogenesis. *Clinical Radiology* **26**: 47–51.

McCredie, J. (1976). Neural crest defects. A neuroanatomic basis for classification of multiple malformations related to phocomelia. *Journal of the Neurological Sciences* **28**: 373–387.

McCredie, J. (1977). Sclerotome subtraction: a radiological interpretation of reduction deformities of the limbs. *Birth Defects: original article series* **XIII 3D**: 65–77.

McCredie, J. and Willert, H.G. (1999). Longitudinal limb deficiencies and the sclerotomes: An analysis of 378 dysmelic malformations induced by thalidomide. *Journal of Bone and Joint Surgery* **81B**: 9–23.

McDermott, L.J. (1943). Development of the human knee joint. *Archives of Surgery* **46**: 705–719.

McDonnell, D., Nouri, M.R. and Todd, M.E. (1994). The mandibular lingual foramen: a consistent arterial foramen in the middle of the mandible. *Journal of Anatomy* **184**: 363–369.

McDougall, A. (1955). The os trigonum. *Journal of Bone and Joint Surgery* **37B**: 257–265.

McFadden, K.D. and Taylor, J.R. (1989). End plate lesions of the lumbar spine. *Spine* **14**: 867–870.

McGahan, J.P., Rab, G.T. and Dublin, A. (1980). Fractures of the scapula. *Journal of Trauma* **20**: 880–883.

McGoey, P.F. (1943). Fracture dislocation of fused triangular and lunate (congenital). *Journal of Bone and Joint Surgery* **25**: 928–929.

McGregor, I.A., Thomson, A.M. and Billewicz, W.Z. (1968). The development of primary teeth in children from a group of Gambian villages, and critical examination of its use for estimating age. *British Journal of Nutrition* **22**: 307–314.

McHenry, H. (1968). Transverse lines in long bones of prehistoric Californian Indians. *American Journal of Physical Anthropology* **29**: 1–17.

McIntosh, N. (1998). The newborn. In: *Forfar and Arneil's Textbook of Pediatrics*, 5th edition (A.G.M. Campbell and N. McIntosh, Eds.), pp. 93–325. Edinburgh: Churchill Livingstone.

McKern, T.W. and Stewart, T.D. (1957). Skeletal age changes in young American males, analysed from the standpoint of age identification. *Headquarters Quartermaster Research and Development Command*, Technical Report EP-45. Natick, MA.

McKusick, V.A. (1990). *Mendelian Inheritance in Man. Catalogs of Autosomal Dominant, Autosomal Recessive and X-linked Phenotypes* 9th edition. Baltimore, MD: Johns Hopkins University Press.

McLean, F.C. and Urist, M.R. (1955). *Bone: An Introduction to the Physiology of Skeletal Tissue.* Chicago, IL: University Press of Chicago.

McMurrich, J.P. (1914). The nomenclature of the carpal bones. *Anatomical Record* **8**: 173–182.

McRae, D.L. (1953). Bony abnormalities in the region of the foramen magnum: correlation of the anatomic and neurologic findings. *Acta Radiologica* **40**: 335–355.

McRae, D.L. and Barnum, A.S. (1953). Occipitalization of the atlas. *American Journal of Roentgenology* **70**: 23–46.

Meals, R.A. and Seeger, L.L. (1991). *An Atlas of Forearm and Hand Cross- sectional Anatomy: With Computed Tomography and Magnetic Resonance Imaging Correction.* London: Dunitz.

Medlar, R.C. and Lyne, E.D. (1978). Sinding-Larson-Johansson disease. *Journal of Bone and Joint Surgery* **60A**: 1113–1116.

Mednick, L.W. (1955). The evolution of the human ilium. *American Journal of Physical Anthropology* **13**: 203–216.

Mehta, L. and Singh, H.M. (1972). Determination of crown – rump length from fetal long bones: humerus and femur. *American Journal of Physical Anthropology* **36**: 165–168.

Meier, S. (1979). Development of the chick embryo mesoblast. Formation of the embryonic axis and establishment of metameric pattern. *Developmental Biology* **73**: 25–45.

Meier, S. (1981). Development of the chick embryo mesoblast: morphogenesis of the prechordal plate and cranial segments. *Developmental Biology* **83**: 49–61.

Meier, S. and Tam, P.P.L. (1982). Metameric pattern development in the embryonic axis of the mouse. I. Differentiation of the cranial segments. *Differentiation* **21**: 95–108.

Meikle, M.C. (1973). The role of the condyle in postnatal growth of the mandible. *American Journal of Orthodontics* **64**: 50–62.

Meindl, R.S., Lovejoy, C.O., Mensforth, R.P. and Walker, R.A. (1985). A revised method of age determination using the os pubis, with a review and tests of accuracy of other current methods of pubis symphyseal ageing. *American Journal of Physical Anthropology* **68**: 29–45.

Melsen, B. (1969). Time of closure of the spheno-occipital synchondrosis determined on dried skulls. *Acta Odontologica Scandinavica* **27**: 73–90.

Melsen, B. (1972). Time and mode of closure of the spheno-occipital synchondrosis determined on human autopsy material. *Acta Anatomica* **83**: 112–118.

Melsen, B. (1975). Palatal growth studied on human autopsy material. *American Journal of Orthodontics* **68**: 42–54.

Menees, T.O. and Holly, L.E. (1932). The ossification in the extremities of the newborn. *American Journal of Roentgenology* **28**: 389–390.

Menkes, B. and Deleanu, M. (1964). Leg differentiation and experimental syndactyly in chick embryo. *Revue Roumaine, Embryology and Cytology* **1**: 69–77.

Mensforth, R.P. (1985). Relative tibia long bone growth in the Libben and Bt-5 prehistoric skeletal populations. *American Journal of Physical Anthropology* **68**: 247–262.

Merbs, C.F. (1989). Spondylolysis: its nature and anthropological significance. *International Journal of Anthropology* **4**: 163–169.

Merbs, C.F. (1996). Spondylolysis of the sacrum in Alaskan and Canadian Inuit skeletons. *American Journal of Physical Anthropology* **101**: 357–367.

Mercer, J. (1931). The secondary os calcis. *Journal of Anatomy* **66**: 84–97.

Mercer, B.M., Sklar, S., Shariatmadar, A., Gillieson, M.S. and D'Alton, M.E. (1987). Fetal foot length as a predictor of gestational age. *American Journal of Obstetrics and Gynecology* **156**: 350–355.

Merchant, V.L. and Ubelaker, D.H. (1977). Skeletal growth of the protohistoric Arikara. *American Journal of Physical Anthropology* **46**: 61–72.

Meredith, H.V. (1944). Human foot length from embryo to adult. *Human Biology* **16**: 207–282.

Meredith, H.V. (1946). Order and age of eruption for the deciduous dentition. *Journal of Dental Research* **25**: 43–66.

Meredith, H.V. (1957). Change in the profile of the osseous chin during childhood. *American Journal of Physical Anthropology* **15**: 247–252.

Meredith, H.V. (1959). Change in a dimension of the frontal bone during childhood and adolescence. *Anatomical Record* **134**: 769–780.

Meschan, I. (1975). *An Atlas of Anatomy Basic to Radiology.* Philadelphia, PA: W.B. Saunders.

Meyer, A.W. (1924a). The 'cervical fossa' of Allen. *American Journal of Physical Anthropology* **7**: 257–269.

Meyer, A.W. (1924b). Patellar supracondylar fossae. *American Journal of Physical Anthropology* **7**: 271–273.

Meyer, A.W. (1928). Spontaneous dislocation and destruction of tendon of long head of biceps brachii. *Archives of Surgery* **17**: 493–506.

Meyer, A.W. (1934). The genesis of the fossa of Allen and associated structures. *American Journal of Anatomy* **55**: 469–510.

Meyer, D.B. (1978). The appearance of 'cervical ribs' during early fetal development. *Anatomical Record* **190**: 481.

Meyer, D.B. and O'Rahilly, R. (1958). Multiple techniques in the study of the onset of prenatal ossification. *Anatomical Record* **132**: 181–193.

Meyer, D.B. and O'Rahilly, R. (1976). The onset of ossification in the human calcaneus. *Anatomy and Embryology* **150**: 19–33.

Mezaros, T. and Kery, L. (1980). Quantitative analysis of growth of the hip. A radiologic study. *Acta Orthopaedica Scandinavica* **51***:* 275–283.

Michaels, L., Prevost, M.J. and Crang, D.F. (1969). Pathological changes in a case of os odontoideum (separate odontoid process). *Journal of Bone and Joint Surgery* **51A**: 965–972.

Michail, J.P., Theodorou, S., Houliaras, K. and Siatis, N. (1958). Two cases of obstetrical separation (epiphysiolysis) of the upper femoral epiphysis. *Journal of Bone and Joint Surgery* **40B**: 477–482.

Michelson, N. (1945). Studies in physical development. V. The ossification time of the os pisiforme. *Human Biology* **17**: 143–146.

Micozzi, M.S. (1982). Skeletal tuberculosis, pelvic contraction and parturition. *American Journal of Physical Anthropology* **58**: 441–445.

Micozzi, M.S. and de la Paz, J.T. (1977). Triad of Naegele's pelvis, Pott's disease and dystocia. *New England Journal of Medicine* **296**: 231–232.

Middleton, S.B., Foley, S.J. and Foy, M.A. (1995). Partial excision of the clavicle for non-union in National Hunt Jockeys. *Journal of Bone and Joint Surgery* **77B**:778–780.

Milch, R.A., Rall, D.P., Tobie, J.E., Albrecht, J.M. and Trivers, G. (1958). Florescence of tetracycline antibiotics in bone. *Journal of Bone and Joint Surgery* **40A**: 897–910.

Miles, M. (1944). Lateral vertebral dimensions and lateral spinal curvature. *Human Biology* **16**: 153–171.

Miles, A.E.W. (1963). Dentition in the estimation of age. *Journal of Dental Research* **42**: 255–263.

Miles, A.E.W. (1994). Non-union of the epiphysis of the acromion in the skeletal remains of a Scottish population of ca. 1700. *International Journal of Osteoarchaeology* **4**: 149–163.

Miles, A.E.W. (1996). Humeral impingement on the acromion in a Scottish island population of *c.*1600 AD. *International Journal of Osteoarchaeology* **6**: 259–288.

Miles, A.E.W. (1998). New light on the acromial attachment of the human coraco-acromial ligament. *International Journal of Osteoarchaeology* **8**: 274–279.

Miles, A.E.W. (1999). Observations on the undersurface of the skeletalized human acromion in two populations. *International Journal of Osteoarchaeology* **9**: 131–145.

Miles, A.E.W. and Bulman, J.S. (1994). Growth curves of immature bones from a Scottish island population of sixteenth to mid-nineteenth century: limb bone diaphyses and some bones of the hand and foot. *International Journal of Osteoarchaeology* **4**: 121–136.

Miles, A.E.W. and Bulman, J.S. (1995). Growth curves of immature bones from a Scottish island population of sixteenth to mid-nineteenth century: shoulder girdle, ilium, pubis and ischium. *International Journal of Osteoarchaeology* **5**: 15–27.

Milgram, J.W. and Lyne, E.D. (1975). Epiphysiolysis of the proximal femur in very young children. *Clinical Orthopaedics and Related Research* **110**: 146–153.

Miller, R.A. (1932). Evolution of the pectoral girdle and fore limb in the primates. *American Journal of Physical Anthropology* **17**: 1–56.

Miller, J.A. (1953). Studies on the location of the lingula, mandibular foramen and mental foramen. *Anatomical Record* **115**: 349.

Miller, S.C. and Roth, H. (1940). Torus palatinus: a statistical study. *Journal of the American Dental Association* **27**: 1950–1957.

Miller, J.Z., Slemenda, C.W., Meany, F.J., Reister, T.K., Hui, S. and Johnston, C.C. (1991). The relationship of bone mineral density and anthropomorphic variables in healthy male and female children. *Bone and Mineral* **14**: 137–152.

Milliken, R.A. (1937). Os subcalcis. *American Journal of Surgery* **37**: 116–117.

Mills, J.L. (1982). Malformation in infants of diabetic mothers. *Teratology* **25**: 385–394.

Milner, C.E. and Soames, R.W. (1998). A comparison of four *in vivo* methods of measuring tibial torsion. *Journal of Anatomy* **193**: 139–144.

Mina, M. and Kollar, E.J. (1987). The induction of odontogenesis in non-dental mesenchyme combined with early murine mandibular arch epithelium. *Archives of Oral Biology* **32**: 123–127.

Mincer, H.H., Harris, E.F. and Berryman, H.E. (1993). The A.B.F.O. study of third molar development and it use as an estimate of chronological age. *Journal of Forensic Sciences* **38**: 379–390.

Ming-Tzu, P. (1935). Septal apertures in the humerus in the Chinese. *American Journal of Physical Anthropology* **20**: 165–170.

Minnaar, A.B.D. (1952). Congenital fusion of the lunate and triquetral bones in the South African Bantu. *Journal of Bone and Joint Surgery* **34B**: 45–48.

Misra, B.D. (1960). Interparietal bone: a case report. *Journal of the Anatomical Society of India* **9**: 39.

Mitchell, G.A.G. (1938). The significance of lumbosacral transitional vertebrae. *British Journal of Surgery* **24**: 147–158.

Mitchell, J. (1998). The incidence and dimensions of the retroarticular canal of the atlas vertebra. *Acta Anatomica* **163**: 113–120.

Mitchell, G.P. and Gibson, J.M.C. (1967). Excision of calcaneo-navicular bar for painful spasmodic flat foot. *Journal of Bone and Joint Surgery* **49B**: 281–287.

Mittler, D.M. and Sheridan, S.G. (1992). Sex determination in subadults using auricular surface morphology: A forensic science perspective. *Journal of Forensic Sciences* **37**: 1068–1075.

Moermann, M. La V. (1981). Proportions of the second metacarpal in normal versus growth impaired children. *Human Biology* **53**: 599–615.

Molleson, T. (1989). Social implications of mortality patterns of juveniles from Poundbury Camp, Romano-British Cemetery. *Anthropologischer Anzeiger* **47**: 27–38.

Molleson, T. and Cox, M. (1993). *The Spitalfields Project. Volume 2 – The Anthropology – The Middling Sort*, Research Report 86. London: Council for British Archaeology.

Molleson, T.I., Oakley, K.P. and Vogel, J.C. (1972). The antiquity of the human footprints of Tana della Basura. *Journal of Human Evolution* **1**: 467–471.

Molleson, T., Cruse, K. and Mays, S. (1998). Some sexually dimorphic features of the human juvenile skull and their value in sex determination in immature juvenile remains. *Journal of Archaeological Science* **25**: 719–728.

Montagu, M.F.A. (1931). On the primate thumb. *American Journal of Physical Anthropology* **15**: 291–314.

Montagu, M.F.A. (1941). Physical anthropology and anatomy. *American Journal of Physical Anthropology* **28**: 261–271.

Monteiro, H., Pinto, S., Ramos, A. and Tavares, A.S. (1957). Aspects morphologiques des sinus para-nasaux. *Acta Anatomica* **30**: 508–522.

Mooney, M.P. and Siegel, M.I. (1986). Developmental relationship between premaxillary-maxillary suture patency and anterior nasal spine morphology. *Cleft Palate Journal* **23**: 101–107.

Moore, W.J. (1981). *The Mammalian Skull.* Cambridge: Cambridge University Press.

Moore, K.L. (1988). *The Developing Human: Clinically Orientated Embryology.* Philadelphia, PA: W.B. Saunders.

Moore, K.L. (1992). *Clinically Oriented Anatomy*, 3rd edition. London: Williams and Wilkins.

Moore, M.K., Stewart, J.H. and McCormick, W.F. (1988). Anomalies of the human chest plate area – radiographic findings in a large autopsy population. *American Journal of Forensic Medicine and Pathology* **9**: 348–355.

Moorrees, C.F.A. and Kent, R.L. (1978). A step function model using tooth counts to assess the developmental timing of the dentition. *Annals of Human Biology* **5**: 55–68.

Moorrees, C.F.A., Fanning, E.A. and Hunt, E.E. (1963a). Formation and resorption of three deciduous teeth in children. *American Journal of Physical Anthropology* **21**; 205–213.

Moorrees, C.F.A., Fanning, E.A. and Hunt, E.E. (1963b). Age variation of formation stages for ten permanent teeth. *Journal of Dental Research* **42**: 1490–1502.

Moradian-Oldak, J., Weiner, S., Addadi, L., Landis, W.J. and Traub, W. (1991). Electron imaging and diffraction study of individual crystals of bone, mineralized tendon and synthetic carbonate apatite. *Connective Tissue Research* **25:** 219–228.

Morant, G.M. (1936). A biometric study of the human mandible. *Biometrika* **28**: 84–122.

Moreno, P., Bardier, M., Roulleau, J. and Gaubert, J. (1982). L'os odontoïde. A propos d'une observation. *Chirurgie Pédiatrique* **23**: 333–337.

Morgan, J.D. and Somerville, E.W. (1960). Normal and abnormal growth at the upper end of the femur. *Journal of Bone and Joint Surgery* **42B**: 264–272.

Morita, S., Hattori, K., Miyazaki, N. and Tanaka, M. (1971). The appearance of primary ossification centres in the Japanese foot phalanges in the later half of fetal life. *Tokyo Jikeikai Medical Journal* **86**: 711–717.

Morreels, C.L., Cherry, J. and Fabrikant, J.I. (1967). Ossified arytenoid cartilage masquerading as a foreign body. *American Journal of Roentgenology* **101**: 837–838.

Morrissey, M.S.C. and Alun-Jones, T. (1989). A case of jaw locking. *Journal of Laryngology and Otology* **103**: 419.

Morton, D.J. (1922). Evolution of the human foot. *American Journal of Physical Anthropology* **5**: 305–325.

Morton, D.G. (1942a). Observations of the development of pelvic conformation. *American Journal of Obstetrics and Gynaecology* **44**: 799–819.

Morton, D.J. (1942b). *The Human Foot. Its Evolution, Physiology and Functional Disorders.* New York: Columbia University Press.

Morton, D.E. (1950). A comparative anatomico-roentgenological study of the cervical spine of twenty cadavers. *American Journal of Radiology* **63**: 523–529.

Morton, D.G. and Gordon, G. (1952). Observations upon the role of sex hormones in the development of bony pelvic conformation. *American Journal of Obstetrics and Gynaecology* **64**: 292–300.

Morton, D.G. and Hayden, C.T. (1941). A comparative study of male and female pelves in children with a consideration of the etiology of pelvic conformations. *American Journal of Obstetrics and Gynecology* **41**: 485–495.

Moseley, H.F. (1968). The clavicle: its anatomy and function. *Clinical Orthopedics and Related Research* **58**: 17–27.

Moser, R.P. and Wagner, G.N. (1990). Nutrient groove of the ilium, a subtle but important forensic radiographic marker in the identification of victims of severe trauma. *Skeletal Radiology* **19**: 15–19.

Moskalewski, S., Oseicka, A. and Maleczyk, J. (1988). Comparison of bone formed intramuscularly after transplantation of scapular and calvarial osteoblasts. *Bone* **9**: 101–106.

Moss, M.L. (1958). The pathogenesis of artificial cranial deformation. *American Journal of Physical Anthropology* **16**: 269–285.

Moss, M.L. (1959). The pathogenesis of premature cranial synostosis in man. *Acta Anatomica* **37**: 351–370.

Moss, M.L. (1963). Morphological variations of the crista galli and medial orbital margin. *American Journal of Physical Anthropology* **21**: 159–164.

Moss, M.L. and Moss-Salentijn, L. (1977). Analysis of developmental processes possibly related to human dental sexual dimorphism in permanent and deciduous canines. *American Journal of Physical Anthropology* **46**: 407–414.

Moss, M.L. and Noback, C.R. (1958). A longitudinal study of digital epiphyseal fusion in adolescence. *Anatomical Record* **131**: 19–32.

Moss, M.L. and Young, R.W. (1960). A functional approach to craniology. *American Journal of Physical Anthropology* **18**: 281–292.

Moss, M.L., Noback, C.R. and Robertson, G.G. (1955). Critical developmental horizons in human fetal long bones. *American Journal of Anatomy* **97**: 155–175.

Moss, M.L., Noback, C.R. and Robertson, G.G. (1956). Growth of certain human fetal cranial bones. *American Journal of Anatomy* **98**: 191–204.

Moss-Salentijn, L. (1975). Cartilage canals in the human spheno-occipital synchondrosis during fetal life. *Acta Anatomica* **92**: 595–606.

Motateanu, M., Gudinchet, F., Sarraj, H. and Schnyder, P. (1991). Case report 665. Congenital absence of posterior arch of atlas. *Skeletal Radiology* **20**: 231–232.

Motwani, R.C. (1937). Some rare abnormalities of bones in the Anatomy Museum of the Grant Medical College, Bombay. *Journal of Anatomy* **71**: 131–133.

Mudge, M.K., Wood, V.E. and Frykman, G.K. (1984). Rotator cuff tears associated with os acromiale. *Journal of Bone and Joint Surgery* **66A**: 427–429.

Mueller, N., Hamilton, S. and Reid, D.G. (1983). Ossified stylohyoid ligament. *Skeletal Radiology* **10**: 273–275.

Muller, T.P. and Mayhall, J.T. (1971). Analysis of contingency table data on torus mandibularis using a log linear model. *American Journal of Physical Anthropology* **34**: 149–153.

Müller, F. and O'Rahilly, R. (1980). The human chondrocranium at the end of the embryonic period, proper, with particular reference to the nervous system. *American Journal of Anatomy* **159**: 33–58.

Müller, F. and O'Rahilly, R. (1986). Somitic-vertebral correlation and vertebral levels in the human embryo. *American Journal of Anatomy* **177**: 3–19.

Müller, F. and O'Rahilly, R. (1994). Occipitocervical segmentation in staged human embryos. *Journal of Anatomy* **185**: 251–258.

Müller, F. and O'Rahilly, R. (1997). The timing and sequence of appearance of neuromeres and their derivatives in staged human embryos. *Acta Anatomica* **158**: 83–99.

Müller, F., O'Rahilly, R. and Tucker, J.A. (1981). The human larynx at the end of the embryonic period proper. 1. The laryngeal and infrahyoid muscles and their innervation. *Acta Otolaryngologica (Stockh.)* **91**: 323–336.

Müller, F., O'Rahilly, R. and Tucker, J.A. (1985). The human larynx at the end of the embryonic period proper. 2. The laryngeal cavity and the innervation of its lining. *Annals of Otology, Rhinology and Laryngology* **94**: 607–617.

Müller, F., O'Rahilly, R. and Benson, D.R. (1986). The early origin of vertebral anomalies as illustrated by a butterfly vertebra. *Journal of Anatomy* **149**: 157–169.

Mundy, G.R. and Martin, T.J. (1993). *Physiology and Pharmacology of Bone. Handbook of Experimental Pharmacology*, Vol. 107. Berlin: Springer.

Murone, L. (1974). The importance of the sagittal diameters of the cervical spinal canal in relation to spondylosis and myelopathy. *Journal of Bone and Joint Surgery* **56B**: 30–36.

Murphy, T. (1955). The spheno-ethmoidal articulation in the anterior cranial fossa of the Australian aborigine. *American Journal of Physical Anthropology* **13**: 285–300.

Murphy, T. (1956). The pterion in the Australian aborigine. *American Journal of Physical Anthropology* **14**: 225–244.

Murphy, T. (1957a). The chin region of the Australian aboriginal mandible. *American Journal of Physical Anthropology* **15**: 517–535.

Murphy, T. (1957b). Changes in mandibular form during postnatal growth. *Australian Dental Journal* **2**: 267–276.

Murphy, J. and Gooding, C.A. (1970). Evolution of persistently enlarged parietal foramina. *Radiology* **97**: 391–392.

Musgrave, J.H. (1971). How dextrous was Neanderthal man? *Nature* **233**: 538–541.

Musgrave, J.H. and Harneja, N.K. (1978). The estimation of adult stature from metacarpal bone length. *American Journal of Physical Anthropology* **48**: 113–120.

Mysorekar, V. R. (1967). Diaphyseal nutrient foramina in human long bones. *Journal of Anatomy* **101**: 813–822.

Mysorekar, V.R. and Nandedkar, A.N. (1987). The groove in the lateral wall of the human orbit. *Journal of Anatomy* **151**: 255–257.

Nabarro, S. (1952). Calcification of the laryngeal and tracheal cartilages associated with congenital stridor in an infant. *Archives of Disease in Childhood* **27**: 185–186.

Nadgir, Y.G. (1917). The supracondylar tubercles of the femur. *Journal of Anatomy* **51**: 375.

Naegele, F.K. (1839). *Das schrägverengte Becken, nebst einem Anhange über die wichtigsten Fehler des weiblichen Beckens überhaupt.* Mainz: Pynson.

Naito, E., Dewa, K., Yamanouchi, H. and Kominami, R. (1994). Sex typing of forensic DNA samples using male- and female-specific probes. *Journal of Forensic Sciences* **39**: 1009–1017.

Nakahara, H., Dennis, J.E., Bruder, S.P., Haynesworth, S.E., Lennon, D.P. and Caplan, A.I. (1991). In vitro differentiation of bone and hypertrophic cartilage from periosteal derived cells. *Experimental Cell Research* **195**: 492–503.

Nalla, S. and Asvat, R. (1995). Incidence of the coracoclavicular joint in South African populations. *Journal of Anatomy* **186**: 645–649.

Napier, J.R. (1955). The form and function of the carpometacarpal joint of the thumb. *Journal of Anatomy* **89**: 362–369.

Napier, J.R. (1956). The prehensile movements of the human hand. *Journal of Bone and Joint Surgery* **38B**: 902–913.

Napier, J.R. (1957). The foot and the shoe. *Physiotherapy* **43**: 65–74.

Napier, J.R. (1980). *Hands.* London: Allen and Unwin.

Nashold, B.S. and Netsky, M.G. (1959). Foramina, fenestrae and thinness of parietal bones. *Journal of Neuropathology and Experimental Neurology* **18**: 432–441.

Nathan, H. (1959). Spondylolysis. Its anatomy and mechanism of development. *Journal of Bone and Joint Surgery* **41A**: 303–320.

Navani, S., Shah, J.R. and Levy, P.S. (1970). Determination of sex by costal cartilages. *American Journal of Roentgenology* **108**: 771–774.

Nayak, U.V. (1931). A case of abnormal atlas and axis vertebra. *Journal of Anatomy* **65**: 399–400.

Neer, C.S. (1960). Non-union of the clavicle. *Journal of the American Medical Association* **172**: 1006–1011.

Neer, C.S. (1968). Fractures of the distal third of the clavicle. *Clinical Orthopedics and Related Research* **58**: 43–50.

Negus, V.E. (1929). *The Mechanism of the Larynx.* London: Heinemann.

Negus, V.E. (1949). *The Comparative Anatomy and Physiology of the Larynx.* London: Heinemann.

Nelson, G.E., Kelly, P.J., Peterson, L.F.A. and Janes, J.M. (1960). Blood supply of the human tibia. *Journal of Bone and Joint Surgery* **42A**: 625–636.

Nemeskéri, J., Harsányi, L. and Acsádi, G. (1960). Methoden zur Diagnose des Lebensalters von Skeletfunden. *Anthropologische Anzeiger* **24**: 70–95.

Nery, E., Kraus, B.S. and Croup, M. (1970). Timing and topography of early human tooth development. *Archives of Oral Biology* **15**: 1315–1326.

Nesbitt, R. (1736). *Human Osteogeny.* London: Wood.

Neuman, W.F. and Neuman, M.W. (1953). The nature of the mineral phase of bone. *Chemical Reviews* **53**: 1–45.

Newell, R.L.M. (1997). The calcar femorale: a tale of historical neglect. *Clinical Anatomy* **10**: 27–33.

Newman, A. (1969). The supracondylar process and its fracture. *American Journal of Roentgenology* **105**: 844–849.

Newman, K.J. and Meredith, H.V. (1956). Individual growth in skeletal bigonial diameter during the childhood period from 5 to 11 years of age. *American Journal of Anatomy* **99**: 157–187.

Nicholson, D.A. and Driscoll, P.A. (1993). The elbow. *British Medical Journal* **307**: 1058–1062.

Nicholson, J.T. and Sherr, H.H. (1968). Anomalies of the occipito-cervical articulation. *Journal of Bone and Joint Surgery* **50A**: 295–304.

Niida, S., Yamamoto, S. and Kodama, H. (1991). Variation in the running pattern of trabeculae in growing human nasal bones. *Journal of Anatomy* **179**: 39–41.

Niida, S., Yamasaki, K. and Kodama, H. (1992). Interference with interparietal growth in the human skull by the tectum synoticum posterior. *Journal of Anatomy* **180**: 197–200.

Nilsson, A., Isgaard, J. and Lindahl, A. (1987). Effects of unilateral arterial infusion of GH and IGF-1 on tibial longitudinal bone growth in hypophysectionized rats. *Calcified Tissue International* **40**: 91–96.

Njio, B.J. and Kjær, I. (1993). The development and morphology of the incisive fissure and the transverse palatine suture in the human fetal palate. *Journal of Craniofacial Genetics and Developmental Biology* **13**: 24–34.

Noakes, T.D. (1981). The aetiology of hallux valgus. *South African Medical Journal* **59**: 362.

Noback, G.J. (1922). Simple methods of correlating crown–rump and crown–heel lengths of the human fetus. *Anatomical Record* **23**: 241–244.

Noback, C.R. (1943). Some gross structural and quantitative aspects of the developmental anatomy of the human embryonic, fetal and circumnatal skeleton. *Anatomical Record* **87**: 29–51.

Noback, C.R. (1944). The developmental anatomy of the human osseous skeleton during the embryonic, fetal and circumnatal periods. *Anatomical Record* **88**: 91–125.

Noback, C.R. (1954). The appearance of ossification centres and fusion of bones. *American Journal of Physical Anthropology* **12**: 63–70.

Noback, C.R. and Moss, M.L. (1953). The topology of the human premaxillary bone. *American Journal of Physical Anthropology* **11**: 181–187.

Noback, C.R. and Robertson, G.G. (1951). Sequences of appearance of ossification centres in the human skeleton during the first five prenatal months. *American Journal of Anatomy* **89**: 1–28.

Noback, C.R., Moss, M.L. and Leszczynska, E. (1960). Digital epiphyseal fusion of the hand in adolescence: a longitudinal study. *American Journal of Physical Anthropology* **18**: 13–16.

Noden, D.M. (1983). The role of the neural crest in patterning of avian cranial skeletal, connective and muscle tissues. *Developmental Biology* **96**: 144–165.

Noden, D.M. (1988). Interactions and fates of avian craniofacial mesenchyme. *Development* **103**(Suppl.): 121–140.

Nolla, C.M. (1960). The development of the permanent teeth. *Journal of Dentistry for Children* **27**: 254–266.

Nomata, N. (1964). A chronological study of crown formation of the human deciduous dentition. *Bulletin of the Tokyo Medical and Dental School* **11**: 55–76.

Nonaka, K., Ichiki, A. and Miura, T. (1990). Changes in the eruption order of the first permanent teeth and their relation to the season of birth in Japan. *American Journal of Physical Anthropology* **82**: 191–198.

Norberg, O. (1960). Studies of the human jaws and teeth during the first years of life. II The premaxillary region. *Zeitschrift für Anatomie und Entwicklungsgeschichte* **122**: 1–21.

Norberg, O. (1963). Studies of the human jaws and teeth during the first years of life. II The premaxillary region. *Zeitschrift für Anatomie und Entwicklungsgeschichte* **124**: 70–82.

Norman, A., Nelson, J. and Green, S. (1985). Fracture of the hook of the hamate: a diagnosis easily missed. *Radiology* **154**: 49–53.

Northcutt, R.G. and Gans, C. (1983). The genesis of neural crest and epidermal placodes: a reinterpretation of vertebrate origins. *Quarterly Review of Biology* **38**: 1–28.

Nortjé, C.J. (1983). The permanent mandibular third molar, its value in age estimation. *Journal of Forensic Odonto-Stomatology* **1**: 27–31.

Nortjé, C.J., Farman, A.G. and Grotepass, F.W. (1977). Variations in the normal anatomy of the dental (mandibular) canal: a retrospective study of panoramic radiographs from 3612 routine dental patients. *British Journal of Oral Surgery* **15**: 55–63.

Novotny, V. (1983). Sex differences of pelvis and sex determination in paleoanthropology. *Anthropologie* **21**: 65–72.

Novotny, V. (1986). Sex determination of the pelvic bone: a systems approach. *Anthropologie* **24**: 197–205.

Nutter, P.D. (1941). Coracoclavicular articulations. *Journal of Bone and Joint Surgery* **23**: 177–179.

Nyström, M., Kilpinen, E. and Kleemola-Kujala, E. (1977). A radiographic study of the formation of some teeth from 0.5 to 3.0 years of age. *Proceedings of the Finnish Dental Society* **73**: 167–172.

Nyström, M., Evälahti, M. and Laine, P.O. (1986a). Times of natural exfoliation of primary teeth in a group of Finnish children. *Journal of Paediatric Dentistry* **2**: 73–77.

Nyström. M., Haataja, J., Kataja, M., Evälahti, M., Peck, L. and Kleemola-Kujala, E. (1986b). Dental maturity in Finnish children, estimated from the development of seven permanent mandibular teeth. *Acta Odontologica Scandinavica* **44**: 193–198.

O'Bannon, R.P. and Grunow, O.H. (1954). The larynx and pharynx radiologically considered. *Southern Medical Journal* **4**: 310–317.

Obletz, B.E. and Halbstein, B.M. (1938). Non-union of the fractures of carpal navicular. *Journal of Bone and Joint Surgery* **20A**: 424–428.

O'Brien, T.O. (1984). Fractures of the hand and wrist region. In: *Fractures in Children* (C.A. Rockwood, K.E. Wilkins and R.E. King, Eds.), pp. 229–299. Philadelphia, PA: Lippincott.

O'Brien, G.D., Queenan, J.T. and Campbell, S. (1981). Assessment of gestational age in the second trimester by real-time ultrasound measurement of the femur length. *American Journal of Obstetrics and Gynecology* **139**: 540–545.

Oda, J., Tanaka, H. and Tsuzuki, N. (1988). Intervertebral disc changes with aging of human cervical vertebrae. From the neonate to the eighties. *Spine* **13**: 1205–1211.

Odgers, P.N.B. (1931). Two details about the neck of the femur: (1) the eminentia. (2) the empreinte. *Journal of Anatomy* **65**: 352–362.

Odita, J.C., Okolo, A.A. and Omene, J.A. (1985). Sternal ossification in normal human newborn infants. *Pediatric Radiology* **15**: 165–167.

Odita, J.C., Okolo, A.A. and Ukoli, F. (1991). Normal values for metacarpal and phalangeal lengths in Nigerian children. *Skeletal Radiology* **20**: 441–445.

O'Donoghue, D.H. and Sell, L.S. (1942). Persistent olecranon epiphyses in adults. *Journal of Bone and Joint Surgery* **24**: 677–680.

O'Donoghue, D.H. and Sell, L.S. (1943). Congenital talonavicular synostosis. *Journal of Bone and Joint Surgery* **25**: 925–927.

Oelrich, T.M. (1978). Pelvic and perinatal anatomy of the male gorilla: selected observations. *Anatomical Record* **191**: 433–446.

Oestreich, A.E., Maze, W.A., Crawford, A.H. and Morgan, R.C. (1987). The anteater's nose – a direct sign of calcaneonavicular coalition on the lateral radiograph. *Journal of Paediatric Orthopaedics* **7**: 709–711.

Oetteking, B. (1922). Anomalous patellae. *Anatomical Record* **23**: 269–279.

Ogata, S. and Uhthoff, H.K. (1990a). The early development and ossification of the human clavicle – an embryological study. *Acta Orthopedica Scandinavica* **61**: 330–334.

Ogata, S. and Uhthoff, H.K. (1990b). Acromial enthesopathy and rotator cuff tear. *Clinical Orthopedics and Related Research* **254**: 39–48.

Ogawa, K., Yoshida, A., Takahashi, M. and Michimasa, U.I. (1997). Fractures of the coracoid process. *Journal of Bone and Joint Surgery* **79B**: 17–19.

Ogden, J.A. (1974a). Changing patterns of proximal femoral vascularity. *Journal of Bone and Joint Surgery* **56A**: 941–950.

Ogden, J.A. (1974b). The anatomy and function of the proximal tibiofibular joint. *Clinical Orthopaedics and Related Research* **101**: 186–191.

Ogden, J.A. (1974c). Dislocation of the proximal tibiofibular joint. *Journal of Bone and Joint Surgery* **56A**: 145–154.

Ogden, J.A. (1979). The development and growth of the musculo-skeletal system. In: *Scientific Basis of Orthopaedics* (J.A. Albright and R. Brands, Eds.), New York: Appleton-Century-Crofts, pp. 41–103.

Ogden, J.A. (1981). Injury to the growth mechanisms of the immature skeleton. *Skeletal Radiology* **6**: 237–253.

Ogden, J.A. (1984a). Growth slowdown and arrest lines. *Journal of Pediatric Orthopaedics* **4**: 409–415.

Ogden, J.A. (1984b). Radiology of postnatal development. XI. The first cervical vertebra. *Skeletal Radiology* **12**: 12–20.

Ogden, J.A. (1984c). Radiology of postnatal development. XII. The second cervical vertebra. *Skeletal Radiology* **12**: 169–177.

Ogden, J.A. (1984d). The uniqueness of growing bones. In: *Fractures in Children* (C.A. Rockwood, K.E. Wilkins and R.E. King, Eds.), pp. 1–86. Philadelphia, PA: Lippincott.

Ogden, J.A. (1984e). Radiology of postnatal development. X. Patella and tibial tuberosity. *Skeletal Radiology* **11**: 246–257.

Ogden, J.A. (1984f). Radiology of postnatal development. IX. Proximal tibia and fibula. *Skeletal Radiology* **11**: 168–177.

Ogden, J.A. and Lee, J. (1990). Accessory ossification patterns and injuries of the malleoli. *Journal of Pediatric Orthopaedics* **10**: 306–316.

Ogden, J.A. and McCarthy, S.M. (1983). Radiology of postnatal development. VIII. Distal tibia and fibula. *Skeletal Radiology* **10**: 209–220.

Ogden, J.A. and Phillips, S.B. (1983). Radiology of postnatal skeletal development. VII. The scapula. *Skeletal Radiology* **9**: 157–169.

Ogden, J.A. and Southwick, W.O. (1976). Osgood-Schlatter's disease and tibial tuberosity development. *Clinical Orthopaedics and Related Research* **116**: 180–189.

Ogden, J.A., Gossling, H.R. and Southwick, W.O. (1975a). Slipped capital femoral epiphysis following ipsilateral femoral fracture. *Clinical Orthopaedics and Related Research* **110**: 167–170.

Ogden, J.A., Hempton, R.F. and Southwick, W.O. (1975b). Development of the tibial tuberosity. *Anatomical Record* **182**: 431–446.

Ogden, J.A., Conlogue, G.J. and Jensen, P. (1978). Radiology of postnatal development: The proximal humerus. *Skeletal Radiology* **2**: 153–160.

Ogden, J.A., Conlogue, G.J., Bronson, M.L. and Jensen, P.S. (1979a). Radiology of postnatal skeletal development. II. The manubrium and sternum. *Skeletal Radiology* **4**: 189–195.

Ogden, J.A., Conlogue, G.J. and Bronson, M.L. (1979b). Radiology of postnatal skeletal development. III. The Clavicle. *Skeletal Radiology* **4**: 196–203.

Ogden, J.A., Conlogue, G.J., Phillips, S.B. and Bronson, M.L. (1979c). Sprengel's deformity. Radiology of the pathological deformation. *Skeletal Radiology* **4**: 204–208.

Ogden, J.A., Tross, R.B. and Murphy, M.J. (1980). Fracture of the tibial tuberosity in adolescents. *Journal of Bone and Joint Surgery* **62A**: 205–215.

Ogden, J.A., Beall, J.K., Conlogue, G.J. and Light, T.R. (1981). Radiology of postnatal development. IV. Distal radius and ulna. *Skeletal Radiology* **6**: 255–266.

Ogden, J.A., McCarthy, S.M. and Jokl, P. (1982). The painful bipartite patella. *Journal of Pediatric Orthopaedics* **2**: 263–269.

Ogden, J., Murphy, M.J., Southwick, W.O. and Ogden, D.A. (1986). Radiology of postnatal development. XIII. C1-C2 inter-relationships. *Skeletal Radiology* **15**: 433–438.

Ogden, J.A., Ganey, T.H., Light, T.R., Belsole, R.J. and Greene, T.L. (1994). Ossification and pseudoepiphyses formation in the 'non-epiphyseal' ends of bones of the hands and feet. *Skeletal Radiology* **23**: 3–13.

O'Halloran, R.L. and Lundy, J.K. (1987). Age and ossification of the hyoid bone: forensic implications. *Journal of Forensic Sciences* **32**: 1655–1659.

Ohtsuki, F. (1977). Developmental changes of the cranial bone thickness in the human fetal period. *American Journal of Physical Anthropology* **46**: 141–154.

Ohtsuki, F. (1980). Areal growth in the human fetal parietal bone. *American Journal of Physical Anthropology* **53**: 5–9.

Olbrantz, K. and Bohrer, S.P. (1984). Fusion of the anterior arch of the atlas and the dens. *Skeletal Radiology* **12**: 21–22.

Oldale, K.N.M. (1990). An investigation into the effects of sex and age related changes on vertebral morphology. Unpublished BSc dissertation, University of London.

Olivares, F.P. and Schuknecht, H.F. (1979). Width of the internal auditory canal. A histological study. *Annals of Otology, Rhinology and Laryngology* **88**: 316–323.

Olivier, G. (1974). Précision sur la détermination de l'âge d'un foetus d'après sa taille ou la longuer de ses diaphyses. *Médicine Légale et Dommage Corporel* **7**: 297–299.

Olivier, G. (1975). Biometry of the human occipital bone. *Journal of Anatomy* **120**: 507–518.

Olivier, G. and Pineau, H. (1957). Biométrie du scapulum; Asymétrie, corrélations et différences sexuelles. *Archives d'Anatomie de Paris* **33**: 67–88.

Olivier, G. and Pineau, H. (1960). Nouvelle détermination de la taille foetalle d'après les longeurs diaphysaires des os longs. *Annales de Médicine Légale* **40**: 141–144.

Onat, T. and Numan-Cebeci, E. (1976). Sesamoid bones of the hand: Relationships to growth, skeletal and sexual development in girls. *Human Biology* **88**: 659–676.

Oner, F.C. and de Vries, H.R. (1994). Isolated capitolunate coalition. *Journal of Bone and Joint Surgery* **76B**: 845–846.

Oon, C.L. (1963). The size of the pituitary fossa in adults. *British Journal of Radiology* **36**: 294–299.

O'Rahilly, R. (1946). Radial hemimelia and the functional anatomy of the carpus. *Journal of Anatomy* **80**: 179–183.

O'Rahilly, R. (1949). Stereographic reconstruction of developing carpus. *Anatomical Record* **103**: 187–193.

O'Rahilly, R. (1951). Morphological patterns in limb deficiencies and duplications. *American Journal of Anatomy* **89**: 135–194.

O'Rahilly, R. (1952). Anomalous occipital apertures. *American Medical Association Archives of Pathology* **53**: 509–519.

O'Rahilly, R. (1953a). A survey of carpal and tarsal anomalies. *Journal of Bone and Joint Surgery* **35A**: 626–642.

O'Rahilly, R. (1953b). Epitriquetrum, hypotriquetrum and lunatotriquetrum. *Acta Radiologica* **39**: 401–410.

O'Rahilly, R. (1954). The prenatal development of the human centrale. *Anatomical Record* **118**: 334–335.

O'Rahilly, R. (1956/57). Developmental deviations in the carpus and tarsus. *Clinical Orthopedics and Related Research* **10**: 9–18.

O'Rahilly, R. (1959). The development and the developmental disturbances of the limbs. *Irish Journal of Medical Sciences* **397**: 30–33.

O'Rahilly, R. (1973). The human foot. Part 1. Prenatal development. In: *Foot Disorders. Medical and Surgical Management*, 2nd edition (N.J. Giannestras, Ed.), pp. 16–23. Philadelphia, PA: Lea and Febiger.

O'Rahilly, R. (1983). The timing and sequence of events in the development of the human eye and ear during the embryonic period proper. *Anatomy and Embryology* **168**: 87–99.

O'Rahilly, R. (1996). Original sources. *Clinical Anatomy* **9**: 355.

O'Rahilly, R. (1997). 'Gestational Age' – letter to the Editor. *Clinical Anatomy* **10**: 367.

O'Rahilly, R. and Benson, D.R. (1985). The development of the vertebral column. In: *The Pediatric Spine* (D.S. Bradford and R.M. Hensinger, Eds.), pp. 3–18. Stuttgart: Thieme.

O'Rahilly, R. and Gardner, E. (1972). The initial appearance of ossification in staged human embryos. *American Journal of Anatomy* **134**: 291–301.

O'Rahilly, R. and Gardner, E. (1975). The timing and sequence of events in the development of the limbs in the human embryo. *Anatomy and Embryology* **148**: 1–23.

O'Rahilly, R. and Meyer, D.B. (1956). Roentgenographic investigation of the human skeleton during early fetal life. *American Journal of Roentgenology* **76**: 455–468.

O'Rahilly, R. and Müller, F. (1984a). The early development of the hypoglossal nerve and occipital somites in staged human embryos. *American Journal of Anatomy* **169**: 237–257.

O'Rahilly, R. and Müller, F. (1984b). Respiratory and alimentary relations in staged human embryos. New embryological data and congenital anomalies. *Annals of Otology, Rhinology and Laryngology* **93**: 421–429.

O'Rahilly, R. and Müller, F. (1986). The meninges in human development. *Journal of Neuropathology and Experimental Neurology* **45**: 588–608.

O'Rahilly, R. and Müller, F. (1987). *Developmental Stages in Human Embryos: Including a Revision of Streeter's 'Horizons' and a Survey of the Carnegie Collection.* Washington, DC: Carnegie Inst.

O'Rahilly, R. and Tucker, J.A. (1973). The early development of the larynx in staged human embryos. Part 1: embryos of the first five weeks (to stage 15). *Annals of Otology, Rhinology and Laryngology* **82**(Suppl. 7): 3–27.

O'Rahilly, R. and Twohig, M.J. (1952). Foramina parietalia permagna. *American Journal of Roentgenology* **67**: 551–561.

O'Rahilly, R., Gardner, E. and Gray D.J. (1956). The ectodermal thickening and ridge in the limbs of staged human embryos. *Journal of Embryology and Experimental Morphology* **4**: 254–264.

O'Rahilly, R., Gray, D.J. and Gardner, E. (1957). Chondrification in the hands and feet of staged human embryos. *Contributions to Embryology* **36**: 183–192.

O'Rahilly, R., Gardner, E. and Gray, D.J. (1959). The skeletal development of the hand. *Clinical Orthopedics and Related Research* **13**: 42–51.

O'Rahilly, R., Gardner, E. and Gray, D.J. (1960). The skeletal development of the foot. *Clinical Orthopaedics and Related Research* **16**: 7–14.

O'Rahilly, R., Müller, F. and Meyer, D.B. (1980). The human vertebral column at the end of the embryonic period proper. 1. The column as a whole. *Journal of Anatomy* **131**: 565–575.

O'Rahilly, R., Müller, F. and Meyer, D.B. (1983). The human vertebral column at the end of the embryonic period proper. 2. The occipitocervical region. *Journal of Anatomy* **136**: 181–195.

O'Rahilly, R., Müller, F. and Meyer, D.B. (1990a). The human vertebral column at The end of the embryonic period proper. 4. The sacro-coccygeal region. *Journal of Anatomy* **168**: 95–111.

O'Rahilly, R., Müller, F. and Meyer, D.B. (1990b). The human vertebral column at the end of the embryonic period proper. 3. The thoracicolumbar region. *Journal of Anatomy* **168**: 81–93.

Orr, T.G. (1918). Fracture of great toe sesamoid bones. *Annals of Surgery* **67**: 609–612.

Ortiz, M.H. and Brodie, A.G. (1949). On the growth of the human head from birth to the third month of life. *Anatomical Record* **103**: 311–333.

Ortner, D.J. and Putschar, W.G.J. (1985). *Identification of Pathological Conditions in Human Skeletal Remains.* Washington, DC: Smithsonian Institute Press.

Ortolani, M. (1948). *La Lussazione Congenita dell'anca. Nuovi Criteri Diagnostici Profilattico Correttivi.* Bologna: Capelli.

Osborne, D. and Effmann, E.L. (1981). Disturbances of trabecular architecture in the upper end of the femur in childhood. *Skeletal Radiology* **6**: 165–173.

Osborne, D.R., Effmann, E.L., Broda, K. and Harrelson, J. (1980). Development of the upper end of the femur with special reference to its internal architecture. *Radiology* **137**: 71–76.

Ossenberg, N.S. (1970). The influence of artificial cranial deformation on discontinuous morphological traits. *American Journal of Physical Anthropology* **33**: 357–371.

Ossenberg, N.S. (1974). The mylohyoid bridge: an anomalous derivative of Meckel's cartilage. *Journal of Dental Research* **53**: 77–82.

Ossenberg, N.S. (1976). Within and between race distances in population studies based on discrete traits of the human skull. *American Journal of Physical Anthropology* **45**: 701–716.

Ossenberg, N.S. (1986). Temporal crest canal: case report and statistics on a rare mandibular variant. *Oral Surgery, Oral Medicine and Oral Pathology* **62**: 10–12.

Ossenberg, N.S. (1987). Retromolar foramen of the human mandible. *American Journal of Physical Anthropology* **73**: 119–128.

Ossenfort, W.F. (1926). The atlas in Whites and Negroes. *American Journal of Physical Anthropology* **9**: 439–443.

Outland, T. and Murphy, I.D. (1953). Relation of tarsal anomalies to spastic and rigid flat foot. *Clinical Orthopaedics and Related Research* **1**: 217–284.

Overton, L.M. and Grossman, J.W. (1952). Anatomical variations in the articulations between the second and third cervical vertebrae. *Journal of Bone and Joint Surgery* **34A**: 155–161.

Owen, S.A. (1901). Note on the superior tibio fibular joint. *Journal of Anatomy and Physiology* **35**: 489–491.

Owen, R. (1970). Congenital pseudoarthrosis of the clavicle. *Journal of Bone and Joint Surgery* **52B**: 644–652.

Owsley, D.W. and Bradtmiller, B. (1983). Mortality of pregnant females in Arikara villages: osteological evidence. *American Journal of Physical Anthropology* **61**: 331–336.

Owsley, D.W. and Jantz, R.L. (1983). Formation of the permanent dentition in Arikara Indians: timing differences that affect dental age assessments. *American Journal of Physical Anthropology* **61**: 467–471.

Owsley, D.W. and Jantz, R.L. (1985). Long bone lengths and gestational age distribution of post-contact period Arikara Indian perinatal infant skeletons. *American Journal of Physical Anthropology* **68**: 321–329.

Owsley, D.W. and Webb, R.S. (1983). Misclassification probability of dental discrimination functions for sex determination. *Journal of Forensic Sciences* **28**: 181–185.

Oxnard, C.E. (1969). Evolution of the human shoulder. Some possible pathways. *American Journal of Physical Anthropology* **30**: 319–332.

Oxorn, H. (1986). *Human Labour and Birth*, 5th edition. Norwalk: Appleton-Century-Crofts.

Oygucu, I.H., Kurt, M.A., Ikiz, I., Erem, T. and Davies, D.C. (1998). Squatting facets on the neck of the talus and extensions of the trochlear surface of the talus in late Byzantine males. *Journal of Anatomy* **192**: 287–291.

Ozaki, I., Fujimoto, S., Nakagawa, Y., Masuhara, K and Tamai, S. (1988). Tears of the rotator cuff of the shoulder associated with pathologic changes in the acromion. *Journal of Bone and Joint Surgery* **70A**: 1224–1230.

Ozonoff, M.B. (1979). *Pediatric Orthopedic Radiology.* Philadelphia, PA: W.B. Saunders.

Ozonoff, M.B. and Ziter, F.M.H. (1985). The upper femoral notch. *Skeletal Radiology* **14**: 198–199.

Ozonoff, M.B. and Ziter, F.M.H. (1987). The femoral head notch. *Skeletal Radiology* **16**: 19–22.

Pais, M.J., Levine, A. and Pais, S.D. (1978). Coccygeal ribs: development and appearance in two cases. *American Journal of Roentgenology* **131**: 164–166.

Pal, G.P. (1987). Variations of the interparietal bone in man. *Journal of Anatomy* **152**: 205–208.

Pal, G.P. (1989). Weight transmission through the sacrum in man. *Journal of Anatomy* **162**: 9–19.

Pal, G.P. and Routal, R.V. (1986). A study of weight transmission through the cervical and upper thoracic region of the vertebral column in man. *Journal of Anatomy* **148**: 245–261.

Pal, G.P. and Routal, R.V. (1987). Transmission of weight through the lower thoracic and the lumbar region of the vertebral column in man. *Journal of Anatomy* **152**: 93–105.

Pal, G.P. and Routal, R.V. (1996). The role of the vertebral laminae in the stability of the cervical spine. *Journal of Anatomy* **188**: 485–489.

Pal, G.P. and Routal, R.V. (1998). Architecture of the cancellous bone of the human talus. *Anatomical Record* **252**: 185–193.

Pal, G.P., Tamankar, B.P., Routal, R.V. and Bhagwat, S.S. (1984). The ossification of the membranous part of the squamous occipital bone in man. *Journal of Anatomy* **138**: 259–266.

Pal, G.P., Cosio, L. and Routal, R.V. (1988). Trajectory architecture of the trabecular bone between the body and the neural arch in human vertebrae. *Anatomical Record* **222**: 418–425.

Panagis, J.S., Gelberman, R.H., Taleisnik, J. and Baumgaertner, M. (1983). The arterial anatomy of the human carpus. Part II: The intraosseous vascularity. *Journal of Hand Surgery* **8**: 375–382.

Pande, B.S. and Singh, I. (1971). One-sided dominance in the upper limbs of human fetuses as evidenced by asymmetry in muscle and bone weight. *Journal of Anatomy* **109**: 457–459.

Panhuysen, R.G.A.M., Coenen, V. and Bruintjes, Tj.D. (1997). Chronic maxillary sinusitis in medieval Maastricht, The Netherlands. *International Journal of Osteoarchaeology* **7**: 610–614.

Panjabi, M.M., Oxland, R.R., Lin, R-M. and McGowen, T.W. (1994). Thoracolumbar burst fracture. A biomechanical investigation of its multidirectional flexibility. *Spine* **19**: 578–585.

Papadopoulos, N., Lykaki-Anastopoulou, G. and Alvanidou, El. (1989). The shape and size of the human hyoid bone and a proposal for an alternative classification. *Journal of Anatomy* **163**: 249–260.

Papangelou, L. (1972). Study of the human internal auditory canal. *Laryngoscope* **82**: 617–624.

Park, E.A. (1964). The imprinting of nutritional disturbances on the growing bone. *Paediatrics* **33**: 815–862.

Park, E.A. and Richter, C.P. (1953). Transverse lines in bone: mechanism of their development. *Bulletin of the Johns Hopkins Hospital* **93**: 234–248.

Parke, W.W. (1975). Development of the spine. In: *The Spine* (F.A. Simeone, Ed.). London: W.B. Saunders.

Parkin, P.J., Wallis, W.E. and Wilson, J.L. (1978). Vertebral artery occlusion following manipulation of the neck. *New Zealand Medical Journal* **88**: 441–443.

Parsons, F.G. (1895). On the movements of the metacarpophalangeal joint of the thumb. *Journal of Anatomy and Physiology* **29**: 446–452.

Parsons, F.G. (1903). On the meaning of some of the epiphyses of the pelvis. *Journal of Anatomy and Physiology* **37**: 315–323.

Parsons, F.G. (1904). Observations on traction epiphyses. *Journal of Anatomy and Physiology* **38**: 248–258.

Parsons, F.G. (1905). On pressure epiphyses. *Journal of Anatomy and Physiology* **39**: 402–412.

Parsons, F.G. (1906). Observations on the head of the tibia. *Journal of Anatomy and Physiology* **41**: 83–87.

Parsons, F.G. (1908). Further remarks on traction epiphyses. *Journal of Anatomy and Physiology* **42**: 388–396.

Parsons, F.G. (1909). The topography and morphology of the human hyoid bone. *Journal of Anatomy and Physiology* **43**: 279–290.

Parsons, F.G. (1914). The characters of the English thigh bone. *Journal of Anatomy and Physiology* **48**: 238–267.

Parsons, F.G. (1915). The characters of the English thigh bone. Part II – the difficulty of sexing. *Journal of Anatomy and Physiology* **49**: 345–361.

Parsons, F.G. (1916). On the proportions and characteristics of the modern English clavicle. *Journal of Anatomy* **51**: 71–93.

Parsons, T.A. (1973). The snapping scapula and subscapular exostoses. *Journal of Bone and Joint Surgery* **55**: 345–348.

Parsons, F.G. and Keith, A. (1897). Seventh Report of the Committee of Collective Investigation of the Anatomical Society of Great Britain and Ireland for the year 1896–1897. *Journal of Anatomy and Physiology* **32**: 182–186.

Paschal, S.O., Hutton, K.S. and Weatherall, P.T. (1995). Isolated avulsion fracture of the lesser tuberosity of the humerus in adolescents. *Journal of Bone and Joint Surgery* **77A**: 1427–1430.

Patake, S.M. and Mysorekar, R. (1977). Diaphyseal nutrient foramina in human metacarpals and metatarsals. *Journal of Anatomy* **124**: 299–304.

Pate, J.R. (1936). An unusual occipito-atloid articulation. *Journal of Anatomy* **71**: 128–129.

Pate, D., Kursunoglu, S., Resnick, D. and Resnik, C.S. (1985). Scapular foramina. *Skeletal Radiology* **14**: 270–275.

Patel, R.B., Barton, P., Salimi, Z. and Molitor, J. (1983). Computer tomography demonstration of distal femoral (trochlear) groove: a normal variant. *Skeletal Radiology* **10**: 170–172.

Paterson, A.M. (1900). The sternum: its early development and ossification in man and mammals. *Journal of Anatomy and Physiology* **35**: 21–32.

Paterson, A.M. (1904). *The Human Sternum.* London: Williams and Norgate.

Paterson, R.S. (1929). A radiological investigation of the epiphyses of the long bones. *Journal of Anatomy* **64**: 28–46.

Paterson, A.M. and Lovegrove, F.T. (1900). Symmetrical perforations of the parietal bone. *Journal of Anatomy and Physiology* **34**: 228–237.

Patte, D. (1990). The subcoracoid impingement. *Clinical Orthopedics and Related Research* **254**: 55–59

Patterson, R.H. (1935). Surgery for cervical ribs. *Annals of Surgery* **102**: 972–979.

Patterson, R. (1937). Multiple sesamoids of the hands and feet. *Journal of Bone and Joint Surgery* **19**: 531–532.

Paturet, G. (1951). *Traité d'Anatomie Humaine.* Tome III. Paris: Masson et Cie.

Payton, C.G. (1935). The growth of the pelvis in the madder fed pig. *Journal of Anatomy* **69**: 326–343.

Peace, K.A.L. (1992). A morphological, radiological and microscopical investigation of costal cartilage calcification in a cadaveric and an archaeological sample. Unpublished BSc dissertation, University of London.

Peacock, A. (1951). Observations on the prenatal development of the intervertebral disc in man. *Journal of Anatomy* **85**: 260–274.

Peacock, A. (1952). Observations on the postnatal structure of the intervertebral disc in man. *Journal of Anatomy* **86**: 162–179.

Pearson, K. and Bell, J. (1919). A study of the long bones of the English skeleton. Part I. The femur. *Drapers' Company Research Memoirs, Biometric Series* **10**: 1–224.

Pedersen, J.F. (1982). Fetal crown–rump length measurement by ultrasound in normal pregnancy. *British Journal of Obstetrics and Gynaecology* **89**: 926–930.

Peele, J.C. (1957). Unusual anatomical variations of the sphenoid sinuses. *Laryngoscope* **67**: 208–237.

Pendergrass, E.P. and Hodes, P.J. (1937). Rhomboid fossa of clavicle. *American Journal of Roentgenology* **38**: 152–155.

Pendergrass, E.P. and Pepper, O.H.P. (1939). Observations on the process of ossification in the formation of persistent enlarged parietal foramina. *American Journal of Roentgenology* **41**: 343–346.

Penning, L. (1988). Functional significance of the uncovertebral joints. *Annals of the Royal College of Surgeons of England* **70**: 164.

Penny, J.N. and Welsh, R.P. (1981). Shoulder impingement syndromes in athletes and their surgical management. *American Journal of Sports Medicine* **9**: 11–15.

Pepper, O.H.P. and Pendergrass, E.P. (1936). Hereditary occurrence of enlarged parietal foramina (their diagnostic importance). *American Journal of Roentgenology* **35**: 1–8.

Persson, M. and Thilander, B. (1977). Palatal suture closure in man from 15 to 35 years of age. *American Journal of Orthodontics* **72**: 41–52.

Peter, K. (1938). Die Nase des Kindes. In: *Handbuch der Anatomie des Kindes*, Band.2 (K. Peter, G. Wetzel, F. Heiderich, Eds), pp. 205–214. Munich: Bergmann.

Peterson, J. (1998). The Natufian hunting conundrum: spears, atlatls or bows? Musculoskeletal and armature evidence. *International Journal of Osteoarchaeology* **8**: 378–389.

Petrtyl, M., Hert, J. and Fiala, P. (1996). Spatial organization in the haversian bone in man. *Journal of Biomechanics* **29**: 161–170.

Peyton, W.T. and Peterson, H.O. (1942). Congenital deformities in the region of foramen magnum: basilar impression. *Radiology* **38**: 131–144.

Pfitzner, W. (1892). Die Sesambeine des menschlichen Körpers. *Morphologische Arbeiten (Schwalbe)* **1**: 517–762.

Pfitzner, W. (1893). Bemerkungen zum Aufbau des menschlichen Carpus. *Anatomischer Anzeiger* **8**(Suppl.): 186–193.

Pfitzner, W. (1895). Beiträge zur Kenntniss des menschlichen Extremitätenskelets. VI. Die Variationen im Aufbauder Handskelets. *Morphologische Arbeiten (Schwalbe)* **4**: 347–570.

Pfitzner, W. (1896). Beiträge zur Kenntniss des menschlichen Extremitätenskelets. VII Die variationen in Aufbaudes Fussskelets. *Morphologische Arbeiten (Jena)* **6**: 245–527.

Pfitzner, W. (1900). Beiträge zur Kenntniss des menschlichen Extremitätenskelets. VII. Die Morphologischen Elemente des menschlichen Handskelets. *Zeitschrift für Morphologische und Anthropologie* **2**: 77–157, 365–678.

Phelan, J.P., Dainer, M.J. and Cowherd, D.W. (1978). Pregnancy complicated by thoracolumbar scoliosis. *Southern Medical Journal* **71**: 76–78.

Phenice, T.W. (1969). Newly developed visual method of sexing the os pubis. *American Journal of Physical Anthropology* **30**: 297–302.

Phillips, C.G. (1986). *Movements of the Hand.* Liverpool: Liverpool University Press.

Pinnell, S.R. and Crelin, E.S. (1963). Fate of pubic bone autotransplanted to the tibia in estrogen treated adult female mice. *Anatomical Record* **145**: 345.

Pirie, A.H. (1921). Extra bones in the wrist and ankle found by Roentgen rays. *American Journal of Roentgenology* **8**: 569–573.

Pitt, M.J. (1982). Radiology of the femoral linea aspera-pilaster complex: the track sign. *Radiology* **142**: 66.

Plaster, R.L., Schoenecker, P.L. and Capelli, A.M. (1991). Premature closure of the triradiate cartilage: a potential complication of pericapsular acetabuloplasty. *Journal of Pediatric Orthopedics* **11**: 676–678.

Plato, C. and Norris, A.H. (1980). Bone measurements of the second metacarpal and grip strength. *Human Biology* **52**: 131–149.

Plato, C.C. and Norris, A.H. (1981). Measurements of the second metacarpal and lateral hand dominance. *Human Biology – Recent Advances* **1**: 159–173.

Plato, C.C. and Purifoy, F. (1982). Age, sex and bilateral variability in cortical bone loss and measurements of the second metacarpal. *Growth* **46**: 100–112.

Plato, C.C., Wood, J. and Norris, A.H. (1980). Bilateral asymmetry in bone measurements of the hand and lateral hand dominance. *American Journal of Physical Anthropology* **52**: 27–31.

Plato, C.C., Garruto, R.M., Yanagihara, R.T., Chen, K.M., Wood, J.L., Gajdusek, D.C. and Norris, A.H. (1982). Cortical bone loss and measurements of the second metacarpal bone. 1. Comparisons between adult Guamanian Chamorros and American Caucasians. *American Journal of Physical Anthropology* **59**: 461–465.

Plato, C.C., Greulich, W.W., Garruto, R.M. and Yanagihara, R. (1984). Cortical bone loss and measurements of the second metacarpal bone. II. Hypodense bone in post-war Guamanian children. *American Journal of Physical Anthropology* **63**: 57–63.

Platt, L.D., Mederis, A.L., Devore, G.R., Horenstein, J.M., Carlsum, D.E. and Brar, H.S. (1988). Fetal foot length: relationship to menstrual age and fetal measurements in the second trimester. *Obstetrics and Gynecology* **71**: 526–531.

Poland, J. (1898). *Skiagraphic Atlas showing the Development of the Bones of the Wrist and Hand.* London: Smith, Elder.

Polig, E. and Jee, W.S.S. (1990). A model of osteon closure in cortical bone. *Calcified Tissue International* **47**: 261–269.

Pollanen, M.S. and Chiasson, D.A. (1996). Fracture of the hyoid bone in strangulation: comparison of fractured and unfractured hyoids from victims of strangulation. *Journal of Forensic Sciences* **41**: 110–113.

Pollanen, M.S., Bulger, B. and Chiasson, D.A. (1995). The location of hyoid fractures in strangulation revealed by xeroradiography. *Journal of Forensic Sciences* **40**: 303–305.

Pollock, F.J. (1959). Pathology of ossicles in chronic otitis media. *Archives of Otolaryngology* **70**: 421–435.

Pollock, A.N. and Reed, M.H. (1989). Shoulder deformities from obstetrical brachial plexus paralysis. *Skeletal Radiology* **18**: 295–297.

Pons, J. (1955). The sexual diagnosis of isolated bones of the skeleton. *Human Biology* **27**: 12–22.

Ponseti, I.V. (1978a). Morphology of the acetabulum in congenital dislocation of the hip: Gross, histological and roentgenographic studies. *Journal of Bone and Joint Surgery* **60A**: 586–599.

Ponseti, I.V. (1978b). Growth and development of the acetabulum in the normal child. *Journal of Bone and Joint Surgery* **60A**: 575–585.

Ponseti, I.V. (1979). Growth and development of the acetabulum in the normal child. *Journal of Bone and Joint Surgery* **60A**: 575–585.

Popich, G.A. and Smith, D.W. (1972). Fontanels: range of normal size. *Journal of Pediatrics* **80**: 749–752.

Porteous, C.J. (1960). The olecranon epiphyses. *Journal of Anatomy* **94**: 286.

Portinaro, N.M.A., Matthews, S.J.E. and Benson, M.K.D. (1994). The acetabular notch in hip dysplasia. *Journal of Bone and Joint Surgery* **76B**: 271–273.

Posener, K., Walker, E. and Weddell, G. (1939). Radiographic studies of the metacarpal and metatarsal bones in children. *Journal of Anatomy* **74**: 76–79.

Posner, A., Bloch, N.R. and Posner, N.S. (1955). The flat sacrum: its importance in obstetrics. *American Journal of Obstetrics and Gynaecology* **70**: 1021–1025.

Post, R.H. (1969). Tear duct size differences of age, sex and race. *American Journal of Physical Anthropology* **30**: 85–88.

Poswillo, D. (1976). Mechanisms and pathogenesis of malformation. *British Medical Bulletin* **32**: 59–64.

Potter, H.P. (1895). The obliquity of the arm of the female in extension. The relation of the forearm with the upper arm in flexion. *Journal of Anatomy and Physiology* **29**: 488–491.

Potter, H.G., Pavlov, H. and Abrahams, T.G. (1992). The hallux sesamoids revisited. *Skeletal Radiology* **21**: 437–444.

Powell, H.D.W. (1961). Extra centre of ossification for the medial malleolus in children. Incidence and significance. *Journal of Bone and Joint Surgery* **43B**: 107–113.

Powell, K.A. (1991). A radiological and histological investigation into the calcification of costal cartilages. Unpublished BSc dissertation, University of London.

Powell, T.V. and Brodie, A.G. (1963). Closure of the spheno-occipital synchondrosis. *Anatomical Record* **147**: 15–23.

Powell, K.A. and MacLaughlin, S.M. (1992). Costal cartilage calcification as an aid to the identification of sex from human skeletal remains. *Journal of Anatomy* **180**: 357.

Powers, J.H. (1934). Traumatic and developmental abnormalities of the sesamoid bones of the great toe. *American Journal of Surgery* **23**: 315–321.

Pöyry, M., Nyström, M. and Ranta, R. (1986). Comparison of two tooth formation rating methods. *Proceedings of the Finnish Dental Society* **82**: 127–133.

Poznanski, A.K. and Holt, J.F. (1971). The carpals in congenital malformation syndromes. *American Journal of Roentgenology* **112**: 443–459.

Poznanski, A.K., Stern, A.M. and Gall, J.C. (1970). Radiographic findings in the hand-foot uterus syndrome (HFUS). *Radiology* **95**: 129–134.

Poznanski, A.K., Garn, S.M. and Holt, J.F. (1971a). The thumb in congenital malformation syndromes. *Radiology* **100**: 115–129.

Poznanski, A.K., Garn, S.M., Kuhns, L.R. and Sandusky, S.T. (1971b). Dysharmonic maturation of the hand in the congenital malformation syndromes. *American Journal of Physical Anthropology* **35**: 417–432.

Poznanski, A.K., Garn, S.M., Nagy, J.M. and Gall, J.C. (1972). Metacarpophalangeal pattern profiles in the evaluation of skeletal malformation. *Radiology* **104**: 1–11.

Prahl-Andersen, B. and Roede, M.J. (1979). The measurement of skeletal and dental maturity. In: *A Mixed-Longitudinal Interdisciplinary Study of Growth and Development* (B. Prahl-Andersen, C.J. Kowalski and P.H.J.M. Heydendael, Eds.), pp. 491–519. New York: Academic Press.

Prakash, S., Chopra, S.R.K. and Jit, I. (1979). Ossification of the human patella. *Journal of the Anatomical Society of India* **28**: 78–83.

Prasad, R., Vettivel, S., Jayaseelan, L., Isaac, B. and Chandi, G. (1996a). Reconstruction of femur lengths from markers at its proximal end. *Clinical Anatomy* **9**: 28–33.

Prasad, R., Vettivel, S., Isaac, B., Jayaseelan, L. and Chandi, G. (1996b). Angle of torsion of the femur and its correlates. *Clinical Anatomy* **9**: 109–117.

Prescher, A. and Klümpen, T. (1995). Does the area of the glenoid cavity of the scapula show sexual dimorphism? *Journal of Anatomy* **186**: 223–226.

Prescher, A. and Klümpen, T. (1997). The glenoid notch and its relation to the shape of the glenoid cavity of the scapula. *Journal of Anatomy* **190**: 457–460.

Presley, R. and Steel, F.L.D. (1976). On the homology of the alisphenoid. *Journal of Anatomy* **121**: 441–459.

Presley, R. and Steel, F.L.D. (1978). The pterygoid and ectopterygoid in mammals. *Anatomy and Embryology* **154**: 95–110.

Price, J.L. and Molleson, T.I. (1974). A radiographic examination of the left temporal bone of Kabwe Man, Broken Hill, Zambia. *Journal of Archaeological Science* **1**: 285–289.

Priman, J. and Etter, L.E. (1959). The pterygospinous and pterygo-alar bars. *Medical Radiography and Photography* **35**: 2–6.

Pritchard, J.A. and MacDonald, P.C. (1980). *William's Obstetrics.* New York: Appleton-Century-Crofts.

Pritchett, J.W. (1988). Growth and predictions of growth in the upper extremity. *Journal of Bone and Joint Surgery* **70A**: 520–525.

Pritchett, J.W. (1991). Growth plate activity in the upper extremity. *Clinical Orthopaedics and Related Research* **268**: 235–242.

Pritchett, J.W. (1992). Longitudinal growth and growth-plate activity in the lower extremity. *Clinical Orthopaedics and Related Research* **275**: 274–279.

Proctor, B. (1964). The development of the middle ear spaces and their surgical significance. *Journal of Laryngology and Otology* **78**: 631–649.

Proctor, B. (1989). *Surgical Anatomy of the Ear and the Temporal Bone.* New York: Thieme.

Protheroe, K. (1969). Avulsion fractures of the calcaneus. *Journal of Bone and Joint Surgery* **51B**: 118–122.

Pruett, B.S. (1928). On the dimensions of the hypophyseal fossa in man. *American Journal of Physical Anthropology* **11**: 205–222.

Pryde, A.W. and Kitabatake, T. (1959). Brachymesophalangism and brachymetapodia of the hand. *Atomic Bomb Casualty Commission Technical Report* 18–59.

Pryke, S.E.R. (1990). An investigation into the ossification of the laryngeal cartilages. Unpublished BSc dissertation, University of London.

Pryke, S.E.R. (1991). Ossification of the laryngeal cartilages. *Journal of Anatomy* **176**: 236.

Pryor, J.W. (1923). Differences in the time of development of centres of ossification in the male and female skeleton. *Anatomical Record* **25**: 257–273.

Pryor, J.W. (1925). Time of ossification of the bones of the hand of the male and female and union of epiphyses with the diaphyses. *American Journal of Physical Anthropology* **8**: 401–410.

Pulvertaft, R.G. (1977). *The Hand,* 3rd edition. London: Butterworth.

Purves, R.K. and Wedin, P.H. (1950). Familial incidence of cervical ribs. *Journal of Thoracic Surgery* **19**: 952–956.

Putschar, W.G.J. (1976). The structure of the human symphysis pubis with special consideration of parturition and its sequelae. *American Journal of Physical Anthropology* **45**: 589–594.

Puyhaubert, A. (1913). Recherchés sur l'ossification des os des membres chez l'homme. *Journal de l'Anatomie et de la Physiologie Normales et Pathologiques de l'homme et des Animaux* **49**: 119–154, 224–268.

Pyle, S.I. and Hoerr, N.L. (1955). *Radiographic Atlas of Skeletal Development of the Knee.* Springfield, IL: C.C. Thomas.

Pyle, S.I. and Sontag, L.W. (1943). Variability in onset of ossification in epiphyses and short bones of the extremities. *American Journal of Roentgenology* **49**: 795–798.

Pyle, S.I., Waterhouse, A.M. and Greulich, W.W. (1971). *A Radiographic Standard of Reference for the Growing Hand and Wrist.* Chicago, IL: Press of Case Western Reserve University.

Pyo, J. and Lowman, R.M. (1959). The 'ponticulus posticus' of the first cervical vertebra. *Radiology* **72**: 850–854.

Quinlan, W.R., Brady, P.G. and Regan, B.F. (1980). Congenital pseudoarthrosis of the clavicle. *Acta Orthopedica Scandinavica* **51**: 489–492.

Qureshi, A.A. and Kuo, K.N. (1999). Posttraumatic cleidoscapular synostosis following a fracture of the clavicle. *Journal of Bone and Joint Surgery* **81A**: 256–258.

Rak, Y. and Clarke, R.J. (1979). Ear ossicle of *Australopithecus robustus*. *Nature* **279**: 62–63.

Rak, Y., Kimbel, W.H. and Johanson, D.C. (1996). The crescent of foramina in *Australopithecus afarensis* and other early hominids. *American Journal of Physical Anthropology* **101**: 93–99.

Ráliš, Z.A. and McKibbin, B. (1973). Changes in shape of the human hip joint during its development and their relationship to its stability. *Journal of Bone and Joint Surgery* **55B**: 780–785.

Ramachandran, C.R. (1986). A simple device for measurement of foot length in neonates. *Journal of Tropical Pediatrics* **32**: 268–269.

Rambaud, A. and Renault, Ch. (1864). *Origine et Dévelopment des Os.* Paris: Librairie de F. Chamerot.

Rang, M. (1969). *The Growth Plate and its Disorders.* Edinburgh: Churchill Livingstone.

Rank, B.J., Wakefield, A.R. and Hueston, J.T. (1973). *Surgery of Repair as Applied to Hand Injuries.* Edinburgh: Churchill Livingstone.

Rao, P.D.P. (1966). Squatting facets on the talus and tibia in Australian Aborigines. *Archaeology and Physical Anthropology in Oceania* **1**: 51–56.

Rao, N.G. and Pai, L.M. (1988). Costal cartilage calcification pattern – A clue for establishing sex identity. *Forensic Science International* **38**: 193–202.

Rao, K.V.S., Gupta, G.D. and Sehgal, V.N. (1989). Determination of length of human upper limb long bones from their fragments. *Forensic Science International* **41**: 219–223.

Ratcliffe, J.F. (1981). The arterial anatomy of the developing human vertebral body. A microarteriographic study. *Journal of Anatomy* **133**: 625–638.

Ratcliffe, J.F. (1982). An evaluation of the intra-osseous arterial anastomoses in the human vertebral body at different ages. A microarteriographic study. *Journal of Anatomy* **134**: 373–382.

Rathbun, T.A. and Buikstra, J.E. (1984). *Human Identification: Case Studies in Forensic Anthropology.* Springfield, IL: C.C. Thomas.

Ratliff, A.H.C. (1968). Traumatic separation of the upper femoral epiphysis in young children. *Journal of Bone and Joint Surgery* **50B**: 757–770.

Ray, C.D. (1955). Configuration and lateral closure of the superior orbital fissure. *American Journal of Physical Anthropology* **13**: 309–321.

Ray, L.J. (1959). Metrical and non-metrical features of the clavicle of the Australian Aborigine. *American Journal of Physical Anthropology* **17**: 217–226.

Redfield, A. (1970). A new aid to aging immature skeletons: development of the occipital bone. *American Journal of Physical Anthropology* **33**: 207–220.

Redlund-Johnell, I. (1986). The costo-clavicular joint. *Skeletal Radiology* **15**: 25–26.

Reed, M.H. (1993). Ossification of the hyoid bone during childhood. *Canadian Association of Radiologists Journal* **44**: 273–276.

Reid, D.G. (1910). The presence of lachrymo-jugal sutures in two human skulls. *Journal of Anatomy and Physiology* **44**: 249–250.

Reilly, J., Yong-Hing, K., MacKay, R. and Kirkaldy, W. (1978). Pathological anatomy of the lumbar spine. In: *Disorders of the Lumbar Spine* (Helfet and Gruebel, Eds.). London: Lippincott.

Reimann, A.F. and Anson, B.J. (1944). Vertebral level of termination of the spinal cord. *Anatomical Record* **88**: 127–138.

Reinberger, J.R. (1933). A Naegele pelvis with coincidental deformities of the genital tract and extremities. *American Journal of Obstetrics and Gynaecology* **25**: 834–839.

Reinhard, R. and Rösing, F.W. (1985). *Ein Literaturüberblick über Definitionen diskreter Merkmale/anatomischer Varianten am Schädel des Menschen.* Ulm: Selbstverlag.

Reiter, A. (1944). Die frühentwicklung der menschlichen wirbelsäule. III mitteilung. Die entwicklung der lumbalsacral und coccygealwirbelsäule. *Zeitschrift für Anatomie und Entwicklungsgeschichte* **113**: 204–212.

Rengachary, S.S., Burr, D., Lucas, S., Hassanein, K.M., Mohn, M.P. and Matzke, H. (1979). Suprascapular entrapment neuropathy: a clinical, anatomical and comparative study. Part 2: Anatomical Study. *Neurosurgery* **5**: 447–451.

Resnick, D., Vinton, V. and Poteshman, N.L. (1981). Sternocostoclavicular hyperostosis. A report of three new cases. *Journal of Bone and Joint Surgery* **63A**: 1329–1332.

Retrum, R.K., Wepfer, J.F., Olen, D.W. and Laney, W.H. (1986). Late fusion of the olecranon epiphysis. *Skeletal Radiology* **15**: 185–187.

Revesz, G. (1958). *The Human Hand: A Psychological Study.* London: Transl. from Dutch.

Reynolds, E.L. (1931). *The Evolution of the Human Pelvis in Relation to the Mechanics of the Erect Posture.* Harvard University: Peabody Museum of American Archaeology and Ethnology.

Reynolds, E.L. (1945). The bony pelvic girdle in early infancy. A roentgenometric study. *American Journal of Physical Anthropology* **3**: 321–354.

Reynolds, E.L. (1947). The bony pelvis in pre-pubertal childhood. *American Journal of Physical Anthropology* **5**: 165–200.

Reynolds, T.R. (1987). Stride length and its determinants in humans, early hominids, primates and mammals. *American Journal of Physical Anthropology* **72**: 101–115.

Rezaian, S.M. (1974). Congenital absence of the dens of the axis. A case report with tetraplegia. *Paraplegia* **11**: 263–267.

Rhine, S. and Sperry, K. (1991). Radiographic identification by mastoid sinus and arterial pattern. *Journal of Forensic Sciences* **36**: 272–279.

Ribot, I. and Roberts, C. (1996). A study of non-specific stress indicators and skeletal growth in two medieval subadult populations. *Journal of Archaeological Science* **23**: 67–79.

Richany, S.F., Bast, T.H. and Anson, B.J. (1954). The development and adult structure of the malleus, incus and stapes. *Annals of Otology, Rhinology and Laryngology* **63**: 394–434.

Richardson, M.L. and Montana, M.A. (1985). Nutrient canals of the ilium: a normal variant simulating disease on computed tomography. *Skeletal Radiology* **14**: 117–120.

Richenbacher, J., Landolt, A.M. and Theiler, K. (1982). *Applied Anatomy of the Back.* Berlin: Springer.

Ridley, M. (1995). Brief communication: pelvic sexual dimorphism and relative neonatal brain size really are related. *American Journal of Physical Anthropology* **97**: 197–200.

Riepert, T., Drechsler, T., Schild, H., Nafe, B. and Mattern, R. (1996). Estimation of sex on the basis of radiographs of the calcaneus. *Forensic Science International* **77**: 133–140.

Riesenfeld, A. (1955). The variability of the temporal lines, its causes and effects. *American Journal of Physical Anthropology* **13**: 599–620.

Riesenfeld, A. (1956). Multiple infraorbital, ethmoidal and mental foramina in the races of man. *American Journal of Physical Anthropology* **14**: 85–100.

Risser, J.C. (1948). Important practical facts in the treatment of scoliosis. *American Academy of Orthopaedic Surgeons Instructional Course Lectures* **5**: 248–260.

Risser, J.C. (1958). The iliac apophysis: an invaluable sign in the management of scoliosis. *Clinical Orthopaedics and Related Research* **11**: 111–118.

Ritter, M.A., DeRosa, G.P. and Babcock, J.L. (1976). Tibial torsion? *Clinical Orthopaedics and Related Research* **120**: 159–163.

Roach, N.A. and Schweitzer, M.E. (1997). Does osteolysis of the distal clavicle occur following spinal cord injury? *Skeletal Radiology* **26**: 16–19.

Robb, J.E. (1998). The interpretation of skeletal muscle sites: a statistical approach. *International Journal of Osteoarchaeology* **8**: 363–377.

Robbins, R.H. (1917). The human pisiform. *Journal of Anatomy* **51**: 150–152.

Robbins, L.M. (1976). The individuality of human footprints. *Journal of Forensic Sciences* **23**: 778–785.

Robbins, L.M. (1985). *Footprints – their Collection, Analysis and Interpretation.* Springfield, IL: C.C. Thomas.

Roberts, D.F. (1976). Environment and the fetus. In: *The Biology of Human Fetal Growth* (D.F. Roberts and A.M. Thomson, Eds.), pp. 267–283. London: Taylor and Francis.

Roberts, J.M. (1984). Fractures and dislocations of the knee. In: *Fractures in Children* (C.A. Rockwood, K.E. Wilkins and R.E. King, Eds.), pp. 891–982. Philadelphia, PA: Lippincott.

Roberts, C. (1987). Bars of bone on hip bones in antiquity; pathological, occupational or genetic? *Human Evolution* **2**: 539–545.

Roberts, C. and Manchester, K. (1995). *The Archaeology of Disease*, 2nd edition. New York: Cornell University Press.

Robertson, W.G.A. (1935). Recovery after judicial hanging. *British Medical Journal* **1**: 121–122.

Robinow, M. (1942). Appearance of ossification centres: grouping obtained from factor analysis. *American Journal of Diseases of Children* **64**: 229–236.

Robinow, M., Richards, T.W. and Anderson, M. (1942). The eruption of deciduous teeth. *Growth* **6**: 127–133.

Robinson, C.M. (1998). Fractures of the clavicle in the adult: epidemiology and classification. *Journal of Bone and Joint Surgery* **80B**: 476–484.

Robinson, R.A., Braun, R.M., Mack, P. and Zadek, R. (1967). The surgical importance of the clavicular component of Sprengel's deformity. *Journal of Bone and Joint Surgery* **49A**: 1481–1484.

Roche, A.F. (1961). Clinodactyly and brachymesophalangia of the fifth finger. *Acta Pediologica* **50**: 387–391.

Roche, A.F. (1962). Lateral comparisons of the skeletal maturity of the human hand and wrist. *American Journal of Roentgenology* **89**: 1272–1280.

Roche, A.F. (1964a). Aural exostoses in Australian aboriginal skulls. *Annals of Otology, Rhinology and Laryngology* **73**: 82–91.

Roche, A.F. (1964b). Epiphyseal ossification and shaft elongation in human metatarsal bones. *Anatomical Record* **149**: 449–452.

Roche, A.F. (1965). The sites of elongation of the human metacarpals and metatarsals. *Acta Anatomica* **61**: 193–202.

Roche, A.F. (1970). Associations between the rates of maturation of the bones of the hand-wrist. *American Journal of Physical Anthropology* **33**: 341–348.

Roche, A.F. (1986). Bone growth and maturation. In: *Human Growth, A Comprehensive Treatise*, Vol. 2, 2nd edition (F. Falkner and J.M. Tanner, Eds.), pp. 25–60. New York: Plenum Press.

Roche, A.F. and Barkla, D.H. (1965). The level of the larynx during childhood. *Annals of Otology, Rhinology and Laryngology* **74**: 645–654.

Roche, A.F. and Hermann, R.F. (1970). Rates of change in width and length-width ratios of the diaphyses of the hand. *American Journal of Physical Anthropology* **32**: 89–96.

Roche, M.B. and Rowe, G.G. (1951). Anomalous centres of ossification for inferior articular processes of the lumbar vertebrae. *Anatomical Record* **109**: 253–259.

Roche, A.F. and Sunderland, S. (1959). Multiple ossification centres in the epiphyses of the long bones of the human hand and foot. *Journal of Bone and Joint Surgery* **41B**: 375–383.

Rodrigues, K.F. (1973). Injury of the acetabular epiphysis. *Injury* **4**: 258–260.

Rodriguez, J.I., Palacios, J. and Rodriguez, S. (1992). Transverse bone growth and cortical bone mass in the human prenatal period. *Biology of the Neonate* **62**: 23–31.

Roede, M.J. and Van Wieringen, J.C. (1985). Growth diagrams 1980–Netherlands third nation-wide survey. *Tijdschrift voor Sociale Geneeskunde* **63**(Suppl. **1**): 1–34.

Rogers, M.H. and Cleaves, E.N. (1935). The adolescent sacro-iliac joint syndrome. *Journal of Bone and Joint Surgery* **17**: 759–768.

Rogers, W.M. and Gladstone, H. (1950). Vascular foramina and arterial supply of the distal end of the femur. *Journal of Bone and Joint Surgery* **32A**: 867–874.

Rojas, M.A. and Montenegro, M.A. (1995). An anatomical and embryological study of the clavicle in cats (Felis domestus) and sheep (Ovis aries) during the prenatal period. *Acta Anatomica* **154**: 128–134.

Romer, A.S. (1959). *The Vertebrate Story*. Chicago, IL: University of Chicago Press.

Romer, A.S. (1966). *Vertebrate Paleontology*, 3rd edition. Chicago, IL: University of Chicago Press.

Romer, A.S. (1970). *The Vertebrate Body*, 4th edition. Philadelphia, PA: W.B. Saunders.

Romer, A.S. and Parsons, T.S. (1986). *The Vertebrate Body*. Philadelphia, PA: Saunders College Publishing.

Romero, R., Pilu, G., Jeanty, P., Ghidini, A. and Hobbins, J.C. (1988). *Prenatal Diagnosis of Congenital Abnormalities*. Norwalk, CT: Appleton and Lange.

Roncallo, P. (1948). Researches about ossification and conformation of the thyroid cartilage in man. *Acta Otolaryngologica* **36**: 110–134.

Rönning, O. and Kantomaa, T. (1988). The growth pattern of the clavicle in the rat. *Journal of Anatomy* **159**: 173–179.

Roos, D.B. (1976). Congenital anomalies associated with thoracic outlet syndrome. *American Journal of Surgery* **132**: 771–778.

Rosen, H. and Sandick, H. (1955). The measurement of tibiofibular torsion. *Journal of Bone and Joint Surgery* **37A**: 847–855.

Rosenberg, K.R. (1992). The evolution of modern human childbirth. *Yearbook of Physical Anthropology* **35**: 89–124.

Rösing, F.W. (1983). Sexing immature skeletons. *Journal of Human Evolution* **12**: 149–155.

Ross, J.P. (1959). The vascular complications of cervical rib. *Annals of Surgery* **150**: 340–345.

Ross, D.M. and Cruess, R.L. (1977). The surgical correction of congenital elevation of the scapula. *Clinical Orthopedics and Related Research* **125**: 17–21.

Ross, C.F. and Hylander, W.L. (1996). *In vivo* and *in vitro* bone strain in the owl monkey circumorbital region and the function of the postorbital septum. *American Journal of Physical Anthropology* **101**: 183–215.

Rossignol, J.C. (1948). Bilateral congenital pseudoarthrosis of the clavicles treated by costo-scapular fusion. *Journal of Bone and Joint Surgery* **30B**: 220.

Rothman, R.H. and Simeone, F.A. (1975). *The Spine*, Vol. 1. Philadelphia, PA: W.B. Saunders.

Routal, R.V. and Pal, G.P. (1990). Transmission of force from ribs to the vertebral column in man. *Journal of the Anatomical Society of India* **39**: 153–160.

Routal, R.R., Pal, G.P., Bhagwat, S.S. and Tamankar, B.P. (1984). Metrical studies with sexual dimorphism in foramen magnum of human crania. *Journal of the Anatomical Society of India* **33**: 85–89.

Rowe, C.R. (1968). An atlas of anatomy and treatment of midclavicular fractures. *Clinical Orthopedics and Related Research* **58**: 29–42.

Royle, G. (1973). A groove in the lateral wall of the orbit. *Journal of Anatomy* **115**: 461–465.

Ruano-Gill, D. (1988). Embryology. In: *The Foot* (B. Helal and D. Wilson, Eds.), pp. 25–30. Edinburgh: Churchill Livingstone.

Ruano-Gill, D., Nardi-Vilardaga, J. and Tejedo-Mateu, A. (1978). Influence of extrinsic factors on the development of the articular system. *Acta Anatomica* **101**: 36–44.

Ruff, C.B. and Jones, H.H. (1981). Bilateral asymmetry in cortical bone of the humerus and tibia–sex and age factors. *Human Biology* **53**: 69–86.

Rushforth, A.F. (1949). A congenital abnormality of the trapezium and first metacarpal bone. *Journal of Bone and Joint Surgery* **31B**: 543–546.

Rushton, M.A. (1933). On the fine contour lines of the enamel of milk teeth. *Dental Record* **53**: 170–171.

Rushton, M.A. (1944). Growth at the mandibular condyle in relation to some deformities. *British Dental Journal* **76**: 57–68.

Russell, K.F. (1939). The presence of a fronto-palatine articulation in aboriginal Australian skulls. *Journal of Anatomy* **74**: 129–130.

Russo, P.E. and Coin, C.G. (1958). Calcification of the hyoid, thyroid and tracheal cartilages in infancy. *American Journal of Roentgenology* **80**: 440–442.

Rutherford, A. (1985). Fractures of the lateral humeral condyle in children. *Journal of Bone and Joint Surgery* **67A**: 851–864.

Rutherfurd, H. (1921). Bifurcate clavicle. *Journal of Anatomy* **55**: 286–287.

Ruwe, P.A., Gage, J.R., Ozonoff, M.B. and De Luca, P.A. (1992). Clinical determination of femoral anteversion: a comparison with established techniques. *Journal of Bone and Joint Surgery* **74A**: 820–830.

Ryan, M.D. and Taylor, T.K.F. (1984). Odontoid fractures. A rational approach to treatment. *Journal of Bone and Joint Surgery* **64B**: 416–421.

Ryder, C.T. and Mellin, G.W. (1966). A prospective epidemiological study of the clinical and roentgenological characteristics of the hip joint in the first year of life. *Journal of Bone and Joint Surgery* **48A**: 1024.

Sahni, D., Jit, I., Neelam, Suri, S. (1998). Time of fusion of the basisphenoid with the basilar part of the occipital bone in northwest Indian subjects. *Forensic Science International* **98**: 41–45.

Sakalinskas, V. and Jankauskas, R. (1991). An otological investigation of Lithuanian skulls. *International Journal of Osteoarchaeology* **1**: 127–134.

Sakellarides, H. (1961). Pseudoarthrosis of the clavicle. *Journal of Bone and Joint Surgery* **43A**: 130–138.

Saleemi, M.A., Hägg, U., Jalil, F. and Zamani, S. (1994). Timing of emergence of individual primary teeth. *Swedish Dental Journal* **18**: 107–112.

Salisbury, J.R. and Isaacson, P.G. (1985). Demonstration of cytokeratins and an epithelial membrane antigen in chordomas and human fetal notochord. *American Journal of Surgical Pathology* **9**: 791–797.

Salmond, R.W.A. (1919). The recognition and significance of fractures of the patellar border. *British Journal of Surgery* **6**: 463–465.

Salter, R.B. and Harris, W.R. (1963). Injuries including the epiphyseal plate. *Journal of Bone and Joint Surgery* **45A**: 587–622.

Saluja, P.G. (1988). The incidence of spina bifida occulta in a historic and a modern London population. *Journal of Anatomy* **158**: 91–95.

Saluja, G., Fitzpatrick, K., Bruce, M. and Cross, J. (1986). Schmorl's nodes (intravertebral herniations of intervertebral tissue) in two historic British populations. *Journal of Anatomy* **146**: 87–96.

Salvatore, J.E. (1968). Sternoclavicular joint dislocation. *Clinical Orthopaedics and Related Research* **58**: 51–55.

Sammarco, J. (1977). Biomechanics of the ankle. I. Surface velocity and instant centre of rotation in the sagittal plant. *American Journal of Sports Medicine* **5**: 231–234.

Sammarco, G.J. (1988). *Anatomy of the Foot.* In: *The Foot* (B. Helal, and D. Wilson, Eds.). Edinburgh: Churchill Livingstone.

Sanders, C.F. (1966). Sexing by costal cartilage calcification. *British Journal of Radiology* **39**: 233.

Sanders, I., Woesner, M.E., Ferguson, R.A. and Noguchi, T.T. (1972). A new application of forensic radiology: identification of deceased from a single clavicle. *American Journal of Roentgenology* **115**: 619–622.

Sandikcioglu, M., Mølsted, K. and Kjær, I. (1994). The prenatal development of the human nasal and vomeral bones. *Journal of Craniofacial Genetics and Developmental Biology* **14**: 124–134.

Sandström, B. and Hedman, G. (1971). Biphalangia of the lateral toes. A study on the incidence in a Swedish population together with some observations on digital sesamoid bones in the foot. *American Journal of Physical Anthropology* **34**: 37–42.

Sandzen, S.G. (1980). *Atlas of Acute Hand Injuries.* New York: McGraw-Hill.

Santo Neto, H., Penteado, C.V. and De Carvalho, V.C. (1984). Presence of a groove in the lateral wall of the human orbit. *Journal of Anatomy* **138**: 631–633.

Sañudo, J.R., Young, R.C. and Abrahams, P. (1996). Brachioradialis muscle inserting on the third metacarpal. *Journal of Anatomy* **188**: 733–734.

Sapherson, D.A. and Mitchell, S.C.M. (1990). Atraumatic sternal fractures secondary to osteoporosis. *Clinical Radiology* **42**: 250–252.

Sarrafian, S.K. (1983). *Anatomy of the Foot and Ankle*, 2nd edition. Philadelphia, PA: Lippincott.

Sarrafian, S.K. and Topouzian, L.K. (1969). Anatomy and physiology of the extensor apparatus of the toes. *Journal of Bone and Joint Surgery* **51A**: 669–679.

Sasaki, H. and Kodama, G. (1976). Developmental studies on the post sphenoid of the human sphenoid bone. In: *Symposium on the Development of the Basicranium* (J.F. Bosma, Ed.), pp. 177–191. Bethesda, MD: US Department of Health, Education and Welfare.

Sashin, D. (1930). A critical analysis of the anatomy and pathologic changes of the sacro-iliac joints. *Journal of Bone and Joint Surgery* **12**: 891–910.

Sataloff, R.T. (1990). Embryology of the facial nerve and its clinical applications. *Laryngoscope* **100:** 969–984.

Sato, T. and Nakazawa, S. (1982). Morphological classification of the muscular tubercles of the vertebrae. *Ojakimas Folia Anatomica Japonica* **58**: 1175–1186.

Sauer, G.R. and Wuthier, R.E. (1988). Fourier transform infrared characterization of mineral phases formed during induction of mineralization by collagenase-released matrix vesicles in vitro. *Journal of Biological Chemistry* **263**: 13718–13724.

Saunders, E. (1837). *Teeth as a Test of Age, Considered with Reference to the Factory Children: Addressed to the Members of both Houses of Parliament.* London: Renshaw.

Saunders, R.L. de C. H. (1942). The os epipyramis or epitriquetrum. *Anatomical Record* **84**: 17–22.

Saunders, J.W. (1948). The proximo-distal sequence of origin of the parts of the chick wing and the role of the ectoderm. *Journal of Experimental Zoology* **108**: 363–404.

Saunders, S.R. (1989). Nonmetric skeletal variation. In: *Reconstruction of Life from the Skeleton* (M.Y. Işcan and K.A.R. Kennedy, Eds.), pp. 95–108. New York: Alan R. Liss.

Saunders, S.R. (1992). Subadult skeletons and growth related studies. In: *Skeletal Biology of Past Peoples: Research Methods* (S.R. Saunders and M.A. Katzenberg, Eds.), pp. 1–20. New York: Wiley-Liss.

Saunders, S.R. and DeVito, C. (1991). Subadult skeletons in the Raymond Dart Anatomical Collection: research potential. *Human Evolution* **6**: 421–434.

Saunders, S.R. and Hoppa, R.D. (1993). Growth deficit in survivors and non-survivors: biological mortality bias in subadult skeletal samples. *Yearbook of Physical Anthropology* **36**: 127–151.

Saunders, S.R. and Melbye, F.J. (1990). Subadult mortality and skeletal indicators of health in Late Woodland Ontario Iroquois. *Canadian Journal of Archaeology* **14**: 61–74.

Saunders, S.R. and Popovich, F. (1978). A family study of two skeletal variants – Atlas bridging and clinoid bridging. *American Journal of Physical Anthropology* **49**: 193–204.

Saunders, S., Hoppa, R. and Southern, R. (1993a). Diaphyseal growth in a nineteenth-century skeletal sample of subadults from St Thomas' Church, Belleville, Ontario. *International Journal of Osteoarchaeology* **3**: 265–281.

Saunders, S., DeVito, C., Herring, A., Southern, R. and Hoppa, R. (1993b). Accuracy tests of tooth formation age estimations for human skeletal remains. *American Journal of Physical Anthropology* **92**: 173–188.

Saupe, H. (1943). Primäre Knochenmarkseiterung der Kniescheibe. *Deutsche Zeitschrift für Chirurgie* **258**: 386–392.

Sawhney, A. and Bahl, I. (1989). Commonly overlooked duplication of foramen transversarium. *Journal of the Anatomical Society of India* **38**: 3–4.

Sawtell, R.O. (1929). Ossification and growth of children from 1–8 years of age. *American Journal of Diseases of Children* **37**: 61–67.

Sawyer, D.R. and Kiely, M.L. (1987). Jugular foramen and mylohyoid bridging in an Asian Indian population. *American Journal of Physical Anthropology* **72**: 473–477.

Sawyer, D.R., Allison, M.J., Elzay, R.P. and Pezzia, A. (1978). The mylohyoid bridge of pre-Columbian Peruvians. *American Journal of Physical Anthropology* **48**: 9–16.

Sawyer, D.R., Allison, M.J., Elzay, R.P. and Pezzia, A. (1979). A study of torus palatinus and torus mandibularis in pre-Columbian Peruvians. *American Journal of Physical Anthropology* **50**: 525–526.

Sawyer, D.R., Allison, M.J. and Pezzia, A. (1980). Elongated styloid process in a Pre-Columbian Peruvian. *Journal of Dental Research* **59:** 79.

Sawyer, D.R., Gianfortune, V., Kiely, M.L. and Allison, M.J. (1990). Mylohyoid and jugular foramen bridging in Pre-Columbian Chileans. *American Journal of Physical Anthropology* **82**: 179–181.

Saxena, S.K., Chowdhary, D.S. and Jain, S.P. (1986). Interparietal bones in Nigerian skulls. *Journal of Anatomy* **144**: 235–237.

Scammon, R.E. and Calkins, L.A. (1923). Simple empirical formulae for expressing the lineal growth of the human fetus. *Proceedings of the Society for Experimental Biology and Medicine* **20**: 353–356.

Scammon, R.E. and Calkins, L.A. (1929). *The Development and Growth of the External Dimensions of the Human Body in the Fetal Period.* Minneapolis, MN: University of Minnesota Press.

Scapinelli, R. (1967). Blood supply of the human patella. Its relation to ischaemic necrosis after fracture. *Journal of Bone and Joint Surgery* **49B**: 563–570.

Schaeffer, J.P. (1910a). On the genesis of air cells in the conchae nasales. *Anatomical Record* **4**: 167–180.

Schaeffer, J.P. (1910b). The sinus maxillaris and its relations in the embryo, child and adult man. *American Journal of Anatomy* **10**: 313–368.

Schaeffer, J.P. (1916). The genesis, development and adult anatomy of the nasofrontal region in man. *American Journal of Anatomy* **20**: 125–146.

Schaeffer, J.P. (1924). Some points in the regional anatomy of the optic pathway, with especial reference to tumours of the hypophysis cerebri and resulting ocular changes. *Anatomical Record* **28**: 243–279.

Schäfer, E.A. and Symington, J. (1898). In: *Quain's Elements of Anatomy.* London: Longmans, Green, and Co.

Schatzker, J. and Pennal, G.F. (1968). Spinal stenosis; A cause of cauda equina compression. *Journal of Bone and Joint Surgery* **50B**: 606–618.

Schejtman, R., Devoto, F.C.H. and Arias, N.H. (1967). The origin and distribution of the elements of the human mandibular retromolar canal. *Archives of Oral Biology* **12**: 1261–1267.

Schell, L.M., Johnston, E.E., Smith, D.R. and Paolone, A.M. (1985). Directional asymmetry of body dimensions among white adolescents. *American Journal of Physical Anthropology* **67**: 317–322.

Scheller, S. (1960). Roentgenographic studies on epiphysial growth and ossification in the knee. *Acta Radiologica Scandinavica* **195**(Suppl.).

Schemner, D., White, P.G. and Friedman, L. (1995). Radiology of the paraglenoid sulcus. *Skeletal Radiology* **24**: 205–209.

Scheuer, J.L. (1998). Age at death and cause of death of the people buried in St Bride's Church, Fleet Street, London. In: *Grave Concerns: Death and Burial in England 1700–1850*, Research Report 113. (M. Cox, Ed.), pp. 100–111. York: Council for British Archaeology.

Scheuer, J.L. and Black, S.M. (1995). *The St Bride's Documented Skeletal Collection*, Research Report. London: St Bride's Church.

Scheuer, J.L. and Bowman, J.E. (1995). Correlation of documentary and skeletal evidence in the St Bride's Crypt population. In: *Grave Reflections: Portraying the Past through Cemetery Studies* (S.R. Saunders and A. Herring, Eds.), pp. 49–70. Toronto: Canadian Scholars'Press.

Scheuer, J.L. and Elkington, N.M. (1993). Sex determination from metacarpals and the first proximal phalanx. *Journal of Forensic Sciences* **38**: 769–778.

Scheuer, J.L. and MacLaughlin-Black, S.M. (1994). Age estimation from the pars basilaris of the fetal and juvenile occipital bone. *International Journal of Osteoarchaeology* **4**: 377–380.

Scheuer, J.L., Musgrave, J.H. and Evans, S.P. (1980). The estimation of late fetal and perinatal age from limb bone length by linear and logarithmic regression. *Annals of Human Biology* **7**: 257–265.

Schier, M.B.A. (1948). The temporomandibular joint – a consideration of its probable functional and dysfunctional sequelae and report: condyle–double head in a living person. *Dental Items of Interest* **70**: 1095–1109.

Schiff, D.C.M. and Parke, W.W. (1973). The arterial supply of the odontoid process. *Journal of Bone and Joint Surgery* **55A**: 1450–1456.

Schlonsky, J. and Olix, M.L. (1972). Functional disability following avulsion fracture of the ischial epiphysis. *Journal of Bone and Joint Surgery* **54A**: 641–644.

Schmid, F. and Moll, H. (1960). *Atlas der normalen und pathologischen Handskeletentwicklung.* Berlin: Springer.

Schofield, G. (1959). Metric and morphological features of the femur of the New Zealand Maori. *Journal of the Royal Anthropological Institute* **89**: 89–105.

Schorstein, G. (1899). A case of congenital absence of both clavicles. *Lancet* **7**: 10–13.

Schour, I. (1936). The neonatal line in the enamel and dentin of the human deciduous teeth and first permanent molar. *Journal of the American Dental Association* **23**: 1946–1955.

Schour, I. and Massler, M. (1941). The development of the human dentition. *Journal of the American Dental Association* **28**: 1153–1160.

Schranz, D. (1959). Age determination from the internal structure of the humerus. *American Journal of Physical Anthropology* **17**: 273–278.

Schreiber, A., Differding, P. and Zollinger, H. (1985). Talus partitus a case report. *Journal of Bone and Joint Surgery* **67B**: 430–431.

Schuller, A. (1943). A note on the identification of skulls by X-ray pictures of the frontal sinuses. *The Medical Journal of Australia* **1**: 554–556.

Schuller, T.C., Kurz, L., Thompson, E., Zemenick, G., Hensinger, R.N. and Herkowitz, H.N. (1991). Natural history of os odontoideum. *Journal of Pediatric Orthopaedics* **11**: 222–225.

Schulter, F.P. (1976). A comparative study of the temporal bone in three populations of man. *American Journal of Physical Anthropology* **44**: 453–468.

Schulter-Ellis, F.P. (1980). Evidence of handedness on documented skeletons. *Journal of Forensic Sciences* **25**: 624–630.

Schulter-Ellis, F.P. and Lazar, G.T. (1984). Internal morphology of human phalanges. *Journal of Hand Surgery* **9**: 490–495.

Schulter-Ellis, F.P., Schmidt, D.J., Hayek, I.A. and Craig, J. (1983). Determination of sex with a discriminant analysis of new pelvic bone measurements. Part 1. *Journal of Forensic Sciences* **28**: 169–180.

Schultz, A.H. (1917). Ein paariger Knocken am unterrand der Squama Occipitalis. *Anatomical Record* **12**: 357–362.

Schultz, A.H. (1918a). Observations on the canalis basilaris chordae. *Anatomical Record* **15**: 225–229.

Schultz, A.H. (1918b). The fontanella metopica and its remnants in an adult skull. *American Journal of Anatomy* **23**: 259–271.

Schultz, A.H. (1918c). Relation of the external nose to the bony nose and the nasal cartilages in whites and negroes. *American Journal of Physical Anthropology* **1**: 329–338.

Schultz, A.H. (1929a). The techniques of measuring the outer body of human fetuses and primates. *Contributions to Embryology* **394**: 215–257.

Schultz, A.H. (1929b). The metopic fontanelle, fissure and suture. *American Journal of Anatomy* **44**: 475–499.

Schultz, A.H. (1930). The skeleton of the trunk and limbs of higher primates. *Human Biology* **2**: 303–456.

Schultz, A.H. (1936). Characters common to higher primates and characters specific for man. *The Quarterly Revue of Biology* **11**: 259–283, 425–455.

Schultz, A.H. (1937). Proportions, variability and asymmetries of the long bones of the limbs and the clavicles in man and apes. *Human Biology* **9**: 281–328.

Schultz, A.H. (1941a). Chevron bones in adult man. *American Journal of Physical Anthropology* **28**: 91–97.

Schultz, A.H. (1941b). Growth and development of the orang-utan. *Contributions to Embryology* **29**: 57–111.

Schultz, A.H. (1963). The relative lengths of the foot skeleton and its main parts in primates. *Symposia of the Zoological Society of London* **10**: 199–206.

Schultz, A.H. (1969). *The Life of Primates*. New York: Universe Books.

Schunke, G.B. (1938). The anatomy and development of the sacro-iliac joint in man. *Anatomical Record* **72**: 313–331.

Schuscik, O. (1918). Zur Verknöcherung der menschlichen Phalangen mit besonderer. Berücksichtigung der Endphalanx. *Anatomischer Anzeiger* **51**: 118–129.

Schutkowski, H. (1987). Sex determination of fetal and neonatal skeletons by means of discriminant analysis. *International Journal of Anthropology* **2**: 347–352.

Schutkowski, H. (1993). Sex determination of infant and juvenile skeletons: 1. Morphognostic features. *American Journal of Physical Anthropology* **90**: 199–205.

Schwartz, J.H. (1982). Dentofacial growth and development in *Homo sapiens*: evidence from perinatal individuals from Punic Carthage. *Anatomica Anzeiger* **152**: 1–26.

Schwartz, A.M., Wechsler, R.J., Landy, M.D., Wetzner, S.M. and Goldstein, S.A. (1982). Posterior arch defects of the cervical spine. *Skeletal Radiology* **8**: 135–139.

Schwarz, G.S. (1957). Bilateral antecubital ossicles (fabellae cubiti) and other rare accessory bones of the elbow. *Radiology* **69**: 730–733.

Schwarz, E. and Rivellini, G. (1963). Symphalangism. *American Journal of Roentgenology* **89**: 1256–1259.

Scoles, P.V., Salvagno, R., Villalba, K. and Riew D. (1988). Relationship of iliac crest maturation to skeletal and chronologic age. *Journal of Pediatric Orthopaedics* **8**: 639–644.

Scott, J.H. (1953). The cartilage of the nasal septum. *British Dental Journal* **95**: 37–43.

Scott, J.H. (1954). The growth of the human face. *Proceedings of the Royal Society of Medicine* **47**: 91–100.

Scott, J.H. (1956). Growth at facial sutures. *American Journal of Orthodontics* **42**: 381–387.

Scott, J.H. (1957). The growth in width of the facial skeleton. *American Journal of Orthodontics* **43**: 366–371.

Scott, J.H. (1958). The cranial base. *American Journal of Physical Anthropology* **16**: 319–348.

Scott, J.H. (1959). Further studies on the growth of the human face. *Proceedings of the Royal Society of Medicine* **52**: 263–268.

Scott, J.H. (1967). *Dento-facial Development and Growth*. London: Pergamon Press.

Scott, C.K. and Hightower, J.A. (1991). The matrix of endochondral bone differs from the matrix of intramembranous bone. *Calcified Tissue International* **49**: 349–354.

Scott, J.E. and Taor, W.S. (1979). The 'small patella' syndrome. *Journal of Bone and Joint Surgery* **61B**: 172–175.

Scranton, P.E. (1988). Osteochondritides. In: *The Foot* (B. Helal and D. Wilson, Eds.), pp. 524–534. Edinburgh: Churchill Livingstone.

Scranton, P.E., McMaster, J.H. and Kelly, E. (1976). Dynamic fibular function. A new concept. *Clinical Orthopaedics and Related Research* **118**: 76–81.

Seddon, H.J. (1932). Calcaneo-scaphoid coalition. *Proceedings of the Royal Society of Medicine* **26**: 419–424.

Seeds, J.W. and Cefalo, R.C. (1982). Relationship of fetal limb lengths to both biparietal diameter and gestational age. *Obstetrics and Gynecology* **60**: 680–685.

Seftel, D.M. (1977). Ear canal hyperostosis – surfer's ear. *Archives of Otolaryngology* **103**: 58–60.

Segebarth-Orban, R. (1980). An evaluation of the sexual dimorphism of the human innominate bone. *Journal of Human Evolution* **9**: 601–607.

Seidemann, R.M., Stojanowski, C.M. and Doran, G.H. (1998). The use of the supero-inferior femoral neck diameter as a sex assessor. *American Journal of Physical Anthropology* **107**: 305–313.

Seidler, H. (1980). Sex diagnosis of isolated Os coxae by discriminant functions. *Journal of Human Evolution* **9**: 597–600.

Sejrsen, B., Kjær, I. and Jakobsen, J. (1993). The human incisal suture and premaxillary area studied on archaeological material. *Acta Odontologica Scandinavica* **51**: 143–151.

Sejrsen, B., Kjær, I. and Jakobsen, J. (1996). Human palatal growth evaluated on medieval crania using nerve canal openings as references. *American Journal of Physical Anthropology* **99**: 603–611.

Sela, J., Schwartz, Z., Swain, L.D. and Boyan, B.D. (1992). The role of matrix vesicles in calcification. In: *Calcification in Biological Systems* (E. Bonucci, Ed.), pp. 73–105. Boca Raton, FL: CRC Press.

Selby, S. (1961). Separate centre of ossification of the tip of the internal malleolus. *American Journal of Roentgenology* **86**: 496–501.

Selby, S., Garn, S.M. and Kanareff, V. (1955). The incidence and familial nature of a bony bridge on the first cervical vertebra. *American Journal of Physical Anthropology* **13**: 129–141.

Sella, E.J., Lawson, J.P. and Ogden, J.A. (1986). The accessory navicular synchondrosis. *Clinical Orthopaedics and Related Research* **209**: 280–285.

Sellars, I.E. and Keen, E.N. (1978). The anatomy and movements of the cricoarytenoid joint. *Laryngoscope* **88**: 667–674.

Selleck, M.A.J. and Stern, C.D. (1991). Fate mapping and cell lineage analysis of Hensen's node in the chick embryo. *Development* **112**: 615–626.

Selvaraj, K.G., Vettivel, S., Indrasingh, I. and Chandi, G. (1998). Handedness identification from intertubercular sulcus of the humerus by discriminant function analysis. *Forensic Science International* **98**: 101–108.

Sendemir, E. and Çimen, A. (1991). Nutrient foramina in the shafts of lower limb long bones: situation and number. *Surgical and Radiologic Anatomy* **13**: 105–108.

Senior, H.D. (1929). The chondrification of the human hand and foot skeleton. *Anatomical Record* **42**: 35.

Seno, T. (1961). The origin and evolution of the sternum. *Anatomischer Anzeiger* **110**: 97–101.

Sensenig, E. (1949). The early development of the human vertebral column. *Contributions to Embryology* **33**: 23–41.

Serafini-Fracassini, A. and Smith, J.W. (1974). *The Structure and Biochemistry of Cartilage.* Edinburgh: Churchill Livingstone.

Serman, N.J. (1989). The mandibular incisive foramen. *Journal of Anatomy* **167**: 195–198.

Sewell, R.B.S. (1904a). A study of the astragalus. Part 1. *Journal of Anatomy and Physiology* **38**: 233–247.

Sewell, R.B.S. (1904b). A study of the astragalus. Part II. *Journal of Anatomy and Physiology* **38**: 423–434.

Sewell, R.B.S. (1905). A study of the astragalus. Part III. *Journal of Anatomy and Physiology* **39**: 74–86.

Shalom, A., Khermosh, O. and Wienbroub, S. (1994). The natural history of congenital pseudoarthrosis of the clavicle. *Journal of Bone and Joint Surgery* **76B**: 846–847.

Shambaugh, G.E. (1967). *Surgery of the Ear*, 2nd edition. Philadelphia, PA: W.B. Saunders.

Shapiro, R. (1972a). Compartmentation of the jugular foramen. *Journal of Neurosurgery* **36**: 340–343.

Shapiro, R. (1972b). Anomalous parietal sutures and the bipartite parietal bone. *American Journal of Roentgenology* **115**: 569–577.

Shapiro, R. and Janzen, A.H. (1960). *The Normal Skull.* New York: Hoeber.

Shapiro, R. and Robinson, F. (1967). The foramina of the middle cranial fossa: a phylogenetic, anatomic and pathologic study. *American Journal of Roentgenology* **101**: 779–794.

Shapiro, R. and Robinson, F. (1976a). The Os Incae. *American Journal of Roentgenology* **127**: 469–471.

Shapiro, R. and Robinson, F. (1976b). Anomalies of the cranio-vertebral border. *American Journal of Roentgenology* **126**: 1063–1068.

Shapiro, R. and Robinson, F. (1976c). Embryogenesis of the human occipital bone. *American Journal of Roentgenology* **127**: 281–287.

Shapiro, R. and Robinson, F. (1980). *The Embryogenesis of the Human Skull.* Massachusetts: Harvard University Press.

Shapiro, F., Holtrop, M.E. and Glimcher, M.J. (1977). Organization and cellular biology of the perichondrial ossification groove of Ranvier. A morphological study in rabbits. *Journal of Bone and Joint Surgery* **59A**: 703–723.

Shaw, J.P. (1993). Pterygospinous and pterygoalar foramina: a role in the etiology of trigeminal neuralgia. *Clinical Anatomy* **6**: 173–178.

Shaw, H.A. and Bohrer, S.P. (1979). The incidence of cone epiphyses and ivory epiphyses of the hand in Nigerian children. *American Journal of Physical Anthropology* **51**: 155–162.

Shea, B.T. (1977). Eskimo craniofacial morphology, cold stress and the maxillary sinus. *American Journal of Physical Anthropology* **77**: 289–300.

Shelby, B. (1992). *Health.* World Press Review, Feb. 4.

Shepard, E. (1951). Tarsal movements. *Journal of Bone and Joint Surgery* **33B**: 258–263.

Shepherd, F.J. (1893). Symmetrical depressions on the exterior surface of the parietal bones (with notes of three cases). *Journal of Anatomy and Physiology* **27**: 501–504.

Shepherd, W.M. and McCarthy, M.D. (1955). Observations on the appearance and ossification of the premaxilla and maxilla in the human embryo. *Anatomical Record* **121**: 13–28.

Shereff, M.J. (1991). Vascular anatomy of the fifth metatarsal. *Foot and Ankle* **11**: 350–353.

Shereff, M.J., Yang, Q.M. and Kummer, F.J. (1987). Extra-osseous and intraosseous arterial supply to the first metatarsal and metatarsophalangeal joint. *Foot and Ankle* **8**: 81–93.

Sherk, H.H. and Dawoud, S. (1981). Congenital os odontoideum with Klippel-Feil anomaly and fatal atlanto-axial instability. *Spine* **6**: 42–45.

Sherk, H.H. and Nicholson, J.T. (1969). Rotary atlanto-axial dislocation associated with ossiculum terminale and mongolism. A case report. *Journal of Bone and Joint Surgery* **51A**: 957–964.

Sherk, H.H., Nicholson, J.T. and Chung, S.M.K. (1978). Fractures of the odontoid process in young children. *Journal of Bone and Joint Surgery* **60A**: 921–924.

Shiller, W.R. and Wiswell, O.B. (1954). Lingual foramina of the mandible. *Anatomical Record* **119**: 387–390.

Shine, I.B. (1965). Incidence of hallux valgus in a partially shoe-wearing community. *British Medical Journal* **1**: 1648–1650.

Shinohara, H. (1997). Changes in the surface of the superior articular joint from the lower thoracic to the upper lumbar vertebrae. *Journal of Anatomy* **190**: 461–465.

Shock, C.C., Noyes, F.R. and Villanueva, A.R. (1972). Measurement of haversian bone remodelling by means of tetracycline labelling in rib of rhesus monkeys. *Henry Ford Hospital Medical Bulletin* **20**: 131–144.

Shopfner, C.E. (1966). Periosteal bone growth in normal infants. *American Journal of Roentgenology* **97**: 154–163.

Shopfner, C.E., Wolfe, T.W. and O'Kell, R.T. (1968). The intersphenoidal synchondrosis. *American Journal of Roentgenology* **104**: 184–193.

Shore, L.R. (1930). Abnormalities of the vertebral column in a series of skeletons of Bantu natives of South Africa. *Journal of Anatomy* **64**: 206–238.

Shore, L.R. (1931). A report on the spinous processes of the cervical vertebrae in the native races of South Africa. *Journal of Anatomy* **65**: 482–505.

Shore, L.R. (1938). A note on the interparietal groove in Egyptian skulls. *Journal of Anatomy* **73**: 1–14.

Shulin, P. and Fangwu, Z. (1983). Estimation of stature from skull, clavicle, scapula and os coxa of male adult of Southern China. *Acta Anthropologica Sinica* **2**: 253–259.

Shulman, S.S. (1941). Rhomboid depression of the clavicle. *Radiology* **37**: 489–490.

Shulman, S.S. (1959). Observation on the nutrient foramina of the human radius and ulna. *Anatomical Record* **134**: 685–697.

Siddiqi, M.A.H. (1934). The lower end of the femur from Indians. *Journal of Anatomy* **68**: 331–337.

Sidhom, G. and Derry, D.E. (1931). The dates of union of some epiphyses in Egyptians from X-ray photographs. *Journal of Anatomy* **65**: 196–211.

Siegler, D. and Zorab, P.A. (1981). Pregnancy in thoracic scoliosis. *British Journal of Diseases of the Chest* **75**: 367–370.

Siegling, J.A. (1941). Growth of the epiphyses. *Journal of Bone and Joint Surgery* **23**: 23–36.

Sigmon, B.A. (1971). Bipedal behaviour and the emergence of erect posture in man. *American Journal of Physical Anthropology* **34**: 55–60.

Silau, A.M., Njio, B., Solow, B. and Kjær, I. (1994). Prenatal sagittal growth of the osseous components of the human palate. *Journal of Craniofacial Genetics and Developmental Biology* **14**: 252–256.

Silau, A.M., Fischer-Hansen, B. and Kjær, I. (1995). Normal prenatal development of the human parietal bone and interparietal suture. *Journal of Craniofacial Genetics and Developmental Biology* **15**: 81–86.

Silberstein, M.J., Brodeur, A.E. and Graviss, E.R. (1979). Some vagaries of the capitellum. *Journal of Bone and Joint Surgery* **61A**: 244–247.

Silberstein, M.J., Brodeur, A.E., Graviss, E.R. and Luisiri, A. (1981a). Some vagaries of the medial epicondyle. *Journal of Bone and Joint Surgery* **63A**: 524–528.

Silberstein, M.J., Brodeur, A.E., Graviss, E.R. and Luisiri, A. (1981b). Some vagaries of the olecranon. *Journal of Bone and Joint Surgery* **63A**: 722–725.

Silberstein, M.J., Brodeur, A.E. and Graviss, E.R. (1982). Some vagaries of the lateral epicondyle. *Journal of Bone and Joint Surgery* **64A**: 444–448.

Silverman, F.N. (1955). A note on the os lunatotriquetrum. *American Journal of Physical Anthropology* **13**: 143–146.

Sim-Fook, L. and Hodgson, A.R. (1958). A comparison of foot forms among the non-shoe and shoe-wearing Chinese population. *Journal of Bone and Joint Surgery* **40A**: 1058–1062.

Simmons, T., Jantz, R.L. and Bass, W.M. (1990). Stature estimation from fragmentary femora: a revision of the Steele method. *Journal of Forensic Sciences* **35**: 628–636.

Simms, D.L. and Neely, J.G. (1989). Growth of the lateral surface of the temporal bone in children. *Laryngoscope* **99**: 795–799.

Simonian, P.T., Vahey, J.W., Rosenbaum, D.M., Mosca, V.S. and Staheli, L.T. (1995). Fracture of the cuboid in children. *Journal of Bone and Joint Surgery* **77B**: 104–106.

Simonton, F.V. (1923). Mental foramen in the anthropoids and in man. *American Journal of Physical Anthropology* **6**: 413–421.

Simpson, D.P. (1969). *Cassell's New Latin–English, English–Latin Dictionary.* London: Cassell.

Simril, W.A. and Trotter, M. (1949). An accessory bone and other bilateral skeletal anomalies of the elbow. *Radiology* **53**: 97–100.

Sinberg, S.E. (1940). Fractures of the sesamoids of the thumb. *Journal of Bone and Joint Surgery* **22B**: 444–445.

Sinclair, D. (1978). *Human Growth after Birth*, 3rd edition. London: Oxford University Press.

Singer, K.P., Jones, T.J. and Breidahl, P.D. (1990). A comparison of radiographic and computer assisted measurements of thoracic and thoracolumbar sagittal curvature. *Skeletal Radiology* **19**: 21–26.

Singh, I. (1959a). Variations in the metacarpal bones. *Journal of Anatomy* **93**: 262–267.

Singh, I. (1959b). Squatting facets on the talus and tibia in Indians. *Journal of Anatomy* **93**: 540–550.

Singh, I. (1960). Variations in the metatarsal bones. *Journal of Anatomy* **94**: 345–350.

Singh, S. (1965). Variations of the superior articular facets of atlas vertebrae. *Journal of Anatomy* **99**: 565–571.

Singh, S. and Gangrade, K.C. (1968). The sexing of the adult clavicles – verification and applicability of the demarking points. *Journal Indian Academy of Forensic Science* **7**: 20–30.

Singh, I.J. and Gunberg, D.L. (1970). Estimation of age at death in human males from quantitative histology of bone fragments. *American Journal of Physical Anthropology* **33**: 373–381.

Singh, S. and Singh, S.P. (1972a). Identification of sex from the humerus. *Indian Journal of Medical Research* **60**: 1060–1066.

Singh, S.P. and Singh, S. (1972b). The sexing of adult femora–demarking points for the Varanasi zone. *Journal of the Indian Academy of Forensic Sciences* **11**: 1–6.

Singh, S. and Singh, S.P. (1975). Identification of sex from tarsal bones. *Acta Anatomica* **93**: 568–573.

Singh, S. and Potturi, B.R. (1978). Greater sciatic notch in sex determination. *Journal of Anatomy* **125**: 619–624.

Singh, M., Nagrath, A.R. and Maini, M.S. (1970). Changes in the trabecular pattern of the upper end of the femur as an index of osteoporosis. *Journal of Bone and Joint Surgery* **52A**: 457–467.

Singh, G., Singh, S.P. and Singh, S. (1974a). Identification of sex from the radius. *Journal of the Indian Academy of Forensic Sciences* **13**: 10–16.

Singh, S., Singh, G. and Singh, S.P. (1974b). Identification of sex from the ulna. *Indian Journal of Medical Research* **62**: 731–735.

Singh, G., Singh, S. and Singh, S.P. (1975). Identification of sex from the tibia. *Journal of the Anatomical Society of India* **24**: 20–24.

Singh, P.J., Gupta, C.D. and Arora, A.K. (1979). Incidence of interparietal bones in adult skulls of Agra region. *Anatomischer Anzeiger* **145**: 528–531.

Singh-Roy, K.K. (1967). On Goethe's vertebral theory of origin of the skull, a recent approach. *Anatomischer Anzeiger* **120**: 250–259.

Sinha, D.N. (1985). Cancellous structure of tarsal bones. *Journal of Anatomy* **140**: 111–117.

Sirang, H. (1973). Ein canalis alae ossis ilii und seine Bedeutung. *Anatomischer Anzeiger* **133**: 225–238.

Skak, S.V. (1993). Fracture of the olecranon through a persistent physis in an adult. *Journal of Bone and Joint Surgery* **75A**: 272–275.

Skawina, A. and Gorczyca, W. (1984). The role of nutrient and periosteal blood vessels in the vascularization of the cortex of shafts of the long bones in human fetuses. *Folia Morphologica (Warszawa)* **43**: 159–164.

Skawina, A. and Miaskiewicz, C. (1982). Nutrient foramina in femoral, tibial and fibular bones in human fetuses. *Folia Morphologica (Warszawa)* **41**: 469–481.

Skawina, A. and Wyczólkowski, M. (1987). Nutrient foramina of humerus, radius and ulna in human fetuses. *Folia Morphologica (Warszawa)* **46**: 17–24.

Skawina, A., Litwin, J.A., Gorczyca, J. and Miodonski, A.J. (1994). The vascular system of human fetal long bones: a scanning electron microscope study of corrosion casts. *Journal of Anatomy* **185**: 369–376.

Skawina, A., Litwin, J.A., Gorczyca, J. and Miodonski, A.J. (1997). The architecture of internal blood vessels in human fetal vertebral bodies. *Journal of Anatomy* **191**: 259–267.

Skeletal Dysplasia Group (1989). Instability of the upper cervical spine. *Archives of Diseases in Childhood* **64**: 283–289.

Skinner, B.M. (1931). Note on the relative lengths of first and second toes of the human foot. *Journal of Anatomy* **66**: 123–124.

Skinner, H.A. (1961). *The Origin of Medical Terms*, 2nd edition. Baltimore, MD: Williams and Wilkins.

Skinner, M. and Dupras, T. (1993). Variation in birth timing and location of the neonatal line in human enamel. *Journal of Forensic Sciences* **38**: 1383–1390.

Slavkin, H.C. (1988). Gene regulation of oral tissues. 1987 Kreshover lecture. *Journal of Dental Research* **67**: 1142–1149.

Slavkin, H.C., Canter, M.R. and Canter, S.R. (1966). An anatomic study of the pterygomaxillary region in the craniums of infants and children. *Oral Surgery, Oral Medicine and Oral Pathology* **21**: 225–235.

Sloane, M.W.M. (1946). A case of anomalous skeletal development in the foot. *Anatomical Record* **96**; 23–26.

Slomann, H.C. (1926). On the demonstration and analysis of calcaneo-navicular coalition by Roentgen examination. *Acta Radiologica* **5**: 304–312.

Smillie, I.S. (1962). *Injuries of the Knee Joint*, 3rd edition. Baltimore, MD: Williams and Wilkins.

Smit, Th. H. (1996). *The Mechanical Significance of the Trabecular Bone Architecture in a Human Vertebra.* Aachen: Shaker.

Smith, T. (1886). A foot having four cuneiforms. *Transactions of the Pathology Society of London* **17**: 222–223.

Smith, G.E. (1907). The causation of the symmetrical thinning of the parietal bones in ancient Egyptians. *Journal of Anatomy and Physiology* **41**: 232–233.

Smith, G.E. (1908a). The significance of fusion of the atlas to the occipital bone and manifestation of occipital vertebrae. *British Medical Journal* **2**: 594–596.

Smith, S.A. (1908b). A case of fusion of the semilunar and cuneiform bones (os lunatotriquetrum) in an Australian Aboriginal. *Journal of Anatomy and Physiology* **42**: 343–346.

Smith, H.D. (1912). Observations on the cranial bone in a series of Egyptian skulls, with especial reference to the persistence of the synchondrosis condylo-squamosa. *Biometrika* **8**: 257–261.

Smith, S. (1925). Notes on the ossification of the scapula. *Journal of Anatomy* **59**: 387.

Smith, A.D. (1941). Congenital elevation of the scapula. *Archives of Surgery* **42**: 529–536.

Smith, C.A. (1947). Effects of maternal undernutrition upon the newborn infant in Holland (1944–1945). *Journal of Pediatrics* **30**: 229–243.

Smith, J.W. (1954). Muscular control of the arches of the foot in standing: an electromyographic assessment. *Journal of Anatomy* **88**: 152–163.

Smith, J.W. (1958). The ligamentous structures in the canalis and sinus tarsi. *Journal of Anatomy* **92**: 616–620.

Smith, L. (1960). Deformity following supracondylar fractures of the humerus. *Journal of Bone and Joint Surgery* **42A**: 235–252.

Smith, J.W. (1962a). The relationship of epiphysial plates to stress in some bones of the lower limb. *Journal of Anatomy* **96**: 58–78.

Smith, J.W. (1962b). The structure and stress relations of fibrous epiphysial plates. *Journal of Anatomy* **96**: 209–225.

Smith, B.H. (1991a). Standards of human tooth formation and dental age assessment. In: *Advances in Dental Anthropology* (M.A. Kelley and C.S. Larsen, Eds.), pp. 143–168. New York: Wiley-Liss.

Smith, K.J. (1991b). A histological and radiological investigation of the manubrio-sternal joint. Unpublished B.Sc. dissertation, University of London.

Smith, S. (1997). Attribution of foot bones to sex and population groups. *Journal of Forensic Sciences* **42**: 186–195.

Smith, J.D. and Abramson, M. (1974). Membranous vs endochondral bone autografts. *Archives of Otolaryngology* **99**: 203–205.

Smith, R.N. and Allcock, J. (1960). Epiphyseal union in the greyhound. *Veterinary Record* **72**: 75–79.

Smith, S. and Boulgakoff, B. (1923). A case of polydactylia shewing certain atavistic characters. *Journal of Anatomy* **58**: 359–367.

Smith, B.H. and Garn, S.M. (1987). Polymorphisms in eruption sequence of permanent teeth in American children. *American Journal of Physical Anthropology* **74**: 289–303.

Smith, D.W. and Töndury, G. (1978). Origin of the calvaria and its sutures. *American Journal of Diseases of Children* **132**: 662–666.

Smith, B.C., Fisher, D.L., Weedn, V.W., Warnock, G.R. and Holland, M.M. (1993). A systematic approach to the sampling of dental DNA. *Journal of Forensic Sciences* **38**: 1194–1209.

Smitham, J.H. (1948). Some observations on certain congenital abnormalities of the hand in African natives. *British Journal of Radiology* **21**: 513–518.

Smithgall, E.B., Johnston, F.E., Malina, R.M. and Galbraith, M.A. (1966). Developmental changes in compact bone relationships in the second metacarpal. *Human Biology* **38**: 141–151.

Sneath, R.S. (1955). The insertion of the biceps femoris. *Journal of Anatomy* **89**: 550–553.

Snell, C. and Donhuysen, H.W.A. (1968). The pelvis in the bipedalism of primates. *American Journal of Physical Anthropology* **28**: 239–246.

Snodgrasse, R.M., Dreizen, S., Currie, C., Parker, G.S. and Spies, T.D. (1955). The association between anomalous ossification centres in the hand skeleton, nutritional status and rate of skeletal maturation in children five to fourteen years of age. *American Journal of Roentgenology* **74**: 1037–1048.

Snow, C.C. (1983). Equations for estimating age at death from the pubic symphysis: A modification of the McKern-Stewart method. *Journal of Forensic Sciences* **28**: 864–870.

Solter, M. and Paljan, D. (1973). Variations in shape and dimensions of the sigmoid groove, venous portion of the jugular foramen, jugular fossa, condylar and mastoid foramina classified by age, sex and body size. *Zeitschrift für Anatomie und Entwicklungsgeschichte* **140**: 319–335.

Solursh, M. (1983). Cell-cell interactions in chondrogenesis. pp 121–141. In: *Cartilage Vol. 2: Development, Differentiation and Growth* (B.K. Hall, Ed.). New York: Academic Press.

Sontag, L.W. (1938). Evidences of disturbed prenatal and neonatal growth in bones of infants aged one month. *American Journal of Diseases of Children* **55**: 1248–1256.

Sontag, L.W., Snell, D. and Anderson, M. (1939). Rate of appearance of ossification centres from birth to the age of 5 years. *American Journal of Diseases of Children* **58**: 949–956.

Soulié, A. and Bardier, E. (1907). Recherches sur le développment du larynx chez l'homme. *Journal d'Anatomie et de al Physiologie Normales et Pathologiques de l'homme et des Animaux* **43**: 137–240.

Souri, S.J. (1959). A morphological study of the fetal pelvis. *Journal of the Anatomical Society of India* **8**: 45–55.

Southam, A.H. and Bythell, W.J.S. (1924). Cervical ribs in children. *British Medical Journal* **2**: 844–845.

Specker, B.L., Brazero, L.W., Tsang, R.C., Levin, R., Searcy, J. and Steichen, J. (1987). Bone mineral content in children 1–6 years of age. *American Journal of Diseases of Children* **141**: 343–344.

Spector, G.T. and Ge, X-X. (1981). Development of the hypotympanum in the human fetus and neonate. *Annals of Otology, Rhinology and Laryngology* **90**(Suppl. **88**): 1–20.

Speer, D.P. (1982). Collagenous architecture of the growth plate and perichondrial ossification groove. *Journal of Bone and Joint Surgery* **64A**: 399–407.

Speijer, B. (1950). *Betekenis en Bepaling van de Skeletleeftijd.* Leiden: Sijthoff.

Spencer, H.R. (1891). Ossification in the head of the humerus at birth. *Journal of Anatomy and Physiology* **25**: 552–556.

Sperber, G.H. (1989). *Craniofacial Embryology*, 4th edition, p. 102. London: Wright, Butterworths.

Spierings, E.L.H. and Braakman, R. (1984). The management of os odontoideum. Analysis of 37 cases. *Journal of Bone and Joint Surgery* **64B**: 422–428.

Spillane, J.D., Pallis, C. and Jones, A.M. (1957). Developmental abnormalities in the region of the foramen magnum. *Brain* **80**: 11–49.

Spoor, C.F. (1993). The human bony labyrinth: a morphometric description. In: The comparative morphology and phylogeny of the human bony labyrinth. Unpublished PhD dissertation, University of Utrecht.

Sprengel, O.G. (1891). Die angeborne Verschiebung des Schulter blattes nach oben. *Archiv fur Klinische Chirurgie* **42**: 545–549.

Spring, D.B., Lovejoy, C.O., Bender, G.N. and Duerr, M. (1989). The radiographic pre-auricular groove: Its non-relationship to past parity. *American Journal of Physical Anthropology* **79**: 247–252.

Sprinz, R. and Kaufman, M.H. (1987). The sphenoidal canal. *Journal of Anatomy* **153**: 47–54.

Spyropoulos, M.N. (1977). The morphogenetic relationship of the temporal muscle to the coronoid process in human embryos and fetuses. *American Journal of Anatomy* **150**: 395–410.

Srivastava, H.C. (1977). Development of the ossification centres in the squamous portion of the occipital bone in man. *Journal of Anatomy* **124**: 643–649.

Srivastava, H.C. (1992). Ossification of the membranous portion of the squamous part of the occipital bone in man. *Journal of Anatomy* **180**: 219–224.

Staaf, V., Mörnstad, H. and Welander, U. (1991). Age estimation based on tooth development: a test of reliability and validity. *Scandinavian Journal of Dental Research* **99**: 281–286.

Stack, H.G. (1962). Muscle function in the fingers. *Journal of Bone and Joint Surgery* **44B**: 899–1022.

Stack, M.V. (1964). A gravimetric study of crown growth rate of the human deciduous dentition. *Biologia Neonatorum* **6**: 197–224.

Stack, M.V. (1967). Vertical growth rate of the deciduous teeth. *Journal of Dental Research* **46**: 879–882.

Stack, M.V. (1968). Relative growth of the deciduous second molar and permanent first molar. *Journal of Dental Research* **47**: 1013–1014.

Stack, M.V. (1971). Relative rates of weight gain in human deciduous teeth. In: *Dental Morphology and Evolution* (A.A. Dahlberg, Ed.), pp. 59–62. Chicago: Chicago University Press.

Stadnicki, G. (1971). Congenital double condyle of the mandible causing temporomandibular joint ankylosis. *Journal of Oral Surgery* **29**: 208–211.

Staheli, L.T. (1977). Torsional deformity. *Pediatric Clinics of North America* **24**: 799–811.

Staheli, L.T. (1984). Fractures of the shaft of the femur. In: *Fractures in Children* (C.A. Rockwood, K.E. Wilkins and R.E. King, Eds.), pp. 845–889. Philadelphia, PA: Lippincott.

Staheli, L.T. and Engel, G.M. (1972). Tibial torsion. A method of assessment and a survey of normal children. *Clinical Orthopaedics and Related Research* **86**: 183–186.

Stallworthy, J.A. (1932). A case of enlarged parietal foramina associated with metopism and irregular synostosis of the coronal suture. *Journal of Anatomy* **67**: 168–174.

Stammel, C.A. (1941). Multiple striae parallel to epiphyses and ring shadows around bone growth centres. *American Journal of Roentgenology* **46**: 497–505.

Standen, V. (1996). External auditory exostoses in prehistoric Chilean populations: a test of chronology and geographic distribution. *Paleopathology Newsletter – Papers in Paleopathology* **94**: 14–15.

Standen, V.G., Arriaza, B.T. and Santoro, C.M. (1997). External auditory exostoses in prehistoric Chilean populations: a test of the cold water hypothesis. *American Journal of Physical Anthropology* **103**: 119–129.

Stark, H.H., Chao, E.K., Zemel, N.P., Rickard, T.A. and Ashworth, C.R. (1989). Fractures of the hook of the hamate. *Journal of Bone and Joint Surgery* **71A**: 1202–1207.

Starkie, C. and Stewart, D. (1931). The intra-mandibular course of the inferior dental nerve. *Journal of Anatomy* **65**: 319–323.

Stauffer, R.N., Chao, E.Y.S. and Brewster, R.C. (1977). Force and motion analysis of the normal, diseased and prosthetic ankle joint. *Clinical Orthopaedics and Related Research* **127**: 189–196.

Steel, F.L.D. (1962). The sexing of the long bones, with reference to the St Bride's series of identified skeletons. *Journal of the Royal Anthropological Institute of Great Britain and Ireland* **92**: 212–222.

Steel, F.L.D. (1966). Further observations on the osteometric discriminant function: the human clavicle. *American Journal of Physical Anthropology* **25**: 319–322.

Steel, F.L.D. and Tomlinson, J.D.W. (1958). The 'carrying angle' of man. *Journal of Anatomy* **92**: 315–317.

Steele, D.G. (1970). Estimation of stature from fragments of long limb bones. In: *Personal Identification in Mass Disasters.* (T.D. Stewart, Ed.), pp. 85–97. Washington, DC: Smithsonian Institute Press.

Steele, D.G. (1976). The estimation of sex on the basis of the talus and calcaneum. *American Journal of Physical Anthropology* **45**: 581–588.

Steele, D.G. and Bramblett, C.A. (1988). *The Anatomy and Biology of the Human Skeleton.* Texas: A&M University Press.

Steele, J. and Mays, S. (1995). Handedness and directional asymmetry in the long bones of the human upper limb. *International Journal of Osteoarchaeology* **5**: 39–49.

Steele, D.G. and McKern, T.W. (1969). A method for assessment of maximum long bone length and living stature from fragmentary long bones. *American Journal of Physical Anthropology* **31**: 215–228.

Steen, S.L. and Lane, R.W. (1998). Evaluation of habitual activities among two Alaskan Eskimo populations based on musculoskeletal stress markers. *International Journal of Osteoarchaeology* **8**: 341–353.

Steggerda, M. and Hill, T.J. (1942). Eruption time of teeth among Whites, Negroes and Indians. *American Journal of Orthodontics and Oral Surgery* **28**: 361–370.

Steinbach, H.L. and Obata, W.G. (1957). The significance of thinning of the parietal bones. *American Journal of Roentgenology* **78**: 39–45.

Steinberg, M.S. (1963). Reconstruction of tissues by dissociated cells. *Science* **141**: 401–408.

Steinbock, R.T. (1976). *Paleopathological Diagnosis and Interpretation. Bone Diseases in Ancient Human Populations.* Springfield, IL: C.C. Thomas.

Steindler, A. (1935). *Mechanics of Normal and Pathological Locomotion in Man.* London: Ballière, Tindall and Cox.

Steiner, H.A. (1943). Roentgenologic manifestations and clinical symptoms of rib abnormalities. *Radiology* **40**: 175–178.

Steinmann, E.P. (1970). A new light on the pathogenesis of the styloid syndrome. *Archives of Otolaryngology* **91**: 171–174.

Stelling, C.B. (1981). Anomalous attachment of the transverse process to the vertebral body: an accessory finding in congenital absence of a lumbar pedicle. *Skeletal Radiology* **6**: 47–50.

Stern, J.T. and Susman, R.L. (1983). The locomotor anatomy of *Australopithecus afarensis. American Journal of Physical Anthropology* **60**: 279–317.

Stevenson, P.H. (1924). Age order of epiphyseal union in man. *American Journal of Physical Anthropology* **7**: 53–93.

Stevenson, P.H. (1929). On racial differences in stature long bone regression formulae with special reference to stature reconstruction formulae for the Chinese. *Biometrika* **21**: 303–321.

Stewart, T.D. (1933). The tympanic plate and external auditory meatus in the Eskimo. *American Journal of Physical Anthropology* **17**: 481–496.

Stewart, T.D. (1934a). Sequence of epiphyseal union, third molar eruption and suture closure in Eskimos and American Indians. *American Journal of Physical Anthropology* **19**: 433–452.

Stewart, T.D. (1934b). Cervical intercostal articulation in a North American Indian. *Journal of Anatomy* **69**: 124–126.

Stewart, T.D. (1938). Accessory sacro-iliac articulations in the higher primates and their significance. *American Journal of Physical Anthropology* **24**: 43–55.

Stewart, S.F. (1951). Club foot: its incidence, cause and treatment. *Journal of Bone and Joint Surgery* **33A**: 577–590.

Stewart, T.D. (1954). Metamorphosis of the joints of the sternum in relation to age changes in other bones. *American Journal of Physical Anthropology* **12**: 519–535.

Stewart, T.D. (1956). Examination of the possibility that certain skeletal characteristics predispose to defects in the lumbar neural arches. *Clinical Orthopedics* **8**: 44–60.

Stewart, T.D. (1957). Distortion of the pubic symphyseal face in females and its effect on age determination. *American Journal of Physical Anthropology* **15**: 9–18.

Stewart, T.D. (1959). Bear paw remains closely resemble human bones. *FBI Law Enforcement Bulletin* **28**: 18–21.

Stewart, T.D. (1962). Anterior femoral curvature: its utility for race identification. *Human Biology* **34**: 49–62.

Stewart, T.D. (1970). *Personal Identification in Mass Disasters.* Washington, DC: Smithsonian Institute Press.

Stewart, T.D. (1979). *Essentials of Forensic Anthropology.* Springfield, IL: C.C. Thomas.

Stewart, D.B. (1984). The pelvis as a passageway. 1. Evolution and adaptations. *British Journal of Obstetrics and Gynaecology* **91**: 611–617.

Steyn, M. and Henneberg, M. (1996). Skeletal growth of children from the Iron Age site at K2 (South Africa). *American Journal of Physical Anthropology* **100**: 389–396.

St Hoyme, L.E. (1965). The nasal index and climate: a spurious case of natural selection in man. *American Journal of Physical Anthropology* **23**: 336.

St Hoyme, L.E. (1984). Sex differentiation in the posterior pelvis. *Collegium Anthropologium* **2**: 139–153.

St Hoyme, L.E. and Işcan, M.Y. (1989). Determination of sex and race: accuracy and assumptions. In: *Reconstruction of Life from the Skeleton* (M.Y. Işcan and K.A.R. Kennedy, Eds.), pp. 53–93. New York: Liss.

Stibbe, E.P. (1929). Skull showing perforations of parietal bone or enlarged parietal foramina. *Journal of Anatomy* **63**: 277–278.

Stillwell, W.T. and Fielding, J.W. (1978). Acquired os odontoideum. *Clinical Orthopaedics* **135**: 71–73.

Stirland, A. (1984). A possible correlation between os acromiale and occupation in the burials from the Mary Rose. *Proceedings of the Fifth European Meeting of the Palaeopathology Association, Sienna, Italy,* pp. 327–334.

Stirland, A. (1991). Diagnosis of occupationally related palaeopathology. Can it be done? In: *Human Palaeopathology: Current Syntheses and Future Opinions* (D.J. Ortner and A.C. Aufderheide, Eds.), pp. 40–47. Washington, DC: Smithsonian Institute Press.

Stirland, A. (1993). Asymmetry and activity-related change in the male humerus. *International Journal of Osteoarchaeology* **3**: 105–113.

Stirland, A. (1994). The angle of femoral torsion: an impossible measurement? *International Journal of Osteoarchaeology* **4**: 31–35.

Stirland, A. (1996). Femoral non-metric traits reconsidered. *Anthropologie* **34**: 249–252.

Stirland, A. (1998). Musculoskeletal evidence for activity: problems of evaluation. *International Journal of Osteoarchaeology* **8**: 354–362.

Stloukal, M. and Hanáková, H. (1978). Die Länge der Längsknochen altslawischer Bevölkerungen, unter besonderer Berücksichtigung von Wachstumsfragen. *Homo* **29**: 53–69.

Stone, A.C., Milner, G.R., Pääbo, S. and Stoneking, M. (1996). Sex determination of ancient human skeletons using DNA. *American Journal of Physical Anthropology* **99**: 231–238.

Stopford, J.S.B. (1914). The supracondylar tubercles of the femur and the attachment of the gastrocnemius muscle to the femoral diaphysis. *Journal of Anatomy and Physiology* **49**: 80–84.

Storey, R. (1986). Perinatal mortality at Pre-Columbian Teotihuacan. *American Journal of Physical Anthropology* **69**: 541–548.

Stott, J.R.R. and Stokes, I.A.F. (1973). Forces under the foot. *Journal of Bone and Joint Surgery* **55B**: 335–344.

Stout, S.D. and Paine, R.R. (1992). Histological age estimation using rib and clavicle. *American Journal of Physical Anthropology* **87**: 111–115.

Stout, S.D., Dietze, W.H., Işcan, M.Y. and Loth, S.R. (1994). Estimation of age at death using cortical histomorphometry of the sternal end of the fourth rib. *Journal of Forensic Sciences* **39**: 778–784.

Stovin, J.J., Lyon, J.A. and Clemmens, R.L. (1960). Mandibulofacial dysostosis. *American Journal of Radiology* **74**: 225–231.

Stratemeier, P.H. and Jensen, S.R. (1980). Partial regressive occipital vertebra. *Neuroradiology* **19**: 47–49.

Straus, W.L. (1926). The development of the human foot and its phylogenetic significance. *American Journal of Physical Anthropology* **9**: 427–438.

Straus, W.L. (1927a). Human ilium – sex and stock. *American Journal of Physical Anthropology* **11**: 1–28.

Straus, W.L. (1927b). Growth of the human foot and its evolutionary significance. *Contributions to Embryology* **19**: 93–134.

Straus, W.L. (1929). Studies on primate ilia. *American Journal of Anatomy* **43**: 403–460.

Straus, W.L. (1942). Rudimentary digits in primates. *The Quarterly Review of Biology* **17**: 228–243.

Streeter, G.L. (1918). The histogenesis and growth of the otic capsule and its contained periotic tissue-spaces in the human embryo. *Contributions to Embryology* **7**: 5–54.

Streeter, G.L. (1920). Weight, sitting height, head size, foot length and menstrual age of the human embryo. *Contributions to Embryology* **11**: 143–170.

Streeter, G.L. (1942). Developmental horizons in human embryos. Description of age group XI 13 to 20 somites and age group XII 21 to 29 somites. *Contributions to Embryology* **30**: 211–245.

Streeter, G.L. (1945). Developmental horizons in human embryos. Description of age group XIII, embryos about 4 or 5 millimeters long, and age group XIV, period of indentation of the lens vesicle. *Contributions to Embryology* **31**: 27–63.

Streeter, G.L. (1948). Description of age groups XV, XVI, XVII and XVIII being the third issue of a survey of the Carnegie collection. *Contributions to Embryology* **32**: 133–203.

Streeter, G.L. (1949). Developmental horizons in human embryos (fourth issue). A review of the histogenesis of cartilage and bone. *Contributions to Embryology* **33**: 149–167.

Streeter, G.L. (1951). Description of age groups XIX, XX, XXI, XXII and XXIII, being the fifth issue of a survey of the Carnegie collection. *Contributions to Embryology* **34**: 165–196.

Stricker, M., Van der Meulen, J.C., Raphael, B. and Mazzola, R. (Eds) (1990). *Craniofacial Malformations*. Edinburgh: Churchill Livingstone.

Stripp, W. and Reynolds, C.P. (1988). Radiography and radiology. In: *The Foot* (B. Helal, and D. Wilson, Eds.), pp. 146–201. Edinburgh: Churchill Livingstone.

Struthers, J. (1848). On a peculiarity of the humerus and the humeral artery. *Monthly Journal of Medical Science* **9**: 264–267.

Struthers, J. (1875). On variations of the vertebrae and ribs in man. *Journal of Anatomy and Physiology* **9**: 17–96.

Struthers, J. (1896). On separate acromion process simulating fracture. *Edinburgh Medical Journal* **42**: 96–114.

Stuart, H.C., Pyle, S.I., Cornoni, J. and Reed, R.B. (1962). Onsets, completions and spans of ossification in the 29 bone growth centres of the hand and wrist. *Pediatrics* **29**: 237–249.

Stuck, W.G. (1933). Fractures of the sternum. *American Journal of Surgery* **22**: 266–270.

Suchey, J.M. (1979). Problems in the ageing of females using the os pubis. *American Journal of Physical Anthropology* **51**: 467–470.

Suchey, J.M. (1986). Skeletal age standards derived from an extensive multi-racial sample of modern Americans. *Paper presented at the Fifty-fifth A.A.P.A. meeting, Albuquerque, New Mexico.*

Suchey, J.M., Wiseley, D.V., Green, R.F. and Noguchi, T.T. (1979). Analysis of dorsal pitting in the os pubis in an extensive sample of modern American females. *American Journal of Physical Anthropology* **51**: 517–540.

Suchey, J.M., Wiseley, D.V. and Katz, D. (1986). Evaluation of the Todd and McKern-Stewart methods for ageing the male os pubis. In: *Forensic Osteology: Advances in Techniques of Human Identification* (K. Reichs, Ed.). Springfield, IL: C.C. Thomas.

Sullivan, D. and Cornwell, W.J. (1974). Pelvic rib. Report of a case. *Radiology* **110**: 355–357.

Sullivan, P. and Lumsden, A.G.S. (1981). Embryology and Development. In: *A Companion to Dental Studies*, Vol. 1, Book 2. (J.W. Osborn, Ed.), pp. 35–46. Oxford: Blackwells.

Sullivan, W.G. and Szwajkun, P. (1991). Membranous vs endochondral bone. *Plastic and Reconstructive Surgery* **87**: 1145.

Sunderland, E.P., Smith, C.J. and Sunderland, R. (1987). A histological study of the chronology of initial mineralization in the human deciduous dentition. *Archives of Oral Biology* **32**: 167–174.

Sundick, R.I. (1977). Age and sex determination of subadult skeletons. *Journal of Forensic Sciences* **22**: 141–144.

Sundick, R.I. (1978). Human skeletal growth and age determination. *Homo* **29**: 228–249.

Suri, R.K. and Tandon, J.K. (1987). Determination of sex from the pubic bone. *Medicine, Science and the Law* **27**: 294–296.

Susman, R.L. (1979). The comparative and functional morphology of the hominoid fingers. *American Journal of Physical Anthropology* **50**: 215–236.

Susman, R.L. (1983). Evolution of the human foot: evidence from plio-pleistocene hominids. *Foot and Ankle* **3**: 365–376.

Susman, R.L. and Creel, N. (1979). Functional and morphological affinities of the sub adult hand (O.H.7) from Olduvai Forge. *American Journal of Physical Anthropology* **51**: 311-332.

Sutow, W.W. and Ohwada, K. (1953). Skeletal maturation in healthy Japanese children 6 to 19 years of age. Skeletal age standards. *Shonika Rinsko* **6**.

Sutow, W.W. and West, E. (1955). Studies on Nagasaki (Japan) children exposed in utero to the atomic bomb. *American Journal of Roentgenology* **74**: 493–499.

Sutro, C.J. (1967). Dentated articular surface of the glenoid – an anomaly. *Bulletin of Hospital Joint Diseases* **28**: 104–115.

Sutton, J.B. (1883). The ossification of the temporal bone. *Journal of Anatomy and Physiology* **17**: 498–508.

Sutton, R.N. (1974). The practical significance of mandibular accessory foramina. *Australian Dental Journal* **19**: 167–173.

Suzuki, R. (1985). Human Adult Walking. In: *Primate Morphophysiology, Locomotor Analysis and Human Bipedalism* (S. Kondo, Ed.), pp. 3–24. Tokyo: University of Tokyo Press.

Suzuki, M. and Sakai, T. (1960). A familial study of torus palatinus and torus mandibularis. *American Journal of Physical Anthropology* **18**: 263–272.

Swanson, P.B. and Logan, B.M. (1999). A survey of nasal conchae in 40 adult human cadaver heads, reviewing typical anatomy and variants. *Clinical Anatomy* **12**: 144.

Sweterlitsch, P.R., Torg, J.S. and Pollack, H. (1969). Entrapment of a sesamoid in the index metacarpophalangeal joint. *Journal of Bone and Joint Surgery* **51A**: 995–998.

Swischuk, L., Hayden, C.K. and Sarwar, M. (1979). The posterior tilted dens. *Pediatric Radiology* **8**: 27–32.

Sycamore, L.K. (1944). Common congenital anomalies of the bony thorax. *American Journal of Roentgenology* **51**: 593–599.

Syftestad, G.T. and Caplan, A.I. (1984). A fraction from extracts of demineralized adult bone stimulates the conversion of mesenchymal cells into chondrocytes. *Developmental Biology* **104**: 348–356.

Symeonides, P.P. (1972). The humerus supracondylar process syndrome. *Clinical Orthopaedics and Related Research* **82**: 141–143.

Symington, J. (1900). On separate acromion process. *Journal of Anatomy and Physiology* **34**: 287–294.

Symmers, W.St.C. (1895). A skull with enormous parietal foramina. *Journal of Anatomy and Physiology* **29**: 329–330.

Symons, N.B.B. (1951). Studies on the growth and form of the mandible. *Dental Record* **71**: 41–53.

Symons, N.B.B. (1952). The development of the human mandibular joint. *Journal of Anatomy* **86**: 326–332.

Szaboky, G.T., Muller, J., Melnick, J. and Tamburro, R. (1969). Anomalous fusion between the lunate and triquetrum. *Journal of Bone and Joint Surgery* **51A**: 1001-1004.

Szaboky, G.T., Anderson, J.J. and Wiltsie, R.A. (1970). Bifid os calcis an anomalous ossification of the calcaneus. *Clinical Orthopaedics and Related Research* **68**: 136–137.

Szilvassy, J. (1980). Age determination on the sternal articular faces of the clavicula. *Journal of Human Evolution* **9**: 609–610.

Tabin, C.J. (1992). Why we have (only) five fingers per hand: *Hox* genes and the evolution of paired limbs. *Development* **116**: 289–296.

Tabin, C.J. (1998). A developmental model for thalidomide defects. *Nature* **396**: 322–323.

Tachdjian, M.O. (1972). *Pediatric Orthopedics*. Philadelphia, PA: W.B. Saunders.

Tachdjian, M.O. (1985). *The Child's Foot*. Philadelphia, PA: W.B. Saunders.

Tague, R.G. (1988). Bone resorption of the pubis and preauricular area in humans and non human primates. *American Journal of Physical Anthropology* **76**: 251–267.

Taitz, C. and Arensburg, B. (1989). Erosion of the foramen transversarium of the axis. *Acta Anatomical* **134**: 12–17.

Taitz, C. and Nathan, H. (1986). Some observations on the posterior and lateral bridge of the atlas. *Acta Anatomica* **127**: 212–217.

Taitz, C., Nathan, H. and Arensburg, B. (1978). Anatomical observations of the foramina transversaria. *Journal of Neurology, Neurosurgery and Psychiatry* **41**: 170–176.

Takahashi, R. (1987). The formation of the nasal septum and the etiology of septal deformity. *Acta Oto-Laryngologica* **443**(Suppl.): 1–160.

Takai, S. (1977). Principal component analysis of the elongation of metacarpal and phalangeal bones. *American Journal of Physical Anthropology* **47**: 301–304.

Takebe, K., Nakagawa, A., Minami, H., Kanazawa, H. and Hirohata, K. (1984). Role of the fibula in weight-bearing. *Clinical Orthopaedics and Related Research* **184**: 289–292.

Tan, K.L. (1971). The third fontanelle. *Acta Pœdiatrica Scandinavica* **60**: 329–332.

Tanagho, E.A. (1978). The anatomy and physiology of micturition. *Clinical Obstetrics and Gynaecology* **5**: 3–26.

Tanaka, T. and Uhthoff, H.K. (1981). Significance of resegmentation in the pathogenesis of vertebral body malformation. *Acta Orthopėdica Scandinavica* **52**: 331–338.

Tanaka, T. and Uhthoff, H.K. (1983). Coronal cleft of vertebrae, a variant of normal enchondral ossification. *Acta Orthopaedica Scandinavica* **54**: 389–395.

Tanguay, R., Buschang, P.H. and Demirjian, A. (1986). Sexual dimorphism in the emergence of deciduous teeth: its relationship with growth components in height. *American Journal of Physical Anthropology* **69**: 511–515.

Tanner, J.M. (1962). *Growth at Adolescence*, 2nd edition. Oxford: Blackwell Scientific.

Tanner, J.M. (1978). *Foetus into Man – Physical Growth from Conception to Maturity.* London: Open Books.

Tanner, J.M. and Whitehouse, R.H. (1959). *Standards for Skeletal Maturity Based On A Study Of 3000 British Children.* London: Institute of Child Health.

Tanner, J.M., Prader, A., Habich, H. and Ferguson-Smith, M.A. (1959). Genes on the Y-chromosome influencing rate of maturation in man: skeletal age studies in children with Klinefelter's (XXY) and Turner's (XO) syndromes. *Lancet* **2**: 141–144.

Tanner, J.M., Whitehouse, R.H., Cameron, N., Marshall, W.A., Healy, M.J.R. and Goldstein, H. (1983). *Assessment of Skeletal Maturity and Prediction of Adult Height (TW2 Method)*, 2nd edition. London: Academic Press.

Tardieu, C. (1998). Short adolescence in early Hominids: infantile and adolescent growth of the human femur. *American Journal of Physical Anthropology* **107**: 163–178.

Tardieu, C. and Trinkaus, E. (1994). Early ontogeny of the human femoral bicondylar angle. *American Journal of Physical Anthropology* **95**: 183–195.

Taxman, R.M. (1963). Incidence and size of the juxtamastoid eminence in modern crania. *American Journal of Physical Anthropology* **21**: 153–157.

Taylor, H.M. (1935). Ossification of cartilages of the larynx and its relationship to some types of laryngeal disease. *Annals of Otology, Rhinology and Laryngology* **44**: 611–625.

Taylor, J.R. and Twomey, L.T. (1984). Sexual dimorphism in human vertebral body shape. *Journal of Anatomy* **138**: 281–286.

Taylor, J.R. and Twomey. L.T. (1986). The role of the notochord and blood vessels in vertebral column development and the aetiology of schmorl's Nodes. In: *Modern Manual Therapy of the Vertebral Column.* (G.P. Grieve, Ed.). Edinburgh: Churchill Livingstone.

Tebo, H.G. and Telford, I.R. (1950). An analysis of the variations in position of the mental foramen. *Anatomical Record* **107**: 61–66.

Telkkä, A. (1950). On the prediction of human stature from the long bones. *Acta Anatomica* **9**: 103–117.

Ten Cate, A.R. (1998). *Oral Histology: Development, Structure and Function*, 5th edition. London: Mosby Yearbook.

Ten Cate, A.R. and Mills, C. (1972). The development of the periodontium: the origin of alveolar bone. *Anatomical Record* **173**: 69–77.

Terry, R.J. (1899). Rudimentary clavicles and other abnormalities of the skeleton of a White woman. *Journal of Anatomy and Physiology* **33**: 413–422.

Terry, R.J. (1921). A study of the supracondylar process in the living. *American Journal of Physical Anthropology* **4**: 129–139.

Terry, R.J. (1923). On the supracondylar process in the Negro. *American Journal of Physical Anthropology* **6**: 401–403.

Terry, R.J. (1930). On the racial distribution of the supracondyloid variation. *American Journal of Physical Anthropology* **14**: 459–462.

Terry, R.J. (1932). The clavicle of the American Negro. *American Journal of Physical Anthropology* **16**: 351–379.

Terry, R.J. (1934). The acromial end of the clavicle in Indians of Illinois. *American Journal of Physical Anthropology* **18**: 437–438.

Terry, R.J. (1943). The inclination of the saddle surface of the trapezium with respect to the angle between the thumb and wrist. *American Journal of Physical Anthropology* **1**: 157–169.

Terry, R.J. (1959). Sprengel's deformity and club foot: an anthropological interpretation. *American Journal of Physical Anthropology* **17**: 251–271.

Thieme, F.P. and Schull, W.J. (1957). Sex determination from the skeleton. *Human Biology* **29**: 242–273.

Thomas, N., Nissen, K.I. and Helal, B. (1988). Disorders of the Lesser Rays. In: *The Foot* (B. Helal and D. Wilson, Eds.), pp. 484–510. Edinburgh: Churchill Livingstone.

Thompson, R. (1907). The relationship between the internal structure of the upper end of the femur and fractures through the base of the neck of the femur. *Journal of Anatomy and Physiology* **42**: 60–68.

Thompson, D.D. (1979). The core technique in the determination of age at death in skeletons. *Journal of Forensic Sciences* **24**: 902–915.

Thompson, F.R. and Bosworth, D.M. (1947). Recurrent dislocation of the patella. *American Journal of Surgery* **73**: 335–339.

Thompson, A. and Buxton, D. (1923). Man's nasal index in relation to certain climatic conditions. *Journal of the Royal Anthropological Institute* **53**: 92–133.

Thompson, G.W., Popovich, F. and Anderson, D.L. (1974). Third molar agenesis in the Burlington Growth Centre in Toronto. *Community Dentistry and Oral Epidemiology* **2**: 187–192.

Thompson, G.W., Anderson, D.L. and Popovich, F. (1975). Sexual dimorphism in dentition mineralization. *Growth* **39**: 289–301.

Thompson, D.A., Flynn, T.C., Miller, P.W. and Fischer, R.P. (1985). The significance of scapular fractures. *Journal of Trauma* **25**: 974–977.

Thompson, T.J., Owens, P.D.A. and Wilson, D.J. (1989). Intramembranous osteogenesis and angiogenesis in the chick embryo. *Journal of Anatomy* **166**: 55–65.

Thoms, H. (1940). Roentgen pelvimetry as a routine prenatal procedure. *American Journal of Obstetrics and Gynaecology* **40**: 891–905.

Thomson, A.T. (1836). Lectures on medical jurisprudence now in course of delivery at London University. *Lancet* **1**: 281–286.

Thomson, A. (1869). On the difference in the mode of ossification of the first and other metacarpal and metatarsal bones. *Journal of Anatomy and Physiology* **3**: 131–146.

Thomson, A. (1885). Notes on some unusual variations in human anatomy. *Journal of Anatomy and Physiology* **19**: 328–332.

Thomson, A. (1889). The influence of posture on the form of the articular surfaces of the tibia and astragalus in the different races of man and the higher apes. *Journal of Anatomy and Physiology* **23**: 616–639.

Thomson, A. (1890). The orbito-maxillary frontal suture in man and the apes with notes on the varieties of the human lachrymal bone. *Journal of Anatomy and Physiology* **24**: 349–357.

Thomson, A. (1899). The sexual differences in the foetal pelvis. *Journal of Anatomy and Physiology* **33**: 359–380.

Thorogood, P. (1987). Mechanisms of morphogenetic specification in skull development. In: *Mesenchymal-Epithelial Interactions in Neural Development* (J.R. Wolff, J. Sievers and M. Berry, Eds.), pp. 141–152. Berlin: Springer.

Thorogood, P. (1988). The developmental specification of the vertebrate skull. *Development* **103**(Suppl.): 141–153.

Tickle, C. (1994). On making a skeleton. *Nature* **368**: 587–588.

Tillmann, B. and Lorenz, R. (1978). The stress at the human atlanto-occipital joint. *Anatomy and Embryology* **153**: 269–277.

Tobin, W.J. (1955). The internal architecture of the femur and its clinical significance. *Journal of Bone and Joint Surgery* **37A**: 57–71.

Todd, T.W. (1912). Cervical rib. Factors controlling its presence and its size. Its bearing on the morphology and development of the shoulder. *Journal of Anatomy and Physiology* **46**: 244–288.

Todd, T.W. (1920). Age changes in the pubic bone. 1. The male white pubis. *American Journal of Physical Anthropology* **3**: 285–334.

Todd, T.W. (1921a). Age changes in the pubic bone. 2. The pubis of the male Negro-White hybrid. *American Journal of Physical Anthropology* **4**: 1–25.

Todd, T.W. (1921b). Age changes in the pubic bone. 3. The pubis of the White female. *American Journal of Physical Anthropology* **4**: 26–39.

Todd, T.W. (1921c). Age changes in the pubic bone. 4. The pubis of the female Negro-White hybrid. *American Journal of Physical Anthropology* **4**: 40–57.

Todd, T.W. (1921d). Age changes in the pubic bone. 5. Mammalian pubic metamorphosis. *American Journal of Physical Anthropology* **4**: 334–406.

Todd, T.W. (1921e). Age changes in the pubic bone. 6. The interpretation of variations in the symphyseal; area. *American Journal of Physical Anthropology* **4**: 407–424.

Todd, T.W. (1922). Numerical significance in the thoracolumbar vertebrae of the mammalia. *Anatomical Record* **24**: 261–286.

Todd, T.W. (1923). Age changes in the pubic symphysis. 7. The anthropoid strain in human pubic symphyses of the third decade. *Journal of Anatomy* **56**: 274–294.

Todd, T.W. (1930a). The anatomical features of epiphyseal union. *Child Development* **1**: 186–194.

Todd, T.W. (1930b). The roentgenographic record of differentiation in the pubic bone. *American Journal of Physical Anthropology* **14**: 255–271.

Todd, T.W. (1937). *Atlas of Skeletal Maturation*. St Louis, MO: Mosby.

Todd, T.W. and D'Errico, J. (1926). The odontoid ossicle of the second cervical vertebra. *Annals of Surgery* **83**: 20–31.

Todd, T.W. and D'Errico, J. (1928). The clavicular epiphysis. *American Journal of Anatomy* **41**: 25–50.

Todd, T.W. and McCally, W.C. (1921). Defects of the patellar border. *Annals of Surgery* **74**; 775–782.

Toldt, C. (1919). *An Atlas of Human Anatomy for Students and Physicians*, English edition, Parts I and II. New York: Rebman.

Tompsett, A.C. and Donaldson, S.W. (1951). The anterior tubercle of the first cervical vertebra and the hyoid bone: their occurrence in newborn infants. *American Journal of Roentgenology* **65**: 582–584.

Töndury, G. and Theiler, K. (1990). *Entwickelungsgeschichte und Fehlbildungen der Wirbelsäule*, 2nd edition. Stuttgart: Hippokrates.

Too-Chung, M.A. and Green, J.R. (1974). The rate of growth of the cricoid cartilage. *Journal of Laryngology and Otology* **88**: 65–70.

Toole, B.P. and Trelstad, R.L. (1971). Hyaluronate production and removal during corneal development in the chick. *Developmental Biology* **26**: 28–35.

Torgersen, J. (1950). A roentgenological study of the metopic suture. *Acta Radiologica* **33**: 1–11.

Torgersen, J. (1951). The developmental genetics and evolutionary meaning of the metopic suture. *American Journal of Physical Anthropology* **9**: 193–210.

Torpin, R. (1951). Roentgenpelvimetric measurements of 3,604 female pelves, White, Negro and Mexican, compared with direct measurements of Todd Anatomic Collection. *American Journal of Obstetrics and Gynaecology* **62**: 279–293.

Townsley, W. (1946). Platymeria. *Journal of Pathology and Bacteriology* **58**: 85–88.

Townsley, W. (1948). The influence of mechanical factors in the development and structure of bone. *American Journal of Physical Anthropology* **6**: 25–45.

Traub, W., Arad, T. and Weiner, S. (1992). Growth of mineral crystals in turkey tendon collagen fibers. *Connective Tissue Research* **28**: 99–111.

Travers, J.T. and Wormley, L.C. (1938). Enlarged parietal foramina. *American Journal of Roentgenology* **40**: 571–579.

Treble, N.J. (1988). Normal variations in radiographs of the clavicle: a brief report. *Journal of Bone and Joint Surgery* **70B**: 490.

Tredgold, A.F. (1897). Variations of ribs in the primates with especial reference to the number of sternal ribs in man. *Journal of Anatomy and Physiology* **31**: 288–302.

Trinkaus, E. (1975). Squatting among the Neandertals: a problem in the behavioral interpretation of skeletal morphology. *Journal of Archaeological Science* **2**: 327–351.

Trinkaus, E. (1983). *The Shanidar Neanderthals*. New York: Academic Press.

Trinkaus, E. (1989). Olduvai hominid 7 trapezial metacarpal one articular morphology: contrasts with recent humans. *American Journal of Physical Anthropology* **80**: 411–416.

Trolle, D. (1948). *Accessory Bones of the Human Foot*, transl. by E. Aagesen. Copenhagen: Munksgaard.

Trotter, M. (1934a). Synostosis between the manubrium and body of the mesosternum in Whites and Negroes. *American Journal of Physical Anthropology* **18**: 439–442.

Trotter, M. (1934b). Septal aperture in the humerus. *American Journal of Physical Anthropology* **19**: 213–227.

Trotter, M. (1937). Accessory sacro-iliac articulations in East African skeletons. *American Journal of Physical Anthropology* **22**: 137–142.

Trotter, M. (1940). A common anatomical variation in the sacro-iliac region. *Journal of Bone and Joint Surgery* **22**: 293–299.

Trotter, M. (1947). Variations in the sacral canal: their significance in the administration of caudal analgesia. *Anaesthetics and Analgesia* **26**: 192–196.

Trotter, M. and Gleser, G.C. (1952). Estimation of stature from long bones of American Whites and Negroes. *American Journal of Physical Anthropology* **10**: 463–514.

Trotter, M. and Gleser, G.C. (1958). A re-evaluation of estimation based on measurements of stature taken during life and of long bones after death. *American Journal of Physical Anthropology* **16**: 79–123.

Trotter, M. and Gleser, G.C. (1977). A corrigenda to 'Estimation of stature from long limb bones of American Whites and Negroes'. *American Journal of Physical Anthropology* **47**: 355–356.

Trotter, M. and Lanier, P.F. (1945). Hiatus canalis sacralis in American Whites and Negroes. *Human Biology* **17**: 368–381.

Trotter, M. and Peterson, R.R. (1969). Weight of bones during the fetal period. *Growth* **33**: 167–184.

Trotter, M., Peterson, R.R. and Wette, R. (1968). The secular trend in the diameter of the femur of American Whites and Negroes. *American Journal of Physical Anthropology* **28**: 65–74.

Trueta, J. (1957). The normal vascular anatomy of the human femoral head during growth. *Journal of Bone and Joint Surgery* **39B**: 358–394.

Trueta, J. and Cavadias, A.X. (1964). A study of the blood supply of the long bones. *Surgery, Gynaecology and Obstetrics* **118**: 485–498.

Trueta, J. and Harrison, M.H.M. (1953). The normal vascular anatomy of the femoral head in adult man. *Journal of Bone and Joint Surgery* **35B**: 442–461.

Trueta, J. and Morgan, J.D. (1960). The vascular contribution to osteogenesis. I. Studies by the injection method. *Journal of Bone and Joint Surgery* **42B**: 97–109.

Tsou, P.M., Yau, A. and Hodgson, A.R. (1980). Embryogenesis and prenatal development of congenital vertebral anomalies and their classification. *Clinical Orthopaedics* **152**: 211–231.

Tucker, F.R. (1949). Arterial supply to the femoral head and its clinical importance. *Journal of Bone and Joint Surgery* **31B**: 82–93.

Tucker, J.A. and O'Rahilly, R. (1972). Observations on the embryology of the human larynx. *Annals of Otology, Rhinology and Laryngology* **81**: 520–523.

Tucker, J.A. and Tucker, G.F. (1975). Some aspects of laryngeal fetal development. *Annals of Otology, Rhinology and Laryngology* **84**: 49–55.

Tucker, G.F., Tucker, J.A. and Vidić, B. (1977). Anatomy and development of the cricoid. Serial-section whole organ study of perinatal larynges. *Annals of Otology, Rhinology and Laryngology* **86**: 1–4.

Tufts, E., Blank, E. and Dickerson, D. (1982). Periosteal thickening as a manifestation of trauma in infancy. *Child Abuse and Neglect* **6**: 359–364.

Tulsi, R.S. (1971). Growth of the human vertebral column. An osteological study. *Acta Anatomica* **79**: 570–580.

Turk, L.M. and Hogg, D.A. (1993). Age changes in the human laryngeal cartilages. *Clinical Anatomy* **6**: 154–162.

Turner, W. (1866). On some congenital deformities of the human cranium. *Edinburgh Medical Journal* **11**: 133–141.

Turner, W. (1869). On supernumerary cervical ribs. *Journal of Anatomy and Physiology* **4**: 130–138.

Turner, W. (1874). Further examples of variations in the arrangement of the nerves of the human body. *Journal of Anatomy and Physiology* **8**: 297–299.

Turner, M.B. (1879). On exostoses within the external auditory meatus. *Journal of Anatomy and Physiology* **13**: 200–203.

Turner, W.A. (1882). A secondary astragalus in the human foot. *Journal of Anatomy and Physiology* **17**: 82–83.

Turner, W. (1885). The infra-orbital suture. *Journal of Anatomy and Physiology* **19**: 218–220.

Turner, W. (1891). Double right parietal bone in an Australian skull. *Journal of Anatomy and Physiology* **25**: 473–474.

Turner, W. (1901). Double left parietal bone in a Scottish skull. *Journal of Anatomy and Physiology* **35**: 496.

Turner, P. (1934). *Aids to Osteology*, 3rd edition. London: Baillière, Tindall and Cox.

Turner, E.P. (1963). Crown development in human deciduous molar teeth. *Archives of Oral Biology* **8**: 523–540.

Turner, A.L. and Porter, W.G. (1922). The structural type of the mastoid process based upon the skiagraphic examination of one thousand crania of various races of mankind. *Journal of Laryngology and Otology* **37**: 115–121.

Turner, M.S. and Smillie, I.S. (1981). The effect of tibial torsion on the pathology of the knee. *Journal of Bone and Joint Surgery* **63B**: 296–398.

Tuttle, R.H. (1967). Knuckle walking and the evolution of hominid hands. *American Journal of Physical Anthropology* **26**: 171–206.

Twigg, H.L. and Rosenbaum, R.C. (1981). Duplication of the clavicle. *Skeletal Radiology* **6**: 281.

Ubelaker, D.H. (1978). *Human Skeletal Remains: Excavation, Analysis and Interpretation*. Washington, DC: Smithsonian Institute Press.

Ubelaker, D.H. (1979). Skeletal evidence of kneeling in prehistoric Ecuador. *American Journal of Physical Anthropology* **51**: 679–686.

Ubelaker, D.H. (1984). Possible identification from radiographic comparison of frontal sinus patterns. In:

Human Identification. Case Studies in Forensic Anthropology (T.A. Rathbun and J.E. Buikstra, Eds.), pp. 399–411. Springfield, IL: C.C. Thomas.

Ubelaker, D.H. (1992). Hyoid fracture and strangulation. *Journal of Forensic Sciences* **37**: 1216–1222.

Ubelaker, D.H. and Pap, I. (1998). Skeletal evidence for health and disease in the Iron Age of northeastern Hungary. *International Journal of Osteoarchaeology* **8**: 231–251.

Uhry, E. (1944). Osgood–Schlatter's disease. *Archives of Surgery* **48**: 406–414.

Uhthoff, H.K. (1990a). The early development of the spine. In: *The Embryology of the Human Locomotor System* (H.K. Uhthoff, Ed.), pp. 34–41. Berlin: Springer.

Uhthoff, H.K. (1990b). The development of the limb buds. In: *The Embryology of the Human Locomotor System* (H.K. Uhthoff, Ed.), pp. 7–14. Berlin: Springer.

Uhthoff, H.K. (1990c). The development of the shoulder. In: *The Embryology of the Human Locomotor System* (H.K. Uhthoff, Ed.), pp. 73–81. Berlin: Springer.

Uhthoff, H.K., Hammond, D.I., Sarkar, K., Hooper, G.J. and Papoff, W.J. (1988). The role of the coraco-acromial ligament in the impingement syndrome. *International Orthopedics* **12**: 97–104.

Ulijaszek, S.J. (1996). Age of eruption of deciduous dentition of Anga children, Papua New Guinea. *Annals of Human Biology* **23**: 495–499.

Ullrich, H. (1975). Estimation of fertility by means of pregnancy and childbirth alterations at the pubis, the ilium and the sacrum. *Ossa* **2**: 23–39.

Underwood, A.S. (1910). An enquiry into the anatomy and pathology of the maxillary sinus. *Journal of Anatomy and Physiology* **44**: 354–369.

Underwood, L.E., Radcliffe, W.B. and Guinto, F.C. (1976). New standards for the assessment of the sella turcica in children. *Radiology* **119**: 651–654.

Upadhyay, S.S., O'Neil, T., Burwell, R.G. and Moulton, A. (1987). A new method using medical ultrasound for measuring femoral anteversion (torsion): technique and reliability. An intra-observer and inter-observer study on dried bones from human adults. *Journal of Anatomy* **155**: 119–132.

Upadhyay, S.S., Burwell, R.G., Moulton, A., Small, P.G. and Wallace, W.A. (1990). Femoral anteversion in healthy children. Application of a new method using ultrasound. *Journal of Anatomy* **169**: 49–61.

Urbaniak, J.R., Schaefer, W.W. and Stelling, F.H. (1976). Iliac apophysis –H.K. prognostic value in idiopathic scoliosis. *Clinical Orthopaedics and Related Research* **116**: 80–85.

Urbantschitsch, V. (1876). Zur Anatomie der Gehörknöchelchen des Menschen. *Archiv für Ohrenheilkunde* **11**: 1–10.

Uri, D.S., Kneeland, J.B. and Herzog, R. (1997). Os acromiale: evaluation of markers for identification on sagittal and coronal oblique MR images. *Skeletal Radiology* **26**: 31–34.

Vallois, H.V. (1926). Les anomalies de l'omoplate chez l'homme. *Bulletin de la Sociétié d'Anthropologie de Paris* **7**: 19–36.

Vallois, H.V. (1928). L'omoplate humaine, étude anatomique et anthropologique. *Bulletin et Mémoirs de la Sociétié d'Anthropologie de Paris* **7**: 129–168.

Vallois, H.V. (1930). Nouvelles preuves de la non-dualité du pré-maxillaire chez l'homme. *Annales d'Anatomie Pathologique et d'Anatomie Normale* **7**: 748–753.

Vallois, H.V. (1946). L'omoplate humaine. *Bulletin de la Sociétié d'Anthropolgie de Paris* **7**: 16–99.

Valvassori, G.E. and Kirdani, M.A. (1967). The abnormal hypoglossal canal. *American Journal of Roentgenology* **99**: 705–711.

Valvassori, G.E. and Pierce, R.H. (1964). The normal internal auditory canal. *American Journal of Roentgenology* **92**: 1232–1241.

Van Alyea, O.E. (1936). The ostium maxillare. Anatomic study of its surgical accessibility. *Archives of Otolaryngology* **24**: 553–569.

Van Alyea, O.E. (1941). Sphenoid sinus. Anatomic study with consideration of the clinical significance of the structural characteristics of the sphenoid sinus. *Archives of Otolaryngology* **34**: 225–253.

Van Beek, G. (1983). *Dental Morphology – an Illustrated Guide*, 2nd edition. Bristol: P.S.G. Wright.

Van der Linden, F.P.G.M. and Duterloo, H.S. (1976). *The Development of the Human Dentition–An Atlas.* Hagerstown, MD: Harper and Row.

Van Dongen, R. (1963). The shoulder girdle and humerus of the Australian Aborigine. *American Journal of Physical Anthropology* **21**: 469–489.

Vanezis, P. (1989). *Pathology of Neck Injury.* London: Butterworths.

Van Gerven, D.P. (1972). The contribution of size and shape variation to patterns of sexual dimorphism of the human femur. *American Journal of Physical Anthropology* **37**: 49–60.

Van Gilse, P.H.G. (1927). The development of the sphenoidal sinus in man and its homology in mammals. *Journal of Anatomy* **61**: 153–166.

Van Gilse, P.H.G. (1938). Des observations ultérieures sur la génèse des exostoses du conduit externe par l'irritation d'eau froide. *Acta Otolaryngologica (Stockholm)* **26**: 343–352.

Vangsness, C.T., Jorgensen, S.S., Watson, T. and Johnson, D.L. (1994). The origin of the long head of the biceps from the scapula and glenoid labrum. *Journal of Bone and Joint Surgery* **76B**: 951–954.

Van Waalwijk, C.V.D. and Boet, J.N. (1949). Lacuna skull and craniofenestria. *American Journal of Diseases of Children* **77**: 315–327.

Vastine, J.H. and Vastine, M.F. (1946). Genetic influence on osseous development with particular reference to the deposition of calcium in the costal cartilages. *American Journal of Roentgenology* **59**: 213–221.

Vastine, J.H. and Vastine, M.F. (1952). Calcification in the laryngeal cartilages. *Archives of Otolaryngology* **55**: 1–7.

Vasudeva, N. and Choudhry, R. (1996). Precondylar tubercles on the basi-occiput of adult human skulls. *Journal of Anatomy* **188**: 207–210.

Vasudeva, N. and Kumar, R. (1995). Absence of foramen transversarium in the human atlas vertebra: a case report. *Acta Anatomica* **152**: 230–233.

Venning, P. (1954). Sibling correlations with respect to the number of phalanges of the fifth toe. *Annals of Eugenics* **18**: 232–254.

Venning, P. (1956). Radiological studies of variations in the segmentation and ossification of the digits of the foot. I. Variation in the number of phalanges and centres of ossification of the toes. *American Journal of Physical Anthropology* **14**: 1–34.

Venning, P. (1960). Variation of the digital skeleton. *Clinical Orthopaedics* **16**: 26–40.

Venning, P. (1961). Radiological studies of variations in the segmentation and ossification of the digits of the foot. III. Cone shaped epiphyses of the proximal phalanges. *American Journal of Physical Anthropology* **19**: 131–136.

Verbout, A.J. (1976). A critical review of the 'Neugliederung' concept in relation to the development of the vertebral column. *Acta Biotheorie (Leiden)* **25**: 219–258.

Verbout, A.J. (1985). The development of the vertebral column. *Advances in Anatomy, Embryology and Cell Biology* **90**.

Verwoerd, C.D.A., Van Loosen, J., Schütte, H.E., Verwoerd-Verhoef, H.L. and Van Velzen, D. (1989). Surgical aspects of the anatomy of the vomer in children and adults. *Rhinology* **9**(Suppl.): 87–96.

Vettivel, S., Indrasingh, I., Chandi, G. and Chandi, S.M. (1992). Variations in the intertubercular sulcus of the humerus related to handedness. *Journal of Anatomy* **180**: 321–326.

Vettivel, S., Selvaraj, K.G., Chandi, S.M., Indrasingh, I. and Chandi, G. (1995). Intertubercular sulcus of the humerus as an indicator of handedness and humeral length. *Clinical Anatomy* **8**: 44–50.

Victoria-Diaz, A. (1979). Embryological contribution to the aetiopathology of idiopathic club foot. *Journal of Bone and Joint Surgery* **61B**: 127.

Vidić, B. (1968a). The postnatal development of the sphenoidal sinus and its spread into the dorsum sellae and posterior clinoid processes. *American Journal of Roentgenology* **104**: 177–183.

Vidić, B. (1968b). The structure of the palatum osseum and its toral overgrowths. *Acta Anatomica* **71**: 94–99.

Vidić, B. (1971). The morphogenesis of the lateral nasal wall in the early prenatal life of man. *American Journal of Anatomy* **130**: 121–139.

Vignaud-Pasquier, J., Lichtenberg, R., Laval-Jeantet, M., Larroche, J.C. and Bernard, J. (1964). Les impressions digitales de la naissance à neuf ans. *Biologia Neonatorum* **6**: 250–276.

Viladot, A. (1988). Local Congenital Disorders. In: *The Foot* (B. Helal and D. Wilson, Eds.), pp. 235–264. Edinburgh: Churchill Livingstone.

Virchow, R. (1854). Über die Involutionskrankheit (Malum senile) der platten Knocken. *Berhandlungen der Physikalich-Medicinischen Gesselschaft in Würtzberg* **4**: 354–382.

Virtama, P. and Helela, T. (1969). Radiographic measurements of cortical bone: variations in a normal population between 1 and 90 years of age. *Acta Radiologica Supplementum* **293**: 1–268.

Visscher, W., Lonstein, J.E. and Hoffman, D.A. (1988). Reproductive outcomes in scoliosis patients. *Spine* **13**: 1096–1098.

Vlček, E. (1975). Morphology of the first metacarpal of Neanderthal individuals from the Crimea. *Bulletins et Mémoirs de la Sociétié d'Anthropologie de Paris* **2**: 257–276.

Vogt, E.C. and Vickers, V.S. (1938). Osseous growth and development. *Radiology* **31**: 441–444.

Vogt, E.C. and Wyatt, G.M. (1941). Craniolacunia (Lückenschädel). A report of 54 cases. *Radiology* **36**: 147–152.

Von Bazan, U.B. (1979). The association between congenital elevation of the scapula and diastematomyelia. *Journal of Bone and Joint Surgery* **61B**: 59–63.

Voorhees, D.R., Daffner, R.H., Nunley, J.A. and Gilula, L.A. (1985). Carpal ligamentous disruptions and negative ulnar variance. *Skeletal Radiology* **13**: 257–262.

Wade, L.J. (1941). Pseudoplatybasia: rupture of the transverse ligament of the axis with displacement of the odontoid process and compression of the cervical cord. *Journal of Bone and Joint Surgery* **23**: 37–43.

Wagner, U.A., Diedrich, V. and Schmitt, O. (1995). Determination of skeletal maturity by ultrasound: a preliminary report. *Skeletal Radiology* **24:** 417–420

Wahby, B. (1903). Abnormal nasal bones. *Journal of Anatomy and Physiology* **38**: 49–51.

Waisbrod, H. (1973). Congenital club foot. An anatomical study. *Journal of Bone and Joint Surgery* **55B**: 796–801.

Wake, M.H. (1979). *Hyman's Comparative Vertebrate Anatomy.* Chicago, IL: University of Chicago Press.

Wakeley, C.P.G. (1924). Bilateral epiphysis at the basal end of the second metacarpal. *Journal of Anatomy* **58**: 340–345.

Wakeley, C.P.G. (1929). A note on the architecture of the ilium. *Journal of Anatomy* **64**: 109–110.

Wakeley, C.P.G. (1931). A case of congenital absence of the radius in a woman. *Journal of Anatomy* **65**: 506–508.

Wakeley, C.J., Johnson, D.P. and Watt, I. (1996). The value of MR imaging in the diagnosis of the os trigonum syndrome. *Skeletal Radiology* **25**: 133–136.

Wakely, J. (1993). Bilateral congenital dislocation of the hip, spina bifida occulta and spondylolysis in a female skeleton from the medieval cemetery at Abingdon, England. *Journal of Paleopathology* **5**: 37–45.

Wakely, J. and Young, I. (1995). A medieval wrist injury. Fracture of the hook of the hamate bone. *Journal of Palaeopathology* **7**: 51–56.

Waldron, T. (1987). The relative survival of the human skeleton: implications for palaeopathology. In: *Death, Decay and Reconstruction* (A. Boddington, A.N. Garland, R.C. Janaway, Eds.), pp. 55–64. Manchester: Manchester University Press.

Waldron, T. (1993). A case-referent study of spondylolysis and spina bifida and transient vertebrae in human skeletal remains. *International Journal of Osteoarchaeology* **3**: 55–58.

Waldron, T. (1994). The nature of the sample. In: *Counting the Dead. The Epidemiology of Skeletal Populations*, pp. 10–27. Chichester: Wiley.

Waldron, T. and Rogers, J. (1990). An epidemiologic study of sacro-iliac fusion in some human skeletal remains. *American Journal of Physical Anthropology* **83**: 123–127.

Walensky, N.A. (1965). A study of anterior femoral curvature in man. *Anatomical Record* **151**: 559–570.

Walker, C. (1917). Absence of premaxilla. *Journal of Anatomy* **51**: 392–395.

Walker, P.L. (1969). The linear growth of long bones in Late Woodland Indian children. *Proceedings of the Indiana Academy of Sciences* **78**: 83–87.

Walker, J.M. (1981). Histological study of the fetal development of the human acetabulum and labrum: Significance in congenital hip disease. *Yale Journal of Biology and Medicine* **34**: 255–263.

Walker, J.M. (1983). Comparison of normal and abnormal human fetal hip joints: a quantitative study with significance to congenital hip disease. *Journal of Pediatric Orthopedics* **3**: 173–183.

Walker, G.F. and Kowalski, C.J. (1972). On the growth of the mandible. *American Journal of Physical Anthropology* **36**: 111–118.

Walker, R.A. and Lovejoy, C.O. (1985). Radiographic changes in the clavicle and proximal femur and their use in the determination of skeletal age at death. *American Journal of Physical Anthropology* **68**: 67–78.

Walker, R.A., Lovejoy, C.O. and Meindl, R.S. (1994). Histomorphological and geometric properties of human femoral cortex in individuals over 50: implications for histomorphological determination of age at death. *American Journal of Human Biology* **6**: 659–667.

Wall, J.J. (1970). Congenital pseudoarthrosis of the clavicle. *Journal of Bone and Joint Surgery* **52A**: 1003–1009.

Wall, C.E. (1991). Evidence of weaning stress and catch-up growth in the long bones of a Central California Amerindian sample. *Annals of Human Biology* **18**: 9–22.

Walling, A.K. and Ogden, J.A. (1991). Case report 666. Bipartite medial sesamoid below the head of the first metatarsal, a developmental variant. *Skeletal Radiology* **20**: 233–235.

Walmsley, T. (1915a). Observations on certain structural details of the neck of the femur. *Journal of Anatomy and Physiology* **49**: 305–313.

Walmsley, T. (1915b). The epiphysis of the head of the femur. *Journal of Anatomy and Physiology* **49**: 434–440.

Walmsley, T. (1918). The reduction of the mammalian fibula. *Journal of Anatomy* **52**: 326–331.

Walmsley, T. (1933). The vertical axes of the femur and their relations. A contribution to the study of posture. *Journal of Anatomy* **67**: 284–300.

Walmsley, R. (1940). The development of the patella. *Journal of Anatomy* **74**: 360–368.

Walters, M. and Price, R. (1998). The anatomy of minimally traumatic femoral neck fractures: natural selection at work in a modern elderly population? *Annals of Human Biology* **25**: 280.

Walther, H.E. (1948). *Krebsmetastasen.* Basel: Schwalbe.

Waltner, J.G. (1944). Anatomic variations of the lateral and sigmoid sinuses. *Archives of Otolaryngology* **39**: 307–312.

Wang, T-M., Shih, C., Liu, J-C. and Kuo, K-J. (1986). A clinical and anatomical study of the location of the mental foramen in adult Chinese mandibles. *Acta Anatomica* **126**: 29–33.

Wang, R-G., Kwok, P. and Hawke, M. (1988). The embryonic development of the human paraseptal cartilage. *Journal of Otolaryngology* **17**: 150–154.

Wanner, J.A. (1977). Variations in the anterior patellar groove of the human femur. *American Journal of Physical Anthropology* **47**: 99–102.

Warkany, J. and Weaver, T.S. (1940). Heredofamilial deviations. II Enlarged parietal foramens combined with obesity, hypogenitalism, microphthalmos and mental retardation. *American Journal of Diseases of Children* **60**: 1147–1154.

Warner, J.J.P., Beim, G.M. and Higgins, L. (1998). The treatment of symptomatic os acromiale. *Journal of Bone and Joint Surgery* **80A**: 1320–1326.

Warwick, R. (1950). The relation of the direction of the mental foramen to the growth of the human mandible. *Journal of Anatomy* **84**: 116–120.

Warwick, R. (1951). A juvenile skull exhibiting duplication of the optic canals and subdivision of the superior orbital fissure. *Journal of Anatomy* **85**: 289–291.

Wasson, W.W. (1933). Changes in the nasal accessory sinuses after birth. *Archives of Otolaryngology* **17**: 197–209.

Watanabe, R.S. (1974). Embryology of the human hip. *Clinical Orthopedics and Related Research* **98**: 8–26.

Watanabe, H., Kurihara, K. and Murai, T. (1982). A morphometrical study of laryngeal cartilages. *Medicine, Science and the Law* **22**: 255–260.

Watanabe, Y., Konishi, M., Shimada, M., Ohara, H. and Iwamoto, S. (1998). Estimation of age from the femur of Japanese cadavers. *Forensic Science International* **98**: 55–65.

Waterman, H.C. (1929). Studies on the evolution of the pelvis of man and other primates. *Bulletin of the American Museum of Natural History* **58**: 585–641.

Waterman, J.K. (1998). The osteological and radiological anatomy of the scaphoid. *Clinical Anatomy* **11**: 358–359.

Watson, D.M.S. (1917). The evolution of tetrapod shoulder girdle and forelimb. *Journal of Anatomy* **52**: 1–63.

Watson, H.K. and Boyes, J.H. (1967). Congenital angular deformity of the digits. *Journal of Bone and Joint Surgery* **49A**: 333–338.

Watts, B.L. (1990). An investigation into sexing the adult human sternum and the incidence of manubrio-costal and manubrio-sternal synostosis. Unpublished BSc dissertation, University of London.

Watts, B.L. (1991). The relationship between age at death and manubrio-costal and manubrio-sternal synostosis. *Journal of Anatomy* **176**: 237.

Watzke, D., and Bast, T.H. (1950). The development and structure of the otic (endolymphatic) sac. *Anatomical Record* **106**: 361–379.

Waugh, R.L. and Sullivan, R.F. (1950). Anomalies of the carpus with particular reference to the bipartite scaphoid (navicular). *Journal of Bone and Joint Surgery* **32A**: 682–686.

Wayman, J., Miller, S. and Shanahan, D. (1993). Anatomical variation of the insertion of scalenus anterior in adult human subjects: implications for clinical practice. *Journal of Anatomy* **183**: 165–167.

Weaver, D.S. (1979). Application of the likelihood ratio test to age estimation using the infant and child temporal bone. *American Journal of Physical Anthropology* **50**: 263–270.

Weaver, D.S. (1980). Sex differences in the ilia of a known sex and age sample of fetal and infant skeletons. *American Journal of Physical Anthropology* **52**: 191–195.

Webb, P.A.O. and Suchey, J.M. (1985). Epiphyseal union of the anterior iliac crest and medial clavicle in a modern sample of American males and females. *American Journal of Physical Anthropology* **68**: 457–466.

Webber, C.E. and Garnett, E.S. (1976). Density of os calcis and limb dominance. *Journal of Anatomy* **121**: 203–205.

Weidenreich, F. (1940). The external tubercle of the human tuber calcanei. *American Journal of Physical Anthropology* **26**: 473–487.

Weiner, D.S. and MacNab, I. (1970). Superior migration of the humeral head. *Journal of Bone and Joint Surgery* **52B**: 524–527.

Weiner, S. and Traub, W. (1989). Crystal size and organization in bone. *Connective Tissue Research* **21**: 259–265.

Weinert, C.R., McMaster, J.H. and Ferguson, R.J. (1973). Dynamic function of the human fibula. *American Journal of Anatomy* **138**: 145–149.

Weinmann, J.P. and Sicher, H. (1947). *Bone and Bones: Fundamentals of Bone Biology.* London: Henry Kimpton.

Weinstein, A.S. and Mueller, C.F. (1965). Intra thoracic rib. *American Journal of Roentgenology* **94**: 587–590.

Weisl H. (1954a). The ligaments of the sacro-iliac joint examined with particular reference to their function. *Acta Anatomica* **20**: 201–213.

Weisl, H. (1954b). The articular surfaces of the sacro-iliac joint and their relation to the movements of the sacrum. *Acta Anatomica* **22**: 1–14.

Weisl, H. (1955). The movements of the sacro-iliac joint. *Acta Anatomica* **23**: 80–91.

Weitzner, I. (1946). Congenital talonavicular synostosis associated with hereditary multiple ankylosing arthropathies. *American Journal of Radiology* **56**: 185–188.

Wells, C. (1968). Osgood-Schlatter's disease in the ninth century. *British Medical Journal* **2**: 623–624.

Wells, C. (1975). Ancient obstetric hazards and female mortality. *Bulletin of the New York Academy of Medicine* **51**: 1235–1249.

Wertheimer, L.G. (1948). Coracoclavicular joint – surgical treatment of a painful syndrome caused by an anomalous joint. *Journal of Bone and Joint Surgery* **30A**: 570–578.

Westhorpe, R.N. (1987). The position of the larynx in children and its relationship to the ease of intubation. *Anaesthesia and Intensive Care* **15**: 384–388.

Westmoreland, E.E. and Blanton, P.L. (1982). An analysis of the variations in position of the greater palatine foramen in the adult human skull. *American Journal of Physical Anthropology* **204**: 383–388.

Weston, W.J. (1956). Genetically determined cervical ribs: a family study. *British Journal of Radiology* **29**: 455–456.

Wetherington, R.K. (1961). A note on the fusion of the lunate and triquetral centres. *American Journal of Physical Anthropology* **19**: 251–254.

Wetherington, R.K. (1982). Cone-shaped epiphyses in Japanese children. *American Journal of Physical Anthropology* **57**: 117–121.

Wetherington, R.K. (1983). Bilateral asymmetry in cone epiphyses of the middle phalanx, fifth finger. *American Journal of Physical Anthropology* **60**: 319–322.

Whillis, J. (1940). The development of synovial joints. *Journal of Anatomy* **74**: 277–283.

White, L.E. (1923). An anatomical and X-ray study of the optic canal in cases of optic nerve involvement. *Boston Medical and Surgical Journal* **189**: 741–748.

White, J.W. (1943). Torsion of Achilles' tendon; its surgical significance. *Archives of Surgery* **46**: 784–787.

White, E.H. (1944). Bilateral congenital fusion of carpal capitate and hamate. *American Journal of Roentgenology* **52**: 406–408.

White, T.D. (1980). Evolutionary implications of Pliocene hominid footprints. *Science* **208**: 175–176.

White, T.D. (1991). *Human Osteology.* London: Academic Press.

White, J.C., Poppel, M.H. and Adams, R. (1945). Congenital malformations of the first rib. *Surgery, Gynaecology and Obstetrics* **81**: 643–659.

Whitehead, R.H. and Waddell, J.A. (1911). The early development of the mammalian sternum. *American Journal of Anatomy* **12**: 89–106.

Whitehouse, W.J. (1977). Cancellous bone in the anterior part of the iliac crest. *Calcified Tissue Research* **23**: 67–76.

Whitehouse, W.J. and Dyson, E.D. (1974). Scanning electron microscope studies of trabecular bone in the proximal end of the human femur. *Journal of Anatomy* **118**: 417–444.

Whitnall, S.E. (1911). On a tubercle on the malar bone and on the lateral attachments of the tarsal plates. *Journal of Anatomy and Physiology* **45**: 426–432.

Whittaker, D.K. (1992). Quantitative studies on age changes in the teeth and surrounding structures in archaeological material: a review. *Journal of the Royal Society of Medicine* **85**: 97–101.

Whittaker, D.K. and MacDonald, D.G. (1989). *A Colour Atlas of Forensic Dentistry.* London: Wolfe.

Whittaker, D.K. and Richards, D. (1978). Scanning electron microscopy of the neonatal line in human enamel. *Archives of Oral Biology* **23**: 45–50.

Wientroub, S., Lloyd-Roberts, G.C. and Fraser, M. (1981). The prognostic significance of the triradiate cartilage in suppurative arthritis of the hip in infancy and early childhood. *Journal of Bone and Joint Surgery* **63B**: 190–193.

Wigh, R. (1951). Air cells in the great wing of the sphenoid bone. *American Journal of Roentgenology* **65**: 916–923.

Wigh, R.E. (1982). The lumbosacral complex. *Skeletal Radiology* **8**: 127–131.

Wigh, R.E. and Anthony, H.F. (1981). Transitional lumbosacral discs: probability of herniation. *Spine* **6**: 168–171.

Wilber, M.C. and Evans, E.B. (1977). Fractures of the scapula. *Journal of Bone and Joint Surgery* **59A**: 358–362.

Wilczak, C.A. (1998). Consideration of sexual dimorphism, age and asymmetry in quantitative measurements of muscle insertion sites. *International Journal of Osteoarchaeology* **8**: 311–325.

Wiley, A.M. (1959). Club foot. An anatomical and experimental study of muscle growth. *Journal of Bone and Joint Surgery* **41B**: 821–835.

Wilgress, J.H.F. (1900). A note on the development of the external malleolus. *Journal of Anatomy and Physiology* **34**: xlii–xliv.

Wilkins, K.E. (1984). Fractures and dislocations of the elbow region. In: *Fractures in Children* (C.A. Rockwood, K.E. Wilkins and R.E. King, Eds), pp. 363–575. Philadelphia, PA: Lippincott.

Wilkinson, J.L. (1951). The anatomy of an oblique proximal septum of the pulp space. *British Journal of Surgery* **38**: 454–459.

Wilkinson, J.L. (1953). The insertions of the flexores pollicis longus et digitorum profundus. *Journal of Anatomy* **87**: 75–88.

Wilkinson, J.L. (1954). The terminal phalanx of the great toe. *Journal of Anatomy* **88**: 537–541.

Willan, P.L.T. and Humpherson, J.R. (1999). Concepts of variation and normality in morphology: important issues at risk of neglect in modern undergraduate medical courses. *Clinical Anatomy* **12**: 186–190.

Willett, A. and Walsham, W.J. (1883). A second case of malformation of the left shoulder girdle with remarks on the probable nature of the deformity. *British Medical Journal* **1**: 513–514.

Williams, G. and Cowell, H. (1981). Köhler's disease of the tarsal navicular. *Clinical Orthopaedics and Related Research* **158**: 53–58.

Williams, P.L., Bannister, L.H., Berry, M.M., Collins, P., Dyson, M. Dussek, J.E. and Ferguson, M.W.J. (1995). *Gray's Anatomy*, 38th edition. Edinburgh: Churchill Livingstone.

Willis, T.A. (1923a). The thoraco-lumbar column in white and Negro stock. *Anatomical Record* **26**: 31–40.

Willis, T.A. (1923b). The lumbo-sacral vertebral column in man. Its stability of form and function. *American Journal of Anatomy* **32**: 95–123.

Willis, T.A. (1929). An analysis of vertebral anomalies. *American Journal of Surgery* **6**: 163–168.

Willis, T.A. (1941). Anatomical variations and roentgenological appearance of the low back in relation to sciatic pain. *Journal of Bone and Joint Surgery* **23**: 410–416.

Willis, T.A. (1949). Nutrient arteries of the vertebral bodies. *Journal of Bone and Joint Surgery* **31A**: 538–540.

Willock, E.F. (1925). An os interfrontale. *Journal of Anatomy* **59**: 439–441.

Willson, J.R., Beecham, C.T. and Corrington, E.R. (1971). *Obstetrics and Geography.* St Louis, MO: Mosby.

Wilsman, N.J. and Van Sickle, D.C. (1972). Cartilage canals, their morphology and distribution. *Anatomical Record* **173**: 79–93.

Wilson, D. (1891). *The Right Hand: Left Handedness.* London: Nature.

Wilson, A.K. (1944). Roentgenological findings in bilateral symmetrical thinness of the parietal bones (senile atrophy). *American Journal of Roentgenology* **51**: 685–696.

Wilson, A.K. (1947). Thinness of parietal bones. Report of a case having predominantly unilateral involvement. *American Journal of Roentgenology* **58**: 724–725.

Wilson, C.L. and Duff, G.L. (1943). Pathologic study of degeneration and rupture of the supraspinatus tendon. *Archives of Surgery* **47**: 121–135.

Wilson, M.J., Michele, A.A. and Jacobson, E.W. (1940). Spontaneous dislocation of the atlanto-axial articulation including a report of a case with quadriplegia. *Journal of Bone and Joint Surgery* **22**: 698–707.

Windle, B.C.A. (1892). The occurrence of an additional phalanx in the human pollex. *Journal of Anatomy and Physiology* **26**: 100–116.

Wise, G.E. (1995). We may have stood on the shoulders of giants but we did not cite them. *Clinical Anatomy* **8**: 235–236.

Witkop, C.J. and Barros, L. (1963). Oral and genetic studies of Chileans 1960. 1. Oral anomalies. *American Journal of Physical Anthropology* **21**: 15–24.

Wolanski, N. (1966). A new method for the evaluation of tooth formation. *Acta Genetica (Basel)* **16**: 186–197.

Wolf, G., Anderhuber, W. and Kuhn, F. (1993). Development of the paranasal sinuses in children: implications for paranasal sinus surgery. *Annals of Otology, Rhinology and Laryngology* **102**: 705–711.

Wolff, J. (1870). Über die innere Architektur der Knochen und ihre Bedeutung für die Frage vom Knochenwachstum. *Archiv für pathologische Anatomie und Physiologie für klinische Medizin* **50**: 389–453.

Wolff, E. (1976). *The Anatomy of the Eye and the Orbit*, 7th edition (R. Warwick, Ed.). London: Lewis.

Wolff, D. and Bellucci, R. (1956). The human ossicular ligaments. *Annals of Otology, Rhinology and Laryngology* **65**: 895–910.

Wolffson, D.M. (1950). Scapula shape and muscle function with special reference to vertebral border. *American Journal of Physical Anthropology* **8**: 331–342.

Wollin, D.G. (1963). The os odontoideum. *Journal of Bone and Joint Surgery* **45A**: 1459–1471.

Wolpert, L. (1976). Mechanisms of limb development and malformation. *British Medical Bulletin* **32**: 65–70.

Wolpoff, M. (1968). Climatic influence on the skeletal nasal aperture. *American Journal of Physical Anthropology* **29**: 405–424.

Wong, M. and Carter, D.R. (1988). Mechanical stress and morphogenetic endochondral ossification in the sternum. *Journal of Bone and Joint Surgery* **70A**: 992–1000.

Woo, T.L. (1937–38). A biometric study of the human malar bone. *Biometrika* **29**: 113–123.

Woo, J-K. (1948). 'Anterior' and 'posterior' medio-palatine bones. *American Journal of Physical Anthropology* **6**: 209–223.

Woo, J-K. (1949a). Racial and sexual differences in the frontal curvature and its relation to metopism. *American Journal of Physical Anthropology* **7**: 215–226.

Woo, J-K. (1949b). Ossification and growth of the human maxilla, premaxilla and palate bone. *Anatomical Record* **105**: 737–761.

Woo, J-K. (1950). Torus palatinus. *American Journal of Physical Anthropology* **8**: 81–111.

Wood, W.Q. (1920). The tibia of the Australian aborigine. *Journal of Anatomy* **54**: 232–257.

Wood, V.E. (1986). The results of total claviculectomy. *Clinical Orthopedics and Related Research* **207**: 186–190.

Wood, B.A. and Chamberlain, A.T. (1986). The primate pelvis: allometry or sexual dimorphism? *Journal of Human Evolution* **15**: 257–263.

Wood, P.J. and Kraus, B.S. (1962). Prenatal development of the human palate. *Archives of Oral Biology* **7**: 137–150.

Wood, N.K., Wragg, L.E. and Stuteville, O.H. (1967). The premaxilla: embryological evidence that it does not exist in man. *Anatomical Record* **158**: 485–490.

Wood, N.K., Wragg, L.E., Stuteville, O.H. and Oglesby, R.J. (1969). Osteogenesis of the human upper jaw: proof of the non-existence of a separate pre-maxillary centre. *Archives of Oral Biology* **14**: 1331–1341.

Wood, N.K., Wragg, L.E., Stuteville, O.H. and Kaminski, E.J. (1970). Prenatal observations on the incisive fissure and the frontal process in man. *Journal of Dental Research* **49**: 1125–1131.

Woodburne, R.T. and Burkel, W.E. (1988). *Essentials of Human Anatomy*, 8th edition. New York: Oxford University Press.

Woodhall, B. (1936). Variations of the cranial venous sinuses in the region of the torcular Herophili. *Archives of Surgery* **33**: 297–314.

Woodhall, B. (1939). Anatomy of the cranial blood sinuses with particular reference to the lateral. *Laryngoscope* **49**: 966–1009.

Wood Jones, F. (1912). On the grooves upon the ossa parietalia commonly said to be caused by the arteria meningea media. *Journal of Anatomy and Physiology* **46**: 228–238.

Wood Jones, F. (1918). *Arboreal Man*. London: Arnold.

Wood Jones, F. (1933). The non-metrical characters of the skull as criteria for racial diagnosis. Part IV. The non-metrical characters of the Northern Chinese skull. *Journal of Anatomy* **68**: 96–108.

Wood Jones, F. (1939). The anterior superior alveolar nerve and vessels. *Journal of Anatomy* **73**: 583–591.

Wood Jones, F. (1941). *Principles of Anatomy as Seen in the Hand*. Baltimore, MD: Williams and Wilkins.

Wood Jones, F. (1947). The premaxilla and the ancestry of man. *Nature* **159**: 439.

Wood Jones, F. (1953). *Buchanan's Manual of Anatomy*, 8th edition. London: Baillière Tindall and Cox.

Woodward, J.W. (1961). Congenital elevation of the scapula. Correction by release and transplantation of muscle origins. *Journal of Bone and Joint Surgery* **43A**: 219–228.

Woolf, A.D. and Dixon, A. (1988). *Osteoporosis: A Clinical Guide*. London: M. Dunitz.

Workshop of European Anthropologists (WEA). (1980). Recommendations for age and sex diagnoses of skeletons. *Journal of Human Evolution* **9**: 517–549.

Wray, J.B. and Herndon, C.N. (1963). Hereditary transmission of congenital coalition of the calcaneus to the navicular. *Journal of Bone and Joint Surgery* **45A**: 365–372.

Wredmark, T., Carlstedt, C.A., Bauer, H. and Saartok, T. (1991). Os trigonum syndrome: a clinical entity in ballet dancers. *Foot and Ankle* **11**: 404–406.

Wright, W. (1903). A case of accessory patellae in the human subject, with remarks on the emargination of the patella. *Journal of Anatomy and Physiology* **38**: 65–67.

Wright, S.M. (1998). Congenital hallux valgus deformity with bilateral absence of the hallucial sesamoids. *Journal of the American Podiatric Association* **88**: 47–48.

Wunderly, J. and Wood-Jones, F. (1933). The non-metrical morphological characters of the Tasmanian skull. *Journal of Anatomy* **67**: 583–595.

Wuthier, R.E. (1989). Mechanism of de novo mineral formation by matrix vesicles. *Connective Tissue Research* **22**: 27–33.

Wyburn, G. (1944). Observations on the development of the human vertebral column. *Journal of Anatomy* **78**: 94–102.

Yamamura, H. (1939). On the fetal pelvis. *Japanese Journal of Obstetrics and Gynaecology* **22**: 268–285.

Yarkoni, S., Schmidt, W., Jeanty, P., Reece, E.A. and Hobbins, J.C. (1985). Clavicular measurement: a new biometric parameter for fetal evaluation. *Journal of Ultrasound Medicine* **4**: 467–470.

Yasuda, Y. (1973). Differentiation of human limb buds *in vitro*. *Anatomical Record* **175**: 561–578.

y'Edynak, G. (1976). Long bone growth in western Eskimo and Aleut skeletons. *American Journal of Physical Anthropology* **45**: 569–574.

Yochum, T.R. and Rowe, L.J. (1987). *Essentials of Skeletal Radiology*. London: Williams and Wilkins.

Yoshikawa, E. (1958). Changes of the laryngeal cartilages during life and application for determination of probable age. *Japanese Journal of Legal Medicine* **12** (Suppl.): 1–40 (Japanese with English summary).

Yoshino, M., Miyasaka, S., Sato, H. and Seta, S. (1987). Classification system of frontal sinus patterns by radiography. Its application to identification of unknown skeletal remains. *Forensic Science International* **34**: 289–299.

Yoshioka, Y., Sin, D. and Cooke, T.D.V. (1987). The anatomy and functional axes of the femur. *Journal of Bone and Joint Surgery* **69A**: 873–880.

Young, R.W. (1957). Postnatal growth of the frontal and parietal bone in white males. *American Journal of Physical Anthropology* **15**: 367–386.

Young, M. and Ince, J.G.H. (1940). Transmutation of vertebrae in the lumbosacral region of the human spine. *Journal of Anatomy* **74**: 369–373.

Young, J.W., Bright, R.W. and Whitley, N.O. (1986). Computed tomography in the evaluation of partial growth plate arrest. *Skeletal Radiology* **15**: 530–535.

Yousefzadeh, D.K., El-Khoury, G.Y. and Smith, W.L. (1982). Normal sagittal diameter and variation in the pediatric cervical spine. *Radiology* **144**: 319–325.

Youssef, E.H. (1964). The development of the human skull in a 34 mm human embryo. *Acta Anatomica* **57**: 72–90.

Zadek, I. (1926). The significance of the accessory tarsal scaphoid. *Journal of Bone and Joint Surgery* **8**: 618–626.

Zadek, I. and Gold, A.M. (1948). The accessory tarsal scaphoid. *Journal of Bone and Joint Surgery* **30A**: 957–968.

Zander, G. (1943). 'Os acetabuli' and other bone nuclei: periarticular calcifications at the hip joint. *Acta Radiologica* **24**: 317–327.

Zaoussis, A.L. and James, J.I.P. (1958). The iliac apophysis and the evolution of curves in scoliosis. *Journal of Bone and Joint Surgery* **40B**: 442–453.

Zawisch, C. (1956). Missverhältniss zwischen den am auf gehellten Ganzembryo und den aus histologisch-embryologischen Schnittserien gewonnenen Ossifikationdaten. *Anatomischer Anzeiger* **102**: 305–316.

Zawisch, C. (1957). Der ossifikationsprozess des Occipitale und die Rolle des tectum posterius beim menschen. *Acta Anatomica* **30**: 988–1007.

Zguricas, J., Snijders, P.J., Hovius, S.E., Heutink, P., Oostra, B.A. and Lindhout, D. (1994). Phenotypic analysis of triphalangeal thumb and associated hand malformations. *Journal of Medical Genetics* **31**: 462–467.

Zeitlin, A. (1935). The traumatic origin of the accessory bones at the elbow. *Journal of Bone and Joint Surgery* **17**: 933–938.

Ziemann-Becker, B., Pirsig, W., Teschler-Nicola, M.E. and Lenders, H. (1994). Stapedial footplate fixation in a 4000 year old temporal bone from Franzhausen II, Austria. *International Journal of Osteoarchaeology* **4**: 241–246.

Zihlman, A. and Brunker, L. (1979). Hominid bipedalism: then and now. *Yearbook of Physical Anthropology* **22**: 132–162.

Zimmerman, C. (1961). Iliac horns: A pathognomic roentgen sign of familial onycho-osteodysplasia. *American Journal of Roentgenology* **86**: 478–483.

Zimmerman, A.W. and Lozzio, C.B. (1989). Intersection between selenium and zinc in the pathogenesis of anencephaly and spina bifida. *Zeitschrift fur Kinderchirurgie* **44**: 48–50.

Zindrick, M.R., Wiltse, L.L. and Widell, E.H. (1987). Analysis of the morphometric characteristics of the thoracic and lumbar pedicles. *Spine* **12**: 160–166.

Zins, J.E. and Whitaker, L.A. (1979). Membranous vs. endochondral bone autografts: implications for craniofacial reconstruction. *Surgical Forum* **30**: 521–523.

Zins, J.E. and Whitaker, L.A. (1983). Membranous vs. endochondral bone: implications for craniofacial reconstruction. *Plastic and Reconstructive Surgery* **72**: 778–784.

Zinsmeister, B.J. and Edelman, R. (1985). Congenital absence of the tibial sesamoid: a report of two cases. *Journal of Foot Surgery* **24**: 260–268.

Zivanovic, S. (1970). The mandibular angle in recent East African Bantu populations. *Archives of Oral Biology* **15**: 1373–1376.

Zoller, H. and Bowie, E.R. (1957). Foreign bodies of food passages versus calcifications of laryngeal cartilages. *Archives of Otolaryngology* **65**: 474–478.

Zongyao, Z. (1982). A preliminary study of estimation of age by morphological changes in the symphysis pubis. *Acta Anthropologica Sinica* **1**: 132–136.

Index

References to illustrations are indicated in **bold** figures.